Splinting the Hand and Upper Extremity: Principles and Process

Splinting the Hand and Upper Extremity: Principles and Process

MaryLynn A. Jacobs, MS, OTR/L, CHT
Partner, Hand Therapist
Performance Rehabilitation of Western New England
Springfield, MA

Noelle M. Austin, MS, PT, CHT
Hand Therapist
Woodbridge, CT

Senior Acquiring Editor: Tim Julet
Managing Editor: Ulita Lushnycky
Development Editor: Nancy Peterson
Senior Marketing Manager: Debby Hartman
Project Editor: Paula C. Williams
Designer: Doug Smock
Compositor: Graphic World, Inc.
Printer: Courier - Kendallville

351 West Camden Street
Baltimore, Maryland 21201-2436 USA

530 Walnut Street
Philadelphia, Pennsylvania 19106-3621 USA

Printed in China

Library of Congress Cataloging-in-Publication Data

Splinting the hand and upper extremity : principles and process / [edited by] MaryLynn Jacobs, Noelle Austin.
p. ; cm
Includes bibliogrphical references and index.
ISBN-13: 978-0-683-30630-9
ISBN-10: 0-683-30630-8
1. Hand--Wounds and injuries--Treatment. 2. Splints (Surgery) I. Jacobs, MaryLynn. II. Austin, Noelle.
[DNLM: 1. Hand. 2. Splints. 3. Arm Injuries--rehabilitation. 4. Arm. 5. Hand Injuries--rehabilitation. WE 26 S761 2002]
RD559 .S795 2002
617.5'7044--dc21
2002016205

The publishers have made every effort to trace the copyright holders for borrowed material. If they have inadvertently overlooked any, they will be pleased to make the necessary arrangements at the first opportunity.

To purchase additional copies of this book call our customer service department at **(800) 638-3030** or fax orders to **(301) 824-7390.** International customers should call **(301) 714-2324.**

Visit Lippincott Williams & Wilkins on the Internet: **http://www.lww.com.** Lippincott Williams & Wilkins customer service representatives are available from 8:30 am to 6:00 pm, EST, Monday through Friday, for telephone access.

10 11 12 13 14
7 8 9 10

CCS1110

Acknowledgments

This Book Is Dedicated
To Our Families

We would like to take this opportunity to thank Ulita Lushnycky, our managing editor for her support, enthusiasm, patience, and gentle approach to keeping us on schedule with this project. In addition, we would also like to extend our thanks to Nancy Peterson, our developmental editor, for her genuine support from the beginning of our project and continued guidance with our manuscript preparation. Also, a sincere thanks to Doug Smock, our design coordinator, for coordinating the overwhelming task of the photography and illustrations for this book.

No book is solely the work of its authors. Thanks to all the patients who were so generous in allowing us to photograph their upper extremities and providing such a plethora of examples for our book. We would like to express our gratitude to the many therapists and physicians we have worked with over the years who have helped expand our knowledge and clinical skills. Many thanks to the following individuals, who have contributed their time and expertise in reviewing various chapters:

Louis Adler MD; Mark P. Altman MD; Gary P. Austin PT, PhD; Cindy Bailey ATC, PT, MS, EMT; Elizabeth Becky MS, OTR/L; Judith Bell-Krotoski OTR/L, FAOTA, CHT; Karen Black OTR/L; Joanne Brown MS, OTR/L, CHT; Mary Ellen Brown MS, OTR/L; Judy Colditz OTR/L, CHT, FAOTA; Janet Cope MS, CAS, OTR/L; Loray Dailey OTR/L; Kelley Emery PTA; Polly Fletcher MS, OTR/L, CHT; Linda Swartz-Grigel OTR/L, PAC; Trudy Hackencamp OTR/L, CHT; Judi Helman MS, OTR/L, CHT; Barry R. Jacobs MD; Melissa Johnson MD; Kenzo Kase DC; Sharon Kovarick OTR/L; Kristina Manniello MS, OTR/L, CHT; Ellen Marcus OTR/L; Amy Marsh; Jenny McConnell BApp Sci (Phty); Laura O'Neil MS; Jodi Quinn COTA/L; Michael L. Rappaport MD; Hazel M. Simin OTR/L, CHT; Joan Simmons MS, OTR/L; Howard Smithline MD; Marlys Staley MS, PT; Donna E. Breger-Stanton MA, OTR/L, CHT; AnnMarie Turo OTR/L; Jim Wallis MSR, ATC; and Steven Wenner MD. We would like to especially thank Kim Kreutzer at Smith+Nephew for the generous support in supplying the majority of splinting materials and components used in Section II for the professional photography. We have thoroughly enjoyed working with TailorSplint. Thanks so much!

Finally, we would like to express our sincere thanks to our families who have been so patient and understanding over the past 4 years. Without their love, support and patience we would not have been able to undertake such a huge task successfully. We love you all very much.

Contents

SECTION III—Optional Methods

SECTION IV—Splinting for Specific Diagnoses and Populations

Contributors

Gary P. Austin, PT, PhD
Assistant Professor of Physical Therapy
Sacred Heart University
Farifield, CT
Physical Therapist
Sacred Heart University Sports Medicine and Rehabilitation Center
Fairfield, CT

Noelle M. Austin, MS, PT, CHT
Hand Therapist
The Orthopaedic Group
Hamden, CT

Elaine Charest, MA, MBA, OTR/L
Director of Rehabilitation Services
Shriners Hospital for Children
Springfield, MA

Ruth Coopee, OTR/L, CHT
Athol Memorial Hospital
Athol, MA
Private practice
Athol, MA

Janet Cope, MS, CAS, OTR/L
Human Anatomy Laboratory Coordinator
Springfield College
Springfield, MA

Lisa M. Cyr, OTR/L, CHT
Hand Therapist
Center for Orthopaedics
New Haven, CT

Christy Halpin, OTR/L, CHT
Senior Hand Therapist
New England Medical Center
Boston, MA

MaryLynn Jacobs, MS, OTR/L, CHT
Partner
Hand Therapist
Performance Rehabilitation of Western New England
Springfield, MA

Nicole Jacobs, OTR/L, CHT
Hand Therapist
New England Medical Center
Boston, MA

Caryl Johnson, OTR/L, CHT
Owner
Johnson Hand Therapy Services
New York, NY
C V Starr Hand Surgery Center
New York, NY

Kristina E. Manniello, MS, OTR/L, CHT
Partner
Hand Therapist
Performance Rehabilitation of Western New England
Springfield, MA

Sue Ann Ordinetz, MS, CAS, OTR/L
Assistant Professor of Occupational Therapy
American International College
Springfield, MA

Reg Richard, MS, PT
Burn Clinical Specialist
Miami Valley Hospital Regional Burn Center
Dayton, OH

Karen Schultz-Johnson, MS, OTR/L, FAOTA, CHT
Director
Hand Therapist
Rocky Mountain Hand Therapy
Vail, CO
Adjunct Faculty
Rocky Mountain University of Health Professions

Lisa Schulz Slowman, MS, OTR/L, CHT
Senior Therapist
Lahey Clinic
Burlington, MA
Spaulding Rehabilitation Hospital
Framingham, MA

Ellen Smithline, RN
Staff Nurse
Emergency Department
Baystate Medical Center
Springfield, MA

Steven Wenner, MD
Hand Surgeon
New England Orthopedic Surgeons
Chief of Orthopedic Surgery
Baystate Medical Center
Springfield, MA

Clinical Pearls

Introduction

Splinting the Hand and Upper Extremity: Principles and Process was inspired by clinicians and students who, in our teaching experience, were requesting one resource that would clarify all appropriate traditional splinting, casting, and taping managements for upper extremity diagnoses. Although an upper extremity therapist tends to fabricate thermoplastic splints the majority of the time, there are many situations when casting, taping, Neoprene splinting, or even a prefabricated splint is a more appropriate choice. This book is unique in that it provides splinting patterns for most upper extremity diagnoses as well as in-depth discussions and instructions for fabricating and choosing these other options. This feature truly distinguishes this book from all others currently on the market. We do not delve into the specifics of rehabilitation techniques and surgical interventions; instead we provide overviews of the various diagnoses described to clarify a particular rationale specific to a splint design or protocol. The reference and suggested reading lists at the end of each chapter guide the student to further study on a particular topic.

This book is divided into four sections. **Section I** focuses on the fundamentals. Much of the mystery surrounding splinting can be eliminated if the therapist has a good working knowledge of appropriate splinting nomenclature (to interpret referrals), upper extremity anatomy, tissue healing guidelines, and a concrete understanding of mechanical principles. This section provides the foundation necessary to plan and create a splint. **Chapter 1** presents and clarifies the ASHT splint nomenclature, which is used consistently throughout the book. **Chapter 2** systematically reviews the bony and neuromuscular anatomy, specifically as it relates to the application of splints. **Chapter 3** describes the stages of healing, factors that influence healing, and the relationship of specific stages of healing to splint selection and application. **Chapter 4** defines the fundamental mechanical terms and concepts pertinent to splint design and fabrication and discusses the clinical relevance and application of these basic principles using specific examples. **Chapter 5** surveys the proper equipment crucial to effective splint fabrication. **Chapter 6** outlines the entire process of creating an accurate splint design from obtaining an appropriate referral to properly dispensing the device. It also introduces the PROCESS concept used in Section II.

Section II is the working section of the book and is organized into four chapters that cover immobilization **(Chapter 7)**, mobilization **(Chapter 8)**, restriction **(Chapter 9)**, and nonarticular **(Chapter 10)** splints. Each chapter includes pattern illustrations and accompanying photography of the splint described. Most of the pattern descriptions include "Clinical Pearls" that apply to that particular splint or other splints throughout this section. These pearls relate to our personal splinting experience. They include fabrication and splint modification tips as well as insight for improving cost containment and maximizing time efficiency. Most splint patterns have alternative splint options in the event that the therapist cannot fabricate a custom splint. Common diagnoses and general positioning are recommended. However, one must appreciate that the diagnoses appropriate for a splint and the recommended positioning can be varied and depend on many factors. The pattern designs illustrated are suggestions of the ones we have found simple to visualize and use. The therapist is encouraged to modify the pattern according to specific patient needs. Section II is meant as a guideline for splint construction—use your creativity to individualize each splint. The included tips of the trade allow for true customization of splints. The clinical pearls are not always unique to a particular splint and many apply to a variety of splints. A list of clinical pearls is provided at the front of the book to help the student locate specific points of interest.

Section III describes alternative interventions for immobilization, mobilization, or restriction of a body part. Because of time constraints, monetary issues, or perhaps lack of product availability, it is not always practical or appropriate to make a splint from thermoplastic materials. The chapters included in this section provide information on alternative means of splinting. Chapter 11 outlines the considerations related to the use of prefabricated splints, including information on how to become an educated consumer on the availability, application, and modification of these splints. It also reviews some of the commonly used and currently available splints. Chapter 12 describes casting as a treatment technique that has the ability to provide outcomes that no other splinting approach can offer. It familiarizes the clinician with the characteristics of casting products so he or she can choose the material that best meets the patient's needs. Chapter 13 provides a brief overview of three popular taping methods: traditional athletic taping, McConnell taping, and Kinesio taping. Each technique is described with specific instructions and multiple clinical examples. Chapter 14 is a noteworthy chapter because Neoprene is becoming increasingly popular. It reviews the basic information regarding the benefits of Neoprene, different types of Neoprene materials, and appropriate diagnoses. Fabrication using a non-sewing technique is also described.

Each chapter in Section IV goes into depth regarding a specific diagnosis or patient population including stiffness, fractures, arthritis, tendon injuries, peripheral nerve injuries, the athlete, adult neyrological dusfunction, the pediatric patient, burns and the musician. After an overview of the topic, the chapters include common splinting interventions and specific considerations. Many chapters include tables that clarify information and decrease redundancy within the text. Case studies accompany each chapter and are meant to stimulate clinical reasoning and synthesize information reviewed in the text.

Appendix A is a list of rehabilitation vendors that offer splinting equipment, materials, prefabricated splints and orthotics. Most offer free catalogs that describe their products. Appendix B provides examples of forms used in a clinical setting. The Splint Index allows the reader to access information about splints by their common names as well as by the ASHT terminology.

This book reviews numerous pattern designs and other options for splinting the upper extremity. Although this endeavor documents a spectrum of splinting management, the possibilities for different options extend far beyond a single text. New challenges face the clinician daily; and it is with each patient that we learn something new, building on our previous knowledge. This book is meant to stimulate clinical skills, encouraging the integration of principles and process from which a clinician can create new splints.

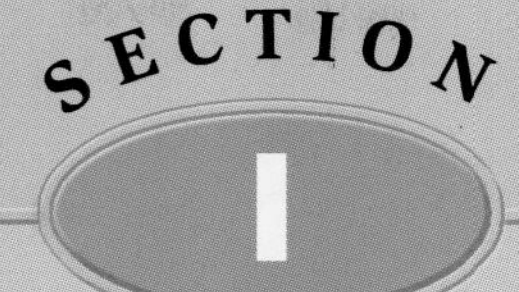

Splinting Fundamentals

CHAPTER

1

Splint Classification

MaryLynn Jacobs, MS, OTR/L, CHT

INTRODUCTION

Splinting the upper extremity requires a unique combination of the therapist's creative abilities and a sound knowledge of anatomic, biomechanical, physiologic, and healing principles as they relate to injury, surgery, and disease. Splinting can be one of the most challenging and most enjoyable aspects of being a therapist. Before delving into the fabrication of splints, one must not only understand proper nomenclature for universal communication but also develop a solid understanding of the clinical reasoning process for selecting the most appropriate splint for the patient.

Owing to the growing recognition of specialists who treat the upper extremity and the increasing use of custom-fabricated splints, it has been necessary to develop a standard language that clearly and uniformly describes splints to those who refer, fabricate, and/or pay for the devices. The **American Society of Hand Therapists (ASHT)** recognized the need to standardize, organize, and simplify traditional splinting terms. ASHT's executive board appointed a splint nomenclature task force composed of well-respected splinting authorities to address this issue. The task force created the first organized system for describing and categorizing splints (American Society of Hand Therapists, 1992). The **Splint Classification System (SCS)** groups splints into progressively more refined categories (Fig. 1–1).

Although the SCS appears to be the most comprehensive classification to date, many clinicians prefer and continue to use the well-accepted common terminology. In Section II of this book, the traditional and universally accepted splint names (e.g., wrist cock-up splint, thumb spica splint) are listed under the heading "Common Names." Note that the SCS is only one method of classifying splints; individual physicians and therapists may not be familiar with this system and may use instead the traditional terminology.

Overview of Splint Classification

In this book, most splints are named according to SCS terms, which includes location, direction (if applicable), and intent (immobilization, mobilization, or restriction). This section summarizes the SCS.

Articular and Nonarticular Splints

The SCS initially divides splints into one of two broad groups: **articular** and **nonarticular.** Articular splints are those that cross one or more joints. Nonarticular splints provide support and protection to a healing bone (e.g., humerus, metacarpal, or phalanx) or to a soft tissue structure (e.g., annular pulley or musculotendinous junction of the medial or lateral epicondyle). There are far fewer nonarticular splints than articular splints.

When interpreting a referral, it is advantageous to distinguish between articular and nonarticular splints so that a joint is not unnecessarily immobilized. For example, if the word *nonarticular* does not precede the words *proximal forearm immobilization splint* on the referral, then the therapist may assume that the elbow or wrist needs to be included in the splint design. By adding the word *nonarticular,* the description becomes more specific. In Section II, the articular splints are separated from the nonarticular splints to aid in pattern location; the term *articular* does not appear in the splint description, because the name of the splint (e.g., wrist immobilization splint) indicates whether a joint is included. However, the term *nonarticular* does appear in the descriptions (e.g., nonarticular humerus splint and nonarticular metacarpal splint), so there is no ambiguity.

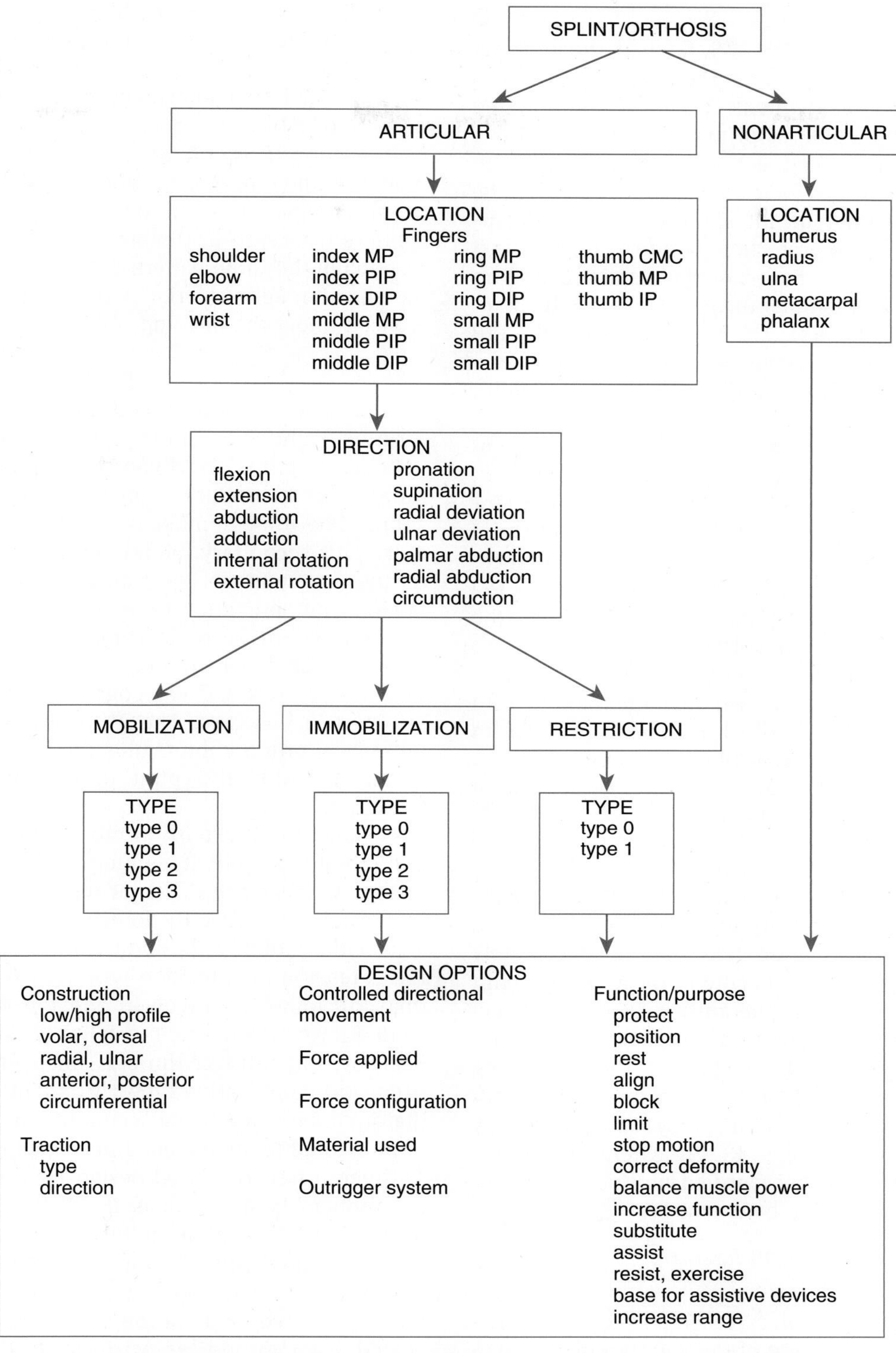

Figure 1–1 *The Splint Classification System. CMC, carpometacarpal; DIP, distal interphalangeal; IP, interphalangeal; MP, metacarpophalangeal; PIP, proximal interphalangeal. Reprinted with permission from American Society of Hand Therapists. (1992). Splint classification system. Garner, NC.*

Location

Location, the next level in the SCS, refers to the joint, set of joints, or body part on which the splint acts, according to the splint's main intent. The SCS refers to the joints included in a splint as primary or secondary. The primary joint is designated as the target joint on which the splint acts and is the focus of the splint's name. The secondary joint is the joint the splint traverses or incorporates for purposes of protection, comfort, and/or maximal splint stabilization. For example, a splint acting on the ring finger (RF) proximal interphalangeal (PIP) joint is named an RF PIP splint. The primary joint is the PIP joint, and the secondary joint may be the RF metacarpophalangeal (MP) joint, incorporated for better splint purchase.

If there are several primary joints involved, as commonly seen after a severe crushing injury to the hand, grouping the joints together may simplify naming. For example, if a crush injury involves all the MP, PIP, and distal interphalangeal (DIP) joints, the splint classification is a hand splint. If the crush injury involves the three joints of only the middle finger (MF), then the splint is described as an MF splint.

Nonarticular splints are described in much the same way. For example, a splint used to immobilize a fifth metacarpal fracture is described as a nonarticular fifth metacarpal splint. Similarly, a splint used to protect a recently reconstructed annular pulley is described as a nonarticular proximal phalanx splint.

Direction

The **direction** descriptor, the next level in the SCS, refers to the position of the primary joint(s) in the splint and provides critical information necessary for accurately fabricating the splint. The specific purpose of the splint must be known before the therapist can add the direction descriptor. Direction defines the position of the involved joints, the desired direction of the mobilizing force (mobilization splint), or the direction in which motion is to be blocked (restriction splint). For example, by adding a direction term—e.g., RF PIP extension splint—the splint's intent is further clarified, in this case by indicating that the joint is to be extended.

Intent: Immobilization, Mobilization, and Restriction

Intent, the next level of the SCS, refers to the overall function or primary purpose of the splint, which is generally **immobilization, mobilization,** or **restriction.** Adding the splint's purpose to the end of the description provides the splint maker with a clearer understanding of what is being requested. For example, a prescription for an RF PIP extension mobilization splint tells the splint fabricator that an extension force needs to be exerted on the PIP joint of the ring finger. The purpose of an RF PIP extension immobilization splint, on the other hand, is to immobilize the PIP joint in extension. Finally, an RF PIP extension restriction splint restricts the full extension of the PIP joint but allows active flexion (as often requested for management of a finger with a swan-neck deformity).

In Section II, splints are organized according to their most common purpose, although additional functions are also defined. For example, the RF PIP immobilization splint is discussed in Chapter 8. However, because it is essentially the same pattern used for a RF PIP extension mobilization splint (serial static design), this use is referenced under the heading "Additional Functions."

Types

Inclusion of the **secondary joint** levels is the final descriptor of the SCS. Immobilization, mobilization, and restriction splints are divided into **types** based on the number of secondary joint levels influenced by the splint. The total number of joint levels included (primary plus secondary joints) is indicated in brackets after the type number. For example, for a posterior elbow flexion immobilization type 1[2] splint, the *1* indicates the number of secondary joint levels involved. The wrist is included to minimize splint migration and to increase comfort and is recognized as the only secondary joint in this case. The *2* (in brackets) refers to the number of primary joints plus the number of secondary joints affected by the splint; in this case, the elbow and the wrist.

For an RF PIP extension mobilization splint, the primary joint is the PIP. If counterforce control is needed to further stabilize the PIP joint within the splint, the MP joint can be included. By doing so, the MP joint becomes a secondary joint. This splint is now classified as an RF PIP extension mobilization type 1[2] splint. When multiple PIP joints are involved and the MP joints are included for counterforce, the splint is classified in a similar way, index finger through small finger (IF–SF) PIP extension mobilization type 1[2] splint. The rationale is that joint *levels* are being accounted for, not the number of individual joints included in the splint.

Given a forearm-based design for the same problem, the proper classification is IF–SF PIP extension mobilization type 2[3] splint. In this example, there is one primary joint level (the PIP) and two secondary joint levels (the MP and wrist). Taking this example one step further, if all three joints of the digits and the wrist are involved (e.g., to address extrinsic flexor tightness after cast immobilization for distal radius fracture), the splint is described as a wrist/hand extension mobilization type 0[4] splint. The wrist, MP, PIP, and DIP joints need to be mobilized in extension to address extrinsic flexor tightness effectively; therefore all are considered primary joints. Another example of a type 0 splint is a simple wrist extension immobilization type 0[1]. See Table 1–1 for a summary of the examples discussed here.

TABLE 1–1 Summary of Examples

Splint	Secondary Level(s)	Total Levels
Posterior elbow flexion wrist immobilization type 1[2]	Wrist	Wrist (secondary) plus elbow (primary)
RF PIP extension mobilization type 1[2]	MP	MP (secondary) plus PIP (primary)
IF–SF PIP extension mobilization type 2[3]	MP and wrist	MP and wrist (secondary) plus PIP (primary)
Wrist/hand extension mobilization type 0[4]		Wrist, MP, PIP, and DIP (primary)
Wrist extension immobilization type 0[1]		Wrist (primary)

When secondary joint levels are included in the prescription, the splint fabricator is prompted to analyze critically the splint's purpose and to consider design options. However, these levels are seldom seen on a referral slip and are often confusing; thus this text does not include secondary levels.

Design Descriptors

The **design descriptor** improves understanding of the type of splint that is requested. In this text, the descriptors are used as an aid whenever necessary. Design descriptors include non-SCS nomenclature that is still widely used by hand surgery and hand therapy specialists; some examples are *static, dynamic, static progressive,* and *serial static.* These terms are discussed separately later in this chapter.

In the SCS, design descriptors, which are selectively included, appear in parentheses after the name of the splint. In this book, however, the descriptors are found at the beginning of the splint's name to help readers with critical-thinking and decision-making processes. The descriptive terms include the following:

- *Digit-based.* Originating from the digit, allowing MP joint motion, and possibly extending to the distal phalanx.
- *Hand-based.* Originating from the hand, allowing wrist motion, and possibly extending to the distal phalanx.
- *Thumb-based.* Originating from the thenar eminence or thumb and incorporating one or more joints of the thumb.
- *Forearm-based.* Originating from the forearm, allowing full elbow motion, and possibly extending to the distal phalanx.
- *Arm-based.* Originating from the upper arm and possibly including the wrist, elbow, and/or shoulder joints.
- *Circumferential.* Encompassing the entire perimeter of a body part.
- *Gutter.* Including only the radial or ulnar portion of a body part.
- *Radial.* Incorporating the radial aspect of a body part.
- *Ulnar.* Incorporating the ulnar aspect of a body part.
- *Dorsal.* Traversing the dorsal aspect of the hand or forearm.
- *Volar.* Traversing the volar aspect of the hand or forearm.
- *Anterior.* Traversing the anterior aspect of a body part.
- *Posterior.* Traversing the posterior aspect of a body part.

Non-SCS Nomenclature

The widely used terms *static, serial static, dynamic,* and *static progressive* are not included in the SCS. These terms designate choices of splint designs that a therapist can incorporate to achieve immobilization, mobilization, or restriction of the intended structure(s). These splint choices are noted under "Common Names" in Section II and are listed in the book's index.

Static Splints

Static splints have a firm base and immobilize the joint(s) they cross. They can be used to facilitate dynamic functions, e.g., by blocking one joint to encourage movement of another. In some cases, a static splint is considered to be nonarticular—having no direct influence on joint mobility—while providing stabilization, protection, and support to a body segment, such as the humerus or metacarpal. Static splints may be the most common splint that therapists are called on to make.

Serial Static Splints

Serial static splints or casts are applied with the tissue at its maximum length; they are worn for long periods to accommodate elongation of soft tissue in the desired direction of correction. They are remolded by the therapist to maintain the joint(s), soft tissue, and muscle–tendon units they cross in a lengthened position. Serial static splints can be constructed to be circumferential and nonremovable. This option provides for greater patient compliance and assures the therapist and physician that the tissue is being continually stressed without the risk of the tissue rebounding, which would happen if the splint were removed.

Dynamic Splints

Dynamic splints generate a mobilizing or supportive force on a targeted tissue that results in passive gains or passive-assisted range of motion (ROM) (Fess & Phillips, 1987). Dynamic splints have a static base that provides the foundation for outrigger attachments. Controlled mobilizing forces are applied via a dynamic (elastic) assist, which may be rubber bands, springs, or wrapped elastic cord. The dynamic force applied through the splint continues as long as the elastic component can contract, even when the shortened tissue reaches the end of its elastic limit (Schultz-Johnson, 1992). A dynamic splint can also be used as an active-resistive exercise modality against its line of pull.

Static Progressive Splints

Static progressive splints achieve mobilization by applying unidirectional, low-load force to the tissue's maximum end ROM until the tissue accommodates. Construction is similar to dynamic splints, except these splints use nonelastic components to deliver the mobilizing force, including nylon cord, strapping materials, screws, hinges, turnbuckles, and nonelastic tape. Once the joint position and tension are set, the splint does not continue to stress the tissue beyond its elastic limit (Schultz-Johnson, 1992). The force can be modified only through progressive splint adjustments. Some patients may tolerate static progressive splinting better than dynamic splinting, perhaps because the joint position is constant while the tissue readily accommodates to the tension and is less subject to the influences of gravity and motion (Schultz-Johnson, 1992, 1996).

Classification of Splints and Objectives for Intervention

This section reviews the objectives for splinting intervention and provides appropriate clinical examples for immobilization, mobilization, and restriction. Remember that not all splints can be simply classified and the primary objective may not always be clear-cut. There may be multiple objectives for splinting intervention. For example a wrist/hand immobilization splint (resting hand splint) for a patient with rheumatoid arthritis may be designed to immobilize inflamed arthritic joints while placing the MP joints in a gentle radially deviated position to minimize ulnar drift and periarticular deformity.

The discussion covers general and common examples to emphasize how critical thinking is necessary when fabricating splints. Experienced therapists recognize that splinting complex injuries requires much overlap and problem solving.

Immobilization Splints

Although the **immobilization splint** is the most common and simplest form of splint fabricated, it can be used for the most complex injuries. Static splints are considered immobilization splints because they do not allow motion of the joints to which they are applied. Immobilization splints can be considered either articular or nonarticular, immobilizing the joints they cross (articular) or stabilizing the structure to which they are applied (nonarticular), as in the case of a humerus splint.

The common objectives for immobilization are as follows:

- Provide symptom relief after injury or overuse.
- Protect and properly position edematous structure(s).
- Aid in maximizing functional use of the hand.
- Maintain tissue length to prevent soft tissue contracture.
- Protect healing structures and surgical procedures.
- Maintain and protect reduction of a fracture.
- Protect and improve joint alignment.
- Block or transfer power of movement to enhance exercise.
- Reduce tone and contracture of a spastic muscle.

These objectives and examples of splinting intervention are discussed in the following sections.

Provide Symptom Relief

An immobilization splint can provide significant pain relief when applied as soon as possible after injury. The injured structures should be splinted in a resting, nonstressed position, minimizing movement that can influence pain. This splint is initially worn day and night and may be removed for only short periods of exercise and hygiene. After the initial symptoms have subsided, splint use is decreased; eventually, the splint may be used only for preventing the risk of re-injury. For example, a person who has sustained a wrist sprain may present with exquisite pain when wrist motion is attempted. The use of a wrist immobilization splint is appropriate for approximately 1 month or until pain subsides. After the period of immobilization, the splint may be used for only sleeping and/or at-risk activities.

EXAMPLE: WRIST/THUMB IMMOBILIZATION SPLINT

A radial wrist/thumb immobilization splint can significantly decrease inflammation and pain within the first dorsal compartment (deQuervain's tenosynovitis) by preventing simultaneous wrist ulnar deviation and thumb flexion. The wrist is splinted in neutral extension with 0 to 5° of ulnar deviation (Eaton, 1992). This position keeps the extensor pollicis brevis and the abductor pollicis longus tendons in alignment with the radius as they exit the pulley about the radial styloid (Eaton, 1992). The thumb carpometacarpal (CMC) joint is positioned in slight abduction, and the MP joint is included in a slightly flexed, comfortable position (Fig. 1–2). The splint is generally worn full time for 3 to 4 weeks, and then use is gradually reduced to nights only once the day symptoms have resolved. The splint is discontinued when the patient is asymptomatic to provocative (painful) positioning.

Protect and Position Edematous Structures

Edema is often the first observable reaction to injury, yet not always the first addressed. Its immediate reduction is

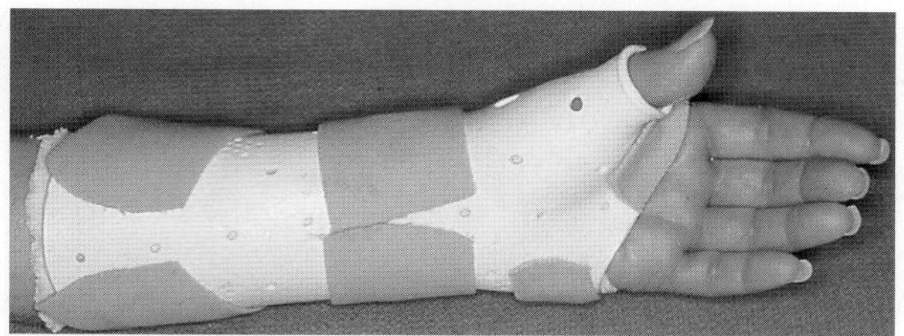

Figure 1–2 Immobilization of the thumb and wrist can provide significant relief for a patient with acute deQuervain's tenosynovitis. Note that the wrist is held in slight ulnar deviation to minimize shear stress of the extensor pollicis brevis and the abductor pollicis longus tendons as they traverse through the retinaculum at the radial styloid area.

critical to facilitate proper healing with minimal complications (such as tight ligaments, which could lead to joint and soft tissue contracture). An edematous hand may be a painful hand that has associated injuries that must be considered before splint application. For example, consider fabricating a splint that places the digital joints in a safe position (MP flexion, IP extension) and can be donned and doffed easily to allow access for wound and pin care. Attention to joint positioning in the splint, elevation, massage, compression wraps, and gentle active ROM of adjacent structures (if appropriate) all contribute to reducing edema and preventing deformity (e.g., MP extension and PIP flexion contractures).

Compression bandages or gloves (e.g., Coban and Isotoner gloves) can be worn under the splint for edema reduction and can complement the splint's effectiveness. However, caution is necessary when donning and doffing these compression devices to avoid injury or re-injury of the healing bones, tendons, and/or ligaments. Furthermore, the therapist must carefully consider the type and placement of the splint straps. A narrow strap placed across an edematous area may cause pooling of edema proximal and distal to the strap and may irritate superficial sensory nerves. Circumferentially wrapping the splint, distal to proximal, with an elasticized wrap (e.g., Ace wrap or Coban) may help distribute pressure evenly along the extremity and aid in minimizing edema.

In addition, patient education regarding the importance of splint use in conjunction with other edema management methods facilitates early reduction of edema.

EXAMPLE: WRIST/HAND/THUMB IMMOBILIZATION SPLINT

Crush injuries are often complex and may involve one or more structures, including bone, ligament, tendon, and nerve. Patients often do well during the initial stages of healing with a simple wrist/hand/thumb immobilization splint to keep the involved structures positioned, supported, and protected. Therapists working with these patients should strive to achieve optimal joint positioning. One of the most important goals is to maintain the antideformity position of the hand (also referred to as the intrinsic plus or safe position): MP flexion, IP extension, and thumb palmar abduction. If this is not accomplished early after injury, MP joint collateral ligament shortening and volar plate contracture may occur, which can result in MP extension and PIP flexion contractures. Optimal joint positions may be difficult to achieve initially owing to stiffness, pain, and significant edema. Be persistant, splint within a comfortable ROM, monitor, and serially adjust the splint as pain allows (Fig. 1–3).

Aid in Maximizing Functional Use

A splint can enhance function by correctly positioning and supporting structures that are injured or unstable. During the day, these supportive, lightweight, functional splints can often help patients use their hands to engage in vocational, academic, or recreational activities. Without support, function is diminished and deforming forces may dominate. These splints can be fabricated to position and support with minimal bulk. The bulkier the splint, the more likely it will interfere with functional use.

EXAMPLE: THUMB CMC IMMOBILIZATION SPLINT

A thumb CMC joint that becomes subluxed and painful when a pinch is attempted may benefit from the use of a well-molded CMC immobilization splint (Colditz, 1995a). Function and comfort are gained by careful attention to molding at the base of the first metacarpal bone. This ensures adequate stabilization of the CMC joint during active use of the thumb and enables the patient to grasp and pinch more effectively (Fig. 1–4).

Maintain Tissue Length

Splints can preserve tissue length when applied carefully and accurately and within the appropriate time frame. Contractures of soft tissue can occur from many sources. One such cause is nerve injury, resulting in muscle–tendon imbalances in the hand. Left untreated, these imbalances often result in tendon–ligament shortening, which in turn may create some degree of joint contracture.

During the initial stages of injury, the splinting goal should be to place the joints in a position that inhibits tissue shortening and enables functional use. During the end stages of scar maturation (3 to 6 months or longer), the splinting goal may be to keep the tissue at its

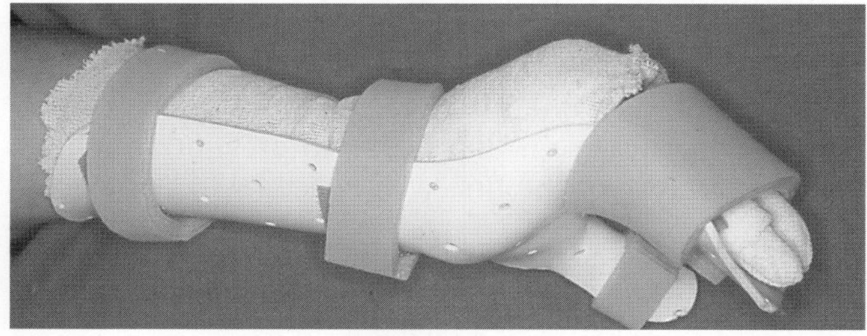

Figure 1–3 A simple wrist/hand/thumb immobilization splint can provide the support, proper positioning (MP flexion, IP extension, thumb palmar abduction), and healing environment that crush injuries require.

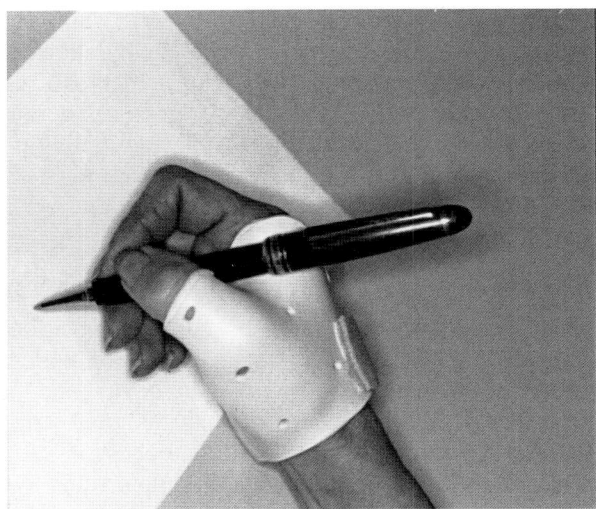

Figure 1–4 A thumb CMC immobilization splint is being used for stabilization of this joint while writing is attempted. This small splint can help prevent subluxation of the CMC joint during functional use.

achieved maximum length to prevent regression of tissue tightness (McFarlane, 1997). At this stage, the splint is not influencing the tissue length but is maintaining the desired and previously achieved ROM. Gains attained in therapy sessions and at home can be maintained with a balanced program of proper immobilization and exercise.

EXAMPLE: WRIST/THUMB CMC PALMAR ABDUCTION IMMOBILIZATION SPLINT

Adduction contractures of the thumb can occur after injury to or repair of the median nerve. To prevent them, a splint should be applied as soon as possible after nerve repair. The splint is forearm-based with the wrist slightly flexed, intimately molded into the first web space, and extending distally to the thumb IP joint crease. Care should be taken to avoid undue stress on the ulnar collateral ligament of the thumb MP joint during fabrication. This splint position maintains the thumb in maximum abduction, preventing a possible adduction contracture while placing the nerve repair in a shortened position to allow for healing (Fig. 1–5**A**). A small spacer can be made to fit over a wrist immobilization splint to be worn for night use only. This may be an option for patients who want to attempt functional use of the hand during the day (Fig. 1–5**B**). Whatever option is chosen, the goal is to prevent an adduction contracture of the first web space.

Protect Healing Structures and Surgical Procedures

A therapist may be called on to fabricate an immobilization splint to rest and protect an extremity that has undergone an operative procedure. This may involve a simple splint or an intricate splint that must immobilize several structures in specific positions because of a complex injury or surgical repair. For postoperative splinting, close communication with the surgeon is critical to guide proper splint selection. Consideration needs to be given to splinting around or over drains, wounds, external pins, or skin grafts. These issues, as well as the pain level and psychological trauma of injury and surgery, make splinting the postoperative extremity a challenge.

EXAMPLE: WRIST IMMOBILIZATION SPLINT

Support, comfort, and protection of the patient's status after closed reduction and external fixation of a distal radius fracture can be achieved using an ulnar wrist immobilization splint with an optional protective covering over the fixator (Fig. 1–6). The external fixator is usually situated along the radial side of the hand, thus lending little or no support to the ulnar side. This wrist splint provides support to the arches of the hand and allows unrestricted motion of the thumb and digits. The splint can be fabricated to include the elbow if forearm rotation is to be limited (Laseter & Carter, 1996). The pin protector keeps the fixator pins from catching on clothing, bedding, etc.; helps keep the pin tracks free from debris; and provides a visual block for patients that are uncomfortable looking at the external pins. The external fixator protector can be made from a thermoplastic material or can be purchased.

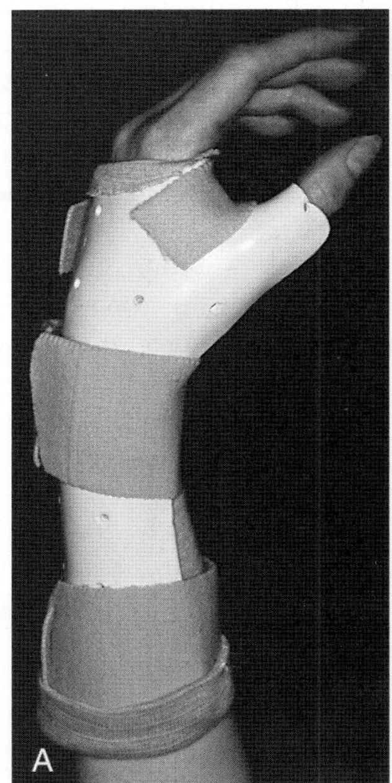

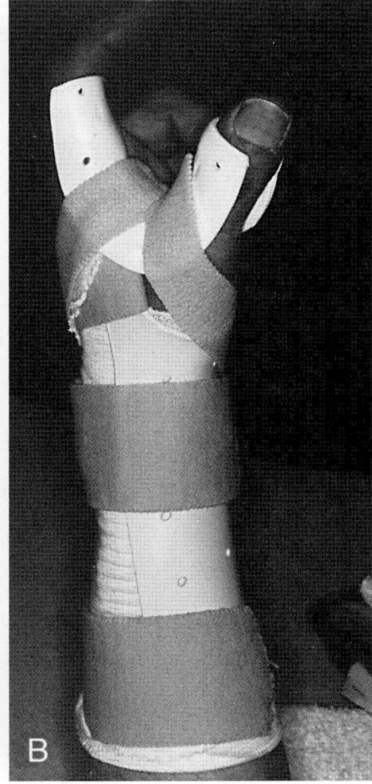

*Figure 1–5 **A,** A wrist/thumb CMC palmar abduction immobilization splint, used to prevent adduction contractures of the first web space after median nerve injury or repair, can be fabricated to incorporate the wrist and first web space. **B,** The splint can also incorporate a removable piece, fabricated over a simple wrist immobilization splint, that is worn at night or when the hand is not being used.*

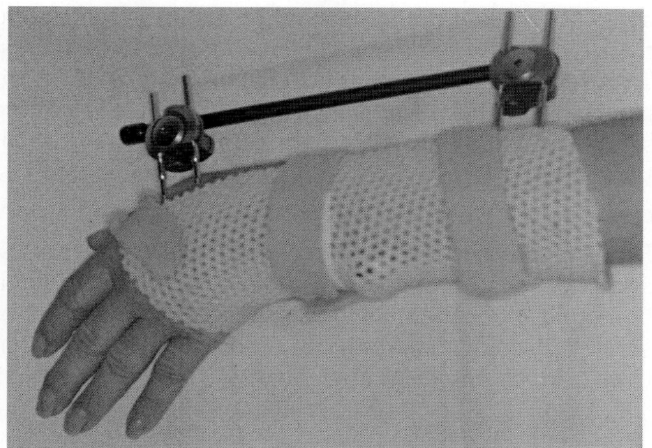

Figure 1–6 An ulnar wrist immobilization splint supports the hand after closed reduction and external fixation of a distal radius fracture.

Maintain and Protect Reduction of a Fracture

A splint can provide fracture stabilization and maintain reduction when applied by an experienced therapist and supervised by a physician. There are times when casting is not appropriate for a patient, but splinting can be used as an alternative. The use of thermoplastic material can often provide an intimate fit around detailed areas, such as the metacarpal heads and phalanges, which may be harder to achieve with traditional casting materials. Some patients are more comfortable with the lighter thermoplastic material and better functional use of the hand that come with splints.

EXAMPLE: RF–SF MP FLEXION IMMOBILIZATION SPLINT

Stable fractures, such as some fifth metacarpal fractures, may be treated effectively with an RF–SF MP immobilization splint (Fig. 1–7). This type of splint, when molded intimately and carefully, provides continued alignment and protection for the healing fracture, maintains the RF–SF MP collateral ligaments in a lengthened position, and allows for active ROM of the proximal and distal joints. The position of the fourth and fifth MP joints is generally 60° of flexion, with the wrist, PIP, and DIP joints often left free. Because the fourth and fifth metacarpals are mobile compared to the second and third metacarpals, the hand portion of the splint should encompass the third metacarpal to improve splint stability and provide adequate purchase of the splint on the hand.

Protect and Improve Joint Alignment

A splint can be fabricated to align subluxed and/or deviated joints to an improved anatomic position. In certain conditions, such as rheumatoid arthritis, joint laxity and/or tendon ruptures may disrupt proper joint mechanics, resulting in significant functional loss. Immobilization splints may work well to provide support and protection; they also redirect and attempt to position ligaments properly during healing (Dell & Dell, 1996; Philips 1995).

EXAMPLE: WRIST/HAND IMMOBILIZATION SPLINT

Patients with arthritis can wear a comfortable and supportive wrist–hand immobilization splint at night; the splint aids in maintaining proper joint alignment, protects against deforming forces, and prevents or minimizes soft tissue contractures. Not only can the splint be molded to support the larger joints involved but strategically directed soft straps can aid in repositioning the small joints of the digits within the splint. Without attention to corrective positioning, joint deformity and limitation of function may occur sooner rather than later. The individual with arthritis often welcomes the rest and support that the immobilization splint provides (Fig. 1–8).

Block or Transfer the Power of Movement

Casting or splinting of individual joints can be used to block or transfer the power of movement to other joints in the same plane of motion. By blocking movement at a particular joint, the power of that movement is then transferred either proximally or distally. This can be especially useful when the goal is to glide a tendon through scar tissue or facilitate movement of a stiff joint. These devices are often used in the field of hand rehabilitation as a home exercise tool.

EXAMPLE: PIP IMMOBILIZATION SPLINT

A circumferential splint or cast to block PIP joint motion, leaving the DIP free, transfers the force of flexion to the DIP joint. The PIP splint acts as a mechanical block, eliminating flexor digitorum superficialis function and encouraging the flexor digitorum profundus tendon to work

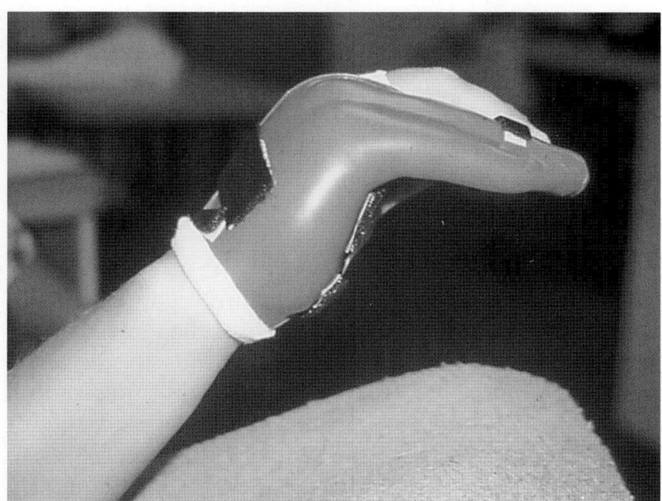

Figure 1–7 A hand immobilization splint for treatment of a fifth metacarpal fracture; the pressure applied through the volar–dorsal nature of this splint during fabrication minimizes the tendency for the bone fragments to shift.

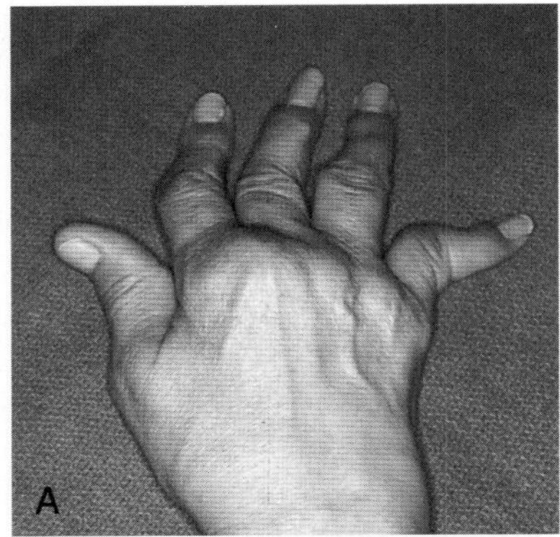

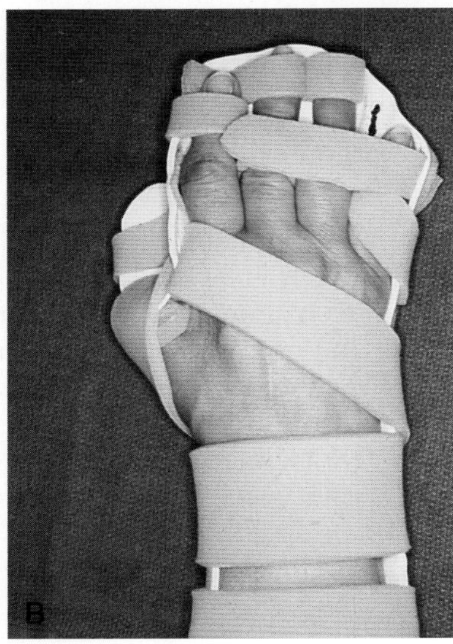

Figure 1–8 ***A,*** *The hand of patient with psoriatic arthritis.* ***B,*** *An immobilization splint with carefully positioned straps provides support to and maintains near optimal positioning of the involved joints during rest periods.*

independently to move the distal phalanx (Fig. 1–9). This same concept can be applied to the DIP joint. If the DIP joint is splinted or casted in extension, the forces of flexion are then transferred to the PIP joint. If the other digits are held in extension, this splint will help block flexor digitorum profundus motion and isolate flexor digitorum superficialis glide.

Reduce Tone and Contracture of a Spastic Muscle

There is controversy in the literature regarding which splint designs and therapeutic approaches are most effective for inhibiting tone in a spastic muscle. However, most therapists agree that early splinting intervention is beneficial for decreasing muscle tone, preventing or reducing contractures, and preventing maceration of skin in the palm (Mathiowetz, Bolding, & Trombley, 1983; McPherson, 1981; Neuhaus, Ascher, & Coullon, 1981; Rose & Shah, 1987).

The choice of splint design is influenced by the severity of the muscle tone, any existing contracture(s), and the ability to position the patient for the actual splint fabrication. Two people may be needed to fabricate these splints. Tone-reducing techniques performed before splint application often helps. See Chapter 21 for details regarding splint options and joint–patient positioning for ease of fabrication.

EXAMPLE: WRIST/HAND/THUMB IMMOBILIZATION SPLINT

For increased flexor muscle tone in the hand, hard cones, attached or incorporated into a ulnar wrist/hand/thumb immobilization splint, control wrist, thumb, and digit position; prevent contracture; and minimize the risk of skin breakdown in the palm (Fig. 1–10).

Mobilization Splints

The rationale of **mobilization splinting** is based on a physiologic theory that controlled tension applied over a long period of time alters cell proliferation. Brand and others have well described and documented the benefits of using different forms of mobilization splinting as a treatment modality (Bell-Krotoski, 1995; Bell-Krotoski & Figarola, 1995; Brand & Thompson, 1993; Colditz, 1995b; Fess, 1995; Fess & McCollum, 1998; Flowers & LaStayo, 1994; Gyovai & Wright Howell, 1992; Prosser, 1996; Rose & Shah, 1987; Tribuzi, 1995). The effectiveness of mobilization splinting is not based on the concept of stretching tissue but relies on actual cell growth. The target tissue lengthens when the living cells of the contracted tissues are stimulated to grow. The stimulation occurs when consistent external tension is applied through the splint over time (Brand & Thompson, 1993). The living cells recognize the tension placed on them, permitting the older cells of collagen to be actively ab-

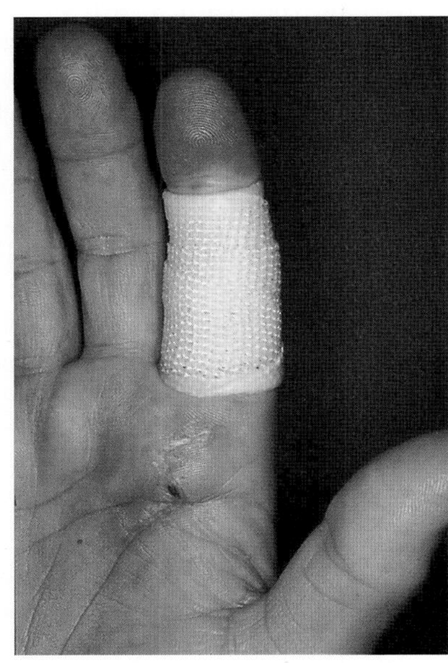

Figure 1–9 A simple cylindrical splint (here fabricated with QuickCast) can be used to isolate and promote flexor digitorum profundus glide.

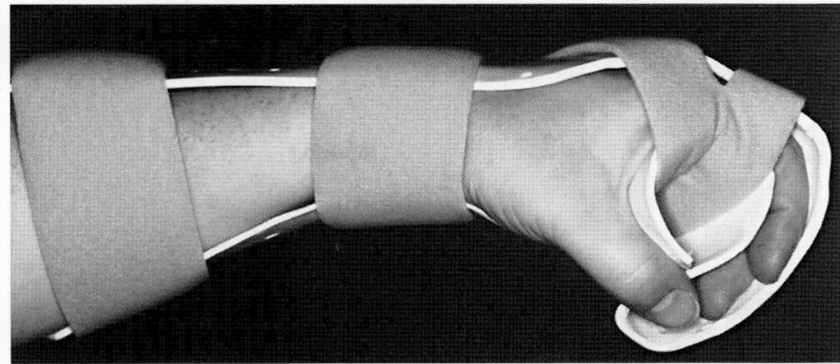

Figure 1–10 A wrist immobilization splint with a palmar cone component is often the splint of choice for reducing tone and preventing skin breakdown.

sorbed and replaced with new collagen cells oriented in the direction of the applied tension.

This concept of tissue growth has been demonstrated in several African groups for whom it is deemed fashionable to stretch out certain body parts, such as earlobes, lips, and necks. For example, a small dowel is placed in the earlobes of a young child; the diameter of the dowel is serially increased as the tissue expands and accommodates to each new size (Fig. 1–11).

Mobilization splints can be challenging to plan and to fabricate. The therapist has many options (dynamic, serial static, static progressive) when contemplating which type of mobilization splint is most appropriate to produce the desired result. The integration of specific information gathered in the initial assessment—e.g., age, motivation, psychological status, associated trauma or disease, avocational or vocational demands, quality of the joint's end ROM (soft, hard, elastic), active versus passive ROM, and function—contributes to the decision-making process. For example, a patient with a dense, long-standing PIP joint flexion contracture may be better served with a serial static or static progressive splint than with a dynamic splint. Serial static or static progressive splints maintain the PIP joint in extension for a set period of time. A dynamic splint may not offer enough elastic force to overcome a dense contracture.

Dynamic and static progressive splints differ only in the way mobilizing forces are applied and delivered to the target tissue. Tension through both types of splints is initially set by the therapist and can be adjusted by the well-informed patient. The patient may be instructed to decrease the tension for night comfort and to increase the tension between treatment sessions. With dynamic splints, the effectiveness of the dynamic forces (especially rubber bands) may diminish over time because of the tendency of the elastic properties of the bands to fatigue under tension. Gravity may also adversely effect the elasticity of the dynamic force by progressively stretching out the bands.

The use of dynamic splints through the night is generally not encouraged. The nature of this splint is to deliver continuous tension to the target structure, even though the tissue may have reached its maximum tolerable length. Most patients cannot endure this persistent tension at night and end up removing the splint (Schultz-Johnson, 1996). Furthermore, sleeping with a dynamic splint may be awkward and cumbersome, and there is a possibility that the line of pull could get caught up in bedding and clothing. When applied properly, static progressive and serial static splints may be worn throughout the night; these splints hold the target structure at or close to maximum tolerable length, but not beyond this position (Schultz-Johnson, 1996).

Patients are able to remove both dynamic and static progressive splints for hygiene, completion of active exercise, and functional use. Serial static casts are generally fabricated to be nonremovable. They can be changed when the tissue has accommodated to the tension placed on them. Generally, this occurs between 3 and 6 days. Some serial static splints are made to be worn for a long period of time (e.g., throughout the night) but allow for periods of exercise and rest. For patients who require an uninterrupted stretch in one direction (as in a PIP flexion contracture secondary to a central tendon injury), a splint that is removable may not be the best choice. Once the splint has been removed, the tissue is able to rebound back to its original resting position and the gains that were achieved may be at least partially lost. A nonremovable circumferential serial static cast should be considered in these situations.

Attempts should be made to measure and document all forces applied to the hand. Too much tension can cause discomfort, edema, and tissue reaction; too little tension may not be effective. Observation and clinical judgment are important means of assessing tension parameters; however, patient education is paramount. Splint wearers should be aware of the signs of too much tension (e.g., blanching skin, pain, numbness, color changes) and what they should perceive (e.g., slight discomfort or a mild stretching sensation). Initially, a gen-

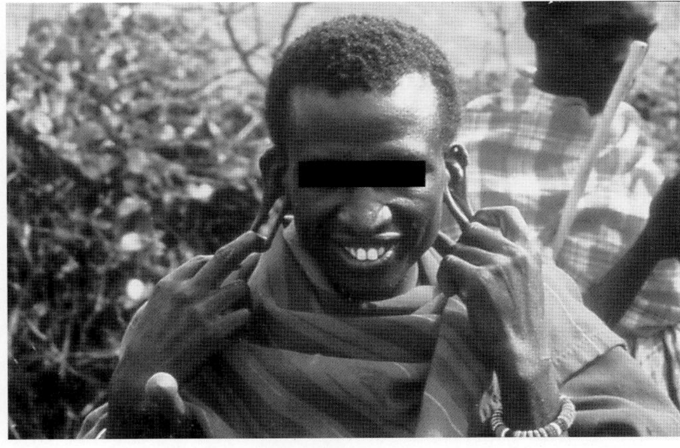

Figure 1–11 The elongated earlobes of this African man are the result of stretching owing to the life-long use of graded dowels.

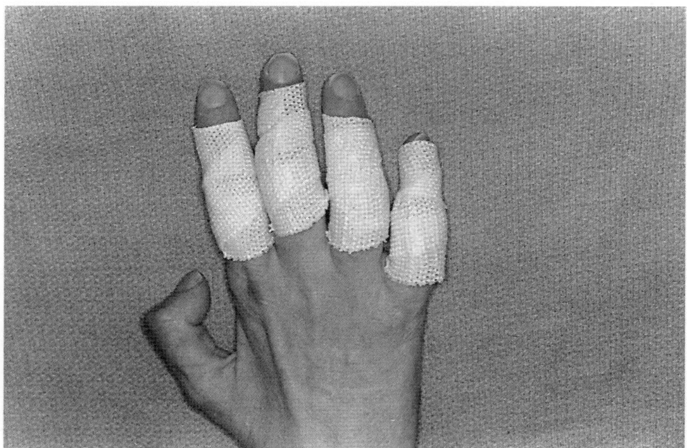

Figure 1–12 Intimately molded casts (here fabricated with QuickCast) can be applied and changed frequently to allow for tissue remodeling. Serial casting can be effective in resolving PIP joint contractures.

eral rule of thumb may be to attempt to wear the splint for 1 hour. If there is no discomfort or sign of tissue distress, gradually increase the time by 1 hour per day. If none of the warning signs is noted, yet the patient perceives a slight stretching sensation, then continue the splinting regimen until the goal time is achieved. Chapter 15 provides more detailed information. The objectives for mobilization splinting are as follows:

- Remodel long-standing, dense, mature scar tissue.
- Elongate soft tissue contractures, adhesions, and musculotendinous tightness.
- Increase passive joint ROM.
- Realign and/or maintain joint and ligament profile.
- Substitute for weak or absent motion.
- Maintain reduction of an intra-articular fracture with preservation of joint mobility.
- Provide resistance for exercise.

These objectives and examples of splinting intervention are discussed in the following sections.

Remodel Long-Standing, Dense, Mature Scar Tissue

A soft tissue contracture can often be addressed with some form of mobilization splinting. The choice of splint types depends on many factors, including information obtained from the physician such as bony union or neurovascular status, maturity of the scar, end feel of the tissue, and the patient's anticipated compliance and motivation level. Mature scar tends to respond well to serial casting or splinting (Schultz-Johnson, 1992). Softer, less mature scar may respond better to dynamic forces, which are applied with proper mechanical principles (Fess & Phillips, 1987; Flowers & LaStayo, 1994). Soft tissue contracture that is associated with Dupuytren's disease and contractures secondary to fibrotic tissue do not respond to mobilization splinting.

EXAMPLE: PIP EXTENSION MOBILIZATION SPLINT

A cylindrical extension mobilization splint (cast) applied to a long-standing, dense PIP flexion contracture may be effective in elongating the contracture and maintaining the desired lengthened position. Therapeutic techniques (e.g., heat, ultrasound, joint mobilization, passive stretching, and massage) used before casting or splinting may aid in preparing the tissue's responsiveness to stretch. As the tissue lengthens or the ROM increases, the serial static splints or casts are changed to support the joint in the new position. Each new device helps remodel the tissue to a further lengthened position. The cast or splint is changed every 3 to 6 days, depending on individual protocols, until the contracture is resolved (Fig. 1–12).

Elongate Soft Tissue Contractures, Adhesions, and Musculotendinous Tightness

Mobilization splinting can be effective in elongating contracted soft tissue and stretching adhesions and tight muscle–tendon units during the proliferative stage of scar formation. Judiciously and incrementally applied tension during this phase of wound healing can greatly enhance tissue accommodation (see Chapter 3 for details). Preparing the tissue—usually by heating and stretching—before splint application maximizes the splint's benefit.

EXAMPLE: WRIST/HAND EXTENSION MOBILIZATION SPLINT

Forearm, wrist, and digit motion can be significantly limited by soft tissue adherence after flexor tendon injury and repair. A wrist/hand extension mobilization splint is one treatment option for addressing flexor tendon adhesions and musculotendinous tightness in the volar forearm (Fig. 1–13). The static progressive nature of the splint holds tension at the wrist's and digit's maximum extension ROM, thereby longitudinally stressing the volar forearm's contracted soft tissue structures. Splint adjustments occur only when the tissue response allows.

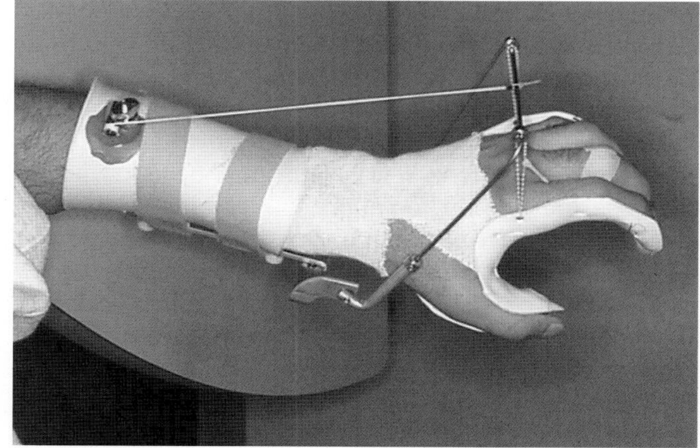

Figure 1–13 A static progressive wrist/hand extension mobilization splint using a Phoenix wrist hinge and MERiT component influences adherent volar forearm soft tissue.

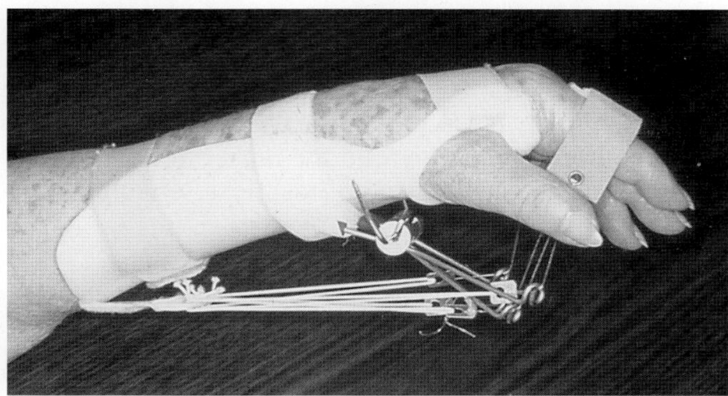

Figure 1–14 A MP flexion mobilization splint using a Rolyan adjustable outrigger kit helps improve MP joint flexion secondary to collateral ligament shortening.

This type of splint can be taken off for hygiene purposes or to work on active and/or passive ROM.

Increase Passive Joint ROM

Splinting is one of the most effective ways of increasing passive mobility of stiff joints. It has been shown that the amount of increase in passive ROM of a stiff joint is proportional to the amount of time the joint is held at its end ROM (Flowers & LaStayo, 1994). Serial static and static progressive mobilization splints may accomplish this goal effectively (Schultz-Johnson, 1996). Both types of splints are applied after the joint has been prepared (warmed and stretched in therapy) at the tissue's near maximum end range and held there until the tissue response allows repositioning to accommodate a change in length. This should be a comfortable, tolerable position for the patient.

EXAMPLE: MP FLEXION MOBILIZATION SPLINT

An MP flexion mobilization splint can be effective in increasing the passive ROM of the MP joints. It can also address MP collateral ligament tightness that can occur after bony or soft tissue injury to the hand or cast immobilization that hinders full MP motion. Before applying dynamic flexion forces to the MP joint(s), check with the physician regarding possible issues such as bony union, neurovascular status, and/or tendon repair strength. This splint applies a gentle flexion force to the tight MP joints. The therapist should be certain that the distal volar border of the splint clears the distal palmar crease, allowing for unrestricted MP flexion (Fig. 1–14).

Realign and/or Maintain Joint and Ligament Profile

When ligaments surrounding a joint become tight, stretched, or damaged from disease or injury, the joint may sublux or deviate. This process causes an alteration of joint mechanics. Patients may experience pain, may note an inability to use the hand, and often develop harmful substitution patterns. Surgical intervention, such as an MP arthroplasty or extensor tendon rebalancing, can be a treatment option for these individuals. After surgery, a therapist may fabricate a mobilization splint. Correctly applied, a postsurgical splint can maintain joint–tendon alignment, thereby decreasing previous substitution patterns and deforming forces, while increasing the functional capabilities of the hand during the course of healing.

EXAMPLE: MP EXTENSION MOBILIZATION SPLINT

An MP extension mobilization splint is often used in the postoperative care of a patient who has undergone MP joint arthroplasty. The splint gives support to the wrist, provides a stable base for outriggers to assist the weakened digital extensors, and prevents undue stress on the reconstructed joints (Swanson, 1995). The splint should be fabricated only after the operative procedure, integrity of the joints and surrounding soft tissue, and ligament reconstruction have been discussed with the surgeon. The purpose of this splint is to provide well-controlled guided motion to the MP joints and to allow for training of the new capsule with proper balance between stability and motion (Fig. 1–15).

The force applied to the MP joints should be just enough to position them in passive extension with some degree of radial deviation, yet allow for gentle active digital flexion. The force used here is much less than the amount used to elongate a soft tissue contracture. Reconstruction of the radial collateral ligament to the index finger MP joint is commonly seen in association with MP arthroplasty. A radially placed outrigger (also known as a supinator attachment) can be added to the splint to correct an IF pronation deformity (DeVore, Muhleman, & Sasarita, 1986; Philips, 1995).

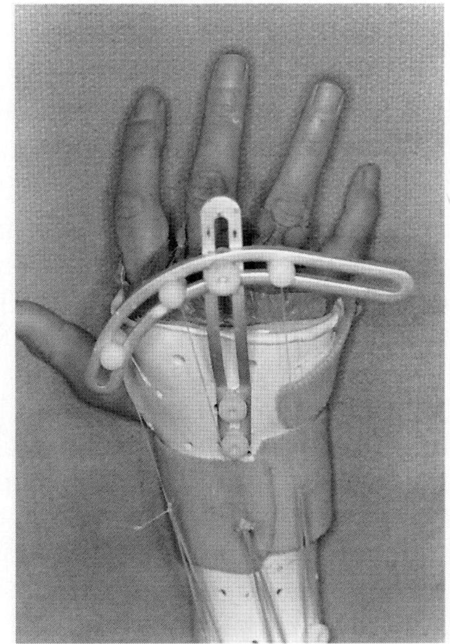

Figure 1–15 The MP extension mobilization splint is used after MP joint arthroplasty. Slings can be adjusted on the outrigger (here, a Base 2 kit) to guide alignment of the MP joints into slight radial deviation.

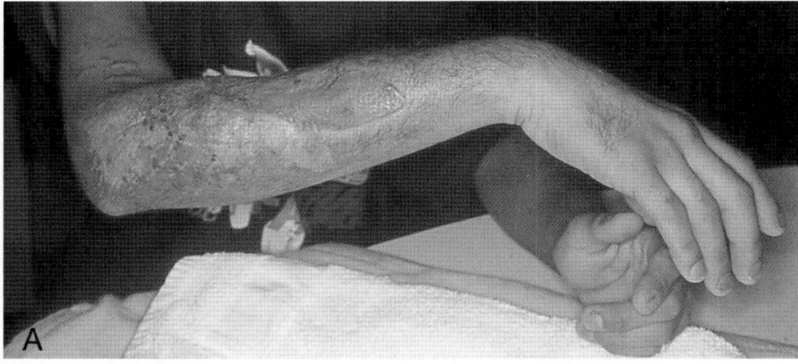

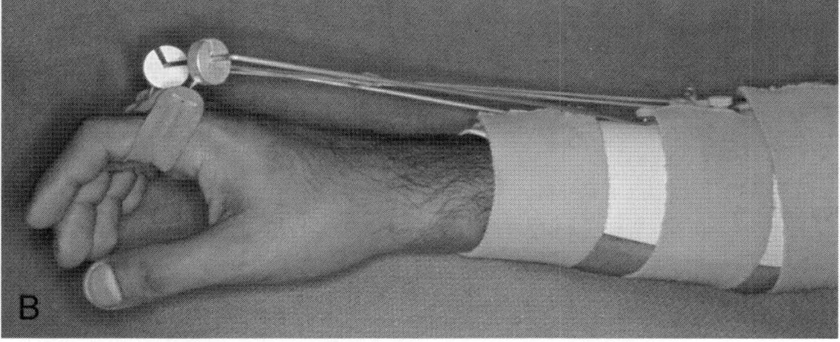

Figure 1–16 ***A,*** *A patient with radial nerve injury.* ***B,*** *A splint that uses the Phoenix outrigger kit allows partial functional use of the hand via tenodesis action.*

Substitute for Weak or Absent Motion

A mobilizing force through a splint may aid functional use of the hand by substituting for absent musculature or assisting in the motion of weak muscles. The dynamic force replaces or assists the motion performed by specific musculature. However, a primary goal when using these splints is to preserve good passive motion (Fess & Phillips, 1987). Splints that take advantage of the natural tenodesis action of the hand are commonly fabricated to assist functional use after nerve injury. Such substitution splints can greatly enhance function, prevent joint contracture, and minimize the overstretching of involved muscle–tendon units (see Chapter 19 for details).

EXAMPLE: WRIST EXTENSION, MP FLEXION/WRIST FLEXION, MP EXTENSION MOBILIZATION SPLINT

A splint that addresses the loss of radial nerve function was first fabricated at the Hand Rehabilitation Center (Chapel Hill, NC) and later described by Colditz (1987). The splint has a thermoplastic component that rests on the dorsum of the forearm, but does not cross the wrist joint. By using a static line directed from the forearm base to the proximal phalanges, the MP joints are suspended in extension. This splint re-creates the tenodesis action of the hand by allowing passive wrist extension through active finger flexion as well as passive finger extension with active wrist flexion. It enables the digits to extend, span, and grasp and release light objects, critical motions for functional use (Fig. 1–16).

Maintain Reduction of an Intra-Articular Fracture

The application of a gentle traction force to a healing intra-articular fracture site during monitored, controlled ROM maintains fracture alignment, facilitates healing, and contributes to the preservation of joint mobility (Dennys, Hurst, & Cox, 1992; Schenck, 1986; Wong, 1995).

Such splints are often fabricated in the operating room or shortly thereafter and are most often created by an experienced therapist who has close, ongoing communication with the surgeon.

EXAMPLE: CIRCULAR TRACTION (SCHENCK DESIGN) PIP INTRA-ARTICULAR MOBILIZATION SPLINT

Intra-articular PIP fractures can be selectively managed with external traction splinting. Schenck (1986) developed and described one such traction splint (Fig. 1–17). The surgeon places a wire horizontally through the middle phalanx leaving the ends of the wire protruding. The wire is bent to hold rubber bands or springs that are then attached to a hoop that extends from the splint base. The rubber band or spring attachment is commonly made with a bent AlumaFoam splint or thermoplastic material that can easily glide along the hoop. The traction from the PIP joint to the hoop can be cautiously moved through a specific degree of motion hourly, or as prescribed by the physician. The completed splint should be checked by the surgeon to ensure proper fracture alignment and force application. This method may be applied to other joints, such as the MP joint.

Provide Resistance for Exercise

Dynamic splints can be used as an exercise tool to apply resistance in the opposite direction of the patient's

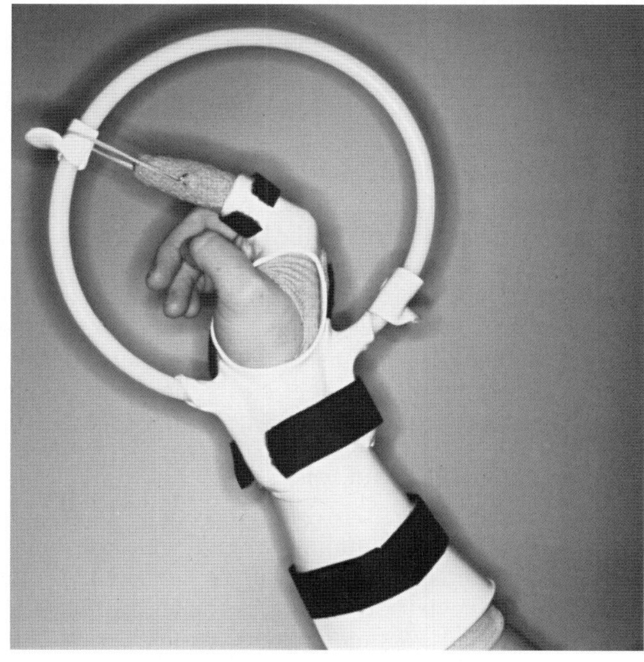

Figure 1–17 *This splint maintains gentle traction and intra-articular fracture alignment while allowing guarded passive motion of the PIP joint.*

active force. This can be a useful way to facilitate tendon excursion through scar, gain tensile strength of specifically targeted muscles, and provide resistance to adherent tendons.

EXAMPLE: PIP EXTENSION MOBILIZATION SPLINT

Providing resistance to an adherent tendon, such as a flexor digitorum superficialis or flexor pollicis longus, can facilitate tendon gliding through scar and contribute to increasing tensile strength once a strengthening program has begun. To facilitate flexor digitorum superficialis glide, the splint is fabricated to position the MP joint in extension, and the DIP is casted in extension. A sling is then applied to the middle phalanx (Fig. 1–18). Resistance to the line of pull is felt when PIP flexion is attempted.

Restriction Splints

Restriction splints limit a specific aspect of joint mobility. These splints can be a challenge to fabricate, especially when made for patients who have multiple injuries with a combination of needs. Static splints, dynamic splints, and forms of taping are considered types of restrictive splints because they can be made to restrict some portion of joint motion while allowing the rest of the joint to move freely. A therapist may be asked to fabricate a splint that completely immobilizes a joint and creatively allows motion or partial motion of other joints. This scenario requires integration of problem-solving skills, clinical judgment, critical thinking, and understanding of how wound healing stages apply to specific tissues. Careful attention to the construction and fit of these splints is crucial because of the expected motion and use of the extremity within the splint.

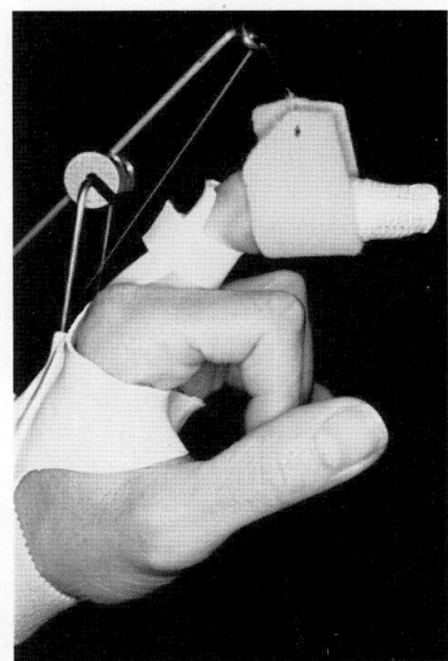

Figure 1–18 A PIP extension mobilization splint being used for controlled resistance to an adherent flexor digitorum superficialis tendon. The DIP is held in extension by a small cast to eliminate the pull of the flexor digitorum profundus tendon. Increasing flexor digitorum superficialis tendon glide and strength are the goals of this splint.

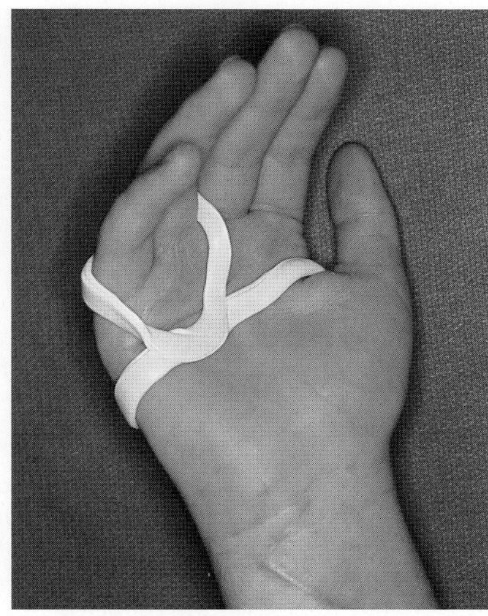

Figure 1–19 After low ulnar nerve injury, preventing hyperextension at the MP joints facilitates extension at the IP joints. The fourth and fifth MP joints are generally positioned between 45 and 70° of flexion.

The objectives for restriction splints are as follows:

- Limit motion after nerve injury or repair.
- Limit motion after tendon injury or repair.
- Limit motion after bone–ligament injury or repair.
- Provide and improve joint stability and alignment.
- Assist in functional use of the hand.

These objectives and examples of splinting intervention are discussed in the following sections.

Limit Motion after Nerve Injury or Repair

Restrictive splints can effectively block potentially deforming and abnormal forces to the hand secondary to nerve injury. They allow the healing nerve or re-innervated nerve to glide within a protected ROM, minimizing tension at the repair site, decreasing the risk of adherence to soft tissue structures, increasing blood flow, and improving the nutritional environment. Chapter 19 provides specific splinting details.

EXAMPLE: RF–SF MP EXTENSION RESTRICTION SPLINT

A restriction splint can prevent the common claw deformity of the ring and small digits that occurs after low ulnar nerve injuries (Fig. 1–19). Such a splint restricts extension motion at the MP joints by applying well-distributed pressure at the dorsum of the proximal phalanxes and allowing the transfer of force from the extrinsic extensors to the dorsal hood mechanism of the digits. By placing the MP joints in some degree of flexion, extension of the interphalangeal (PIP and DIP) joints is made possible in the absence of the ulnar innervated intrinsic muscles by means of the extrinsic extensors. This position provides the extensor tendons with a mechanical advantage that greatly enhances composite grasp and release, which is quite awkward and difficult without the splint.

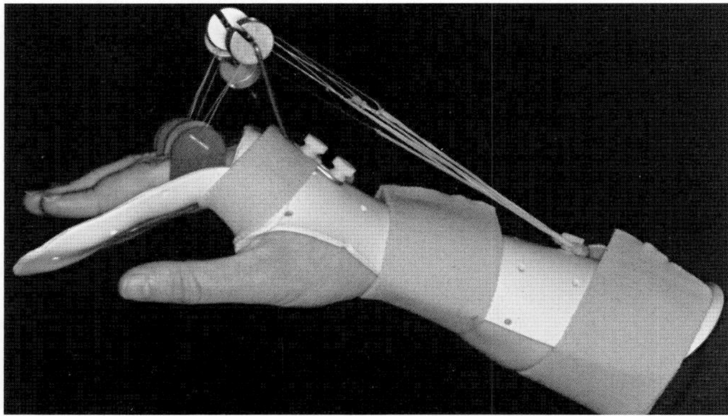

Figure 1–20 This restrictive splint (using a Phoenix outrigger kit) immobilizes the wrist in static extension while providing dynamic MP flexion to a predetermined range. The patient actively flexes the digits to the volar block, allowing passive excursion of the extensor tendons. Dynamic forces, via the rubber bands, return the digits to full extension.

Limit Motion after Tendon Injury or Repair

After soft tissue injury or surgical repair, limited motion is often necessary to promote tissue healing, prevent joint contractures, maintain tissue length, and facilitate gliding of structures to minimize adhesion formation. There are numerous protocols that address splinting these types of injuries, and only one technique is discussed here. Refer to Chapter 20 for a discussion of a variety of tendon protocols.

EXAMPLE: WRIST EXTENSION IMMOBILIZATION, DIGIT EXTENSION MOBILIZATION/FLEXION RESTRICTION SPLINT

Extensor tendon injuries in zones V to VII can be managed with a restrictive splint (Fig. 1–20). The wrist is held in static extension (35 to 45°) while the MP joints are passively extended using rubber band traction. Active MP flexion against the rubber bands can be performed to a set volar block. Initially, the block is restricted to approximately 30° of MP joint motion. Gradually, as healing progresses, the block is adjusted to allow greater MP flexion. The adjustments are generally done each week, as long as the tendon healing allows (Evans & Burkhalter, 1986; Thomas, Moutet, & Guinard, 1996). This type of splint promotes early protected motion and tendon excursion for optimal healing with less risk of adhesion formation and tendon rupture.

Limit Motion after Bone–Ligament Injury or Repair

After fracture reduction or surgical fixation, a splint that allows a restricted ROM can be used to promote bone growth, healing of associated ligaments, joint mobility, and soft tissue and tendon gliding. The initial amount of joint restriction depends on the surgical procedure, the severity of the fracture-dislocation, the extent of ligament involvement, and the physician protocol. The therapist and/or physician monitors the amount and degree of allowed extension or flexion exercise and gradually may increase the limits of motion as healing progresses. The permitted, restricted arc of motion promotes healing of the injury or repair and aids in minimizing tendon adherence (Schenck, 1986).

EXAMPLE: ELBOW EXTENSION RESTRICTION SPLINT

Limiting full extension after a posterior elbow dislocation is the key to preventing re-injury. A static or dynamic splint can minimize lateral movement of the elbow, decrease motions of pronation and supination, and restrict elbow extension. The degree of elbow extension restriction is determined by the severity of the fracture dislocation and the position required to prevent subluxation. The position may be altered as the involved structures heal and the physician permits. Care is taken to minimize the risk of flexion contracture by carefully extending the splint limits as soon as timing allows. By applying a posterior elbow extension restriction splint, the distal forearm straps may be removed to allow unrestricted functional elbow flexion while limiting elbow extension to the confines of the splint (Fig. 1–21**A**). A hinged extension re-

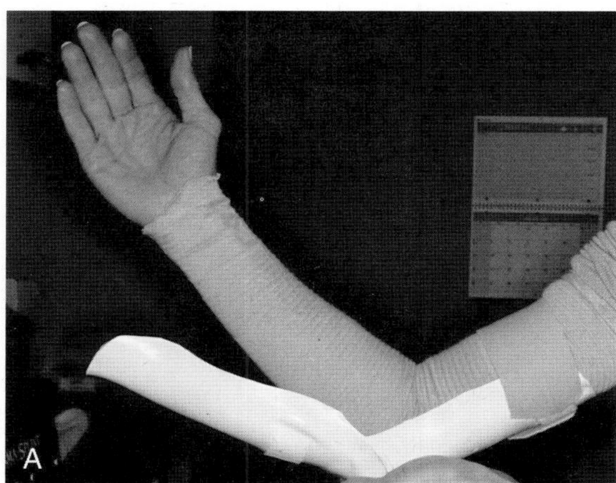

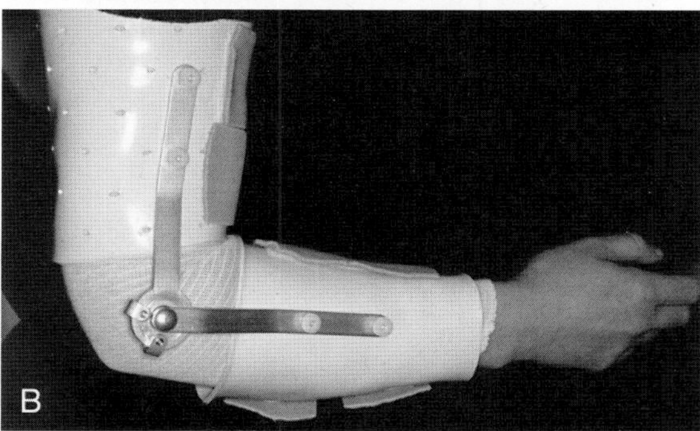

*Figure 1–21 **A,** When this elbow extension restriction splint's distal straps are removed, the patient is able to flex the elbow within the splint's parameters. **B,** This elbow extension restriction splint (with a Phoenix elbow hinge component) limits the amount of elbow extension yet allows unimpeded flexion.*

striction splint includes an elbow hinge applied to a forearm and humerus splint. The hinge is locked to prevent a specific degree of extension while allowing unrestricted elbow flexion (Fig. 1–21**B**).

Provide and Improve Joint Stability and Alignment

A restrictive splint, such as an IF–SF MP ulnar deviation splint, can help support and realign subluxed and/or deviated joints to an improved anatomic position while preserving some functional use of the extremity. Such restrictive splints can block or restrict harmful movement patterns that place undue stress on joints, ligaments, and tendons. Functional splints often allow patients to use their hands in a natural way, while limiting pain and edema and without contributing to further joint or soft tissue breakdown.

EXAMPLE: THUMB IP EXTENSION/LATERAL DEVIATION RESTRICTION SPLINT

A small dorsal thumb IP joint splint can limit the IP hyperextension and lateral IP deviation deformities sometimes seen in the patient with rheumatoid arthritis (Fig. 1–22). This splint creates an extension block with lateral borders (a hood) to allow IP flexion. This positioning greatly improves stability during pinch. An elastic wrap is recommended for securing the proximal portion of the splint about the proximal phalanx of the thumb, the distal hood can be left free (Terrono, Nalebuff, & Philips, 1995). Applied in this way, the splint allows functional IP flexion with minimal deforming forces. Therapy should also include gentle ROM exercises to avoid soft tissue contractures, intrinsic muscle tightness, and collateral ligament shortening.

Assist in Functional Use of the Hand

Splints are an excellent way to assist and ready the hand for functional use. Chronic, improper positioning as a result of a poorly fit splint can lead to contractures, functional lengthening or shortening of tendons, pain, and prolonged edema. Splinting can be used advantageously to position joints and tendons while preventing the possible consequences. The key to independence is maintaining function for as long as possible.

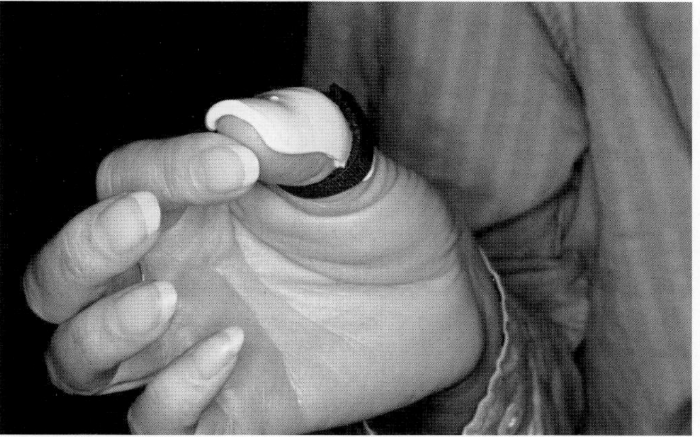

Figure 1–22 This thumb IP extension restriction splint provides stability and protection to an unstable IP joint. The block prevents deviation and hyperextension at the joint but allows limited flexion for light activities that require pinching.

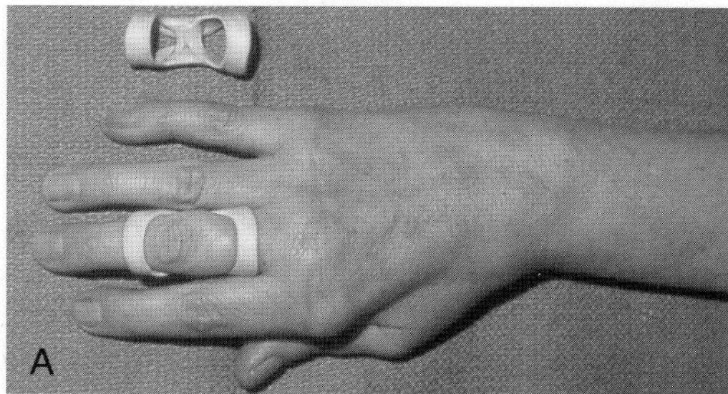

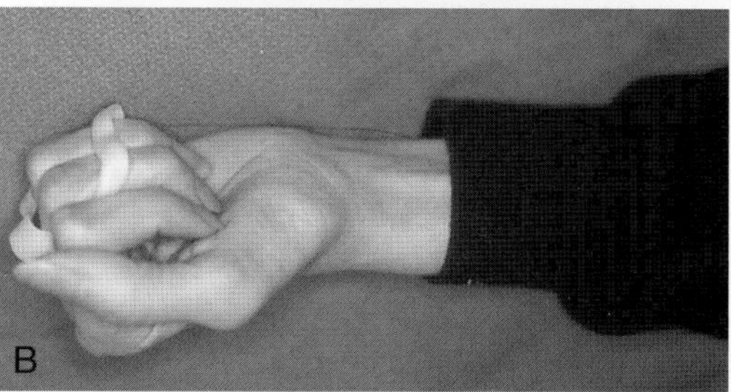

*Figure 1–23 A small PIP extension restrict splint worn during digit extension (**A**) and flexion (**B**).*

EXAMPLE: PIP EXTENSION RESTRICTION SPLINT

A small lightweight splint can be used to manage a supple swan-neck deformity (PIP hyperextension, DIP flexion). Such a splint balances digital extension by applying three-point pressure about the PIP joint (Fig. 1–23). Dorsal pressure applied proximal and distal to the PIP joint limits the joint's extension; volar pressure directly supports the joint. Hyperextension is not permitted; however, flexion of the digit is preserved. Intervention should also include a program of intrinsic stretching and ROM exercises for the wrist and uninvolved joints. Patients can manage quite well with these small devices, which allow them to have better stability during pinching and grasping activities.

CONCLUSION

This chapter describes the splint nomenclature developed by ASHT and provides practical clinical examples of splints and their uses. The SCS provides a mechanism to describe splints through a sequence of analytic steps. This chapter clarifies splint classification, outlines common objectives for splinting intervention, and discusses practical examples.

Splinting the injured extremity is one part of a comprehensive rehabilitation program. For a successful

splinting program, the patient must understand the importance of compliance, must be aware of the splint's function, and must know how to use the splint. The patient should be physically able to apply the splint to the extremity, otherwise the splint may have a detrimental effect. The greater the therapist's understanding of the choices available, the more creative and effective he or she can be with the modality of splinting.

REFERENCES

American Society of Hand Therapists. (1992). *Splint classification system.* Garner, NC.

Bell-Krotoski, J. A. (1995). Plaster cylinder casting for contractures of the interphalangeal joints. In J. M. Hunter, E. J. Mackin, & A. D. Callahan AD (Eds.). *Rehabilitation of the hand* (4th ed., pp. 1609–1616). St. Louis: Mosby.

Bell-Krotoski, J. A., & Figarola, F. (1995). Biomechanics of soft tissue growth and remodeling with plaster casting. *Journal of Hand Therapy, 8,* 131–137.

Brand, P. W., & Thompson, D. E. (1993). Mechanical resistance. In P. W. Brand & A. Hollister (Eds.). *Clinical mechanics of the hand* (2nd ed., pp. 92–127). St. Louis: Mosby.

Colditz, J. C. (1987). Splinting for radial nerve palsy. *Journal of Hand Therapy, 1,* 18–23.

Colditz, J. C. (1995a). Anatomic considerations for splinting the thumb. In J. M. Hunter, E. J. Mackin, & A. D. Callahan AD (Eds.). *Rehabilitation of the hand* (4th ed., pp. 1161–1172). St. Louis: Mosby.

Colditz, J. C. (1995b). Therapist's management of the stiff hand. In J. M. Hunter, E. J. Mackin, & A. D. Callahan AD (Eds.). *Rehabilitation of the hand* (4th ed., pp. 1142–1159). St. Louis: Mosby.

Dell, P. C., & Dell, R. B. (1996). Management of rheumatoid arthritis of the wrist. *Journal of Hand Therapy, 9,* 157–164.

Dennys, L. J., Hurst, L. N., & Cox, J. (1992). Management of proximal interphalangeal joint fractures using a new dynamic traction splint and early active movement. *Journal of Hand Therapy, 5,* 16–2422.

DeVore, G. L. , Muhleman, C. A., & Sasarita, S. G. (1986). Management of the pronation deformity in metacarpophalangeal joint implant arthroplasty. *The Journal of Hand Surgery, 11,* 859–861.

Eaton, E. G. (1992). Entrapment syndromes in musicians. *Journal of Hand Therapy, 5,* 91–96.

Evans, R. B. & Burkhalter, W. E. (1986). A study of the dynamic anatomy of the extensor tendons and implications for treatment. *The Journal of Hand Surgery, 11,* 774–779.

Fess, E. W. (1995). Principles and methods of splinting for mobilization of joints. In J. M. Hunter, E. J. Mackin, & A. D. Callahan (Eds). *Rehabilitation of the hand* (4th ed., pp. 1589–1598). St. Louis: Mosby.

Fess, E. W., & McCollum, M. (1998). The influence of splinting on healing tissue. *Journal of Hand Therapy, 11,* 157–161.

Fess, E. W., & Phillips, C. A. (1987). Classification and nomenclature of splints and splint components. In *Hand splinting: Principles and methods* (2nd ed., pp. 71–102). St. Louis: Mosby.

Flowers, K. R., & LaStayo, P. (1994). Effect of total end range time on improving passive range of motion. *Journal of Hand Therapy, 7,* 150–157.

Gyovai, J. E., & Wright Howell, J. (1992). Validation of spring forces applied in dynamic outrigger splinting. *Journal of Hand Therapy, 5,* 8–15.

Laseter, G. F., & Carter, P. R. (1996). Management of distal radius fractures. *Journal of Hand Therapy, 9,* 122–126.

Mathiowetz, V., Bolding. D. J., & Trombley, C. A. (1983). The immediate effects of positioning devices on normal and spastic hand measured by electromyography. *American Journal of Occupational Therapy, 37,* 247–254.

McFarlane, R. (1997). Dupuytren's disease. *Journal of Hand Therapy, 10,* 8–13.

McPherson, J. J. (1981). Objective evaluation of a splint designed to reduce hypertonicity. *American Journal of Occupational Therapy, 35,* 189–194.

Neuhaus, B. E., Ascher, E. R., & Coullon, B. A. (1981). A survey of rationales for and against hand splinting in hemiplegia. *American Journal of Occupational Therapy, 35,* 83–90.

Philips, C. A. (1995). Therapist's management of patients with rheumatoid arthritis. In J. M. Hunter, E. J. Mackin, & A. D. Callahan AD (Eds). *Rehabilitation of the hand* (4th ed., pp. 1348–1350). St. Louis: Mosby.

Prosser, R. (1996). Splinting in the management of proximal interphalangeal joint flexion contracture. *Journal of Hand Therapy, 9,* 378–386.

Rose, V., & Shah, S. (1987). A comparative study on the immediate effects of hand orthoses on reduction of hypertonus. *Australian Occupational Therapy Journal, 34,* 444–449.

Schenck, R. R. (1987). Dynamic traction and early passive movement for fractures of the proximal interphalangeal joint. *The Journal of Hand Surgery, 11,* 850–858.

Schultz-Johnson, K. S. (1992). Splinting: A problem solving approach. In B. G. Stanley, & S. M. Tribuzi (Eds.). *Concepts in hand rehabilitation* (pp. 238–271). Philadelphia: FA Davis.

Schultz-Johnson, K. (1996). Splinting the wrist: Mobilization and protection. *Journal of Hand Therapy, 9,* 165–175.

Swanson, A. B. (1995). Postoperative rehabilitation programs in flexible implant arthroplasty of the digits. In J. M. Hunter, E. J. Mackin, & A. D. Callahan (Eds.). *Rehabilitation of the hand* (4th ed., pp. 1364–1371). St. Louis: Mosby.

Terrono, A., Nalebuff, E., & Philips, C. (1995). The rheumatoid thumb. In J. M. Hunter, E. J. Mackin, & A. D. Callahan (Eds.). *Rehabilitation of the hand* (4th ed., pp. 1329–1336). St. Louis: Mosby.

Thomas, D., Moutet, F., Guinard, D. (1996). Postoperative management of extensor tendon repairs in zones V, VI, VII. *Journal of Hand Therapy, 9,* 309–314.

Tribuzi, S. M. (1995). Serial plaster splinting. In J. M. Hunter, E. J. Mackin, & A. D. Callahan (Eds.). *Rehabilitation of the hand* (4th ed., pp. 1600–1608). St. Louis: Mosby.

Wong, S. (1995). Combination splint for distal interphalangeal joint stability and protected proximal interphalangeal joint mobility. *Journal of Hand Therapy, 5,* 269–270.

SUGGESTED READING

Coppard, B. M., Lohman, H. (1996). *Introduction to splinting.* St. Louis: Mosby.

Hunter, J. M., Mackin, E. J., & Callahan, A. D. (Eds). *Rehabilitation of the hand* (4th ed.). St. Louis: Mosby.

Hurov, J. R., & Concannon, M. J. (1999). Management of a metacarpophalangeal joint fracture using a dynamic traction splint and early motion. *Journal of Hand Therapy, 12,* 219–227.

Jacobs, M. L. (1995). Low profile dynamic wrist splint. *Journal of Hand Therapy, 8,* 39–40.

McKee, P., & Morgan, L. (1998). *Orthotics in rehabilitation.* Philadelphia: Davis.

Veldhoven, G. V. (1995). The proximal interphalangeal joint swing traction splint. *Journal of Hand Therapy, 8,* 265–268.

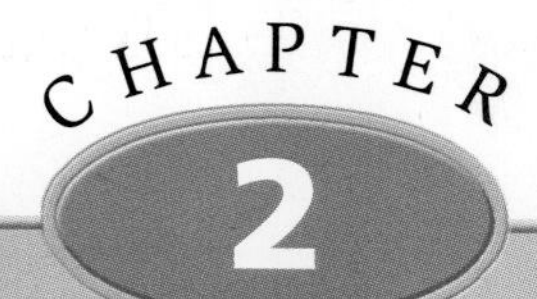

Anatomical Principles

Noelle M. Austin, MS, PT, CHT

INTRODUCTION

The anatomy of the upper extremity is composed of a complex arrangement of bones, joints, nerves, muscles, and vascular structures, which work together to permit a wide range of functional capabilities. To be effective as clinicians, therapists must have a comprehensive understanding of how these structures function conjointly under normal and abnormal conditions, such as injury and disease. This chapter focuses on the anatomic structures of the upper extremity and notes how they are specifically related to issues of splinting.

The Bones and Joints of the Upper Extremity

The skeletal structure of the upper extremity is defined proximally by the shoulder girdle and distally by the finger joints (Fig. 2–1). This complex configuration of bones allows each joint to move in specific ways, permitting mobility and function of the hand in space. Dysfunction of even one joint in the upper extremity can affect the ability of the other joints to function normally (Calliet, 1994).

Except for the scapulothoracic joint, the joints of the upper extremity are considered **synovial joints,** which have a **joint cavity, articular cartilage** lining the bony ends, and an **articular capsule** containing synovial fluid (Fig. 2–2) (Moore, 1992; Moore & Agur, 1995). Synovial joints are categorized by their bony configuration and the amount of motion they allow. Each type of synovial joint is represented in the upper extremity (Fig. 2–3) (Moore, 1992; Moore & Agur, 1995). **Ligaments** are composed of thick connective tissue that emanates from the joint capsule; they provide stability to the joint. The ligaments of each joint are shown in the figures throughout this chapter.

Wherever the patient's problem lies—from the shoulder to the distal interphalangeal (DIP) joint—the therapist's goal is to appreciate normal joint mechanics; to preserve, as much as possible, the normal anatomic alignment; and to provide the opportunity for maximal functional use. Therapists must understand how the upper extremity structures interact under normal and abnormal conditions and must ultimately be aware of how therapy intervention can influence the final outcome.

The Shoulder

In the proximal upper extremity, the **shoulder complex** includes the **sternoclavicular, acromioclavicular, scapulothoracic,** and **glenohumeral** joints. The first three of these joints are discussed here because they link the upper extremity to the trunk and their status can affect the ultimate function of the limb. The sternoclavicular joint is a **saddle joint** consisting of the medial end of the clavicle and the lateral aspect of the manubrium; it allows motion in several directions (Fig. 2–4) (Moore, 1992; Moore & Agur, 1995). The acromioclavicular joint is a **plane joint** formed by the lateral end of the clavicle and medial portion of the acromion; it permits rotation and anterior to posterior movement of the acromion on the clavicle (Fig. 2–5) (Moore, 1992; Moore & Agur, 1995). The articulation between the scapula and thorax is considered a **pseudo joint** (false joint); it allows the scapula to glide along the thoracic wall as the arm moves in space (Fig. 2–6) (Kapandji, 1982). The **ball-and-socket** arrangement of the glenohumeral joint is formed by an articulation between the glenoid fossa of the scapula and the head of the humerus. This loose configuration provides a highly mobile arrangement; however, mobility is achieved by sacrificing stability. The joint allows the arm to move freely in extension and flexion, abduction and adduction, and in-

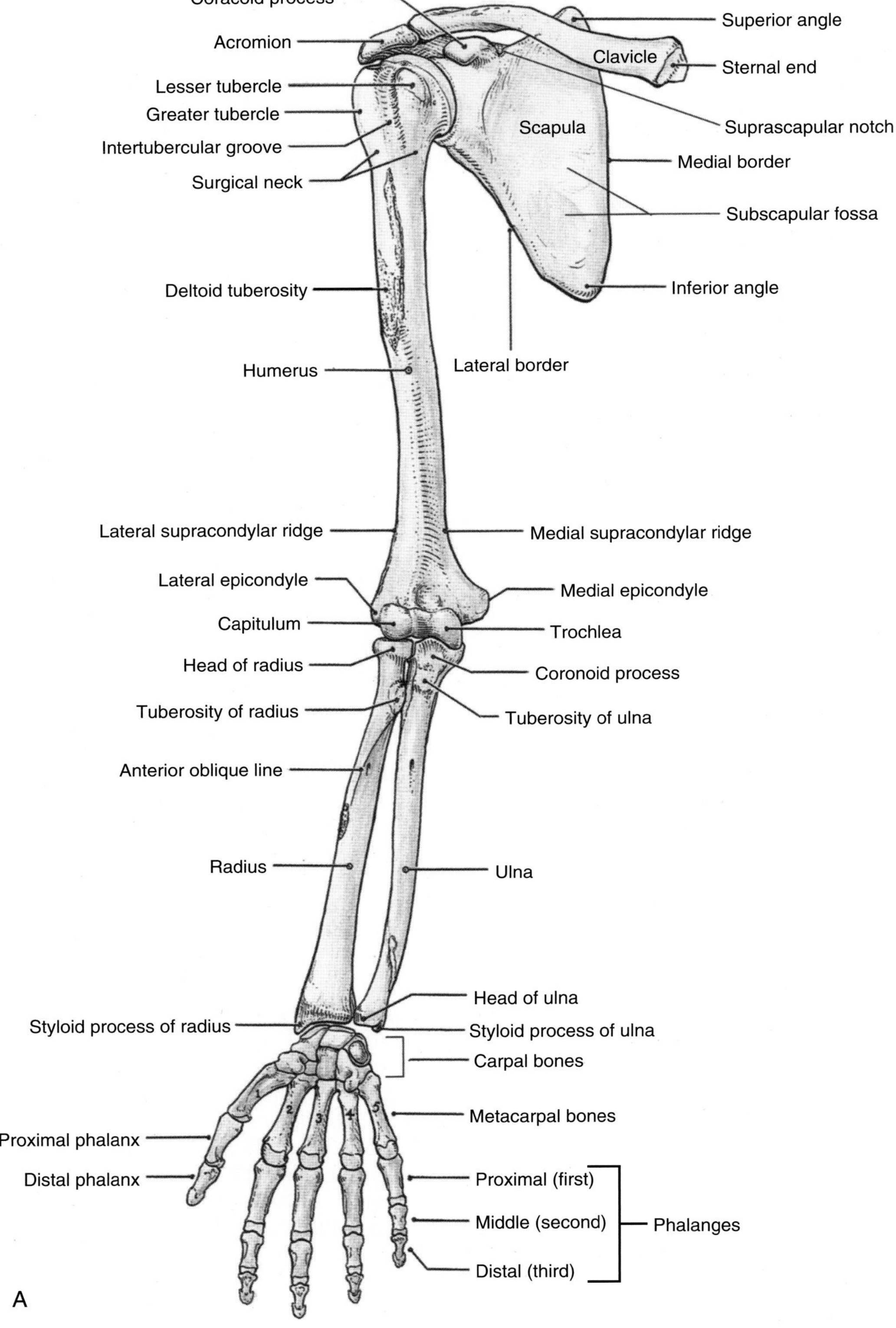

Figure 2–1 *Anterior **(A)** and posterior **(B)** views of the skeletal structure of the upper extremity. **C,** Anterior and posterior views of the skeletal structure of the hand. Reprinted with permission from Moore, K. L., & Agur, A. M. (1995).* Essential clinical anatomy. *Baltimore: Williams & Wilkins.*

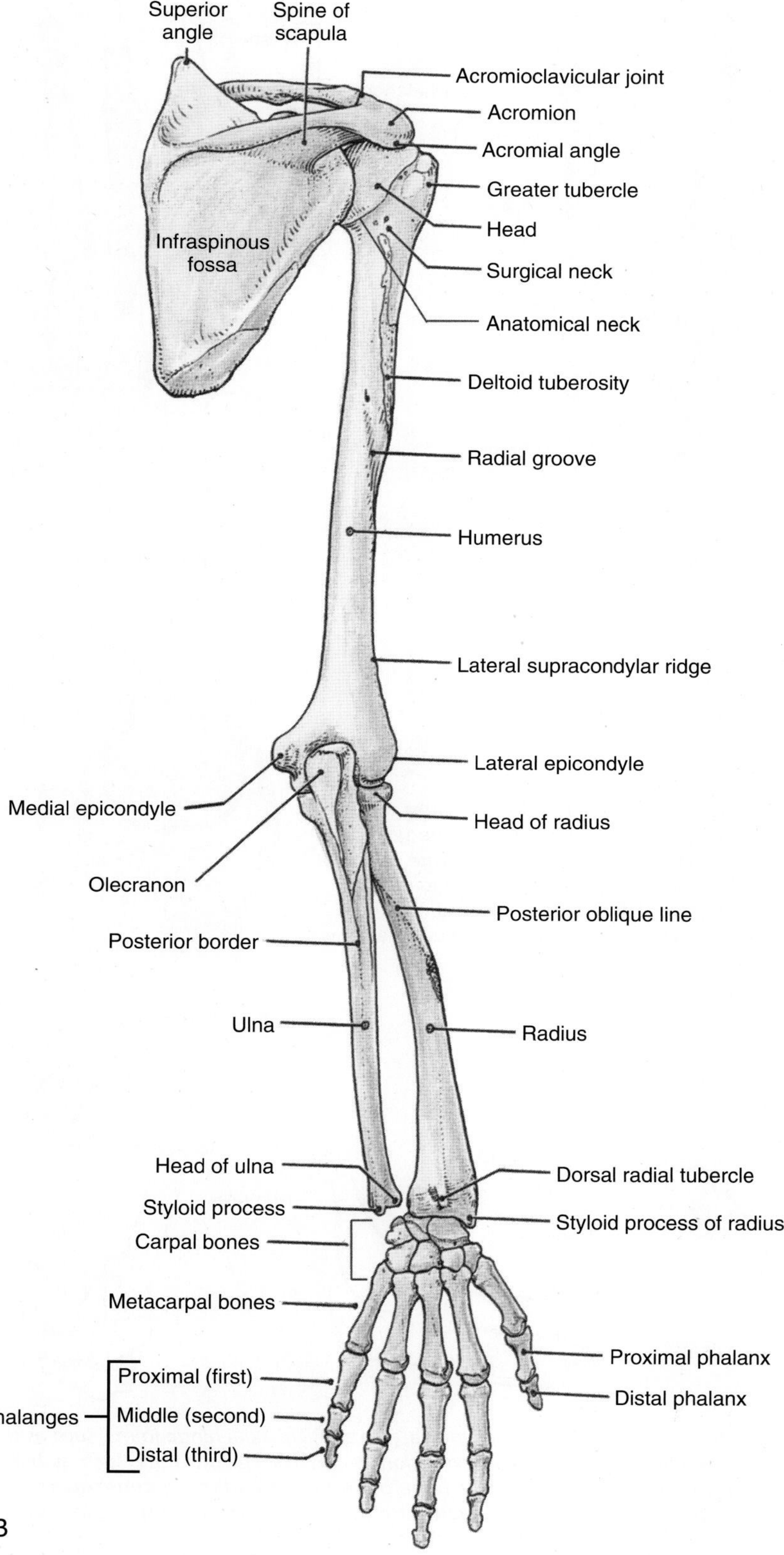

Figure 2–1 Continued.

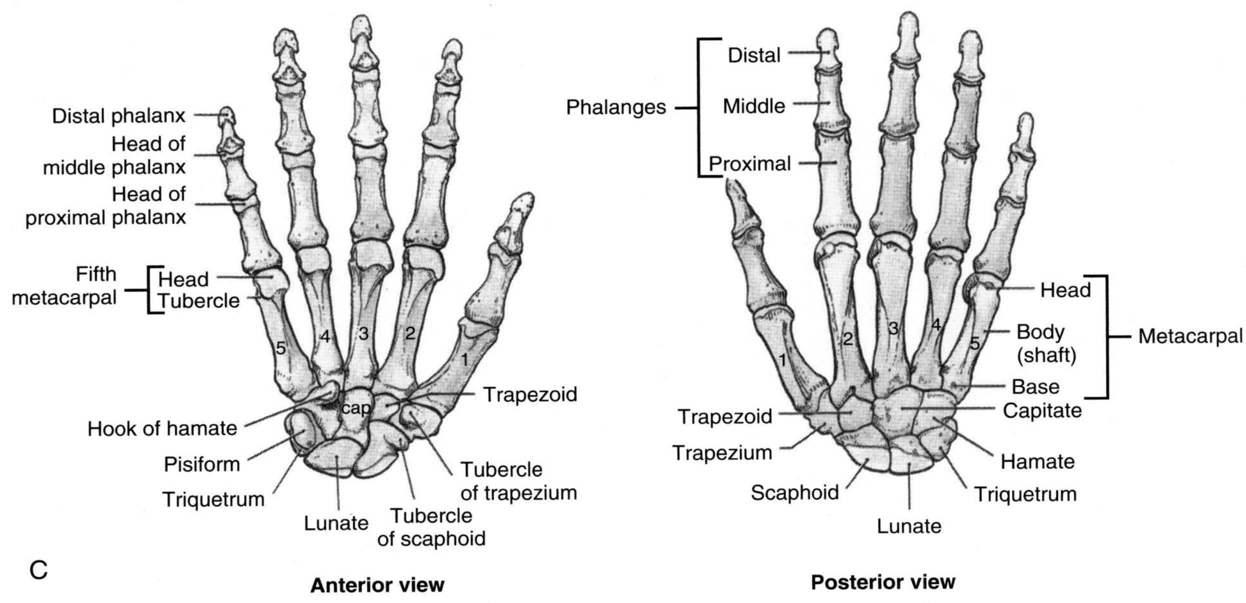

Figure 2–1 *Continued.*

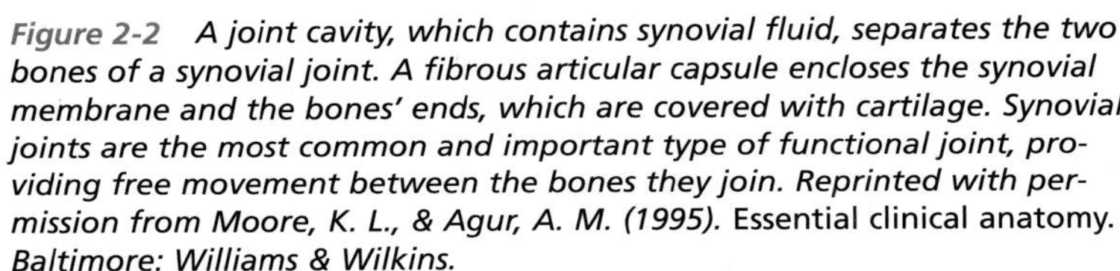

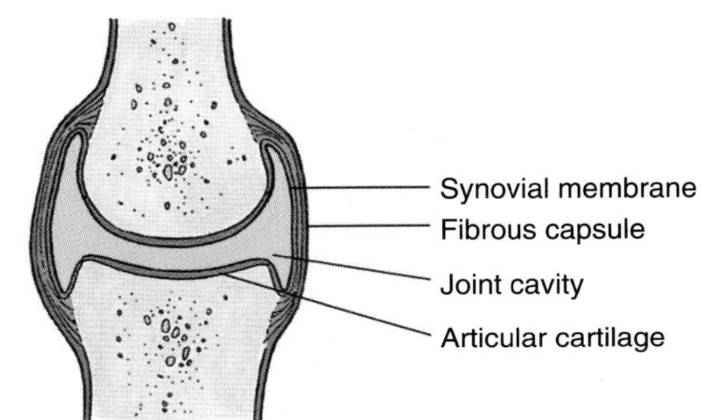

Figure 2-2 A joint cavity, which contains synovial fluid, separates the two bones of a synovial joint. A fibrous articular capsule encloses the synovial membrane and the bones' ends, which are covered with cartilage. Synovial joints are the most common and important type of functional joint, providing free movement between the bones they join. Reprinted with permission from Moore, K. L., & Agur, A. M. (1995). Essential clinical anatomy. *Baltimore: Williams & Wilkins.*

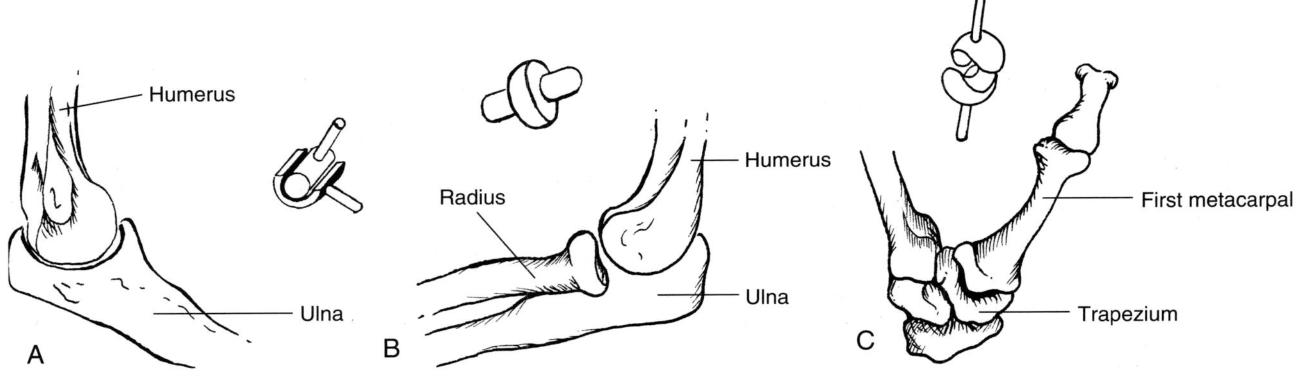

Figure 2–3 Types of upper extremity synovial joints. ***A,*** *Uniaxial hinge joints, such as the humeroulnar joint, permit only flexion and extension.* ***B,*** *Uniaxial pivot joints, such as humeroradial joint, allow rotation. A round process on one bone fits into a ligamentous socket in the other bone.* ***C,*** *One bone of a biaxial saddle joint, such as the trapeziometacarpal joint, is concave and the other is convex at the point of articulation.*

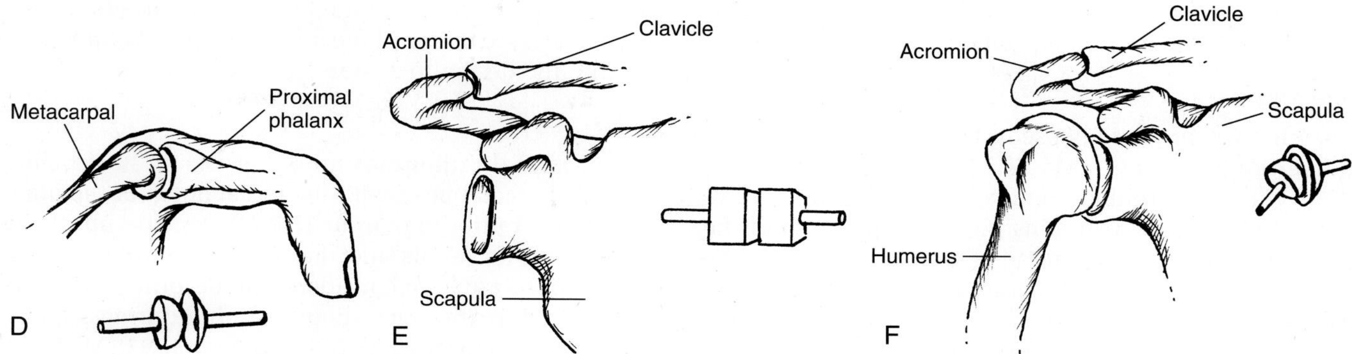

Figure 2–3 *Continued.* ***D,*** *Biaxial condyloid joints, such as the metacarpophalangeal joint, permit flexion and extension, abduction and adduction, and circumduction.* ***E,*** *Plane joints, such as the acromioclavicular joint, permit gliding or sliding movements.* ***F,*** *Multiaxial ball-and-socket joints, such as the glenohumeral joint, permit flexion and extension, abduction and adduction, medial and lateral rotation, and circumduction. The rounded head of one bone fits into a concavity in the other bone. Adapted with permission from Moore, K. L., & Agur, A. M. (1995).* Essential clinical anatomy. *Baltimore: Williams & Wilkins.*

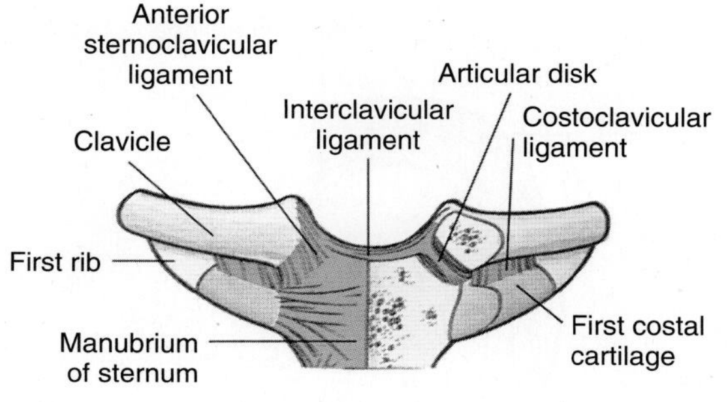

Figure 2–4 *The sternoclavicular joint. Reprinted with permission from Moore, K. L., & Agur, A. M. (1995).* Essential clinical anatomy. *Baltimore: Williams & Wilkins.*

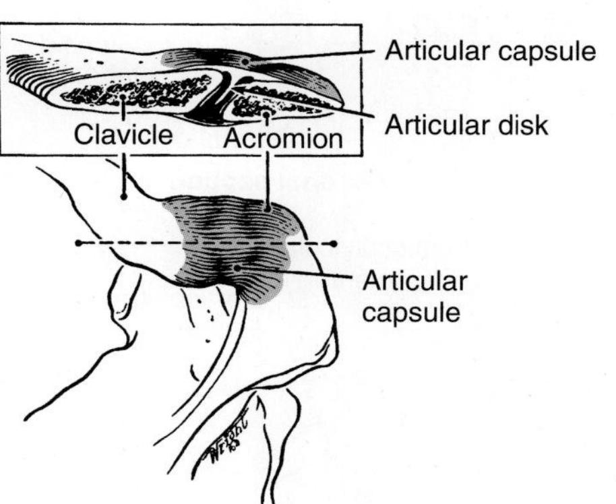

Figure 2–5 *Acromioclavicular joint. Reprinted with permission from Moore, K. L., & Agur, A. M. (1995).* Essential clinical anatomy. *Baltimore: Williams & Wilkins.*

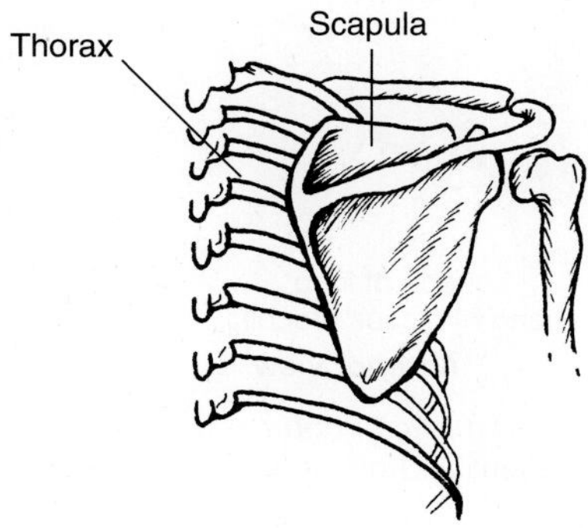

Figure 2–6 *The scapulothoracic joint.*

ternal and external rotation (Fig. 2–7) (Kapandji, 1982; Moore, 1992, Moore & Agur, 1995).

The Elbow

The **elbow joint** is composed of the **humeroulnar** and **humeroradial** joints (Moore, 1992; Moore & Agur, 1995). The humeroulnar joint consists of the trochlea of the distal humerus as it joins the trochlear notch of the proximal ulna. The humeroradial joint is made up of the capitulum of the distal humerus and the head of the radius. The elbow joint is generally considered a **hinge joint,** which allows extension and flexion (Fig. 2–8). There is a normal valgus **carrying angle** of 5°in males and 10 to 15°in females (Hoppenfeld, 1976). When fabricating elbow splints with the forearm positioned in supination, the therapist must incorporate the valgus angle into the design to ensure an appropriate fit.

The Forearm

The **proximal radioulnar joint** consists of the articulation of the radial head with the radial notch of the ulna. The **distal radioulnar joint** (DRUJ) is made up of the ulnar notch of radius and the head of the ulna. These articulations are both considered **pivot joints;** they permit the radius to rotate about the ulna during supination and pronation (Fig. 2–9) (Moore, 1992; Moore & Agur, 1995). Stability is provided proximally by the anular and quadrate ligaments and distally by the anterior

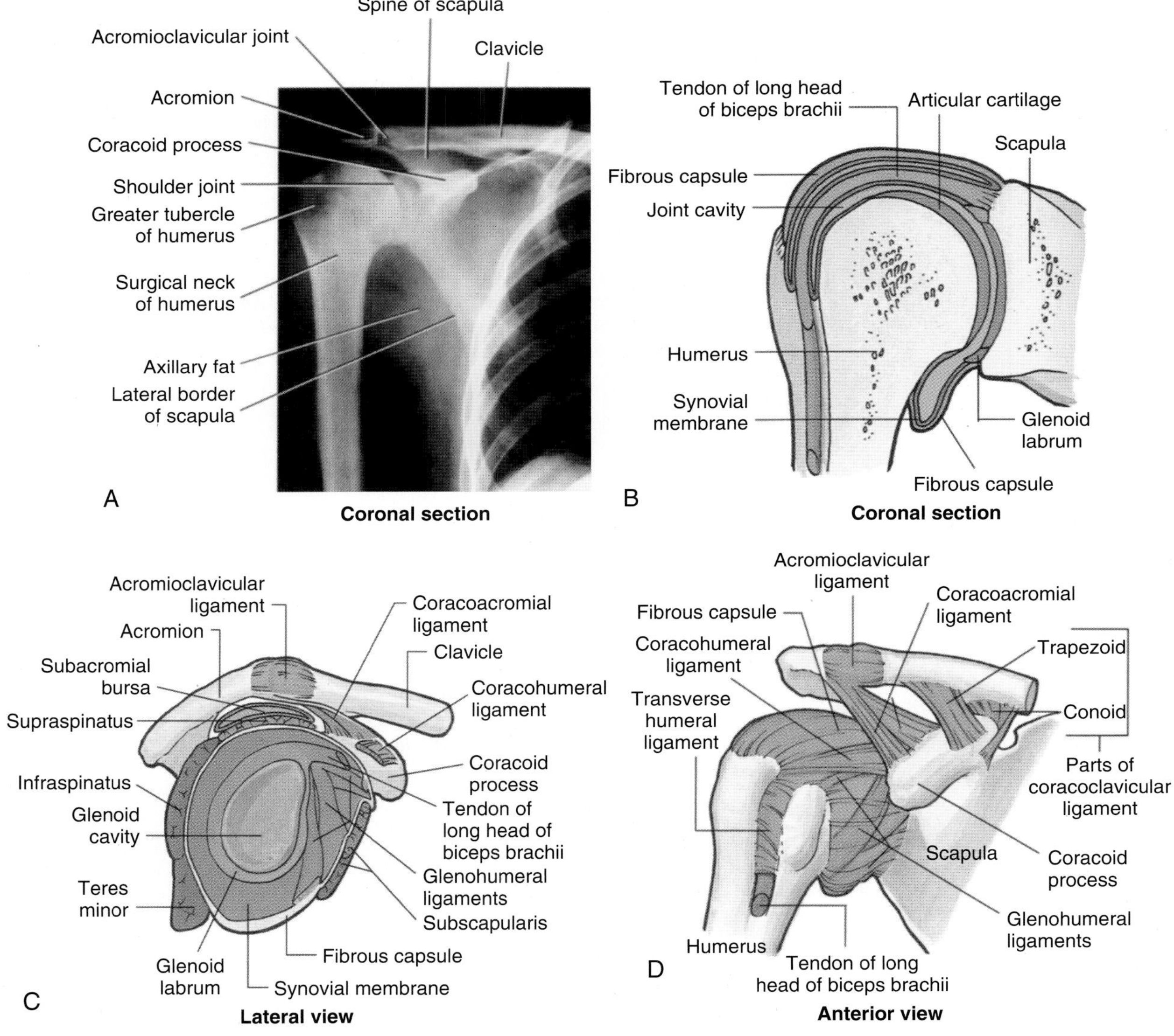

*Figure 2–7 Coronal **(A and B)**, lateral **(C)**, and anterior **(D)** views of the glenohumeral joint. Reprinted with permission from Moore, K. L., & Agur, A. M. (1995).* Essential clinical anatomy. *Baltimore: Williams & Wilkins.*

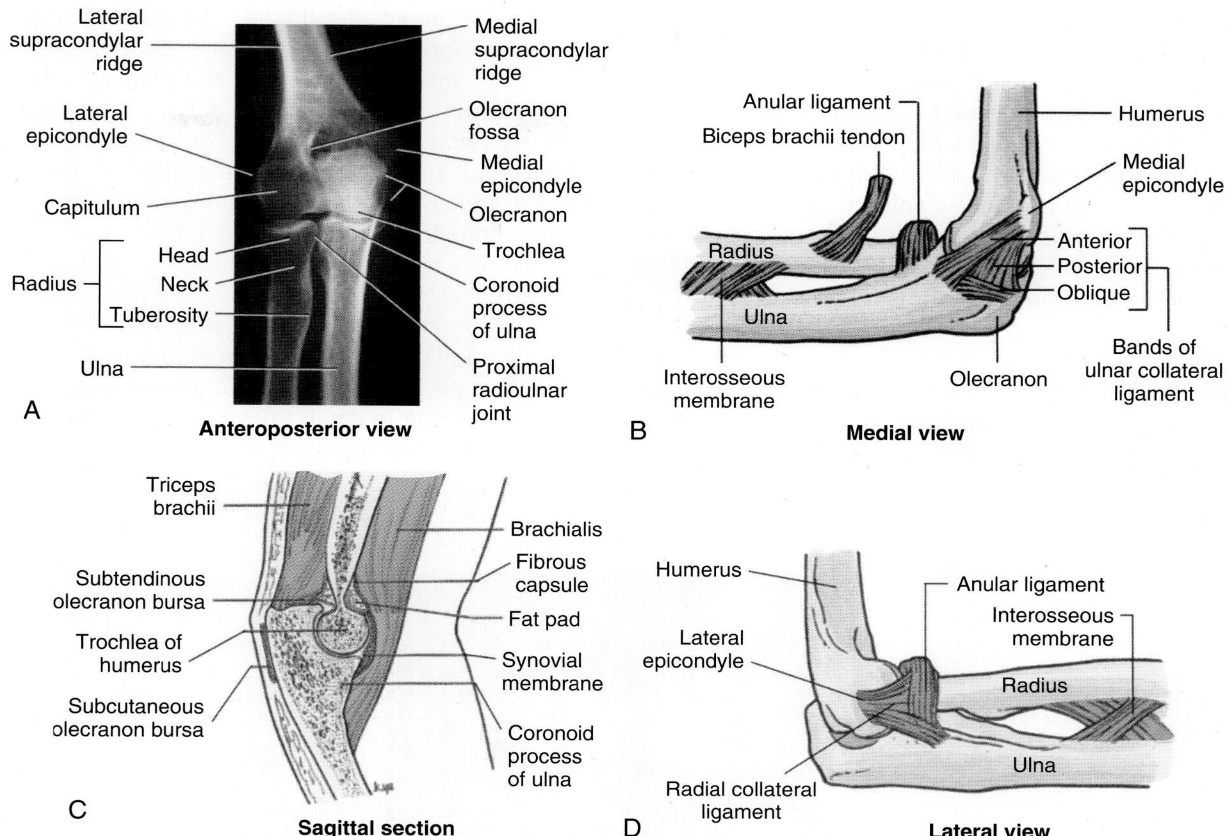

Figure 2–8 *Anteroposterior **(A)**, medial **(B)**, sagittal **(C)**, and lateral **(D)** views of the elbow joint. Reprinted with permission from Moore, K. L., & Agur, A. M. (1995).* Essential clinical anatomy. *Baltimore: Williams & Wilkins.*

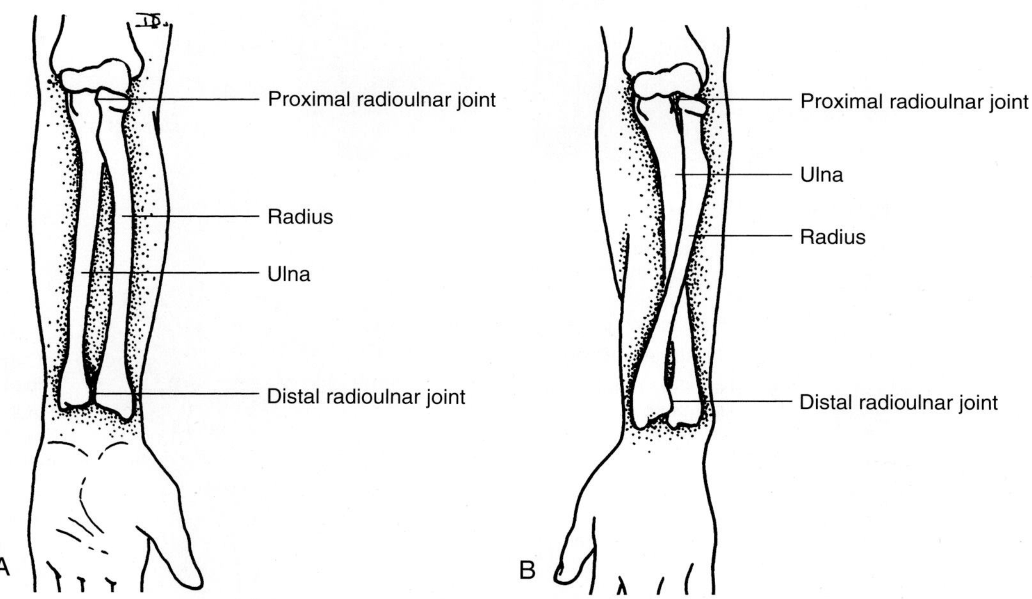

Figure 2–9 *Supination **(A)** and pronation **(B)** of the proximal and distal radioulnar joints. Reprinted with permission from Moore, K. L., & Agur, A. M. (1995).* Essential clinical anatomy. *Baltimore: Williams & Wilkins.*

and posterior radioulnar ligaments along with the **triangular fibrocartilage complex** (TFCC) (Norkin & Levangie, 1992; Tubiana, Thomine, & Mackin, 1996). The **interosseous membrane** helps bind the radius and ulna together by virtue of its fiber orientation from the radius to the ulna (Norkin & Levangie, 1992). Therapists applying forearm-based splints must appreciate the variation in muscle bulk during forearm rotation and compensate for this by rotating the forearm at the end of the molding process to ensure adequate fit.

The Wrist

The **wrist complex** incorporates the **radiocarpal** and **midcarpal** joints. The radiocarpal joint is a **condyloid joint** created by the connection between the distal radius with the scaphoid and lunate. The midcarpal joint is a plane joint formed by the intimate union of the proximal (scaphoid, lunate, triquetrum, and pisiform) and distal (trapezium, trapezoid, capitate, and hamate) carpal rows (Moore, 1992; Moore & Agur, 1995). In combination, the radiocarpal and midcarpal joints allow extension and flexion, radial and ulnar deviation, and a small amount of circumduction (Fig. 2–10 and Table 2–1).

The Hand

The **carpometacarpal (CMC) joints** of the digits are considered plane joints; they provide minimal motion at the index and middle fingers and progressively more mobility in the ring to small fingers (Moore, 1992; Moore & Agur, 1995). This arrangement allows humans to grasp

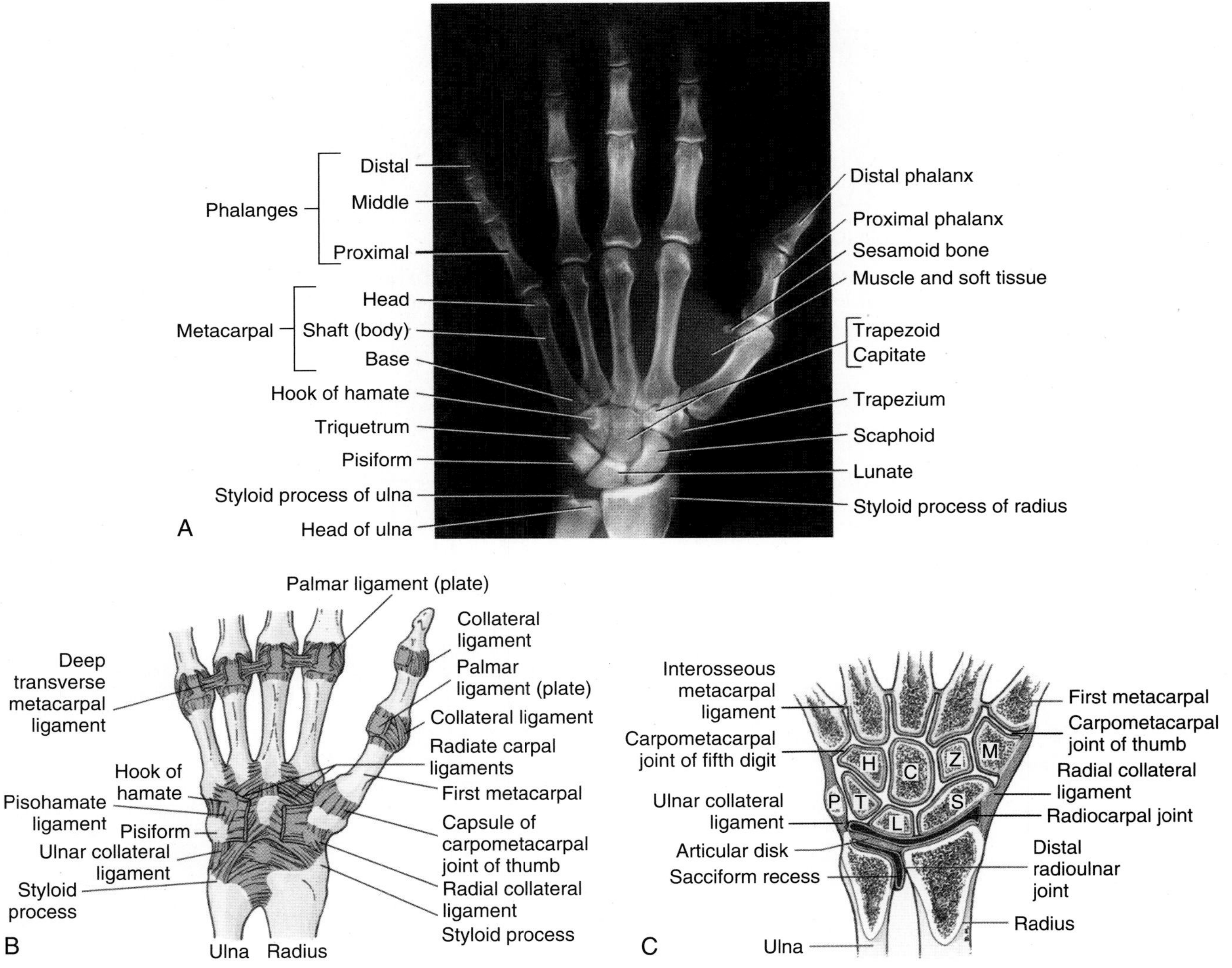

Figure 2–10 ***A,*** *Bony anatomy of the hand and wrist.* ***B,*** *Ligamentous structures of the hand and wrist.* ***C,*** *bony anatomy of the wrist.* C, *capitate;* H, *hamate;* L, *lunate;* M, *trapezium;* P, *pisiform;* S, *scaphoid;* T, *triquetrum;* Z, *trapezoid. Reprinted with permission from Moore KL, Agur AM.* Essential clinical anatomy. *Baltimore: Williams and Wilkins, 1995:339–340.*

TABLE 2–1 Joints of the Wrist and Hand

Characteristic	Wrist Joint	Carpometacarpal and Intercarpal Joints	Intermetacarpal Joints
Type	Condyloid synovial	Plane synovial	Carpometacarpal joint of the thumb: saddle synovial; all others: plane synovial
Articulation	Distal end of radius and articular disk superiorly; articulate with scaphoid, lunate, and triquetral bones inferiorly	Midcarpal joint is between proximal and distal rows of carpals; individual carpals articulate with each other	Carpals and metacarpals articulate with each other, as do metacarpals; carpometacarpal joint of thumb is between trapezium and base of first metacarpal
Articular (fibrous) capsule	Surrounds joint and is attached to distal ends of radius and ulna and proximal row of carpals	Surrounds joint	Surrounds joint
Ligaments	Anterior and posterior ligaments strengthen the capsule; ulnar collateral ligament is attached to styloid process of ulna and triquetrum; radial collateral ligament is attached to styloid process of radius and scaphoid	Carpals are united by anterior, posterior, and interosseous ligaments	Bones are united by anterior, posterior, and interosseous ligaments
Movements	Flexion and extension, abduction and adduction, circumduction	Small amount of gliding; flexion and abduction at the midcarpal joint	Carpometacarpal joints: first digit—flexion and extension, abduction and adduction; second and third digits—almost no movement; fourth digit—slightly more mobile; fifth digit—more mobile
Blood supply	Dorsal and palmar carpal arterial arches	Dorsal and palmar carpal arterial arches	Dorsal and palmar metacarpal arteries and deep carpal and deep palmar arterial arches
Nerve supply	Anterior interosseous branch of median nerve; posterior interosseous branch of radial nerve; dorsal and deep branches of ulnar nerve	Anterior interosseous branch of median nerve; posterior interosseous branch of radial nerve; dorsal and deep branches of ulnar nerve	Anterior interosseous branch of median nerve; posterior interosseous branch of radial nerve; dorsal and deep branches of ulnar nerve

Reprinted with permission from Moore, K. L., & Agur, A. M. (1995). *Essential clinical anatomy.* Baltimore: Williams & Wilkins.

objects tightly (Fig. 2–10). The CMC joint of the thumb, formed by the articulation of the trapezium with the base of the first metacarpal, is considered a saddle joint. It permits radial abduction and adduction, palmar abduction and adduction, and opposition (Fig. 2–10) (Moore, 1992; Moore & Agur, 1995).

The digital **metacarpophalangeal** (MP) **joints** are condyloid joints formed by the union of the metacarpal heads with the base of the proximal phalanges. They allow flexion and extension, abduction and adduction, and circumduction (Fig. 2–11 and Table 2–2) (Moore, 1992; Moore & Agur, 1995). The thumb MP joint is unique in its ability to allow a few degrees of abduction and rotation, which improves precision pinch function (Fess & Philips, 1987).

Distally, the **digital proximal interphalangeal** (PIP), and **distal interphalangeal** (DIP), and **thumb interphalangeal** (IP) joints are considered simple hinge joints, allowing only extension and flexion (Fig. 2–11) (Moore, 1992; Moore & Agur, 1995). Therapists must appreciate the tension placed on the ligamentous structures when splinting the digits. The MP joint **collateral ligaments** are taut in flexion and slack in extension, but the opposite is true for the palmar plate (taut in extension; slack in extension). Therefore, the MP joints should be positioned in flexion to place these ligaments at maximal length and to prevent shortening and extension contractures (Fig. 2–11C) (Chase, 1995; Fess & Philips, 1987). Similarly, when addressing the IP joints, the therapist must remember that the volar plate is taut in extension

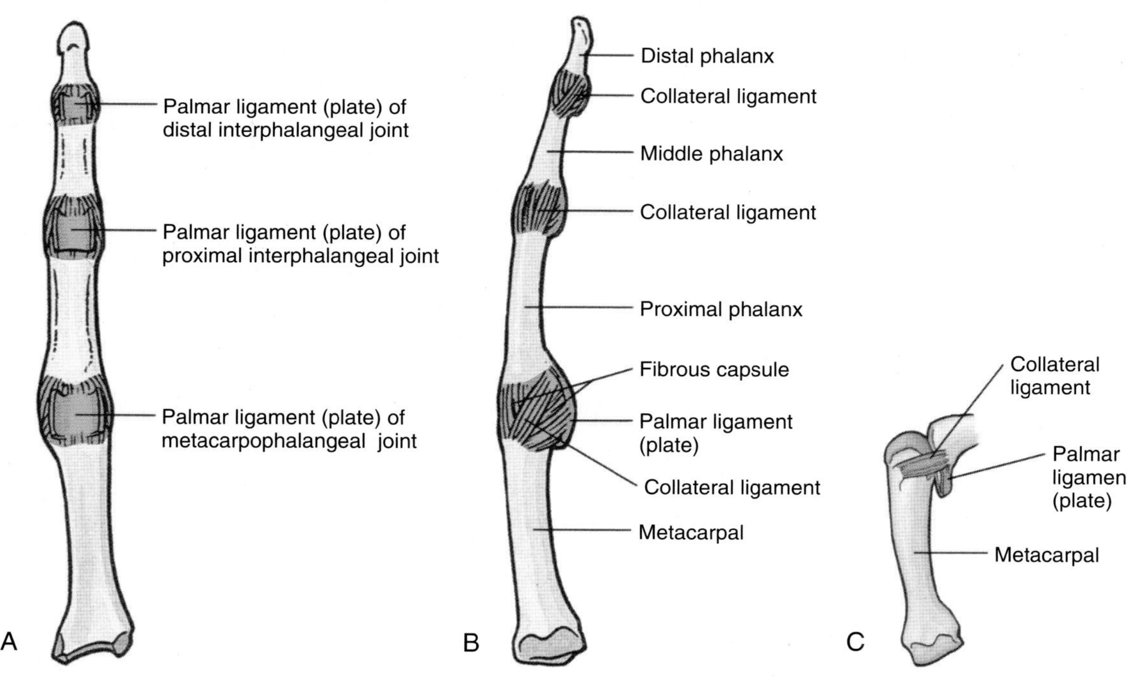

*Figure 2–11 Volar **(A)** and lateral **(B)** views of the metacarpophalangeal and interphalangeal joints. **C**, Tension on soft tissue structures in the metacarpophalangeal joint. Reprinted with permission from Moore, K. L., & Agur, A. M. (1995).* Essential clinical anatomy. *Baltimore: Williams & Wilkins.*

TABLE 2–2 Joints of the Digits

Characteristic	Metacarpophalangeal Joints	Interphalangeal Joints
Type	Condyloid synovial	Hinge synovial
Articulation	Heads of metacarpals articulate with bases of proximal phalanges	Heads of phalanges articulate with bases of more distally located phalanges
Articular (fibrous) capsule	Encloses each joint	Encloses each joint
Ligaments	Strong palmar ligaments are attached to phalanges and metacarpals; deep transverse metacarpal ligaments unite second to fifth joints that hold heads of metacarpals together; collateral ligaments pass from heads of metacarpals to bases of phalanges	Similar to metacarpophalangeal joints, except they unite phalanges
Movements	*Second to fifth digits:* flexion and extension, abduction and adduction, circumduction; *thumb:* flexion and extension, limited abduction and adduction	Flexion and extension
Blood supply	Deep digital arteries arise from superficial palmar arches	Digital arteries
Nerve supply	Digital nerves arise from ulnar and median nerves	Digital nerves arise from ulnar and median nerves

Reprinted with permission from Moore, K. L., & Agur, A. M. (1995). *Essential clinical anatomy.* Baltimore: Williams & Wilkins.

and slack in flexion. Ideally these joints are positioned in full extension to prevent shortening and flexion contractures (Fig. 2–12).

Arches of the Hand

The bony architecture, along with the muscles of the hand, contributes to the formation and maintenance of the arches in the hand (Fig. 2–13) (Bowers & Tribuzi, 1992; Chase, 1995; Fess & Philips, 1987; Tubiana et al., 1996). The **proximal transverse arch** is a rigid arrangement at the level of the distal carpal bones. In comparison, the **distal transverse** and **longitudinal** arches are mobile and add depth to the hand. The distal transverse arch is located at the level of the metacarpal heads and provides the ability

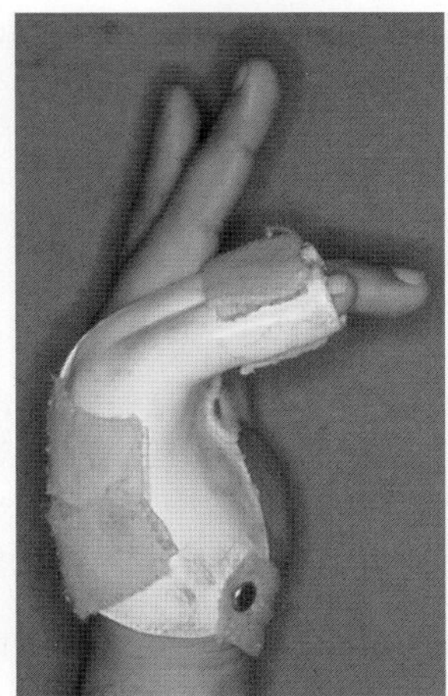

Figure 2–12 In the antideformity position, the MP joints are flexed and the IP joints are extended.

of the hand to grasp objects of different sizes. The mobility afforded by the ring and small finger CMC joints allows for this mobile arch. The longitudinal arch courses from the carpal level through the four digital rays. This highly mobile arch adapts to meet the needs of specific grasping activities. When splinting for metacarpal fractures, the therapist must appreciated the differences in mobility of the CMC joints. For example, splinting small finger metacarpal fractures requires inclusion of the middle and ring finger metacarpals to gain adequate purchase, stability and immobilization of the fracture.

When the hand is injured, the arch system can be compromised, altering hand function. For example, ulnar nerve injury and the subsequent loss of intrinsic function (active MP flexion/IP extension) disrupts the normal arch system, causing virtual collapse (Fig. 2–14). Therapists must appreciate the mobility and stability that the arches

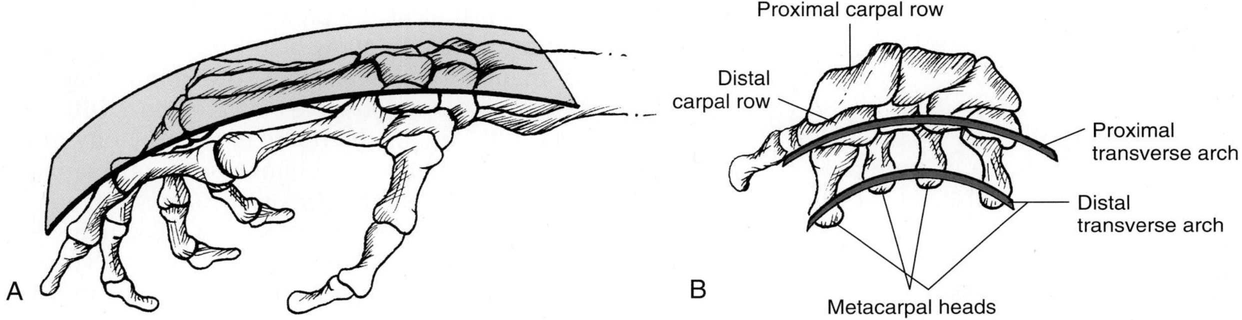

Figure 2–13 ***A,*** *The longitudinal arch of the hand spans the length of the rays and carpus.* ***B,*** *The proximal and distal transverse arches of the hand.*

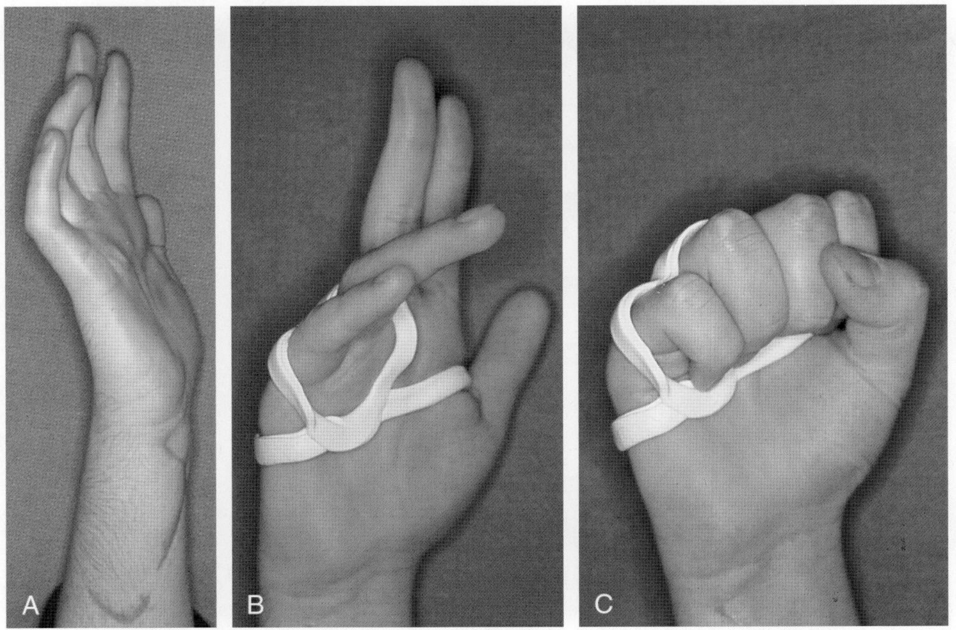

Figure 2–14 ***A,*** *After ulnar nerve injury, there is a loss of the arch system. MP extension restriction splint during active digit extension* ***(B)*** *and active digit flexion* ***(C).***

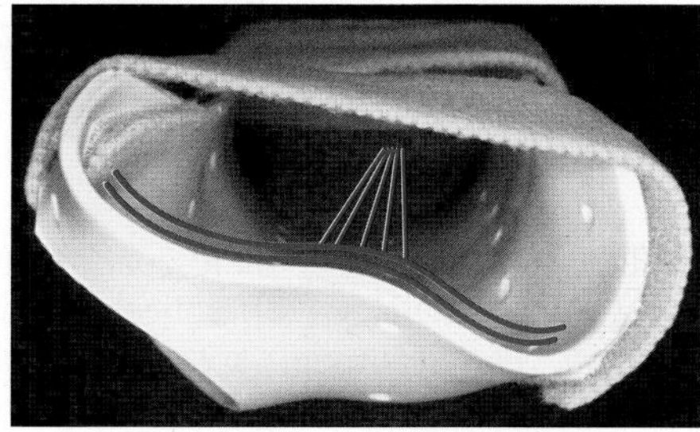

Figure 2–15 A wrist immobilization splint that includes the transverse and longitudinal arches to ensure a stable fit.

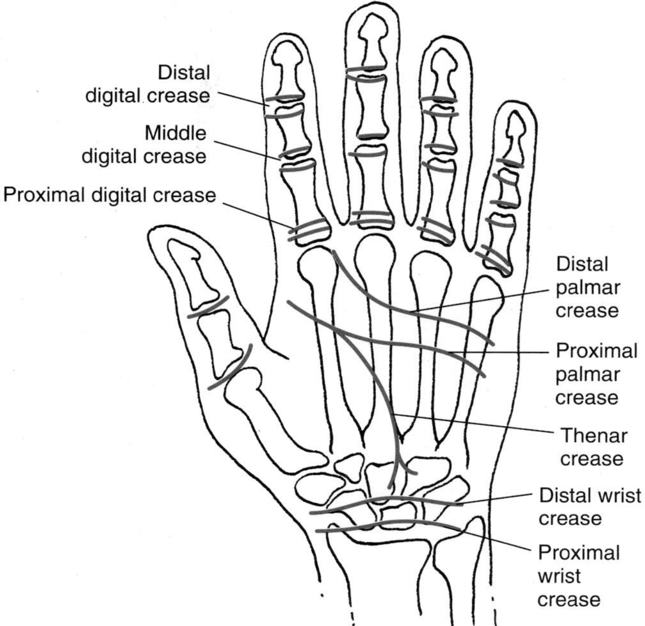

Figure 2–16 The relationship between the palmar creases and their underlying joints.

provide and should incorporate them into each splint to maximize the functional potential of the hand. In addition, a well-contoured splint that incorporates the arches minimizes migration of the splint on the body and better stabilizes a mobilization splint on the extremity when force is applied (Fig. 2–15).

Creases of the Hand

Palmar creases are distributed throughout the hand in a relatively consistent pattern (Bowers & Tribuzi, 1992; Chase, 1995; Fess & Philips, 1987). These creases form in direct relation to the underlying structures and the functional demands placed on those structures. To splint the hand appropriately, the therapist must gain an appreciation for which specific joints underlie each crease (Fig. 2–16). The therapist can use the creases as boundaries when making patterns and fabricating splints. To permit motion distally, the splint must clear the creases proximally (Fig. 2–17). For example, wrist splints must clear the proximal (PPC) and distal (DPC) palmar creases to allow a full digital range of motion. (To maintain wrist position, the splint should extend distally as far as possible in the palm.) Differences in metacarpal length contribute to the obliquity of the PPC and DPC, requiring an oblique angle at the distal edge of a volar wrist splint (Fig. 2–18). An additional consideration involves the importance of recognizing each patient's individual anatomic characteristics. For example, in one patient, clearing for the DPC on the radial side of the palm may be enough to allow full motion of the MP joints; but in another patient, the splint must clear the PPC to allow full motion.

Splinting Implications

Bony prominences exist throughout the upper extremity skeleton, and they must be taken into consideration

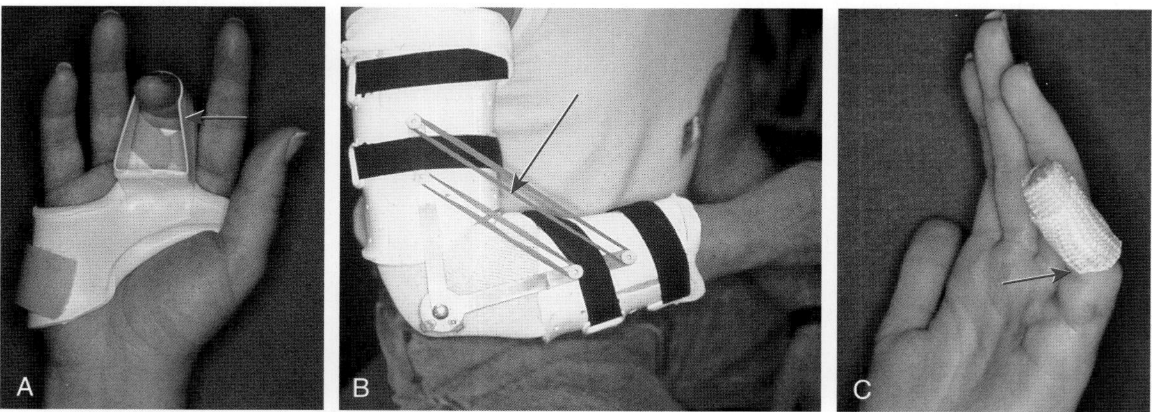

*Figure 2–17 **A,** A PIP flexion mobilization splint that clears the middle digital crease to allow unimpeded PIP flexion. **B,** An elbow flexion mobilization splint with clearance at the anterior aspect. **C,** A DIP immobilization splint that extends too far proximally to allow full flexion of the PIP joint.*

when molding a splint (Fess & Philips, 1987; Pratt, 1995). These areas tend to be vulnerable because of minimal soft tissue covering. Avoiding excess pressure over these areas by the splinting material or by strapping is of extreme importance. Excessive pressure can cause pain, redness, and possible skin necrosis (breakdown) from ischemia. The primary prominences to consider include the following (Fig. 2–19):

- Clavicle
- Spine of scapula
- Acromion
- Olecranon
- Medial and late
- Radial and ulr
- Base of first
- Dorsal thu
- Dorsal MP, PIP,
- Pisiform

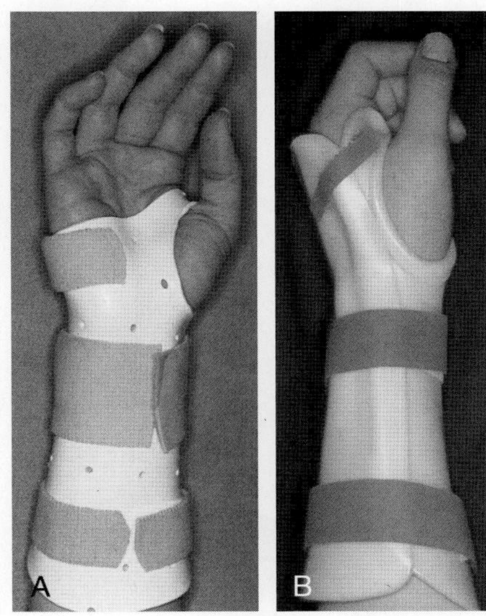

Figure 2–18 ***A,*** *A wrist immobilization splint that clears the DPC and PPC to allow the digits full range of motion.* ***B,*** *A wrist immobilization splint with inadequate clearance of the PPC, impeding the range of motion at the index MP joint.*

Clinical Example

A well-molded splint can prevent the ai plications by providing a custom fit with acc such as padding or flaring of the splint's edges risk areas (Fig. 2–20A–C). For example, when molding ulnar border of a volar wrist support, the therapist should flare the edge adjacent to the ulnar styloid process to help prevent the bone from abutting the hard splinting material during forearm rotation motions (Fig. 2–20D).

Nerves and Muscles of the Upper Extremity

The nerve supply to the upper extremity arises from the **brachial plexus** (Fig. 2–21 and Table 2–3) (Moore, 1992; Moore & Agur, 1995). The plexus originates from the cervical level of the spinal cord via the brachial plexus, receiving contributions from the ventral rami of spinal nerves C5–T1. Variations may exist with some contribution from C4 and T2. These five nerve roots combine to form the **superior, middle,** and **inferior trunks.** Posterior to the clavicle, the three trunks in turn divide into the three **anterior divisions** and three **posterior divisions.** The divisions then give rise to the **posterior, lateral,** and **medial cords** of the plexus. The cords are named according to

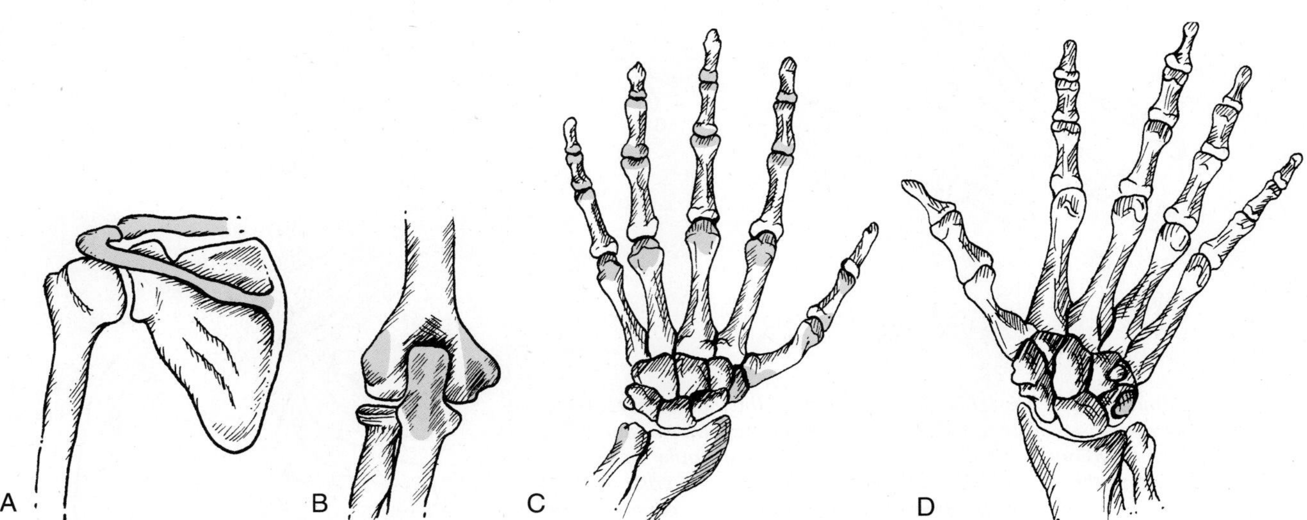

Figure 2–19 *Bony prominences of the shoulder* ***(A)****, elbow* ***(B)****, dorsal wrist and hand* ***(C)****, and volar wrist and hand* ***(D)****.*

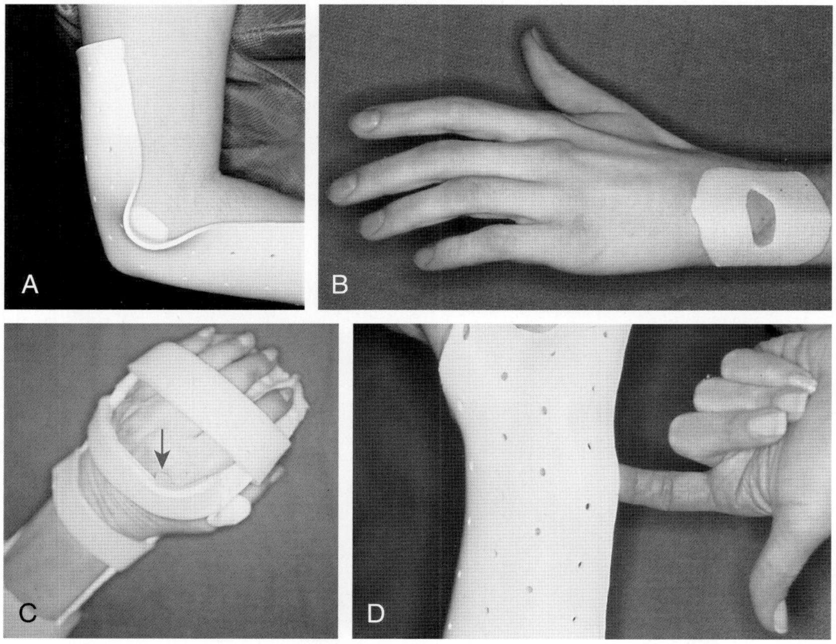

Figure 2–20 *Accommodations for bony prominences.* ***A,*** *Prepadding at lateral epicondyle for a posterior elbow immobilization splint.* ***B,*** *Prepadding with a donut at the distal ulna.* ***C,*** *Padding of the strap that traverses the index MP joint.* ***D,*** *Flaring at the distal ulna on a wrist immobilization splint.*

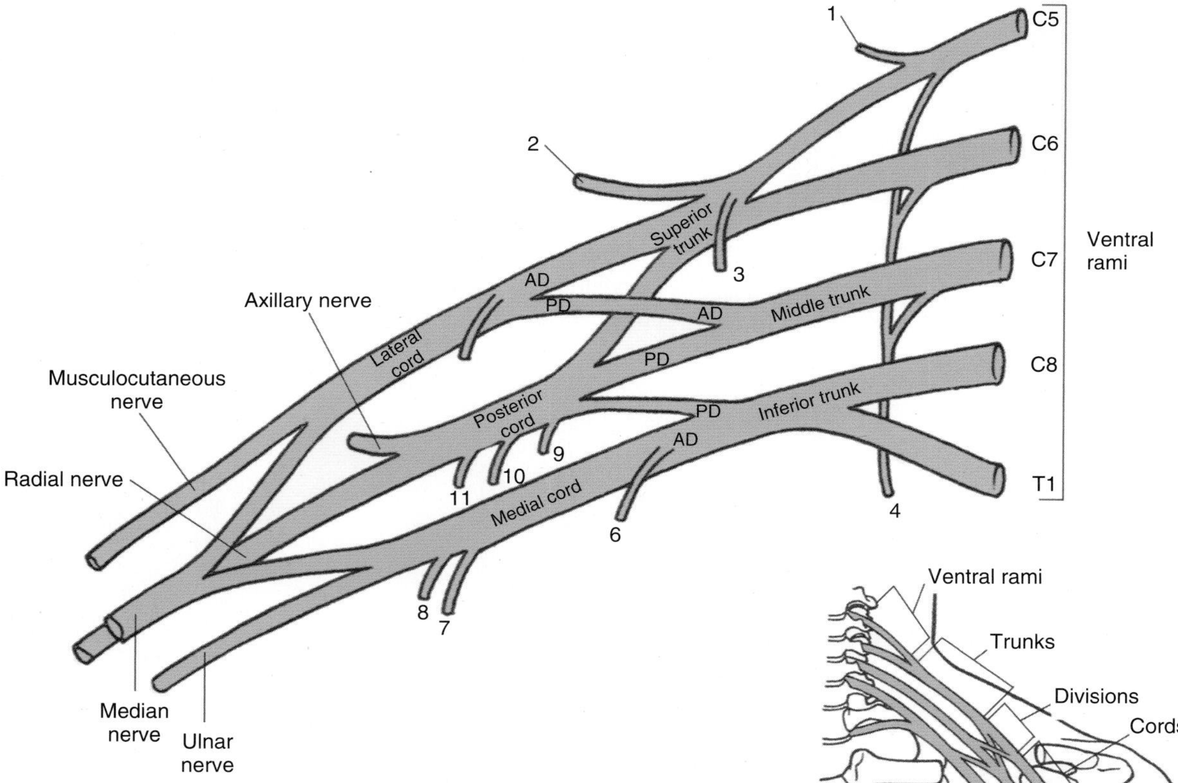

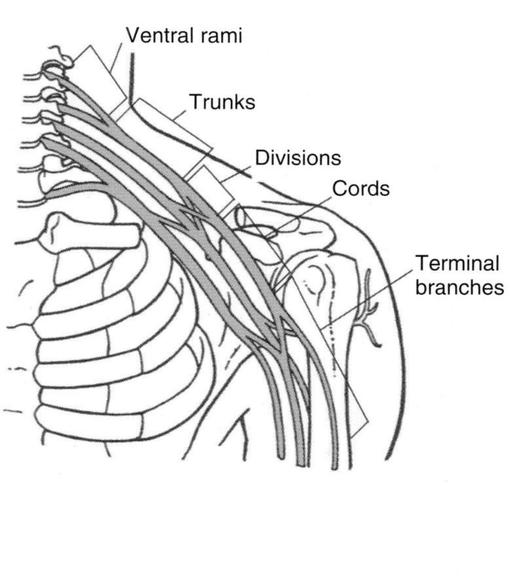

Figure 2–21 *Branches of the brachial plexus. Note that the musculocutaneous, median, and ulnar nerves are arranged like the limbs of a capital M.* AD, *anterior division;* PD, *posterior division;* 1, *Dorsal scapular nerve;* 2, *suprascapular nerve;* 3, *nerve to subclavius;* 4, *long thoracic nerve;* 5, *lateral pectoral nerve;* 6, *medial pectoral nerve;* 7, *medial brachial cutaneous nerve;* 8, *medial antebrachial cutaneous nerve;* 9, *upper subscapular nerve;* 10, *thoracodorsal nerve;* 11, *lower subscapular nerve. Reprinted with permission from Moore KL, Agur AM.* Essential clinical anatomy. *Baltimore: Williams and Wilkins, 1995: 298–299.*

TABLE 2–3 Nerves of the Brachial Plexus

Nerve	Origin	Course	Distribution
Supraclavicular branches			
Dorsal scapular	Ventral ramus of C5 with a frequent contribution from C4	Pierces scalenus medius, descends deep to levator scapulae, and enters deep surface of rhomboids	Innervates rhomboids and occasionally supplies levator scapulae
Long thoracic	Ventral rami of C5–C7	Descends posterior to C8 and T1 rami and passes distally on external surface of serratus anterior	Innervates serratus anterior
Nerve to subclavius	Superior trunk receiving fibers from C5 and C6 and often C4	Descends posterior to clavicle and anterior to brachial plexus and subclavian artery	Innervates subclavius and sternoclavicular joint
Suprascapular	Superior trunk receiving fibers from C5 and C6 and often C4	Passes laterally across posterior triangle of neck, through scapular notch under superior transverse scapular ligament	Innervates supraspinatus, infraspinatus, and shoulder joint
Infraclavicular branches			
Lateral pectoral	Lateral cord receiving fibers from C5–C7	Pierces clavipectoral fascia to reach deep surface of pectoral muscles	Primarily supplies pectoralis major but sends a loop to medial pectoral nerve that innervates pectoralis minor
Musculocutaneous	Lateral cord receiving fibers from C5–C7	Enters deep surface of coracobrachialis and descends between biceps brachii and brachialis	Innervates coracobrachialis, biceps brachii, and brachialis; continues as lateral antebrachial cutaneous nerve
Median	Lateral root is a continuation of lateral cord, receiving fibers from C6 and C7; medial root is a continuation of medial cord receiving fibers from C8 and T1	Lateral root joins medial root to form median nerve lateral to axillary artery	Innervates flexor muscles in forearm, except flexor carpi ulnaris, ulnar half of flexor digitorum profundus, and five hand muscles
Medial pectoral	Medial cord receiving fibers from C8 and T1	Passes between axillary artery and vein and enters deep surface of pectoralis minor	Innervates pectoralis minor and part of pectoralis major
Medial brachial cutaneous	Medial cord receiving fibers from C8 and T1	Runs along the medial side of axillary vein and communicates with intercostobrachial nerve	Supplies skin on medial side of arm
Medial antebrachial cutaneous	Medial cord receiving fibers from C8 and T1	Runs between axillary artery and vein	Supplies skin over medial side of forearm
Ulnar	A terminal branch of medial cord receiving fibers from C8 and T1 and often C7	Passes down medial aspect of arm and runs posterior to medial epicondyle to enter forearm	Innervates one and a half flexor muscles in forearm, most small muscles in hand, and skin of hand medial to a line bisecting ring finger
Upper subscapular	Branch of posterior cord receiving fibers from C5 and C6	Passes posteriorly and enters subscapularis	Innervates superior portion of subscapularis
Thoracodorsal	Branch of posterior cord receiving fibers from C6–C8	Arises between upper and lower subscapular nerves and runs inferolaterally to latissimus dorsi	Innervates latissimus dorsi
Lower subscapular	Branch of posterior cord receiving fibers from C5 and C6	Passes inferolaterally, deep to subscapular artery and vein, to subscapularis and teres major	Innervates inferior portion of subscapularis and teres major
Axillary	Terminal branch of posterior cord receiving fibers from C5 and C6	Passes to posterior aspect of arm through quadrangular space[a] in company with posterior circumflex humeral artery and then winds around surgical neck of humerus; gives rise to lateral brachial cutaneous nerve	Innervates teres minor and deltoid, shoulder joint, and skin over inferior part of deltoid
Radial	Terminal branch of posterior cord receiving fibers from C5–C8 and T1	Descends posterior to axillary artery; enters radial groove with deep brachial artery to pass between long and medial heads of triceps	Innervates triceps brachii, anconeus, brachioradialis, and extensor muscles of forearm; supplies skin on posterior aspect of arm and forearm via posterior cutaneous nerves of arm and forearm

[a]Quadrangular space is bounded superiorly by subscapularis and teres minor, inferiorly by teres major, and medially by long head of triceps, and laterally by humerus.

Modified with permission from Moore, K. L., & Agur, A. M. (1995). *Essential clinical anatomy.* Baltimore: Williams & Wilkins.

their relationship to the axillary artery. The cords provide the origin for the **terminal nerve branches: musculocutaneous, axillary, radial, median,** and **ulnar nerves.** Figure 2–21 and Table 2–3 outline the specific origins of the small branches throughout the plexus.

Each terminal nerve branch traverses through the upper extremity, passing through and innervating specific muscles along its path toward the hand (Fig. 2–22 and Table 2–4) (Green, 1988; "Nerve Compression Syndromes,"* 1992; Spinner, 1995). (Chapter 19 includes a

TABLE 2–4 Nerves of the Upper Extremity

Nerve[a]	Origin	Course
Median	By two roots from lateral (C6 and C7) and medial (C8 and T1) cords of brachial plexus	Enters cubital fossa medial to brachial artery, passes between heads of pronator teres, descends between flexor digitorum superficialis and flexor digitorum profundus, and passes close to flexor retinaculum as it passes through carpal tunnel to reach hand
Recurrent branch of median	Arises from median nerve as soon as it passes distal to flexor retinaculum	Loops around distal border of flexor retinaculum to reach thenar muscles
Lateral branch of median (1)	Lateral division of median nerve as it enters palm of hand	Runs laterally, supplying first lumbrical and cutaneous branches to anterior surface of thumb and lateral side of index finger
Medial branch of median (1)	Medial division of the median nerve as it enters the palm of the hand	Runs medially to second lumbrical muscle and sends cutaneous branches to adjacent sides of index and middle fingers and adjacent sides of middle and ring fingers
Palmar cutaneous branch of median (2)	Medial nerve just proximal to flexor retinaculum	Passes between tendons of palmaris longus and flexor carpi radialis and runs superficial to flexor retinaculum
Anterior interosseous	Medial nerve in distal part of cubital fossa	Passes inferiorly on interosseous membrane to supply flexor digitorum profundus, flexor pollicis longus, and pronator quadratus
Ulnar (3)	Medial cord of brachial plexus (C8 and T1), but often receives fibers from ventral ramus of C7	Passes posterior to medial epicondyle of humerus and enters forearm between heads of flexor carpi ulnaris; descends through forearm between flexor carpi ulnaris and flexor digitorum profundus; becomes superficial in distal part of forearm and passes superficial to flexor retinaculum
Superficial branch of ulnar	Arises from ulnar nerve at wrist as it passes between pisiform and hamate bones	Passes to palmaris brevis and to skin of medial one and a half digits

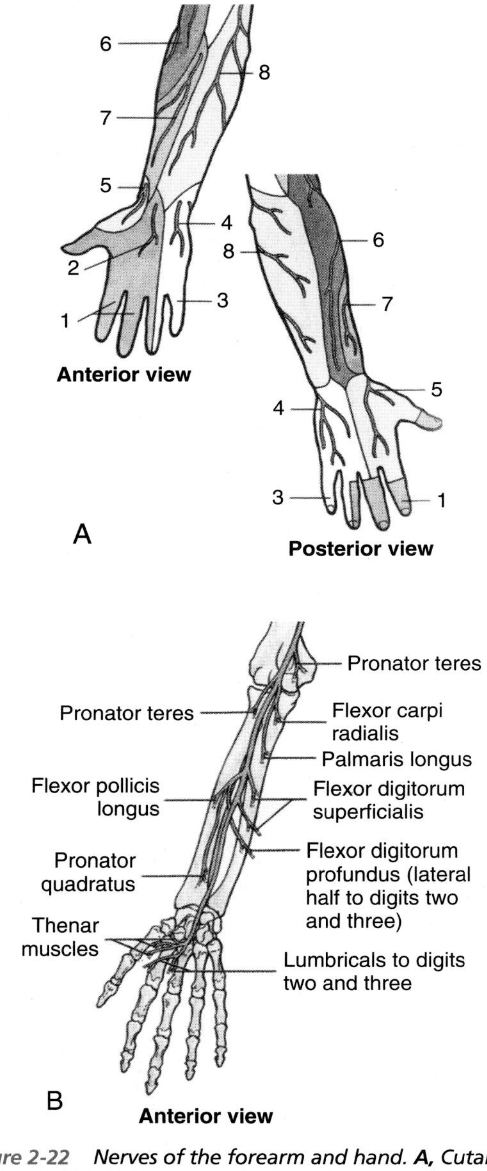

Figure 2-22 *Nerves of the forearm and hand.* ***A,*** *Cutaneous nerves. 1, Lateral and medial branches of median nerve; 2, palmar cutaneous branch of median nerve; 3, ulnar nerve; 4, palmar cutaneous branch of the ulnar nerve; 5, superficial branch of the radial nerve; 6, posterior antebrachial cutaneous nerve; 7, lateral antebrachial cutaneous nerve; 8, medial antebrachial cutaneous nerve.* ***B,*** *Median nerve.*

[a]Numbers in parentheses refer to Figure 2.22A.
Modified with permission from Moore, K. L., & Agur, A. M. (1995). *Essential clinical anatomy.* Baltimore: Williams & Wilkins.

TABLE 2–4 Continued

Nerve[a]	Origin	Course
Deep branch of ulnar	Arises from ulnar nerve as described above	Supplies muscles of hypothenar eminence and then curves around inferior edge of hamate to pass deeply in palm to supply muscles shown in Figure 2-22C
Palmar cutaneous branch of ulnar (4)	Ulnar nerve near middle of forearm	Descends on ulnar artery and perforates deep fascia in the distal third of forearm
Radial	Posterior cord of brachial plexus (C5–C8 and T1)	Passes into cubital fossa and descends between brachialis and brachioradialis; at level of lateral epicondyle of humerus, it divides into superficial and deep branches
Superficial branch of radial (5)	Continuation of radial nerve after deep branch is given off	Passes distally, anterior to pronator teres and deep to brachioradialis; pierces deep fascia at wrist and passes onto dorsum of hand
Deep branch of radial	Arises from radial nerve just distal to elbow	Winds around neck of radius in supinator; enters posterior compartment to supply muscles shown in Figure 2-22D
Posterior interosseus	Terminal branch of deep branch of radial nerve	Passes deep to extensor pollicis longus and lies on interosseous membrane
Posterior antebrachial cutaneous (6)	Arises in arm from radial nerve	Perforates lateral head of triceps and descends along lateral side of arm and posterior aspect of forearm to wrist
Lateral antebrachial cutaneous (7)	Continuation of musculocutaneous nerve	Descends along lateral border of forearm to wrist
Medial antebrachial cutaneous (8)	Medial cord of brachial plexus, receiving fibers from C8 and T1	Runs down arm on medial side of brachial artery; pierces deep fascia in cubital fossa and runs along medial aspect of forearm

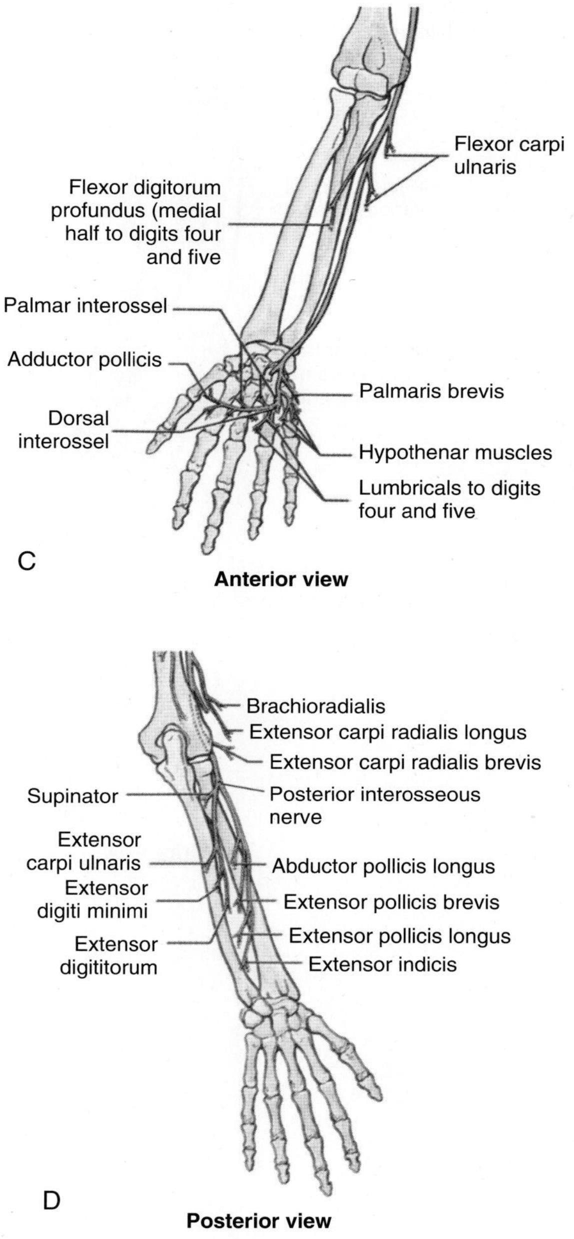

C Anterior view

D Posterior view

*Figure 2–22 Continued. **C,** Ulnar nerve. **D,** Radial nerve.*

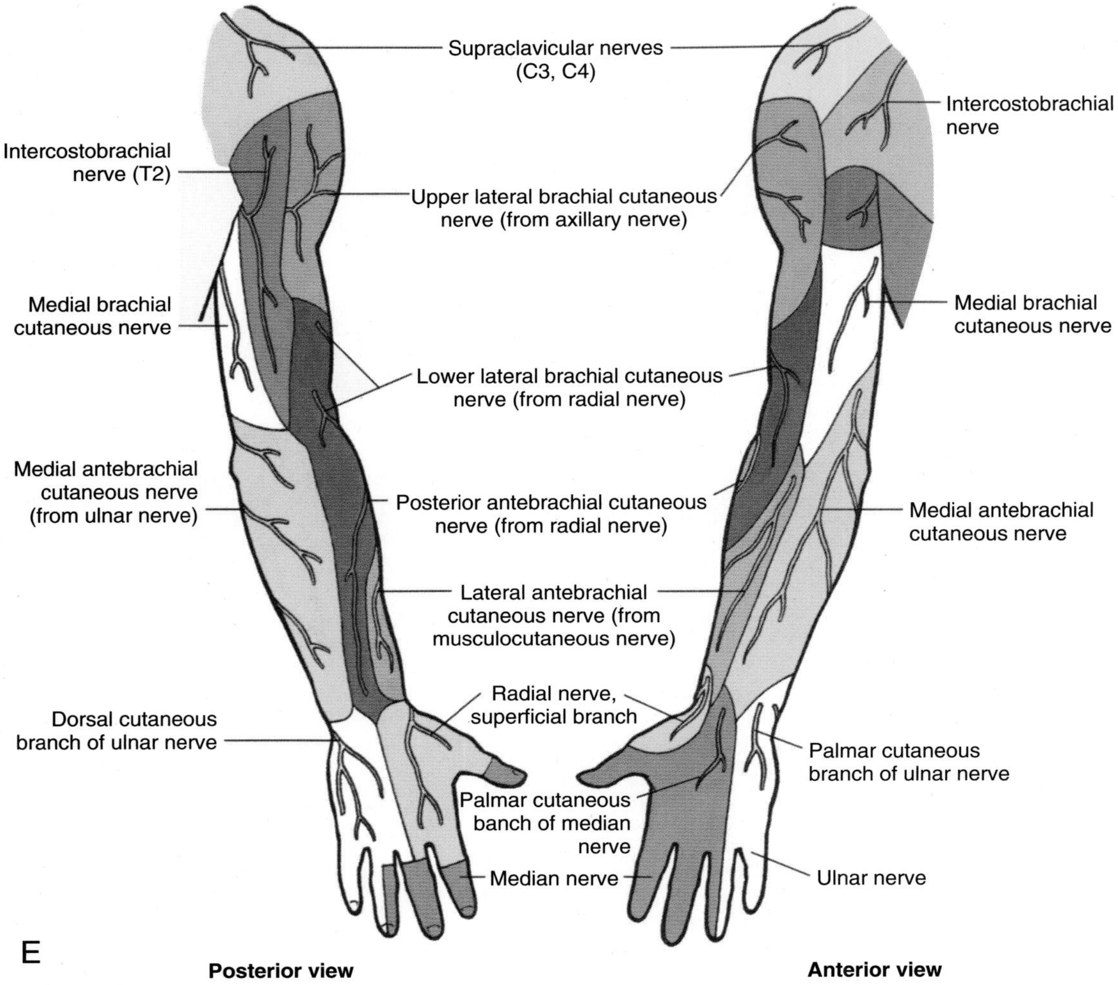

Supraclavicular nerves
(C3, C4)
Intercostobrachial nerve (T2)
Intercostobrachial nerve
Upper lateral brachial cutaneous nerve (from axillary nerve)
Medial brachial cutaneous nerve
Medial brachial cutaneous nerve
Lower lateral brachial cutaneous nerve (from radial nerve)
Medial antebrachial cutaneous nerve (from ulnar nerve)
Posterior antebrachial cutaneous nerve (from radial nerve)
Medial antebrachial cutaneous nerve
Lateral antebrachial cutaneous nerve (from musculocutaneous nerve)
Radial nerve, superficial branch
Dorsal cutaneous branch of ulnar nerve
Palmar cutaneous branch of ulnar nerve
Palmar cutaneous banch of median nerve
Median nerve
Ulnar nerve
E
Posterior view
Anterior view

C4
C5
C6
C7
C8
T1
T2
C4
C5
T1
T2
C5
C6
T1
C8
C6
C7
C8
C7
F
Posterior view
Anterior view

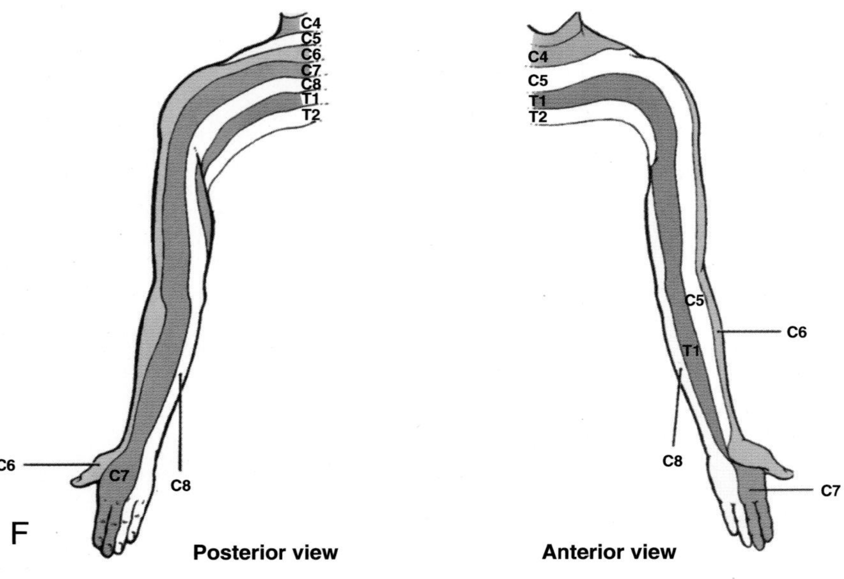

Figure 2–22 *Continued.* ***E,*** *Distribution of cutaneous nerves in the upper extremity.* ***F,*** *Dermatomes of the upper extremity. Reprinted with permission from Moore, K. L., & Agur, A. M. (1995).* Essential clinical anatomy. *Baltimore: Williams & Wilkins.*

detailed discussion of nerve anatomy, including pathways, innervations, and compression sites.) In general, the radial nerve innervates the dorsal extensor muscles of the elbow, forearm, wrist, and hand. The median and ulnar nerves provide innervation to the volar flexor muscles and the intrinsic muscles of the hand. Sensation of the upper extremity is provided by various cutaneous nerves. Throughout each nerve's individual pathway, areas exist in which the nerves are vulnerable to compression by other anatomic structures, such as muscles and ligaments. These nerves are also vulnerable to external forces, such as from splints.

Therapists must have a working knowledge of peripheral neuroanatomy, along with full comprehension of the muscular and cutaneous innervations in the upper extremity. Table 2–5 lists the muscular attachments, innervations, and actions and serves as a handy reference when making decisions about splinting and rehabilitation of a patient. Chapter 18 provides a detailed discussion of the muscular anatomy of the forearm and hand.

TABLE 2–5 Muscles of the Upper Extremity

Muscle	Proximal Attachment	Distal Attachment	Innervation[a]	Main Actions
Pectoral Muscles				
Pectoralis major	*Clavicular head:* anterior surface of medial half of clavicle; *sternocostal head:* anterior surface of sternum, superior six costal cartilages, and aponeurosis of external oblique muscle	Lateral lip of intertubercular groove of humerus	Lateral and medial pectoral nerves: clavicular head (C5 and **C6**), sternocostal head (**C7, C8,** and T1)	Adducts and medially rotates humerus; draws scapula anteriorly and inferiorly; acting alone: clavicular head flexes humerus and sternocostal head extends it
Pectoralis minor	Third to fifth ribs near their costal cartilages	Medial border and superior surface of coracoid process of scapula	Medial pectoral nerve (C8 and T1)	Stabilizes scapula by drawing it inferiorly and anteriorly against thoracic wall
Subclavius	Junction of first rib and its costal cartilage	Inferior surface of middle third of clavicle	Nerve to subclavius (**C5** and C6)	Anchors and depresses clavicle
Serratus anterior	External surfaces of lateral parts of first to eighth ribs	Anterior surface of medial border of scapula	Long thoracic nerve (C5, **C6,** and **C7**)	Protracts scapula and holds it against thoracic wall; rotates scapula
Superficial Back, Scapular, and Arm Muscles				
Trapezius	Medial third of superior nuchal line; external occipital protuberance, ligamentum nuchae, and spinous processes of C7-T12 vertebrae	Lateral third of clavicle, acromion, and spine of scapula	Spinal root of accessory nerve (CN XI) and cervical nerves (C3 and C4)	Elevates, retracts, and rotates scapula, superior fibers elevate, middle fibers retract, and inferior fibers depress scapula; superior and inferior fibers act together in superior rotation of scapula
Latissimus dorsi	Spinous processes of inferior six thoracic vertebrae, thoracolumbar fascia, iliac crest, and inferior three or four ribs	Floor of intertubercular groove of humerus	Thoracodorsal nerve (**C6, C7,** and C8)	Extends, adducts, and medially rotates humerus; raises body toward arms during climbing
Levator scapulae	Posterior tubercles of transverse processes of C1-C4 vertebrae	Superior part of medial border of scapula	Dorsal scapular (C5) and cervical (C3 and C4) nerves	Elevates scapula and tilts its glenoid cavity inferiorly by rotating scapula

[a]Boldface indicates main segmental innervation; damage to these segments or to motor nerve roots arising from them results in paralysis of muscles concerned.

CN, cranial nerve.

Modified with permission from Moore, K. L., & Agur, A. M. (1995). *Essential clinical anatomy.* Baltimore: Williams & Wilkins.

Continued

TABLE 2–5 Continued

Muscle	Proximal Attachment	Distal Attachment	Innervation[a]	Main Actions
Rhomboid minor and major	*Minor:* ligamentum nuchae and spinous processes of C7 and T1 vertebrae; *major:* spinous processes of T2-T5 vertebrae	Medial border of scapula form level of spine to inferior angle	Dorsal scapular nerve (C4 and **C5**) rotate	Retracts scapula and rotates it to depress glenoid cavity; fixes scapula to thoracic wall
Deltoid	Lateral third of clavicle, acromion, and spine of scapula	Deltoid tuberosity of humerus	Axillary nerve (**C5** and C6)	*Anterior:* flexes and medially rotates arm; *middle:* abducts arm; *posterior:* extends and laterally rotates arm
Supraspinatus[b]	Supraspinous fossa of scapula	Superior facet on greater tubercle of humerus	Suprascapular nerve (C4, **C5,** and C6)	Helps deltoid abduct arm and acts with rotator cuff muscle
Infraspinatus[b]	Infraspinous fossa of scapula	Middle facet on greater tubercle of humerus	Suprascapular nerve (**C5** and C6)	Laterally rotates arm; helps hold humeral head in glenoid cavity of scapula
Teres minor[b]	Superior part of lateral border of scapula	Inferior facet on greater tubercle of humerus	Axillary nerve (**C5** and C6)	Laterally rotates arm; helps hold humeral head in glenoid cavity of scapula
Teres major	Dorsal surface of inferior angle of scapula	Medial lip of intertubercular groove of humerus	Lower subscapular nerve (**C6** and C7)	Adducts and medially rotates arm
Subscapularis[b]	Subscapular fossa	Lesser tubercle of humerus	Upper and lower subscapular nerves (C5, **C6,** and C7)	Medially rotates and adducts arm; helps hold humeral head in glenoid cavity
Biceps brachii	*Short head:* tip of coracoid process of scapula; *long head:* supraglenoid tubercle of scapula	Tuberosity of radius and fascia of forearm via bicipital aponeurosis	Musculocutaneous nerve (C5 and **C6**)	Supinates forearm and, when it is supine, flexes forearm
Brachialis	Distal half of anterior surface of humerus	Coronoid process and tuberosity of ulna	Musculocutaneous nerve (C5 and **C6**)	Flexes forearm in all positions
Coracobrachialis	Tip of coracoid process of scapula	Middle third of medial surface of humerus	Musculocutaneous nerve (C5, **C6,** and C7)	Helps flex and adduct arm
Triceps brachii	*Long head:* infraglenoid tubercle of scapula; *lateral head:* posterior surface of humerus, superior to radial groove; *medial head:* posterior surface of humerus, inferior to radial groove	Proximal end of olecranon of ulna and fascia of forearm	Radial nerve (C6, **C7,** and **C8**)	Chief extensor of forearm; long head steadies head of abducted humerus
Anconeus	Lateral epicondyle of humerus	Lateral surface of olecranon and superior part of posterior surface of ulna	Radial nerve (C7, C8, and T1)	Assists triceps in extending forearm; stabilizes elbow joint; abducts ulna during pronation

[a]Boldface indicates main segmental innervation; damage to these segments or to motor nerve roots arising from them results in paralysis of muscles concerned.

[b]Collectively, the supraspinatus, infraspinatus, teres minor, and subscapularis muscles are referred to as the rotator cuff muscles, the prime function of these muscles is to hold the head of the humerus in the glenoid cavity of the scapula during all shoulder joint movements.

CN, cranial nerve.

Modified with permission from Moore, K. L., & Agur, A. M. (1995). *Essential clinical anatomy.* Baltimore: Williams & Wilkins.

TABLE 2–5 Continued

Muscle	Proximal Attachment	Distal Attachment	Innervation[a]	Main Actions
Muscles of Anterior Surface of Forearm				
Pronator teres	Medial epicondyle of humerus and coronoid process of ulna	Middle of lateral surface of radius	Median nerve (C6 and **C7**)	Pronates and flexes forearm
Flexor carpi radialis	Medial epicondyle of humerus	Base of second metacarpal bone	Median nerve (C6 and **C7**)	Flexes and abducts hand
Palmaris longus	Medial epicondyle of humerus	Distal half of flexor retinaculum and palmar aponeurosis	Median nerve (C7 and C8)	Flexes hand and tightens palmar aponeurosis
Flexor carpi ulnaris	*Humeral head:* medial epicondyle of humerus; *ulnar head:* olecranon and posterior border of ulna	Pisiform bone, hook of hamate bone, and fifth metacarpal bone	Ulnar nerve (C7 and **C8**)	Flexes and adducts hand
Flexor digitorum superficialis	*Humeroulnar head:* medial epicondyle of humerus, ulnar collateral ligament, and coronoid process of ulna; *radial head:* superior half of anterior border of radius	Bodies of middle phalanges of medial four digits	Median nerve (C7, **C8,** and T1)	Flexes middle phalanges of medial four digits; acting more strongly, it flexes proximal phalanges and hand
Flexor digitorum profundus	Proximal three-quarters of medial and anterior surfaces of ulna and interosseous membrane	Bases of distal phalanges of medial four digits	*Medial part:* ulnar nerve (**C8** and T1); *lateral part:* median nerve (**C8** and T1)	Flexes distal phalanges of medial four digits; assists with flexion of hand
Flexor pollicis longus	Anterior surface of radius and adjacent interosseous membrane	Base of distal phalanx of thumb	Anterior interosseous n. from median (**C8** and T1)	Flexes phalanges of first digit (thumb)
Pronator quadratus	Distal quarter of anterior surface of ulna	Distal quarter of anterior surface of radius	Anterior interosseous n. from median (**C8** and T1)	Pronates forearm; deep fibers bind radius and ulna together
Muscles of Posterior Surface of Forearm				
Brachioradialis	Proximal two thirds of lateral supracondylar ridge of humerus	Lateral surface of distal end of radius	Radial nerve (C5, **C6,** and C7)	Flexes forearm
Extensor carpi radialis longus	Lateral epicondyle of humerus	Base of second metacarpal bone	Radial nerve (C6 and C7)	Extends and abducts hand at wrist joint
Extensor carpi radialis brevis	Lateral epicondyle of humerus	Base of third metacarpal bone	Deep branch of radial nerve (**C7** and C8)	Extends and abducts hand at wrist joint
Extensor digitorum	Lateral epicondyle of humerus	Extensor expansions of medial four digits	Posterior interosseous nerve (**C7** and C8), a branch of the radial nerve	Extends medial four digits at metacarpophalangeal joints; extends hand at wrist joint
Extensor digit minimi	Lateral epicondyle of humerus	Extensor expansion of fifth digit	Posterior interosseous nerve (**C7** and C8), a branch of the radial nerve	Extends fifth digit at metacarpophalangeal and interphalangeal joints
Extensor carpi ulnaris	Lateral epicondyle of humerus and posterior border of ulna	Base of fifth metacarpal bone	Posterior interosseous nerve (**C7** and C8), a branch of the radial nerve	Extends and adducts hand at wrist joint

Continued

TABLE 2–5 Continued

Muscle	Proximal Attachment	Distal Attachment	Innervation[a]	Main Actions
Anconeus	Lateral epicondyle humerus	Lateral surface of olecranon and superior part of posterior surface of ulna	Radial nerve (C7, C8, and T1)	Assists triceps in extending elbow joint; stabilizes elbow joint; abducts ulna during pronation
Supinator	Lateral epicondyle of humerus, radial collateral and anular ligaments, supinator fossa, and crest of ulna	Lateral, posterior, and anterior surfaces of proximal third of radius	Deep branch of radial nerve (C5 and **C6**)	Supinates forearm (i.e., rotates radius to turn palm anteriorly)
Abductor pollicis longus	Posterior surfaces of ulna, radius, and interosseous membrane	Base of first metacarpal bone	Posterior interosseous nerve (C7 and **C8**)	Abducts thumb and extends it at carpometacarpal joint
Extensor pollicis brevis	Posterior surface of radius and interosseous membrane	Base of proximal phalanx of thumb	Posterior interosseous nerve (C7 and **C8**)	Extends proximal phalanx of thumb at carpometacarpal joint
Extensor pollicis longus	Posterior surface of middle third of ulna and interosseous membrane	Base of distal phalanx of thumb	Posterior interosseous nerve (C7 and **C8**)	Extends distal phalanx of thumb at metacarpophalangeal and interphalangeal joints
Extensor indicis	Posterior surface of ulna and interosseous membrane	Extensor expansion of second digit	Posterior interosseous nerve (C7 and **C8**)	Extends second digit and helps extend hand
Muscles of Hand				
Abductor pollicis brevis	Flexor retinaculum and tubercles of scaphoid and trapezium bones	Lateral side of base of proximal phalanx of thumb	Recurrent branch of median nerve (**C8** and T1)	Abducts and helps oppose thumb
Flexor pollicis brevis	Flexor retinaculum and tubercle of trapezium bone	Lateral side of base of proximal phalanx of thumb	Recurrent branch of median nerve (**C8** and T1)	Flexes thumb
Opponens pollicis	Flexor retinaculum and tubercle of trapezium bone	Lateral side of first metacarpal bone	Recurrent branch of median nerve (**C8** and T1)	Opposes thumb toward center of palm and rotates it medially
Adductor pollicis	*Oblique head:* bases of second and third metacarpals, capitate, and adjacent carpal bones; *transverse head:* anterior surface of body of third metacarpal bone	Medial side of base of proximal phalanx of thumb	Deep branch of ulnar nerve (C8 and **T1**)	Adducts thumb toward middle digit
Abductor digiti minimi	Pisiform bone	Medial side of base of proximal phalanx of fifth digit	Deep branch of ulnar nerve (C8 and **T1**)	Abducts fifth digit
Flexor digiti minimi brevis	Hook of hamate bone and flexor retinaculum	Medial side of base of proximal phalanx of fifth digit	Deep branch of ulnar nerve (C8 and **T1**)	Flexes proximal phalanx of fifth digit

[a]Boldface indicates main segmental innervation; damage to these segments or to motor nerve roots arising from them results in paralysis of muscles concerned.

CN, cranial nerve.

Modified with permission from Moore, K. L., & Agur, A. M. (1995). *Essential clinical anatomy.* Baltimore: Williams & Wilkins.

TABLE 2–5 Continued

Muscle	Proximal Attachment	Distal Attachment	Innervation[a]	Main Actions
Opponens digiti minimi	Hook of hamate bone and flexor retinaculum	Medial border of fifth metacarpal bone	Deep branch of ulnar nerve (C8 and ***T1***)	Draws fifth metacarpal bone anteriorly and rotates it, bringing fifth digit into opposition with thumb
Lumbricals one and two	Lateral two tendons of flexor digitorum profundus	Lateral sides of extensor expansions of second to fifth digits	Median nerve (C8 and **T1**)	Flex digits at metacarpophalangeal joints and extend interphalangeal joints
Lumbricals three and four	Medial three tendons of flexor digitorum profundus	Lateral sides of extensor expansions of second to fifth digits	Deep branch of ulnar nerve (C8 and **T1**)	Flex digits at metacarpophalangeal joints and extend interphalangeal joints
Dorsal interossei one to four	Adjacent sides of two metacarpal bones	Extensor expansions and bases of proximal phalanges of second to fourth digits	Deep branch of ulnar nerve (C8 and **T1**)	Abduct digits and assist lumbricals
Palmar interossei one to three	Palmar surfaces of second, fourth, and fifth metacarpal bones	Extensor expansions of digits and bases of proximal phalanges of second, fourth, and fifth digits	Deep branch of ulnar nerve (C8 and **T1**)	Adduct digits and assist lumbricals

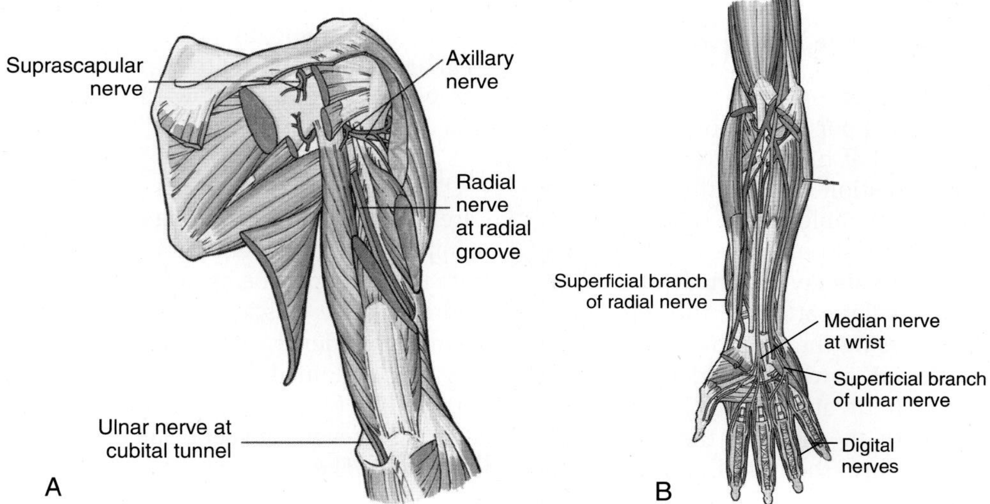

*Figure 2–23 Nerves of the upper **(A)** and lower **(B)** arm that are highly susceptible to compression. Reprinted with permission from Moore, K. L., & Agur, A. M. (1995).* Essential clinical anatomy. *Baltimore: Williams & Wilkins.*

Splinting Implications

Therapists must avoid compression of the superficial nerves while molding the splint and again when applying straps and mobilization components (Fess & Philips, 1987). Symptoms of nerve irritation include complaints of numbness, paresthesias, burning, motor control changes, and/or pain. Timely splint modification or strap adjustment is necessary if the patient reports any of these signs. Patient education regarding this matter is the key to preventing long-term nerve damage and ensuring maximal compliance with splint wearing. Patients are more inclined to wear a comfortable splint than one that is causing undue symptoms. Specific nerves that are vulnerable to compression because of their superficial location include the following (Fig. 2–23):

- Suprascapular nerve
- Axillary nerve
- Radial nerve at radial groove

- Ulnar nerve at cubital tunnel
- Superficial branch of ulnar nerve
- Superficial branch of radial nerve
- Median nerve at wrist
- Digital nerves

Clinical Example

When fabricating a splint, the therapist must be aware of potential nerve irritation to prevent the aforementioned complications. Accommodations include applying padding, flaring the splint edges, and using straps and slings of adequate width to disperse pressure about the at-risk areas (Fig. 2–24A-B). For example, when applying a dorsal protective splint to a patient who has sustained a flexor tendon injury, the therapist must recognize that the dorsal sensory branch of the radial nerve is highly susceptible to irritation. The nerve may be affected by both the wrist flexion position and the splinting material that is applied to the dorsal surface of the forearm and hand. Furthermore, the splint must be worn on a full-time basis. The therapist must be sure there is no excess pressure along the dorsal and radial forearm over the path of this nerve. Any signs of skin redness or patient complaints of numbness or paresthesias in the dorsoradial hand indicate the need for timely intervention by the therapist (Fig. 2–24C).

Vascular Supply of the Upper Extremity

The blood supply to the upper extremity arises proximally from larger vessels that bifurcate to form smaller vessels that provide circulation distally throughout the extremity (Fig. 2–25 and Table 2–6) (Moore, 1992; Moore & Agur, 1995). In the shoulder area, the **axillary artery** originates from the **subclavian artery** at the border of the first rib. The axillary artery in turn continues as the brachial artery, passing the inferior border of the teres major. The **brachial artery** provides the main blood supply to the arm. In the inferior portion of the cubital fossa, at the level of the neck of the radius, the brachial artery divides to form the **radial artery** and the larger **ulnar artery.** These arteries descend through the forearm into the hand to unite and form the **superficial** and **deep palmar arterial arches.** The ulnar artery primarily forms the superficial arch, whereas the radial artery primarily forms the deep arch. The superficial and deep palmar arches provide circulation to the hand and give rise to the digital arteries.

Superficial and **deep venous arches** lie close in relation to the superficial and deep arterial arches. The **dorsal digital veins** drain into the **dorsal metacarpal veins,** forming the **dorsal venous network.** This network continues as the **cephalic** and **basilic veins** proximally (Fig. 2–26). The therapist must be familiar with the circulation of the upper extremity when forming splints, especially for patients with injury to, surgical repair of, or compromise of these structures.

Splinting Implications

When splints, straps, casts, or edema wraps are applied too tightly, circulation to a tissue may be compromised (Fess & Philips, 1987). Therapists must educate their patients on the signs of impaired blood flow: color changes (deep red, blue, or blanched), temperature changes (cool/cold or extreme warmth), or an excessive throbbing sensation. Prompt alterations must be made to correct the problem. There may also be vascular problems related solely to the position of the body part in the splint. For example, in a patient who has undergone surgical arterial repair, the therapist must carefully position the joints above and below the repair to prevent undue tension at the surgical site.

Clinical Example

Careful application of circumferential wraps and straps is imperative to prevent disruption of blood flow to and from the body part being splinted (Fig. 2–27). Therapists commonly use elasticized compression wraps for management of edema. Edema most likely results in a digit that has sustained a trauma (from injury, surgery, or both). One of the therapist's primary goals is to decrease edema to prevent the sequelae of stiffness and adhesion formation. The therapist must judiciously apply these

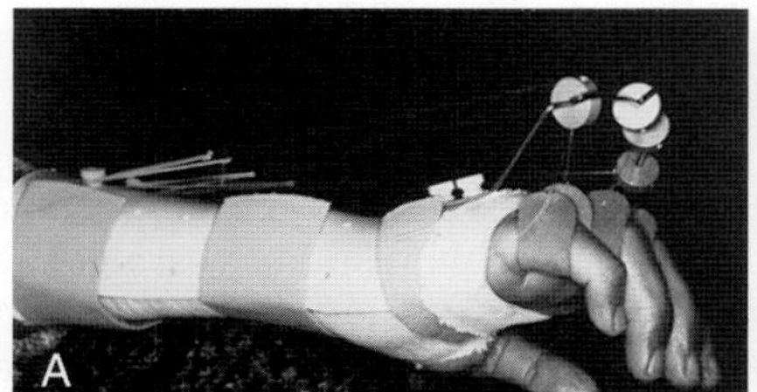

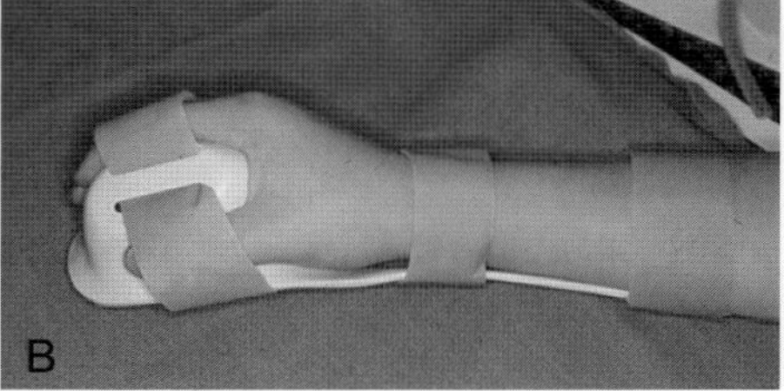

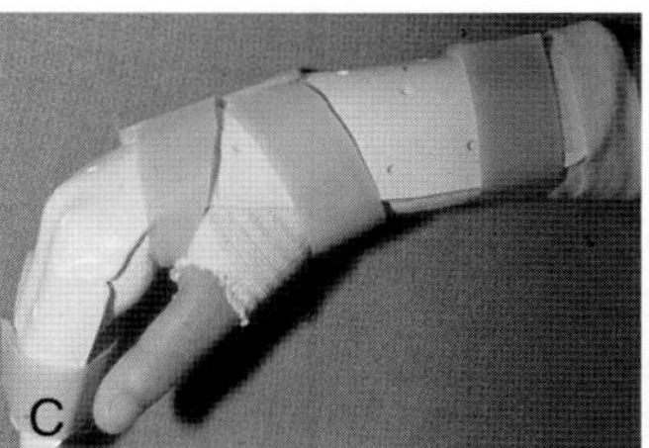

Figure 2–24 ***A,*** *This splint puts the digital nerves at risk for compression volarly as the weight of the fingers pulls the slings.* ***B,*** *The wrist strap on this antispasticity splint is not wide enough; thus the radial sensory nerve is at risk for irritation.* ***C,*** *The radial border of this wrist–digit extension restriction splint crosses over the path of the radial sensory nerve, putting the nerve at risk for irritation.*

TABLE 2–6 Blood Supply of the Upper Extremity

Artery	Origin	Course
Branches of subclavian, axillary, and brachial arteries		
Vertebral	Superior aspect of first part of subclavian artery	Ascends through transverse foramina of cervical vertebrae (except C7) and enters skull through foramen magnum
Internal thoracic	Inferior surface of subclavian artery	Descends, inclining anteromedially, posterior to sternal end of clavicle and first costal cartilage, and enters thorax
Thyrocervical trunk	Anterior aspect of first part of subclavian artery	Ascends as a short, wide trunk and gives rise to three branches: inferior, suprascapular, and transverse cervical
Suprascapular	Thyrocervical trunk	Passes inferolaterally over anterior scalene muscle and phrenic nerve, crosses subclavian artery and brachial plexus, and runs laterally posterior and parallel to clavicle; it then passes to posterior aspect of scapula and supplies supraspinatus and infraspinatus muscles
Superior thoracic	Only branch of first part of axillary artery	Runs anteromedially along superior border of pectoralis minor; then passes between it and pectoralis major to thoracic wall
Thoracoacromial	Second part of axillary artery, deep to pectoralis minor	Curls around superomedial border of pectoralis minor, pierces clavipectoral fascia, and divides into four branches
Lateral thoracic	Second part of axillary artery	Descends along axillary border of pectoralis minor and follows it onto thoracic wall
Subscapular	Third part of axillary artery	Descends along lateral border of subscapularis and axillary border of scapula to its inferior angle, where it passes onto thoracic wall
Circumflex scapular	Subscapular artery	Curves around axillary border of scapula and enters infraspinous fossa
Thoracodorsal	Subscapular artery	Continues course of subscapular artery and accompanies thoracodorsal nerve
Anterior and posterior circumflex humeral	Third part of axillary artery	These arteries anastomose to form a circle around surgical neck of humerus; *posterior:* passes through quadrangular space with axillary nerve
Deep brachial	Brachial artery near its origin	Accompanies radial nerve through groove in humerus and takes part in anastomosis around elbow joint
Superior and inferior ulnar collateral	*Superior:* arises from brachial artery near middle of arm; *inferior:* arises from brachial artery just superior to elbow	*Superior:* accompanies ulnar nerve to posterior aspect of elbow; *inferior:* divides into anterior and posterior branches; *both:* take part in anastomosis around elbow joint
Arteries of the Forearm		
Radial	Smaller terminal division of brachial in cubital fossa	Runs inferolaterally under cover of brachioradialis and distally lies lateral to flexor carpi radialis tendon; winds around lateral aspect of radius and crosses floor of anatomical snuff box to pierce fascia; ends by forming deep palmar arch with deep branch of ulnar artery
Ulnar	Larger terminal branch of brachial in cubital fossa	Passes inferomedially and then directly inferiorly, deep to pronator teres, palmaris longus, and flexor digitorum superficialis to reach medial side of forearm; passes superficial to flexor retinaculum at wrist and gives a deep palmar branch to deep arch and continues as superficial palmar arch
Radial recurrent	Lateral side of radial, just distal to its origin	Ascends on supinator and then passes between brachioradialis and brachialis
Anterior and posterior ulnar recurrent	Ulnar, just distal to elbow joint	*Anterior* passes superiorly and *posterior* passes posteriorly to anastomose with ulnar collateral and interosseous recurrent arteries

Modified with permission from Moore, K. L., & Agur, A. M. (1995). *Essential clinical anatomy.* Baltimore: Williams & Wilkins.

Continued

TABLE 2–6 Continued

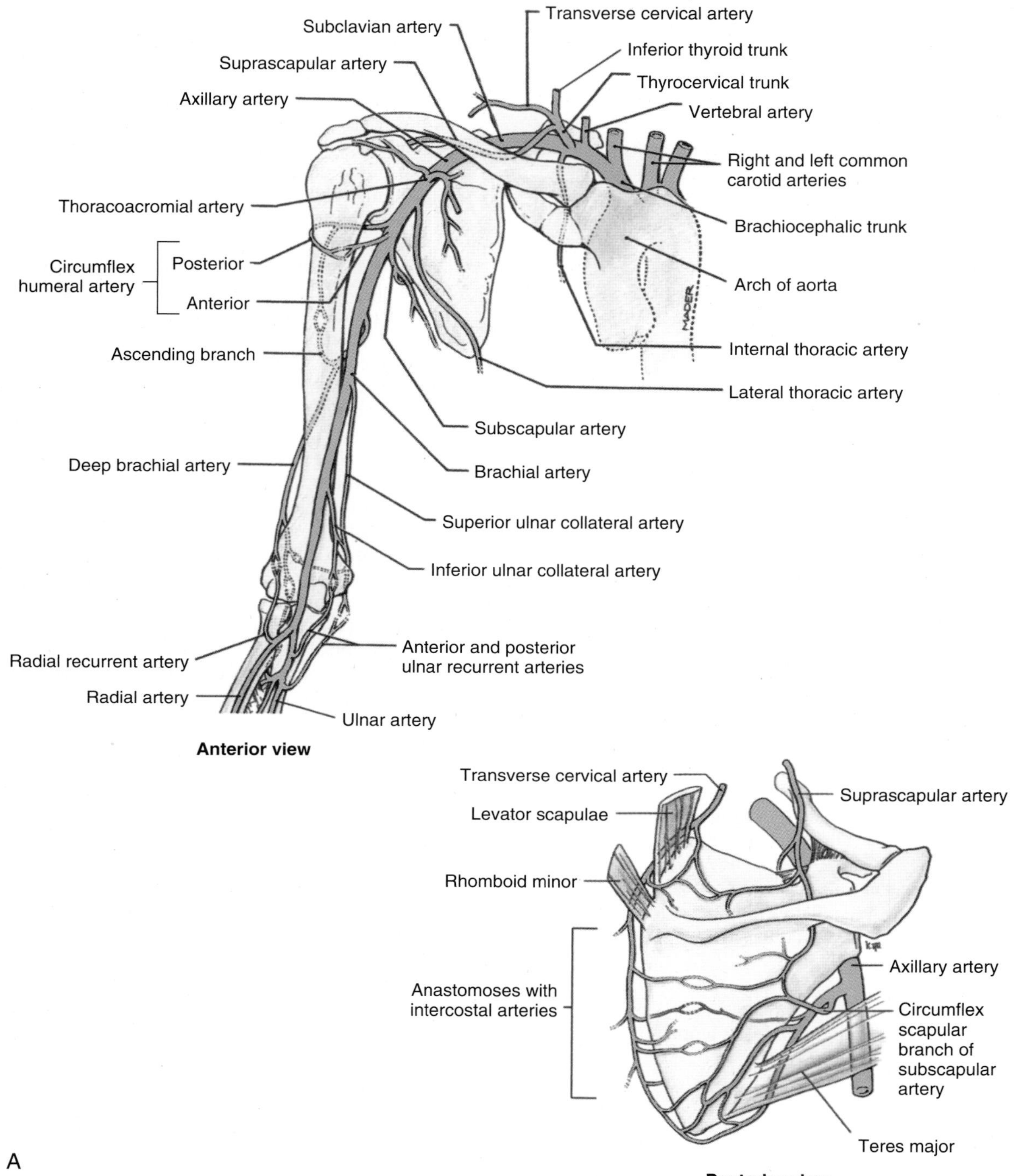

Figure 2–25 Arteries of the shoulder and upper arm ***(A)****, forearm* ***(B)****, and hand* ***(C)****. Reprinted with permission from Moore, K. L., & Agur, A. M. (1995).* Essential clinical anatomy. *Baltimore: Williams & Wilkins.*

TABLE 2–6 Continued

Artery	Origin	Course
Common interosseous	Ulnar, just distal to bifurcation of brachial	After a short course, terminates by dividing into anterior and posterior interosseous arteries
Anterior and posterior interosseous	Common interosseous artery	Pass to anterior and posterior sides of interosseous membrane
Arteries of the Hand		
Superficial palmar arch	Direct continuation of ulnar artery; arch is completed on lateral side by superficial branch of radial artery or another of its branches	Curves laterally deep to palmar aponeurosis and superficial to long flexor tendons; curve of arch lies across palm at level of distal border of extended thumb
Deep palmar arch	Direct continuation of radial artery; arch is completed on medial side by deep branch of ulnar artery	Curves medially deep to long flexor tendons and is in contact with bases of metacarpals
Common palmar digitals	Superficial palmar arch	Pass distally on lumbricals to webbings of digits
Proper palmar digitals	Common palmar digital arteries	Run along sides of the second to fifth digits
Princeps pollicis	Radial artery as it turns into palm	Descends on palmar aspect of first metacarpal and divides at the base of proximal phalanx into two branches that run along sides of thumb
Radialis indicis	Radial artery, but may arise from principes pollicis artery	Passes along lateral side of index finger to its distal end
Dorsal carpal arch	Radial and ulnar arteries	Arches within fascia on dorsum of hand

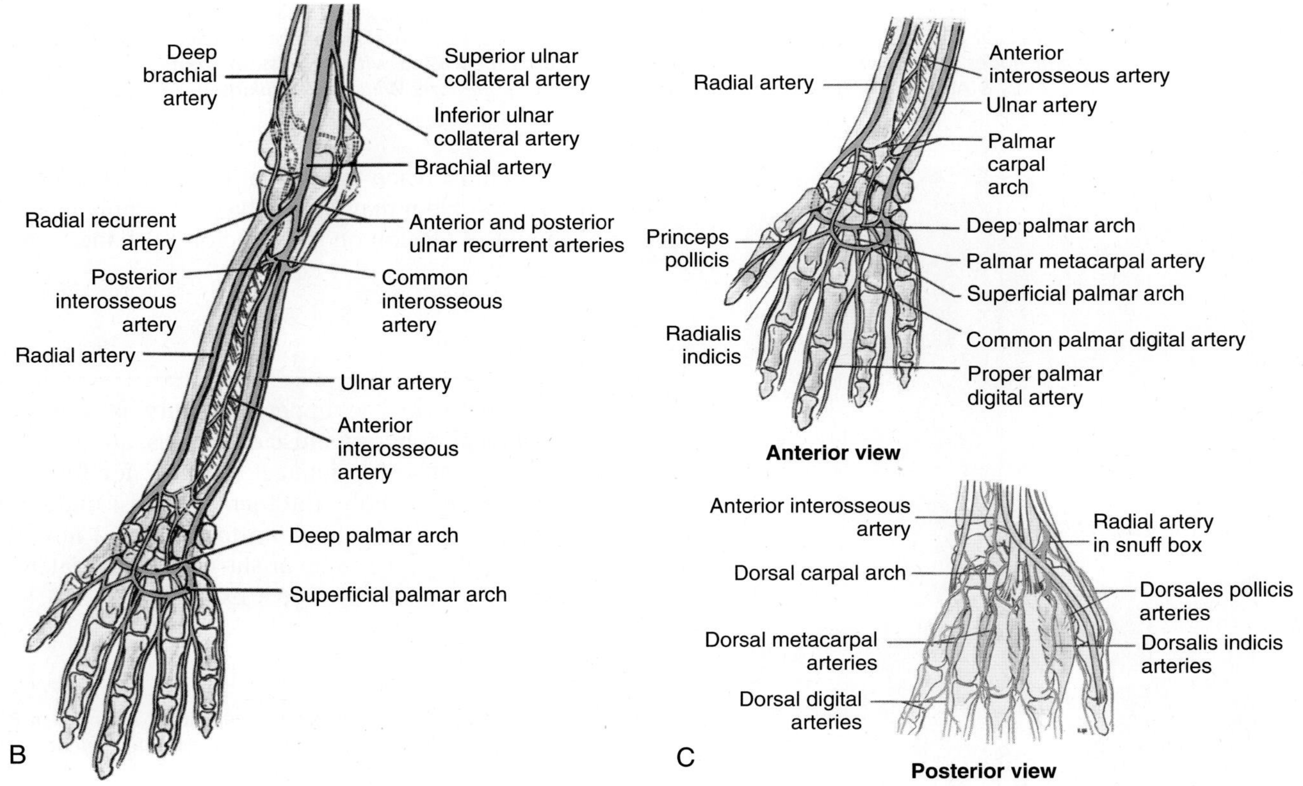

Figure 2–25 Continued.

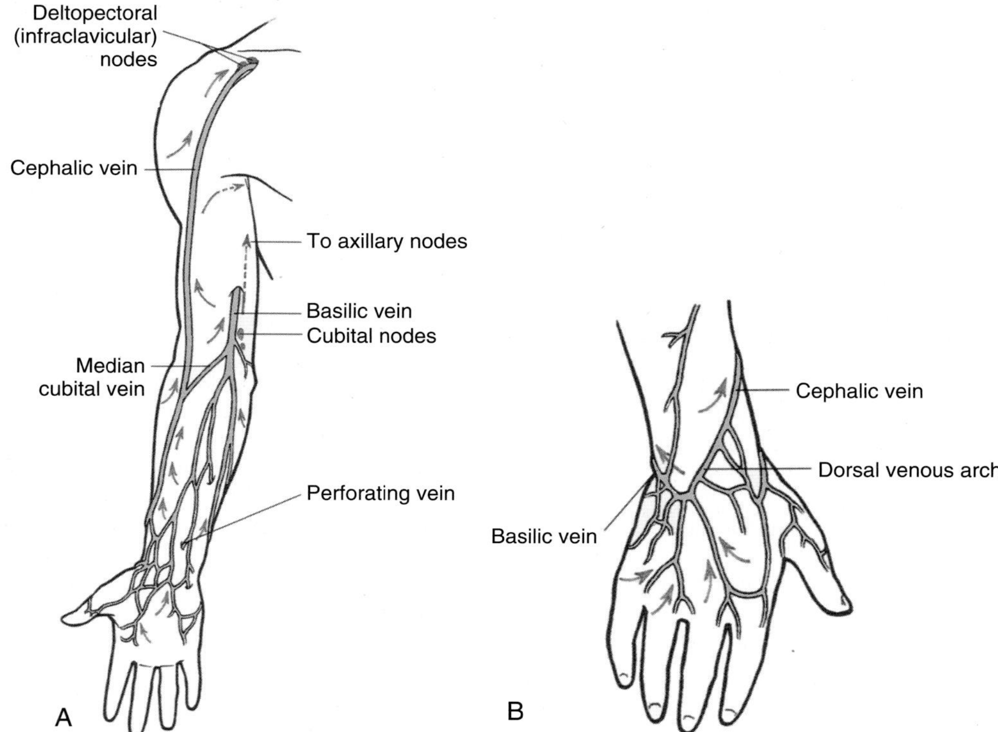

Figure 2–26 Superficial venous and lymphatic drainage of upper limb. ***A,*** *Anterior view showing the cephalic and basilic veins and their tributaries.* Red arrows, *superficial lymphatic drainage to lymph nodes.* ***B,*** *Dorsal view showing dorsal venous arch. Reprinted with permission from Moore, K. L., & Agur, A. M. (1995).* Essential clinical anatomy. *Baltimore: Williams & Wilkins.*

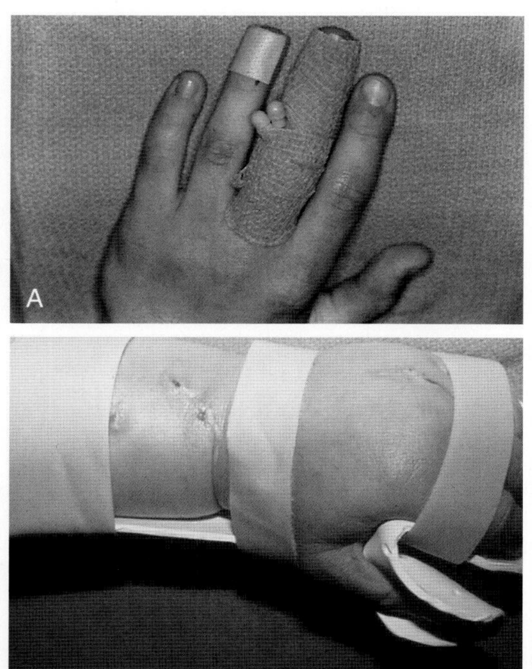

Figure 2–27 ***A,*** *The compressive wrap on this digit has the potential to compress the vessels.* ***B,*** *Note the high compression forces applied by the straps traversing the forearm and hand.*

wraps and must teach the patient to be aware of adverse signs. The problem may be resolved by simply changing the amount of tension on the wrap or by changing to intermittent use.

CONCLUSION

The anatomy of the upper extremity is a intricate arrangement of bones, muscles, vessels, and other soft tissue structures that interact to allow for functional use of the upper limb. The therapist must understand how these structures function together and how they interact with splints so he or she can appropriately apply these devices to the upper extremity.

REFERENCES

Bowers, W. H., & Tribuzi, S. M. (1992). Functional anatomy. In B. G. Stanley & S. M. Tribuzi (Eds.). *Concepts in hand rehabilitation* (pp. 3–34). Philadelphia: F.A. Davis Company.

Calliet, R. (1994). *Hand pain and impairment* (4th ed.). Philadelphia: F.A. Davis Company.

Chase, R. A. (1995). Anatomy and kinesiology of the hand. In J. M. Hunter, E. J. Mackin, & A. D. Callahan (Eds.). *Rehabilitation of the hand* (4th ed., pp. 23–39). St. Louis: Mosby Year Book.

Fess, E. E., & Philips, C. (1987). *Hand splinting: Principles and methods* (2nd ed.). St. Louis: Mosby Year Book.

Green, D. P. (1988). *Operative hand surgery* (2nd ed.). New York: Churchill Livingstone.

Hoppenfeld, S. (1976). *Physical examination of the spine and extremities.* Norwalk, CT: Appleton-Century-Crofts.

Kapandji, I. A. (1982). *The physiology of the joints: Vol. 1. Upper Limb* (5th ed.). New York: Churchill Livingstone.

Moore, K. L. (1992). *Clinically oriented anatomy* (4th ed.). Baltimore: Williams & Wilkins.

Moore, K. L., & Agur, A. M. (1995). *Essential clinical anatomy.* Baltimore: Williams & Wilkins.

Nerve compression syndromes. (1992). *Hand Clinics, 8,* 201–395.

Norkin, C. C., & Levangie, P. K. (1992). *Joint structure and function: A comprehensive analysis* (2nd ed.). Philadelphia: Davis.

Pratt, N. E. (1995). Surface anatomy of the upper extremity. In J. M. Hunter, E. J. Mackin, & A. D. Callahan (Eds.). *Rehabilitation of the hand* (4th ed., pp. 41–50). St. Louis: Mosby Year Book.

Spinner, M. (1995). Nerve lesions in continuity. In J. M. Hunter, E. J. Mackin, & A. D. Callahan (Eds.). *Rehabilitation of the hand* (4th ed., pp. 627–634). St. Louis: Mosby Year Book.

Tubiana, R., Thomine, J. M., & Mackin, E. (1996). *Examination of the hand and wrist* (2nd ed.). St. Louis: Mosby.

SUGGESTED READING

Agur, A. M. (1992). *Grant's atlas of anatomy* (9th ed.). Baltimore: Williams & Wilkins.

Brand, P. W., & Hollister, A. (1993). *Clinical mechanics of the hand* (2nd ed.). St. Louis: Mosby Year Book.

Clemente, C. D. (1997). *Anatomy: A regional atlas of the human body* (4th ed.). Baltimore: Williams & Wilkins.

Cooney, W. P., Dobyns, J. H., & Linscheid, R. L. (1997). *The wrist.* St. Louis: Mosby.

Hollinshead, W. H., & Jenkins, D. B. (1981). *Functional anatomy of the limbs and back* (5th ed.). Philadelphia: Saunders.

Kendall, F. P., McCreary, E. K., & Provance, P. G. (1993). *Muscles: Testing and function* (4th ed.). Baltimore: Williams & Wilkins.

Lampe, E. W. (1988). *Clinical symposia: Surgical anatomy of the hand.* West Caldwell, NJ: Ciba-Geigy.

Lichtman, D. M. (1988). *The wrist and its disorders.* Philadelphia: Saunders.

McMinn, R. M., & Hutchings, R. T. (1988). *Color atlas of human anatomy* (2nd ed.). Chicago: Yearbook Medical.

Morrey, B. F. (1985). *The elbow and its disorders.* Philadelphia: Saunders.

Netter, F. H. (1997). *Atlas of human anatomy* (2nd ed.). East Hanover, NJ: Novartis.

Pick, T. P., & Howden, R. (1977). *Gray's anatomy.* New York: Bounty.

Putz, R., Pabst, R., & Taylor, A. N. (1997). *Sobotta: Atlas of human anatomy* (12th ed.). Baltimore: Williams & Wilkins.

Rohen, J. W., Yokochi, C., & Lutjen-Drecoll, E. (1998). *Color atlas of anatomy: A photographic study of the human body* (4th ed.). Baltimore: Williams & Wilkins.

Soderberg, G. L. (1986). *Kinesiology: Application to pathological motion.* Baltimore: Williams & Wilkins.

Taleisnik, J. (1985). *The Wrist.* New York: Churchill Livingstone.

Zancolli, E. A. (2001). Advances in hand anatomy. *Hand Clinics, 17.*

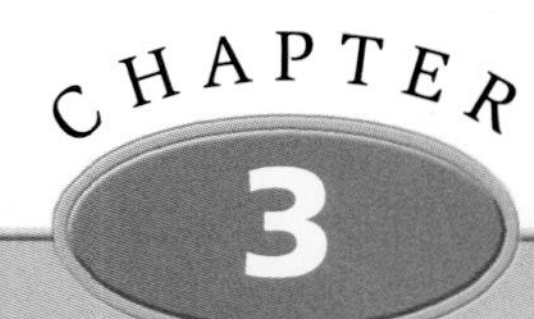

Tissue Healing

Steven Wenner, MD, and Ellen Smithline, RN

INTRODUCTION

Surgeons and therapists who care for patients who have undergone upper extremity injury or surgery must understand the biology of tissue healing to know how and when to use the modalities of treatment in their armamentarium, including splinting. This chapter reviews the stages of tissue healing, the factors that influence healing, and how they relate to splint application. The status and stage of a healing wound directs the specifics of splint selection, fabrication, and patient use. The surgeon and therapist must keep this in mind when splints are prescribed and constructed and must realize that these treatment decisions influence the healing tissue's response (Fess & McCollum, 1998). The latter part of this chapter describes how splint management depends on the healing characteristics particular to specific tissues.

Stages of Wound Healing

The stages of tissue healing are inflammation, fibroplasia (proliferative), and scar maturation (chronic stage or remodeling). To recognize the differences among these stages, one first must understand the role of oxygen. Tissue oxygenation is essential for wound healing. Oxygen is carried in the blood, dissolved in the plasma, and bound to hemoglobin. It is the fuel for the healing of injury or infection. Oxygen is responsible for collagen synthesis, angiogenesis (increased blood flow), and epithelialization (Stotts & Wipke-Tevis, 1997). Wounds heal more predictably and more rapidly when the tissue is oxygenated; conversely, inadequate oxygenation decreases the ability of the wounds to heal in both the acute and chronic phases. Appropriate splint selection and design depend on the stage of the wound. Each stage is described below.

Inflammatory Stage

The **stage of inflammation,** which usually lasts for less than 1 week, is characterized by an influx of white blood cells, especially macrophages, and an increase in local vascularity (Fig. 3–1). The injured area is cleansed of bacteria, necrotic debris, and foreign material. Edema typically lasts for several days, unless there is persistent contamination (Smith & Dean, 1998; Strickland, 1987).

At this stage of tissue healing, rest is more important than exercise; immobilization splints are useful for protecting, supporting, and resting the injured part (Fig. 3–2). Splints may also be used to decrease the stress or tension on a surgically repaired structure, such as a tendon or nerve (Fig. 3–3). The splint should maintain the injured part in the position that is most advantageous for rapid healing and subsequent restoration of function. Simultaneously, adjacent structures should be positioned to prevent unwanted deformity and to facilitate prompt return to function (Smith & Dean, 1998).

Fibroplasia and Proliferative Stage

The **stage of fibroplasia** begins 4 or 5 days after the injury occurs and lasts for 2 to 6 weeks (Fig. 3–4). Fibroblasts enter the wound and begin synthesizing collagen, which ultimately becomes scar tissue. The growth of granulation tissue, the foundation of the wound, depends on adequate angiogenesis (development of blood vessels) and neurogenesis (nerve regeneration). Early in this stage, immobilization prevents disruption of newly deposited immature collagen fibers and thereby facilitates an increase in tensile strength of the wound. Between weeks 3 and 6, cellularity diminishes, and the extracellular matrix, largely collagen, increases both in volume and in tensile strength (Smith & Dean, 1998; Strickland, 1987).

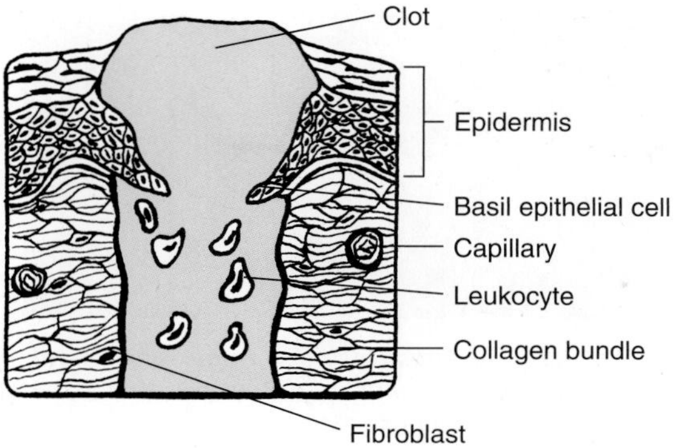

Figure 3–1 Fibrin is deposited during the inflammatory stage and forms the initial gel of the wound matrix.

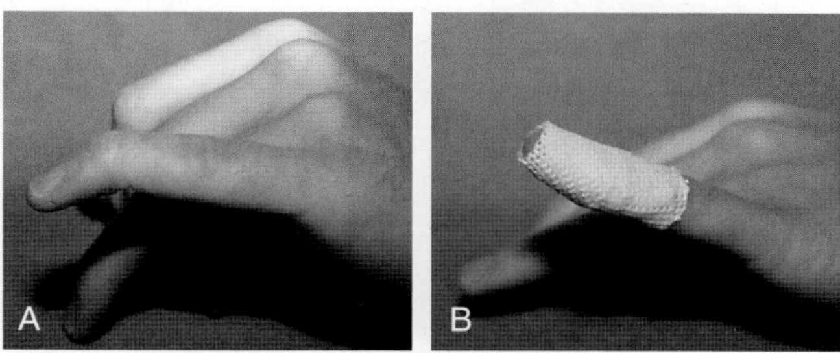

*Figure 3–2 **A,** Traumatic disruption of the terminal extensor tendon (mallet finger). **B,** A DIP joint immobilization splint (fabricated from QuickCast) was used for 6 weeks to promote healing of the tendon and to maintain function of the proximal joints.*

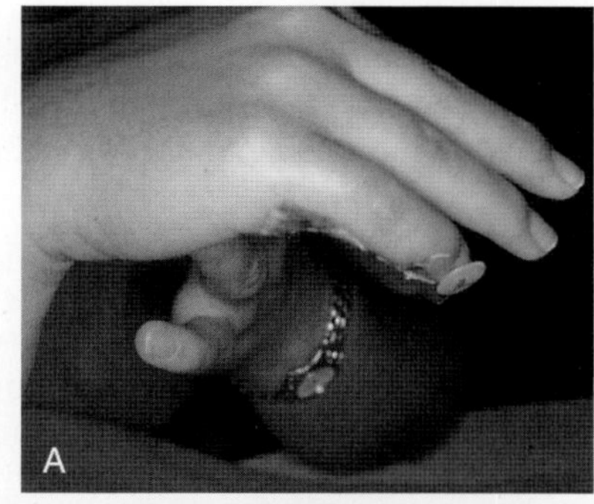

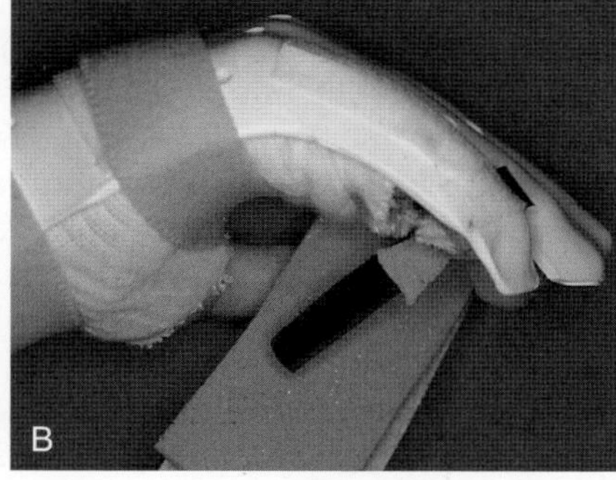

*Figure 3–3 **A,** Repair of the flexor digitorum profundus of the small finger. **B,** A wrist/digit extension restriction splint was used to provide protection to the repaired structure.*

During this stage, gently and judiciously applied stress can facilitate tissue growth. Mobilization splints, which take advantage of tissue's elasticity and responsiveness to external stress, are useful at this stage (Fig. 3–5). A balance must be achieved between applying enough stress to influence scar remodeling favorably and avoiding excessive stress, which could cause further tissue damage.

Maturation and Remodeling Stage

The **stage of scar maturation** is next (Fig. 3–6). Collagen is organized as it remodels along the lines of stress; this enhances the tensile strength of the healing wound. The load per cross-sectional area that can be sustained by the wound is referred to as *tensile strength.* The strength accelerates at a rate equal to the pace of collagen synthesis; this influences decisions concerning splinting and therapy (Fess & McCollum, 1998 & Strickland, 1987). Therefore, a tissue's tensile strength should be considered when developing a rehabilitation plan for patients who have undergone procedures such as tendon or nerve repair. Healing related to specific tissues is discussed later in this chapter.

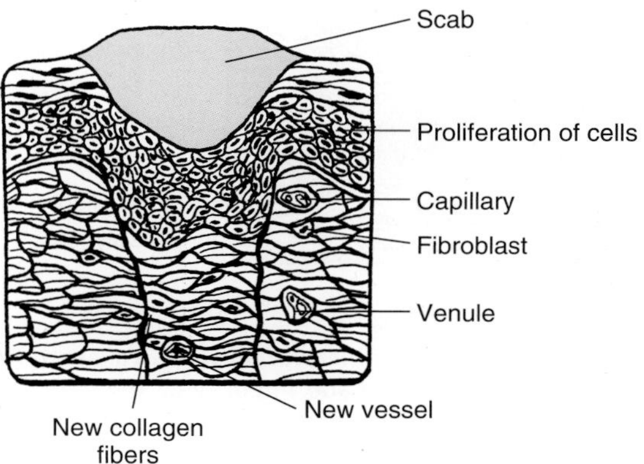

Figure 3–4 During the proliferative stage, collagen is laid down, which gives strength to the wound.

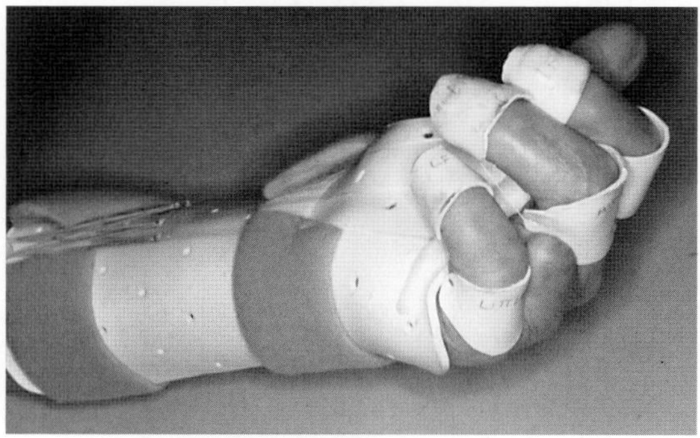

Figure 3–5 A composite index finger, middle finger, and small finger flexion mobilization splint was applied at approximately 4 weeks after a crush injury to gently mobilize the finger joints. (Notice amputation of ring finger.)

In a well-nourished immunocompetent patient, a surgically repaired wound that is held by sutures is at its weakest at 2 weeks postsurgery. Tensile strength is 30% in 3 weeks, 60% in 6 weeks, and 90% in 6 months (Fig. 3–7). Therefore, the recommendation is to wait 6 weeks before subjecting the wound to aggressive tension (Kane, 1997).

Although scars soften during the maturation and remodeling stage, they also shorten. This shortening is accompanied by a decrease in the scar's elasticity; thus stretching is valuable for preventing unwanted contractures (Fig. 3–8). The length of the maturation phase depends on several factors, including age, genetic background, location of the wound, and length and intensity of the inflammatory phase (Smith & Dean, 1998). This process may last for many months (Smith & Dean, 1998; Strickland, 1987).

Although the three stages of tissue healing were described as sequential, there is overlap in their occurrence (Fig. 3–9). Just as the healing stages overlap, so do the time frames for using specific splint types. For example, immobilization splints may be indicated throughout the healing process but are most commonly used in the inflammatory stage (Colditz, 1995; Fess & Phillips, 1987).

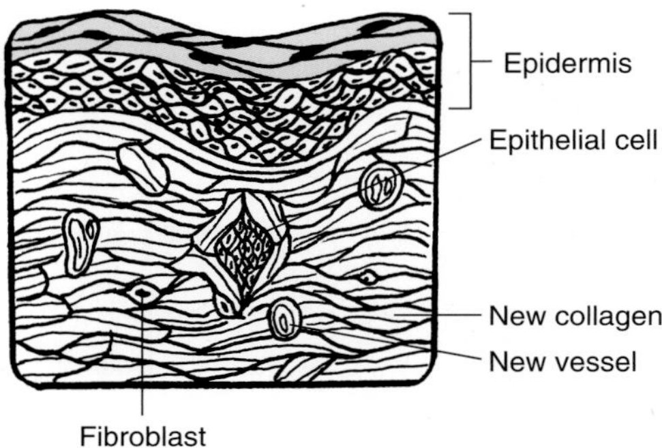

Figure 3–6 During the scar maturation stage, collagen, which is responsible for the structure and integrity of the wound, is deposited in a generally random manner.

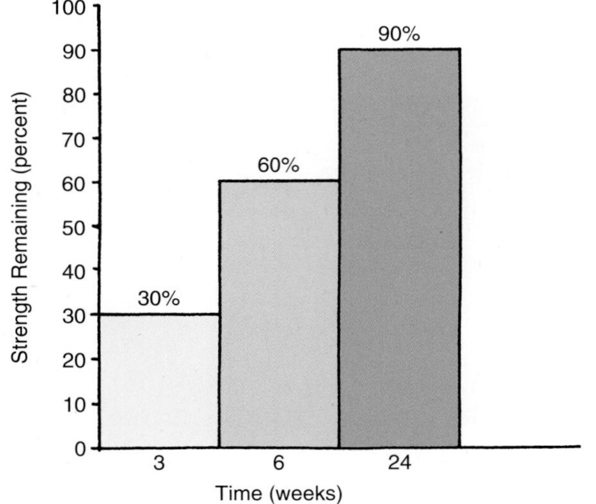

Figure 3–7 Tensile strength at 3 weeks, 6 weeks, and 6 months.

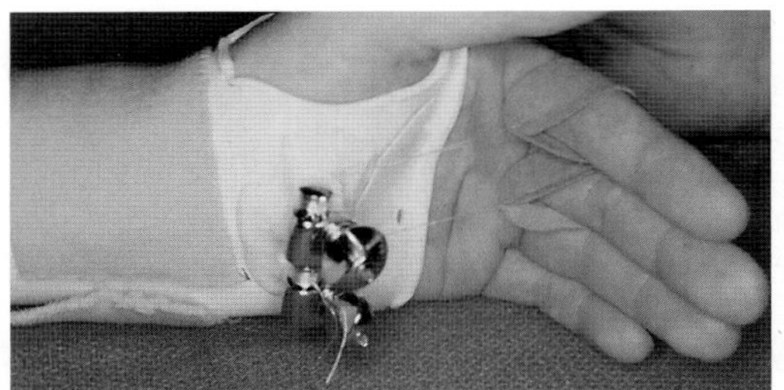

Figure 3–8 Static progressive index finger and middle finger MP flexion mobilization splint used 8 weeks after a metacarpal fracture. The MERiT components provide the static progressive stretch.

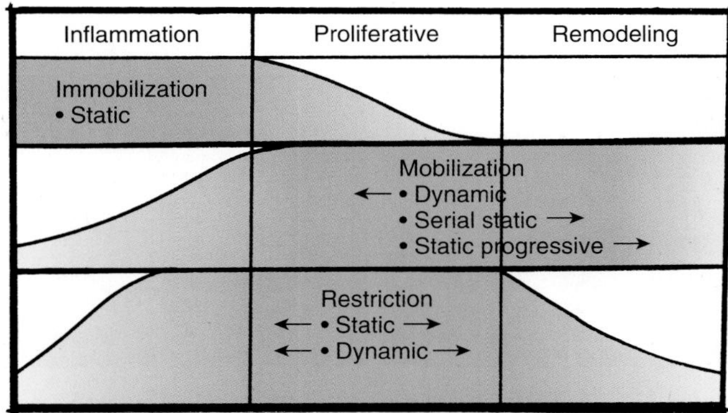

Figure 3–9 Splinting management for the patient should be based on the current stage of healing. The most common splinting intervention is shown here; however special conditions may require deviation from these guidelines.

Effect of Splinting on Tissue Healing

Wound healing during the inflammatory and early fibroplastic stages is best managed with immobilization splints. During that time, rest is more important than exercise (Fig. 3–10). When edema subsides and acute pain lessens, the fibroplastic or proliferative stage has begun. At that point, mobilization splints are appropriate. Stress should be applied to the healing tissue to the degree that it favorably influences scar remodeling, but not so much that it further damages tissues. Various insults, such as severe tissue trauma or persistent contamination, can prolong the inflammatory phase and retard healing.

Tissue that is not susceptible to prolonged inflammation and is not readily re-injured will tolerate repetitively or continuously applied gentle stress. If edema decreases and motion increases while the patient is using a mobilizing splint, the splint is having a beneficial effect. However, the overly aggressive use of mobilization splints (dynamic, static progressive, or serial static) during the fibroplastic stage, or their premature use (during the inflammatory stage), may re-injure healing tissues and retard recovery. For example, unstable fractures and torn collateral ligaments are injuries for which active range of motion (ROM) and accompanying mobilizing splints should be delayed until the likelihood of disruption of healing owing to a repeat injury is diminished. This usually means deferring such a regimen until the latter half of the fibroplastic stage or until the stage of scar remodeling (Fess & McCollum, 1998; Strickland, 1987).

For most tissues, the stress that can be safely applied and the degree and duration of the force increase at approximately 6 weeks after injury. This is when the scar maturation or remodeling stage commences, and it is the sensible time to introduce serial static or static progressive splints.

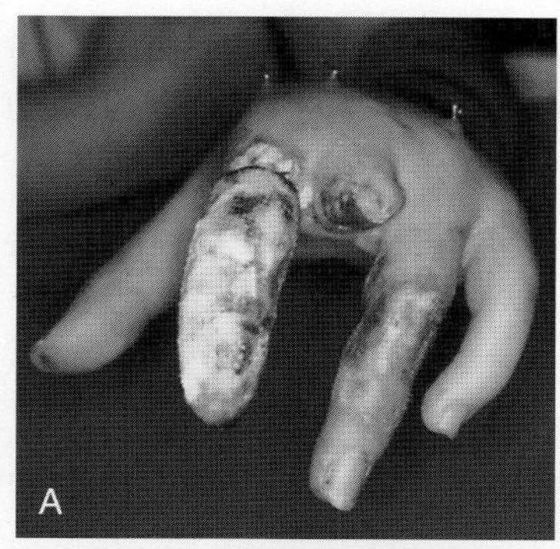

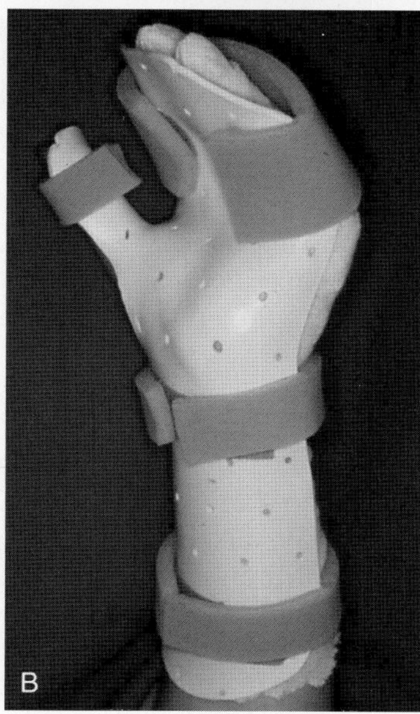

Figure 3–10 ***A,*** *A press injury led to the amputation of the middle finger and replantation of the index and ring fingers.* ***B,*** *A simple immobilization splint promotes healing by providing a safe position for the joints. Note the wrist extension, metacarpophalangeal flexion, interphalangeal extension, and thumb palmar abduction.*

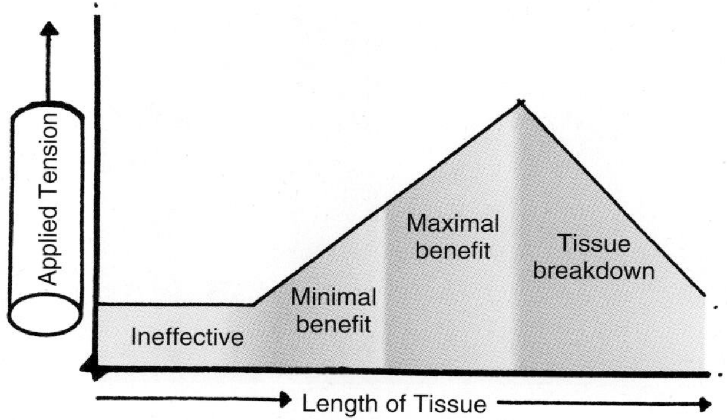

Figure 3–11 *Length–tension curve depicting elastic and plastic behaviors of tissue.*

Tissue Remodeling

A brief description of **tissue remodeling** and its clinical implications will aid the reader in understanding the outcome of applying splints on healing tissue. Soft tissue is alive and possesses viscoelastic properties that allow it to lengthen and shorten within a certain range. When soft tissue has shortened, perhaps as a consequence of scar contracture, splinting and casting techniques are useful for stretching the tight tissue.

Tissue remodeling may be induced by gentle stretching over a period of time, causing an alteration in cellular structure and alignment in response to the applied forces. Old cells are phagocytosed, and new cells are created, orienting themselves in the direction of the tension. By this process, the length of the previously contracted tissue increases; this is called *elastic behavior* (Brand & Thompson, 1993). Tissue fibers that are stretched beyond their elastic limits will tear or rupture (*plastic behavior*). When the tissue and cells are injured in this manner, protein is released from the cells and more scarring occurs (Fig. 3–11).

Clinical Considerations

The goal in gaining length of contracted tissue is to do so without causing microscopic tearing, which results in inflammation, hemorrhage, and further scarring. This may occur when a therapist or physician is too aggressive in the passive stretching program or uses excessive force in splinting. Such tissues become reactive, stiff, and painful, possibly leading to problems such as reflex sympathetic dystrophy (RSD). If tissue is held stretched to its tolerable limit, for a longer time, it has a greater chance of undergoing permanent remodeling and lengthening (Brand & Thompson, 1993). Patients who are prescribed mobilization splints should be advised that increasing the tension (high stress) for short periods of time is not as beneficial as wearing the splint at a tolerable tension (lower stress) for a longer period of time (Fig. 3–12) (Brand & Thompson, 1993; Colditz, 1995; Fess & Phillips, 1987).

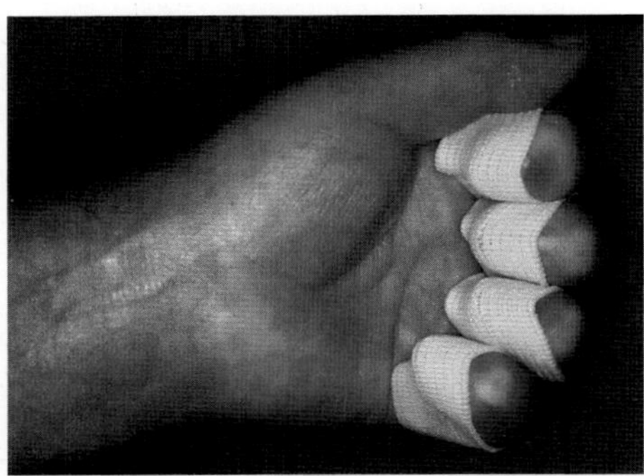

Figure 3–12 Simple PIP/DIP mobilization straps can provide a gentle stretch simultaneously to the PIP and DIP joints of the same finger. Note the blanching at the DIP joints: Too much tension is not tolerated for long and may cause significant tissue irritation.

Conditions and Factors That Influence Tissue Healing

Tissue healing and remodeling are influenced by several factors. As mentioned previously, the most common impediment to satisfactory healing is oxygen deprivation. These factors should be considered in the ongoing assessment of a patient's progress and may warrant modifications in the therapeutic plan. Any one, or combination of the conditions and characteristics briefly described in the following sections may influence the length of time a splint is used. For example, poor oxygenation usually increases a tissue's healing time and, therefore, increases the duration of time a splint needs to be worn.

When treating patients with conditions that may lead to sensory changes in the distal extremities, monitor them closely for possible skin irritation or breakdown caused by the splint. Since such patients cannot fully appreciate the splint's contact with the skin (pressure areas), carefully instruct them or their caregivers to inspect the skin. These patients and/or caregivers should be told to call the therapist promptly if signs of undue pressure or friction are noted. For these patients, consider fabricating splints that are lighter weight, incorporate protective padding, or are made with gel-lined materials to aid in protecting the at-risk tissue.

Sharp or jagged splint borders can be minimized by using materials that provide a smooth, well-contoured edge. Wide, soft, and strategically placed straps may aid in minimizing sheer and compression stresses along the splint–skin interface. This is of particular importance when splinting an individual with vascular insufficiency.

Age

Age strongly influences the healing process. As Stotts and Wipke-Tevis (1997) noted, "fetal wound healing is virtually scarless." The younger the patient, the more likely the tissue(s) involved will heal quickly and without complications. In general, younger patients wear splints and casts for shorter periods of time and ROM is initiated earlier than for older patients.

Lifestyle Factors

Nutrition

A **poor diet** that lacks essential nutrients impedes the stages of wound healing. Proteins, carbohydrates, vitamins, and minerals are all needed to allow tissues to heal. A deficient diet may also contribute to weight loss, an increased risk of infection, poor wound closure, and reduction in subcutaneous fat (which can increase tension over bony prominences) (Pinchocofsky-Devin, 1997). For thin, bony areas, consider using soft prefabricated splints or splint materials made of Neoprene. Use caution when applying straps to avoid friction over bony prominences.

Tobacco Use

Smoking **tobacco** markedly diminishes the body's ability to heal. Nicotine, carbon monoxide, and hydrogen cyanide are inhaled with each puff. It is well documented that nicotine causes delayed wound healing (Jenson, 1991; Silverstein, 1992; Smith & Feske, 1996). Because it is a vasoconstrictor, nicotine restricts blood flow to the skin, thereby creating low oxygen levels. Embolization (obstruction of blood flow) at the microvascular level occurs as a result of increased blood viscosity and platelet aggregation. Nicotine decreases the formation of red blood cells, fibroblasts, and macrophages (the cellular elements required to repair wounds). Carbon monoxide has 300 times the affinity for hemoglobin than does oxygen. When it binds with hemoglobin, oxygen transport is decreased and thus there is less oxygen within the tissues. As discussed earlier, this leads directly to slower wound-healing times; therefore, smokers may need to wear splints for a longer time than nonsmokers. Therapists should review with each patient the effects of continued nicotine use on healing rates.

Alcohol Use

Excessive **alcohol** intake can impair the immune system, lead to malnourishment, and cause liver damage (Rund, 1997). Alcoholics may also have multiorgan involvement, which can contribute to poor wound healing. As with tobacco use, patient education is paramount.

Medical Conditions

Connective tissue disorders (CTDs) and **systemic diseases** not only have a generalized effect on the body but also may be associated with impaired tissue oxygenation, which can delay local tissue healing (LeRoy, 1996). With any of the medical conditions mentioned in this chapter, splinting should be only one aspect of the medical and therapeutic intervention. When a splint is fabricated for a patient that has a medical condition that effects tissue healing, neurovascular status, and/or sensation, both the therapist and the patient should inspect the skin frequently. The therapist should adjust the splint and modify the straps as soon as any signs of redness or irritation occur. Affected patients may not perceive the discomfort of the splint on the body part owing to nerve and/or vascular involvement.

Buerger's Disease

Buerger's disease is associated with tobacco smoking. Affected individuals frequently have nonhealing ulcers of the hands and/or feet. Arterial and venous occlusion may occur. Unfortunately, many of these patients cannot stop smoking because nicotine dependency is a serious addiction. If vascular problems persist, these individuals may have to undergo amputation later in the course of the disease.

Raynaud's Phenomenon

Raynaud's phenomenon or disease is caused by spasticity or occlusion of the digital arteries, with blanching and numbness in the digits (Fig. 3–13). In the advanced stages, the skin may become firm, thickened, and leathery. Flexion contractures can develop because of skin that is tightly bound to the underlying subcutaneous tissue. Cold temperatures, strong emotions, and repetitive movements are among the many factors that precipitate the onset of symptoms. These factors should be taken into account when splinting is considered (LeRoy, 1996). Splinting materials that are soft, flexible, and contribute to retaining warmth (e.g., Neoprene) may be a sensible option for these patients.

Systemic Lupus Erythematosus

Systemic lupus erythematosus (SLE) is a disease that effects the major body organs. It may produce inflammation of joints and dermal vasculitis and may lead to the development of Buerger disease. SLE occurs predominately in women and its course is variable (LeRoy, 1996).

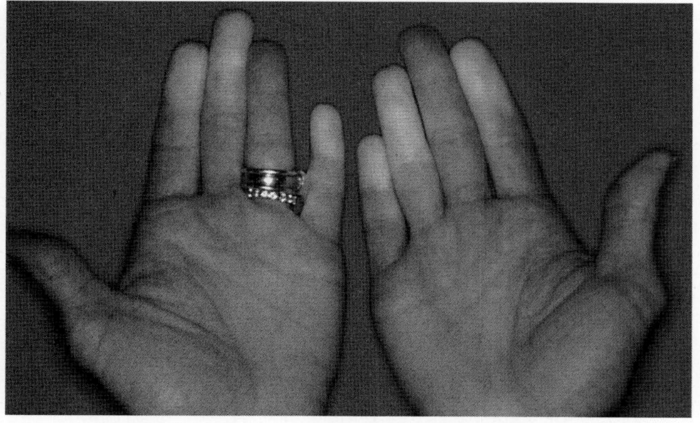

Figure 3–13 Note the blanching of the digits caused by Raynaud phenomenon.

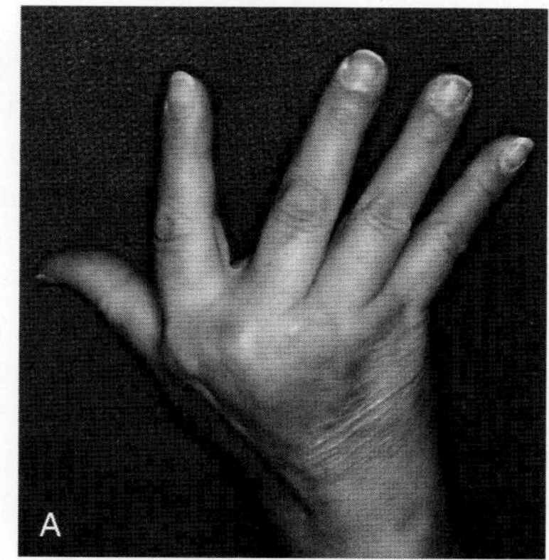

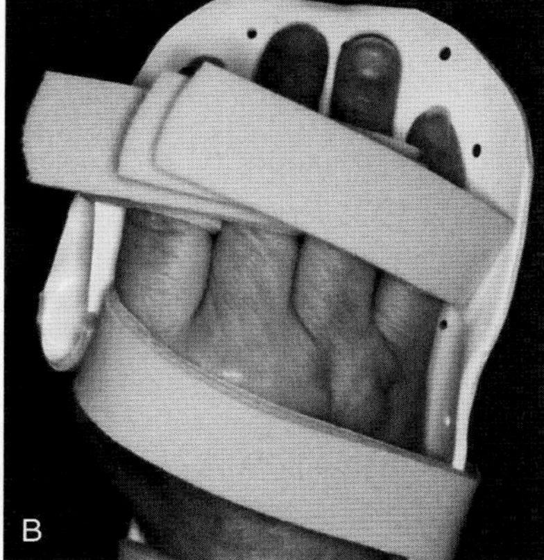

*Figure 3–14 **A,** Rheumatoid arthritis. **B,** A night wrist–digit immobilization splint maintains the metacarpophalangeal joints in a neutral position and supports the wrist and thumb.*

Diabetes

Patients with **diabetes** may present with nonhealing wounds owing to ischemia, neuropathy, or both (Davidson, 1999). Diabetic neuropathy demands attention to the details of splinting. Patients may lack protective sensation; splint pressure may, therefore, cause unnoticed skin injury. It is important that the patient and therapist perform frequent, regular inspection of the splinted area for early signs of pressure and redness.

Rheumatoid Arthritis

Rheumatoid arthritis (RA) is a systemic immunologic disorder that primarily effects the synovial joints. Frequently, the small joints of the hand are involved, as are the wrists. Splinting has an important role in the treatment of these patients (Fig. 3–14). Splints are used to protect inflamed, painful joints and to help prevent further joint deformity.

Patients who have rheumatologic disease may use medications that retard healing; corticosteroids for instance, inhibit the normal development of tensile strength in a healing wound by interfering with the inflammatory phase of healing (discussed further later in this chapter). The prolonged healing time should be taken into account when formulating a treatment plan. Sutures may need to stay in longer than normal to ensure adequate epithelialization. When possible, thin, lightweight materials and/or materials that are soft and flexible should be used to fabricate the splint. Many of these patients have fragile skin and require additional protection at the splint–skin interface. Chapter 17 discusses the selection of appropriate splinting materials for this condition.

Sickle Cell Disease

Sickle cell disease is a group of inherited blood diseases that can cause severe pain, damage to vital organs, and occasionally death in childhood or early adulthood (Sickle Cell Disease Research Foundation, 1999). The deformed red blood cells cannot pass easily through the blood vessels, creating a sludging effect and preventing oxygen from reaching the tissues. This results in severe pain and damage to the organs; wound healing is also inhibited. Splints fabricated for these patients should be made with caution. The therapist must ensure that the straps and other materials do not compress tissue, which could further impede vascular flow.

Peripheral Vascular Disease

Patients with **peripheral vascular disease** (PVD) are at risk for impaired wound healing because of tissue hypoxia. Improvement in arterial circulation and/or venous drainage improves wound healing; therefore, any signs of compression with the use of a splint should be addressed promptly. For example, splint straps should be applied firmly enough to secure the splint on the body part but not so tight that circulation is effected.

Medical Treatment and Complications

Radiation Therapy

Radiation therapy may be beneficial in curing or controlling cancer, but it may also have a damaging effect on previously healthy tissue. Vascular deterioration occurs, creating an hypoxic environment for the tissue. This adverse consequence of radiation therapy may not become apparent until several years after treatment. Management of these wounds is difficult because of the circulatory compromise. Hyperbaric oxygen therapy may be considered (Mark, 1994). Splints and strapping should be applied cautiously to these areas for the reasons described previously.

Steroids

Corticosteroid use can impair all phases of wound healing. Because these drugs slow the healing process, they increase the risk of infection and make it difficult to diagnose infection; signs and symptoms may be masked by the suppressed inflammatory response (Stotts & Wipke-Tevis, 1997). It is especially important for therapists to evaluate potential areas of friction or pressure when splinting patients who are using steroid medications. Steroids, like tobacco and alcohol, slow the healing process and increase the risk of skin breakdown. Daily skin inspection and timely splint modification can accommodate the risks associated with steroid use.

Edema

Edema, an increase of interstitial fluid, may decrease oxygen diffusion to the tissues. Worsening edema may limit the oxygen available to the healing tissue by increasing congestion and decreasing capillary blood flow. Edema sometimes results from the overly aggressive manipulation of healing tissue by manual techniques or splinting methods; thus it may indicate a change in the therapy protocol. Caution should be taken when applying a mobilization splint to a severely edematous part (Fess & Phillips, 1987). Rest, by use of an immobilization splint, may be a better plan until the edema has subsided enough to allow the use of more aggressive techniques.

To reduce edema before splint application, the therapist may use elevation, massage, and other therapeutic techniques. Compression garments (Isotoner gloves) and circumferential bandages (Ace or Coban wraps) can be worn under splints, and strapping can be modified to prevent window edema (swelling between straps) (Fig. 3–15). However, too much compression may decrease arterial blood flow, thereby creating vascular compromise to the limb. Circulation should be monitored after application of compression garments and circumferential bandages, and patients should be informed about the signs and symptoms of diminished arterial blood flow (e.g., dusky or blue nail beds; numbness, tingling, or

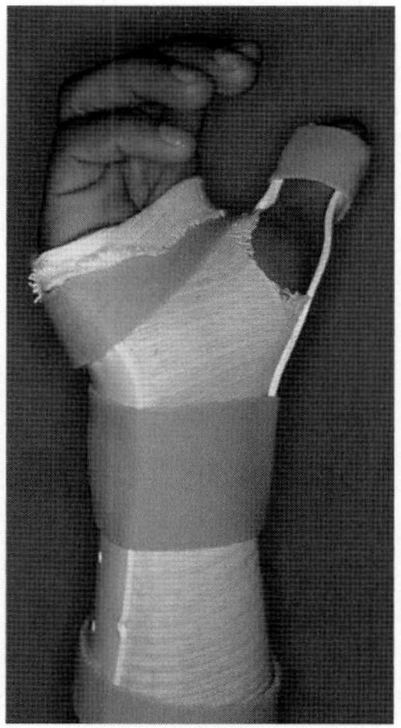

Figure 3–15 A compressive stockinette is used under the splint to control edema after extensor pollicis longus repair.

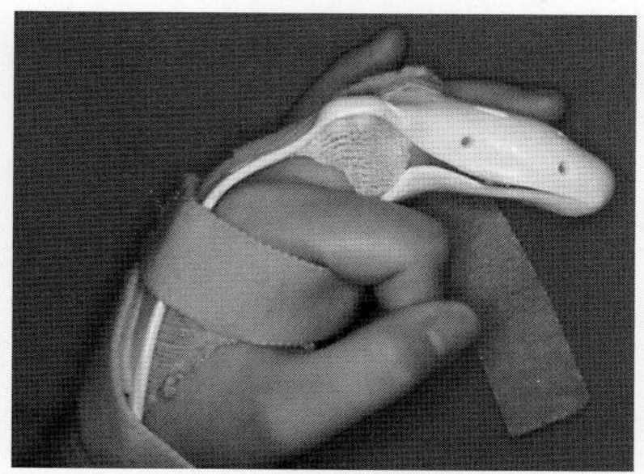

Figure 3–16 A hand-based immobilization splint is used to protect the protruding pins used after the repair of an intra-articular fracture of the proximal phalanx of the middle finger. The splint design shown here allows easy donning and doffing for pin site care, and the perforations allow air exchange to promote healing of the soft tissue injuries.

coolness of skin). As edema diminishes, the splint will need to be remolded to ensure an adequate fit.

Edema itself can cause significant restriction in the ROM of the joint. Reactive, stiff, painful, edematous tissue does not permit motion; the therapeutic program must be modified to restore tissue homeostasis (Brand & Thompson, 1993). More rest and less movement of the injured part are usually appropriate, and the stress applied to the healing tissue by the splint should be less than normal.

Infection

Infection is defined as the invasion and multiplication of microorganisms in body tissues; it may be acute, subacute, or chronic (Thompson & Taddonio, 1997). Infection increases oxygen demand and decreases oxygen delivery to tissues secondary to edema and collagen breakdown. These changes prolong the inflammatory phase of wound healing. In addition to the common signs of infection (erythema and wound drainage), other signs include wound discoloration, granulation tissue that bleeds easily (friable), unexpected pain or tenderness, pocketing at the base of the wound, and delayed wound healing (vanRijswidk, 1997). The infection must be treated before wound healing can occur. Splints that are applied to an area that is infected should be fabricated to allow for easy donning and doffing for wound care (e.g., whirlpools and pin care) (Fig. 3–16). Consider using perforated thermoplastic materials to increase air exchange under splints that have dressings.

Splinting for Specific Tissues

For the therapist and surgeon to determine the cause of a joint's immobility and to correct it, they must understand the integrity of the articular surfaces, bones, ligaments, joint capsules, tendons, skin, and subcutaneous tissues. The type of splinting (static, serial static, static progressive, or dynamic), the technical considerations for designing the splint, and the pattern used depend on the specifics of the tissue pathology (Strickland, 1987).

Skin

Wounds heal by either primary or secondary intention. Primary closure, or healing by **primary intention,** occurs when wound edges are aligned by suture material or, for superficial wounds, Steri-strips or skin glue. This allows collagen synthesis to bind the edges together, accelerating the healing curve. A surgical wound will seal within 24 to 48 hours after the repair.

Healing by **secondary intention** refers to the process of a wound closing from the inside out. The wound base fills with granulation tissue and is then covered with epithelial cells. As this process occurs, the wound edges are gradually drawn centripetally until closure has been achieved. This method may be chosen if the wound is contaminated or infected and when there may be inadequate skin coverage, as is sometimes seen with an open palm Dupuytren's release (Fig. 3–17).

Skin grafts and **flaps** demand specific dressing and splinting measures to ensure their survival. A partial- or full-thickness skin graft obtains its nutrition by diffusion from the surrounding tissues. Vascularized granulation tissue enters the graft from its bed and allows its incorporation as living skin. This takes approximately 2 weeks, during which time the graft must be held close to the underlying bed. The dressings and splints should maintain immobilization of the graft. If movement of adjacent joints is desirable, and can be achieved without disrupting the graft–bed relationship, then the splint should permit it. For example, a skin graft used for Dupuytren's release should be permitted to heal in place and become revascularized; the simultaneous motion of recently released joints should be allowed, but without disturbing the graft.

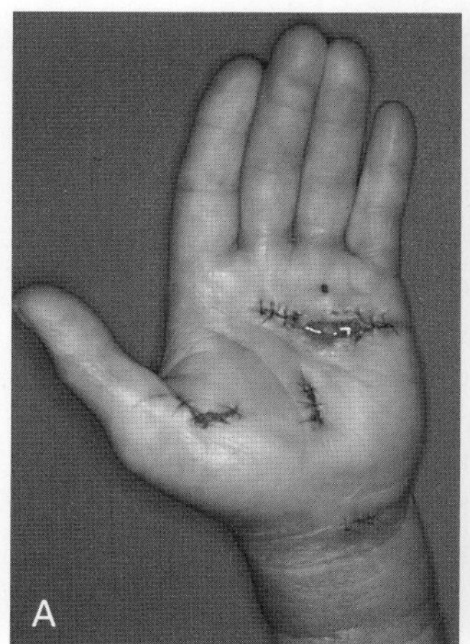

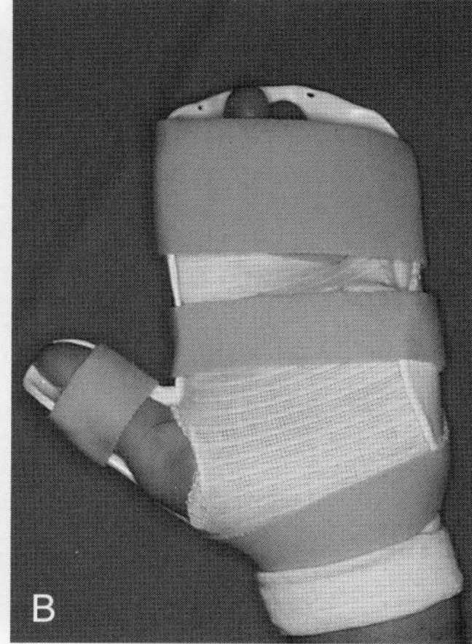

*Figure 3–17 **A,** Dupuytren's disease after open palm release. **B,** A dorsal hand immobilization splint is used to maintain digit extension.*

Skin and soft tissue flaps require specific attention to their pedicles. Through the pedicle, circulation enters and exits the flap. It must not be compromised, compressed, or kinked by the position of the operated site (hand or digit) in the splint or by the splint straps.

Tendon

Tendon healing occurs because of intrinsic and extrinsic contributions. Intrinsic healing, which depends on cells bridging the injury site directly, relies on vincular blood flow, blood flow from the proximal synovial fold in the palm and the bone insertion distally, and diffusion of synovial fluid (and the nutrients it contains). Extrinsic healing depends on the ingrowth of fibroblasts and neovascular tissue, which together form adhesions. These adhesions cause scar bridging or a scar collar at the site of tendon injury; if the adhesions are too thick or inelastic, they may restrict tendon gliding (Wang, 1998).

The stages of tendon healing are the same as for other wounds—inflammatory, fibroplastic, and remodeling—and the timing is also similar. However, the critical need to restore tendon gliding to regain active digital motion and the confounding nature of the healing process (the formation of adhesions as a natural part of the healing process that, however, limit tendon mobility) present challenges to the surgeon and therapist. The surgeon must create a repair that has maximum strength, permits early motion, and minimizes bulk to ease gliding. The therapist must then initiate an early ROM program to establish gliding of the tendon in its canal, especially at the site of injury, and fabricate a splint that facilitates exercise but limits stress on the repair (Wang, 1998). Tendons that are mobilized soon after repair, heal with fewer and less restrictive adhesions, achieve greater tensile strength sooner, and establish better gliding than immobilized tendons. Clinical results reflect this favorable biology of healing.

Note that the precise early rehabilitation program after, for example, a flexor tendon repair depends on the surgeon's and therapist's experience, the nature of the injury, technical factors of the tendon repair (integrity of repair, suture strength), and presence of associated injuries. The health-care team may choose an entirely passive exercise program, a passive flexion–active extension program, or a (gentle) active flexion–active extension program. Common to all three protocols though, is the focus on reestablishing early tendon gliding. Splints are employed in each protocol, sometimes as a static device (passive program) and sometimes as a dynamic one (passive flexion–active extension) (Fig. 3–18). Chapter 18 provides more detailed information on tendon protocols and proper splinting regimes.

Periarticular Soft Tissue

Joint stiffness results either from direct injury to the articular surfaces, capsule, and ligament apparatus or sec-

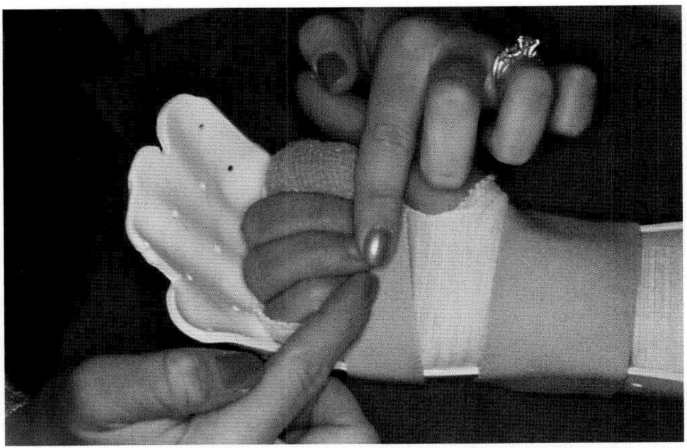

Figure 3–18 A wrist–digit extension restriction splint used after a flexor tendon repair. The therapist performs passive flexion, after which the patient actively extends to the splint's dorsal block. Note that this is but one of several flexor tendon protocols.

ondarily from edema, scar formation, and contracture affecting the soft tissues of the joint and its motivating muscle–tendon units. Anatomic restoration of joint congruity and soft tissue support, and the elimination of edema help prevent such joint stiffness.

A number of questions must be addressed by the surgeon and therapist to achieve successful mobilization of a stiff joint: Has articular congruity been restored? Is there periarticular scarring of, for example, the capsule and ligaments? Are the tendons that move the joint adherent? Does the posture of a proximal joint adversely influence the joint that the splint is designed to improve? Is the scar still amenable to remodeling? In addition, the therapist must be acutely observant of the initial response of the joint and scar to a mobilization splinting. Recurrent inflammation may demand a less aggressive approach, whereas improvement in the contracture may necessitate a change in the precise configuration of the splint (Brand & Thompson, 1993; Fess & McCollum, 1998; Strickland, 1987; Wang, 1998). In certain instances, a contracted ligament will lengthen just so much; further increases in joint motion may be the result of a hinge-open effect rather than to concentric articular gliding. The therapist must be wary of this unwanted outcome (Brand & Thompson, 1993; Strickland, 1987).

Commonly encountered contractures include elbow flexion, MP joint extension, PIP joint flexion, and thumb adduction. Such contractures may be the result of direct joint trauma (e.g., intra-articular fractures), periarticular crushing, sprains, articular surface contusions (e.g., jammed finger), and other injuries. However, contractures may also occur secondarily from edema and subsequent soft tissue contracture that follow injury elsewhere in the upper extremity. These and other contractures may respond to a therapy program that includes edema control, exercise, and mobilization splint-

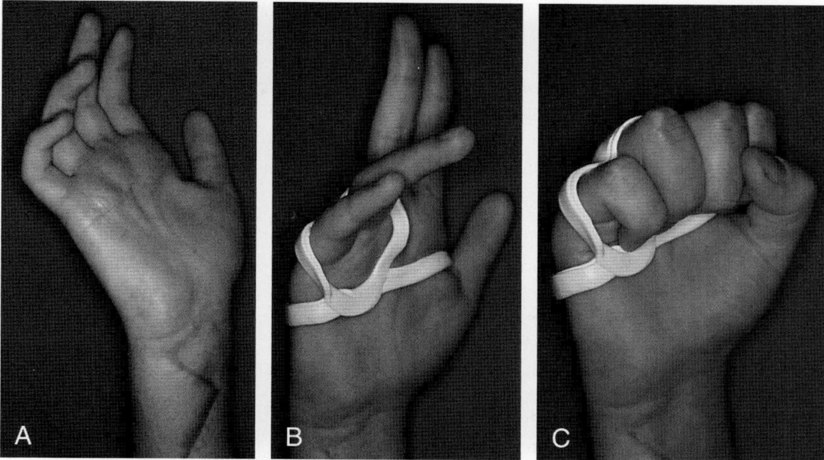

Figure 3–19 ***A,*** *A patient with claw deformity 6 weeks after a flexor tendon and ulnar nerve repair.* ***B,*** *A ring finger to small finger MP extension restriction splint allows the extrinsic extensors to extend the IP joints.* ***C,*** *The splint allows full flexion.*

ing (usually dynamic, static progressive, or serial static). However, surgical release is sometimes required, after which a resumption of therapy, with splinting, is indicated (Slade & Chou, 1998). Chapter 15 discusses splinting for stiffness in more detail.

Bone and Cartilage

Fracture healing follows the same sequence as the healing of other tissues. Inflammation and edema with marrow cavity hemorrhage occur at the time of injury. The next, fibroplastic, stage, is characterized cellularly by migration of osteoprogenitor cells from their endosteal and periosteal origins to the fracture site. The collagen matrix that is deposited by these cells eventually calcifies. The developing callus remodels during the scar maturation stage. This process of remodeling of cells responds to the controlled application of stress. Splints rigidly immobilize the fractured bone early in the fibroplastic stage but are remolded to permit more stress on the bone during callus maturation and remodeling (Slade & Chou, 1998).

Splints are usually less bulky and can be contoured more precisely than casts. Their use with fractures permits earlier and more complete mobilization of nearby joints. This lessens fracture site, distal limb, and digit edema, with its concomitant fibrosis, ligament and capsular contracture, and tendon adherence (Slade & Chou, 1998). Chapter 16 discusses splinting for fractures.

Nerve

Nerve injury results in degeneration of the axon and the myelin sheath distal to the wound and for a short distance proximally. During the stage of inflammation in **nerve healing,** macrophages clear the cellular debris. Axon buds then migrate through the endoneural tube, and Schwann cells envelop the axon in a new myelin sheath as the stage of fibroplasia progresses (Dagum, 1998).

During the fibroplastic stage, protection of the nerve repair against tensile forces is crucial. The surgeon must observe intraoperatively the effect of movement of nearby joints on tension at the site of the repair, because this guides the early postoperative rehabilitation program of the nearby joints. If only a nerve repair was performed, then immobilization for 3 to 4 weeks, followed by controlled mobilization, is appropriate. If, however, tendons were repaired simultaneously and if early restoration of tendon gliding is desirable (wrist-level injuries), then the considerations described for tendon injuries are also pertinent (Fig. 3–19) (Dagum, 1998). Chapter 19 offers detailed information on therapy management.

CONCLUSION

Knowledge of the sequence of events of tissue healing is critical for understanding how and when to intervene—both surgically and conservatively. The selection of a particular treatment program by the surgeon and therapist, including the timely use of specific splints, is determined by the nature of the injury and its repair, the stage of tissue healing, factors that may influence the healing process, and the response of the tissues to previous therapeutic measures.

REFERENCES

Brand, P. W., & Thompson, D. E. (1993). Mechanical resistance. In P. W. Brand & A. Hollister (Eds.). *Clinical mechanics of the hand* (2nd ed., pp. 92–128). St. Louis: Mosby.

Colditz, J. C. (1995). Therapist's management of the stiff hand. In J. M. Hunter, E. J. Mackin, & A. D. Callahan (Eds.). *Rehabilitation of the hand* (4th ed., pp. 1141–115). St. Louis: Mosby.

Dagum, A. B. (1998). Peripheral nerve regeneration, repair, and grafting. *Journal of Hand Therapy, 11,* 111–117.

Davidson, M. B. (1999). The dangerous toll of diabetes. Available at: http://www.diabetes.org/ada/facts/asp. No longer available.

Fess, E. W., & McCollum, M. (1998). The influence of splinting on healing tissue. *Journal of Hand Therapy, 11,* 157–161.

Fess, E. W., & Phillips, C. (Eds.). (1987). *Hand splinting: Principles and methods* (2nd ed.). St. Louis: Mosby.

Jenson, J. A. (1991). Cigarette smoking decreases tissue oxygen. *Archives of Surgery, 126,* 1131–1134.

Kane, D. P. (1997). Surgical repair. In D. Krasner, & D. Kane (Eds.). *Chronic wound care: A clinical source book for healthcare professionals* (2nd ed., pp. 235–244). Wayne, PA: Health Management Publishing.

LeRoy, E. C. (1996). Systemic sclerosis: A vascular perspective. *Rheumatic Diseases Clinics of North America, 22,* 674–694.

Marx, R. Radiation injury to tissue. (1994). In E. Kindwall (Ed.). Hyperbaric medicine practice (pp. 447–503). Flagstaff, AZ: Best Publishing.

Pinchocofsky-Devin, G. (1997). Nutritional assessment and intervention. In D. Krasner, & D. Kane (Eds.). *Chronic wound care: A clinical source book for healthcare professionals* (2nd ed., pp. 73–83). Wayne, PA: Health Management Publishing.

Rund C. (1997). Postoperative care of skin graft, donor sites, and myocutaneous flaps. In D. Krasner, & D. Kane (Eds.). *Chronic wound care: A clinical source book for healthcare professionals* (2nd ed., pp. 245–250). Wayne, PA: Health Management Publishing.

Sickle Cell Disease Research Foundation. (2001). What Is Sickle Cell Disease? Available at: http//www.scdrf.org. Accessed November 10, 2001.

Silverstein, P. (1992). Smoking and wound healing. *American Journal of Medicine, 93,* 22s–24s.

Slade, J. F., & Chou, K. H. (1988). Bony tissue repair. *Journal of Hand Therapy, 11,* 118–124.

Smith, J., & Feske, N. (1996). Cutaneous manifestations and consequences of smoking. *Journal of the American Academy of Dermatology, 34,* 717–726.

Smith, K. L., & Dean, S. J. (1998). Tissue repair of the epidermis and dermis. *Journal of Hand Therapy, 11,* 95–104.

Stotts, N., & Wipke-Tevis, D. (1997) Cofactor in impaired wound healing. In D. Krasner, & D. Kane (Eds.). *Chronic wound care: A clinical source book for healthcare professionals* (2nd ed., pp. 64–72). Wayne, PA: Health Management Publishing.

Strickland, J. W. (1987). Biologic basis for hand splinting. In F. W. Fess & C. Phillips (Eds.). *Hand splinting: Principles and methods* (2nd ed., pp. 43–70). St. Louis: Mosby.

Thompson, P. D., & Taddonio, T. E. (1997). Wound infection. In D. Krasner, & D. Kane (Eds.). *Chronic wound care: A clinical source book for healthcare professionals* (2nd ed., pp. 84–89). Wayne, PA: Health Management Publishing.

vanRijswidk, L. (1997). Wound assessment and documentation. In D. Krasner, & D. Kane (Eds.). *Chronic wound care: A clinical source book for healthcare professionals* (2nd ed., pp. 16–28). Wayne, PA: Health Management Publishing.

Wang, E. D. (1998), Tendon repair. *Journal of Hand Therapy, 11,* 105–109.

SUGGESTED READING

(1998). [Special issue]. *Journal of Hand Therapy, 11.*

Akeson, W., Ameil, D., Abel M. F., Garfin, S. R., & Woo, S. L. (1987). Effects of immobilization on joints. *Clinical Orthopaedics and Related Research, 219,* 28–37.

Brand, P. W, & Hollister, A. (1993). *Clinical mechanics of the hand* (2nd ed.). St. Louis: Mosby.

Buckwalter, J. (1996). Effects of early motion on healing of musculoskeletal tissues. *Hand Clinics, 12,* 13–24.

Dellon, A. L. (1990). Wound healing in nerve. *Clinics in Plastic Surgery, 17 (3),* 545–570.

Evans, R. B., & Thompson, D. E. (1993). The application of stress to the healing tendon. *Journal of Hand Therapy, 4,* 262–280.

Flowers, K. R., & LaStayo, P. (1994). Effect of total end range time on improving passive range of motion. *Journal of Hand Therapy, 7,* 150–157.

McClure, P., Blackburn L, Dusold, C. (1994). The use of splints in the treatment of joint stiffness: Biologic rationale and an algorithm for making clinical decisions. *Physical Therapy, 74,* 1101–1107.

Peacock, E., & Van Winkle, W. (1976). *Wound repair.* Philadelphia: Saunders.

Smith, K. L. (1992). Wound healing. In B. G. Stanley & S. M. Tribuzi (Eds.). *Concepts in hand rehabilitation* (pp. 35–56). Philadelphia: Davis.

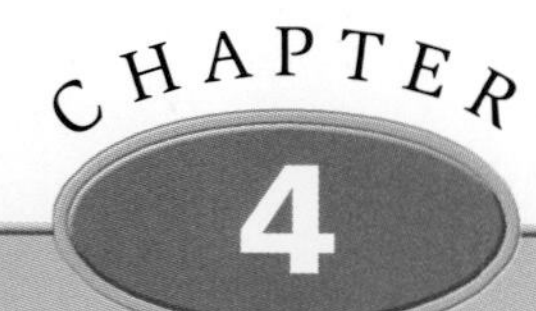

Mechanical Principles

Gary P. Austin, PT, PhD, and
MaryLynn Jacobs, MS, OTR/L, CHT

INTRODUCTION

Splinting is the intentional application of external loads to specific anatomic structures to manipulate the internal reaction forces and thus enhance or restore function of the extremity. **Mechanics** is the science that addresses the effects of forces on structures. Ideally, the effective therapist integrates basic mechanical concepts into all facets of design and fabrication of a splint. A potential barrier to understanding and incorporating these concepts is the confusing mechanical terminology. Therefore, the purposes of this chapter are twofold: to define the fundamental mechanical terms and concepts pertinent to splint design and fabrication and to discuss the clinical relevance and application of these basic principles using specific examples.

Force

As clinicians and students interested in the therapeutic application of **force,** it is essential that the concept of force be clearly defined. Force is an action or influence that either arrests, produces, or changes the direction of motion (LeVeau, 1992). A force can be sufficiently described using the following parameters:

- **Nature:** The type or kind of force (e.g., push or pull).
- **Magnitude:** The amount or quantity of influence present.
- **Line or angle of application:** The path or direction along which the force acts.
- **Point of application:** The location on the structure at which the line of force acts.

An unbalanced force with a point of application other than the center of the object results in the rotation of an object around a fixed axis. Such a force is referred to as a **moment of force,** or **torque.** An example of torque is pulling down on a lever to open a door (Fig. 4–1A). A force with a point of application directly through the center of the object results in the translation of an object along a straight or curvilinear path. This is referred to as **linear force.** An example of linear force is the act of pushing a box along a floor (Fig. 4–1B). Although it may appear that **rotational force** should be the principal focus when discussing splinting, in fact most motions incorporate both rotational and **translational** components.

As will become evident, a splint is fundamentally the sum of translational and rotational forces acting on anatomic structures for a specific therapeutic purpose. Thus the different applications of force and force systems must be appreciated. Although at first glance it appears that two forces equal in magnitude would have the same therapeutic effect, this is rarely the case. Furthermore, therapists must understand that the system with the greater force does not always yield the greatest benefit.

There are different forms or types of force. The most pertinent forces for the design and fabrication of splints are torque (moment of force), elastic force, and friction force.

Torque

The vast majority of articulations in the human body consist of segments or levers assembled around an **axis of rotation,** i.e., the proximal and distal segments rotate around a joint axis. By virtue of this structure, the point of application of force is at a distance from the joint axis, producing joint motion that is rotational in nature. Rotational motion is produced, changed, or halted by force applied in the form of torque. Torque, or the moment of force, is the potential for a force to produce the rotation of a lever around an axis.

The magnitude of torque is a function of two components: the magnitude of applied force and the perpendicular distance from the axis of rotation to the point of application of the force, otherwise known as the moment arm. More specifically:

$$\tau = F \times d$$

where τ is torque, F is force, and d is the perpendicular distance from the axis of rotation to the point of application (Fig. 4–2**A**). It is important to note that the torque about an axis, or joint, can be modified by manipulating either the distance from the axis of rotation at which the force is applied (Fig. 4–2**B**) or the quantity of the applied force (Fig. 4–2**C**). Increases in the force and/or distance produce increases in torque; in other words, torque is directly proportional to both force and distance.

Lever Systems and Mechanical Advantage

For splints, torque is commonly applied to a joint via leverage. **Levers** are rigid structures through which a force can be applied to produce rotational motion about a fixed axis. A lever system is composed of a **fulcrum,** or fixed axis, and two arms: the **effort arm** (EA) and the **resistance arm** (RA). The effort arm, also referred to as the force arm, is the segment of the lever between the fulcrum and the effort force (EF) that is attempting to stabilize or mobilize a structure. The relation to splinting is as follows: The fulcrum typically coincides with the anatomic axis of the target joint, the effort arm is the segment of the splint that applies the effort force, and the resistance arm is the segment of the limb that resists the effort force. The effort force and resistance force (RF), in acting about a fixed axis, create opposing torques about the fulcrum (Fig. 4–3).

The components of the lever system can be arranged to create different types, or classes, of levers, each with a characteristic mechanical advantage or efficiency. The **mechanical advantage** (MA) of a lever system is defined by the relation between the length of the effort arm and the length of the resistance arm:

$$MA = EA/RA$$

Thus there are three possible relations and three classes of lever systems (Fig. 4–4A-C). Examples of a **first-class**

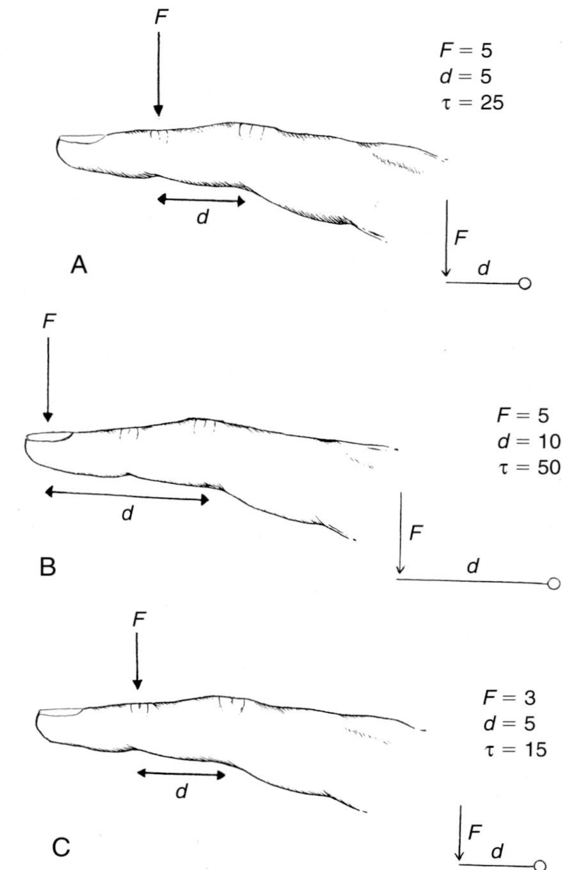

*Figure 4–2 The torque (τ), or moment of force, can be affected by changes in either the distance (d) from the axis of rotation at which the force (F) is applied or the magnitude of the force applied. **A,** F = 5, d = 5, τ = 25. **B,** F = 5, d = 10, τ = 50. **C,** F = 3, d = 5, τ = 15.*

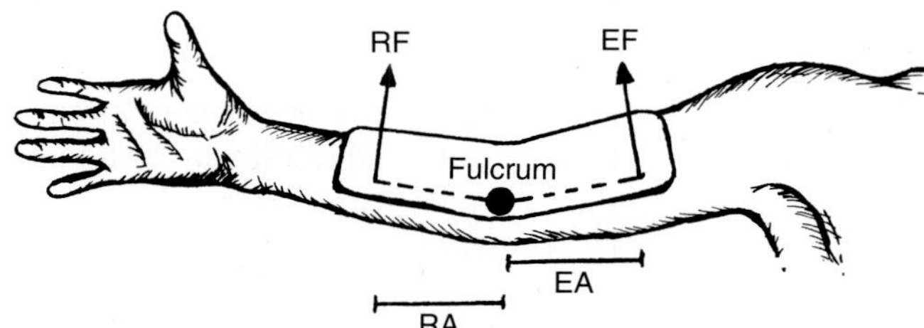

Figure 4–3 In this anterior elbow immobilization splint, the effort arm (EA) is the proximal segment of the splint, which applies the effort force (EF); and the resistance arm (RA) is the distal segment of the limb, which applies the resistance force (RF). These forces, acting about the elbow joint axis, create opposing torques.

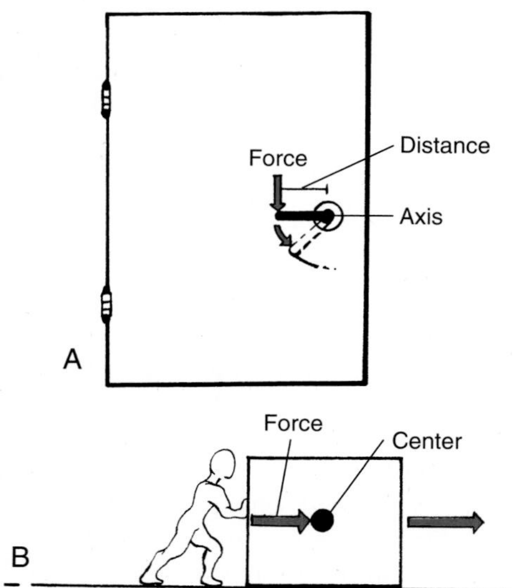

*Figure 4–1 **A,** Force is applied at a distance from the axis, causing a rotation of the lever. **B,** Linear force is applied directly through the center of the box, causing a translation across the surface.*

lever system are a seesaw, a pair of scissors, pliers, and a crow bar. Because the fulcrum is between the effort and the resistance arms, the mechanical advantage can be greater than, less than, or equal to 1. Common **second-class lever** systems include the wheelbarrow and the nutcracker. In each of these, the mechanical advantage is greater than 1, because the resistance is between the effort force and the fulcrum. Examples of **third-class lever** systems are a spoon, a fork, tweezers, a shovel, and a fishing rod. In this case, the effort force is applied between the fulcrum and the resistance force; because the effort arm is shorter than the resistance arm, the mechanical advantage is less than 1. Note that the majority of splints are first-class lever systems.

Clinical Considerations

The goal when designing a lever system, or splint, is to generate the most efficient work. The length of the resistance arm greatly influences the mechanical advantage of the applied force. The effort arm of the splint can also affect the mechanical advantage by the manner in which it is molded to the body part. Both the effort and the resistance arms should conform to the structures they touch and should incorporate enough surface area for adequate pressure distribution. When forces act on a joint, there must be a balance–counterbalance effect. If the opposing force (effort arm) is not distributed well enough to counterbalance the distal force (resistance arm), the splint may become uncomfortable and thus ineffective. Therapists can create mechanical advantages through meticulous splinting techniques and the judicious application of basic mechanical principles.

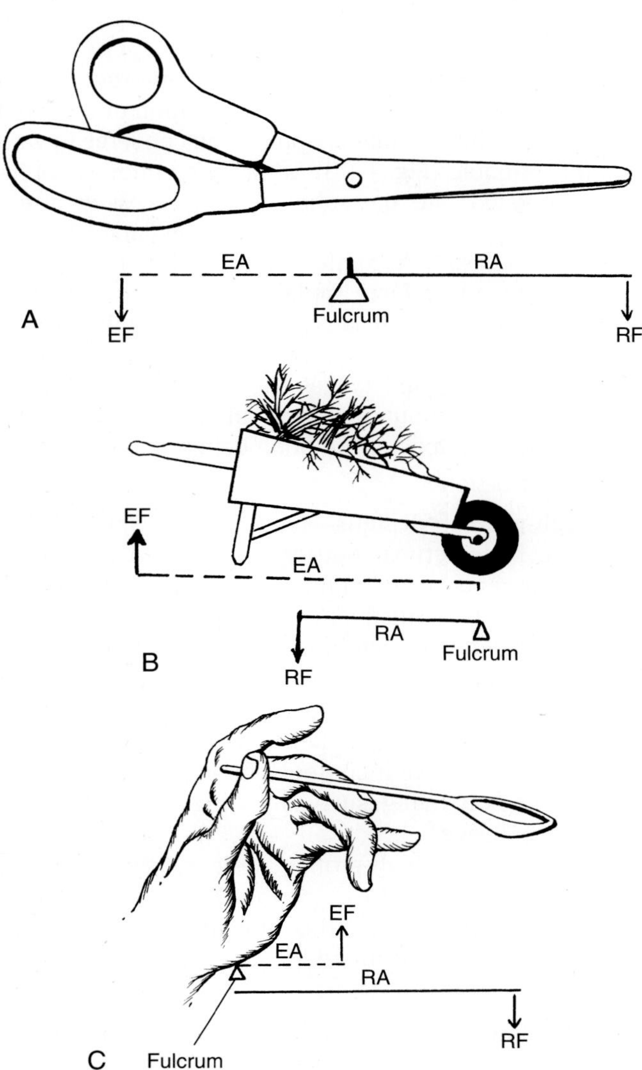

Figure 4–4 ***A,*** *A first-class lever system.* ***B,*** *A second-class lever system.* ***C,*** *A third-class lever system.*

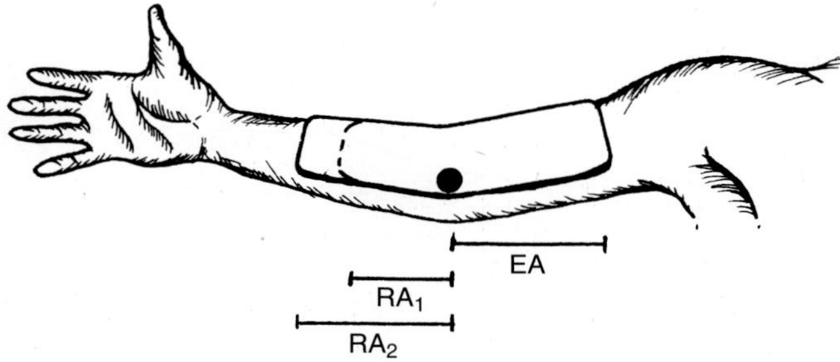

Figure 4–5 When the resistance arm (RA_2) is lengthened, less force is required to generate sufficient torque to prevent elbow joint movement. When the resistance arm (RA_1) is shortened, greater force is required to immobilize the elbow joint.

- The longer the resistance arm, the less force required to generate sufficient torque (Fig. 4–5). And, conversely, the shorter the resistance arm, the more force required to produce sufficient torque.
- The effort arm is most comfortable when adequate length and depth are incorporated into the splint (Fig. 4–6). A short, narrow, and shallow effort arm is likely to cause pressure and discomfort; a well-molded effort arm dissipates pressure.
- The greater the force generated through the resistance arm, the broader and longer the effort arm required as a counterbalance.

As a clinical example, consider fabricating a splint to mobilize a stiff proximal interphalangeal (PIP) joint in the direction of flexion. For counterbalance, the effort arm (on the volar proximal phalanx) is fabricated in the direction of extension. If the surface contact area of the effort arm is not of adequate length, circumference, and contour, localized shear and compression stress and migration of the splint may result (shear and compression stress are discussed later in this chapter). When the proximal segment migrates or shifts, the resistance arm is not able to provide a perpendicular angle of pull to the PIP joint axis of rotation, causing the resistance arm to alter the sling's fit on the middle phalanx (Fig. 4–7).

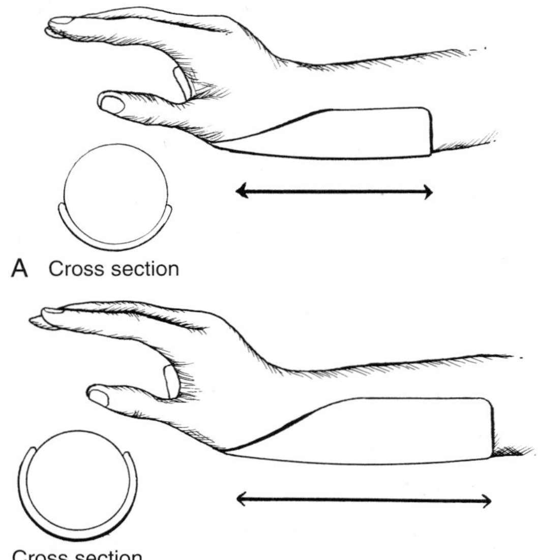

Figure 4–6 ***A,*** *A splint with a short, narrow, and shallow effort arm is likely to cause discomfort from inadequate pressure distribution.* ***B,*** *A splint with a longer, broader, and deeper effort arm adequately distributes pressure and thus increases comfort. The depth of the splint should encompass two thirds of the circumference of the body part, not only adding strength but also allowing for adequate placement of straps without the risk of compressing soft tissue.*

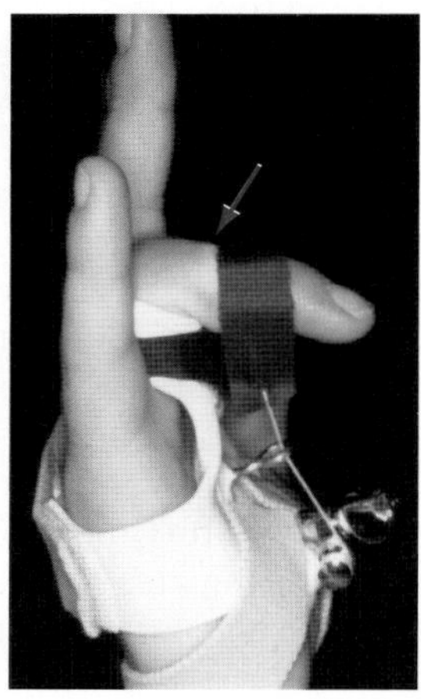

Figure 4–7 Shear stress is created on the proximal dorsal edge of this sling, secondary to a change in the angle of pull. In addition, improper fit and shifting of the effort arm in the proximal segment of the splint contribute to the loss of the 90° angle of application.

Angle of Application

The **angle of application** of the moment of force or torque is critical to the proper design and fabrication of splints. Ideally, the force should be applied so that the angle of application is oriented 90° to the lever. This maximizes the therapeutic effect of the external force because the total force influencing the target segment acts in the intended direction. When the force is applied in a purely perpendicular orientation to the target segment, there are no forces in other directions (Fig. 4–8A-C). However, at an angle other than 90°, a portion of the force acting on the segment is applied in a direction other than the desired trajectory (either compression or tension), thereby effectively diminishing the perpendicular component and decreasing the therapeutic torque (Fig. 4–8D-E). Thus, when the angle of application is either greater or less than 90°, the beneficial effect of the application of torque cannot be optimized, and potentially damaging compression and/or sheer stress is applied.

Design Considerations

GENERAL

- To achieve a near 90° angle of application, use line guides and pulleys to aid in the orientation (Fig. 4–9A).
- To prevent undue torque or stress on the surrounding soft tissues, view the splint from all angles to ensure that the pull of the line is directed centrally over the digit or limb and oriented properly in all planes (Fig. 4–9B).
- When using a mobilization splint to improve flexion of the digits, the anatomic configuration of the hand requires that the line of application converge toward the scaphoid (Fig. 4–9B). If this orientation is not incorporated into the splint design, excessive stress will be placed on the metacarpophalangeal (MP) joints, causing discomfort and potential harm.
- Occasionally, a force applied in either a radial or ulnar direction is indicated, e.g, after MP joint arthroplasties or sagittal band repairs (Fig. 4–10). (Except for special circumstances such as these, the line of application should be centrally located over the longitudinal axis of the bone being mobilized.)

HIGH-PROFILE DESIGN

- **High-profile designs**—mobilization splints that have high vertical outriggers—may require fewer adjustments to maintain the optimal 90° angle of application. Adjustments must be made when improvements are seen in joint motion; otherwise the line of pull will no longer be at 90°.
- Patient compliance is often a challenge because the splint is large. The dimensions of the high-profile design can make it cumbersome to engage in activities of daily living, such as putting the arm through a shirt sleeve.
- When using high-profile designs, the therapist should be careful to attach the outrigger sturdily on the splint base since this attachment site has the potential of low stability.

LOW-PROFILE DESIGN

- With **low-profile designs**—mobilization splints that have low, close to the surface outriggers—the force required to mobilize a joint may be uncomfortable and difficult to tolerate for extended periods of time.

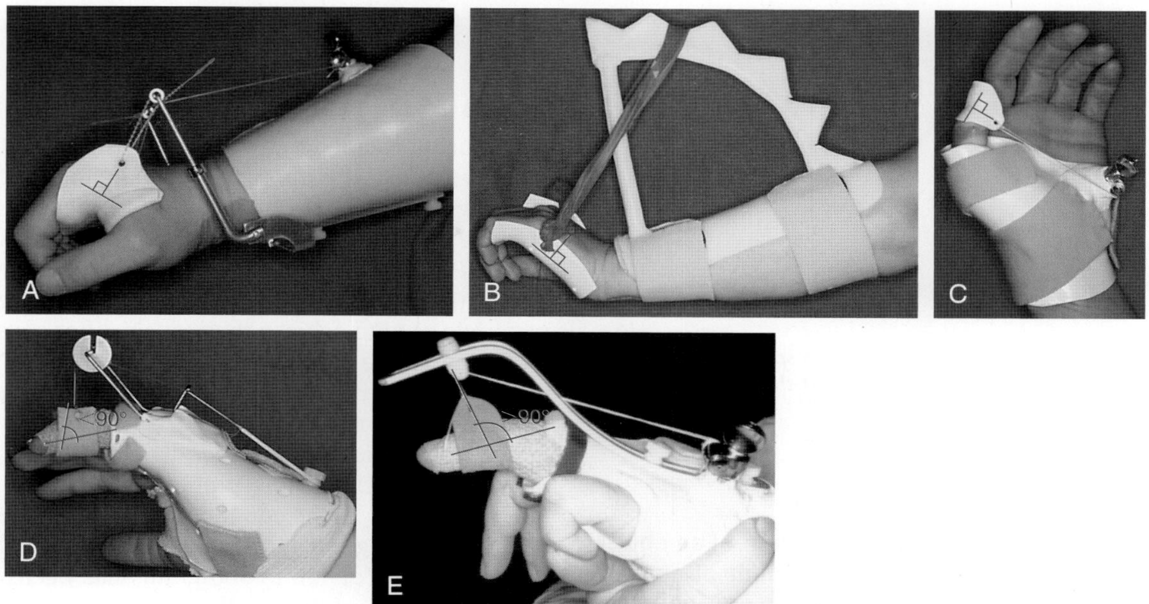

Figure 4–8 *The optimal 90° angle of application, demonstrated by a Phoenix wrist hinge (**A**), a wrist extension mobilization splint (**B**), and a thumb IP flexion mobilization splint (**C**). **D,** The angle of force application is less than 90° in this hand-based PIP extension mobilization splint, causing shear stress at the distal volar edge of the sling. **E,** The angle of force application is greater than 90° in this splint, leading to shear stress at the proximal volar edge of the sling.*

- Low-profile designs may be cosmetically appealing. However, when greater resistance is necessary, such as when mobilizing a dense 60° PIP flexion contracture, it may be more appropriate to incorporate a higher outrigger into the splint design. In such a situation, the force is applied at a greater distance from the joint axis to produce a greater amount of torque on the contracture.
- A low-profile design is an excellent choice for a splint that is used to substitute for weak or absent musculature, as seen when managing a radial nerve injury. Typically, less torque is needed to hold the distal segments (wrist and MP joints in this case) in the proper position to substitute for the loss of muscle action than is needed to try to mobilize a stiff joint. For this purpose, only minimal adjustments are necessary, and the low-profile design tends to enhance function.
- Although dynamic splints require periodic adjustments to maintain an optimal 90° angle of pull, many make the unsubstantiated claim that high-profile dynamic splints require less frequent adjustment of the outrigger than do low-profile dynamic splints. However, it is best to assume that both low- and high-profile splints require adjustments at the same frequency to maintain the optimal 90° line of pull on the target segment.
- Low-profile splint designs can be less cumbersome for performance of activities of daily living and often fit under loose clothing.

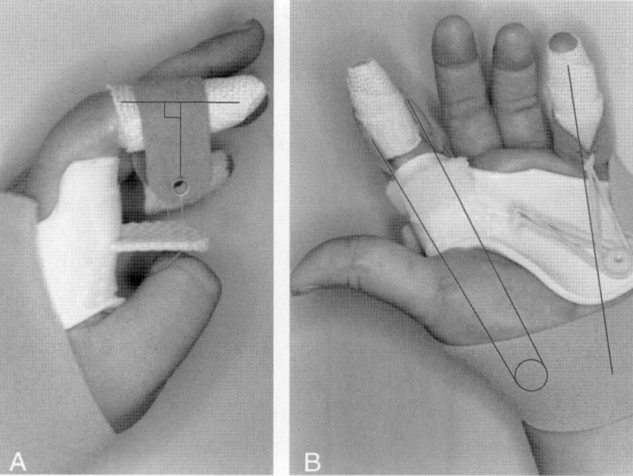

Figure 4–9 ***A,** Lateral view of the 90° angle of application of a hand-based index finger PIP flexion mobilization splint. The thermoplastic line guide (perforated material) allows for simple splint adjustments as the range of motion improves. Note the small cast that aids in distributing pressure across the middle phalanx. **B,** Volar view highlighting the line of application directed toward the scaphoid. Note the two monofilament lines originating from the index finger sling and traveling through the perforated material. The small finger loop is addressing a stiff MP joint. Because of the relative shortness of the small finger, a cast applied to the IP joints creates a longer, more effective, lever arm to concentrate the flexion force to the MP joint.*

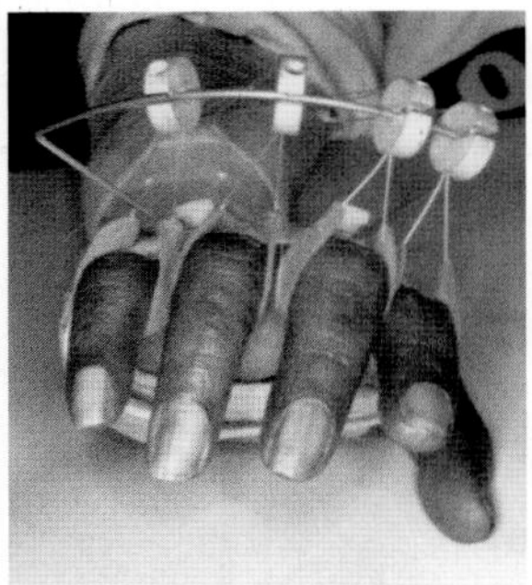

Figure 4–10 This MP extension mobilization splint has a radially directed pull to protect the reconstruction of the radial collateral ligaments of the MP joints.

Elastic Force

Elastic force is that influence on the motion of an object or segment that is the result of the amount of applied stretch. Elastic force is directly proportional to both the **stiffness** of a structure and the amount of displacement present. Specifically:

$$F = -k\Delta l$$

where F is elastic force, k is stiffness, and Δl is the change in length or displacement. Elastic force can be increased by increasing the stiffness of the structure and/or increasing the amount of displacement or stretch. Stiffness is the relationship between the amount of force produced and the applied stretch:

$$-k = \frac{F}{\Delta l}$$

In other words, a stiffer structure produces a large amount of resistance to a small stretch, whereas a less stiff structure offers little resistance in response to the same stretch.

Clinically, when a therapist fabricates a splint to influence tissue response, he or she must consider the elastic nature of both the target tissues and the materials used to make the splint. The therapist should be familiar with the properties of the materials, including such factors as resistance to stretch, rigidity, and conformability (see Chapter 5 for more information).

Torque-Angle Measurement

The notion of elastic force and stiffness applies not only to the materials used to produce external loads (e.g., rubber bands, elastic cord, and spring coils) but also to the internal reaction forces of the limb. An example is the torque-angle measurement proposed by Brand and Hollister (1993), in which torque is measured at several joint angles. These measurements provide the clinician with information regarding the magnitude of resistance to motion at particular joint angles throughout an arc of movement. A stiff hand, for example, offers more resistance at different angles than does a "normal" hand.

Clinical Considerations

When using elastic force to mobilize stiff structures, the therapist must take into account the clinical objectives. Is the goal mobilization of a mature, dense joint contracture or the stabilization of the MP joints in extension after MP joint arthroplasty? Both situations may employ an elastic force; however, the amount of force and the materials used to achieve these goals differ considerably.

To date, there is no documented ideal amount of elastic force for optimal mobilization of a specific structure. However, the amount of force applied depends on such factors as individual tolerance, diagnosis, stage of tissue healing, chronicity of the problem, severity of the contracture, density of the contracture, patient's age, lifestyle factors (smoking, alcohol use), and other health-related issues. A range of 100 to 300 grams has been suggested for mobilization of the small joints of the hand, whereas higher parameters (350+ grams) seem to be more effective for larger structures (Bell-Krotoski & Figarola, 1995; Brand & Hollister, 1993; Flowers & LaStayo, 1994; Giurintano, 1995). The estimate of 300 grams is based on what is tolerated per unit of surface area of the skin, not on the tolerance of the contracted tissue to tension. Therefore, in most cases, skin tolerance becomes the limiting factor in determining appropriate splint tension, not the specific targeted tissue. "While the optimum force has yet to be calculated, the amount of force applied to the tissues must be determined relative to the tissues that are contracted. A force of 800 grams may be on the high end of the spectrum for the PIP joint but is a relatively small amount when considering remodeling at the elbow or shoulder" (Bell-Krotoski & Figarola, 1995).

The therapist can almost always rely on the tissue's response to the tension to help determine the effectiveness of the mobilizing forces. Signs of too much stress include edema, skin blanching, vascular changes, and complaints of pain. With tools such as tension gauges (e.g., Haldex gauge), the therapist can obtain a general estimate of the amount of tension a dynamic splint is applying to the involved area (Fig. 4–11). A few of the common devices a therapist can use to generate an elastic force for mobilizing soft tissue are discussed in the next sections.

RUBBER BANDS

A **rubber band's** length and thickness help determine its effectiveness when used for mobilization splinting. Thinner (narrow) rubber bands tend to elongate more easily than do thicker ones. The therapist must consider the purpose of the splint before selecting the rubber band. For example, a narrow rubber band may not be stiff enough to aid in mobilizing a dense PIP flexion contracture but may generate adequate force to maintain a PIP joint in extension after an extensor tendon repair. Over time, rubber bands may become brittle and lose some of their elasticity; the clinician must monitor this closely.

WRAPPED ELASTIC CORD

Wrapped elastic cord is made of a light layer of cotton wrapped around an elastic cord. It provides a greater degree of resistance or stiffness when stretched. With this type of material, less stretch is required to generate movement of a stiff joint than with a rubber band; therefore, caution should be used.

SPRING COILS

Spring coils can produce an elastic force as well. they are available in a variety of sizes (diameters and lengths) that offer different degrees of resistance. The composition, stiffness, and length of the coil aid the therapist in the appropriate selection for the tissue involved. Spring coils produce a consistent controlled force with little material breakdown, an advantage over rubber bands. However, they are more costly and less readily available than rubber bands.

Friction Force

Friction force is a type of translational force, sometimes referred to as either static friction or kinetic friction. Friction opposes movement between two surfaces and acts parallel to the surfaces. The force of friction (F_x) is proportional to the coefficient of friction (μ) and the contact force (F_c):

$$F_x = \mu F_c$$

The coefficient of friction is specific to each material. At rest, the opposing force of friction is categorized as static and depends on the coefficient of static friction (μs) and F_c. As soon as motion occurs, friction is classified as kinetic, or moving, friction. and depends on the coefficient of kinetic friction (μ_k) and F_c.

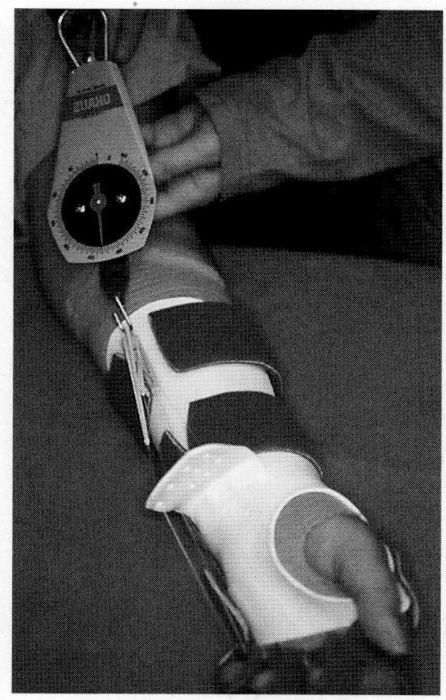

Figure 4–11 A tension gauge applied to a mobilization splint determines the approximate forces on the intended tissue.

In situations of either motion or equilibrium, friction is directly proportional to (1) the coefficient of friction specific to the material(s) and (2) the amount of contact force. The therapist, therefore, can minimize friction by using materials with lower coefficients of friction, such as smooth, nonperforated thermoplastics (instead of gel or foam-lined thermoplastic materials). In addition, friction can be reduced by decreasing the contact force generated by rubber bands and straps. Often friction must be minimized to prevent skin irritation or breakdown, such as chaffing or blistering. Sources of potential harmful friction include splint borders, poor-fitting straps, attachments that rub against the skin (e.g., the underside of rivets or rubber band posts), and edges that extend beyond joint creases.

Clinical Considerations

Friction may be desired to prevent the migration of a splint along the skin. In such cases, friction can be increased by applying straps to increase the contact force or by simply lining the splint with thin foam strips or a tape (e.g., Microfoam) to increase the coefficient of friction.

At times a small amount of splint migration is inevitable; for example, a wrist immobilization splint causes some degree of friction along the splint–skin interface as the patient moves the digits and elbow. An attempt must be made to decrease this friction force; it can be lessened by covering the involved area with materials such as cotton stockinette, Tubigrip or Tubipad.

Friction, also referred to as drag, may be present in the pulley systems used for dynamic mobilization splints. As the monofilament line passes through the line guide (pulleys or outriggers), the point of contact can be a source of friction, increasing unwanted resistance through the splint. This can be the result of the coefficient of friction of the monofilament, the splint line, or the line guide itself (Fig. 4–12). The amount of friction present is increased when the angle at which the monofilament line enters one of these devices is increased.

Most manufactures of splinting components have attempted to address these issues. For example, the Phoenix outrigger has a tubular plastic insert in which the monofilament line passes, and the Rolyan adjustable outrigger is completely rounded and smooth to reduce dragging of the line as it traverses over and through the outrigger (see Chapter 5 for additional information). Therapists should be aware of this problem when fabricating home-made line guides. Friction can be minimized by smoothing and rounding the edges and by carefully monitoring the angles of force application.

Stress

When designing and fabricating splints, the therapist must understand the **stress** produced by external forces. By definition, stress is the response of, or resistance offered by, a surface to the deformation caused by an ex-

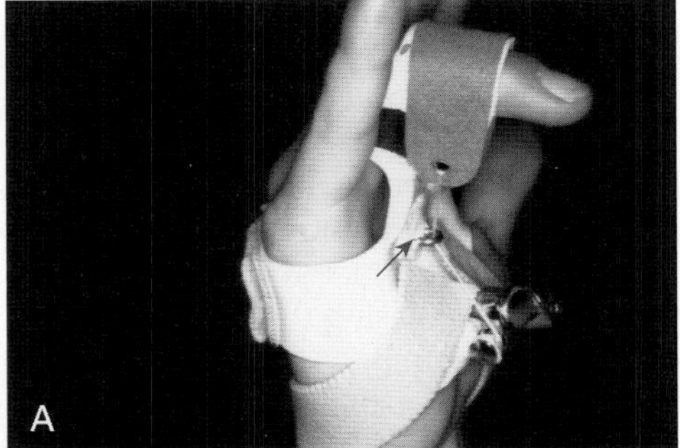

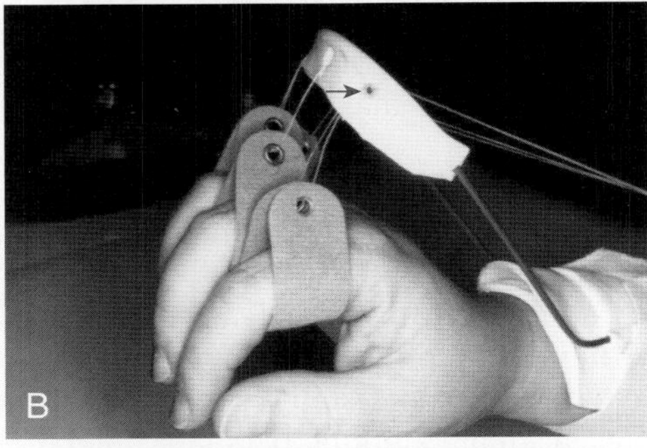

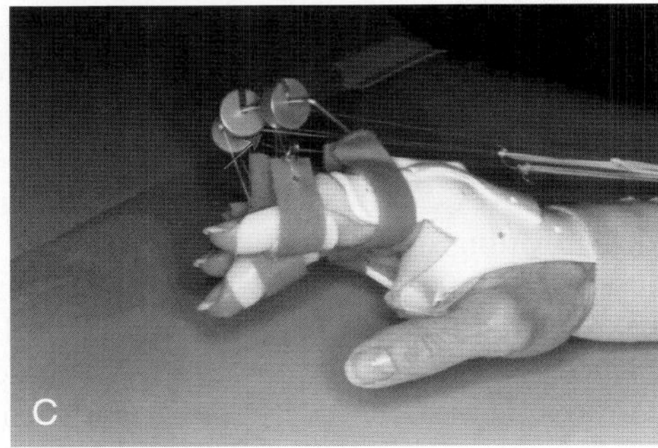

*Figure 4–12 Examples of monofilament line guides that approach at different angles. Note the point of contact and potential sites of friction: commercial line guide (**A**), thermoplastic material with punched hole (**B**), and Phoenix outrigger (**C**).*

ternally applied force or moment (Nordin & Frankel, 2001; Soderberg, 1986). Stress (σ), often simply referred to as pressure, is described according to the amount of force (F) per unit area (A), specifically:

$$\sigma = \frac{F}{A}$$

Stress, therefore, is directly proportional to F, and inversely proportional to A. In other words, stress is increased when either the magnitude of the force applied to the surface area is increased or the amount of area over which the force is applied is decreased (Fig. 4–13). Stress can occur in different forms, the most important of which are compression, shear, tensile, bending, and torsion.

Compression

Compression, often mistakenly referred to simply as **pressure,** is the special case of stress in which opposing loads push toward one another along the same line of application (Fig. 4–14). A compressive stress (σ) is distinguished by the perpendicular angle of application of the load. Usually, compression results in a squeezing type of force, causing a broadening and flattening of the object (Nordin & Frankel, 19??). Compressive stress is maximized by the perpendicular nature of the force application. Notably, pure compression lacks a force component parallel to the surface (defined as shear). Compression is proportional to the perpendicular force (F_{perp}) and inversely proportional to the surface area:

$$\sigma_c = \frac{F_{perp}}{A}$$

For a constant magnitude of force, compression can be minimized by increasing the surface area over which the force can be distributed. For a constant surface area, compression can be reduced by decreasing the perpendicular force.

Clinical Considerations

The therapist must be sure to fabricate splint bases that are of sufficient length, depth, and contour. In addition

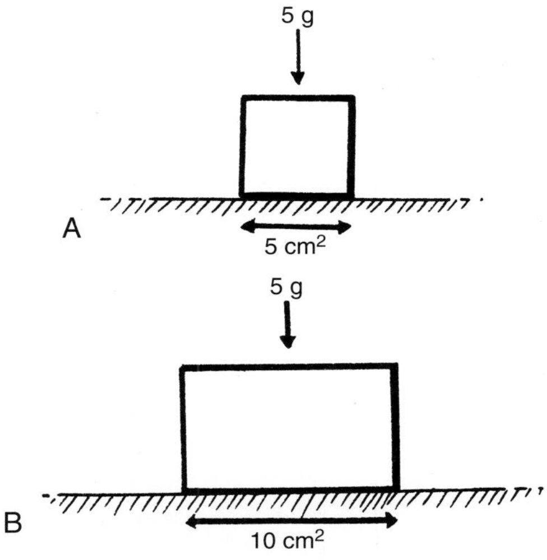

*Figure 4–13 Different magnitudes of stress (g/cm^2) can result from the application of a 5-g force to different sized areas. **A,** Small area (5 cm^2): stress = 1 g/cm^2. **B,** Large area (10 cm^2): stress = 0.5 g/cm^2.*

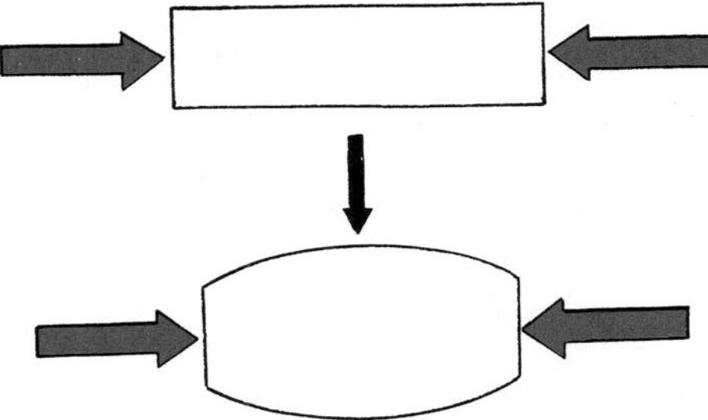

Figure 4–14 To maximize compressive stress, force should be applied in a perpendicular fashion.

to offering greater mechanical advantage, a longer splint base provides greater surface area over which to distribute the contact force. A wider and deeper splint base is not only stronger but minimizes shear stress and maximizes pressure distribution.

Optimizing the conformity of materials to the shapes, contours, and curvatures of the body part being splinted can minimize compressive stress. If care is not taken to meticulously pad vulnerable areas such as the ulnar or radial styloid and pin sites, increased compressive stress can result in discomfort, possible pin migration, and probable noncompliance.

Straps—although necessary to secure the splint firmly on the extremity—can be sources of compressive stress. Narrow strap width, especially in conjunction with shallow splints (less than two thirds of the circumference), can produce high compressive stresses on the soft tissue. This can lead to an uncomfortable, ill-fitting splint (Fig. 4–15). Increasing the width and conformability of the straps distributes the compressive forces over a greater surface area and helps minimize splint migration.

Splint borders should be fabricated so that they lie flush with the skin surface that the strap traverses. The strap should not bridge the two borders of the splint; it should, in fact, actually come in contact with the skin. For example, the lateral borders of a volar forearm splint base should be just at the level of the dorsal forearm. The strap(s) can then be applied to rest lightly on the dorsal forearm.

High splint borders that cause bridging of the straps will not adequately secure the splint onto the extremity. There will be too much room left between the splint strap and the skin, allowing unwanted movement of the splinted part (Fig. 4–16).

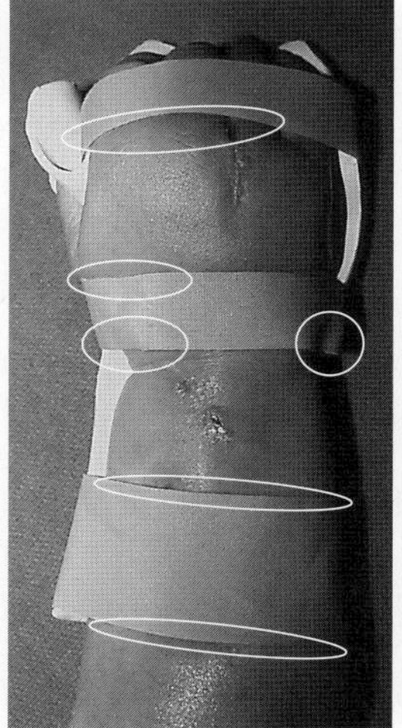

Figure 4–15 Improper selection and placement of straps can create high and uncomfortable compressive and shear forces. The borders of this splint are inadequate to support the bulk of the hand and forearm. The narrow straps are also a source of high compressive stress.

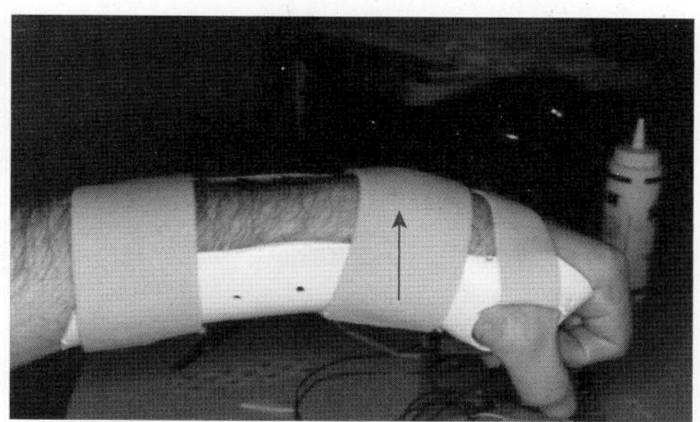

Figure 4–16 When the splint borders are too generous, the straps float above the skin, leaving room for unintended motion. Although the therapist chose the proper strap for this wrist immobilization splint, the wrist can separate from the splint with functional use of the hand.

The therapist should remember that slings and loops can also be sources of compression stress. Several techniques help the splint fabricator avoid compression to the lateral, dorsal, or volar aspects of the digit (or body part in the sling or loop). One splint line can be attached to each side of a sling (two pieces of line) and then joined after they pass through the pulley. This prevents the circumferential compression created when one line is thread through both ends of the loop, an important consideration when splinting a digit with edema or neurovascular issues (Fig. 4–17A). Alternatively, a well-contoured cuff fabricated from thermoplastic, plaster, or QuickCast may be placed under the sling as a support. The cuff disperses the compressive forces applied through the sling by lifting the borders away from the skin and increasing the area of force application (Fig. 4–17B). Circumferential cuffs can also be fabricated to maximize pressure distribution (Fig. 4–17C).

Shear

Shear stress results from force being applied parallel to the surface and produces a tendency for an object either to deform or to slide along the surface. This can occur in two instances: when two parallel opposing forces are applied in the same plane (coplanar) but not along the same line (noncollinear) and when two oblique opposing forces share the same point of application but are neither parallel nor perpendicular (Fig. 4–18). In the first case, shear stress is high owing to the parallel force and compressive stress is negligible in the absence of perpendicular force. In the second case, in which the angle of application does not equal 90°, there exists both a parallel component (shear) and a perpendicular component (compression). Although difficult to measure, the amount of shear in the latter case can be inferred from the angle of application. Shear is inversely proportional to the angle of application: As the angle approaches 0° (as in the former case), the shear dominates; and as it becomes more perpendicular, it decreases.

Shear is often accompanied by other stresses, e.g., compression, tension, and torsion (as seen in splints that attempt to mobilize forearm rotation). In addition, static or kinetic friction may be present as a counterforce to the shear stress. If static friction is high, it may impart high shear stresses to the subcutaneous tissue interfaces.

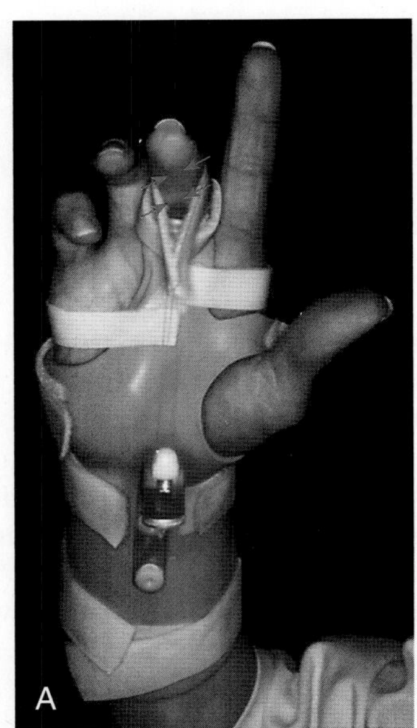

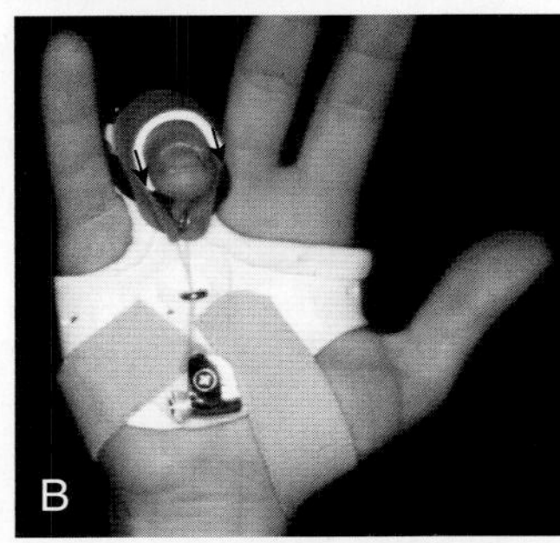

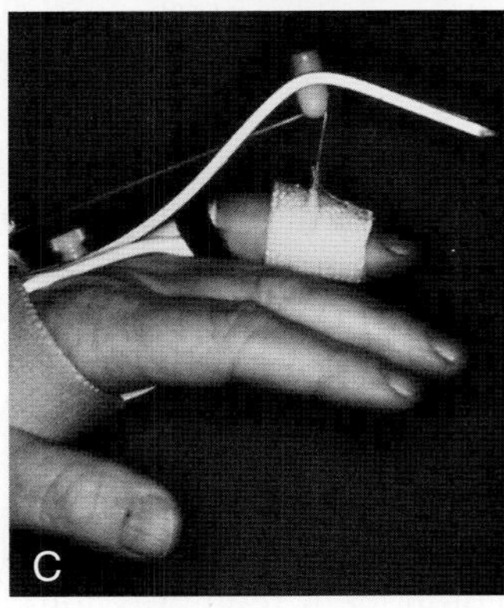

Figure 4–17 ***A,*** *A forearm-based PIP flexion mobilization splint with one monofilament line converging at the volar aspect of the digit creates compressive stress along the dorsum and lateral aspect of the digit.* ***B,*** *A hand-based PIP flexion mobilization splint with a sling over a digital cuff to decrease compression by lifting the sling borders off the middle phalanx.* ***C,*** *Circumferential slings constructed with QuickCast can maximize surface area.*

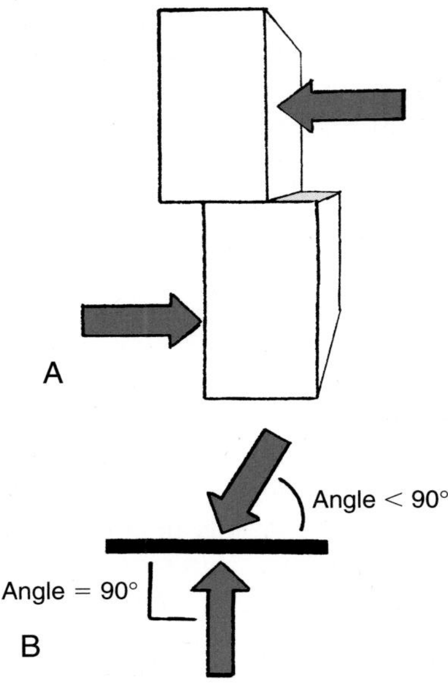

Figure 4–18 *Shear stress results force being applied parallel to the surface and can occur when two parallel opposing forces are applied in the same plane (coplanar) but not along the same line (noncollinear)* ***(A)*** *and when two oblique opposing forces share the same point of application but are neither parallel nor perpendicular* ***(B)****.*

For example, ineffective strapping on a posterior elbow immobilization splint may quickly lead to noncompliance because of discomfort. If 1" traditional loop straps (instead of conforming soft or elasticized straps) are applied in an oblique fashion to secure the anterior elbow into the splint, the loop strap edges are likely to rub along the skin. Rather than applying a direct compressive stress (i.e., perpendicular), the straps impart an oblique compressive stress and produce shear stress in the tissues over which they traverse (especially in the presence of high static friction) (Fig. 4–19). In such cases, the therapist should consider using soft, conforming 2" straps (e.g., made from Neoprene, Betapile, or Velfoam) or a circumferential wrap that is applied along the entire length of the splint for even compression.

Clinical Considerations

The therapist should use care to smooth out, roll, and/or flare uneven or sharp splint edges. This is especially important near joint creases where movement will occur (e.g., the volar distal portion of a wrist immobilization splint where the MP joints are free to move).

When using circumferential bandages or wraps to assist in the molding of a splint (e.g., when a second set of hands is needed), the therapist should avoid applying them too tightly. During the wrapping process, splint borders may inevitably be pushed in toward the body part. This makes it difficult to smooth the borders away from the skin and may cause shear stress along the entire length of the splint–skin interface (Fig. 4–20).

When fabricating a mobilization splint, the therapist must consider both compression and shear stresses. Mobilizing forces, which are attached to the proximal splint base, usually traverse the length of the splint and terminate distally to the intended joint(s). If the proximal base of the splint is not adequately secured to the limb, motion at the distal joints will result in an undesirable migration or dragging and shearing of the proximal base over the skin. The amount of shear stress depends on the coefficient of friction of the materials used and the direction and amount of force necessary to make the change at the intended joint(s) (Fig. 4–21).

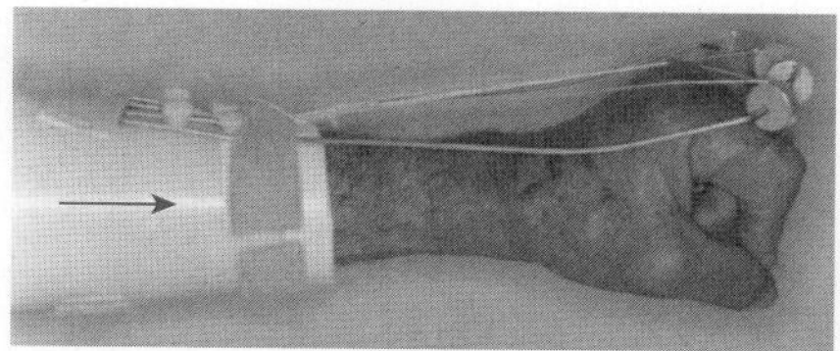

Figure 4–21 Mobilizing forces terminate at the distal end of this radial nerve splint, increasing shear stress proximally. The mobilizing force drags the splint base distally. If the splint is not adequately secured, the base will translate distally.

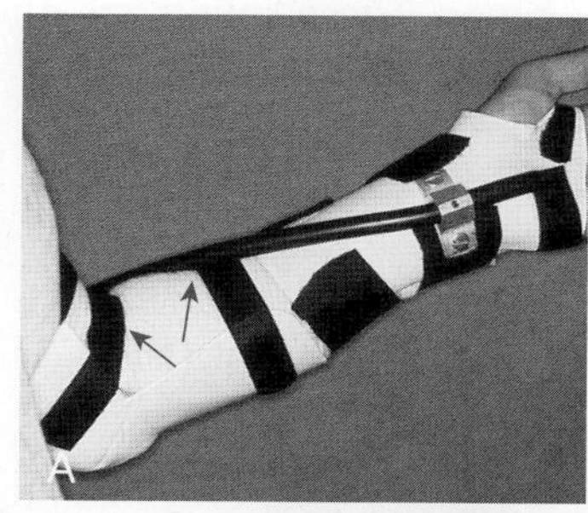

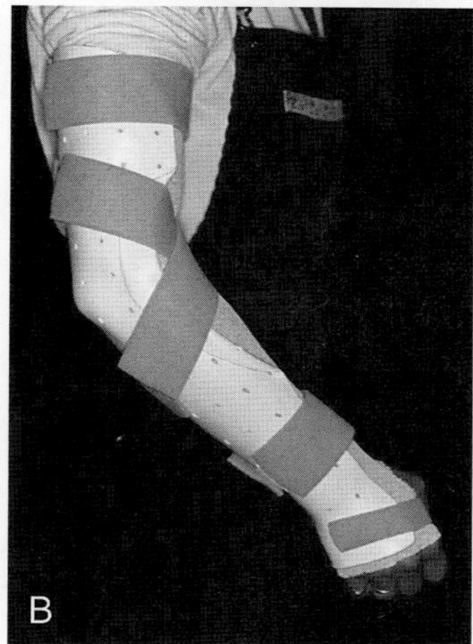

*Figure 4–19 **A,** The 1" straps, placed just proximal and distal to the elbow crease, place high shear and compression stress to the tissue beneath. **B,** Conforming, soft 2" straps better distribute the force and improve patient comfort.*

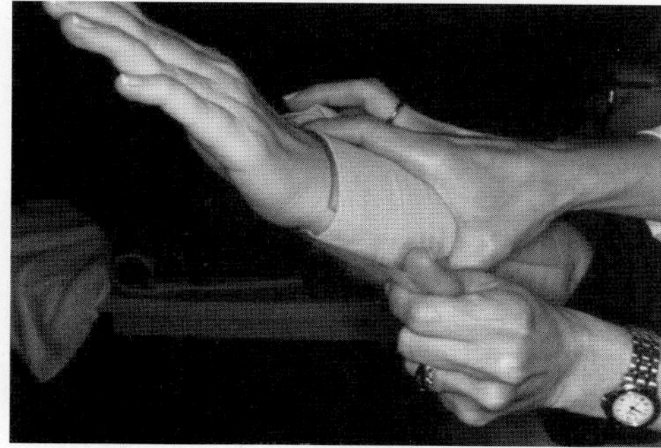

Figure 4–20 Use caution when applying an Ace wrap to secure a splint while molding. The wrap can cause shear at the borders if not applied carefully; this can be avoided by leaving a small piece of thermoplastic material outside the wrap so that it will not be pushed in by the bandage. Wrap the splint lightly and uniformly.

The therapeutic effect of a mobilization splint is to increase the range of motion, thereby causing the angle of application to shift from 90° (Fig. 4–8E). Alterations in the angle of application through a sling can create an uneven pull, resulting in shear stress proximally on the splint base and distally on the sling. The patient may cease to use the splint because of discomfort. When tissue is changing rapidly owing to mobilization splinting, the patient should visit the clinic frequently so the therapist can adequately monitor the splint line and adjust it as necessary to ensure a 90° angle of force application. Commercially available outriggers make adjustment simple.

Splint bases must be fabricated to the correct length and circumference. The proximal splint border of a short forearm-based splint is likely to pivot on the volar aspect of the forearm (because of attempted distal movement by the patient), causing shear stress at the proximal splint border and irritation of the superficial sensory nerves and skin (Fig. 4–22).

Tensile

Tensile stress is opposite in nature to compressive stress and is the result of opposing loads pulling away from a surface along the same line of application (Fig. 4–23). Tensile stress, also referred to as tension and distraction, results in stretching, as evidenced by the lengthening and narrowing of an object to which is applied. As is true with compression, tensile stress is the greatest when the force is applied perpendicular to the surface. Thus to optimize the effect of tensile stress, the pulling force should be applied at a 90° orientation to the target surface.

Clinical Considerations

When splinting to gain thumb abduction, the therapist may find it challenging to optimize tensile stress. Force applied to the proximal phalanx does not deliver tensile stress to the tight first dorsal interossei or to the adductor pollicis (thumb web); rather it produces excessive stress at the ulnar collateral ligament of the thumb MP joint. The therapist should take care when fabricating a

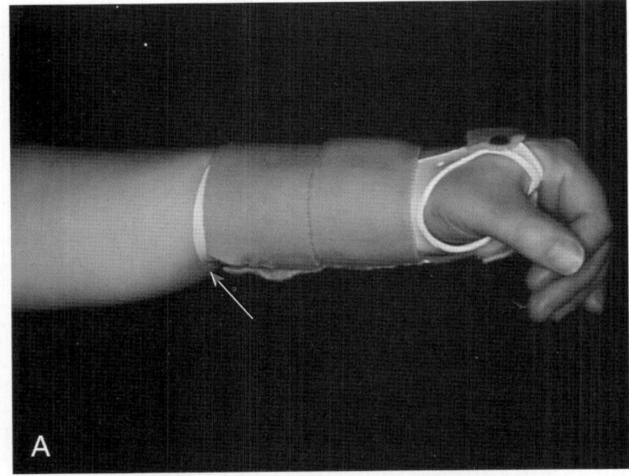

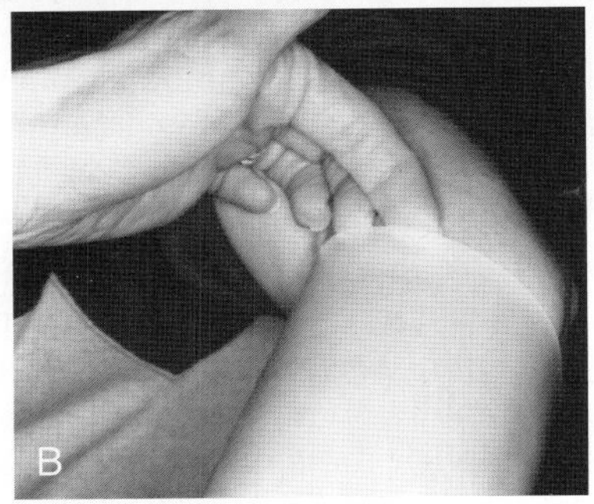

Figure 4–22 ***A,*** *The proximal border of this short forearm-based splint is pivoting on the volar aspect of the forearm and digging into the skin.* ***B,*** *The proximal borders should be flared away from the skin as they are cooling during the fabrication process.*

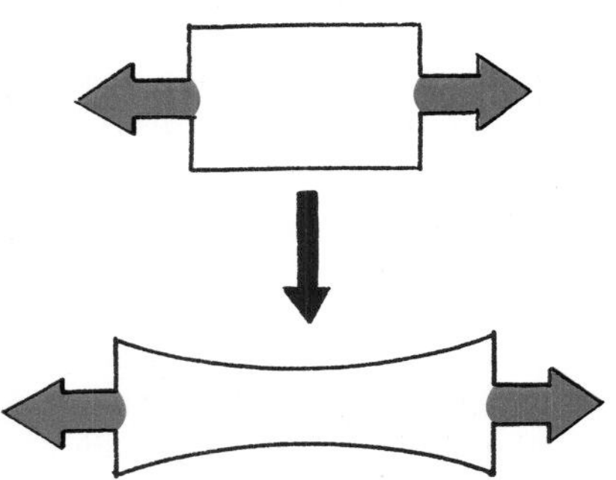

Figure 4–23 *Tensile stress results from opposing forces pulling away from a surface along the same line of application. It is also referred to as tension, distraction, and stretching.*

splint that delivers tensile stress directly to the distal aspect of the first metacarpal. The sling should conform around the head of the first metacarpal (which may cause discomfort in the web space if not molded well), and the angle of application should be directed 90° from the long axis of the first metacarpal (Fig. 4–24).

Tensile stress can be used to maintain reduction of an intra-articular fracture while preserving joint mobility. The application of a gentle traction force to a healing intra-articular fracture site can help maintain bone alignment, facilitate healing, and preserve joint range of motion. An example is the circular traction PIP intra-articular mobilization splint designed by Schenck (1986) (see Fig. 1–17). The surgeon places a wire horizontally through the bone proximal to the fracture site, leaving the ends of the wire protruding. The wire is bent to place rubber bands or springs, which are then attached to a hoop extending from the splint base. Tensile stress is then delivered from the wire to the hoop via the rubber band or spring. The hoop allows for segmental changes in range of motion while maintaining consistent stress throughout the range. These splints are often fabricated during the immediate postoperative period (Fig. 4–25).

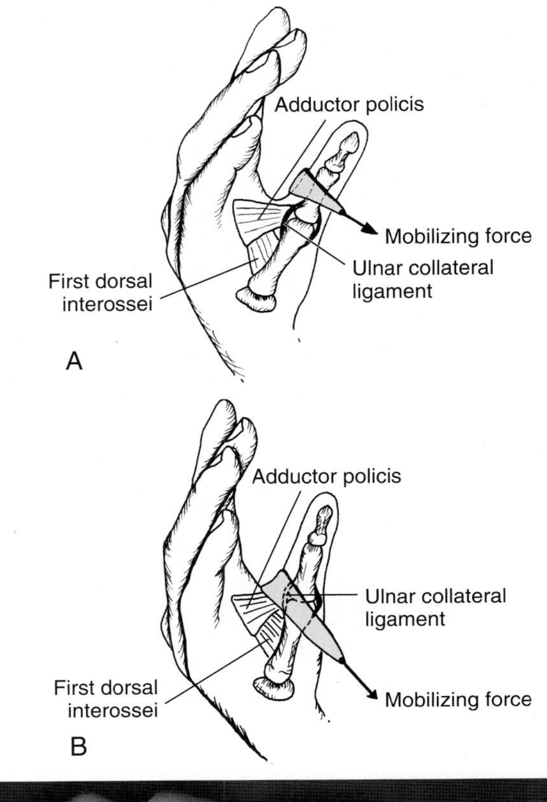

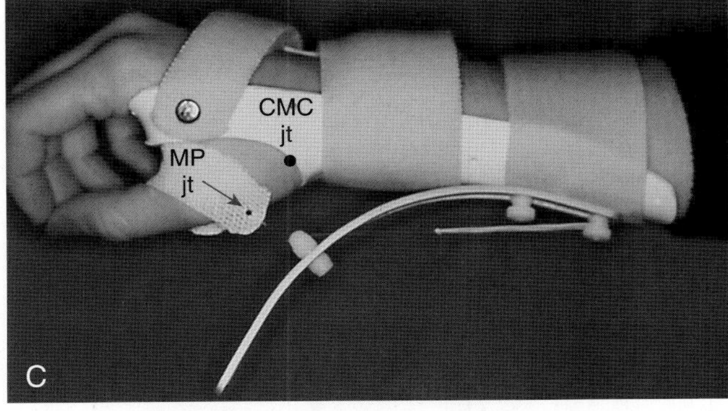

Figure 4–24 ***A,*** *An incorrectly applied thumb sling stressed the ulnar collateral ligament at the thumb MP joint.* ***B,*** *A correctly applied thumb sling mobilizes the first dorsal interossei and the adductor pollicis muscles.* ***C,*** *A QuickCast sling was molded to orient stress to the distal portion of the first metacarpal instead of the ulnar collateral ligament.*

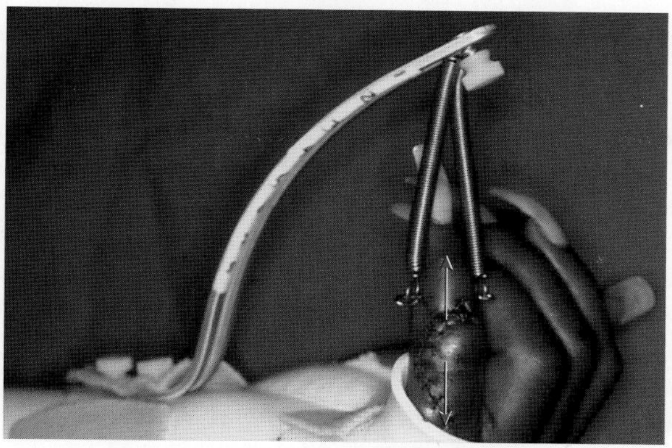

Figure 4–25 *Variation of a PIP intra-articular splint. Note the perpendicular line of application via the spring coils attached to a surgically placed horizontal wire through the middle phalanx. Gentle tension is applied to the PIP joint, maintaining ligament length and bone alignment while providing supervised periods of limited joint range of motion.*

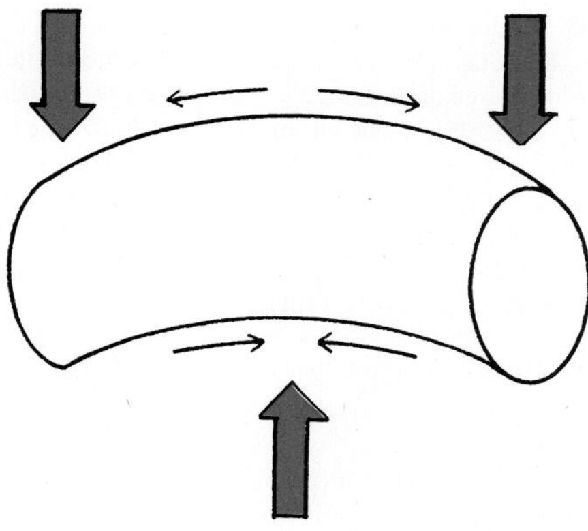

Figure 4–26 *Bending is the application of force in such a manner that the object simultaneously undergoes tension, compression, and shear as it bends about a transverse axis.*

Bending and Torsion

Compression, shear, and tensile stresses can be present in two particular combinations. **Bending** is the application of loads to a structure in such a manner that the object simultaneously undergoes tension, compression, and shear as it bends about a transverse axis (Fig. 4–26). Compression develops on the concave aspect of the structure, and tension forms across the convex aspect. In addition, shear stress develops as a result of the opposing parallel forces producing the bending (LeVeau, 1992). The bending stress is directly proportional to both the magnitude of the force and the distance from the transverse axis at which it is applied.

Torsion is stress produced when a rotational force is applied to a rod or cylinder, causing a portion of the structure to turn around the longitudinal axis (Fig. 4–27) (Nordin & Frankel, 19??). Torsion, also referred to as twisting, is directly proportional to the distance from the longitudinal to the point of application of the force. To generate greater torsion, apply the force farther from the axis about which the intended twisting will occur. Torsion results in the simultaneous generation of compression, tension, and shear forces.

Clinical Considerations

BENDING

A clinical example of the effects of bending stress is when a therapist attempts to elongate an elbow extension contracture by using an elbow flexion mobilization splint. The therapist must appreciate the tensile stress present along the posterior aspect of the elbow while compression stress is applied to the soft tissue structures along the anterior aspect of the elbow (Fig. 4–28). Shear stress simultaneously may occur at the skin–splint interface of both the humeral and forearm cuffs owing to splint migration. The force applied through the splint attempts to mobilize the distal segment (forearm cuff) in the direction of elbow flexion. In doing so, the proximal segment tends to migrate distally, while the distal segment migrates proximally. This shifting of the splint can cause shear stress along the splint–skin interface.

TORSION

The concept of torsion stress is demonstrated by a supination–pronation mobilization splint used to gain forearm rotation. To appreciate this concept, the therapist must first understand that forearm rotation is created by the simultaneous effort of both the proximal and the distal radioulnar joints. The nature of this splint design imparts a torsion stress along the entire length of the forearm, which is considered the axis of rotation. Therefore, the principles of adequate splint length, pressure distribution, and precise splint molding along the entire forearm are critical for the construction of these splints (Fig. 4–29). The potential pressure points include the proximal and distal ends of the splint where the force originates and terminates (elbow and wrist joints). With this splint, compression and shear stresses and distal migration (the result of a linear force) are inevitably present at the splint–skin interface during force application. The effectiveness of this type of splint depends on proper splint fit, which requires careful monitoring by the therapist along with education of the patient.

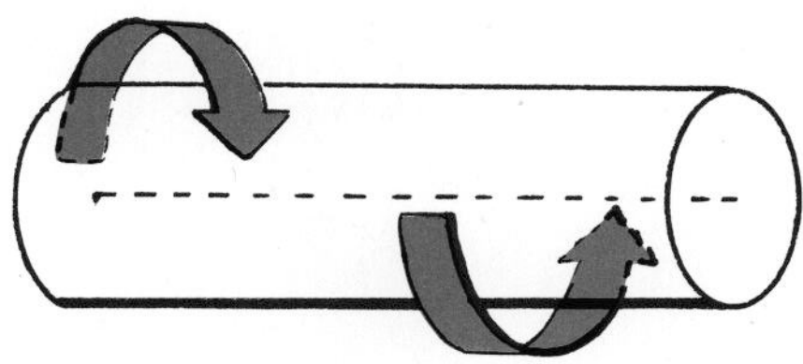

Figure 4–27 *Torsion stress, or twisting, is produced when a rotational force is applied to a rod or cylinder, causing a portion of the structure to turn around the longitudinal axis.*

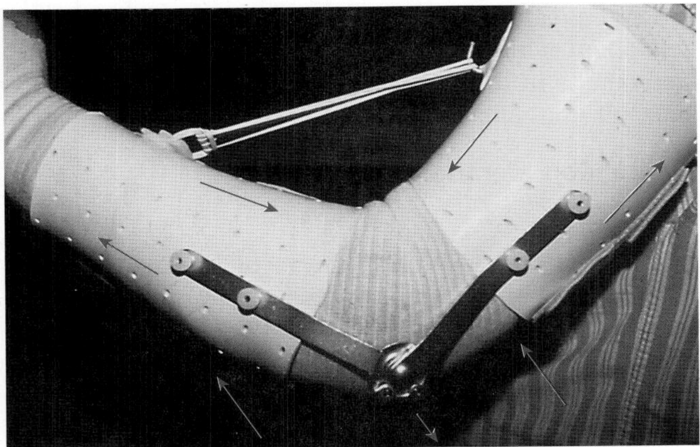

Figure 4–28 An elbow flexion mobilization splint uses bending stress to increase elbow flexion.

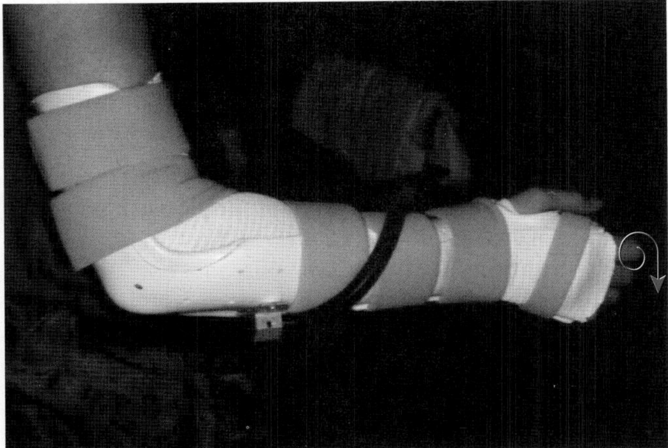

Figure 4–29 A forearm supination–pronation mobilization splint uses torsion stress to increase the supination of the forearm.

CONCLUSION

Splinting enhances or restores function of the extremity via the intentional application of external loads to manipulate the internal reaction forces of specific anatomic structures. This chapter defined and clarified the fundamental mechanical terms and concepts pertaining to the design and fabrication of splints. In addition, the clinical relevance of these terms and concepts were discussed in light of specific clinical application. The effective therapist successfully integrates basic mechanical concepts into all facets of splint design and fabrication.

REFERENCES

Bell-Krotoski, J. A., & Figarola, J. H. (1995). Biomechanics of soft tissue growth and remodeling with plaster casting. *Journal of Hand Therapy, 6,* 131–137.

Brand, P. W., & Hollister, A. (1993). *Clinical mechanics of the hand* (2nd ed.). St. Louis: Mosby.

Flowers, K. R., & LaStayo, P. (1994). Effect of total end range time on improving passive range of motion. *Journal of Hand Therapy, 7,* 150–157.

Giurintano, D. J. (1995). Basic biomechanics. *Journal of Hand Therapy, 8,* 79–84.

LeVeau, B. F. (1992). *Biomechanics of human motion* (3rd ed.). Philadelphia: Saunders.

Nordin, M., & Frankel, V.H. (2001). Basic biomechanics of the musculoskeletal system (3rd ed.). Philadelphia: Lippincott Williams & Wilkins.

Schenck, R. R. (1986). Dynamic traction and early passive movement for fractures of the proximal interphalangeal joint. *Journal of Hand Surgery, 1A,* 850–858.

Soderberg, G. L. (1986) *Kinesiology: Application to pathological motion.* Baltimore: Williams & Wilkins.

SUGGESTED READING

Fess, E. E. (1995). Splints: mechanics versus convention. *Journal of Hand Therapy, 8,* 124–130.

Fess, E. E., & Philips, C. A. (1987). *Hand splinting: Principles and methods* (2nd ed.). St. Louis: Mosby.

Gyovai, J. E., & Wright Howell, J. (1992). Validation of spring forces applied in dynamic outrigger splinting. *Journal of Hand Therapy, 7,* 8–15.

CHAPTER 5

Equipment and Materials

Noelle M. Austin, MS, PT, CHT

INTRODUCTION

This chapter presents the fundamentals of splinting, including reviews of the equipment and materials needed to create splints effectively and efficiently. With today's rising health care costs, it has become increasingly important to be economical. Thus therapists have been forced to change the way they buy and use rehabilitation products. They must educate themselves about what is available and ask sales representatives to conduct inservices to present new products. Such measures can help therapists make more fiscally prudent decisions. If therapists take the time to research a particular item, they will usually be able to find a lower cost or less-expensive substitute. The constant innovation in splinting techniques and methods has spurred the need for consumers to be discriminating when purchasing products. Experimenting with new materials and providing feedback to vendors can promote positive changes in the available rehabilitation materials.

Before fabricating a splint, the therapist must be sure to have the necessary equipment, tools, materials, and accessories readily accessible. These products can be purchased from rehabilitation vendors (see Appendix A for contact information). To provide patients with the best splinting options, therapists must be aware of what is currently available. Therapists should be familiar with the major rehabilitation catalogs and should spend some time in local hardware and hobby stores. When attending continuing education courses, therapists should visit vendors' booths and make an effort to obtain hands-on experience with new or unfamiliar products; these measures increase the therapists' comfort with using rehabilitation materials. Note that each vendor has its own version of common rehabilitation items and mobilization component kits.

Essential Equipment

This section discusses the equipment needed to fabricate upper extremity splints effectively. In Section II, "Clinical Pearls" provide detailed information and helpful hints on how to use specific products and offer alternative and cost-effective techniques.

Heating Sources

Thermoplastic materials need to be heated to a soften condition before they can be molded to the body part. Splint pans and heat guns provide the means to warm the material for splint fabrication.

Splint Pans

Ideally, **splint pans** are used to heat materials; however, if they are not available, hot pack heaters or electric frying pans will suffice. Although hot pack heaters are readily available in most clinics, their use includes the following disadvantages: inability to control water temperature, difficult to remove materials without overstretching (especially if attempted in a vertical manner), and possibility of contamination from dirty water.

Splint pans are available in several sizes, ranging from a pan that is large enough to accommodate big pieces of splint material to a small household electric frying pan

(Fig. 5–1). Each type of splinting material must be heated to a specific temperature per the manufacturer's specifications to take advantage of that material's specific properties. The water temperature should be adjusted accordingly. Some of the newer pan designs have thermal regulators, a thermometer can also be used to check the temperature before heating the material. Be aware that, owing to the location of the heating coils, materials may be heated unevenly when using a splint pan. This can be avoided by moving the material around the pan during the heating process.

There are a number of ways to prevent splint material from sticking to the bottom and sides of the pan, including the addition of a drop of liquid hand soap, dish washing liquid, or lotion to the water. Another trick is to employ the use of splint pan netting. Not only does this stop material from sticking to the pan but it also protects the hands from being burned, prevents the overstretching of softened materials, and eases the task of removing the heated material from the water. Remember that netting may leave an imprint in the plastic material. An alternative is to layer the bottom of the pan with paper towels. Spatulas help when removing heated material from the pan and prevent imprints in the material. Consider adding a liquid disinfectant when changing the splint water to prevent contamination.

Heat Guns

Heat guns are a source of dry heat that can be used to spot warm specific areas of thermoplastic material. Special nozzles are available to direct the heat to a small area, preventing the overheating of the adjacent regions of the splint. Minor changes in splint contour and edge finishing can be accomplished with a heat gun. Care must be taken when using this device to adjust a splint, inadvertent overheating of adjacent regions can cause irregular surfaces and the loss of contour or fit of the splint.

The heat gun can be used to prepare the surface of the thermoplastic material for bonding, as when applying components such as outriggers. These guns are particularly useful when heating components before applying them to the splint (Fig. 5–2). In addition, heating self-adhesive hook can ensure that it will be adequately attached to the splint.

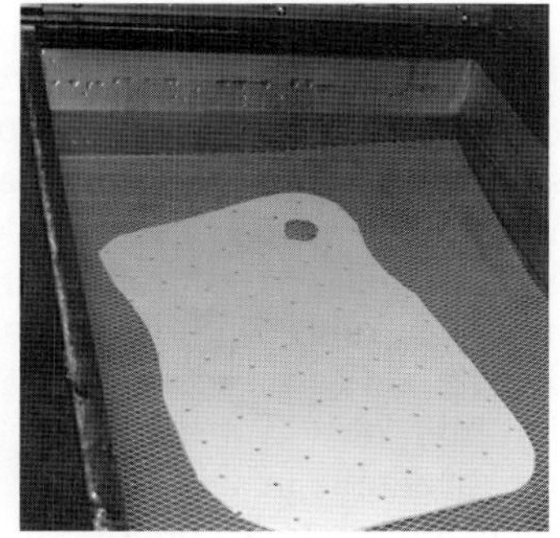

Figure 5–1 *A large splint pan.*

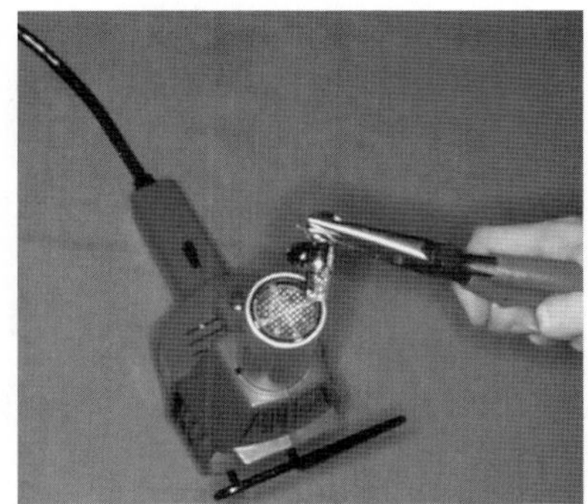

Figure 5–2 *A heat gun and needle-nose pliers are used to prepare a MERiT component for attachment onto a splint base.*

Splinting Tools

It is extremely important to use high-quality tools when splinting. Using tools that are not appropriate for the specific task can be frustrating and ineffective, making the fabrication process more difficult than otherwise. In the long run, an initial investment in quality products saves time and money. Well-maintained tools help avoid the need for replacement tools and guard the therapist against developing a repetitive stress injury.

In addition to cutting devices, other mandatory tools include pliers, hole punches, hand drills, and wire cutters and benders. Many other tools can assist in making the splinting process easier. The therapist should read through rehabilitation catalogs to learn about these tools and how they are used in the fabrication process.

Cutting Devices

Splint materials are available in large sheets, which need to be cut into specific shapes or patterns for a particular design. Many types of cutting devices are found in manufacturers' catalogs. When cutting unheated materials, use a utility knife or heavy-duty shears or snips. Some distributors offer time-saving precut thermoplastic materials, eliminating the need to cut up large sheets; some of these materials are ready to be warmed in the water and molded onto the body part.

Using dull, improperly chosen **scissors** to cut out splint patterns from warmed material can be frustrating. Invest in a quality pair of scissors (e.g., Gingher) that are comfortable to use (Fig. 5–3). Designating a "splint-material only" pair of scissors can help prevent adhesive from sticking to the blades, which causes the warm splint material to stick to the scissors' blades. Assign the use of other, less-expensive scissors for cutting adhesive-backed materials, such as hook, lining, and padding. Adhesive can be removed from the blades with splinting solvent, rubbing alcohol, or nail polish remover. It is necessary to sharpen the blades frequently to maintain sharp, smooth edges; ask a local fabric or craft store about sharpening services. Furthermore sharp blades may help protect the therapist from developing overuse syndromes, which may result from making the repetitive, forceful strokes needed to operate dull scissors.

When cutting with scissors, practice using *smooth, long strokes* rather than short snips, which cause multiple irregular sharp edges and lead to an uncomfortable, unsightly splint. All borders and corners should be smooth and slightly rounded to maximize patient comfort, provide an aesthetically pleasing result, and add strength and rigidity to the splint.

Other scissors may be useful in the clinic. Bandage scissors, which remove surgical or wound dressings, have a protective blunt tip to prevent injury to the patient. Small bandage or cast scissors, designed to remove casts, are essential when using serial casting techniques (Fig. 5–4). They provide a safe way to remove a finger cast effectively and without cutting the digit. Self-opening spring-loaded scissors decrease the stress placed on the therapist's joints.

Pliers

Pliers are important for a variety of splinting tasks, including bending wire for outriggers, embedding small components such as eyelets into warm splint material, setting speedy rivets in place, and holding components or adhesive hooks when using a heat gun. Various types of pliers are available in a range of styles and sizes, although the most common are blunt- and needle-nose pliers (Fig. 5–2). It is essential to have both types on hand in the clinic to manipulate a variety of splinting components.

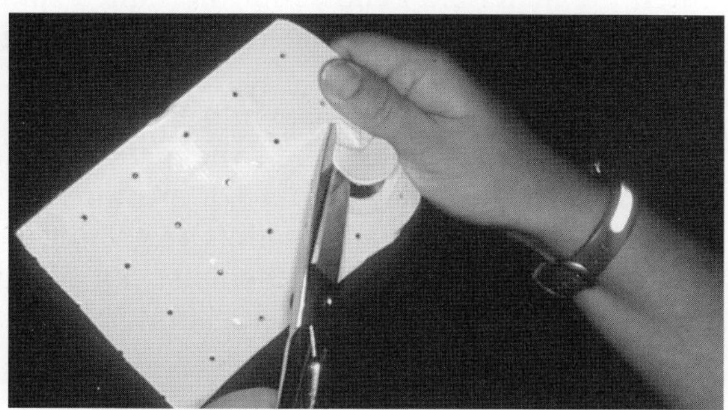

Figure 5–3 *To obtain a smooth cut edge, the scissors should be sharp and the material should be warm.*

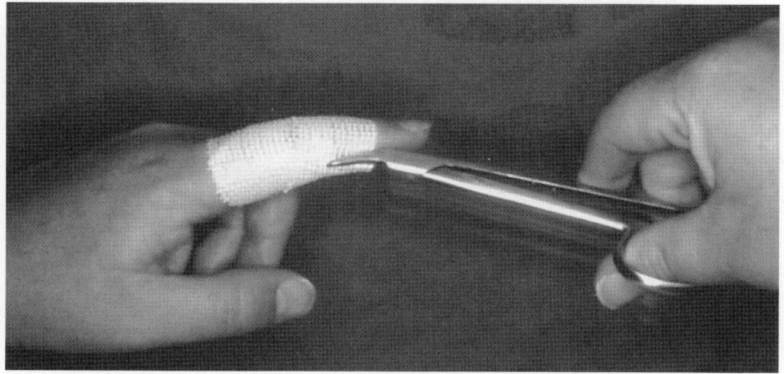

Figure 5–4 *A splint/cast trimmer is used to remove a serial static finger cast.*

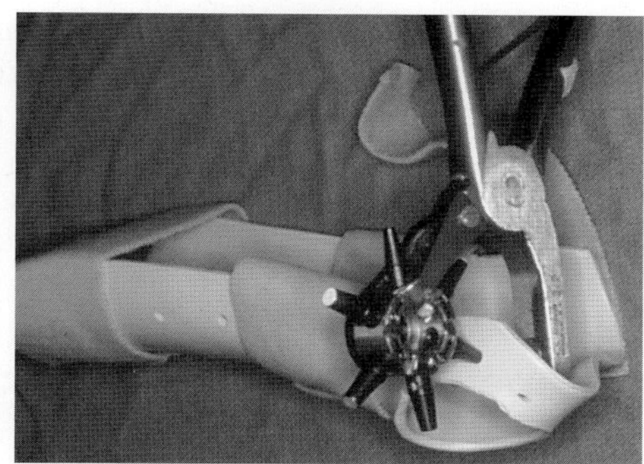

Figure 5–5 *A hole punch is needed to prepare material for a rivet.*

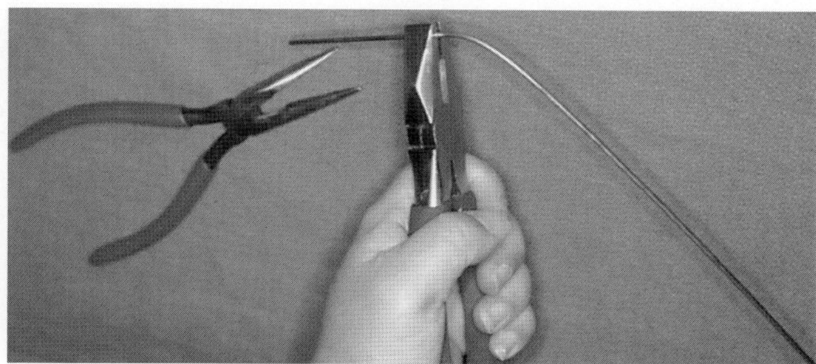

Figure 5–6 *Blunt-nose pliers help bend wires to create homemade outriggers.*

Hole Punches

A high-quality **hole punch** with a range of hole sizes is necessary for adding holes to soft materials for strapping or finger loops/slings and to hard thermoplastic materials for straps, outriggers, and hinge components (Fig. 5–5). When the tubes on the tool grow dull, it becomes difficult to punch a hole; therefore, it is wise to buy a heavy-duty tool with replaceable tubes.

Hand Drills

Hand drills are used to make holes in a splint in locations that the hole punch cannot reach, such as applying an elbow hinge to a humeral and/or forearm cuff. The drill can also be used to add perforations to specific regions of a splint, which help prevent skin maceration or rash caused by excess perspiration.

Wire Cutters and Benders

Wire cutters and **benders** provide a way to customize an outrigger for specific anatomic requirements (Fig. 5–6). When component kits are not available or appropriate for a patient, the therapist must fabricate the splint from scratch, using outrigger wire and ingenuity to create the desired effect. By bending the wire, the therapist can create a customized splint to accommodate a difficult anatomic configuration or situation, for example, splinting over postsurgical dressings, wounds, casts, or external pins or fixators.

Low-Temperature Thermoplastic Splinting Materials

Numerous types of **low-temperature thermoplastic splinting materials** are available through rehabilitation vendors (Alimed, Inc., 2000; DeRoyal/LMD, 1997; North Coast Medical, Inc., 2001; Sammons Preston, 2000; Smith + Nephew, Inc., 2001; see Appendix A for contact information). Many therapists are justifiably confused about how to choose the right material for a specific splint. Unfortunately, there is no easy answer. Therapists must use their clinical knowledge and experience when making these decisions.

A single type of material is not suitable for all splints or for all patients; there are many factors that must be taken into account when it comes to selecting the appropriate material. Therapists must recognize each material's unique characteristics (e.g., conformability and resistance to stretch) and understand the desired function of the splint in terms of the required rigidity and ventilation. In addition, they need to appreciate the particular nuances of each patient in terms of diagnosis, compliance, and age as well as recognize the limitation of their own splinting skills and experience.

The beginning splinter should develop a comfort level with a few types of materials before venturing on to others. The more experienced splinter who is comfortable using only a few types of materials, however, should broaden his or her selection choices by experimenting with other available materials. Expanding one's splinting options ultimately benefits the patients. Remember, however, that material selection may also be limited by other factors, including availability, budgetary constraints, and physician preferences.

To help the therapist begin to understand the multitude of splint material options, the following sections introduce the terms used to describe the materials' characteristics (e.g., drapability and resistance to stretch). Later sections discuss the general categories of splint materials (e.g., plastic and rubber-like). Specific brand-name materials are not examined in depth because the availability of materials often changes; refer to manufacturers' catalogs for current availability. If the therapist understands the particular characteristics and general categories of splinting materials, he or she should be able to select the correct one from almost any catalog.

Unfortunately, there is little agreement among the material manufacturers, the distributors, and the therapists in terms of nomenclature. For example, some distributors describe a material's conformability, whereas others label this same factor as drape or moldablility. This can be confusing for a therapist who is trying to decide which material to use. The following sections simplify the nomenclature as much as possible and present broad concepts and key points to aid the selection of a particular splint material.

Handling Characteristics

Comformability and Resistance to Stretch

To meet the requirements of a specific patient, the therapist must choose a material with the correct conformability and resistance to stretch. **Conformability** or **drape** is the degree to which a heated material is able to mold well and produce an intimate fit that encompasses the contours and irregularities of the splinted part (North Coast Medical, Inc.; Smith + Nephew, Inc.). **Resistance to stretch** is the degree to which a heated material is able to counteract being stretched or pulled (North Coast Medical, Inc.; Smith + Nephew, Inc.). Resistance to stretch is generally inversely related to the degree of conformability (Breger Lee & Buford, 1992).

HIGH CONFORMABILITY/LOW RESISTANCE TO STRETCH

- Requires only light handling during the molding process to achieve a precisely formed splint.
- Best used when gravity can assist in the splinting process (Fig. 5–7).
- Often the material of choice for the skilled splinter, because little handling is needed during the molding process.
- Recommended when the patient is best approached with minimal handling (e.g., the patient who is postsurgical, extremely painful, or arthritic.
- Recommended for smaller splints (e.g., finger and hand supports) because the therapist can achieve a precise fit, maximizing patient comfort and preventing splint migration.

LOW CONFORMABILITY/HIGH RESISTANCE TO STRETCH

- Requires firm handling during the molding process to obtain a well-conformed splint.

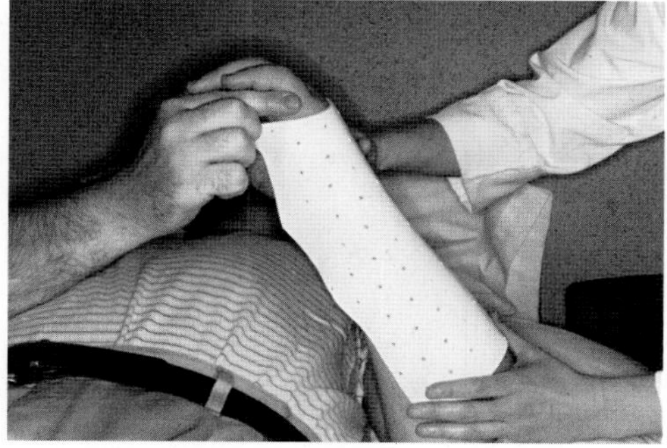

Figure 5–7 A forearm-based ulnar wrist splint is molded with the assistance of gravity.

- Can be used when the splint cannot be formed with the assistance of gravity.
- Comfortable for the novice splinter, who may feel more in control with a hands-on approach.
- Circumferential wraps may be used to aid in the molding process when splinting without an assistant, molding against gravity, or splinting a large area. Wrapping too tightly may cause the splint borders to dig and results in skin irritation. (Fig 5–8)
- Recommended for larger splints (e.g., forearm, elbow, and shoulder) for which an intimate fit is not crucial and a greater degree of control may be needed.

Memory

Memory is the degree to which a material is able to return to its original shape once molded and then reheated (DeRoyal/LMB; North Coast Medical, Inc.; Sammons Preston; Smith + Nephew, Inc.). This quality ranges from 100 to 0% (no) memory.

HIGH-MEMORY MATERIAL

- Recommended when fabricating a splint that will require frequent remolding (e.g., a serial static splint); once the material is reheated, it tends to return to the shape of the original pattern.
- Cost-efficient to remold an existing splint instead of making a new splint to accommodate for each change in tissue status.
- Recommended for novice splinters; they can place the material back in the water and start over if a mistake is made during the molding process.
- Do not remove the molded splint from the body part until it is completely set, or it will return to its original shape. This may alter the final fit of the splint, which is especially consequential when the material is wrapped circumferentially, as in a thumb immobilization splint. If the material is removed too soon, the patient may not be able to don the splint after setting is complete.
- Be careful when using a heat gun for spot heating; ridges can form, which may adversely effect the comfort and fit of the splint.

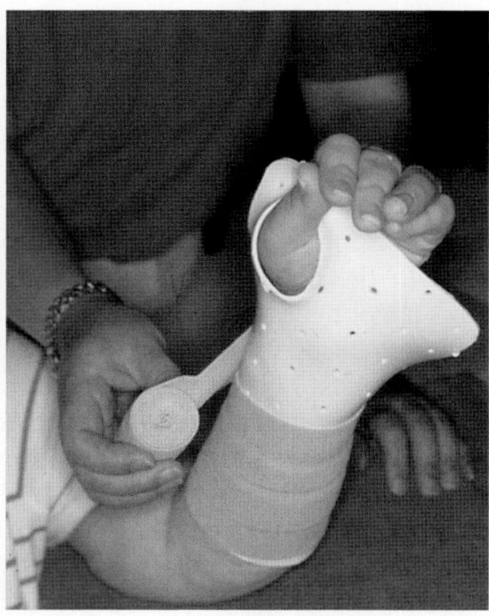

Figure 5–8 *A forearm-based wrist splint is molded with a proximal wrap to allow hands-on positioning distally.*

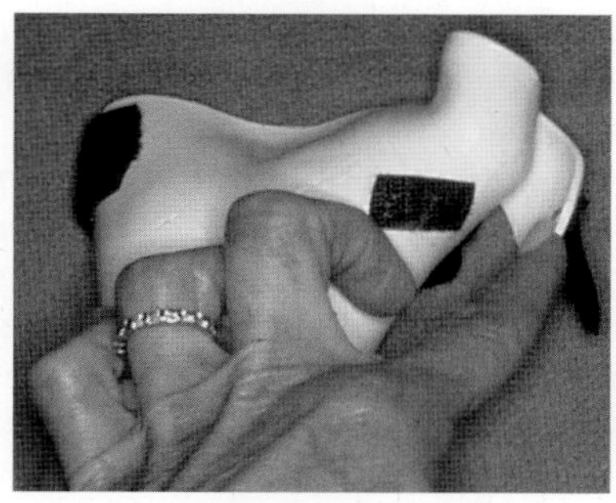

Figure 5–9 *Coated material allows overlapped pieces to pop open, which can accommodate, e.g., an enlarged thumb IP joint.*

Rigidity

Rigidity is the ultimate stiffness or strength of a material or the degree to which a molded splint is able to resist deformation when external forces are applied (DeRoyal/LMB; North Coast Medical, Inc.). This quality ranges from highly rigid to highly flexible.

- High-rigidity materials are recommended when the potential forces placed on the splint will be significant (e.g., a hand splint for a construction worker who applies excessive force to the hands).
- Thicker materials ($^1/_8$") are more rigid than thinner materials ($^1/_{16}$").
- Overstretching during the fabrication process, creates weakened areas in the splint, which may decrease rigidity.
- Specific diagnoses (e.g., metacarpal fractures) require more rigid materials to support the healing structures.
- A circumferential design provides a more rigid support than a volar or dorsal approach, even if the material is thin.

Bonding

Bonding is the ability of a material to adhere to itself once heated (DeRoyal/LMB; North Coast Medical, Inc.; Smith + Nephew, Inc.).

- Coated material does not bond to itself when heated. For example, fabricating this helps with thumb immobilization splints and allows the therapist to create a trap door to ease splint removal (Fig. 5–9).
- Coated material has a reduced tendency to adhere to the patient's skin, hair, and wound dressings.
- Coated material is easier to clean than noncoated material because it is less porous; this is especially helpful for patients who require long-term splint use.

- Do not overstretch coated material; this weakens the coating bond and may allow the material to adhere to itself.
- The coating may be removed with a splint solvent or by aggressively scratching the surface if adherence to another piece of material is required.
- Uncoated material adheres to itself, which is especially helpful when attaching outriggers or when using an extra piece of material to reinforce a particular area of the splint.
- Use a stockinette liner over the dressing when molding with uncoated material to prevent sticking to dressings and superficial skin.
- When coated material is unavailable, use a wet paper towel or hand lotion between two pieces of uncoated material to prevent adherence (Fig. 5–10).

Heating and Working Times

Each material has an optimal heating temperature (ranging from 140 to 170°F), **heating time** (ranging from 0.5 to 2 minutes), and **working time** (from 1 to 7 minutes). Specific information can be found in manufacturers' catalogs (Alimed, Inc.; DeRoyal/LMB; North Coast Medical, Inc.; Sammons Preston; Smith + Nephew, Inc.) (see Appendix A). The working time refers to the time in which the heated material can be molded onto the body part before the splint sets.

- All materials should be partially heated (about 30 seconds) before the specific pattern is cut. Material is heated partially when lifting the edge with scissors or spatula reveals moderate stiffness with slight bending.
- Some materials provide a self-sealing edge for a smooth finish after being cut while warm.
- When making large splints, the novice therapist may want to hold one edge of the material while the other edge is partially heated for cutting; this allows the splinter to maintain control of the material at all times.
- Thin or highly perforated materials have a shorter working time; thick solid materials have a longer working time.

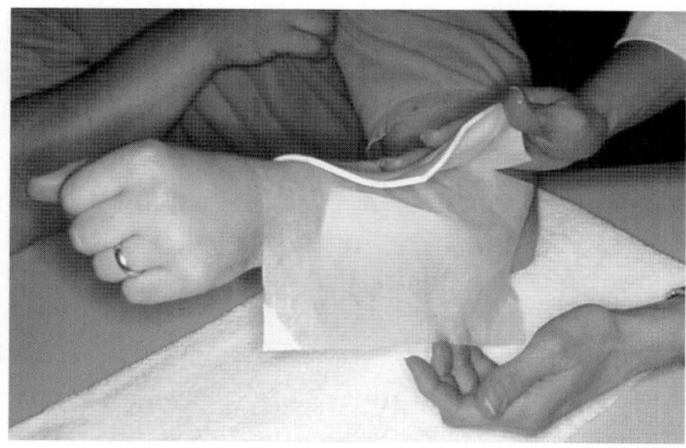

Figure 5–10 A wet paper towel placed between uncoated material prevents adherence.

- Elastic and rubber-like materials tend to have longer working times than plastic materials.
- Do not remove the splint from the body part too soon, or the splint's shape and fit may be lost.
- Materials with longer working times are recommended for complex splints requiring specific positions of immobilization, such as commonly encountered for neurologically involved patients.
- Materials with shorter working times are recommended for patients that are unable to hold a specific position for a long period (e.g., pediatric patients).
- Sometimes it is necessary to hasten the setting time (e.g., for a patient who is in pain). Note that this cannot be done with high-memory material because the final fit may be altered.
- Accelerate the cooling by wrapping the material with an elastic wrap that has been soaked in ice water or with a TheraBand that has been stored in the freezer. Note that wrapping may cause irritation if it causes the splint edges to dig into the skin.
- Accelerate the cooling by using cold spray or by removing a partially set splint and placing it under cold running water. Note that the cold spray technique may irritate the skin or eyes.
- Avoid overheating the material, which can alter its properties and lead to overstretching, thinning, and fatigue, which in turn can decrease the rigidity of the completed splint.
- Always dry off any excess water on the material.
- Before applying the material to the patient's body part, check the material's temperature against the therapist's skin.
- Be extra careful to avoid overheating or burning the skin of patients who have any sensory involvement including loss of sensation or skin hypersensitivity (commonly seen after cast removal).

Physical Characteristics

Thickness

Materials are available in several **thicknesses,** most commonly $^{1}/_{16}$", $^{3}/_{32}$", $^{1}/_{8}$", and $^{3}/_{16}$" thick (Fig. 5–11) (Alimed, Inc.; DeRoyal/LMB; North Coast Medical, Inc.; Sammons Preston; Smith + Nephew, Inc.). It is not uncommon for splinters to get in the habit of using $^{1}/_{8}$" material for all splints, but this is not necessary. The therapist may choose a specific thickness based on the splint's function. To create the lightest and least bulky splint, the therapist should choose the thinnest material possible that provides the required support. Thicker materials tend to provide more rigid support. Thinner materials offer a less bulky, lighterweight alternative. When thin materials are used for circumferential splints, they can create adequate rigidity if the therapist takes advantage of contouring. For example, circumferential forearm fracture splints may be best created with $^{3}/_{32}$" or $^{1}/_{16}$" material instead of $^{1}/_{8}$" material,

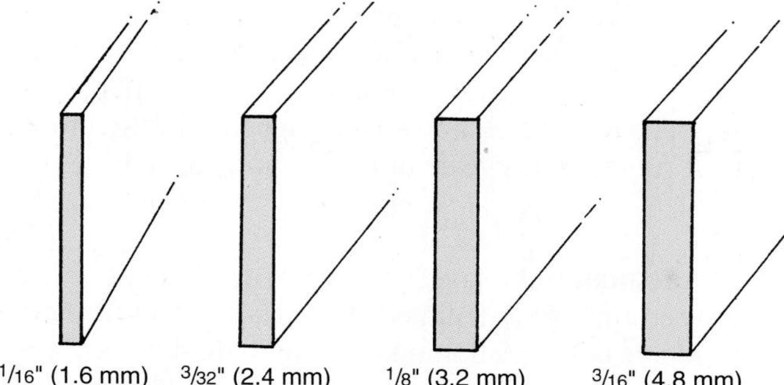

Figure 5–11 Materials of different thicknesses.

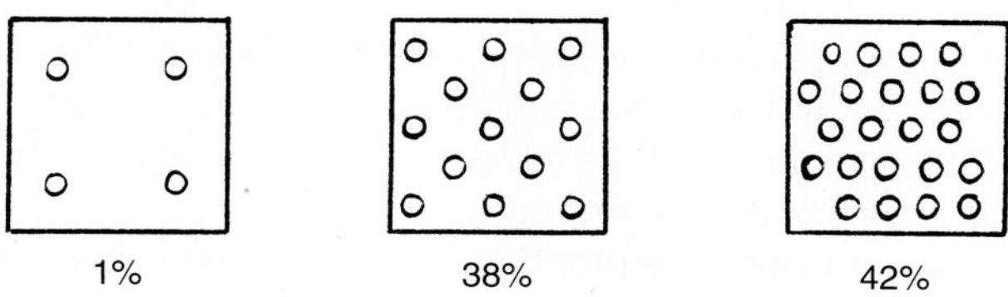

Figure 5–12 Density of perforations.

which creates a bulky splint that can impede function. Thinner materials can be cut more easily, which can decrease the strain on the therapist's hands.

Perforations

Almost all thickness and types of material are available in **perforated** and **nonperforated** forms. The density of perforations can range from 1 to 42% (Fig. 5–12) (Alimed, Inc.; DeRoyal/LMB; North Coast Medical, Inc.; Sammons Preston; Smith + Nephew, Inc.). Perforated materials allow air exchange, which helps decrease the incidence of skin problems, such as rash, excessive sweating, and/or maceration (Breger Lee & Buford, 1991, 1992).

The therapist must decide whether providing a lightweight splint with increased ventilation is worth the sacrifice in splint strength. This downside must be weighed carefully to ensure that the splint provides an adequate amount of rigidity or support. For example, a splint to support a fracture requires a more rigid support than one applied for tendinitis. In most cases a 3/32" lightly perforated material in a circumferential design can adequately support a distal radius fracture while allowing air exchange.

Because perforations help decrease the splint's weight, they can increase splint compliance. Superperforated materials may need to be edged with extra-thin material to provide a smooth, reinforced border. Do not overstretch heated perforated materials, because the holes elongate and the material may thin out unevenly (Fig. 5–13).

Colors

Splint materials are available in an assortment of **colors.** Bright colors may help maximize compliance in a young patient or aid in a quick retrieval among bed linens in a nursing home. On the other hand, some patients may feel the colors draw unwanted attention to themselves and their condition. In these cases, skin tones are the more appropriate choice. Darker colors, such as black, help hide dirt and are best worn by patients who work in an industrial environment.

Categories

The most commonly used thermoplastic materials can be categorized in and described by the following terms: plastic, rubber or rubber-like, combination plastic and rubber-like, and elastic (Sammons Preston). These groupings help the therapist keep track of each type of material and its workable characteristics.

Thermoplastic materials are traditionally sold in 18" by 24" sheets; however, some manufacturers now sell materials in easy-to-use precut forms. Precut materials can help save time and money and decrease material waste. These precut forms and blanks come in variety of material types to satisfy most splinting needs. Other options include preformed splints (prefabricated into a specific shape and size) that are offered in a range of sizes and splint material types. Once heated, most of these can be modified to provide a custom fit.

Plastic

Plastic materials are generally highly conformable and have minimal resistance to stretch (e.g., Polyform and Multiform) (Berger Lee & Buford, 1992; Alimed, Inc.; DeRoyal/LMB; North Coast Medical, Inc.; Sammons Preston; Smith + Nephew, Inc.). These materials are best used with gravity's assistance and by an experienced splinter, because the material can be challenging to control. The ability to make minor adjustments in a splint pattern by

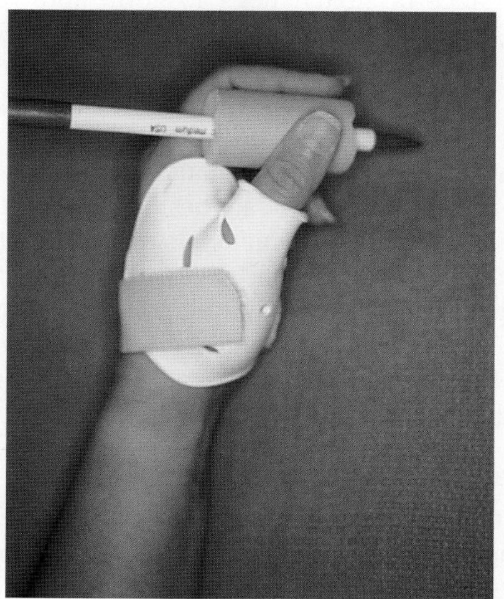

Figure 5–13 Because the material was overstretched when this thumb splint was fabricated, there is a weakened area at the ulnar MP joint.

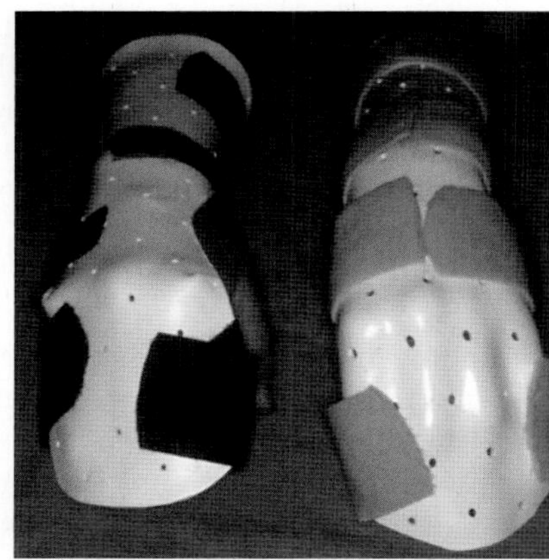

Figure 5–14 An intimate fit can be achieved with plastic materials (right); *note the detail of the contours obtained across the dorsum of the MP joints. Rubber-like materials tend to mold to the shape of the hand with less detail* (left).

stretching the material can help ensure a better fit (Fig. 5–14). Small splints requiring a well-molded precise fit are best made with these materials. Plastic materials contour nicely when splinting over pins or bony prominences.

The therapist may leave fingerprints in the material if he or she uses a too aggressive hands-on approach during the molding process. Gentle handling with smooth, light strokes is the best way to work with these materials. Overheating can make plastic materials too soft, leading to overstretching and making them difficult to control. To minimize overstretching, handle these materials horizontally on splint pan netting rather than vertically.

Rubber or Rubber-Like

Rubber or **rubber-like materials** offer a good degree of control at the expense of conformability, owing to their high resistance to stretch (e.g., Ezeform and Kay-Prene) (DeRoyal/LMB; North Coast Medical, Inc.; Sammons Preston; Smith + Nephew). These materials do not drape and contour as well as plastic materials; thus the final fit is sometimes less detailed. Larger splints that do not require an intimate fit, such as a wrist/hand immobilization splint worn over wound dressings, are best made with these materials (Fig. 5–14). Rubber materials offer a significant degree of control with minimal stretching or fingerprinting. Beginning splinters may find these materials easy to work with use because they are forgiving and tolerate repeated handling and manipulation. Cut rubber-like materials when still slightly warm to obtain extremely smooth edges.

Combination Plastic and Rubber-Like

Combination plastic and rubber-like materials tend to offer the best of both worlds in terms of conformity and stretch (e.g., NCM Preferred and LMB Blend) (DeRoyal/LMB; North Coast Medical, Inc.; Sammons Preston; Smith + Nephew). These materials produce a splint with a well-molded fit while allowing the therapist some degree of control during the molding process. Many therapists find these materials to be useful for a wide variety of splints, including forearm- and hand-based splints (large and small). The specific characteristics depend on the proportions of rubber and plastic in the thermoplastic base.

Elastic

All **elastic materials** have some amount of memory (e.g., Aquaplast and Orfit) (Alimed, Inc.; DeRoyal/LMB; North Coast Medical, Inc.; Sammons Preston; Smith + Nephew). As noted earlier, this characteristic is best used in situations in which there is a need for frequent remolding to accommodate for changes in tissue. Some of these materials are available uncoated, which allows them to adhere to the part being splinted, this may help in achieving a precise, intimate fit by acting as a second pair of hands. The degree of conformability and stretch depends on the specific material's chemical composition.

When pinched together lightly, coated elastic materials can provide a temporary bond that can be popped apart once the splint is set. This technique can be helpful when splinting without the assistance of gravity (Fig. 5–15). It is easy to determine when most elastic materials are heated fully, because they turn transparent (except for some colored elastic materials, which turn opaque). This transparency provides visualization of sites where potential irritation can occur and allows for accommodations of these hot spots during the molding process. Therapists generally deem these materials as quite versatile and use them successfully for a multitude of splints.

Elastic materials do have some disadvantages. If the molded splint is removed when the material is still slightly warm, the material will continue to set, causing further tightening or shrinking and altering the final fit. Obtaining a well-contoured splint with $\frac{1}{8}$" material may be troublesome because of the material's tendency to bounce back during its setup time. Elastic materials have a longer setup time than plastic materials and can be frustrating when time efficiency is an issue. In addition, the novice splinter may find it difficult to achieve a smooth edge with these materials.

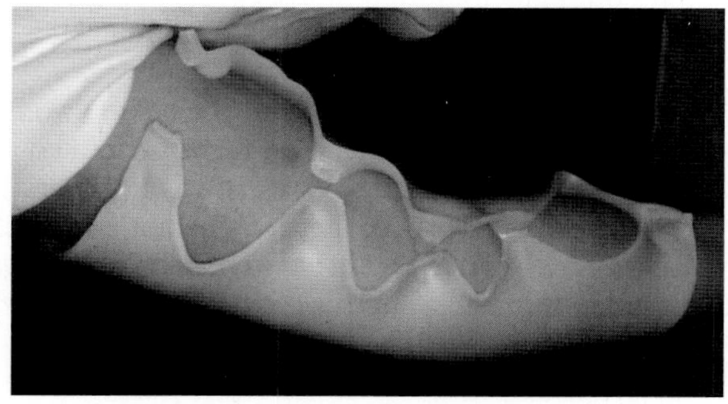

Figure 5–15 A posterior elbow immobilization splint applied with the pinch-and-pop technique. The edges will be trimmed to form smooth borders anteriorly.

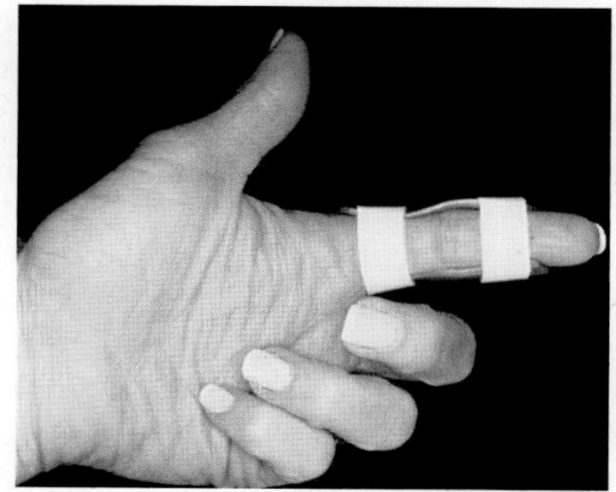

Figure 5–16 Thin loop strapping used for a finger splint.

Other

Other material choices currently available include lined materials (e.g., Gel-Cush, Orfilined), mesh-type thermoplastic materials (e.g., Hexcelite), foam materials (e.g., Plastazote) that require dry heating, and Neoprene–Lycra for soft restrictive splints (see Chapter 14 for splinting with Neoprene). Casting techniques provide an option for some forms of splinting. Casts require the use of plaster, fiberglass, or QuickCast materials (see Chapter 12 for details). Taping techniques are gaining popularity for immobilizing or restricting a joint or body part (see Chapter 13 for more information). As noted earlier, therapists must be diligent in keeping up with new materials and techniques.

Additional Equipment

Strapping Materials

The most common way to secure a splint to a body part is with **hook-and-loop straps.** Velcro is the most familiar brand name; however, other versions are available (Alimed, Inc.; DeRoyal/LMB; North Coast Medical, Inc.; Sammons Preston; Smith + Nephew, Inc.). Usually, the adhesive-backed hook strip is attached to the splint and the loop strip is wrapped around the body part. Hook-and-loop straps are available in several widths ($^1/_2$" to 2") and colors. Precut strapping is convenient, reducing waste and speeding up the fabrication process. Adhesive-backed hook strips are available in precut lengths, which can eliminate sticky scissors. Many patients, especially children, enjoy choosing their own strap colors, and involving the patient can help maximize compliance. Thin loop helps decrease the bulk when splinting a digit (Fig. 5–16). Spot heating the adhesive-backed hook before applying it to the splint increases adherence and provides a firm attachment.

When a hook strip is used to secure a circumferential loop strap, the therapist must decide whether to use one or two pieces of hook strip (Fig. 5–17). A disadvantage of using two smaller pieces is the increased risk of detachment with repeated donning and doffing of the splint. Two pieces, however, may better accommodate a bulky splint, as when strapping a proximal forearm splint. An advantage of one longer strip of hook material is the increased surface area of attachment, lowering the chance that the strap will come off the splint. However, this method requires more hook-and-loop material, which can be costly. Remember to allow enough loop strip to cover the hook strip fully; otherwise, the hook strip tends to stick to clothing and bedding. Round the edges of the loop strip to prevent snagging and inadvertent detachment on clothing; in addition, rounded edges are more aesthetically pleasing.

In addition to the conventional hook-and-loop material, therapists can use **elasticized loop** to secure the splint firmly to the patient. **Soft foam** and **Neoprene straps** are available; they may be more comfortable against the skin than traditional hook-and-loop tape. These materials conform nicely to the contours of the extremity and allow for some fluctuations owing to edema. These straps are not as durable as hook-and-loop material and thus may increase the cost of a splint. One way to prolong the life of foam straps is to use the reverse side once the original side does not provide a secure attachment.

Many other strapping systems exist, including hook-and-loop strips combined on one strap. This material works well for patients with limited use of an extremity. For the pediatric population, systems are available that provide the extra strength needed to secure splints adequately to active children (e.g., Dual-Lock fastening system). D-rings and buckles are options for securing straps that need to control the tension; these are especially beneficial for circumferential splints used as fracture bracing.

A rivet can be used to secure one end of the strap permanently to a small area of the splint, where an adhesive-backed hook strip would be inefficient. Riveting one end may also help patients from losing the straps (Fig. 5–18). Be sure to cover the underside of the rivet with a small piece of lining to protect the skin; rusting can occur as a result of excessive moisture.

Therapists must be creative when designing strapping systems for a splint, taking into account each pa-

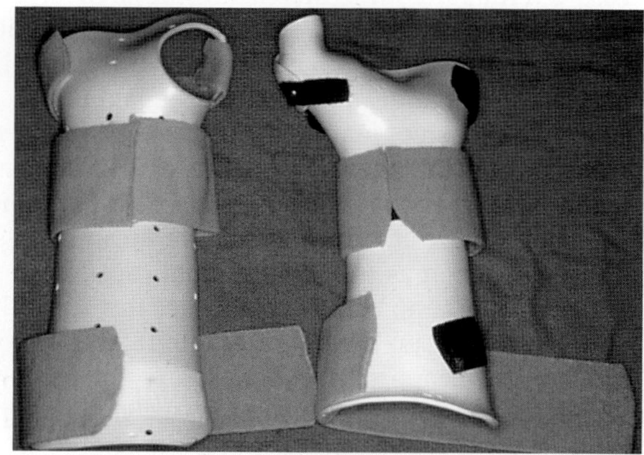

Figure 5–17 Methods of applying adhesive-backed hook strips to a wrist splint.

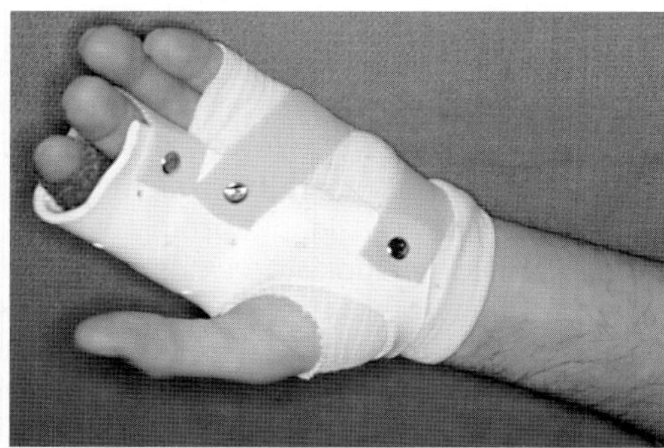

Figure 5–18 *This hand splint includes rivets to secure the straps volarly.*

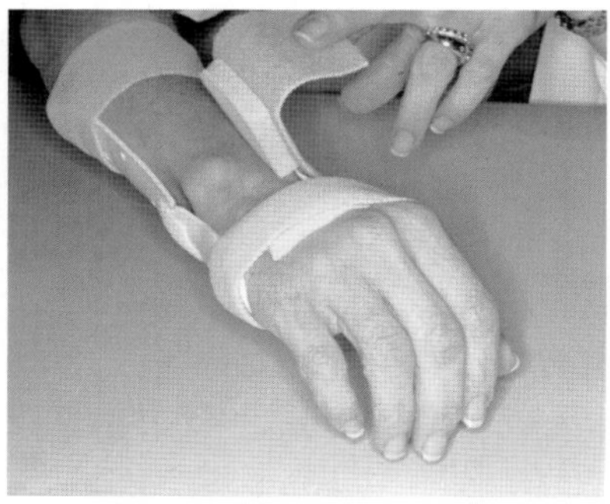

Figure 5–19 *Foam placed across the wrist strap can prevent irritation of bony prominences.*

tient's unique needs. For example, a patient with severe arthritis may benefit from specialized loops on the straps to ease donning and doffing of the splint and the strategic placement of the straps to aid in improving joint alignment.

Helpful hints are provided throughout Section II to highlight where and why straps should be placed in specific areas. Keep the following general principles in mind when considering where to place straps on a splint.

- Wider straps offer better force distribution than narrow ones (Brand, 1995; Brand & Hollister, 1993; Fess & Philips, 1987). Increasing the area of pressure contact helps prevent soft tissue irritation. However, straps should not be so wide that they impair the range of motion at unaffected joints.
- Use self-adhesive foam in conjunction with the strap to prevent uneven pressure distribution and tenderness at bony regions (Fig. 5–19). Uneven pressure can result from placing a strap across a bony area, such as the ulnar styloid process.
- To make the straps sit flush against the skin, they must be placed on the splint at an angle to accommodate the shape of the body part. For example, when applying straps to a forearm, the therapist must take into account the tapered shape of the body part. This is especially applicable when splinting a patient with large forearms.
- Straps should be tight enough to hold the splint securely in place but not so tight that circulation is impaired. Pinching the skin against the splint borders can irritate superficial sensory nerves and should be avoided. Educating the patient regarding signs of neurovascular compromise is imperative.
- Remember to maximize the mechanical advantage of a splint by securing straps in specific areas (Brand & Hollister, 1993; Fess & Philips, 1987). For example, the proximal strap on a wrist support should be placed as close to the proximal edge as possible and the middle strap should be attached just proximal to the axis of the immobilized wrist joint to prevent the patient from bowing out of the splint.
- To make the splint less likely to be removed by a questionably compliant patient, use a circumferencial bandage to secure the splint.
- If the straps have caused window edema (swelling between the straps), try applying a bias-cut wrap (commercially available nonelasticized material cut on the bias) from distal to proximal as well as elevation to decrease swelling (Fig. 5–20). This technique provides a more even pressure distribution across the entire splinted area. When the edema subsides, the wrap can be replaced with traditional hook-and-loop strips.
- Soft straps can be fringed to improve pressure distribution, increase comfort, and aid in edema control. Patients should always be told to watch for signs of swelling (especially distal to and between straps), vascular compromise, sensory changes, and improper fit. They should be instructed to loosen the straps appropriately.

Lining and Padding Materials

Occasionally therapists find it beneficial to line the inside of a splint partially or completely with a **lining material** to improve comfort, especially for older patients with thin skin. Be judicious with linings, because they cannot be

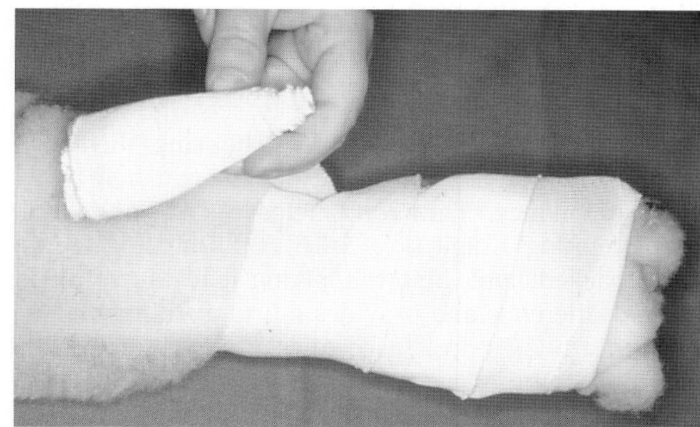

Figure 5–20 *A bias-cut wrap secures resting support for a patient with severe edema. The lining of Dacron batting helps maintain a dry environment within the splint.*

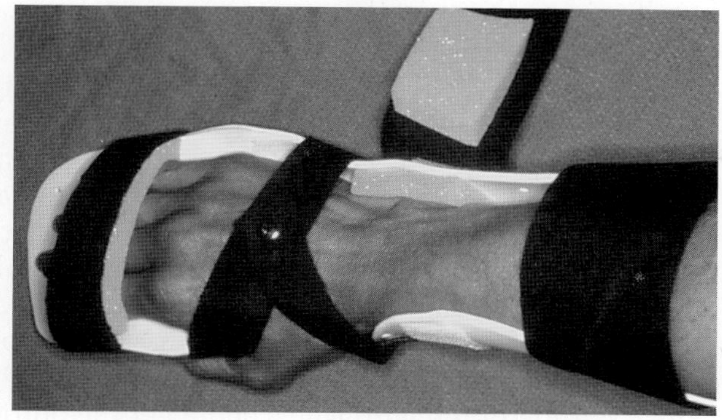

Figure 5–21 The padding on the ulnar border of this wrist support could cause the splint to shift radially, irritating the radial sensory nerve.

washed. Linings often become malodorous and discolored from the perspiration that inevitably occurs when the splint prevents airflow. Skin integrity can be compromised when subjected to a prolonged moist environment; rashes, macerations, or actual skin breakdown may be seen. Adhesive-backed liners are difficult to remove and frequent changes can be frustrating and expensive.

Alternatives include washable cotton stockinette or polypropylene liners. Removable polyester (e.g., Dacron) batting effectively wicks the moisture away from the skin (Fig. 5–20). Do not use cotton batting, which allows the wetness to remain against the skin. Batting can be especially helpful for patients who are required to wear splints on a full time basis, especially in hot and humid climates. The batting should be changed at least daily to prevent skin problems. Patients can purchase their own quilt batting from almost any fabric store.

Disposable liners can improve the comfort within a splint and control edema (e.g., Tubigrip). Patients usually do not like the feel of hard thermoplastic directly against their skin. Therapists can choose from cotton or polypropylene stockinette or an elasticized tubular bandage (e.g., Tubigrip and Tubipad). Cotton liners cut from a roll often fray and need to be replaced, which can be costly. Cotton liners are also available in precut sizes that have finished edges. Instruct patients to change the liner daily, wash by hand, and air dry. Polypropylene offers a more durable alternative and is also effective in wicking moisture away from the skin; however, it is more expensive than cotton. Foam- and gel-lined stockinette liners are available to improve the comfort of a splint, aid in scar management, and decrease vibratory stress. These products are more expensive than the standard liners.

Use **splint padding** sparingly, if at all. Remember, a properly fitting splint does not need padding. There is no substitute for a well-molded splint; therefore, it is not appropriate to pad a splint to make it fit better after the molding process (Fig. 5–21). Adding padding after fabrication alters the splint fit and can create shear and compression stresses to adjacent areas (Brand and Holister, 1993; Fess & Philips, 1987). The increased bulk over the padded area may cause an increase in pressure. On the other hand, padding in splints can be beneficial if used correctly. The best way is to apply it before molding so the splint will accommodate the lining's dimensions. Adhesive-backed Dycem and Microfoam tape linings prevent splint migration and keep the body part from sliding around in the splint. To create a bubble to prevent splint material from touching the skin or external pins, try placing a small piece of therapy putty or foam over the area before heating, then remove the piece once the splint has cooled.

The therapist must weigh the costs and benefits when deciding whether lining or padding a splint is appropriate. Many materials are available through rehabilitation catalogs, including closed- and open-cell products. Closed-cell materials (e.g., Polycushion and SplintCushion) are impermeable to water and easy to clean, but they do not permit air exchange. Open-cell materials (e.g., Moleskin and Molestick), on the other hand, are somewhat breathable; however, the material can absorb water, which may lead to bacteria growth and problems with infection control. Padding and lining materials are available in a variety of thickness and textures, keeping a few in the clinic's inventory should be sufficient.

Scar management techniques can be incorporated directly into a splint design by employing the use of gel, elastomer, or Otoform products. Gel is available in sheets or pads. Form the heated material over the scar mold to allow for accommodation of the product within the confines of the splint (Fig. 5–22). These products need to be reformed as the scar changes, at which time the splint must be remolded to adjust for this alteration in dimension. Using a splint material that is conducive to frequent reheating, such as one from the elastic group, is the best choice. Some materials on the market have a layer of gel laminated to the thermoplastic material (e.g., Gel-Cush), providing another means of scar management.

Components

This section presents the **splint components** needed to fabricate a mobilization splint. The specific systems are discussed in Section II. Because there are frequent innovations in splinting techniques and products, it is important to read current catalogs and journals to stay abreast of what is on the market.

Outrigger Systems

The outrigger portion of a splint is an extension from the splint base that acts as an anchor for apply a mobilizing force (Fig. 5–23). **Outrigger systems** must be adjustable devices that allow the therapist to maintain the optimal 90° angle of pull. Each rehabilitation catalog offers numerous outrigger systems to meet specific therapy needs (Alimed, Inc.; DeRoyal/LMB; North Coast Medical, Inc.; Sammons Preston; Smith + Nephew, Inc.) (see Appendix A).

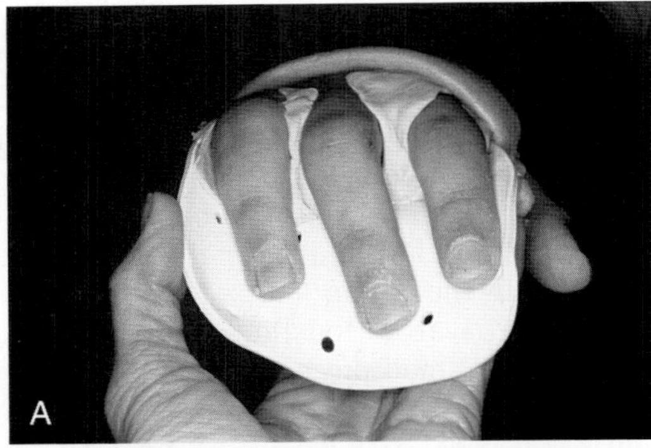

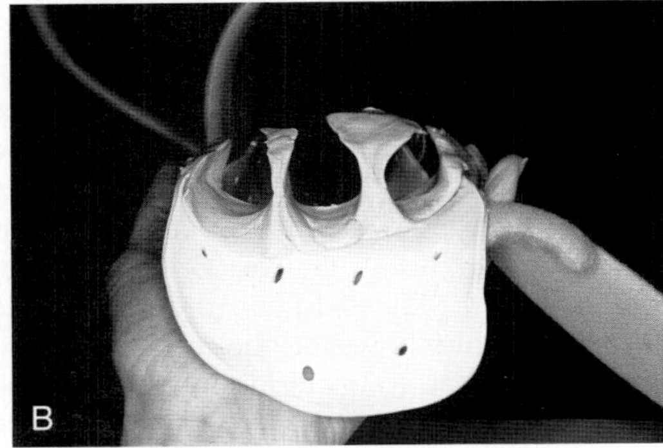

Figure 5–22 This volar splint has an incorporated scar mold for a patient with a contracted palmar scar.

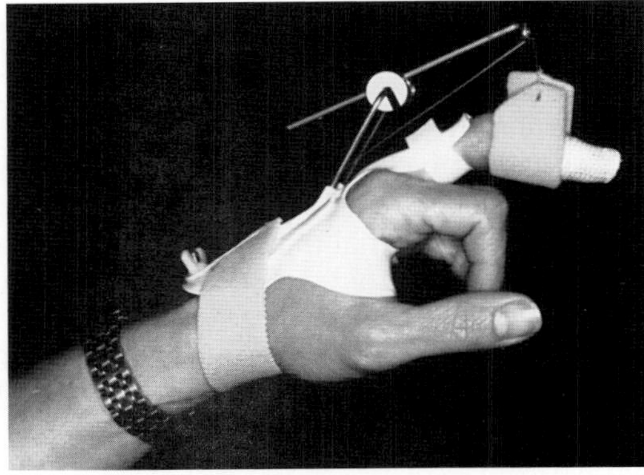

Figure 5–23 Hand-based PIP extension mobilization splint with a dorsal Roylan adjustable outrigger kit.

To determine which is the most appropriate option for a given patient, the therapist must carefully consider many factors: the therapist's preference, the patient's unique needs, and product availability. For example, when presented with a patient who needs a digit extension mobilization splint, the therapist must determine which design to use: hand or forearm-based; single or multiple digits; high or low profile; and static progressive, serial static, or dynamic. In general, the accessories for a specific system—line guides, pulleys, and proximal attachment devices—can be purchased separately to allow custom-fabricated splints.

When a commercial outrigger kit is not appropriate or available, the outrigger can be easily made from wire or thermoplastic tubing (see Section II for details) (Fig. 5–24). Copper or aluminum wire can be cut with pliers or snips and bent using a vice, pliers, or a bending bar. A small piece of perforated thermoplastic material can be molded to the frame to allow the line to glide through. Thermoplastic tubes can be easily shaped into outriggers after they have been softened in warm water. To attach a custom outrigger to the splint base, use a big enough piece of splint material to adequately cover the proximal portion of the outrigger. The higher the outrigger, the less stable the attachment site; be sure to provide adequate proximal length for attaching to the splint base. To form a strong bond, use solvent to remove any coating on the material. If no wire or tubing is available, heat a strip of thermoplastic material and create a rolled tube, which can then be formed into an outrigger.

Hinges

Rehabilitation catalogs offer **hinges** for splinting the wrist and elbow joints. Hinges allow motion in one plane of movement. They are extremely versatile, satisfying a variety of splinting needs (Fig. 5–25). They can be used for immobilization, by creating a static situation when locked to prevent motion; restriction, by blocking a portion of the available range of motion; and mobilization, by using a dynamic component or static line to stretch the joint or

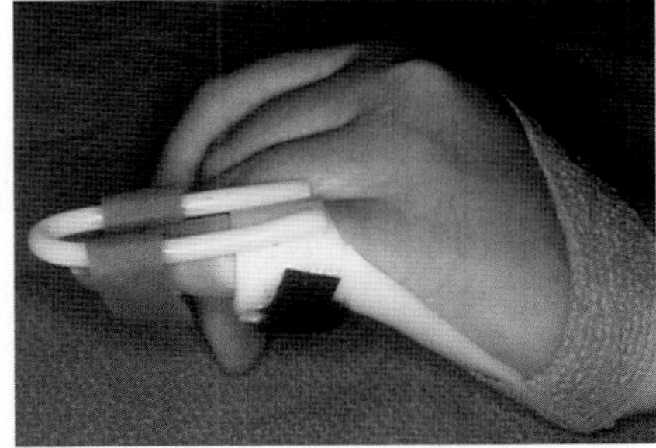

Figure 5–24 Hand-based PIP extension mobilization splint; Aquatube was used to form the outrigger.

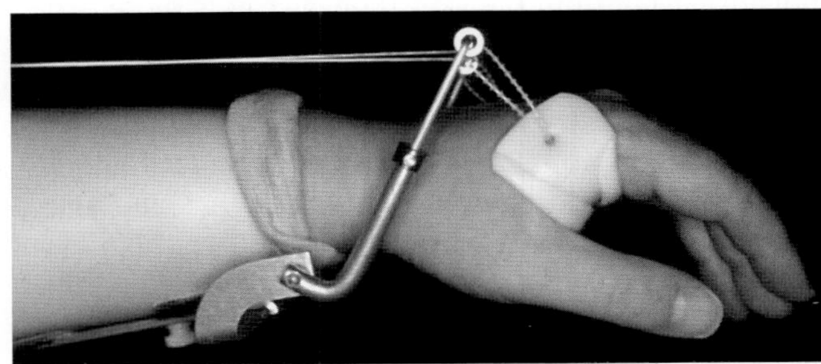

Figure 5–25 The Phoenix wrist hinge for wrist extension mobilization.

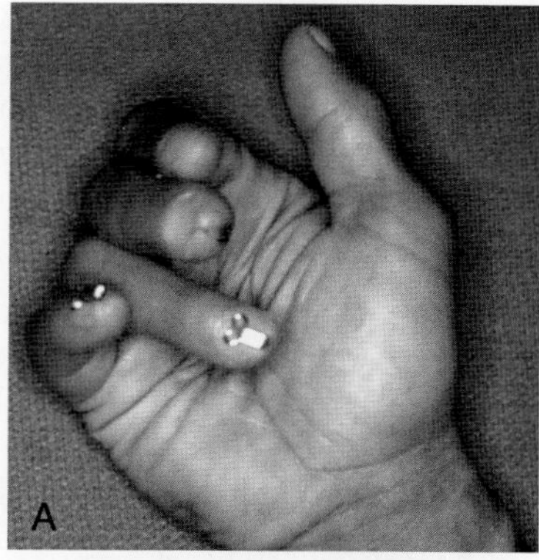

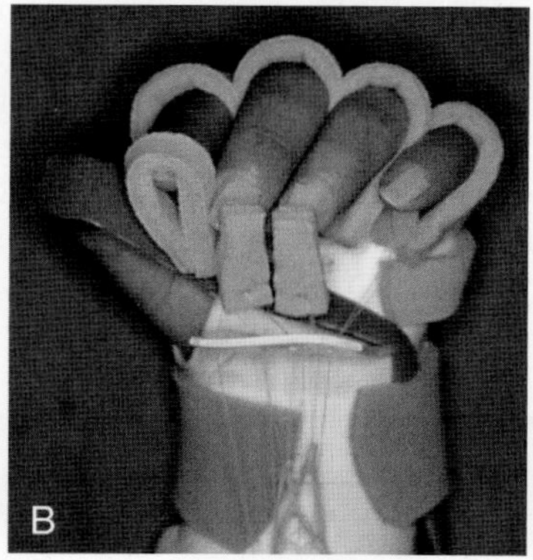

*Figure 5–26 Fingertip attachments for the application of mobilization forces include dress hooks glued to the nails **(A)** and hook material glued to the nails **(B).***

soft tissue structures. Hinges are helpful for mobilization splinting to prevent splint migration; for example, in a dynamic elbow flexion splint, the hinge prevents the proximal and distal cuffs from being drawn together by the rubber band traction. If kits are not available, hand-made versions can be fashioned from a crimped piece of thermoplastic tubing or by loosely attaching two pieces of thermoplastic material together with a large rivet or rubber band post (Thomes & Thomes, 1999).

Accessories

FINGERTIP ATTACHMENTS

Mobilization splinting of the digits frequently requires a way to apply force directly from the fingertips via a **fingertip attachment.** The options available include fingernail hooks, adhesive-backed hooks, and wrap-on hooks (Trueman, 1998) (Fig. 5-26). Fingernail hooks and adhesive-backed hooks require the use of glue on the nail to provide a secure attachment. To prepare the surface of the nail for a secure bond, scratch with an emery board and then clean with alcohol. The devices are detached by using nail polish remover. Removable wrap-on hooks provide a means of attaching a mobilization force without the disrupting the nail; they are lined with a slip-resistant material. When using these products, do not compress the digit's neurovascular structures.

FINGER SLINGS AND LOOPS

Finger slings and **loops** can be purchased in a variety of materials, including suede, leather, and soft material, the choice of which depends on patient preference. For cost containment, use strap material scraps to make custom slings and loops. A sling is an open trough in which each end of the fabric has its own line; those lines may or may not converge. A loop is a closed trough in which the two ends of the fabric converge to a single line (Fig. 5–27). Loops are easier and quicker to apply because only one line needs to be secured, whereas a sling requires two lines. Caution should be taken not to compromise vascularity in the digit when applying finger slings and loops. Slings decrease the compressive forces on the digit. Educate the patient on the signs and symptoms of impaired circulation. See Chapter 4 for details about designing line attachments to minimize compressive and shear forces on the digit (Brand, 1995; Brand & Hollister, 1993; Fess & Philips, 1987). A digital cuff fabricated from splint material can also help prevent unnecessary forces under the sling. The same mechanical principles are applicable when designing a mobilization splint for the wrist or elbow; the distal cuff is analogous to the finger sling or loop.

LINES

Static **lines,** which connect the distal attachment to the more proximal connection, can be fashioned using nonelastic monofilament or nylon cord (Fig. 5–28). These materials create a line that is resistant to drag, which is especially important when they are gliding through line guides or pulleys. The length should be sufficient to allow unobstructed gliding through the pulleys. Because these lines are nonelastic, they can be effectively used for fabricating static progressive splints.

LINE GUIDES

A **line guide** or **pulley** gives the therapist a means to change the direction of a force. Maximizing the angle of application, ideally at 90°, improves the effectiveness of the splint (Brand, 1995; Brand & Hollister, 1993; Fess & Phillips, 1987); see Chapter 4 for details. There are many types of commercially available guides. The therapist can fashion one by using a scrap piece of thermoplastic material and punching a hole in it to allow the line to pass through. Superperforated materials are user friendly; the

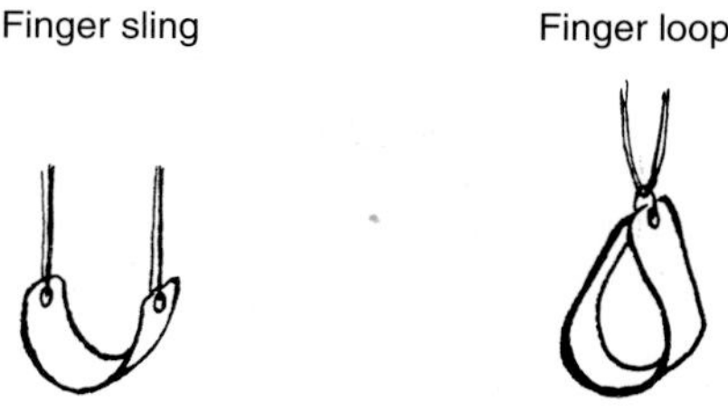

Figure 5–27 A finger sling and finger loop.

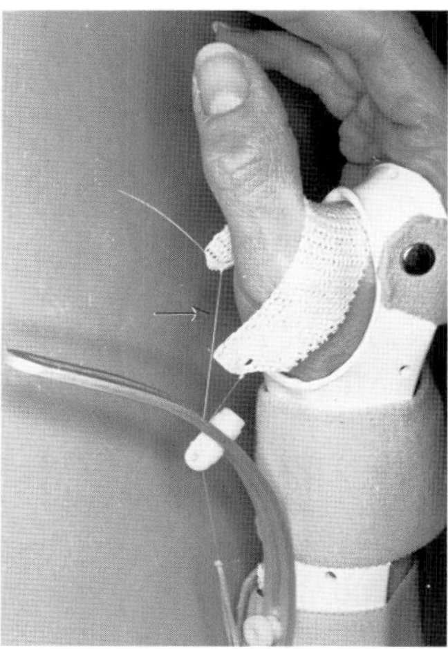

Figure 5–28 A static line is used to attach a QuickCast sling to the elastic force for a first web space mobilization splint with a Base2 outrigger kit.

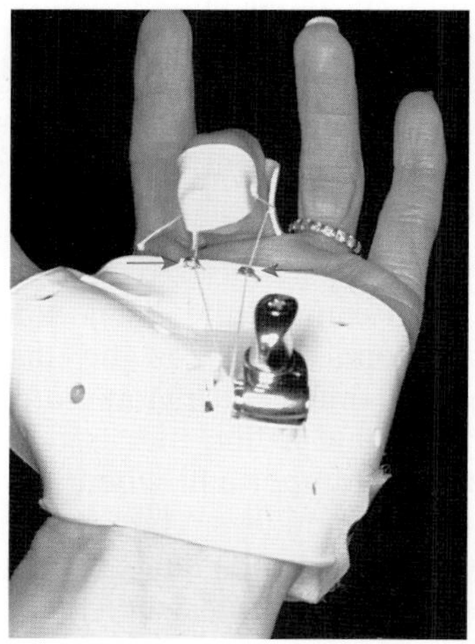

Figure 5–29 Safety pins were bent, heated, and imbedded into the thermoplastic material to act as line guides for the static progressive force applied via the MERiT component.

therapist can easily change the angle of pull by choosing from the many existing holes. Metal eyelets and safety pins offer yet more options, they are inexpensive and can be easily bent, heated, and imbedded in the thermoplastic material (Fig. 5–29). Thermoplastic tubes can also be used to create a frictionless glide.

LINE CONNECTORS AND STOPS

Line connectors provide an alternative to knots for attaching the line to slings or mobilization forces. They allow the therapist to adjust tension in a dynamic splint easily by changing the placement of the connector rather than becoming frustrated with tying and retying knots that frequently loosen. Connectors are simply crimped with pliers.

Line stops provide a means to control the available range of motion allowed in a restrictive-type splint (Fig. 5–30). Stops are applied to the splinting line proximal to the line guides or pulleys at a specific point, determined by the desired motion restricted. They can be removed and reapplied to change the available range. Tape can also be used on the line to restrict the range of motion.

MOBILIZATION FORCES

The therapist can apply a **mobilization force** to a body part in a number of ways. For dynamic splinting, choose from stretchy forces, such as graded rubber bands, wrapped elastic cord, elastic thread, graded springs, and TheraBand or TheraTubing products (Mildenberger, Amadio, & An, 1986) (Fig. 5-31). It may be necessary to replace elastic products frequently to ensure an accurate generation of force on the tissue. These force-generating components may be connected distally by means of a static line. It is important to use a force or tension gauge to measure the applied force to prevent the sling from being too aggressive with the tissue. Static progressive splints use a nonelastic nylon cord to provide the mobilization force.

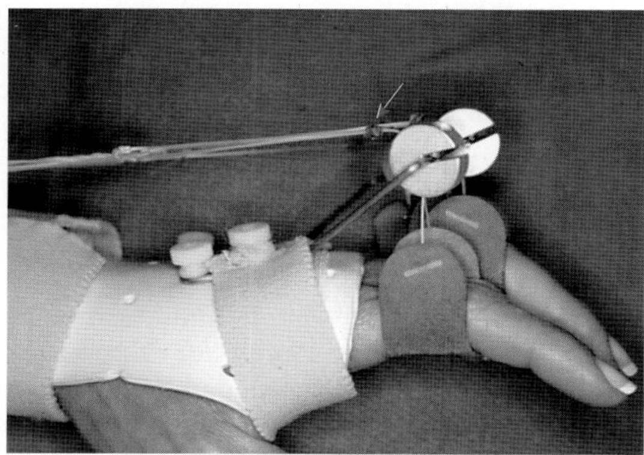

Figure 5–30 When rehabilitating an extensor tendon repair, line stops can be used with a dynamic digit extension splint to restrict MP flexion.

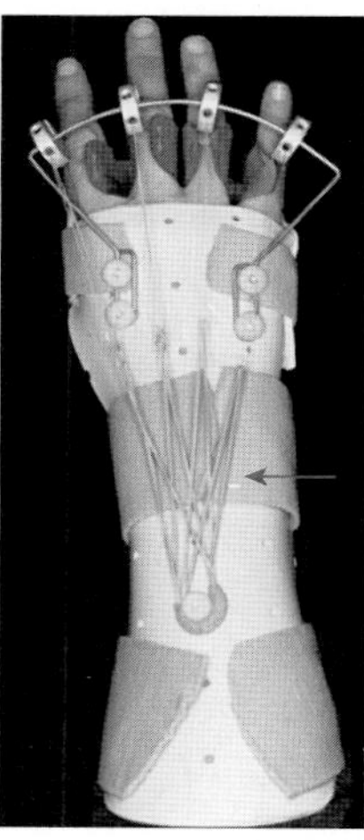

Figure 5–31 Rubber bands provide the MP extension mobilization force on this Phoenix outrigger kit.

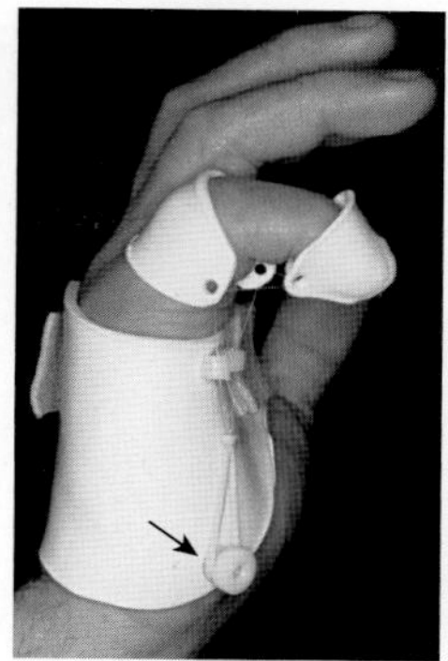

Figure 5–32 A rubber band post acts as convenient proximal attachment device for this low-profile final-flexion splint. Note the Aquatube line guides.

PROXIMAL ATTACHMENT DEVICES

A distally applied dynamic or static force requires a **proximal attachment device** for connecting to the splint (Fig. 5-32). Dynamic forces can be attached with rubber band posts or hooks made from thermoplastic material. Static forces can be secured through the use of a tuning device (e.g., MERiT component) or strips of loop strapping material. A thumb screw on the tuning device provides a way to progressively change the static tension. Loop strips allow easy adjustment: the strip is simply attached to a different place on the hook material to alter the tension.

CONCLUSION

It is imperative for the therapist to keep abreast of current available equipment and materials to provide patients with the most effective splinting intervention. Therapists with the knowledge and skills required for splinting are able to respond to the individual needs of each patient by their creatively fabricating the most appropriate splint.

REFERENCES

Alimed, Inc. (2000). Orthopedic rehabilitation products catalog. Dedham, Massachusetts.

Brand, P. W. (1995). The forces of dynamic splinting: Ten questions before applying a dynamic splint to the hand. In J. M. Hunter, E. J. Mackin, & A. D. Callahan (Eds.). *Rehabilitation of the hand* (4th ed., pp. 1581–1588). St. Louis: Mosby Year Book.

Brand, P. W., & Hollister, A. (1993). *Clinical mechanics of the hand* (2nd ed.). St. Louis: Mosby Year Book.

Breger Lee, D. E., & Buford, W. L. (1992). Properties of thermoplastic splinting materials. *Journal of Hand Therapy, 5,* 202–211.

Breger Lee, D. E., Buford, W.L. (1991). Update in splinting materials and methods. *Hand Clinics, 7,* 569–585.

DeRoyal/LMB. (1997). Product catalog. Powell, Tennessee.

Fess, E. E., & Philips, C. A. (1987). *Hand splinting: Principles and methods.* St. Louis: Mosby Year Book.

Mildenberger, L. A., Amadio, P. C., & An, K. N. (1986). Dynamic splinting: A systematic approach to the selection of elastic traction. *Archives of Physical Medicine, 67,* 241–244.

North Coast Medical, Inc. (2001). Hand therapy catalog. San Jose, California.

Sammons Preston catalog. (2000). Bolingbrook, Illinois.

Smith + Nephew, Inc. (2000). Rehabilitation division catalog. Germantown, Wisconsin.

Thomes, L. J., & Thomes, B. J. (1999). Making hinges with thermoplastic tubing. *Journal of Hand Therapy, 12,* 228–229.

Trueman, S. (1998). Bio-dynamic finger component. *Journal of Hand Therapy, 11,* 209–211.

SUGGESTED READING

American Society of Hand Therapists. (1992). *Splint classification system.* Chicago.

Barr, N. R., Swan, D. (1988). *The hand: Principles and techniques of splintmaking* (2nd ed.). Boston: Butterworth-Heinemann.

Belkin, J., & English, C. B. (1996). Hand splinting: Principles, practice, and decision-making. In L. W. Pedretti (Ed.). *Occupational therapy—Practice skills for physical dysfunction* (4th ed., pp. 319–343). St. Louis: Mosby Year Book.

Breger Lee, D. E. (1995). Objective and subjective observations of low-temperature thermoplastic materials. *Journal of Hand Therapy, 8,* 138–143.

Cannon, N. M., Foltz, R. W., Koepfer, J., Lauer, M.R., Simpson, D.M., Bromley, R.S. (1985). *Manual of hand splinting.* New York: Churchill Livingstone.

Coppard, B. M., Lohman, H. (2001). *Introduction to splinting: A critical-thinking & problem-solving approach* (2nd ed.). St. Louis: Mosby Year Book.

Duncan, R. M. (1989). Basic principles of splinting the hand. *Physical Therapy, 69,* 112–124.

Fess, E. E. (1995). Principles and methods of splinting for mobilization of joints. In J. M. Hunter, E. J. Mackin, & A. D. Callahan (Eds.). *Rehabilitation of the hand* (4th ed., pp. 1589–1598). St. Louis: Mosby Year Book.

Fess, E. E. (1995). Splints: Mechanics versus convention. *Journal of Hand Therapy, 8,* 124–130.

Fess, E. E., & Kiel, J. H. (1997). Neuromuscular treatment: Upper extremity splinting. In H. L. Hopkins, & H. D. Smith (Eds.). *Willard and Spackman's occupational therapy* (9th ed., pp. 406–421). Baltimore: Lippincott, Williams & Wilkins.

Fess, E. E., & McCollum, M. (1998). The influence of splinting on healing tissues. *Journal of Hand Therapy, 11,* 157–161.

Kiel, J. (1983). *Basic hand splinting: A pattern designing approach.* Boston: Little, Brown.

Lee, D. B. (1995). Objective and subjective observations of low-temperature thermoplastic materials. *Journal of Hand Therapy, 3,* 138–143.

Linden CA, Trombley CA (1995). Orthoses: Kinds and purposes. In C. A. Trombley (Ed.). *Occupational therapy for physical dysfunction* (4th ed., pp. 551–581). Baltimore: Williams & Wilkins.

Lowe, C. T. (1995). Construction of hand splints. In C. A. Trombley (Ed.). *Occupational therapy for physical dysfunction* (4th ed., pp. 583–597). Baltimore: Williams & Wilkins.

Malick, M. H. (1978). *Manual on dynamic hand splinting with thermoplastic material* (2nd ed.). Pittsburgh: Harmaville Rehabilitation Center.

Malick, M. H. (1979). *Manual on static splinting* (5th ed.). Pittsburgh: Harmaville Rehabilitation Center.

McKee, P., & Morgan, L. (1998). *Orthotics in rehabilitation.* Philadelphia: Davis.

Melvin, J. L. (1989). *Rheumatic disease in the adult and child: Occupational therapy and rehabilitation* (3rd ed.). Philadelphia: Davis.

Schultz-Johnson, K. (1992). Splinting: A problem-solving approach. In B. G. Stanley & S. M. Tribuzi (Eds.). *Concepts in hand rehabilitation* (pp. 238–271). Philadelphia: Davis.

Shafer, A. (1986). Common problems, useful solutions. *Hand Rehabilitation [AliMed], 4.*

Shafer. A. (1988–1989). Demystifying splinting materials. *OT Products News [AliMed], 1.*

Swan, D. (1984). Low temperature hand splinting with thermoplastic materials. *Physiotherapy, 70,* 341.

Tenney, C. G., & Lisak, J. M. (1986). *Atlas of hand splinting.* Boston: Little, Brown.

Wilton, J. C. (1997). *Hand splinting: Principles of design and fabrication.* Philadelphia: Saunders.

CHAPTER 6

Process of Splinting

Noelle M. Austin, MS, PT, CHT

INTRODUCTION

This chapter presents the process of splinting, from receiving the physician's orders to issuing the splint to the patient. Discussion includes information needed from the physician, items to include on the upper extremity evaluation, interpretation of the findings, and establishment of an appropriate treatment plan. Finally, this chapter introduces the unique style of Section II of this book, which details splint fabrication. This format uses the acronym **PROCESS,** which provides the reader with a systematic approach to splinting and makes the description of each splint simple to follow and easy to understand. All the chapters in Section II follow this format; therefore, it is critical for the reader to be familiar with the PROCESS concept.

Referral

A patient is generally referred to the therapist by a physician for fabrication of a splint and/or therapy. An example of a **referral** form is included in Appendix B. The referral should include as much of the following information as possible:

- Patient name
- Diagnosis and/or surgical procedure
- Date of injury and/or date of surgery
- Precautions
- Splint specifications
  - **Purpose** (e.g., immobilization)
  - **Type** (e.g., immobilization splint to rest a body part)
  - **Desired joint position(s)** (e.g., wrist at 30° extension, metacarpophalangeals [MP] at 40° flexion, proximal interphalangeals [PIP] and distal interphalangeals [DIP] at 0°)
  - **Goal** (e.g., allow tendons to heal)
  - **Wearing schedule** (e.g., at all times, except bathing and exercise)

It is extremely helpful to obtain a copy of the operative report, especially for complicated cases in which multiple procedures were performed that require protection in specific positions. Understanding what structures were injured and how they were repaired dictates the postoperative rehabilitation and splinting/management approach. It also is beneficial to view the radiographs and other special studies (e.g, MRIs, CT scans, and nerve conduction velocity studies) to gain a greater insight about the patient's condition.

Although the therapist may not always have the opportunity to see test results or operative reports before examining the patient, it remains imperative that one has a full understanding of the diagnosis and prescribed intervention before rendering treatment. If there are questions or concerns, do not hesitate to call the physician's office to receive clarification of orders. When in doubt, be conservative with positioning, splints can always be modified once the physician is contacted.

Ideally, therapists should strive to establish a strong relationship with their referring physicians. It is important to appreciate that each doctor has his or her own philosophy on treatment approach. Communicating effectively with the referral source promotes a professional relationship full of mutual respect and trust. Physicians are more apt to return phone calls and respond to requests when they have thoughtful interactions with the therapist. Always organize thoughts, questions, and concerns before speaking with the physician; his or her time is valuable and often limited. Asking intelligent, relevant questions helps instill confidence in the therapist's skills and provides for optimum patient treatment.

Sometimes general referrals are sent, giving the therapists some latitude to decide on the splint to be made. Therapists are then challenged to use their clinical skills to provide patients with the most appropriate splint. Whenever possible, attempt to contact the physician with suggestions and to receive verbal orders. As patients' conditions evolve, their splinting needs most likely change. It then becomes essential for patients to follow-up with their doctor to receive an updated referral with new splint orders that reflect the change in status.

Evaluation

The **evaluation** provides the basis for all critical thinking and therapy intervention. All patients must be evaluated so the most appropriate splint can be chosen. Appendix B includes a sample upper extremity evaluation. Splinting should not be approached as a rote intervention; each patient should be viewed as a unique case, and the therapist should appreciate that no two patients are alike in terms of rehabilitation and splinting needs, despite similar diagnoses. Even when patients are referred for a one-time visit, therapists must perform at least an abbreviated, yet comprehensive, version of an evaluation. Therapists are challenged to gather and integrate all the pertinent information that will allow them to make decisions that are in the best interest of their patients.

During the evaluation process, the therapist not only establishes a rapport with the patient but also gains some insight into the issues of compliance and motivation. Note the resting posture of the injured part and how freely the patient uses or moves the extremity. It is essential to address signs of neglect early on to prevent long-term disuse. At the other extreme, the overzealous patient should be cautioned when the diagnosis requires complete rest or limited use. Keep in mind that some patients, owing to diagnostic precautions, may not tolerate a complete evaluation; thus portions of the evaluation (e.g., range of motion [ROM] and strength) may not be appropriate to assess (e.g., status post multiple flexor tendon repairs). As healing progresses, these segments of the evaluation should be addressed.

This section briefly reviews the subjective and objective information that the therapist should obtain from the patient as part of the evaluation process, highlighting some key points related to splint application. For more details, see one of the many available upper extremity rehabilitation texts. The sources listed as suggested reading for this chapter offer more in-depth studies.

Subjective Information

Age

The therapist must take into consideration the **age** of the patient, because the approach to splinting differs for an infant, child, young adult, middle-aged adult, and older patient. For example, when splinting infants, it is important to be sure that there are no small parts that can potentially loosen and present a choking hazard. Thin splint material—3/32" or 1/16"—generally provides sufficient strength for their small hands. Consider taking advantage of the available hard-to-remove strapping systems when designing a splint for a pediatric patient. Compliance of the older child may be enhanced if he or she is given a splint that is colored or decorated to the child's taste (Fig. 6–1). Chapter 22 gives more specific information on splinting the pediatric patient.

A strong, durable material that is easy to clean is generally the appropriate choice for a young athlete. When splinting geriatric patients who have fragile, sensitive skin, consider using lightweight, perforated materials. Strapping systems for the older population should be constructed to allow for easy, independent donning and doffing.

Hand Dominance

Hand dominance becomes especially important when considering the functional needs of a patient. Patients may require instruction and specific training on how to modify activities of daily living (ADLs) to compensate for splint constraints. Adaptations to the splint can be incorporated during fabrication, e.g., to build up the handles for use in combination with the splint to maintain function of the dominant hand.

Past Medical History

Consideration should be given to **past medical history,** including unrelated medical conditions and how they can influence the present upper extremity diagnosis. A listing of current conditions and medications should be obtained for the medical record. For example, a patient with diabetes may suffer from decreased circulation, which can lead to prolonged healing times and sensory changes. This condition mandates frequent and vigilant inspection of the skin under the thermoplastic material and straps to check for skin changes. Chapter 3 provides further information on how specific diseases can effect the healing process.

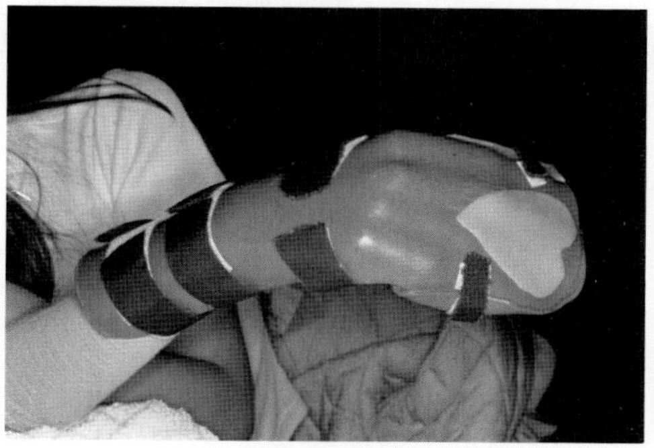

Figure 6–1 Pediatric dorsal wrist and hand immobilization splint used after a flexor tendon repair. Note the thermoplastic heart applied to the distal portion of the splint.

History of Present Condition

Questioning the patient regarding the **history of the present condition** should include factors such as the onset of symptoms, mechanism of injury, previous therapeutic intervention, surgical history, and postoperative management. This information can guide the therapist in making decisions about how to treat the patient most effectively. During the interview process, the therapist should begin to think about the rehabilitation options. However, the therapist must realize that a splint is only one part of the treatment regime and is best complemented by other modalities, such as exercise and patient education. For example, a patient with nonoperative carpal tunnel syndrome may benefit from a splint to position the wrist in neutral while sleeping. But if that patient does not make complementary lifestyle changes, such as creating an ergonomic workstation, the symptoms of the syndrome will likely remain problematic.

Social and Vocational History

The **home environment** can affect a patient's ability to comply with a rehabilitation regime. Obtaining information regarding the level of assistance a patient has at home (from family members or other caregivers) becomes pertinent when there is a question about the patient's ability to don and doff the splint independently and to follow through with a home program or activity limitations. For example, a patient that is supposed to wear a splint full time while acting as the sole caretaker of three children may have difficulty functioning within the constraints of a splint. Therapists need to consider the patient as a whole person, not just a diagnosis.

Interviewing the patient regarding his or her **work environment,** including work tasks, is also important, especially if the patient must wear the splint during work hours. Functional demands help dictate the material and design of the splint. In regard to splint selection, for example, thicker materials (1/8") may be the most appropriate choice for individuals who work at labor-intensive jobs. Splint adaptations may be needed to allow maximal function (Fig. 6–2). The same is true when considering a patient's avocational interests. For example, if the patient participates in athletic competition, the splint must abide by sports-specific regulations to be acceptable during play. Exterior padding may be required to prevent injury to others.

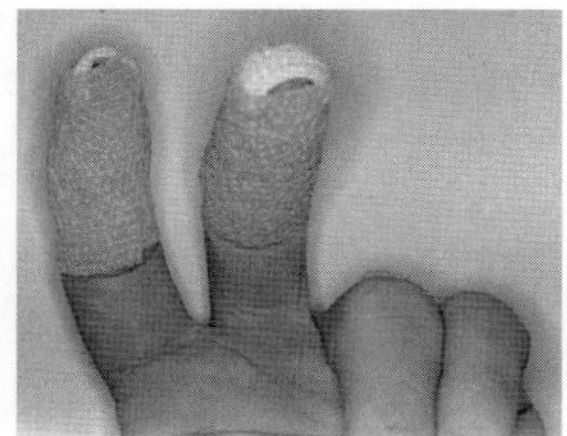

Figure 6–2 *Dorsal DIP immobilization splints for treatment of crush injuries allows sensory input to the fingertips to encourage functional use of the splinted digits.*

Functional Level

Discussing the patient's current **functional level** is important to ascertain how the injury or surgery has affected his or her life. In addition to the detailed history, standardized testing of dexterity and coordination can help the therapist assess functional performance (Apfel, 1990; Jebson, Taylor, Trieschmann, Trotter, & Howard, 1969; McPhee, 1987; Smith, 1973; Tiffin & Asher, 1948; Totten & Flinn-Wagner, 1992). Completion of a simple questionnaire that asks the patient to grade his or her functional ability to complete specific tasks (e.g., no assistance through minimal, moderate, or maximal assistance or unable to complete), is another way to gather information. These data help the therapist establish functional goals and provide a means to mark progress.

Involve the patient in setting up functional goals. Integrating personal goals into the treatment plan is a great way to maximize compliance. For example, a patient may be discouraged with his or her inability to play the piano after a trigger finger release. Acknowledging this frustration and establishing goals that include the return to playing the piano may make the patient more apt to follow the prescribed treatment regime.

Patients must have a clear understanding of their limitations while wearing a splint. For example, a patient who underwent an extensor tendon repair requires full-time immobilization and is thus unable to use that hand during the early stages of healing. This patient may require assistance with tasks such as bathing, dressing, and food preparation. The therapist must fully discuss with the patient the precautions and risks associated with the diagnosis, surgical procedure, and therapy program (including splinting) to maximize compliance and reduce chance of rupture or attenuation of the surgical repair.

Therapists can offer patients helpful hints on how to improve independence and function for ADLs. Simple modifications, such as using kitchen utensils with built-up handles, can ease the stress and pain of arthritic joints. These modifications can be used simultaneously with a splint or a splint can be fabricated to be used for a specific functional task. For example, cylindrical foam, Elastomer, or thermoplastic material can be used to modify writing utensils.

Pain

The therapist should ask the patient to describe **pain** in terms of quality, degree, and location (Chapman, Schimek, Colpitts, Gerlach, & Dong, 1985; Echternach, 1993; Melzack, 1975; Schultz-Johnson, 1988a). Changes in degree can be determined by using a scale (e.g., 1 to 10). Mapping out the pain on a illustration of the upper extremity may help define the location. Avoid placing patients with moderate to severe pain in mobilization splints. Aggressive mobilization may aggravate pain and increase edema. If mobilization splinting is ordered for such a patient, contact the physician to discuss any concerns. Pain may also dictate the choice of materials used; highly drapable materials may be easier to apply, because they conform without much hands-on manipulation. Splints can be made to accommodate the electrode pads often used to modify pain (e.g., transcutaneous electrical nerve stimulation; TENS).

Objective Information

Edema

Quantify **edema** whenever possible by measuring volume or circumference. Use a **volumeter** to measure the volume of the limb or a **measuring tape** to quantify circumference (Fig. 6–3) (Brand & Wood, 1977; Hunter & Mackin, 1995; Schultz-Johson, 1988b). The therapist must fully describe the quality (e.g., pitting, brawny) and location. In the early stages of healing of an acutely injured or postoperative extremity, edema is frequently an issue that requires therapy intervention. Edema may be reduced by a splint that correctly positions the extremity; compression garments (e.g., gloves, elasticized tubular bandages); and education regarding elevation, ice, and exercise (if appropriate) (Fig. 6–4).

Edema may increase after the use of splints, especially with mobilization splints. Consistent, repeated evaluation provides the therapist with information about how the tissue is tolerating the splinting regime. If the extremity becomes edematous and reactive, the splinting approach should be modified. For example, if edema is aggravated by a mobilization splint, consider resting the body part in an immobilization splint for a few days. Once the edema has decreased, cautiously reintroduce the mobilization splint, monitoring for edema changes.

Fluctuations in edema can affect the strapping choice. Window-type edema, which occurs between two straps, may be avoided by wrapping the limb circumferentially.

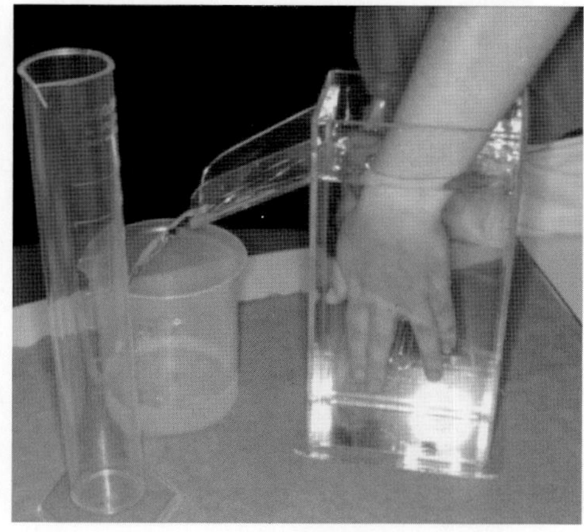

Figure 6–3 A volumeter quantifies edema. Measure the contralateral limb for comparison.

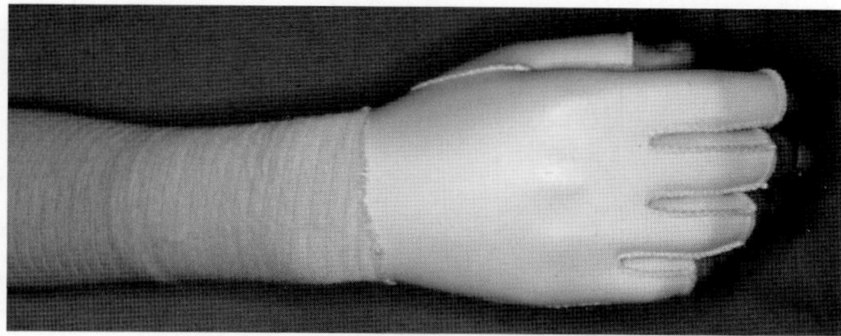

Figure 6–4 Edema management may include the use of a compression glove and an elasticized tubular bandage, such as Tubigrip.

These wraps (e.g., Coban or Ace wraps), applied distal to proximal, impart an even pressure to an edematous limb. Circumferential splints should be used cautiously with patients who have an edematous extremity; if applied too tightly, problematic pooling of edema distal to the splint can occur. In select cases, these splints may help reduce edema; Chapter 12 provides more information.

Sensibility

Assessing **sensibility** is essential when conducting an upper extremity evaluation (Bell-Krotoski, 1991, 1995; Bell-Krotoski, Weinstein, & Weinstein, 1993; Callahan, 1995; Dellon, 1981; Moberg, 1958; Novak, Mackinnon, Williams, & Kelly, 1993; Tan, 1992). **Monofilament** examination and **two-point discrimination** testing are the most common methods for evaluating sensibility (Fig. 6–5). A monofilament examination, considered a threshold test, is administered by applying graded forces of filaments to the testing area (Bell-Krotoski & Tomancik, 1987). Two-point discrimination, considered an innervation density test, involves the ability to distinguish between two stimuli applied to the skin at specific locations (Dellon, 1978; Dellon, Mackinnon, & Crosby, 1987; Mackinnon & Dellon, 1985). Quick screening for light touch may be adequate if the patient has no complaints or signs of nerve involvement.

The therapist must consider impaired sensation in order to provide the patient with a properly fitting splint and to prevent tissue irritation. Every effort should be made to increase the surface area of application to disperse the pressures on sensory-impaired regions. When applying a splint to a limb with impaired sensation, the therapist must review the precautions with the patient. Any complaints of numbness or paresthesias should be dealt with immediately. Because they lack complete sensory feedback, such patients must learn to perform frequent visual examinations of the splinted extremity, looking for any signs of excess pressure.

Soft Tissue and Wound Status

Therapists should assess the **soft tissue** and **wound status.** Document any wounds or surgical incisions and quantify with measurements and descriptions (Evans,

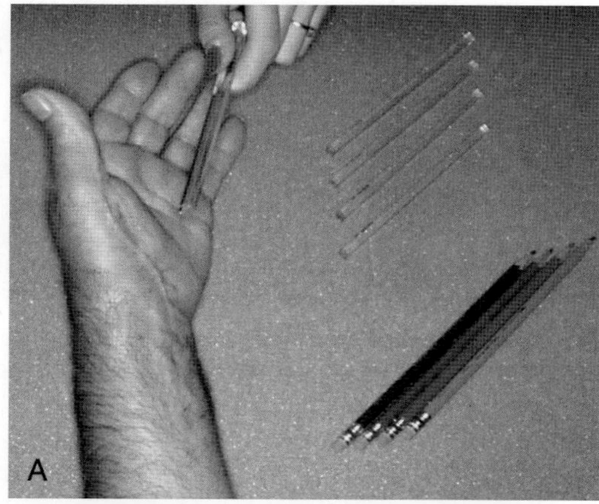

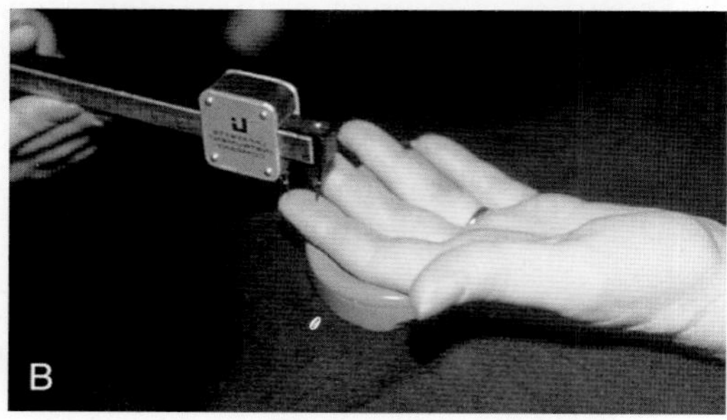

Figure 6–5 ***A,*** *A monofilament set.* ***B,*** *A two-point discriminator.*

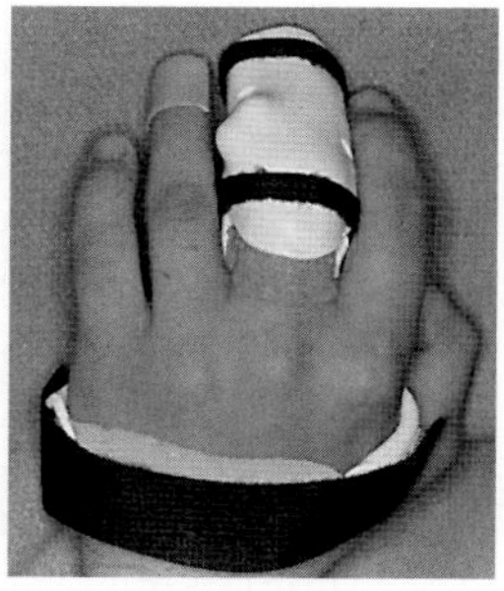

Figure 6–6 A clamshell splint designed to protect the external pins that protrude dorsally. The thermoplastic material was carefully molded over the prepadded pins.

1991; Evans & McAuliffe, 1995; McCulloch & Kloth, 1990). Maceration, rashes, and skin breakdown can result when the skin is subjected to prolonged splint wear or excessive moisture. Perforated materials are a good choice for splinting over wounds, because they allow air exchange between the splint and skin.

Therapists frequently need to be creative when splinting over wound dressings and/or surgical hardware, such as pins or external fixators. To splint directly over exposed pins, prepad the area, and then apply the warm thermoplastic material. Consider using solid highly drapable material for this type of splint (Fig. 6–6). Sensitive scars can be splinted over with a gel-lined material. Scars can also be prepadded with gel or an Elastomer or Otoform-type product (Fig. 6–7).

Vascularity

Color and temperature differences between the involved and uninvolved side should also be noted to address the **vascular status** of the limb. Altered sympathetic response may present with color and temperature changes of the skin. Assessment becomes of extreme importance when vascular structures have been injured or surgically repaired (Ashbell, Kutz, & Kleinert, 1967; Levinsohn, Gordon, and Sessler, 1991). Straps or slings that are applied too tightly may impede circulation, manifested by a change in color and/or temperature. Wide straps and slings may dissipate pressure on the affected part by increasing the area of force application (Brand & Hollister, 1993; Fess & Phillips, 1987). Chapter 4 provides a more detailed discussion of these matters.

Circumferential splints are not the best choice for patients who have undergone vascular repair or who have possible vascular compromise. Such splints may not provide enough room for fluctuations in edema. When edema increases, the pressure within the splint may also increase, leading to impaired circulation.

Range of Motion

Goniometers are used to measure active and passive **range of motion** (ROM) (Fig. 6–8) (Boone, Azen, Lin, Spence, Baron, & Lee, 1978; Cambridge-Keeling, 1995; Hamilton & Lachenbruch, 1969). Active ROM provides information about a patient's willingness or ability to move. Gaining insight regarding the soft tissue and joint status of the musculotendinous unit is important (e.g., tendon adherence, tendon continuity, and nerve innervation). Joint stiffness and musculotendinous tightness can be assessed with passive ROM measurements.

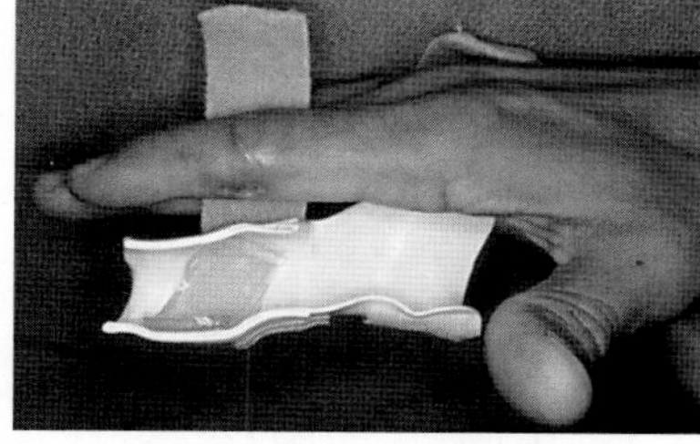

Figure 6–7 Elastomer was incorporated into this splint to provide compression for scar management.

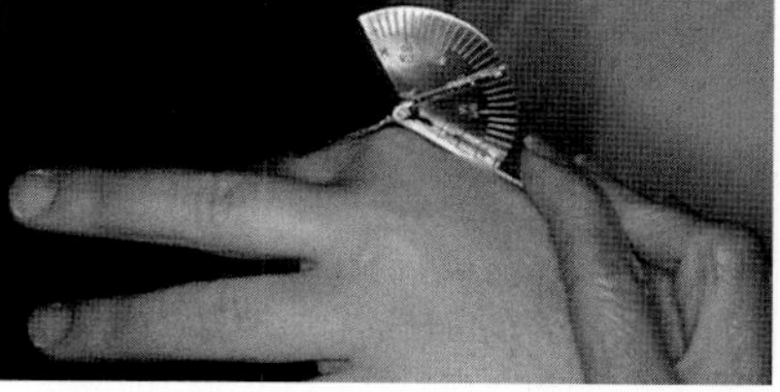

Figure 6–8 A small finger goniometer is a convenient way to measure the small joints of the hand.

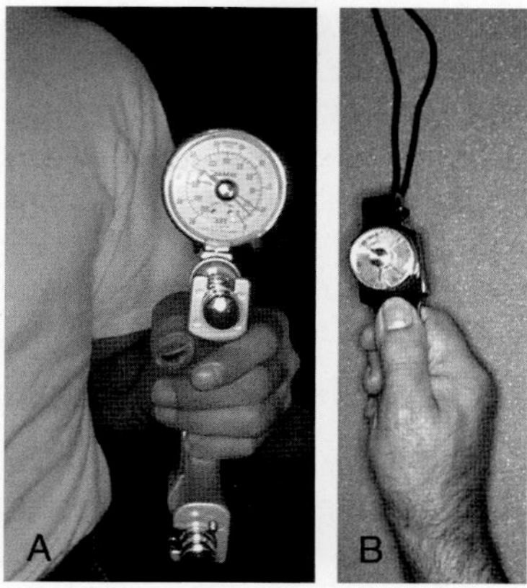

Figure 6–9 *Grip (**A**) and pinch (**B**) dynamometers.*

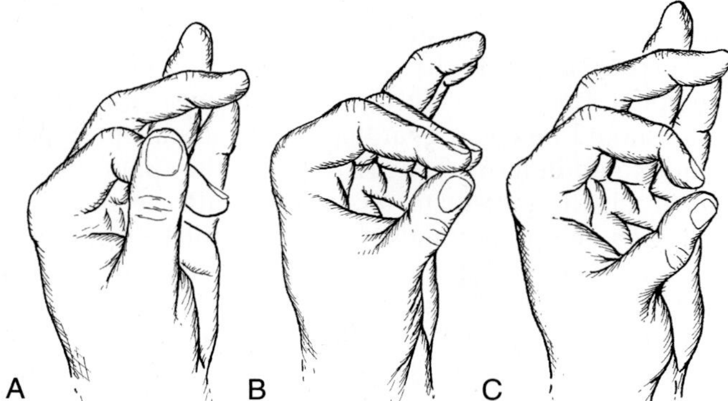

Figure 6–10 *Three types of pinches: lateral (**A**), three point (**B**), and thumb to index-finger tip (**C**).*

Ongoing evaluation of ROM becomes imperative when introducing a splint to mobilize tissue. ROM is a way of measuring gains and provides feedback for the splinting effort. If no improvements are evident, the splinting regime must be changed accordingly. For example, if no gains are made from use of a dynamic PIP extension splint, the therapist should consider changing to a serial static treatment approach. ROM measurements can also indicate that joints are getting tighter, as is sometimes seen at the MP joints when a wrist cast extends too far distally, impeding full MP motion.

Strength

Grip dynamometers, pinch gauges, and **manual muscle testing** (MMT) provide ways to assess muscle function and nerve innervation (Fig. 6–9B) (Bechtol, 1954; Daniels & Worthingham, 1986; Kendall, McCreary, & Provance, 1993; Mathiowetz, Volland, Kashman, & Weber, 1985; Mathiowetz, Weber, Volland, & Kashman, 1984; Schmidt & Toews, 1970). Three types of pinch may be tested: lateral or key pinch, three point (three-jaw chuck), and thumb tip to index-finger tip (tip pinch) (Fig. 6–10) (Casanova & Grunert, 1989). Quantifying changes in strength is helpful when justifying the need for continued therapy.

Strength testing may be contraindicated in many cases, depending on the diagnosis and healing time. For example, elbow flexion strength testing should be deferred in the early stages of healing after a biceps tendon repair owing to the high risk of rupture immediately after surgery. Strength can be safely assessed once the physician has approved the initiation of progressive resistive exercise.

MMT provides the means for monitoring recovery from a nerve injury. As the nerve reinnervates muscles, patients present with higher muscle grades (0 to 5). This change in status alters the therapy and splinting plans. For example, the splint must be modified for a patient with a radial nerve palsy once the wrist extensors become innervated. Because the splint no longer needs to incorporate the wrist, the therapist should choose a hand-based MP extension mobilization splint to allow the newly innervated wrist extensors to function while regaining strength.

Exercise splints can be fabricated to provide resistance to movement through the use of graded rubber bands, wrapped elastic cord, elastic thread, graded springs, and TheraBand or TheraTubing products. The patient can use the splint for frequent daily exercise sessions to improve strength in the targeted muscle group(s). When treating patients with adherent tendon repairs, adding resistance may aid in improving tendon glide through scar tissue.

Problem Solving and Goal Setting

From the findings of the evaluation and the information gathered from the patient interview, the therapist is able to establish treatment goals. Therapists must appreciate that splinting is only one way problems can be addressed. The therapist must first define a **list of problems.** Table 6–1 outlines the problems and corresponding goals for a patient at 1 week postsurgery for carpal tunnel release.

Note that for each problem, there is a short- and long-term goal. Although this is a relatively simple example, this method of creating an appropriate treatment plan is applicable to all patients. The critical thinking process allows the therapist to organize the findings of the evaluation and begin to plan the therapy intervention. The therapist must then prioritize the problems. It can be overwhelming to treat a patient with multiple injuries; setting priorities is mandatory (although sometimes difficult to do). All treatment problems and interventions are interrelated. For example, when edema has been successfully addressed, ROM is usually also improved.

TABLE 6–1 Approach to Goal Setting

Therapy Problems	Short-Term Goals (2–3 weeks)	Long-Term Goals (1–2 months)
Healing incision	Healed incision	Soft, mobile scar
Moderate edema in hand	Minimal edema	No edema
Pain level 2[a]	Pain level: 1	Pain level: 0
Decreased ROM of wrist and digits	Increase ROM of digits to normal and of wrist to 75%	Normal ROM
Decreased grip and pinch strength	Increase grip to 5 lb and pinch to 2 lb	Strength 75% of normal
Impaired ability to complete ADLs[b]	Independent for self-care and driving; minimal difficulty with cooking and cleaning	Full functional use

[a]On a scale of 0 to 10.
[b]Includes self-care, driving, cooking, and cleaning.

After the problems are defined, the therapist should establish **short-** and **long-term goals.** For example, when applying a mobilization splint, the therapist should set reasonable short-term ROM goals that can be reached in 1 week; this encourages the patient to follow the splint-wearing schedule and therapy program. Each time the patient reaches a goal, a new goal should be established. As mentioned previously, the patient's own goals should be integrated within the therapy goals (when appropriate).

Therapy intervention is a dynamic process, limited only by the lack of imagination on the part of the therapist. The therapist needs to take the time to interpret the evaluative findings and appreciate that as the patient progresses, the problems and priorities also change, as should the treatment goals. Ideally, all problems should be addressed. But, it is unrealistic to think that one treatment modality is going to satisfy all the deficits. A **comprehensive treatment plan** should be instituted, of which splinting may or may not be a part. Therapists must use critical reasoning skills, based on knowledge and experience, to devise the best treatment regime, taking into account the patient's individual needs. Each time a patient returns to the clinic, he or she should be reevaluated to determine if changes in therapy management must be made.

A skilled therapist would never approach two patients in the same way. Therapists need to be responsive to the specific and changing needs of their patients, altering the therapy treatment in response to changes in tissue status. For example, when considering the stage of healing of a particular tissue, therapists must apply the most appropriate splint for that stage. A splint that is appropriate for a patient one week, may not be the best choice a month or even a week later. In general, immobilization splinting is appropriate for resting an acutely injured body part; this is followed by a more aggressive approach, such as mobilization splinting, during the later stages of healing. Refer to Chapter 3 for a more detailed discussion.

Patient Education and Precautions

Educating the patient is essential for deriving the greatest benefit from the splinting effort. A sample patient education handout is given in Appendix B. An opportune time to educate the patient is during a trial wearing of the splint (20 to 30 minutes) in the clinic to check for any immediate problems. Patients must understand the purpose of the splint, which relates to understanding the diagnosis and treatment approach. The patient and caregiver should be made aware of how to don and doff the splint, what to expect and what to look out for while wearing the splint, and when and how long to wear it. Instructions should be clear regarding what the patient is permitted to do in terms of activities with the splint on and off. Teach the patient to monitor for adverse reactions such as skin redness and irritation, circulatory compromise, and nerve compression. Educating the caregivers is mandatory, especially when splinting a child or an older individual with cognitive or physical impairments.

Proper care of the splint is necessary for hygiene and to ensure greatest function. Patients need to wash the splint with warm water and soap or rubbing alcohol and replace the liners and strapping when needed. If the splint is exposed to heat sources it may soften and distort; thus the patient must keep the splint away from stoves, radiators, fireplaces, and direct sunlight (e.g., the car dashboard). Therapists must give the patient and caregiver written instructions along with a means to contact the clinic if any problems or questions arise.

Ideally, schedule the patient for a follow-up visit to check splint tolerance and to review the instructions. If patients are not scheduled to return to the clinic, they often do not report problems of discomfort or ineffectiveness. There is nothing worse than getting a phone call from a physician about a patient who has not worn a splint because it wasn't comfortable or, worse yet, was harmful to the patient in some way. If the patient is unable to return to the clinic for follow-up because he or she lives far away, the therapist should attempt to call the patient to obtain verbal feedback and/or to offer a referral to a facility closer to his or her home, if appropriate.

Splint Pricing and Insurance Reimbursement

Reimbursement for splinting depends on the insurance carrier. Patients should be made aware of their coverage and encouraged to contact their customer service representative for clarification of benefits. The pricing of splints depends on the facility and their individual reimbursement policy; there is no universally accepted system. Each facility determines its reimbursement schedule based on several factors. The cost of a splint may include fabrication time, thermoplastic materials, strapping, lining and padding, stockinettes, and components.

Cost constraints have forced therapists to be more judicious with splinting intervention. Less costly options that do not compromise appropriate treatment standards should be offered to patients. For example, perhaps a prefabricated splint purchased at a medical-supply store could serve the same purpose as a custom wrist support. Casting may be a less costly option, when compared to the price of thermoplastic materials. Home-made outriggers from wire and scrap thermoplastic material may be less expensive than the commercially available component kits. The Clinical Pearls included in Section II note ways to decrease the costs of splints. Therapists should take a proactive role in their state organizations by educating insurance companies to promote and maximize reimbursement of therapy services.

Splint-Making Process

The chapters in Section II are organized first by purpose (immobilization, mobilization, and restriction) and then by the body part of origin (digit, hand, forearm, arm). For example, a static wrist support (wrist immobilization splint) is described under immobilization (Chapter 7) and then within the section that focuses on forearm-based splints. The description of each splint includes common names, alternative options, primary functions, additional functions, and common diagnoses and optimal positions. Positions are suggested as only a guide; the therapist must always be sure to contact the referring physician to determine positioning. Finally, the fabrication process is detailed for each splint, using the PROCESS concept.

PROCESS

The PROCESS format, used throughout Section II, provides a highly organized, systematic approach to splinting. The PROCESS acronym is defined as follows:

P—pattern creation
R—refine pattern
O—options for materials
C—cut and heat
E—evaluate fit while molding
S—strapping and components
S—splint finishing touches

The steps for the fabrication of each splint are organized in this manner. Each step consists of a list of information unique to the specific splint discussed. The basic principles applicable to all splints and a summary are included in the pull-out sleeve at the back of the book. Use the pull-out sleeve as a bookmark when splinting, and refer to the universal points when fabricating each splint. Keep the book open to the appropriate page for handy reference during the fabrication process. Section II has been conveniently designed so that the photographs and pattern can be viewed simultaneously, to improve comprehension and usability.

Clinical Pearls are presented throughout Section II. These include helpful hints regarding splint fabrication and creative modifications that the authors have found extremely effective in clinical practice. These tricks of the trade allow the reader to create truly customized splints. There is no cookbook method that can be used with every patient. Therapists must individualize their splinting approach according to the specific needs of each patient.

When splinting a patient with an injury that does not allow optimal positioning for pattern tracing or splint molding, the therapist must make modifications. For example, positioning the hand flat on a table is contraindicated for patients recovering from flexor tendon repairs, because this position puts the repaired structures at risk for attenuation or rupture. As an appropriate alternative, trace the pattern on the uninvolved extremity. When checking the fit of the pattern, use the uninvolved side, if needed, to eliminate unnecessary movement of the injured extremity. Other positioning techniques include lying a patient on a plinth, using foam arm supports, and getting assistance from another therapist.

The following sections introduce the general instructions for fabricating splints.

Pattern Creation

- Obtain referral with specific splinting information from physician.
- Perform upper extremity evaluation.
- Determine splinting needs and decide on type of splint(s) to fabricate.
- Trace pattern on paper towel per splint diagram, and cut it out. Use anatomic landmarks highlighted on pattern to aid in accurate pattern creation.

Refine Pattern

- Check fit of pattern by trying it on patient's extremity.
- Mark any areas that need adjustment (by adding or deleting material).

Options for Material

- Decide on type of splint and strapping material.
- Transfer pattern to splint material using wax pencil or pen.

Cut and Heat

- Partially heat splint material until soft enough to cut, and trim pattern accordingly.

- Place patient's extremity in desired position and heat thermoplastic material to appropriate temperature.
- Apply any desired padding to high-risk areas before molding.
- Dry water off material and check temperature on your own skin before applying to patient.

Evaluate Fit While Molding

- Mold splint to patient, and remember to
  * Use gravity to assist whenever possible.
  * Incorporate arches.
  * Provide adequate length and width.
  * Evenly distribute pressure while molding.
  * Handle materials gently.
- Mark areas to be trimmed with fingernail edge or pen, and carefully remove splint from patient.
- Trim designated areas.

Strapping and Components

- Determine optimal means of securing splint to extremity.
- Place splint on patient's limb and apply appropriate strapping.
- Affix specific components—such as hinges or outriggers—per pattern instructions, if appropriate.

Splint Finishing Touches

- Flare edges and round sharp corners of splint. (Best completed by selectively dipping 1 to 2 mm of material's edge into splinting pan.) Round corners of strapping.
- Provide patient with written handouts describing purpose, precautions, wearing schedule and proper care of splint.
- Check that patient is able to don and doff splint independently.
- Provide extra stockinette, straps, or other items that may require replacement.
- Schedule follow-up visit to reevaluate and modify splint as appropriate.

CONCLUSION

This chapter provides an overview of the splinting process. A comprehensive evaluation is necessary to gather the information required to make sound clinical decisions regarding specific treatment interventions. The therapist must appreciate the phases of tissue healing and how therapy and splinting are applied appropriately in order to do no harm. Effective communication with the patient and physician helps maximize the patient's final outcome.

REFERENCES

Apfel, E. (1990). Preliminary development of a standardized hand function test. *Journal of Hand Therapy, 3,* 191.

Ashbell, T., Kutz, J., & Kleinert, H. (1967). The digital Allen test. *Plastic and Reconstructive Surgery, 39,* 311–312.

Bechtol, C. O. (1954). Grip test: use of a dynamometer with adjustable handle spacing. *Journal of Bone and Joint Surgery (American volume), 36,* 820.

Bell-Krotoski, J. A. (1991). Advances in sensibility evaluation. *Hand Clinics, 7,* 527–546.

Bell-Krotoski, J. A. (1995). Sensibility testing: Current concepts. In J. M. Hunter, E. J. Mackin, & A. D. Callahan (Eds.). *Rehabilitation of the hand* (4th ed., pp. 109–128). St. Louis: Mosby Year Book.

Bell-Krotoski, J. A., & Tomancik, E. (1987). Repeatability of testing with Semmes-Weinstein monofilaments. *The Journal of Hand Surgery (American), 12,* 155–162.

Bell-Krotoski, J. A., Weinstein, S., & Weinstein, C. (1993). Testing sensibility, including touch-pressure, two-point discrimination, point localization, and vibration. *Journal of Hand Therapy, 6,* 114–123.

Boone, D. C., Azen, S. P., Lin, C. M., Spence, C., Baron, C. & Lee, L. (1978). Reliability of goniometric measurements. *Physical Therapy, 58,* 1355–1390.

Brand, P. W., & Hollister, A. (1993). *Clinical mechanics of the hand* (2nd ed.). St. Louis: Mosby Year Book.

Brand, P., & Wood, H. (1977). *Hand volumeter instruction sheet.* Carville, LA: U.S. Public Health Service Hospital.

Callahan, A. D. (1995). Sensibility assessment: Prerequisites and techniques for nerve lesions in continuity and nerve lacerations. In J. M. Hunter, E. J. Mackin, & A. D. Callahan (Eds.). *Rehabilitation of the hand* (4th ed., pp. 129–152). St. Louis: Mosby Year Book.

Cambridge-Keeling, C. A. (1995). Range-of-motion measurement of the hand. In J. M. Hunter, E. J. Mackin, & A. D. Callahan (Eds.). *Rehabilitation of the hand* (4th ed., pp. 93–107). St. Louis: Mosby Year Book.

Casanova, J. S., & Grunert, B. K. (1989). Adult prehension: Patterns and nomenclature for pinches. *Journal of Hand Therapy, 2,* 231–244.

Chapman, C. R., Schimek, F., Colpitts, Y. H., Gerlach, R., & Dong, W. K. (1985). Pain measurement: An overview. *Pain, 22,* 1–31.

Daniels, L., & Worthingham, C. (1986). *Muscle testing techniques of muscle examination* (5th ed.). Philadelphia: Saunders.

Dellon, A. L. (1981). *Evaluation of sensibility and re-education of sensation in the hand.* Baltimore: Williams & Wilkins.

Dellon, A. L. (1978). The moving two-point discrimination test: Clinical evaluation of the quickly adapting fiber/receptor system. *The Journal of Hand Surgery (American), 3,* 474–481.

Dellon, A. L. , Mackinnon, S. E., & Crosby, P. M. (1987). Reliability of two-point discrimination measurements. *The Journal of Hand Surgery (American), 12,* 693–696.

Echternach, J. L. (1993). Clinical evaluation of pain. *Physical Therapy Practice, 2,* 14–26.

Evans, R. B. (1991). An update on wound management. *Hand Clinics, 7,* 409–432.

Evans, R. B., & McAuliffe, J. A. (1995). Wound classification and management. In J. M. Hunter, E. J. Mackin, & A. D. Callahan (Eds.). *Rehabilitation of the hand* (4th ed., pp. 217–235). St. Louis: Mosby Year Book.

Fess, E. E., & Philips, C. (1987). *Hand splinting: Principles and methods* (2nd ed.). St. Louis: Mosby Year Book.

Hamilton, G. F., & Lachenbruch, P. A. (1969). Reliability of goniometers in assessing finger joint angle. *Physical Therapy, 49,* 465–469.

Hunter, J. M., & Mackin, E. J. (1995). Edema: Techniques of evaluation and management. In J. M. Hunter, E. J. Mackin, & A. D. Callahan (Eds.). *Rehabilitation of the hand* (4th ed., pp. 77–85). St. Louis: Mosby Year Book.

Jebson, R. H., Taylor, N., Trieschmann, R. B., Trotter, M. J., & Howard, L. A. (1969). An objective and standardized test of hand function. *Archives of Physical Medicine and Rehabilitation, 50,* 311–319.

Kendall, F. P., McCreary, E. K., & Provance, P. G. (1993). *Muscles: Testing and function* (4th ed.). Baltimore: Williams & Wilkins.

Levinsohn, D. G., Gordon, L., & Sessler, D. I. (1991). The Allen's test: Analysis of four methods. *The Journal of Hand Surgery (American), 16,* 279–282.

Mackinnon, S. E., & Dellon, A. L. (1985). Two-point discriminator tester. *The Journal of Hand Surgery (American), 10,* 906–907.

Mathiowetz, V., Volland, G., Kashman, N., & Weber, K. (1985). Grip and pinch strength: Normative data for adults. *Archives of Physical Medicine and Rehabilitation, 66,* 69–74.

Mathiowetz, V., Weber, K., Volland, G., & Kashman, N. (1984). Reliability and validity of grip and pinch strength evaluation. *The Journal of Hand Surgery (American), 9,* 222–226.

McCulloch, J. M., & Kloth, L. C. (1990). Evaluation of patients with open wounds. In L. C. Kloth, J. M. McCulloch, & J. A. Feedar (Eds.). *Wound healing: alternatives in management* (pp. 97–118). Philadelphia: Davis.

McPhee, S. D. (1987). Functional hand evaluations: A review. *American Journal of Occupational Therapy, 41,* 158–163.

Melzack, R. (1975). The McGill Pain Questionnaire: Major properties and scoring methods. Pain 1, 277–299.

Moberg, E. (1958). Objective methods of determining the functional value of sensibility in the hand. *Journal of Bone and Joint Surgery (British volume), 40,* 454–476.

Novak, C. B., Mackinnon, S. E., Williams, J. I., & Kelly, L. (1992). Establishment of reliability in the evaluation of hand sensibility. *Journal of Plastic and Reconstructive Surgery, 17B,* 102.

Schmidt, R. T., & Toews, J. V. (1970). Grip strength as measured by the Jamar dynamometer. *Archives of Physical Medicine and Rehabilitation, 51,* 321–327.

Schultz-Johnson, K. (1988a). *Schultz upper extremity pain assessment.* Colorado Springs, CO: Upper Extremity Technology.

Schultz-Johnson, K. (1988b). *Volumetrics: A literature review.* Glenwood Springs, CO: Upper Extremity Technology.

Smith, H. B. (1973). Smith hand function evaluation. *American Journal of Occupational Therapy, 27,* 244–251.

Tan, A. M. (1992). Sensibility testing. In B. G. Stanley, & S. M. Tribuzi (Eds.). *Concepts in hand rehabilitation* (pp. 92–112). Philadelphia: Davis.

Tiffin, J., & Asher, E. (1948). The Purdue Pegboard: Norms and studies of reliability and validity. *Journal of Applied Psychology, 32,* 234.

Totten, P. A., & Flinn-Wagner, S. (1992). Functional evaluation. In B. G. Stanley, & S. M. Tribuzi (Eds.). *Concepts in hand rehabilitation* (pp. 113–149). Philadelphia: Davis.

SUGGESTED READING

American Society of Hand Therapists. (1992). *Clinical assessment recommendations* (2nd ed.). Chicago.

American Society for Surgery of the Hand. (1990). *The hand: Examination and diagnosis* (3rd ed.). New York: Churchill Livingstone.

Aulicino, P. L. (1995). Clinical examination of the hand. In J. M. Hunter, E. J. Mackin, & A. D. Callahan (Eds.). *Rehabilitation of the hand* (4th ed., pp. 53–75). St. Louis: Mosby Year Book.

Bear-Lehman, J., & Abreu, B. C. (1989). Evaluating the hand: Issues in reliability and validity. *Physical Therapy, 69,* 1025–1033.

Bell-Krotoski, J. A., Breger-Lee, D. E., & Beach, R. B. (1995). Biomechanics and evaluation of the hand. In J. M. Hunter, E. J. Mackin, & A. D. Callahan (Eds.). *Rehabilitation of the hand* (4th ed., pp. 153–184). St. Louis: Mosby Year Book.

Donatelli, R. A. (Ed.). (1997). *Clinics in physical therapy: Physical therapy of the shoulder* (3rd ed.). New York: Churchill Livingstone.

Fess, E. E. (1995). Documentation: Essential elements of an upper extremity assessment battery. In J. M. Hunter, E. J. Mackin, & A. D. Callahan (Eds.). *Rehabilitation of the hand* (4th ed., pp. 185–214). St. Louis: Mosby Year Book.

Fess, E. E. (1986). The need for reliability and validity in hand assessment instruments. *The Journal of Hand Surgery (American), 11,* 621–623.

Groth, G. N., & Ehretsman, R. L. (2001). Goniometry of the proximal and distal interphalangeal joints, Part I: A survey of instrumentation and placement preferences. *Journal of Hand Therapy, 14,* 18–22.

Groth, G. N., Van Deven, K. M., Phillips, E. C., & Ehretsman, R. C. (2001). Goniometry of the proximal and distal interphalangeal joints, Part II: Placement preferences, interrater reliability, and concurrent validity. *Journal of Hand Therapy, 14,* 23–29.

Hoppenfeld, S. (1976). *Physical examination of the spine and extremities.* Norwalk, CT: Appleton-Century-Crofts.

Ianotti, J. P. (1994). Evaluation of the painful shoulder. *Journal of Hand Therapy, 7,* 77–83.

MacDermid, J. C., Evenhuis, W., & Louzon, M. (2001). Inter-instrument reliability of pinch strength scores. *Journal of Hand Therapy, 14,* 36–42.

Malick, M. H., & Kasch, M. C. (Eds.). (1984). *Manual on management of specific hand problems.* Pittsburgh, PA: AREN.

Morrey, B. F. (1993). *The elbow and its disorders* (2nd ed.). Philadelphia: Saunders.

Nicholson, B. (1992). Clinical evaluation. In B. G. Stanley, & S. M. Tribuzi (Eds.). *Concepts in hand rehabilitation* (pp. 57–91). Philadelphia: Davis.

Rockwood, C. A., & Matsen, F. A. (Eds.). (1990). *The shoulder.* Philadelphia: Saunders.

Tubiana, R., Thomine. J. M., & Mackin, E. J. (1996). *Examination of the hand and wrist* (2nd ed.). St. Louis: Mosby Year Book.

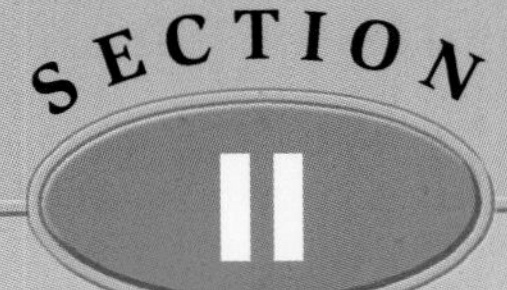

Splint Fabrication

MaryLynn Jacobs, MS, OTR/L, CHT,
and Noelle Austin, MS, PT, CHT

This section contains the directions for splint fabrication. The splints have been organized into four chapters according to splint type: immobilization (Chapter 7), mobilization (Chapter 8), restriction (Chapter 9), and nonarticular (Chapter 10). Before delving into splint fabrication, it is important to note that the patterns given here should not be approached as if they were a cookbook recipe, blindly used for every patient. The patterns are a collection of designs that are used frequently. They are intended to be modified to meet each specific patient's needs and diagnosis requirements; therapists must individualize their splinting approaches according to the unique needs of each patient. Again, these patterns are to be used as basic guidelines only. Detailed information about splinting specific patient populations and diagnoses can be found in Section IV.

The description of each splint includes a list of **Common Names** that are used by the hand community. To be consistent, the American Society of Hand Therapists (ASHT) nomenclature is used; however, inclusion of the common names allows the reader to cross-reference and use the terms preferred in his or her clinical setting. Under the heading **Alternative Splint Options,** other splints are noted that may be used as a substitute or alternative if for some reason the described splint is not appropriate because of the specific circumstances of the patient or diagnosis.

The ASHT Splint Classification System (SCS) defines splints in terms of the primary function they perform on the body part rather than the diagnosis for which the splint was ordered. This may not always be clear to the reader who wants to locate a particular pattern. Several of the patterns can be used for splints that have different functions. These splint patterns are categorized by their most common application, **Primary Function,** and their other uses are listed under the heading **Additional Functions.** The reader may use the cross-reference index (found in the back of the book) to locate a specific pattern.

Common Diagnoses and General Optimal Positions are outlined for each splint. As noted, these lists are intended to be general guidelines. For example, only the most common diagnoses for each splint are noted. The fabrication method of each splint follows the **PROCESS** acronym, which is described in detail in Chapter 6. **Clinical Pearls** are found throughout Section II. Remember that many of these "tricks of the trade" and clinical tips can be applied to a variety of splints not just the splint they are located adjacent to in the text. See the list of Clinical Pearls at the beginning of the book to locate a specific point of interest.

Most of the splints shown in Section II (except for the Clinical Pearls) were fabricated from TailorSplint thermoplastic material (Smith+Nephew). A nonperforated material was used for the photographed splints to minimize distractions and improve visualization of details. The therapist is encouraged to use the most appropriate material for the diagnosis and patient; more information may be found under the heading **Options for Materials** and Chapter 5.

Chapter 7: Immobilization Splints

1 • Digit- and Thumb-Based Splints

Distal Interphalangeal (DIP) Immobilization Splint (Fig. 7–1)

Common Names

- DIP extension splint
- DIP resting splint
- Static DIP extension splint
- Mallet finger splint

Alternative Splint Options

- Aluminum padded splint
- Stax finger splint
- Finger cast

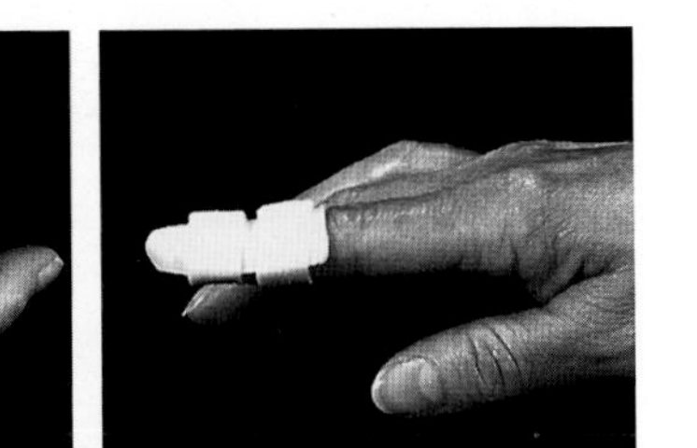

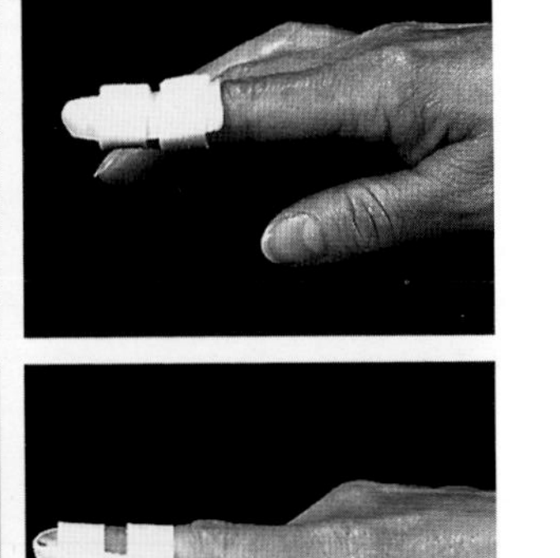

Figure 7–1

Primary Functions

- Immobilize DIP joint to allow healing of involved structure(s).
- Rest a painful and/or inflamed DIP joint.

Additional Functions

- Promote gliding of flexor digitorum superficialis (FDS) tendon by restricting movement of DIP joint during active flexion exercises.
- Statically position DIP joint flexion contracture at maximum extension to facilitate lengthening of tissue (mobilization splint).

Common Diagnoses and General Optimal Positions

Diagnosis	Position
• Zone I extensor tendon injury and/or repair (mallet finger)	0 to +10° hyperextension
• Distal phalanx fracture	Tolerable ext
• Partial fingertip amputation	Tolerable ext
• Crush injury to distal phalanx	Tolerable ext
• Nailbed injury and repair	Tolerable ext
• DIP jt osteoarthritis	Position of comfort

CLINICAL PEARL
Management of Mallet Finger

When treating a mallet finger, the DIP joint should be positioned in neutral to slight hyperextension uninterrupted for approximately 6 weeks during the healing process. Preventing skin breakdown on the dorsum of the DIP joint is imperative. Reliable patients may be instructed to carefully remove the splint for hygiene and skin inspection while maintaining DIP extension; all other patients should be seen regularly by the therapist for skin inspection. Consider a circumferential splint design using thermoplastic material, plaster, or QuickCast. Plaster or QuickCast used circumferentially, may help eliminate bulk at the fingertip, control edema, and deter removal of the splint when compliance is questionable. QuickCast, used without a liner, can be worn while bathing without risk of material breakdown, making it a good choice for children and athletes. (See Chapters 12 and 18 for more specific information.)

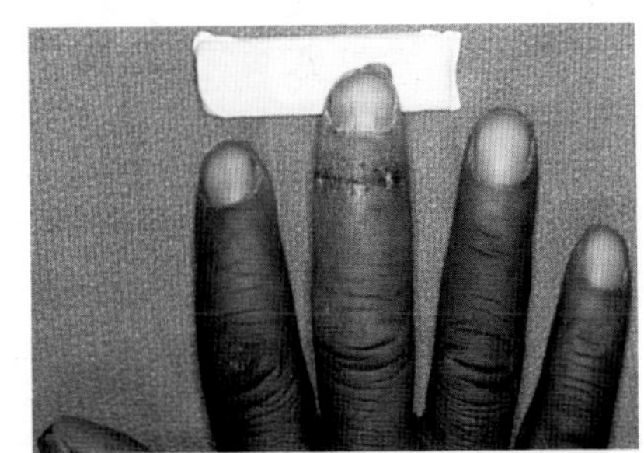

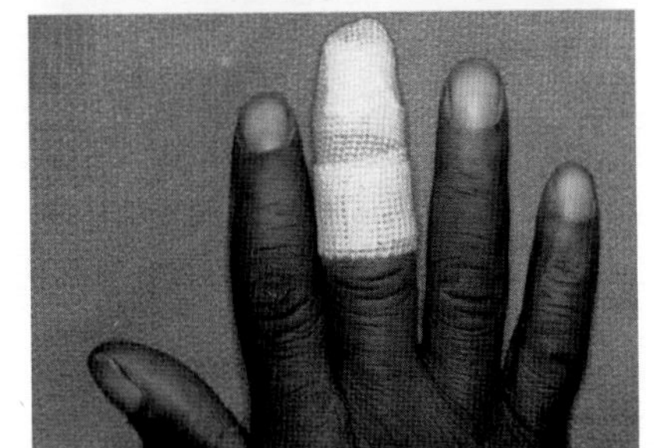

Fabrication Process

Pattern Creation (Fig. 7–2)

- Mark for proximal border distal to middle digital crease.
- Allow extra ¼" to ½" of material around borders, depending on digit circumference.

Refine Pattern

- Proximal border should allow nearly full proximal interphalangeal (PIP) joint motion.
- Lateral borders should encompass two thirds of circumference of digit to prevent undue compressive stress from straps.

Options for Material

- Consider nonremovable circumferential splint or cast for young children or questionably compliant patients.

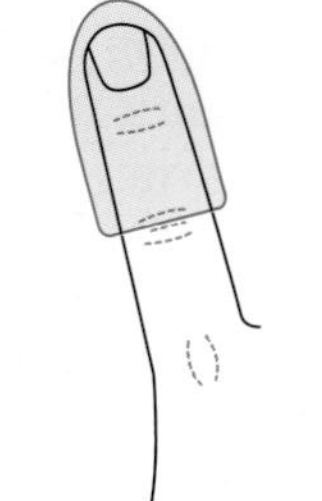

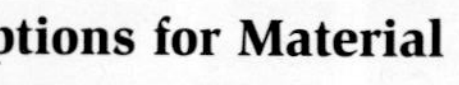

Figure 7–2

- Perforated thermoplastics may prevent skin maceration; consider using them for patients who require full-time splint use.
- Use thinnest material possible that provides necessary strength, to decrease splint bulk.
- Materials that can be reheated and remolded several times are a good option if ongoing splint modifications become necessary to accommodate for fluctuations in edema or changes in desired joint position.

Cut and Heat

- If possible, position patient's forearm supinated for volar design and pronated for dorsal design.
- If using elasticized wrap (Coban) or dressings under splint, apply to digit before heating splint material.

Evaluate Fit While Molding

DORSAL DESIGN

- Place material on dorsal aspect of digit, just distal to PIP joint. The longer the proximal border, the more stable the splint on the digit.
- Avoid applying direct pressure over dorsum of DIP joint while molding; it may cause pressure areas on splint. Incorporate thin padding, if necessary.

VOLAR DESIGN

- Place material on volar aspect of digit, just distal to PIP joint crease.
- Apply slight DIP extension force (patient may aid in extending tip by using his or her other hand to gently position tip by fingernail).
- Pinch together excess material distally; then trim to shape of fingertip to aid in further protection of a sensitive or painful tip.

Strapping and Components

- Use two ½" straps or one 1" strap to secure splint.
- Extra-thin ½" strapping material can help decrease bulk between digits.

DORSAL DESIGN

- Place straps at proximal border and over distal phalanx.

VOLAR DESIGN

- Place straps at proximal splint border and directly over DIP joint.
- Light padding under distal strap may reduce splint migration and improve comfort.

Splint Finishing Touches

- Smooth material borders and avoid rolling and flaring, which may irritate adjacent soft tissues or interfere with PIP joint movement.
- Check for mobility of uninvolved joints.

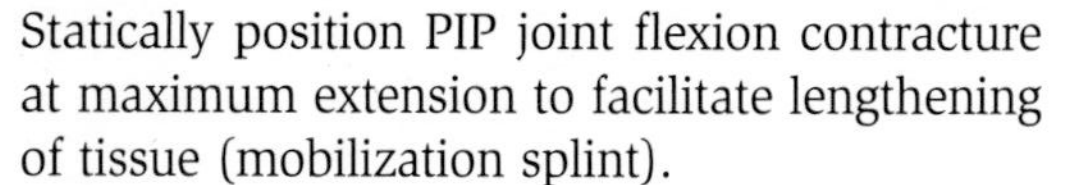

PIP Immobilization Splint (Fig. 7–3)

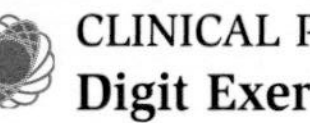

Common Names

- Finger splint
- PIP resting splint
- Static PIP extension splint
- Finger gutter splint

Alternative Splint Options

- Aluminum padded splint
- Finger cast

Primary Functions

- Immobilize PIP joint to allow healing of involved structure(s).
- Rest a painful and/or inflamed PIP joint.

Additional Functions

- Promote gliding of flexor digitorum profundus (FDP) tendon by restricting movement of PIP joint during active flexion exercises.
- Statically position PIP joint flexion contracture at maximum extension to facilitate lengthening of tissue (mobilization splint).
- Restrict specific amount of extension (e.g., dorsal dislocation of PIP joint) or flexion (e.g., zone II and III extensor tendon injury) to protect healing structures (restriction splint).

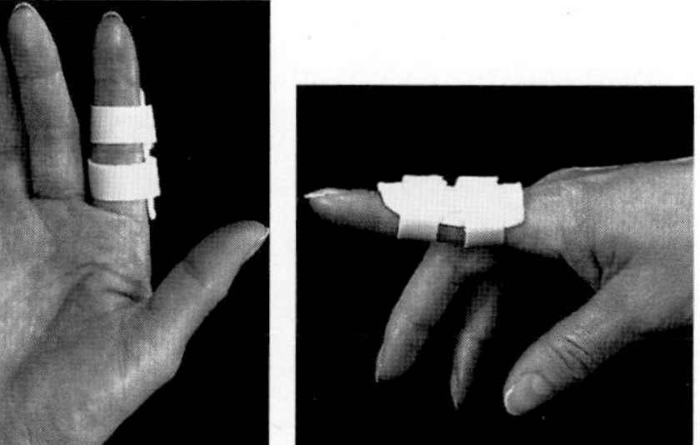
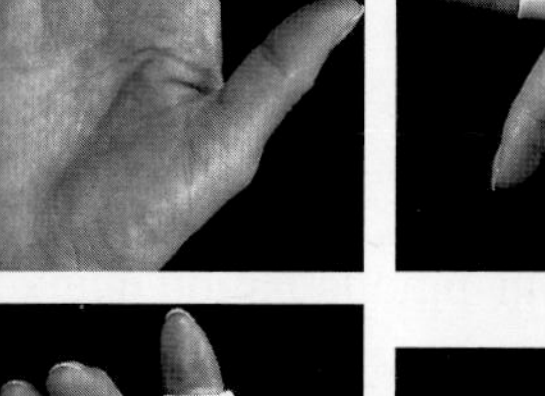
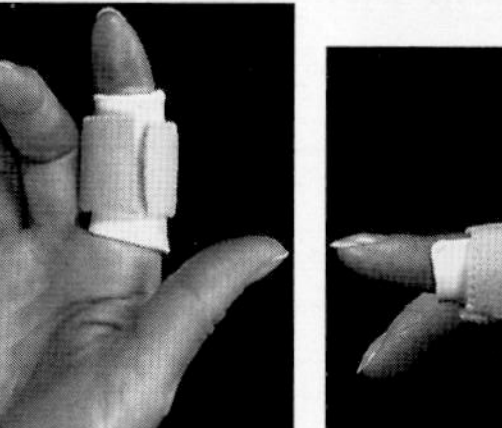
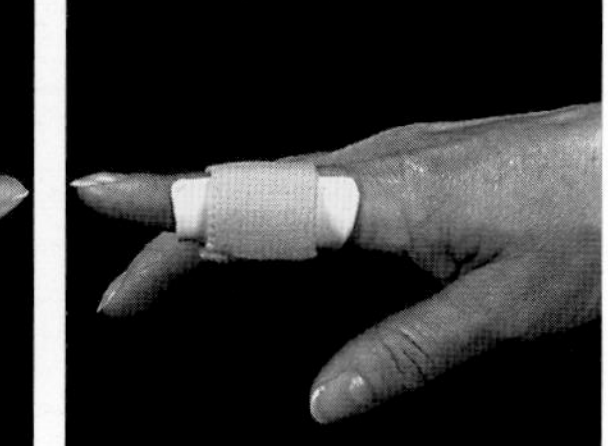
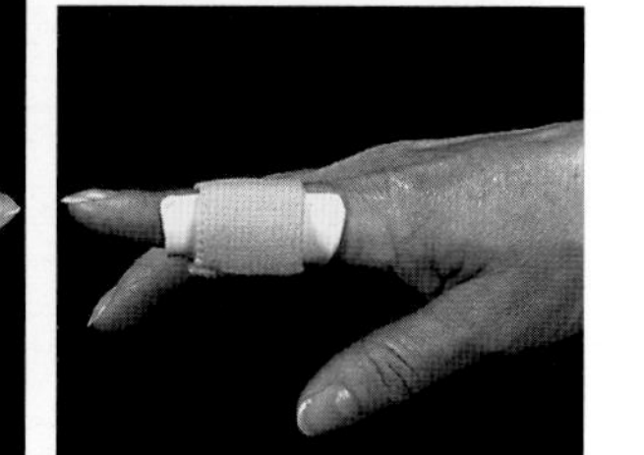

Figure 7–3

Common Diagnoses and General Optimal Positions

Diagnosis	Position
Zone III and IV extensor tendon injury	0°
Boutonniere deformity	0°
PIP jt sprain	0°
PIP jt intra-articular fracture	0°
PIP jt arthritis	Position of comfort
PIP jt arthroplasty	0°

CLINICAL PEARL
Incorporation of DIP Joint into PIP Splint

The DIP joint can easily be incorporated into either the dorsal or the volar splint design.

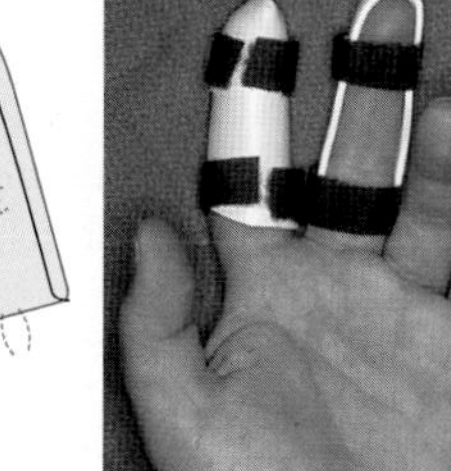
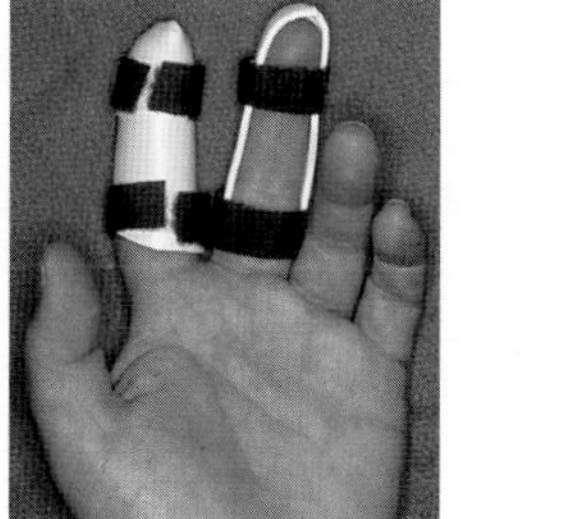

CLINICAL PEARL
Digit Exercise Splints

A splint that immobilizes all the PIP and DIP joints in extension can aid in directing the forces of flexion to the MP joints during active flexion exercises (A). This type of splint can be used as an exercise tool to increase active MP flexion, which is often necessary after MP joint arthroplasty. A splint that immobilizes the PIP joint in extension can aid in directing the force of flexion to the DIP joint during active flexion exercises (B). This splint can be used as an exercise tool to increase active DIP flexion, to maximize FDP tendon glide, and/or to stretch tight oblique retinacular ligaments.

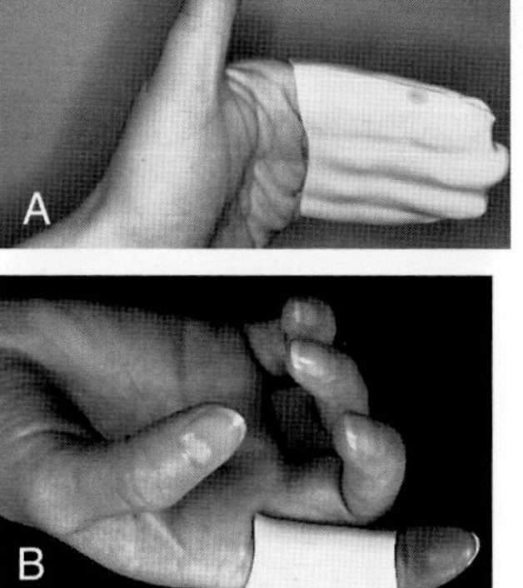

Fabrication Process

Pattern Creation (Fig. 7–4)

- Mark for proximal border at proximal digital crease and distal border at distal digital crease.
- Allow extra $^1/_4$" to $^1/_2$" of material around borders, depending on digit circumference.
- Consider including DIP joint if splinted digit is small (children, small adults) to improve ability of splint to secure desired PIP joint position.

Refine Pattern

- Proximal border should allow unrestricted MP joint motion.
- Distal border should allow unrestricted DIP joint motion.
- Lateral borders should encompass two thirds of circumference of digit to prevent undue compressive stress from straps.
- Web space areas should have adequate rooms to allow unrestricted motion of adjacent digits.
- May extend pattern distally to include DIP joint.

Options for Materials

- Consider using $^3/_{32}$" thermoplastic material (perforated or nonperforated); it is light and thin but still provides stability to PIP joint.
- Materials that can be reheated and remolded several times are a good option if ongoing splint modifications become necessary to accommodate for fluctuations in edema or changes in desired joint position.
- A circumferential design fabricated with plaster, QuickCast, or thermoplastic material can help when splinting the small finger PIP joint. Small surface area can make it difficult for the traditional design to obtain adequate purchase.

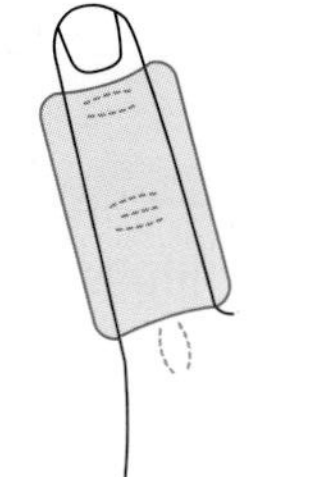

Figure 7–4

Cut and Heat

- Position patient forearm supinated for volar design and pronated for dorsal design.
- If using elasticized wrap (Coban) under splint, apply to digit before heating splint material.
- Thin padding over PIP joint may be incorporated into dorsal design if necessary; apply to digit before heating splint material.

Evaluate Fit While Molding

DORSAL DESIGN

- Place material on dorsal aspect of digit, just proximal to dorsal DIP joint skin folds and distal to MP joint. The longer the longitudinal borders, the more stable the splint on the digit.
- Allow gravity to form lateral borders of splint. Avoid grabbing or wrapping material around digit.
- Avoid applying direct pressure over dorsum of PIP joint while molding, which may cause pressure areas.

VOLAR DESIGN

- Place material on volar aspect of digit, just clearing DIP joint crease and slightly distal to MP joint crease.
- Allow gravity to form lateral borders of splint. Avoid grabbing or wrapping material around digit.
- If used to address flexion contracture, carefully mold with even, gentle pressure throughout length of splint in direction of extension.

Strapping and Components

- Use two $^1/_2$" straps or one 1" strap to secure splint directly over PIP joint.
- Extra-thin $^1/_2$" strapping material can help decrease bulk between digits.

DORSAL DESIGN

- Place straps at proximal border and over middle phalanx.

VOLAR DESIGN

- Place straps over proximal and middle phalanx.
- Place one strap with piece of foam directly over PIP joint, if maintaining PIP extension is an issue.
- Light padding under distal strap may reduce splint migration and improve comfort.

Splint Finishing Touches

- Smooth material borders and avoid rolling or flaring, which may irritate adjacent soft tissues and web spaces or may interfere with MP and/or DIP joint movement.
- Check for mobility of uninvolved joints.

Thumb Interphalangeal (IP) Immobilization Splint (Fig. 7–5)

Common Names

- Thumb IP extension splint
- Static thumb splint

Alternative Splint Options

- Aluminum padded splint
- Stax splint
- Thumb cast

Primary Functions

- Immobilize thumb IP joint to allow healing of involved structure(s).
- Rest a painful and/or inflamed thumb IP joint.

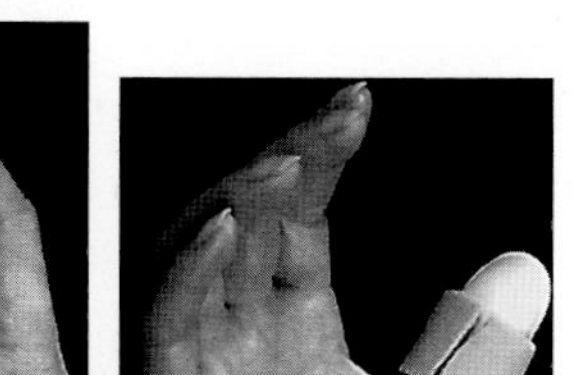

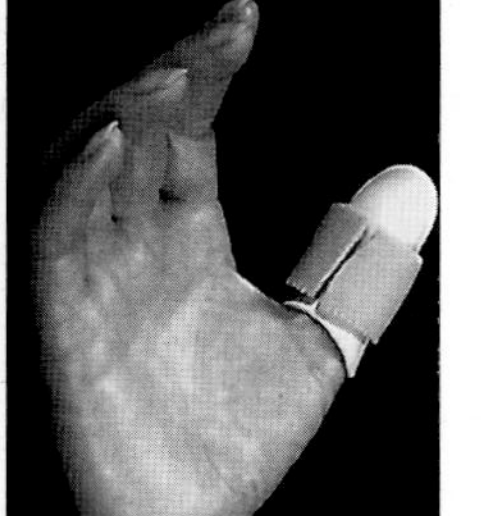

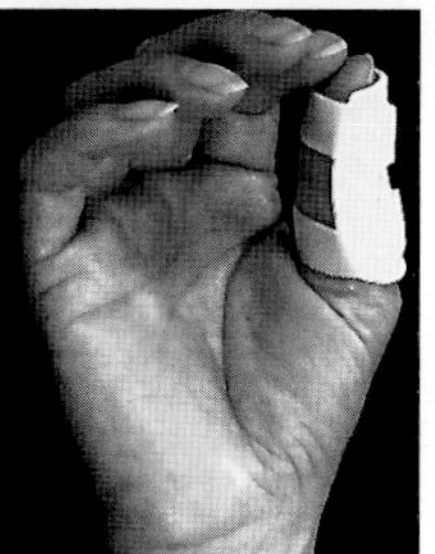

Figure 7–5

Additional Functions

- Statically position IP joint flexion contracture at maximum extension to facilitate lengthening of tissue (mobilization splint).

Common Diagnoses and General Optimal Positions

Diagnosis	Position
• Zone TI extensor tendon injury (mallet th)	+5 to +15° hyperextension
• Distal phalanx fracture	0 to +15° hyperextension (depends on flexor pollicis longus [FPL] status)
• Crush injury to distal phalanx	0° to slight hyperextension
• Nail bed injury and repair	0°
• Partial tip amputation	Tolerable ext
• IP jt sprain	0° to slight hyperextension
• IP jt arthritis	Position of comfort

CLINICAL PEARL
Protective Fingertip Splint Caps

To mold the distal end of a digit splint, pinch the excess distal material together; then cut to the shape of the tip, forming a protective cap. Carefully smooth the seam while the material is warm to prevent separation. This closed-tip design protects the tip post crush or nailbed injury.

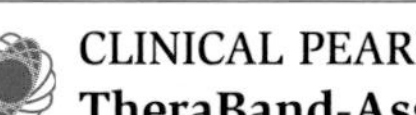

CLINICAL PEARL
Thumb Splint with Tab

The overlapping tabs of a volar design should encompass the majority of the proximal phalanx dorsally, allowing approximately ½" overlap. Use a thin coated material (preferably $^{3}/_{32}$" or $^{1}/_{16}$") to prevent inadvertent bonding of the dorsal tabs. Use one ½" strap on the most superficial tab and secure it to hook material.

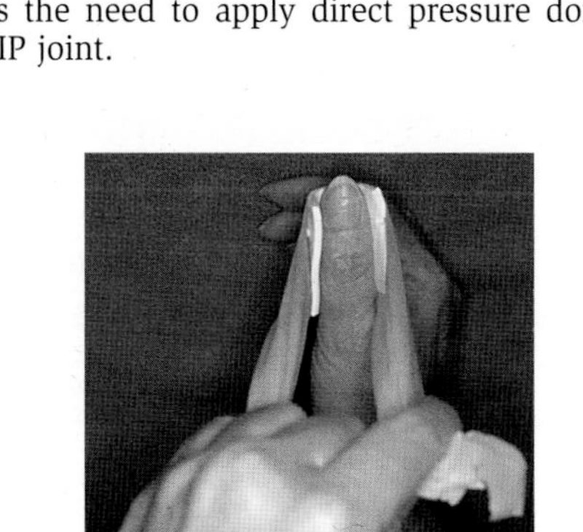

CLINICAL PEARL
TheraBand-Assisted Molding

TheraBand can be applied volarly to the distal phalanx while molding a volar DIP splint. This technique aids in positioning the DIP in hyperextension and precludes the need to apply direct pressure dorsally at the DIP joint.

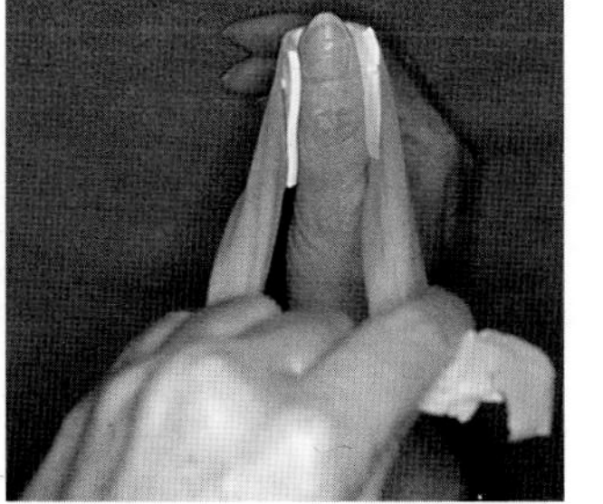

Fabrication Process

Pattern Creation (Fig. 7–6)

- Mark for proximal border at proximal thumb crease.
- Allow extra 1/4" to 1/2" of material around borders, depending on thumb circumference.
- Dorsal design may improve function of thumb by providing partial sensory input.

Refine Pattern

DORSAL DESIGN

- Extend proximal border to middle of dorsal MP joint skinfolds.
- Lateral borders should encompass two thirds of circumference of thumb to prevent undue compressive stress from straps.
- Taper lateral borders slightly volar and distal to avoid irritation at first web space.

VOLAR DESIGN

- Extend proximal border just distal to volar MP joint crease.
- Taper lateral borders slightly dorsal and proximal.

Options for Materials

- Consider nonremovable circumferential splint or cast for young children or questionably compliant patients.

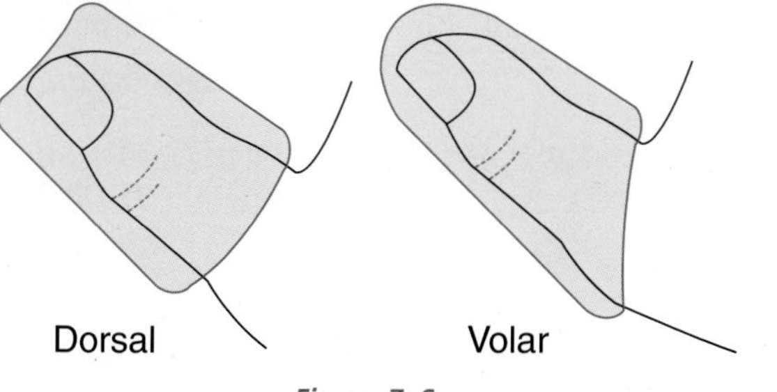

Figure 7–6

- Perforated thermoplastics may prevent skin maceration; consider using them for patients who require full-time splint use.
- Use thinnest material possible that provides necessary strength, to decrease splint bulk.
- Materials that can be reheated and remolded several times are a good option if ongoing splint modifications become necessary to accommodate for fluctuations in edema or changes in desired joint position.

Cut and Heat

- Position patient's forearm supinated for volar design and pronated for dorsal design.
- IP joint position depends on diagnosis.
- If using elasticized wrap (Coban) or dressings under splint, apply to thumb before heating splint material.

Evaluate Fit While Molding

DORSAL DESIGN

- Place material on dorsal aspect of thumb to middle of dorsal MP joint skinfolds. The longer the proximal border, the more stable the splint on the thumb.
- Avoid applying direct pressure over dorsum of IP joint while molding, which may create pressure spots. Thin padding may be incorporated if necessary.
- Allow gravity to contour lateral sides of small splint, otherwise keep hands lightly moving along material to provide intimate contouring.
- Slightly flare material about the MP joint.

VOLAR DESIGN

- Place material on volar aspect of thumb, just clearing volar MP joint crease.
- Apply slight IP extension pressure (patient may aid in extending tip by using his or her other hand to gently lift tip by fingernail).

Strapping and Components

- Use one or two straps to secure splint.
- Apply straps proximally as close to MP flexion crease as possible without interfering with MP joint flexion.
- May use fork or Y-type straps or elasticized wrap to secure splint to thumb.

Splint Finishing Touches

- Smooth material borders and avoid rolling or flaring, which may irritate adjacent soft tissues or may interfere with thumb MP joint movement.

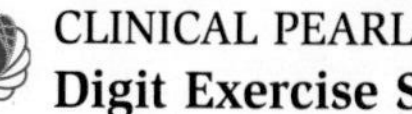

CLINICAL PEARL

Digit Exercise Splint

A splint that immobilizes the DIP joint in extension can aid in directing the force of flexion to the PIP joint during active exercises. This splint can be used as an exercise tool to increase active PIP flexion and/or maximize FDS tendon glide. Note the self-sealing edge on the volar surface of the circumferential splint design shown; it was created by cutting the thermoplastic material while it was still warm.

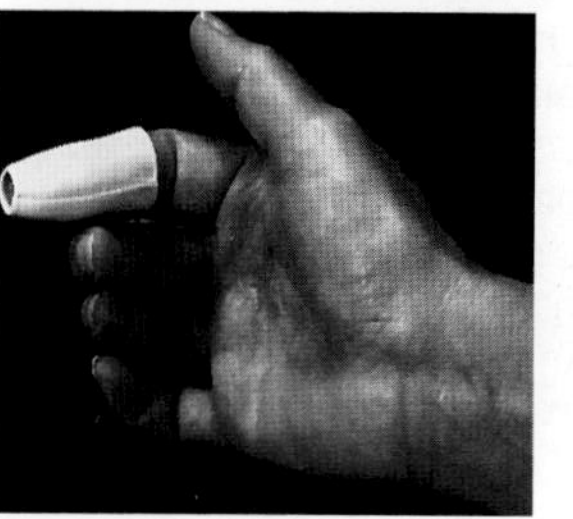

2 • Hand-Based Splints

Dorsal MP/PIP/DIP Immobilization Splint (Fig. 7–7)

Common Names

- Hand-based digit extension splint
- Hand-based digit resting splint
- Static finger splint
- Dorsal hand splint

Primary Functions

- Immobilize the MP, PIP, and/or DIP joint(s) to allow healing or rest of the involved structure(s).

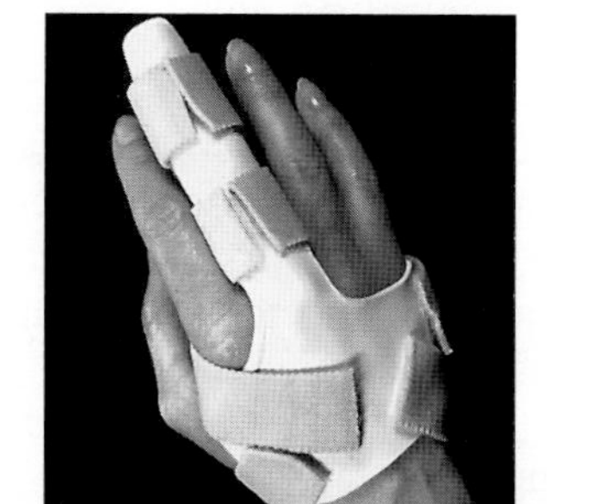

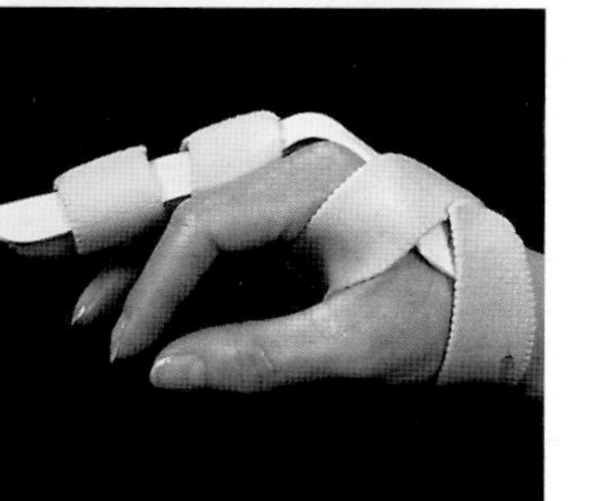

Figure 7–7

Additional Functions

- Restrict specific amount of extension (e.g., after digital nerve repair) to protect healing structures (restriction splint).

Common Diagnoses and General Optimal Positions

Diagnosis	Position
• Intra-articular fracture of PIP/DIP jt	MP: 60° flex, PIP/DIP: 0°
• Dupuytren's surgical release	Postsurgery: all jts maximal ext; 3 to 6+ months: maximum ext at night only
• Trigger finger	MP: 0°; PIP/DIP: free
• Tenosynovitis	Position of comfort, intrinsic plus
• Infection	Position of comfort, intrinsic plus
• MP/PIP jt volar plate injury	MP/PIP: 20 to 30° flex

CLINICAL PEARL
Tab Through Web Space

Using a pattern that extends a tab through the first web space can help prevent splint migration and add stability to the splint. The use of a rivet provides a secure means of attaching strapping to a small area.

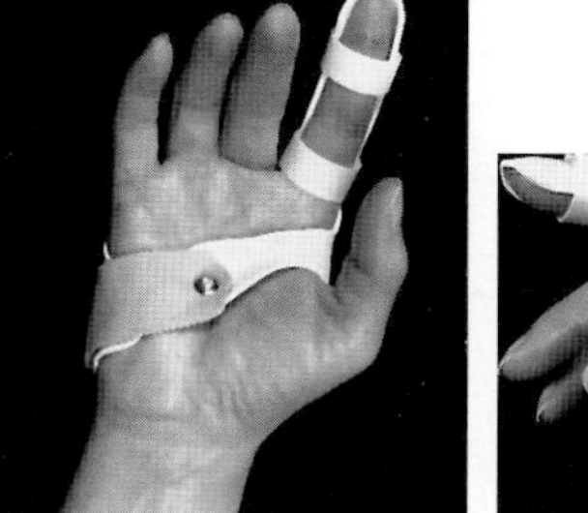

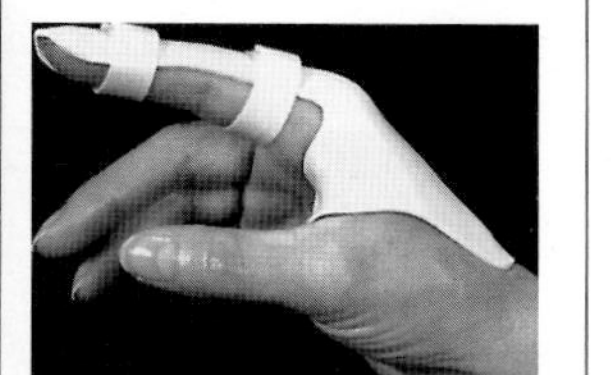

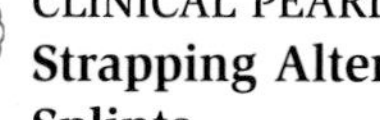

CLINICAL PEARL
Strapping Alternatives for Small-Digit Splints

Instead of traditional straps, an elasticized wrap, such as Coban, can be applied circumferentially over small thermoplastic splints. This wrap helps secure the splint to the digit, prevents splint migration, and helps control edema. Elasticized wraps can also be used over finger casts to keep them clean and/or to better secure the proximal portion of the cast, if the therapist is concerned that the cast will become loose if edema subsides. If elasticized wrap is applied beneath the splint, use tape (e.g., Transpore or Microfoam) to secure the splint to the digit. As shown, a split strap design can be used to increase the surface area for attachment of the loop material onto the hook (A). Or use tape to secure a dorsal AlumaFoam splint (B).

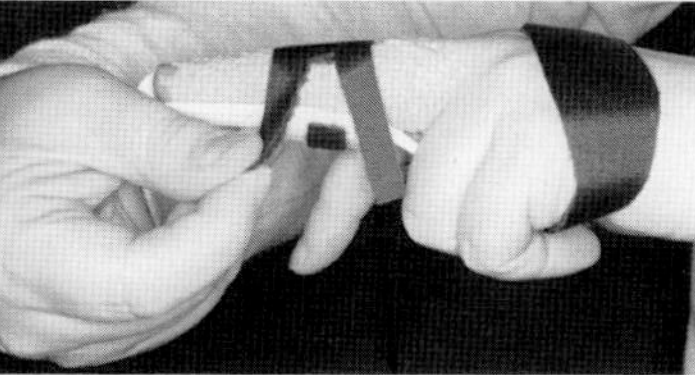

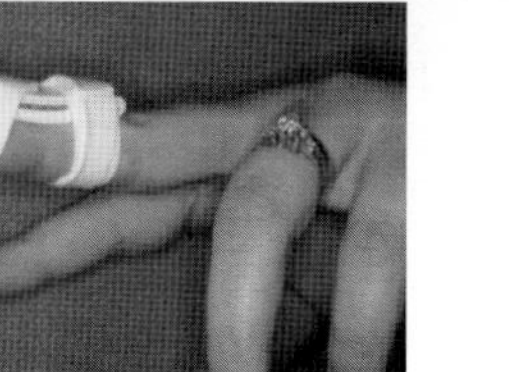

Fabrication Process

Pattern Creation (Fig. 7–8)

- Consider dorsal design if patient presents with volar wound, skin graft, or incision to allow for air circulation.
- Mark for proximal border at wrist crease.
- Allow extra 1/4" to 1/2" of material around borders, depending on digit circumference.
- Be sure the proximal portion of the splint has adequate surface area for strap application.
- For small finger (SF), consider splinting together with ring finger (RF) to provide greater protection, better splint stabilization, and improved comfort.
- If MP is to be flexed, allow extra material distally to accommodate for flexion angle. If material must be stretched over MP joint, a weakened and unstable splint may result.
- Draw pattern with fingers slightly abducted. Be sure to provide enough surface area to accommodate all immobilized digits. Remember, material can always be trimmed away after initial molding is completed.

Refine Pattern

- Proximal border should allow full wrist motion and clearance of ulnar styloid.

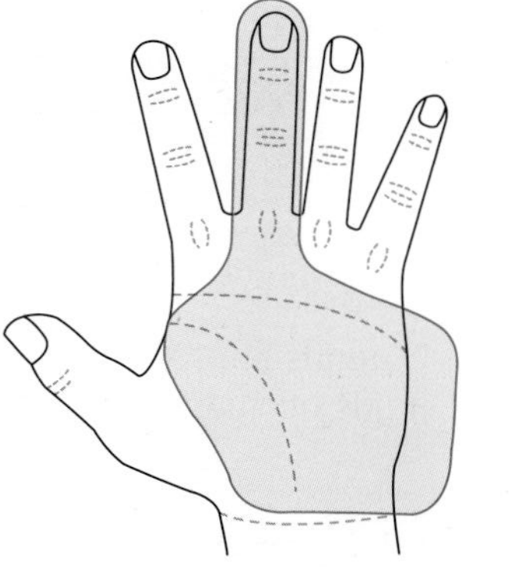

Figure 7–8

- Lateral digit borders should form trough to prevent undue compressive stress from straps; however, if lateral borders of splint are too generous, digit may have too much mobility within splint.
- Allow adequate room in digit web space areas to allow unrestricted motion of unaffected digits.

Options for Materials

- Use highly drapable material to achieve intimate fit over MP joints to prevent splint migration and improve comfort.
- Perforated thermoplastics may help prevent skin maceration; consider using them for patients who require full-time splint use.
- Materials that can be reheated and remolded several times are a good option if ongoing splint modifications become necessary to accommodate for fluctuations in edema, changes in motion, or bulk of dressings.

Cut and Heat

- Position patient's forearm pronated for gravity-assisted molding.
- If using elasticized wrap (Coban) or dressings under splint, apply to digit before heating splint material.
- Thin padding may be incorporated dorsally across MP joints if necessary; apply before heating splint material.

Evaluate Fit While Molding

- Lateral borders should form trough, instead of flat pan, to strengthen molded splint.
- Contour dorsal MP area well. If more than one digit is included in splint, make sure contours of dorsal MP joints are well defined.
- Avoid applying direct pressure over dorsum of MP and PIP joints while molding.

Strapping and Components

- Apply straps at DIP joint, around proximal phalanx, through first web space to ulnar border, and about wrist to prevent splint migration.
- Soft or elasticized strap works well around wrist.
- Consider using rivets to secure one end of proximal strap to minimize space needed for hook material.

Splint Finishing Touches

- Smooth material borders and avoid rolling or flaring, which may irritate adjacent soft tissues and web spaces or may interfere with unaffected joint movement.
- Check for unrestricted movement of uninvolved joints.

CLINICAL PEARL

Strapping Through Web Spaces

Trim strapping material to contour through the web spaces to prevent the borders from irritating these sensitive areas. Notice how inadequate splint length may lead to a pressure point at the proximal border (A). Ideally, the splint should incorporate the ulnar border of the hand and extend proximally just distal to the wrist crease. Note that elasticized strapping material tends to fray if trimmed. An alternative is to use thin strapping material to decrease the bulk between the digits (B).

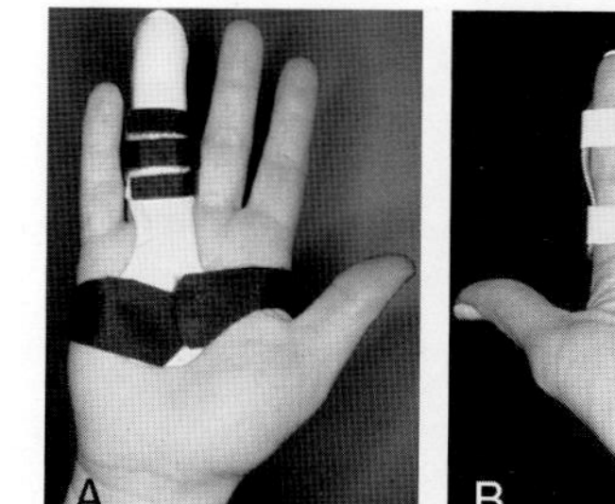

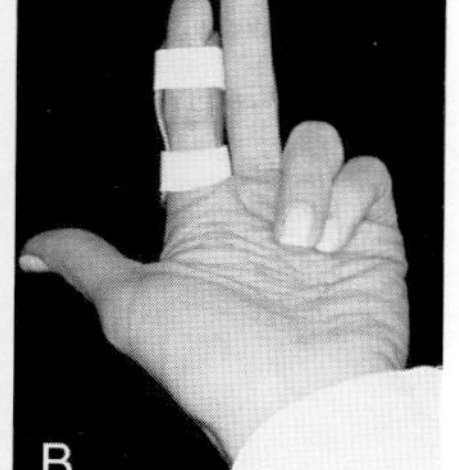

Volar MP/PIP/DIP Immobilization Splint (Fig. 7–9)

Common Names

- Hand-based digit extension splint
- Hand-based digit resting splint
- Static finger splint
- Volar resting splint
- Volar hand splint

Primary Functions

- Immobilize the MP, PIP, and/or DIP joint(s) to allow healing or rest of the involved structure(s).

Additional Functions

- Promote gliding of flexor digitorum superficialis (FDS) and flexor digitorum profundus (FDP) tendons and actively stretch intrinsic muscles by restricting movement of MP joint during active flexion exercises.
- Statically position MP joint contracture at maximum flexion or extension to facilitate lengthening of tissue (mobilization splint).
- Restrict specific amount of flexion (e.g., after zone IV extensor tendon repair) to protect healing structures (restriction splint).

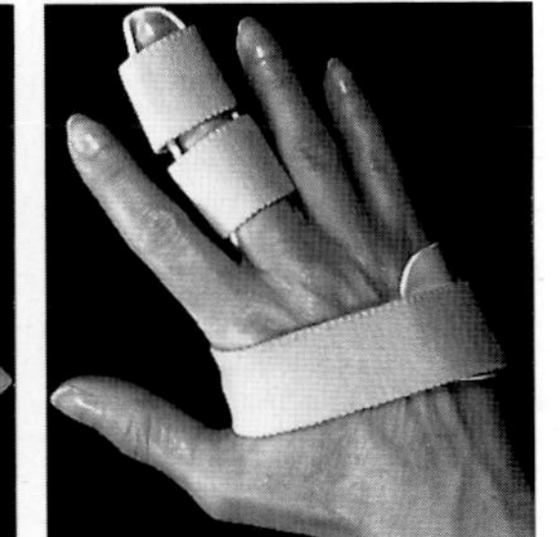
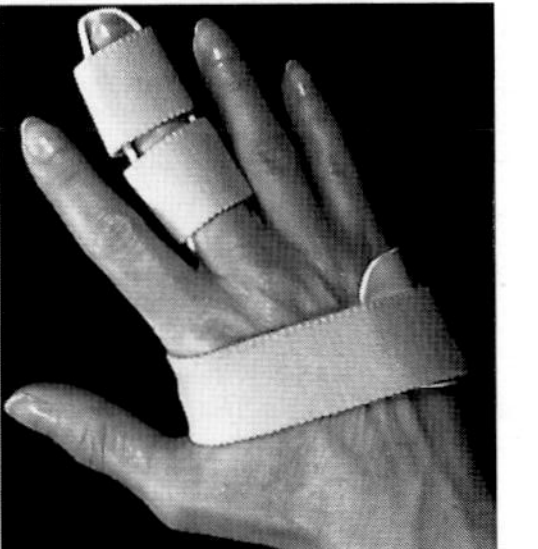

Figure 7–9

Common Diagnoses and General Optimal Positions

Diagnosis	Position
• Intra-articular fracture of PIP or DIP jt	MP: 60° flex; PIP/DIP: 0°
• Fracture of proximal and/or middle phalanx	MP: slight flex; PIP/DIP: 0°
• Dupuytren's surgical release	Postsurgery: all jts maximal ext; 3 to 6+ months: maximum ext at night only
• MP jt sprain	MP: 60 to 80° flex; PIP/DIP: 0°
• Trigger finger release	MP: 0°; PIP/DIP: free
• Tenosynovitis	Position of comfort, intrinsic plus
• Infection	Position of comfort, intrinsic plus
• Crush injury	MP: 60 to 80° flex; PIP/DIP: 0°
• Zone IV extensor tendon injury	MP/PIP/DIP: 0°
• Sagittal band injury and repair	MP: 0° with slight deviation to side of injury or repair; PIP/DIP: free

CLINICAL PEARL

Rolling Material Through Web Spaces

Avoid cutting splint material to accommodate for web space areas. This may significantly alter the rigidity of the splint. Instead, carefully roll and flatten a small border of the warm material back onto itself, just enough to clear for mobility of the adjacent digits.

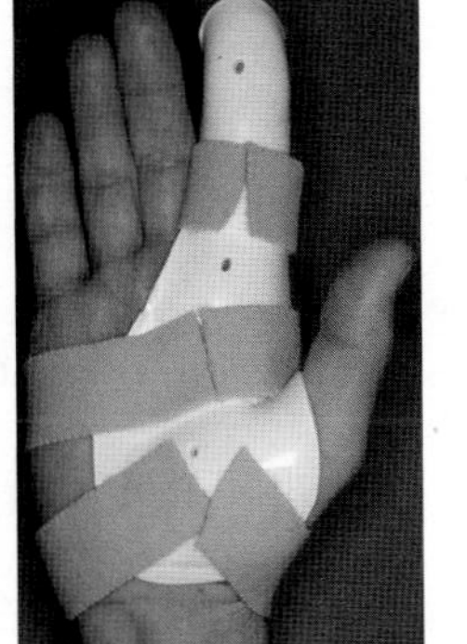

CLINICAL PEARL

Contouring Around Thumb to Increase IF Stability

Allowing unimpeded thumb mobility when immobilizing the IF is challenging, because to adequately stabilize this digit, a portion of the thenar eminence must be included in the splint. The contouring technique shown provides good stability to the splint along the radial volar aspect of the splint and allows maximal thumb mobility.

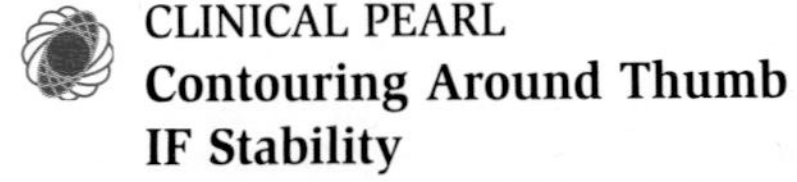

Fabrication Process

Pattern Creation (Fig. 7–10)

- Consider volar design if patient has dorsal wound, extruding pins, or incision to allow for better air circulation.
- Mark for proximal border at wrist crease.
- Allow extra 1/4" to 1/2" of material around borders, depending on digit circumference.
- Be sure proximal portion of the splint has adequate surface area for strap application.
- If SF is involved, consider splinting together with RF finger to provide greater protection, better splint stabilization, and improved comfort.
- Draw pattern with fingers slightly abducted. Be sure to provide enough surface area to accommodate all immobilized digits. Remember, material can always be trimmed away after initial molding is completed.

Refine Pattern

- Proximal border should allow full wrist motion.
- Radial border should allow nearly full thumb motion.
- Lateral borders should form trough to prevent undue compressive stress from straps.

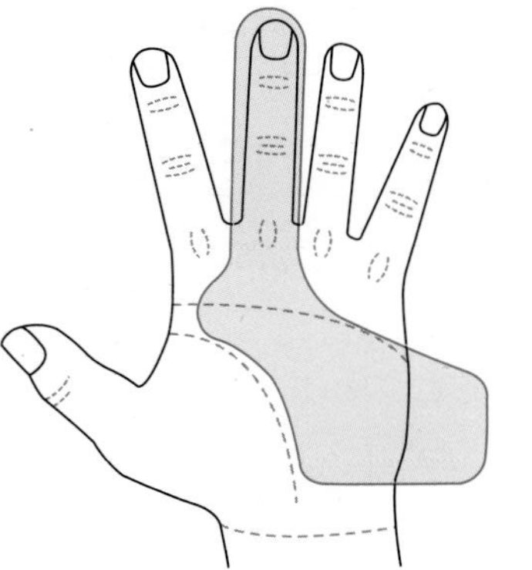

Figure 7–10

- Allow adequate room in web space areas to allow unrestricted motion of unaffected digits.
- May modify pattern to exclude PIP and/or DIP joints if necessary.

Options for Materials

- Perforated thermoplastics may prevent skin maceration; consider using them for patients who require full-time splint use.
- Materials that can be reheated and remolded several times are a good option if ongoing splint modifications become necessary to accommodate for fluctuations in edema, changes in motion, or bulk of dressings.

Cut and Heat

- Position patient with hand supinated for gravity assisted molding.
- If using elasticized wrap (Coban) or dressings under splint, apply to digit before heating splint material.

Evaluate Fit While Molding

- Lateral borders should form trough, instead of flat pan, to strengthen molded splint.
- Remember that when splinting index finger (IF), thumb mobility is somewhat hindered owing to necessary contouring about thumb web to obtain proper fit.

Strapping and Components

- Apply straps at DIP joint, around proximal phalanx, and through web space to ulnar border.
- Additional strap around wrist may be necessary to prevent migration and aid in proper fit.
- Consider using rivets to secure one end of proximal strap to minimize space needed for hook material.
- Padding under proximal phalanx strap may reduce splint migration and rotation, maintain MP joint position, and improve comfort.
- A customized soft foam strap used through first web space can improve comfort and prevent skin irritation caused by friction from traditional loop material.

Splint Finishing Touches

- Smooth material borders and avoid rolling or flaring, which may irritate adjacent soft tissues and web spaces or may interfere with unaffected joint movement.
- Check for unrestricted movement of uninvolved joints.

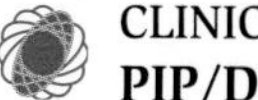

CLINICAL PEARL
PIP/DIP Exercise Splint

A splint that immobilizes the MP joints in extension can aid in directing the force of flexion to the PIP or DIP joints during active exercises. This splint can be used as an exercise tool to increase active PIP and DIP flexion, to maximize FDS and FDP tendon glide, and/or to stretch tight intrinsic muscles.

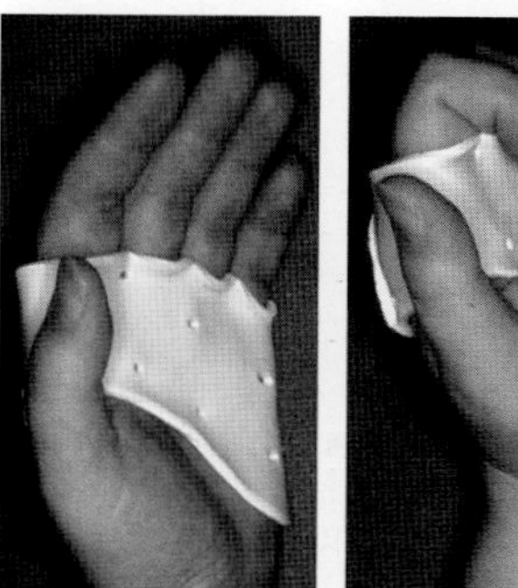

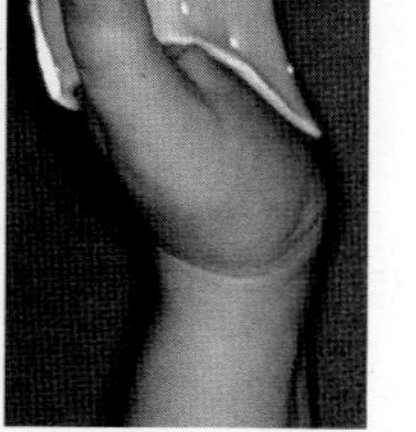

Ulnar MP/PIP/DIP Immobilization Splint (Fig. 7–11)

Common Names

- Hand-based ulnar gutter splint
- Hand-based ulnar fracture brace
- Metacarpal fracture brace
- Clamdigger splint

Alternative Splint Options

- Plaster cast

Primary Functions

- Immobilize proximal phalanxes and metacarpals of RF and SF to allow healing and/or protection of involved structure(s).

Additional Functions

- Restrict MP joint extension secondary to low ulnar nerve injury (restriction splint).

Common Diagnoses and General Optimal Positions

- Metacarpal head or neck fracture — MP: 60 to 90° flex (may include PIP/DIP: 0°)
- Proximal phalanx fracture — MP: 60 to 90° flex; PIP/DIP: 0°
- Complicated middle phalanx fracture — MP: 60 to 90° flex; PIP/DIP: 0°
- MP capsulectomy — MP: 60 to 90° flex; PIP/DIP: 0°

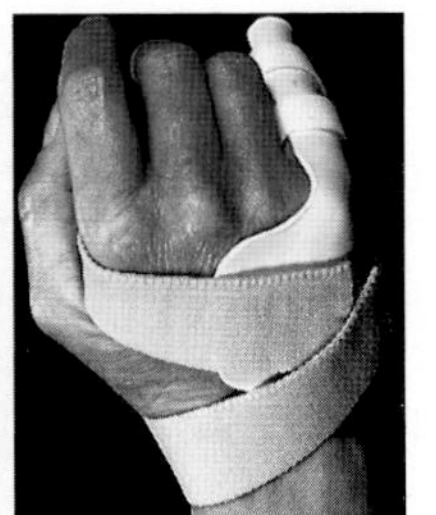
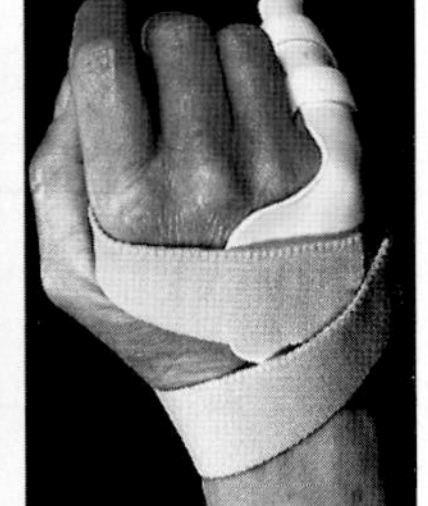

Figure 7–11

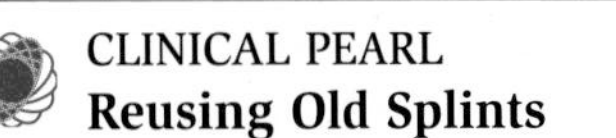

CLINICAL PEARL
Rivets to Secure Straps

Riveting straps on the splint helps secure and maintain the strap position, especially in small areas where it may be difficult to adhere hook material. Always apply a thin lining material, such as Moleskin, on the under side of the rivet to avoid skin irritation. Another method is to attach the strap on the skin side of the splint to prevent irritation from the underside of the rivet.

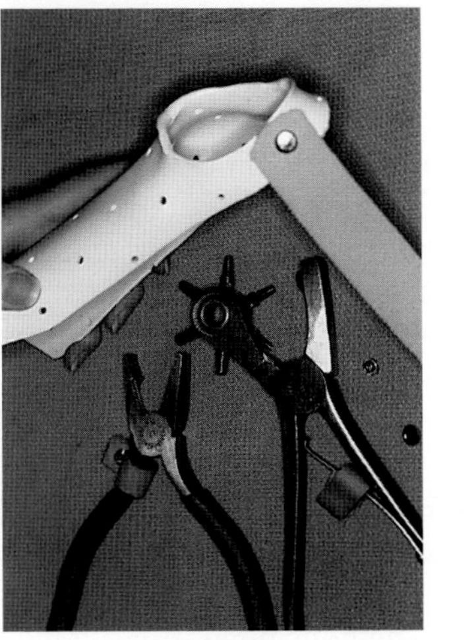

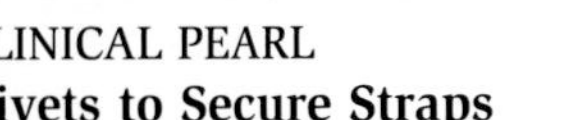

CLINICAL PEARL
Reusing Old Splints

To save money, reuse old splints to fabricate new splints, when appropriate. For example, during the initial phases of healing after a scaphoid fracture, the patient may require a wrist and thumb immobilization splint for protection. Once the fracture has healed, the patient may experience joint stiffness at the thumb MP and/or IP joints that requires mobilization splinting. The original immobilization splint can be remolded into a mobilization splint by simply trimming the thumb region and attaching components.

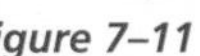

CLINICAL PEARL
Forearm-Based Ulnar MP/PIP/DIP Immobilization Splint

The wrist can be incorporated into a hand-based design. The ulnar styloid should be prepadded for comfort. The PIP and DIP joints of the involved digits may be included, depending on the diagnosis (i.e., location of the fracture). This splint was lined with 1/16" material to provide increased splint stability. Commonly, a forearm-based splint can be remolded and modified to a hand-based design as healing progresses.

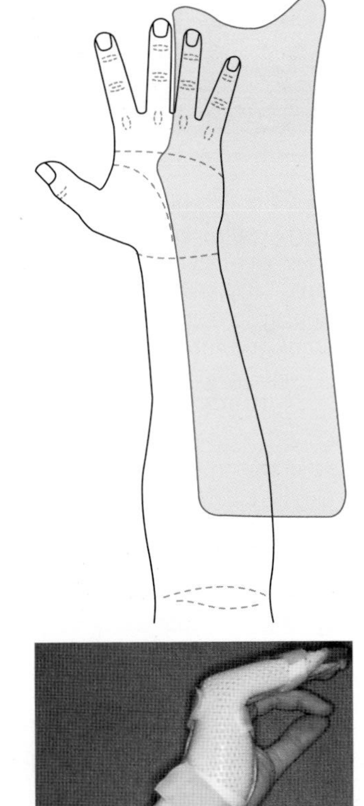

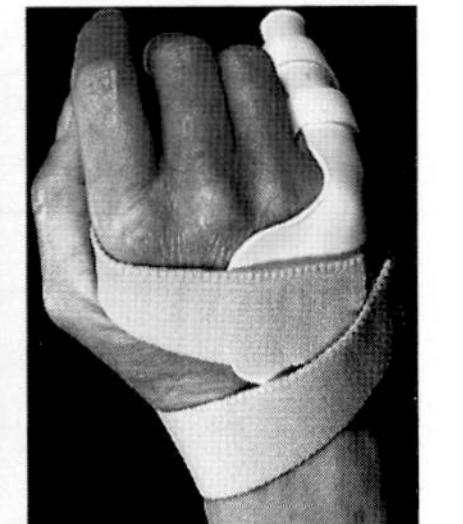

Fabrication Process

Pattern Creation (Fig. 7–12)

- Mark for proximal border at wrist crease, clearing ulnar styloid.
- Allow extra ½" to 1" of material distally, because dorsal material must stretch over flexed MP joints.

Refine Pattern

- Proximal border should allow full wrist motion.
- Radial border should allow full thumb, IF, middle finger (MF), and RF motion.
- Make sure pattern encompasses third metacarpal proximal to MP joint. Remember fourth and fifth metacarpals are mobile—thus if goal is to immobilize metacarpal fracture, splint must be anchored to stable third metacarpal.
- Allow unimpeded motion of RF by keeping splint design accurate.

Options for Materials

- Use drapable material to achieve intimate fit about MP joints to prevent splint migration and improve comfort.
- Materials that can be reheated and remolded several times are a good option if ongoing splint modifications become necessary to accommodate for fluctuations in edema and changes in MP joint motion.
- Perforated thermoplastics may prevent skin maceration; consider using them for patients who require full-time splint use.

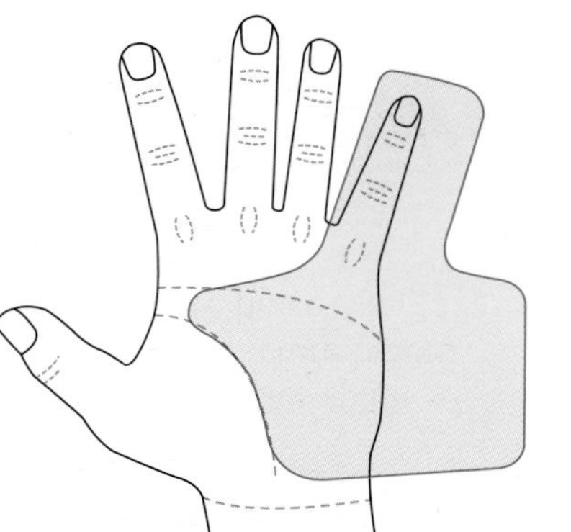

Figure 7–12

Cut and Heat

- Position extremity with shoulder and elbow flexed with forearm pronation to achieve gravity-assist position (ulnar border of hand should face upward).
- Place MP joint in appropriate amount of flexion.
- If included, position PIP and/or DIP joints as per diagnosis.
- If using thin padding dorsally across MP joints, apply to the area before heating splint material.

Evaluate Fit While Molding

- Place material on ulnar aspect of hand just distal to wrist.
- Gently stretch dorsal material over MP joints while maintaining arches of hand.
- Allow gravity to assist while gently contouring and encompassing SF and MP joint proximally.
- Incorporate natural descent of fifth MP below fourth MP.
- Be sure to maintain desired joint positions as material sets.
- Avoid applying direct pressure over dorsum of MP and PIP joints while molding.
- Do not seal off splint distally; allow for ability to check for vascular compromise and provide some air exchange.
- Amount of MP flexion desired may be difficult to achieve initially due to pain, stiffness, and/or dorsal edema; serial splinting into flexion may be necessary.

Strapping and Components

- Soft or elasticized strap works well around wrist to prevent slippage.
- Use customized soft foam strap through first web space to improve comfort and prevent skin irritation caused by friction from traditional loop material.
- Consider using rivets to secure one end of proximal strap to minimize space needed for hook material.
- Traditional straps will suffice to secure digits; be sure to trim straps between digit web spaces to prevent skin irritation.

Splint Finishing Touches

- Smooth material borders, making sure there are no sharp edges, especially at ulnar styloid.
- If PIP and DIP joints are included, trim excess material from distal splint to allow for visualization of fingertips.
- Check clearance of wrist and RF, making sure there is no abutment with splint material.

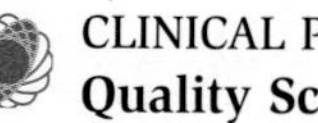

CLINICAL PEARL

Quality Scissors

Not all scissors are appropriate for every task. Having various types of scissors on hand can make the splint fabrication process a lot easier. For example, large scissors, such as Gingher heavy-duty scissors, are best used for cutting out splint patterns on warm thermoplastic material and may not be effective for small detailed cutting. Joyce Chen scissors are an excellent alternative for detailed cutting in small areas. When serial static finger splints fabricated from plaster or QuickCast are required, splint/cast trimmers are extremely helpful for removing the casts as shown.

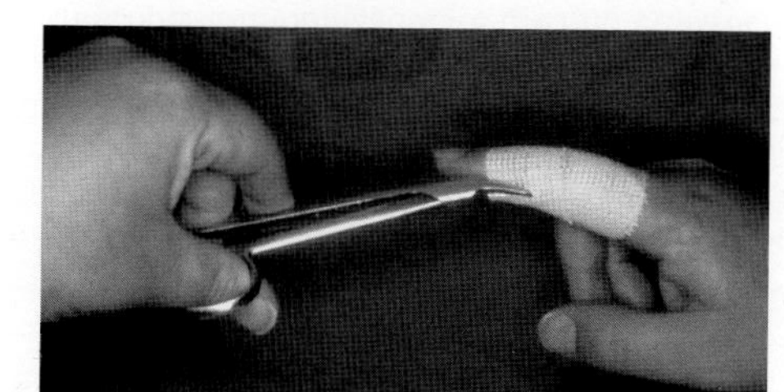

Radial MP/PIP/DIP Immobilization Splint (Fig. 7–13)

Common Names

- Hand-based radial gutter splint
- Hand-based radial fracture brace
- Metacarpal fracture brace
- Clamdigger splint

Alternative Splint Options

- Plaster cast

Primary Functions

- Immobilize proximal phalanxes and metacarpals of IF and MF to allow healing and/or protection of involved structure(s).

Common Diagnoses and General Optimal Positions

Diagnosis	Position
• Metacarpal head or neck fracture	MP: 60 to 90° flex (may include PIP/DIP: 0°)
• Proximal phalanx fracture	MP: 60 to 90° flex; PIP/DIP: 0°
• Complicated middle phalanx fracture	MP: 60 to 90° flex; PIP/DIP: 0°
• MP capsulectomy	MP: 60 to 90° flex; PIP/DIP: 0°
• Sagittal band injury or repair	MP: 0° with slight deviation to affected side; PIP/DIP: free

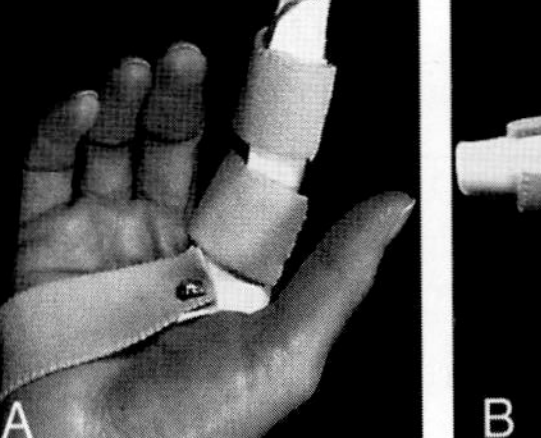
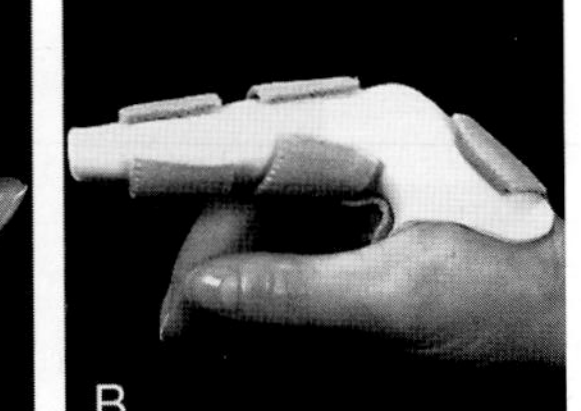
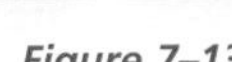

Figure 7–13

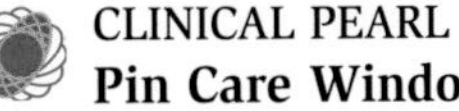

CLINICAL PEARL
Pin Care Window

For patients with complicated injuries that require pin care during the immobilization period, consider fabricating a removable window for easy access to the pins. This technique eliminates the need to remove the entire splint when inspecting pin sites. While molding the splint material over the pin(s), use a piece of gauze or cotton batting to prevent the thermoplastic material from adhering to the pins; this also provides a protective bubble to ensure the material will not place undue pressure directly over the area.

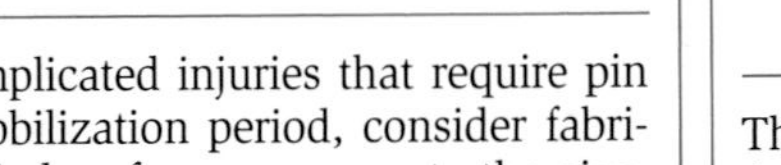
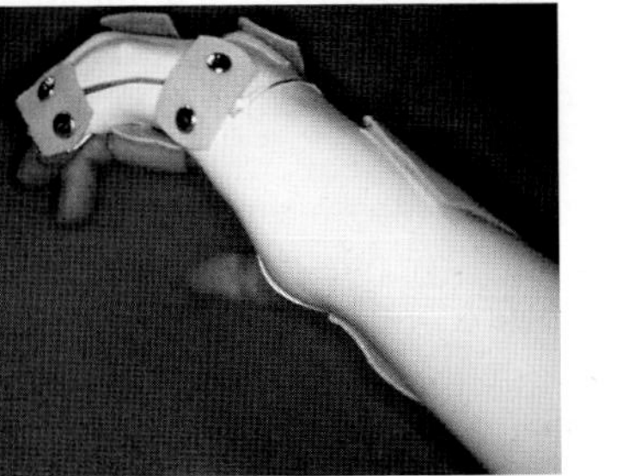
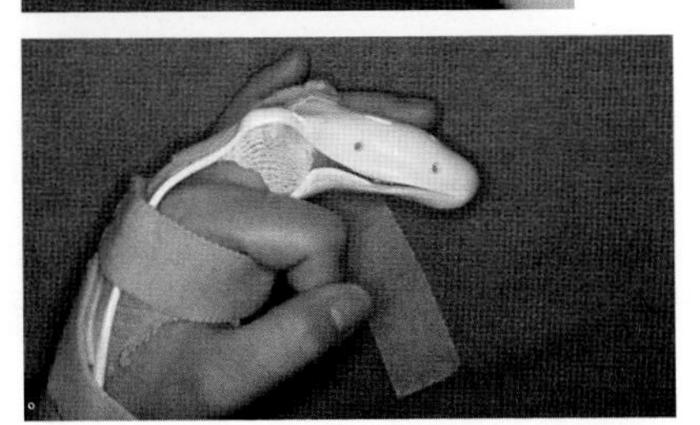

CLINICAL PEARL
Forearm-Based Radial Wrist/MP Immobilization Splint

The wrist can be incorporated into a hand-based splint design. The PIP or DIP joints of the involved digits may be included, depending on the diagnosis (i.e., location of the fracture). Take caution not to cut the thenar hole too big, which decreases the stability of the splint and risks improper immobilization of the injured structures. With the forearm-based design, be careful not to apply pressure over the superficial radial sensory nerve. Commonly, a forearm-based splint needs to be modified to a hand-based design as healing progresses.

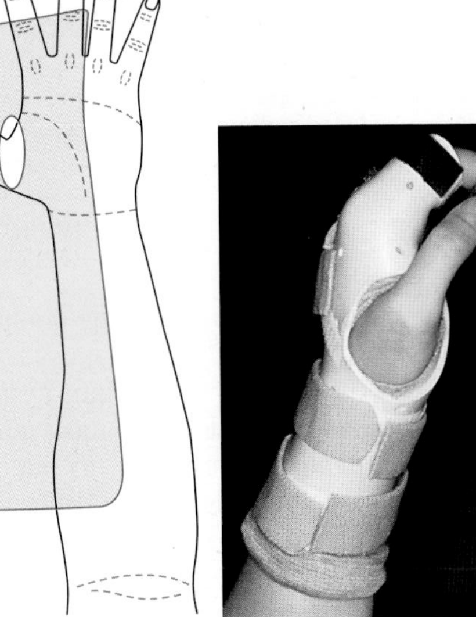
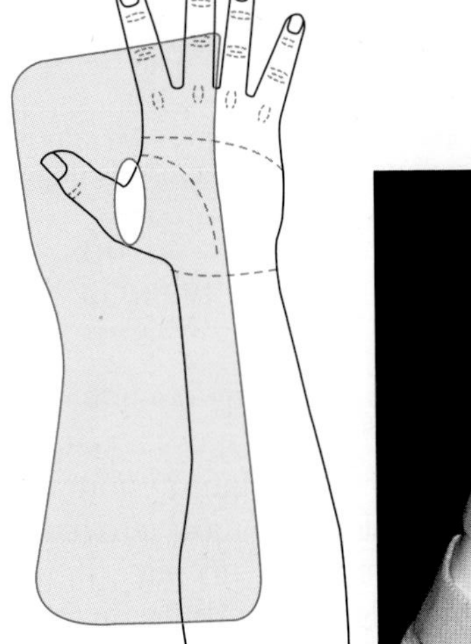

Fabrication Process

Pattern Creation (Fig. 7–14)

- Mark for proximal border at wrist crease.
- Allow extra ½" to 1" of material distally, because dorsal material must stretch over flexed MP joints.

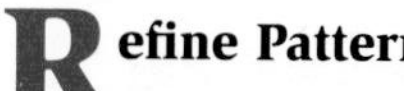

Refine Pattern

- Proximal border should allow full wrist motion.
- Ulnar border should allow full MF motion.
- Make sure pattern encompasses third metacarpal dorsally.

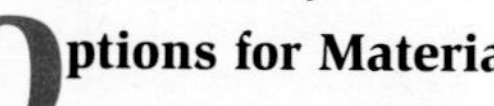

Options for Materials

- Use drapable material to achieve intimate fit about MP joints, to prevent splint migration and improve comfort.
- Materials that can be reheated and remolded several times are a good option if ongoing splint modifications become necessary to accommodate for fluctuations in edema and changes MP joint motion.

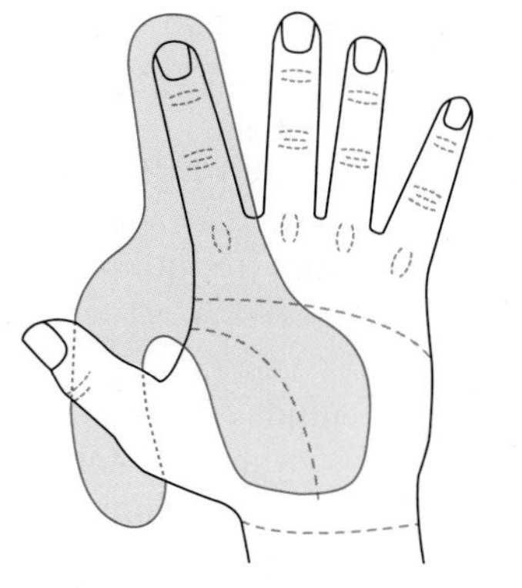

Figure 7–14

- Perforated thermoplastics may prevent skin maceration; consider using them for patients who require full-time splint use.

Cut and Heat

- Position forearm in neutral rotation to achieve gravity assist position.
- Place MP joints in appropriate amount of flexion.
- Position PIP and DIP joints as per diagnosis; place thumb in palmar abduction and opposition.
- If using thin padding dorsally across MP joints, apply to area before heating splint material.

Evaluate Fit While Molding

- Place material on radial aspect of hand just distal to wrist.
- Gently stretch dorsal material over MP joint while maintaining arches of hand.
- Allow gravity to assist while gently contouring and encompassing IF and MP joint proximally.
- Be sure to maintain desired joint positions as material sets.
- Avoid applying direct pressure over dorsum of MP and PIP joints while molding.
- Do not seal off splint distally; allow for ability to check for vascular compromise and provide some air exchange.
- Amount of MP flexion requested may be difficult to achieve initially due to pain, dorsal edema, or stiffness; serial static splinting into flexion may be necessary.

Strapping and Components

- Soft or elasticized strap works well around wrist to prevent splint migration.
- Consider using rivets to secure one end of proximal strap to minimize space needed for hook material.
- Traditional straps suffice to secure digits; be sure to trim straps in between digit web spaces to prevent irritation.

Splint Finishing Touches

- Smooth around first web space, making sure there is no irritation from material with thumb motion.
- If PIP and DIP joints are included, trim excess material from distal splint to allow for visualization of fingertips.
- Check clearance of wrist and MF, making sure there is no abutment with splint material.

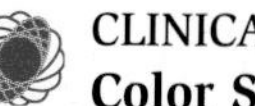

CLINICAL PEARL

Color Stain Test

When a patient complains of irritation from a splint, have him mark the area on his skin using a washable marker or lipstick; then put the splint back. When the splint is removed again, the color from the marker can be seen on the splint. Thus the therapist can identify the specific part of the splint that needs to be adjusted.

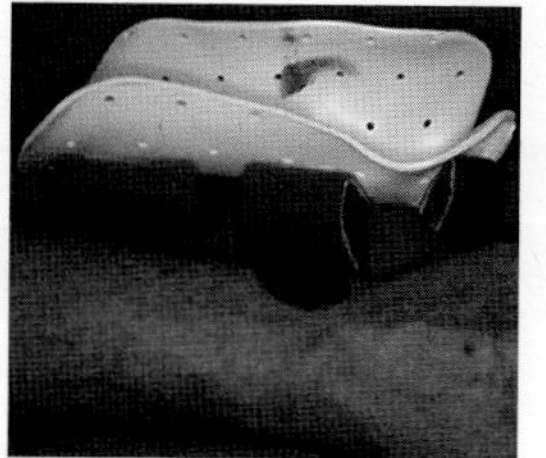

Thumb MP Immobilization Splint (Fig. 7–15)

Common Names

- Short opponens splint
- MP splint
- Basal joint splint
- Mickey Stanley (Detroit)
- Gamekeeper's thumb splint

Primary Functions

- Immobilize thumb MP joint to allow for healing of involved structure(s).
- Rest painful and/or inflamed MP joint.

Additional Functions

- Promote gliding of FPL tendon by restricting movement of MP joint during active thumb flexion exercises.

Common Diagnoses and General Optimal Positions

Diagnosis	Position
• Ulnar collateral ligament (UCL) injury (grade 1 to 3)	Slight flex MP with UD
• Radial collateral ligament (RCL) injury (grade 1 to 3)	Slight MP flex with RD
• Trapeziometacarpal (TM) jt arthritis	MP: slight flex; carpometacarpal (CMC): neutral
• MP jt arthritis	Position of comfort
• MP jt arthroplasty	Near full ext
• MP jt dorsal dislocation	20 to 30° MP flex

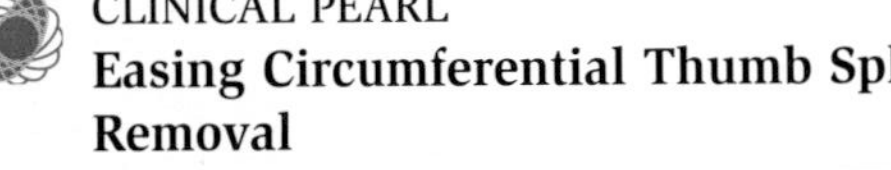
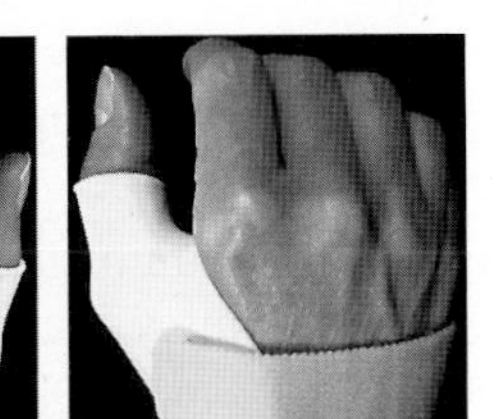

Figure 7–15

CLINICAL PEARL
Easing Circumferential Thumb Splint Removal

If thumb splint needs to come off for exercise sessions, make sure the patient can indeed remove the splint. Often the circumference of the IP joint is larger than that of the proximal phalanx, making it difficult to remove the splint. Wrapping tape or Coban around the proximal phalanx before molding can help. One disadvantage is that this technique may cause some looseness in fit proximally. Another method involves applying a thin layer of lotion to the thumb area before molding. Consider using the trap door method (see page 116, "Clinical Pearl: Trap Door for Circumferential Thumb Splints").

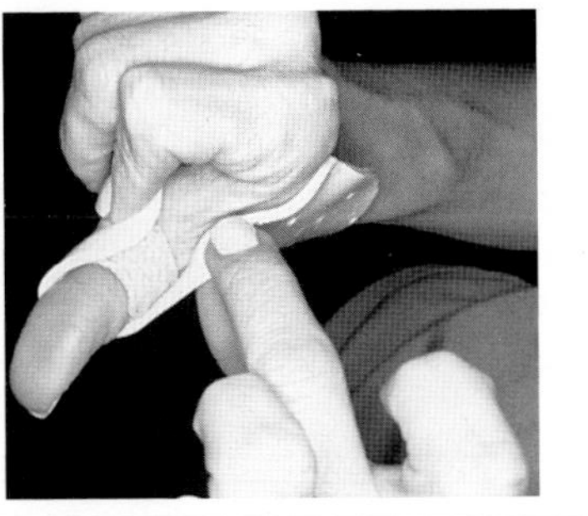

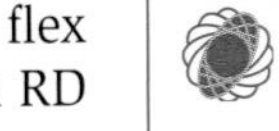

CLINICAL PEARL
Exercise Splint to Facilitate FPL Glide or Thumb IP Motion

A splint that immobilizes the thumb MP joint in extension can help direct the force of flexion to the IP joint during active exercises. This can be used as an exercise tool to increase active IP flexion and/or maximize FPL tendon glide.

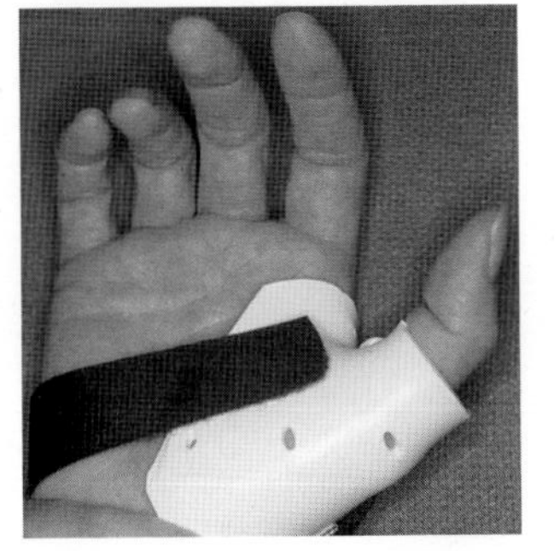

Fabrication Process

Pattern Creation (Fig. 7–16)

- Mark for proximal border just distal to wrist crease.
- Mark for ulnar border at third metacarpal.

Refine Pattern

- Proximal border should allow full wrist motion.
- Remember to allow unimpeded motion of wrist, index finger MP, and thumb IP joints by keeping splint design accurate.
- Ulnar border should allow full mobility of distal transverse arch.
- Radial portion of splint should be generous enough to be pulled through first web space and adequately cover dorsum of web space.
- May extend pattern distally to include IP joint, if necessary.

Options for Materials

- Use drapable material to achieve intimate fit at MP joint, prevent splint migration and improve comfort.

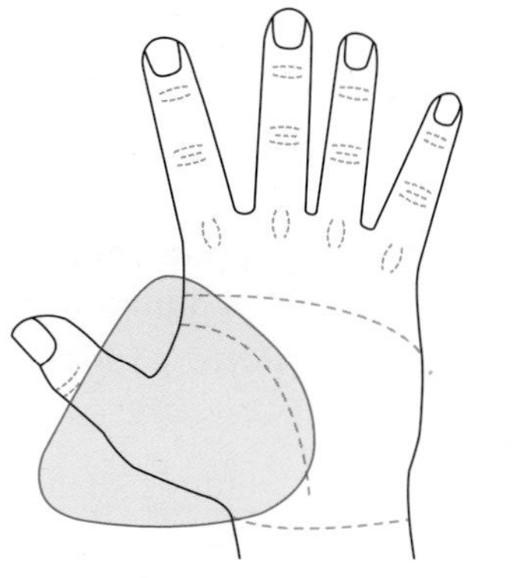

Figure 7–16

- Consider using coated material so circumferential thumb piece can be popped open without permanent bonding.
- Use thinnest material possible that provides necessary strength, to decrease splint bulk.
- Remember that elastic materials tend to shrink around proximal phalanx of thumb (making splint difficult to don and doff); do not remove until splint is completely set.

Cut and Heat

- Position patient's forearm in slight supination.
- Place thumb in palmar abduction and MP joint in appropriate flexion and deviation.
- Consider placing light layer of lotion on thumb before molding to ease removal of splint.

Evaluate Fit While Molding

- Proximally, place and mold material across thenar eminence to thenar crease.
- Distally, carefully wrap material through first web space from dorsal to volar.
- Mold through web space and overlap material onto itself by approximately 1".
- Be sure to maintain desired thumb CMC and MP joint positions as material sets.
- Avoid applying direct pressure over dorsum of MP joint while molding.
- Clear IP joint flexion crease; avoid rolling material.

Strapping and Components

- One 1" strap around wrist provides secure fit. Place strap either across hypothenar eminence or about wrist (per patient preference).
- Consider using rivets to secure strap.
- Elasticized straps are preferred across mid-hypothenar area to allow mobility of ulnar two digits.

- If circumferential portion of splint needs to be popped apart for donning and doffing over IP joint, small strap must be applied at this opening.

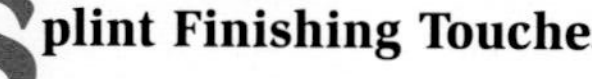

Splint Finishing Touches

- Smooth distal and proximal borders.
- Gently flare proximal to thumb IP joint.
- Check clearance of wrist, thumb IP, and index finger MP joints, making sure there is no abutment with splint material.

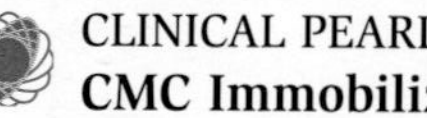

CLINICAL PEARL

CMC Immobilization Splint

The pattern for the MP joint immobilization splint can be adjusted to provide support to only the CMC joint. This allows for unimpeded MP joint mobility and may be a more functional alternative to the other designs described.

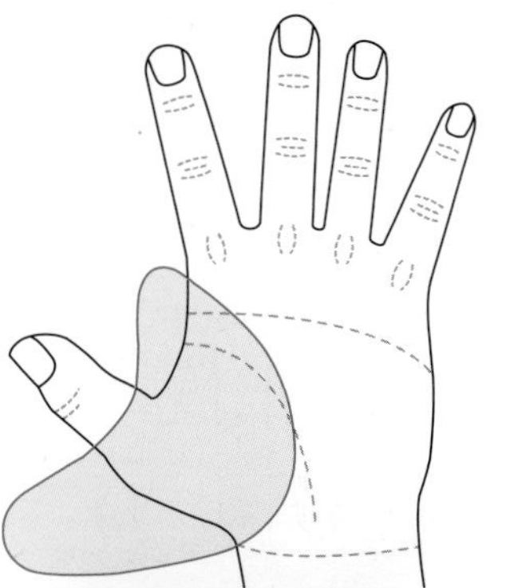

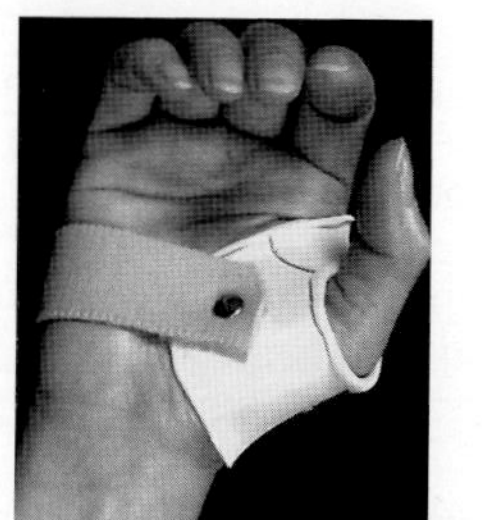

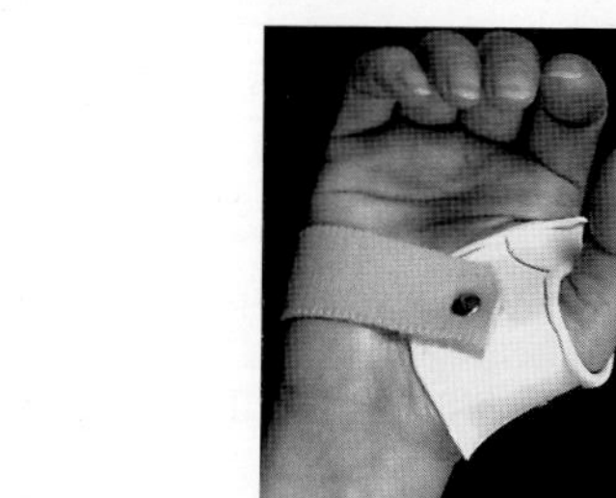

Thumb CMC Immobilization Splint (Fig. 7–17)

Common Names

- CMC palmar abduction splint
- Short thumb spica splint
- Short opponens splint
- MP splint

Alternative Splint Options

- Prefabricated thumb support
- Neoprene thumb and wrist wrap
- Plaster cast
- QuickCast short thumb kit

Primary Functions

- Immobilize thumb CMC and MP joints to allow healing, rest, and/or protection of involved structure(s).

Additional Functions

- Improve functional use by positioning thumb in functional opposition.
- Promote gliding of FPL or extensor pollicis longus (EPL) tendon by restricting movement of MP joint during active flexion and extension exercises.

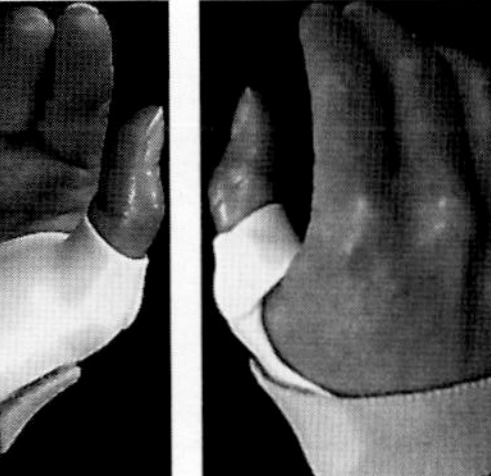

Figure 7–17

Common Diagnoses and General Optimal Positions

• TM jt arthritis	Slight MP flex with palm abd and th opp
• Lax or mildly subluxed TM jt	Slight MP flex with palm abd and th opp
• UCL injury (grade 1 to 3)	Slight MP flex with UD
• RCL injury (grade 1 to 3)	Slight MP flex with RD
• Low median nerve injury	Slight MP flex with palm abd and th opp

CLINICAL PEARL

Trap Door for Circumferential Thumb Splints

To ease donning and doffing of a circumferential thumb splint, use a coated material (which will not adhere to itself). Once the material is completely cool, pop apart the overlapped segment and create a trap door. This technique helps when there is an enlarged joint or fluctuating edema about the thumb MP or IP joint.

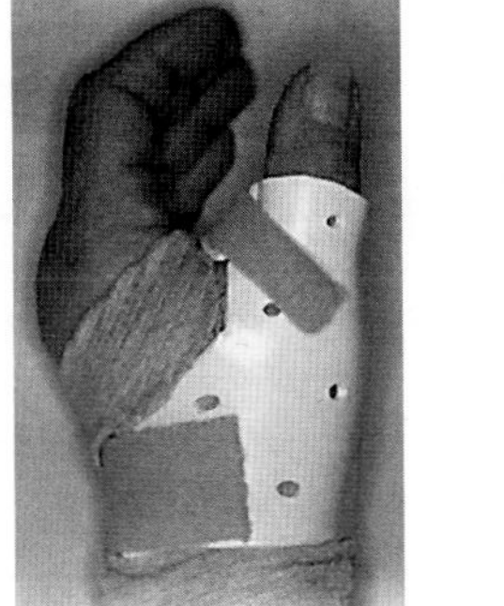

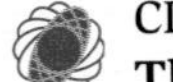

CLINICAL PEARL

Thumb MP/IP Immobilization Splint

To include the IP joint in the splint design, extend the pattern distally. This can be helpful when splinting an injury that needs more support than the thenar-based design provides. Make sure to use coated material for ease of removal. Try not to enclose the tip, because it is important to be able to monitor vascular changes. This splint was used after a MP joint fusion.

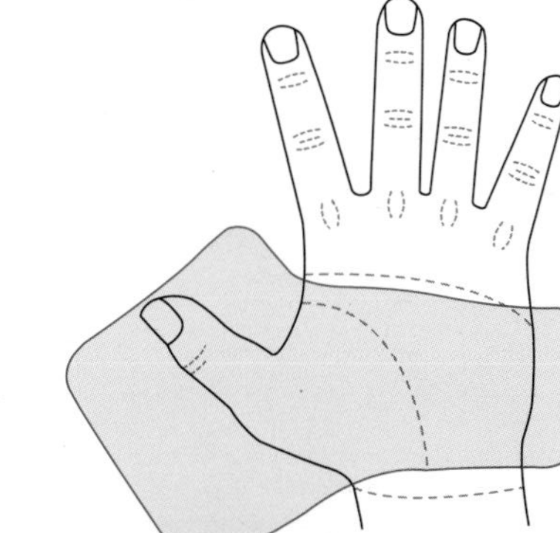

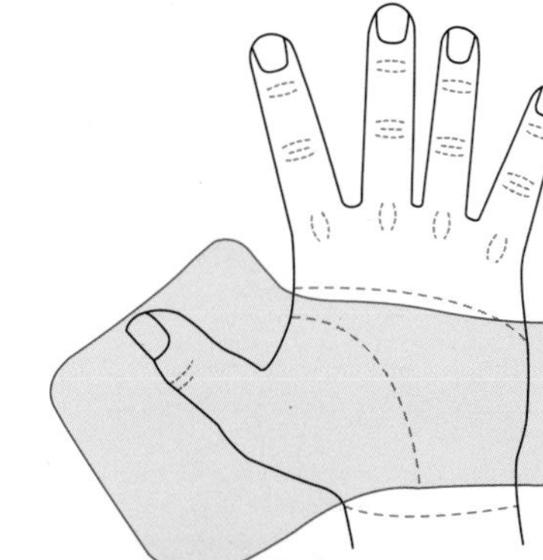

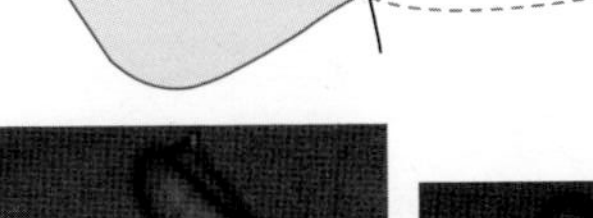

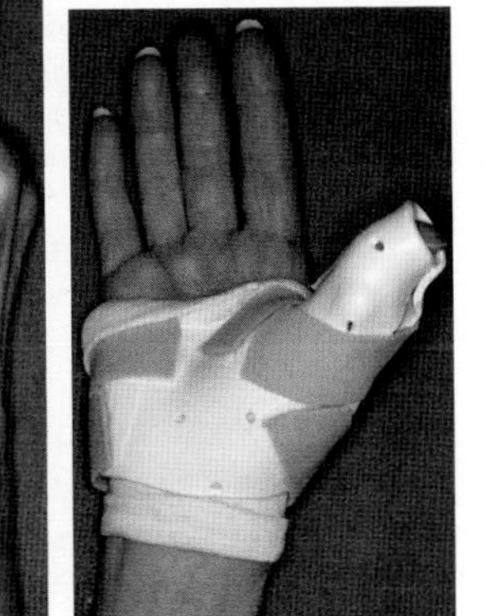

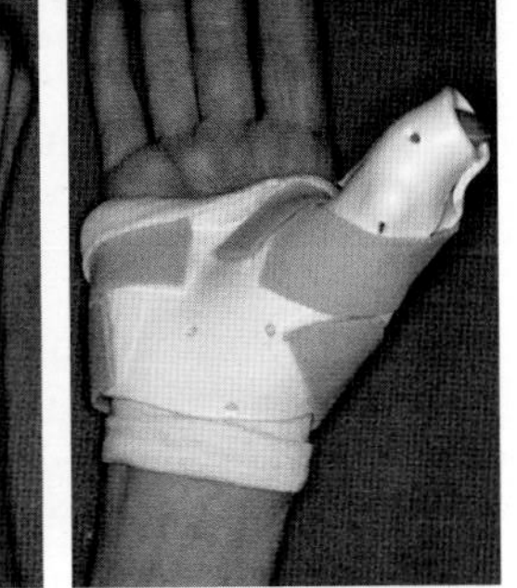

Fabrication Process

Pattern Creation (Fig. 7–18)

- Mark for proximal border just distal to wrist crease.
- Mark for distal border at thumb IP flexion crease and distal palmar crease.

Refine Pattern

- Allow unimpeded motion of wrist, thumb IP, and digit MP joints by keeping splint design accurate.
- Provide ample material within web space to support palmar abduction position adequately.
- Allow enough material to mold around ulnar border without overlapping dorsally.
- May extend pattern distally to include IP joint or trim pattern to omit MP joint. if necessary.

Options for Materials

- Use drapable material to achieve intimate fit about CMC and MP joints, to prevent splint migration and improve comfort.

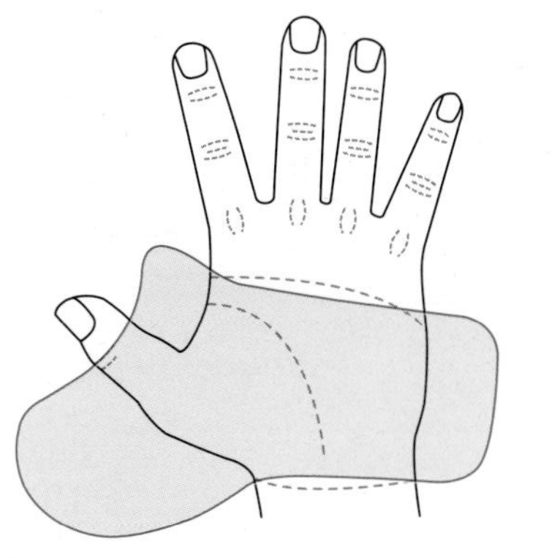

Figure 7–18

- Use coated material so circumferential thumb piece can be popped open without permanent sealing.
- Use thinnest material possible that provides necessary strength to minimize splint bulk.
- Remember that elastic materials tend to shrink around thumb (making splint difficult to don and doff); do not remove until splint is completely set.

Cut and Heat

- Position patient's forearm in slight supination to achieve gravity-assist position.
- Place thumb MP joint in appropriate amount of flexion and CMC joint in desired amount of palmar abduction and opposition.
- Consider placing light layer of lotion on thumb before molding to ease removal of splint.

Evaluate Fit While Molding

- Place material on volar aspect of hand and thumb while maintaining desired joint positions; at the same time gently contour palmar arches.
- Radially, carefully wrap material through first web space from volar to dorsal.
- Mold through web space and overlap material onto itself by approximately 1".
- Proximally, mold well around base of CMC joint.
- Ulnarly, wrap material around ulnar border to fourth metacarpal dorsally.
- Maintain desired thumb CMC and MP joint positions as material sets by having patient lightly oppose thumb to index finger tip.
- Avoid applying direct pressure over dorsum of MP joint while molding.
- Clear IP joint flexion crease; avoid rolling material.

Strapping and Components

- One 1" strap attached dorsally to radial and ulnar segments suffices.
- Consider using rivets to secure dorsal strap.
- If circumferential portion of splint needs to be popped apart for donning and doffing over IP joint, small strap must be applied at opening.

Splint Finishing Touches

- Smooth distal and proximal borders.
- Gently flare proximal to thumb IP joint.
- Do not apply pressure directly over superficial branches of radial and ulnar sensory nerves.
- Check for clearance of wrist, thumb IP, and digit MP joints. Make sure there is no abutment with splint material.

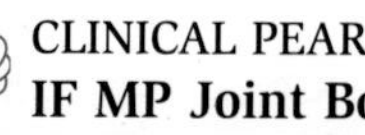

CLINICAL PEARL
IF MP Joint Border

It is imperative when splinting around the first web space to be sure the index border is not too high. The splint shown here has an overgenerous border that impedes IF MP joint motion; this may cause tissue irritation.

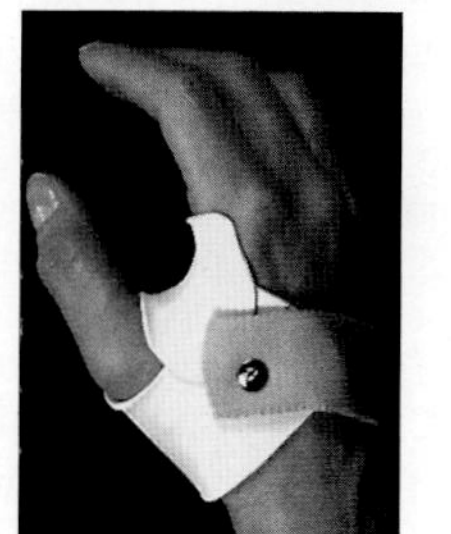

Thumb Abduction Immobilization Splint (Fig. 7–19)

Common Names

- CMC splint
- Web stretcher
- C-bar splint

Alternative Splint Options

- Plaster cast

Primary Functions

- Prevent soft tissue contracture of first web space as result of median nerve injury or disease.

Additional Functions

- Statically position first web space contracture at maximum palmar abduction to facilitate lengthening of tissue (mobilization splint).

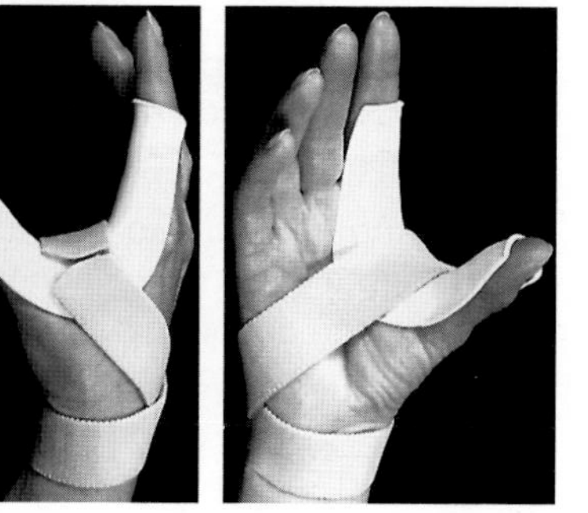

Figure 7–19

Common Diagnoses and General Optimal Positions

• Median nerve injury	Maximum palm and rad abd
• Postoperative contracture release	Maximum palm and rad abd

CLINICAL PEARL
Thumb Positioning

Always check thumb position before, during, and after the molding process. When splinting the thumb in a position for function, the CMC joint should be placed midway between palmar and radial abduction, and the MP joint should be in slight flexion (20 to 30°) (A). This allows for effective pinch to the index and middle fingers. If the therapist is not careful, as the patient relaxes his or her hand during the molding process, the wrist will tend to flex, which promotes thumb extension, and radial abduction (B). This places the thumb in a poor position for function.

CLINICAL PEARL
Thumb Post Splint

For patients without a thumb (congenital or traumatic), this splint provides a functional pinch for light activities of daily living (ADLs) or may act as a temporary mold (preprosthesis) to allow the patient to adjust to the use of a prosthetic. This temporary mold helps determine the correct length and position of a permanent prosthetic. The pattern depends on the level the amputation or congenital anomaly (A). Products such as Elastomer or prosthetic foam, instead of thermoplastic material, can be used to fabricate the internal roll (B). The length and width of the roll are determined by the amount of amputated thumb—use the unaffected side as a guide. Use $^1/_8$" material that has much rigidity and durability. Remember that this is a functional splint and must be able to withstand the rigors of ADLs (C). While molding, maintain the desired thumb post position as the material sets to allow for effective three-point pinch. Since the prosthetic thumb has no sensation, tell the patient to use vision with all thumb activities.

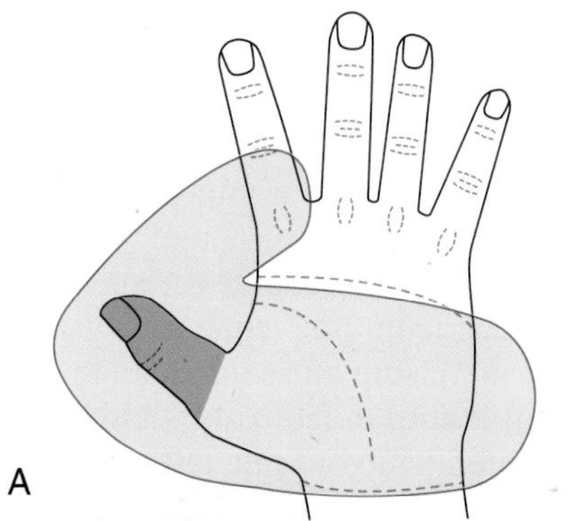

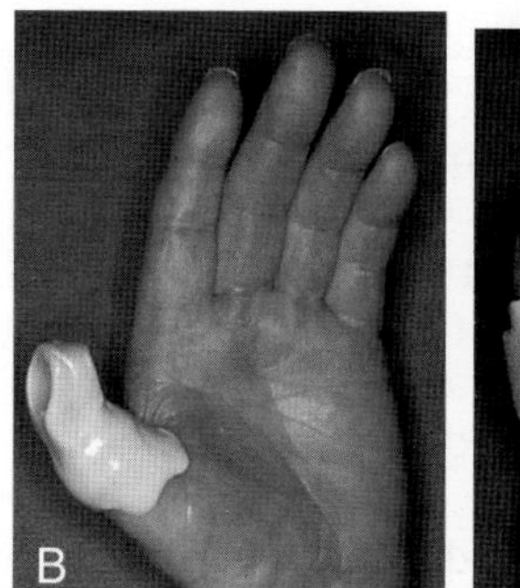
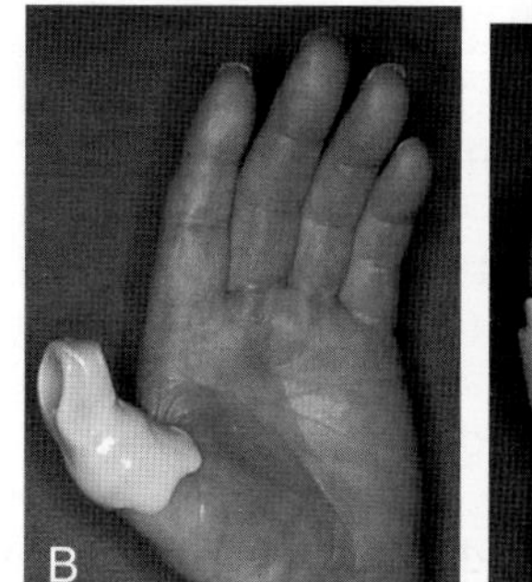
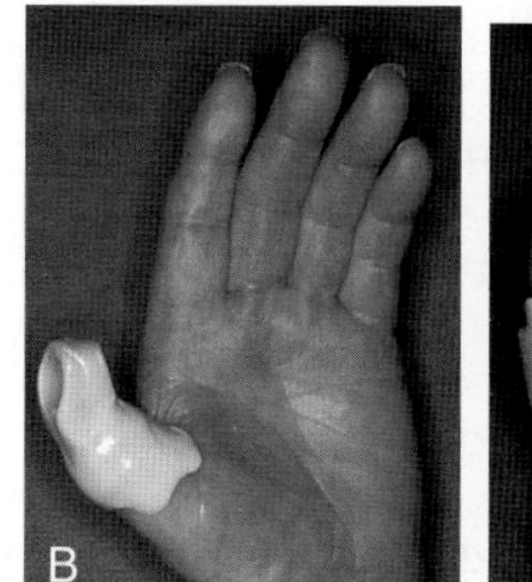

Fabrication Process

Pattern Creation (Fig. 7–20)

- Mark for proximal border just distal to wrist crease.
- Mark for distal borders at tip of thumb and just proximal to IF middle phalanx.
- Allow enough material to encompass three quarters of thumb circumference ulnarly and three quarters of IF phalanx radially.

Refine Pattern

- Proximal border should allow full wrist motion.
- Provide ample material within web space to support palmar and radial abduction position adequately and to allow enough surface area for strap application.

Options for Materials

- Use $^1/_8$" thermoplastic material to provide rigidity needed to maintain position of tissue.
- Use highly drapable material to achieve intimate fit about CMC and MP joints, to prevent splint migration and improve comfort.
- Consider perforated material when splint will be used in conjunction with scar management products such Elastomer or silicone gel.

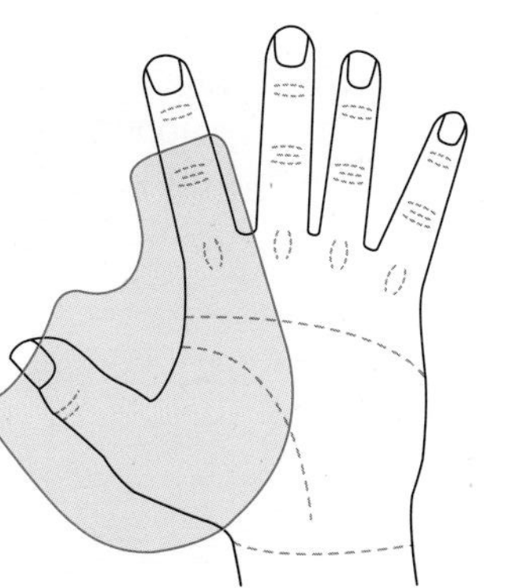

Figure 7–20

- Materials that can be reheated and remolded several times are a good option if ongoing splint modifications become necessary to accommodate for changes in motion (a common issue because it is difficult to achieve desired joint position initially).

Cut and Heat

- Position patient with elbow resting on table and forearm in slight supination to achieve gravity-assist position.
- Place thumb in appropriate amount of palmar and radial abduction.

Evaluate Fit While Molding

- Place warm material along thumb and IF while maintaining desired position.
- Mold with even pressure throughout length of splint, focusing on gentle abduction pressure to distal portions of first and second metacarpals.
- Flare around bony thumb and IF MP joints.
- Maintain desired thumb position as material sets.

Strapping and Components

- Apply one 1" elasticized strap directed from volar web space, around wrist $1^1/_2$ times and attach to dorsal aspect.

Splint Finishing Touches

- Smooth distal and proximal borders.
- Check clearance of wrist, making sure there is no abutment with splint material.
- Define consistent wearing schedule for patient. Many therapists suggest patients wear these splints at night only, allowing functional use during day.

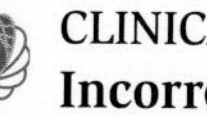

CLINICAL PEARL

Incorrect Pressure Application to Address First Web Tightness

If pressure is applied distal to the MP joint, stress is placed on the ulnar collateral ligament instead of the intended first web space (as shown here). This force may eventually disrupt the MP ulnar collateral ligament. Make sure pressure is applied to the most proximal ulnar portion of the first metacarpal and avoid applying pressure distal to the MP joint.

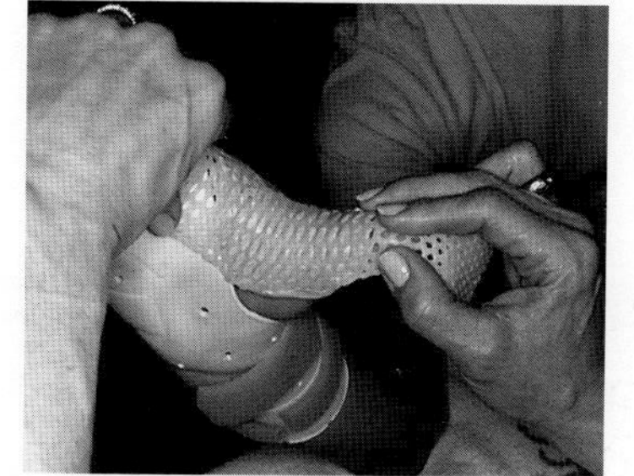

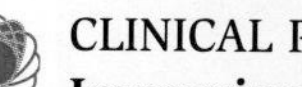

CLINICAL PEARL

Improving Pressure Distribution beneath First Web Immobilization Splint

Elastomer-type products can be used to achieve better pressure distribution in difficult areas such as the first web space. Here, a $^3/_{32}$" material is being applied over Elastomer. Such curing materials can be made to seep through the holes in a perforated material, providing a way to secure the product onto the thermoplastic. These products work well for splinting patients who have undergone a first web space surgical release by incorporating the known benefits of scar management and maintaining the desired range of motion.

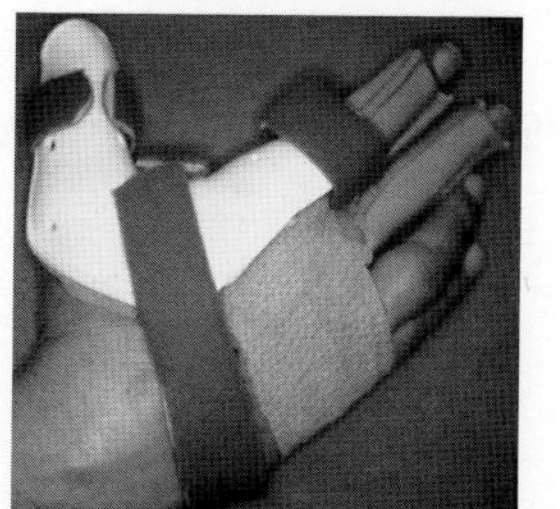

3 • Forearm-Based Splints

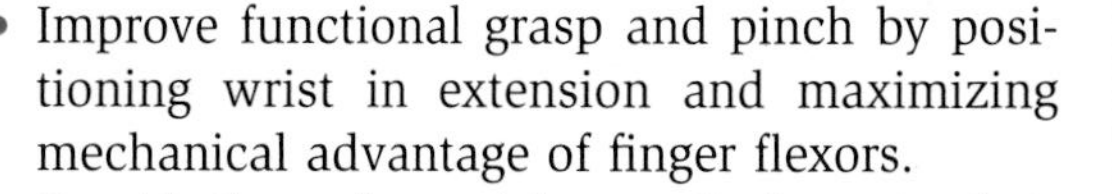
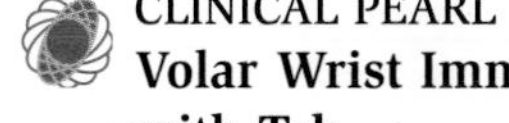

Dorsal Wrist Immobilization Splint (Fig. 7–21)

Common Names

- Dorsal wrist cock-up splint
- Dorsal wrist support
- Wrist extension splint
- Static wrist splint
- Radial bar wrist splint

Alternative Splint Options

- Prefabricated wrist splint
- Cast

Primary Functions

- Immobilize wrist joint to allow healing, rest, or protection of involved structures(s).

Additional Functions

- Substitute for weak or absent wrist extensor muscle function.
- Improve functional grasp and pinch by positioning wrist in extension and maximizing mechanical advantage of finger flexors.
- Provide base for outrigger attachment when fabricating digit extension mobilization splints.

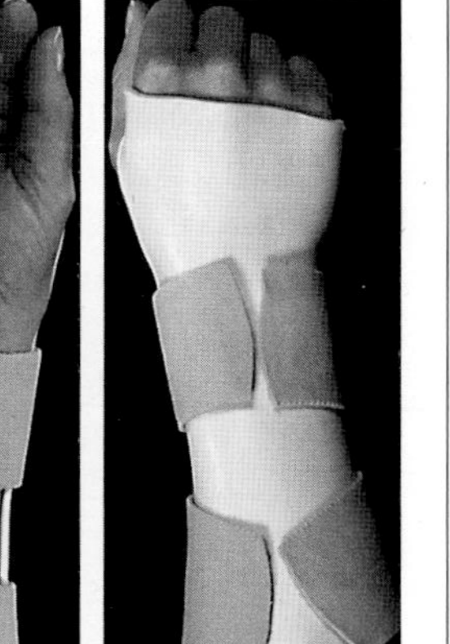
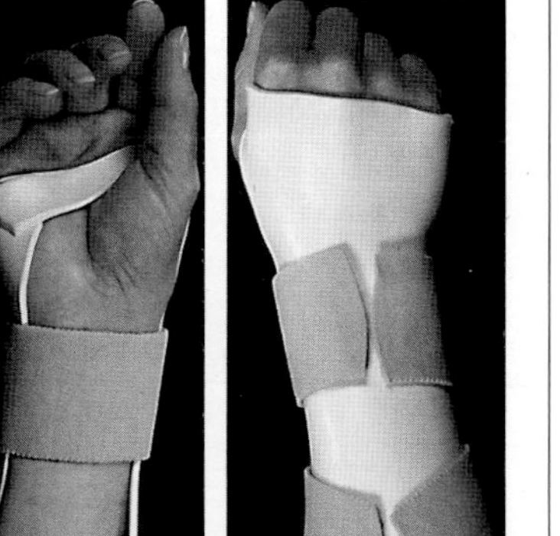
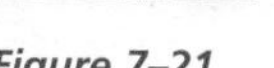

Figure 7–21

Common Diagnoses and General Optimal Positions

• Carpal tunnel syndrome	0°
• Median and/or ulnar nerve repair	0 to 15° flex
• Radial nerve palsy	20 to 35° ext

CLINICAL PEARL
Proximal Strap Design for Forearm-Based Splints

To apply a strap appropriately around the forearm, the therapist must appreciate the tapered shape of this region. Straps should be applied with a slight angle to avoid sheer stress on the forearm tissue. Soft or elasticized straps may contour and accommodate for forearm bulk better than rigid straps.

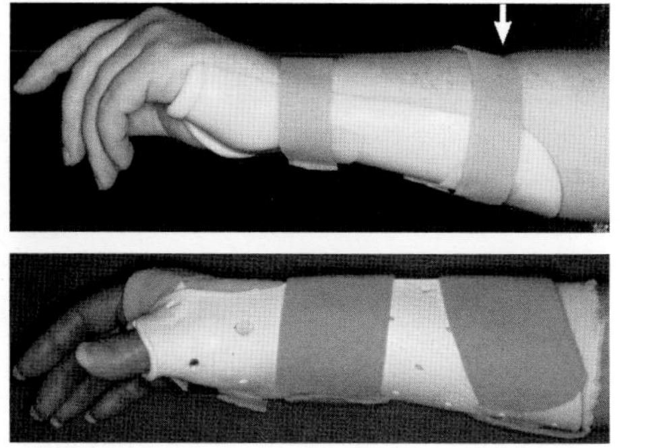

CLINICAL PEARL
Volar Wrist Immobilization Splint with Tab

The dorsal splint pattern can be used to fabricate a volar-based design. The major difference is the width of the dorsal tab in the volar design. The increased width accommodating the majority of the metacarpals surface area can add rigidity to the splint, providing more stable positioning into wrist extension.

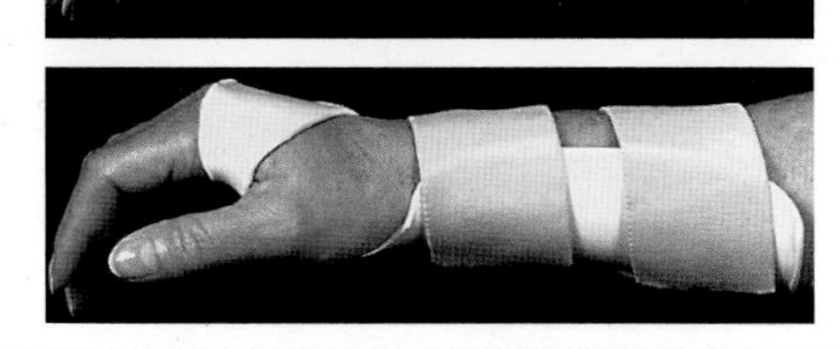

Fabrication Process

Pattern Creation (Fig. 7–22)

- Consider dorsal design for patients who are not comfortable in volar splint.
- Dorsal design allows for better sensory input to palm than does volar design.
- Good design for patients with volar skin grafts, wounds, pins, or hypersensitive scars.
- Remember that this design may not provide necessary strength to immobilize wrist completely; volar thumbhole design is better option for maximizing wrist immobilization.
- Mark for proximal border two thirds length of forearm.
- Mark distal border just proximal to MP joints.
- Distal radial tab (palmar bar) should be long enough (approximately 3") to traverse through palm and secure on distal ulnar border.
- Tab should incorporate oblique angle that traverses from index to small metacarpal heads.
- Mark thumb clearance by making arc from thumb MP to base of first CMC joint.

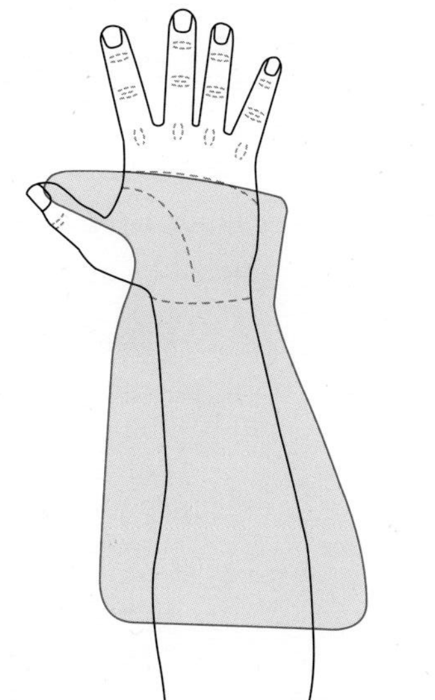

Figure 7–22

- Allow enough material to encompass half to two thirds circumference of forearm, remembering that forearm tapers distally.

Refine Pattern

- Proximal border should allow full elbow motion.
- Distal border should allow unimpeded motion of digital MP and thumb joints.
- Provide appropriate amount of material within palmar surface to support arches adequately.

Options for Materials

- Consider 1/8" thermoplastic material to provide needed rigidity to maintain wrist position.
- If patient has difficulty maintaining wrist extension (e.g., secondary to radial nerve injury), consider uncoated materials or those that are slightly tacky to help prevent material from slipping and to make it easier to position patient and mold splint.
- Gel- or foam-lined materials help provide dorsal wrist scar compression, decrease distal migration, and increase comfort.
- Consider perforated material when splint will be used during activity or in conjunction with scar-management products such as Elastomer. Scar products seep through perforations, which helps anchor them into splint.

Cut and Heat

- Position patient with elbow resting on table and forearm pronated for gravity-assisted molding. Position thumb in palmar abduction.
- Prepad ulnar styloid with adhesive-backed foam, putty, cotton ball, or silicone gel.

Evaluate Fit While Molding

- Position material on dorsum of involved hand and wrist just proximal to MP joints.
- Place radial bar through thumb web and guide rest of bar along palmar surface just proximal to distal palmar crease, overlapping and securing on distal ulnar border (pull material if needed for increased length).
- Carefully incorporate arches of hand by using smooth, even strokes and constantly redirecting material into arches. Continual molding over volar bar is mandatory to prevent negative effects of gravity.
- Do not grab proximal splint or try to secure with tight circumferential bandage. This may cause borders of splint to irritate skin. Instead, allow gravity to assist in forming forearm trough.
- Make sure desired wrist position is maintained. Some patients tend to flex and deviate wrist while splint is being formed.

Strapping and Components

- Distal strap: 1" strap connecting radial bar to distal ulnar border.
- Middle strap: 2" strap just proximal to dorsal wrist crease; use piece of adhesive foam to further stabilize wrist in splint and prevent migration. Foam should not overlap splint edges.
- Proximal strap: 2" soft or elasticized strap is good choice, especially if patient will use splint for functional purposes. Such straps can better accommodate changes in forearm bulk during movement than traditional loop strap.

Splint Finishing Touches

- Smooth and slightly flare borders.
- Gently flare around dorsal thumb region; avoid rolling, which can make future splint modifications difficult.
- Check clearance of elbow, radial and ulnar styloid processes, thumb, and MP joints.
- Pay careful attention to index metacarpal, which frequently abuts radial portion of splint as it traverses through first web space.
- Check for compression over radial and ulnar sensory nerve branches.

Volar Wrist Immobilization Splint (Fig. 7–23)

Common Names

- Wrist cock-up splint
- Thumbhole wrist splint
- Wrist gauntlet splint
- Palmar wrist cock-up splint
- Static wrist splint
- Wrist drop splint

Alternative Splint Options

- Prefabricated wrist splint
- Cast

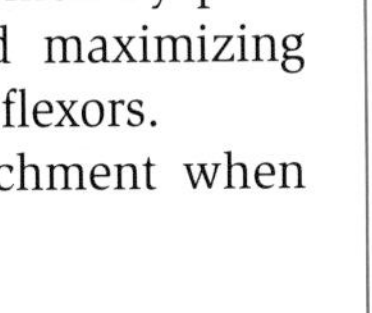

Figure 7–23

Primary Functions

- Immobilize wrist joint to allow healing, rest, and/or protection of involved structures(s).

Additional Functions

- Statically position wrist flexion contracture at maximum extension to facilitate lengthening of tissue (mobilization splint).
- Substitute for weak or absent wrist extensor muscle function.
- Improve functional grasp and pinch by positioning wrist in extension and maximizing mechanical advantage of finger flexors.
- Provide base for outrigger attachment when fabricating mobilization splints.

Common Diagnoses and General Optimal Positions

• Carpal tunnel syndrome	0°
• Carpal tunnel release	20 to 35° ext
• Wr tenosynovitis and post-tenosynovectomy	Flexors: 0°; extensor: 20 to 40° ext
• Rheumatoid arthritis or osteoarthritis	Position of comfort
• Wr arthroplasty	0°
• Wr arthrodesis	Dictated by fusion
• Ganglion excision	20 to 35° ext
• Wr sprain or instability	Dictated by structures involved
• Distal radius and/or ulna fracture (post cast)	Maximal ext
• Carpal fracture	Dictated by structures involved
• Metacarpal fracture or dislocation (base)	Slight ext
• Epicondylitis	Medial: 0°; lateral: 20 to 35° ext
• Radial nerve palsy	20 to 35° ext

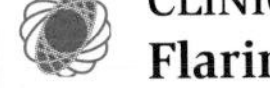

CLINICAL PEARL

Flaring Versus Rolling of Edges

Flaring force should be gently applied to the warmed splint edge (approximately $^1/_4$" should be warmed) by the therapist's thenar and hypothenar regions. When deciding how to finish the edges of a splint, consider the advantages of flaring and the disadvantages of rolling: (1) rolling does not allow for simple splint modifications, such as widening the opening for the thumb or shortening the distal border to allow unimpeded MP joint motion; (2) rolling back of a previously rolled region may lead to a bulky, unsightly splint; and (3) flaring provides for a neater looking splint.

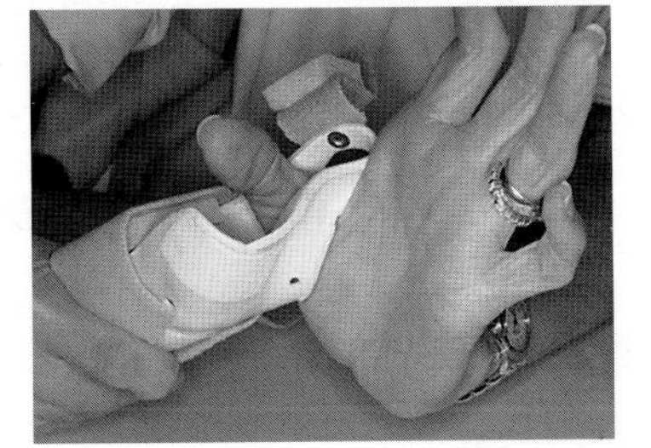

Fabrication Process

Pattern Creation (Fig. 7–24)

- Mark for proximal border two thirds length of forearm.
- Mark for distal border just proximal to distal palmar crease.
- Incorporate oblique angle that traverses from index to small metacarpal heads.
- Mark for thumbhole in distal radial portion of pattern, approximately 1" down and in.
- Allow enough material to encompass half to two thirds circumference of forearm, remembering that forearm tapers distally.

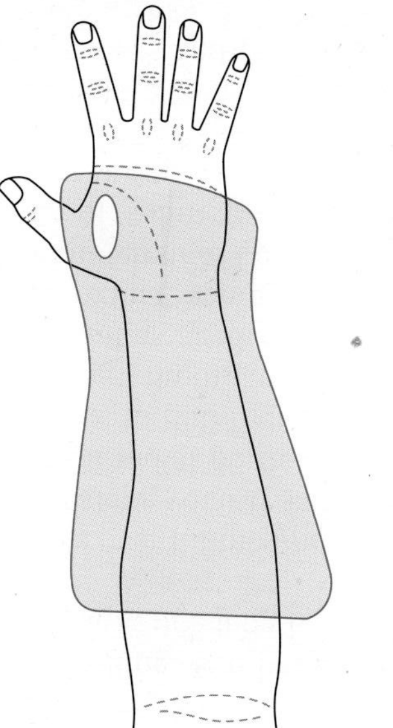
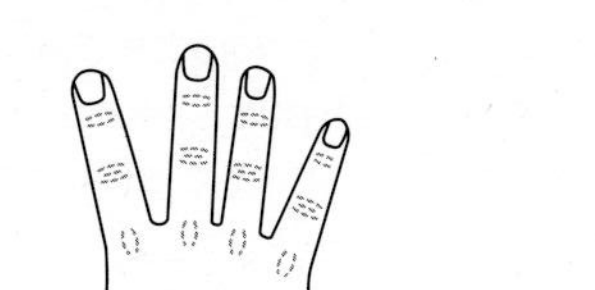

Figure 7–24

Refine Pattern

- Proximal border should allow full elbow motion.
- Distal border should allow unimpeded motion of MP joints and nearly full thumb mobility (thumb mobility may depend on splint's goal).
- For average adult, thumbhole should be about size of elongated half dollar. When measuring pattern on patient, hole should lie approximately over thumb MP joint.
- Provide appropriate amount of material within first web space to support thumb position and provide adequate surface area for strap application dorsally.

Options for Materials

- Material selection depends on splint requirements.
- Consider $\frac{1}{8}$" thermoplastic material to provide needed rigidity to support an unstable ligamentous injury or postoperative repair.
- Consider $\frac{1}{16}$" material for immobilizing wrist that does not require rigid support or for patients who will not place high demands on splint (e.g., patient with arthritis).
- If patient has difficulty maintaining wrist extension (e.g., secondary to radial nerve injury), consider uncoated materials or those that are slightly tacky to help prevent material from slipping and to make it easier to position patient and mold splint.
- Materials that can be reheated and remolded several times are a good option if ongoing splint modifications become necessary to accommodate for fluctuations in edema or changes in desired joint position.
- Gel- or foam-lined materials help provide volar wrist scar compression, decrease distal migration, and increase comfort.
- Consider perforated material when splint will be used during activity or in conjunction with scar-management products such as Elastomer. Scar products seep through perforations, which helps anchor them into splint.

Cut and Heat

- Position patient with elbow resting on table and forearm supinated for gravity-assisted molding. Position thumb in gentle palmar abduction and opposition.
- If patient has difficulty supinating forearm (e.g., distal radius fractures after cast immobilization), have patient flex elbow on table and adduct shoulder toward midline or lie patient supine with shoulder abducted and externally rotated 90° with elbow flexed.
- Cut out thumbhole in material either by making series of holes with hole punch before heating or by carefully piercing the slightly warm material with sharp scissors.

Volar Wrist Immobilization Splint *(Continued)*

Evaluate Fit While Molding

- Lay warm material on towel, positioning thumbhole on correct side of material as if material were to be placed on supinated forearm.
- Using index fingers, gently open hole, slightly enlarging and elongating it (making it egg shaped); avoid rolling. Use borders of thenar crease as landmarks for length and width of hole.
- Place thumbhole over thumb and guide rest of material evenly along volar wrist and forearm.
- Remember dorsal radial portion of splint and how gravity tends to pull material away from hand (elongating thumbhole); continually reposition material as needed.
- Do not grab proximal splint or try to secure with tight circumferential bandage. This may cause borders of splint to irritate skin. Instead, allow gravity to assist in forming forearm trough.
- Carefully incorporate arches of hand by using smooth, even strokes and constantly redirecting material into arches. Avoid strongly molding into arches, which may cause significant discomfort in palm once material has set.
- Rotate forearm into pronated position at end of molding to check for clearance of ulnar and radial styloid processes; flare about styloids as necessary.
- Make sure desired wrist position is maintained. Some patients tend to flex and ulnarly deviate wrist while splint is being formed.

Strapping and Components

- Distal strap: 1" strap directed from radial dorsal web area to distal ulnar border. Strip of adhesive foam can be used under strap to further stabilize metacarpals.
- Middle strap: 2" strap just proximal to dorsal wrist crease; use piece of adhesive foam to further stabilize wrist in splint and prevent migration. Foam should lie directly over ulnar styloid and should not overlap splint edges.
- Proximal strap: Depending on size of forearm, 1" or 2" strap may suffice; strap should have slight volar to dorsal angle.

Splint Finishing Touches

- Smooth and slightly flare distal and proximal borders.
- Gently flare around thenar hole; avoid rolling, which can make future splint modifications difficult.
- Check clearance of elbow, radial and ulnar styloid processes, thumb, and finger MP joints.
- Pay careful attention to index metacarpal, which frequently abuts radial portion of splint as it traverses through first web space.

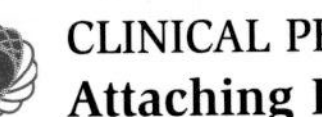

CLINICAL PEARL

Attaching Distal Straps

There are several methods for attaching the distal straps. (A) Loop material can be riveted to the thermoplastic material. Remember to cover the surface of the rivet that contacts the skin with a thin adhesive lining material to prevent skin irritation. Adhesive hook can be applied volar and dorsal on the radial web segment. (B) Direct the strap from the volar hook to the dorsal hook and then over to the ulnar border. Fabricate a homemade rivet out of splint material by forming a scrap piece of heated thermoplastic into a small ball the size of a pea and then hyperheating it over a heat gun. (C) Prepare the attachment site on splint's surface by scratching and/or brushing with solvent. Make a hole through the strap and apply the warm ball through the hole and onto the splint. Be careful to correctly position and align the strap, because once the material hardens, it is not easily adjusted.

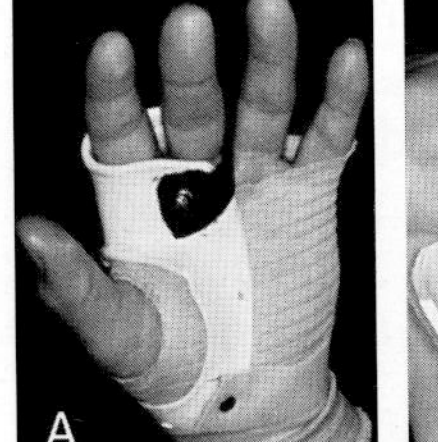

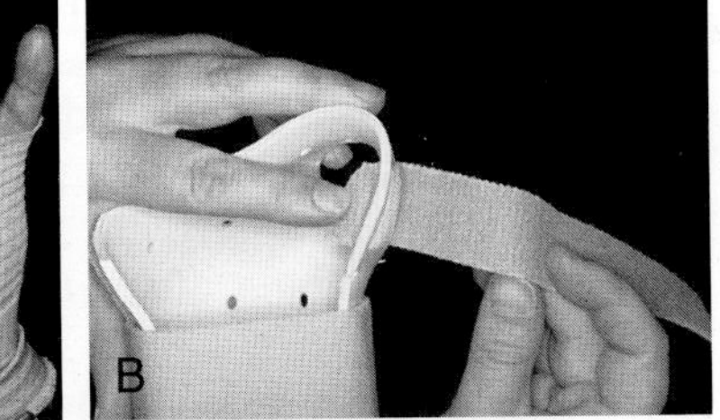

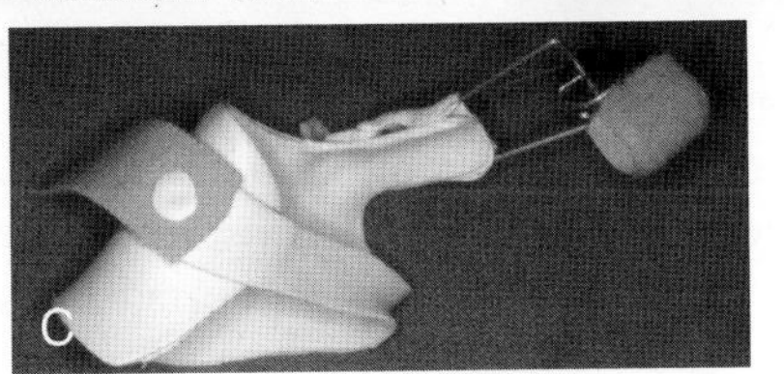

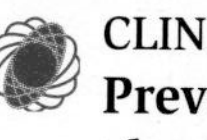

CLINICAL PEARL

Preventing Buckling of Splint Material about the Thumb

To prevent buckling of splint material dorsally when fabricating the thumbhole wrist splint, consider the following points: (1) Do not overheat the thermoplastic material; (2) do not make the thumbhole too big; (3) when placing the heated material on the hand, do not position the thumbhole too far radially (the hole should allow visualization of nearly the entire thenar eminence); and (4) during the molding process, gently and continually reposition the dorsal piece against the skin to counteract the effects of gravity.

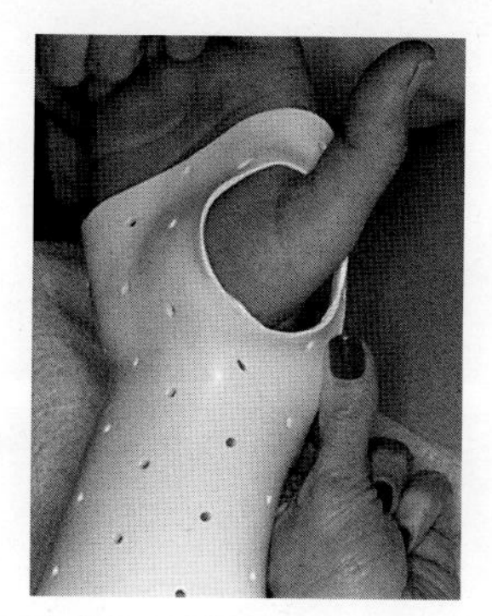

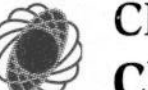

CLINICAL PEARL

Clamshell Wrist Immobilization Splint

The volar wrist immobilization splint can be modified by molding an additional piece of thermoplastic material dorsally to create a clamshell effect (A and B). This modification can provide additional protection and more effective immobilization of the wrist. First, fabricate the volar splint per the instructions given in the text, but do not apply the strapping. Next, create the pattern for the dorsal piece, allowing approximately $1/2$" of overlap of the dorsal piece over the molded volar splint. Prepad the ulnar styloid process to help prevent irritation. Use a coated material to prevent unwanted adherence of the two thermoplastic pieces. If uncoated material is the only choice, use a stockinette or a wet paper towel over the volar splint while molding the dorsal piece (C). To incorporate the thumb, use the forearm-based thumb immobilization splint pattern and add the dorsal piece in the same way.

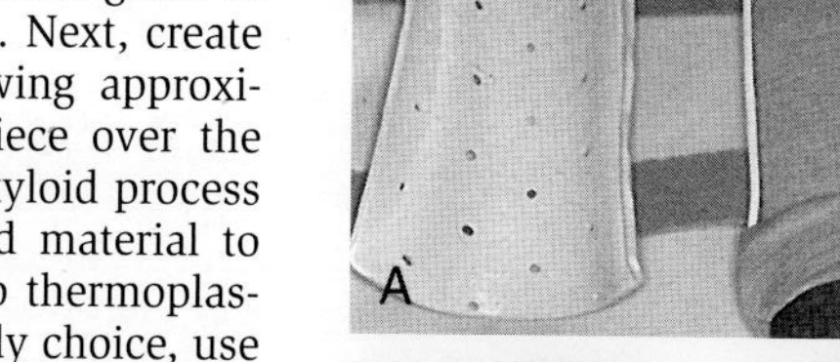

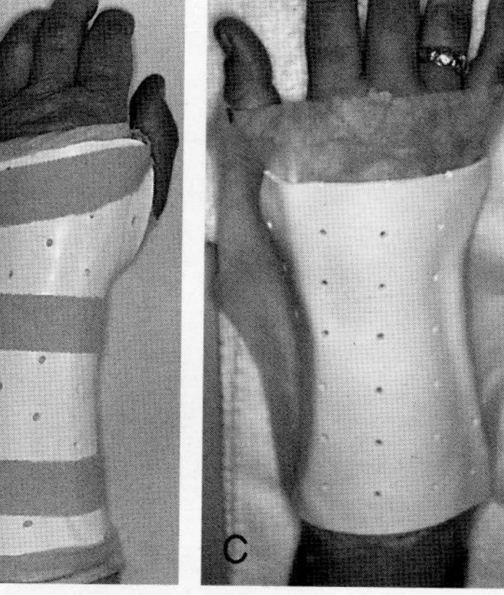

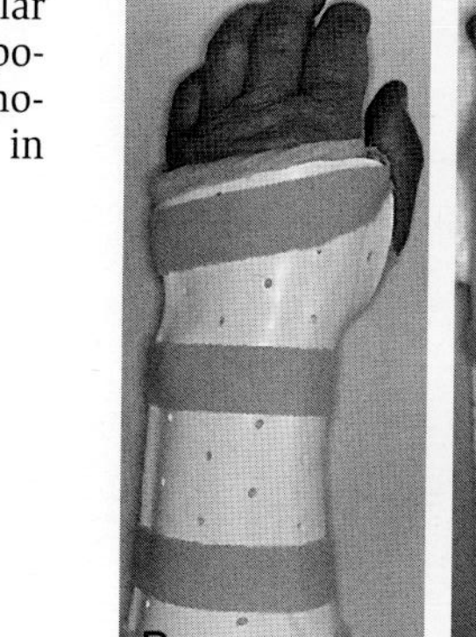

A B C

CLINICAL PEARL

Light Tip Pinch to Incorporate Palmar Arches

To improve incorporation of the arches of the hand within a splint, have the patient lightly hold a piece of cotton or material between the thumb and index finger. This technique can be used with many volar and circumferential splints to help achieve an intimate fit in the hand, improving comfort and maximizing functional use. Do not let patient pinch too hard, since this may exaggerate thumb opposition.

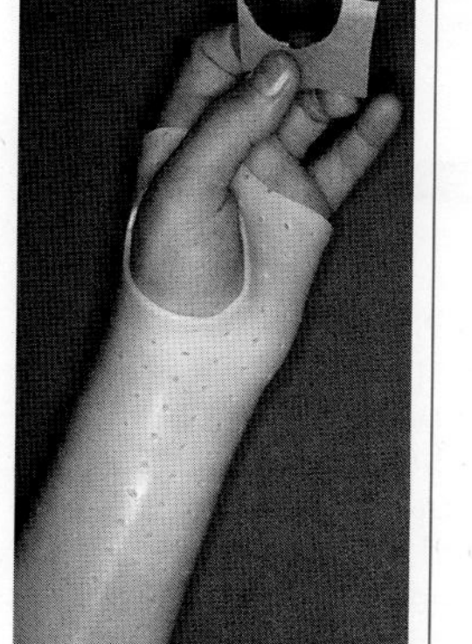

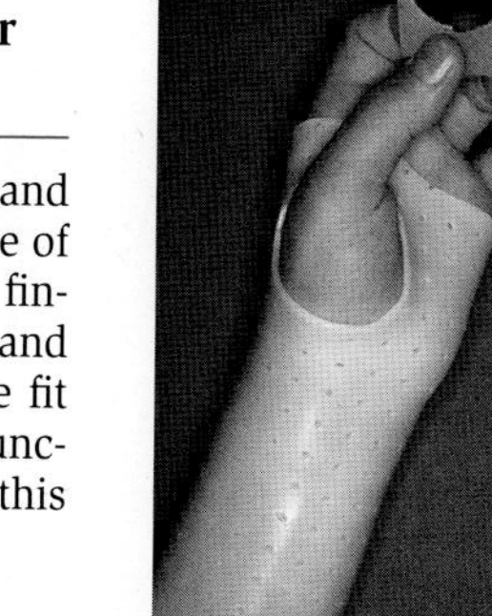

Ulnar Wrist Immobilization Splint (Fig. 7–25)

Common Names

- Ulnar gutter splint

Alternative Splint Options

- Prefabricated wrist splint
- Cast

Primary Functions

- Immobilize wrist joint to allow healing of involved structure(s).

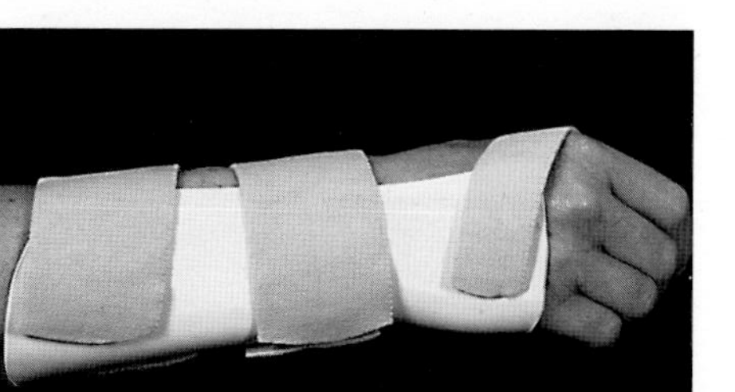

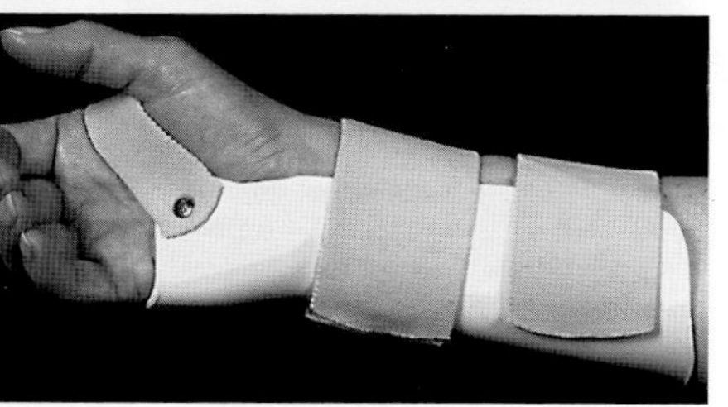

Figure 7–25

Additional Functions

- Maximize radial hand function while immobilizing ulnar side of hand.

Common Diagnoses and General Optimal Positions

Diagnosis	Position
• RF or SF metacarpal fracture (base)	Wr: 0 to 20° ext; RD and UD: 0°
• Lunate, triquetrum, or hamate instability or fracture	Wr: 0 to 20° ext; RD and UD 0°
• Triangular fibrocartilage complex (TFCC) injury or repair	Wr: 0°; RD and UD: 0°
• Extensor carpi ulnaris tenosynovitis	Wr: 0 to 20° ext with slight UD
• Flexor carpi ulnaris tenosynovitis	Wr: 0° with slight UD
• Ulnar nerve compression at Guyon's canal	Wr: 0° with slight UD

CLINICAL PEARL

Ulnar Wrist Immobilization Splint for External Fixator

Commonly, patients are referred for a wrist splint to be worn in conjunction with an external fixator to provide added support to the wrist, improve comfort, and protect the arm from inadvertent external forces. Because the patient is probably unable to rotate the arm freely to achieve a gravity-assist position, the therapist must have an alternative approach. Lay the patient supine with the elbow and shoulder flexed to achieve the desired position for molding (A). Straps should be applied carefully and thoughtfully. Avoid strap contact with the pin sites, which can be sensitive and prone to skin irritation and infection (B). Be creative when trimming the straps to obtain a comfortable fit. As an alternative, circumferential wraps can be used to secure the splint on the arm, this is especially beneficial if edema is an issue.

Fabrication Process

Pattern Creation (Fig. 7–26)

- Mark for proximal border two thirds length of forearm.
- Mark distal border just proximal to distal palmar crease of MF to SF.
- Incorporate oblique angle that traverses from index to small metacarpal heads.
- Mark for thenar crease from MP flexion crease between IF and MF, and base of CMC joint.
- Allow enough material to encompass half to two thirds circumference of forearm, remembering that forearm tapers distally.

Refine Pattern

- Proximal border should allow full elbow motion.

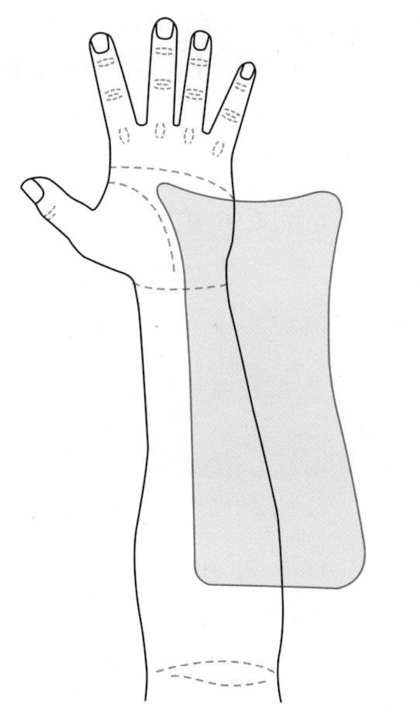

Figure 7–26

- Distal border should allow unimpeded motion of MP joints and full thumb mobility.

Options for Materials

- Consider 1/8" thermoplastic material to provide needed rigidity to support unstable ligamentous injury or healing fracture.
- If patient has difficulty achieving gravity-assist position, consider uncoated materials or those that are slightly tacky to help prevent material from slipping and to make it easier to position patient and mold splint.
- Gel- or foam-lined materials may help with molding over ulnar styloid and bony dorsum, decrease distal migration, and increase comfort.

Cut and Heat

- While material is heating, prepad ulnar styloid using self-adhesive padding or silicone gel.
- Position extremity with patient supine with shoulder and elbow flexed to 90° (ulnar aspect of hand facing ceiling) or with patient sitting with shoulder flexed to 90° and elbow flexed fully; radial side of hand (thumb) should be pointing toward floor.

Evaluate Fit While Molding

- Drape warm material centrally over ulnar border of forearm and hand, making sure palmar material lies along thenar crease and just proximal to distal palmar crease.
- Gently flare material along distal borders.
- If splinting RF or SF proximal metacarpal fracture, completely incorporate MF metacarpal to anchor splint and prevent mobility of ulnar two metacarpals.
- Do not grab proximal splint or try to secure with tight circumferential bandage. This may cause borders of splint to irritate skin. Instead, allow gravity to assist in forming forearm trough.
- Carefully incorporate arches of hand by using smooth, even strokes and constantly redirecting material into arches.
- When material is almost set, gently rotate forearm to check for clearance of ulnar styloid. Styloid becomes more prominent with forearm rotation; if space is not incorporated into splint when molding, ulnar styloid irritation may occur during functional use. If patient complains of abutment, carefully push out material, forming small bubble.
- Make sure desired wrist position is maintained. Some patients tend to flex and deviate wrist while splint is being formed.

Strapping and Components

- Distal strap: 1" strap, trimmed to contour around first web space, is directed from volar radial to dorsal radial border. Consider riveting strap on volar surface to secure strap firmly and decrease bulk within palm.
- Middle strap: 2" strap just proximal to dorsal wrist crease; use piece of adhesive foam to further stabilize wrist in splint and prevent migration (avoid excessive compression over radial sensory nerve).
- Proximal strap: depending on size of forearm, 1" or 2" strap may suffice; strap should have slight volar to dorsal angle.

Splint Finishing Touches

- Smooth and slightly flare all borders.
- Check clearance of elbow, thumb, and MP joints.

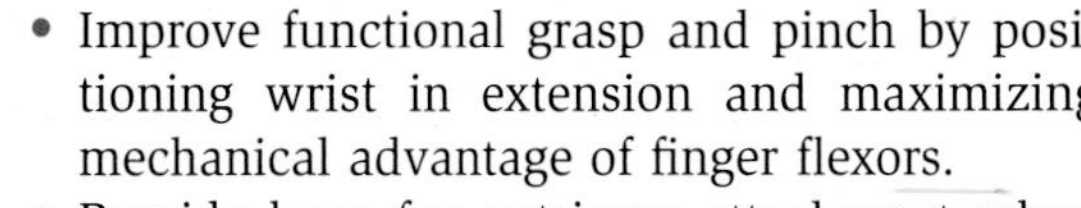

Circumferential Wrist Immobilization Splint (Fig. 7–27)

Common Names

- Wrist fracture brace
- Circumferential wrist splint
- Circumferential wrist cock-up splint
- Circumferential thumbhole wrist splint
- Wrist gauntlet splint

Alternative Splint Options

- Clamshell wrist splint
- Cast
- Prefabricated splint

Primary Functions

- Immobilize wrist joint to allow healing, rest, and/or protection of involved structures(s).

Additional Functions

- Statically position wrist flexion or extension contracture at maximum length to facilitate lengthening of tissue (mobilization splint).
- Substitute for weak or absent wrist extensor muscle function.
- Improve functional grasp and pinch by positioning wrist in extension and maximizing mechanical advantage of finger flexors.
- Provide base for outrigger attachment when fabricating mobilization splints.

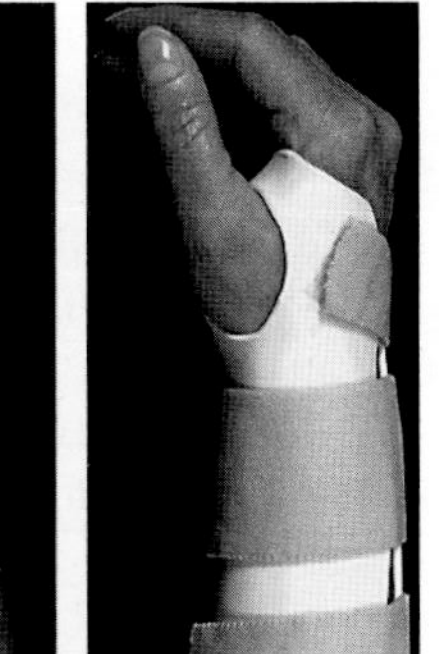

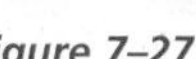

Figure 7–27

Common Diagnoses and General Optimal Positions

• Wr sprain or instability	Dictated by structures involved
• Distal radius and/or ulna fracture (post cast)	Maximal ext
• Carpal fracture	Dictated by structures involved
• Metacarpal fracture or dislocation (base)	Slight ext

CLINICAL PEARL

Zippered Circumferential Wrist Splint

The Rolyan AquaForm zippered wrist splint provides another option for a circumferential splint. Choose the appropriate size and length per catalog instructions. Prepad the ulnar styloid process and position the patient with the elbow resting on a table. Heat and apply the warmed splint to the arm with the zippered edge along the dorsal ulnar border, zip it up, and gently place wrist in the desired position. This is an excellent option for patients who require continued immobilization (e.g., fractures, after dorsal capsulodesis) yet need to remove the splint for protected exercises and hygiene. Be careful not to catch the patient's skin in the zipper; use a stockinette beneath the splint to prevent this.

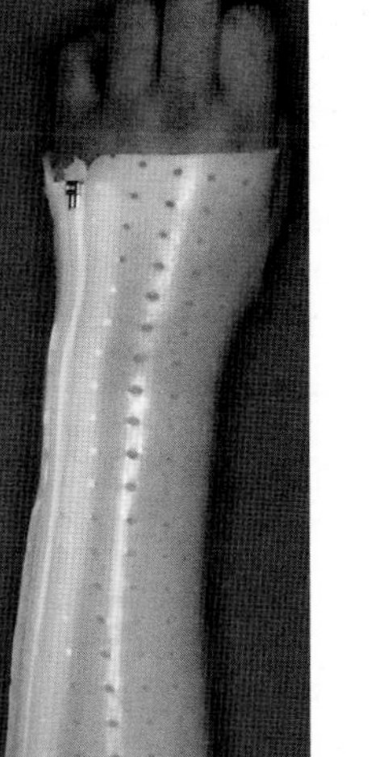

CLINICAL PEARL

Circumferential Splint As a Base for Mobilization Components

Circumferential designs provide a stable base for attaching mobilizing components. Because of the intimate fit provided with this all-encompassing design, splint migration can be minimized. Here a flexion glove was used over the Rolyan AquaForm zippered wrist splint to provide a flexion mobilization force to the digits while the wrist remains stabilized in extension. This prevents the common problem of the wrist flexing to reduce the stretch on tight digits caused by the flexion glove's corrective force.

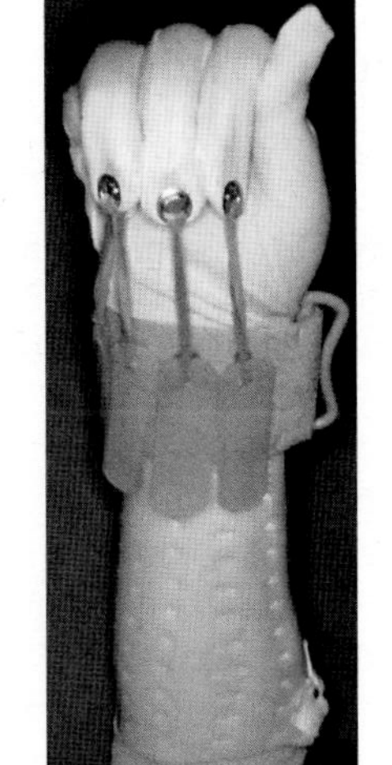

Fabrication Process

Pattern Creation (Fig. 7–28)

- Alternative to clamshell wrist immobilization splint.
- Mark for proximal border two thirds length of forearm.
- Mark for distal border just proximal to distal palmar crease.
- Widen pattern proximally, remembering that forearm tapers distally.
- Incorporate oblique angle that traverses from index to small metacarpal heads.
- Mark for thumbhole, located distally and approximately two thirds from ulnar border; position hole down 1 in. from this point.

Refine Pattern

- Proximal border should allow full elbow motion.

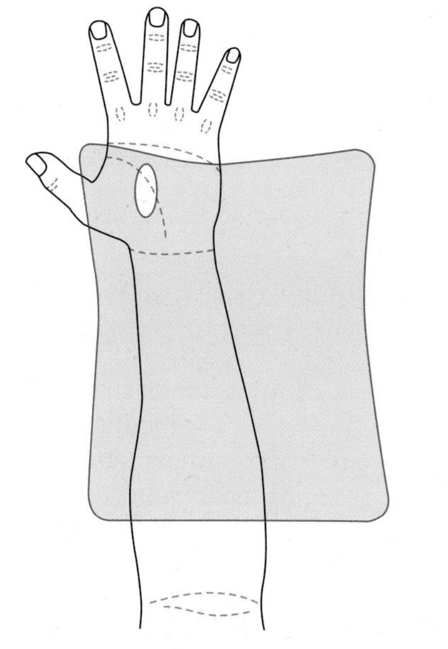

Figure 7–28

- Distal border should allow unimpeded motion of MP joints and nearly full thumb mobility.
- For average adult, thumbhole should be about size of elongated half dollar. When measuring pattern on patient, hole should lie approximately over thumb MP joint.

Options for Materials

- Elastic materials are an excellent choice because they tend to stretch easily when heated and provide an intimate fit. Remember that elastic materials tend to shrink around the splinted part; do not remove until splint is completely set.
- Use $^3/_{32}$" material, which is adequate for stabilizing forearm; circumferential nature of this splint makes it rigid.
- Although $^1/_8$" material can be used, its thickness increases splint's rigidity, making it difficult to remove.
- May use $^1/_{16}$" material for young children and older adults.
- Lightly perforated materials allow air exchange and increase splint flexibility, making donning and doffing easier.

Cut and Heat

- Position patient with elbow resting on table and forearm supinated for gravity-assisted molding. Position thumb in palmar abduction and opposition.
- If patient has difficulty supinating forearm, have patient flex elbow on table and adduct shoulder toward midline or lie patient supine with shoulder abducted and externally rotated 90° with elbow flexed.
- Cut out thumbhole in material either by making series of holes with hole punch before heating or by carefully piercing the slightly warm material with sharp scissors.
- Prepad ulna styloid (and radial styloid, if necessary) with adhesive-backed padding or gel.

Evaluate Fit While Molding

- Lay warm material on towel, positioning thumbhole on correct side of material as if it were to be placed on forearm.
- Using index fingers, gently open hole, slightly enlarging and elongating it.
- Place thumbhole over thumb (using thenar crease as guide) and gently stretch and guide rest of material evenly.
- Do not grab proximal splint or try to secure with tight circumferential bandage.
- Gently redirect antigravity surface of splint by applying smooth strokes over area.
- Carefully incorporate arches of hand by using smooth, even strokes and constantly redirecting material into arches. Avoid strongly molding into arches, which may cause significant discomfort in palm once material has set.
- Rotate forearm into pronated position at end of molding to check for clearance of ulnar and radial styloid processes.
- Make sure desired wrist position is maintained. Some patients tend to flex and deviate wrist while splint is being formed.

Strapping and Components

- Self-adhesive D-ring straps: 1" straps distally and 2" straps proximally work well, because they allow firm and easy closure. Patient can make adjustments according to comfort.

Splint Finishing Touches

- Smooth and slightly flare distal and proximal borders as well as thenar hole.
- Check clearance of elbow, radial and ulnar styloid processes, thumb, and finger MP joints.
- Pay careful attention to index metacarpal, which frequently abuts radial portion of splint as it traverses through first web space.

Radial Wrist/Thumb Immobilization Splint (Fig. 7–29)

Common Names

- Radial gutter splint
- Radial gutter thumb spica splint
- Thumb gauntlet splint
- Radial wrist support
- Long Opponens splint

Alternative Splint Options

- Prefabricated wrist and thumb support
- QuickCast
- Cast

Primary Functions

- Immobilize wrist and thumb joint(s) to allow healing, rest, and/or protection of involved structure(s).

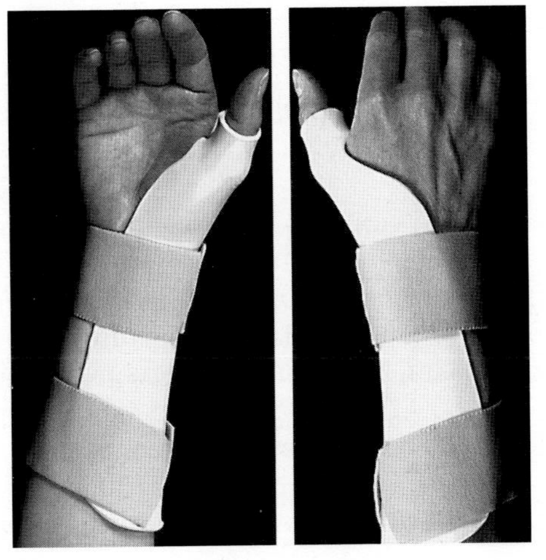

Figure 7–29

Additional Functions

- Improve functional pinch by positioning wrist and thumb in optimal positions.

Common Diagnoses and General Optimal Positions

- deQuervain's tenosynovitis — Wr: 20° ext; th CMC: between rad and palm abd; MP: slight flex; IP: included or free, depending on severity
- Th UCL reconstruction — Wr: 20° ext; th CMC: palm abd; MP: 5° flex and slight UD
- Th RCL reconstruction — Wr: 20° ext; th CMC: palm abd; MP: 5° flex and slight RD
- Th STT or CMC jt arthritis — Wr: 0 to 20° ext; th CMC: between rad and palm abd; MP: 5 to 10° flex
- EPL repair — Wr: 25 to 30° ext; th CMC: rad abd; MP: ext; IP: slight hyperextension
- Tendon transfers for th ext — Wr: 25 to 30° ext; th CMC: rad abd; IP: slight hyperextension

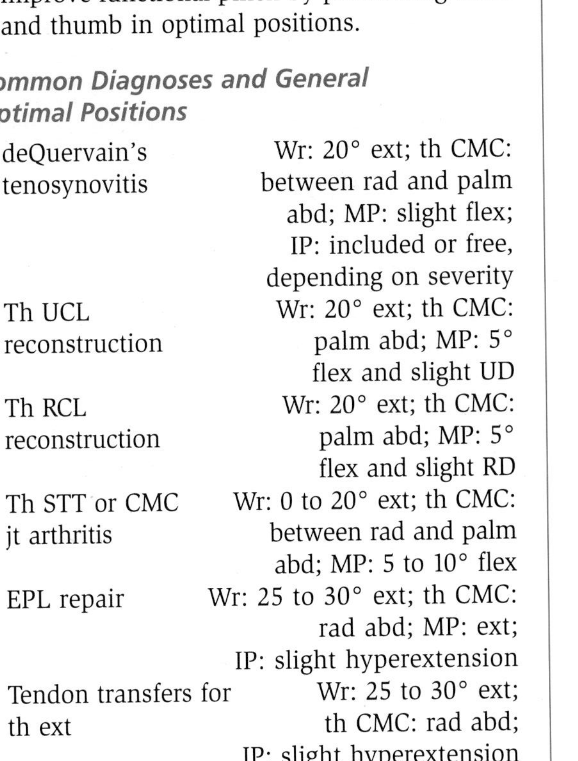

CLINICAL PEARL

Adjustments of Thumb Immobilization Splint

To splint the CMC joint only, refine the radial thumb immobilization splint pattern by ending just proximal to the MP joint (A and B). While molding, apply gentle counter pressure to the first metacarpal (dorsal pressure proximally and volar pressure distally). The pattern can also be adjusted to include the IP joint of the thumb by allowing for additional material distally at the thumb (C and D).

Fabrication Process

Pattern Creation (Fig. 7–30)

- Mark proximal border two thirds length of forearm.
- Mark distal border at IF and MF proximal palmar crease.
- Mark ulnar and radial sides of thumb IP joint.
- Allow enough material to encompass $\frac{1}{2}$ to $\frac{2}{3}$ circumference of forearm, remembering that forearm tapers distally.

Refine Pattern

- Proximal border should allow full elbow motion.
- Distal border should allow unimpeded motion of MP joints and thumb IP flexion.
- Circumferential thumb portion should allow enough material to overlap $\frac{1}{2}$" to 1".

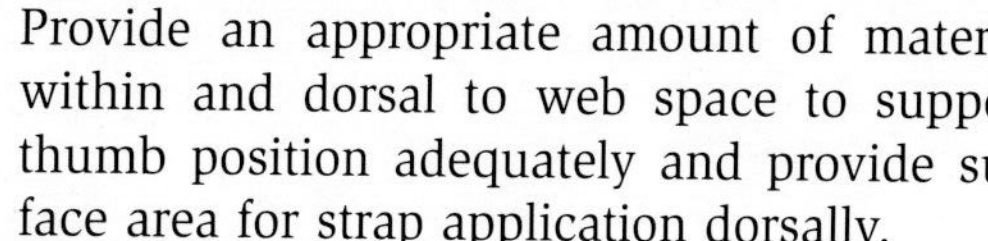

Figure 7–30

- Provide an appropriate amount of material within and dorsal to web space to support thumb position adequately and provide surface area for strap application dorsally.

Options for Materials

- Remember that materials with memory tend to shrink around proximal phalanx; do not remove until splint is completely set.
- Use coated material so material will pop apart once completely cooled, forming trap door to allow for easy donning and doffing of splint.
- Use $\frac{1}{16}$" or $\frac{3}{32}$" material for immobilizing patients with arthritis; this makes for lightweight splint with adequate rigidity.
- Gel- or foam-lined materials may help provide radial styloid scar compression, decrease distal migration, and increase comfort.

Cut and Heat

- While material is heating, prepad (with soft adhesive foam, silicone gels) at first dorsal compartment if tender.
- Consider placing light layer of lotion on thumb before molding to ease removal of splint.
- Position patient with elbow resting on table with forearm slightly supinated for gravity-assisted molding.
- Thumb should be positioned per diagnosis. Commonly, position of function is palmar abduction and opposition.

Evaluate Fit While Molding

- Place thumb portion of material on radial proximal phalanx and guide rest of material evenly along radial forearm.
- Carefully contour dorsal section of distal thumb material through web space.
- Gently pull and overlap dorsal thumb material through web space to support proximal phalanx, and lightly overlap onto volar piece.
- Avoid direct pressure over radial styloid, STT joint, and dorsal MP joint.
- Do not grab proximal splint or try to secure with tight circumferential bandage. This may cause borders of splint to irritate skin. Instead, allow gravity to assist in forming forearm trough.
- Carefully incorporate arches of hand by using smooth, even strokes and constantly redirecting material into arches.
- Make sure desired wrist position is maintained. Some patients tend to flex and deviate wrist while splint is being formed.

Strapping and Components

- Distal strap: 1" strap directed from dorsal web area to volar ulnar border.
- Middle strap: 2" strap just proximal to dorsal wrist crease; use piece of adhesive foam to further stabilize wrist in splint and prevent migration. Foam should lie directly over ulnar styloid and should not overlap splint edges.
- Proximal strap: depending on size of forearm, 1" or 2" strap may suffice; strap should have slight volar to dorsal angle.

Splint Finishing Touches

- Smooth and slightly flare all borders and around thumb opening.
- Check clearance of elbow, thumb IP joint, and IF MP joint flexion.

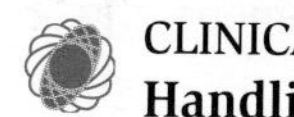

CLINICAL PEARL
Handling Warm Splint Material

The surface used to dry off warmed plastic material after removal from the splint pan can cause unsightly ridges or markings. To prevent towel markings, place the warm material on a pillow case before molding it onto the patient's extremity.

Volar Wrist/Thumb Immobilization Splint (Fig. 7–31)

Common Names

- Thumb spica splint
- Long opponens splint
- Radial gutter splint

Alternative Splint Options

- Prefabricated wrist and thumb splints
- QuickCast
- Cast
- Silicone rubber splint

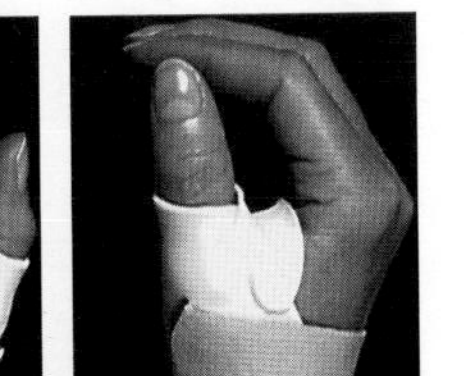
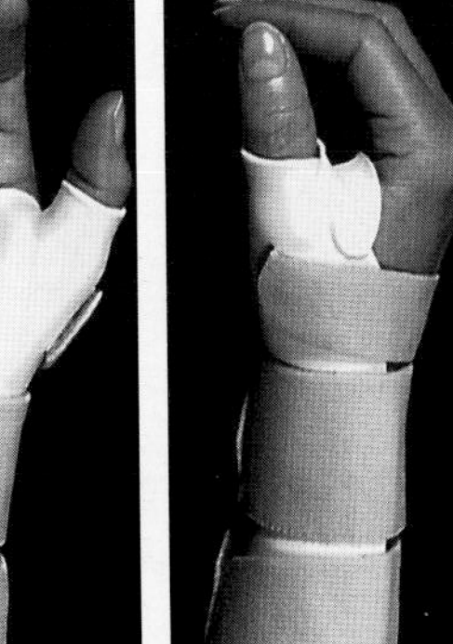

Figure 7–31

Primary Functions

- Immobilize wrist and thumb joint(s) to allow healing, rest, and/or protection of involved structure(s).

Additional Functions

- Improve functional pinch by positioning wrist and thumb in optimal positions.

Common Diagnoses and General Optimal Positions

Diagnosis	Position
• Scaphoid fracture (after cast immobilization)	Wr: 0 to 20° ext; RD and UD: 0°; th: between rad and palm abd; MP: 10° flex; IP: free
• Bennett fracture (after cast immobilization)	Wr: 0 to 20° ext; RD: 5°; th: 45° rad abd; MP: 5 to 10° flex
• deQuervain's tenosynovitis	Wr: 20° ext; th CMC: between rad and palm abd; MP: slight flex; IP: included or free (depends on severity)
• Intersection syndrome	Wr: 20° ext; RD and UD 0°; th CMC: rad abd; MP: 5 to 10° flex
• Th STT or CMC jt arthritis	Wr: 0 to 20° ext; th CMC: between rad and palm abd; MP: 5 to 10° flex
• STT or CMC/TM arthroplasty	Wr: 20° ext; RD and UD: 0°; th: between rad and palm abd; MP: 5 to 10° flex
• Lax or mildly subluxed STT jt	Wr: 0 to 20° ext; th CMC: medium palm abd; MP: slight flex
• EPL repair	Wr: 20 to 40° ext; th CMC: slight rad abd; MP: 0°; IP: 0+°
• Extensor pollicis brevis (EPB) or abductor pollicis longus (APL) repair	Wr: 20 to 40° ext; th CMC: slight rad abd; MP: 0°
• Tendon transfers (opponensplasty)	Wr: 0°; th CMC: medium palm abd; MP: 5 to 10° flex
• Th UCL reconstruction	Wr: 20° ext; th CMC: palm abd; MP: 5° flexion with slight UD
• Th RCL reconstruction	Wr: 20° ext; th CMC: palm abd; MP: 5° flex with slight RD

Fabrication Process

Pattern Creation (Fig. 7–32)

- Mark proximal border two thirds length of forearm.
- Mark distal border at thumb IP flexion crease and distal palmar crease.
- Allow enough material to encompass half to two thirds circumference of forearm, remembering that forearm tapers distally.

Refine Pattern

- Proximal border should allow full elbow motion.
- Distal border should allow unimpeded motion of IF to SF MP and thumb IP joint.
- Provide an appropriate amount of material within and dorsal to web space to support thumb position adequately and provide surface area for strap application dorsally.

Options for Materials

- Use drapable material to achieve intimate fit about thumb STT and MP joints, to prevent splint migration and improve comfort.

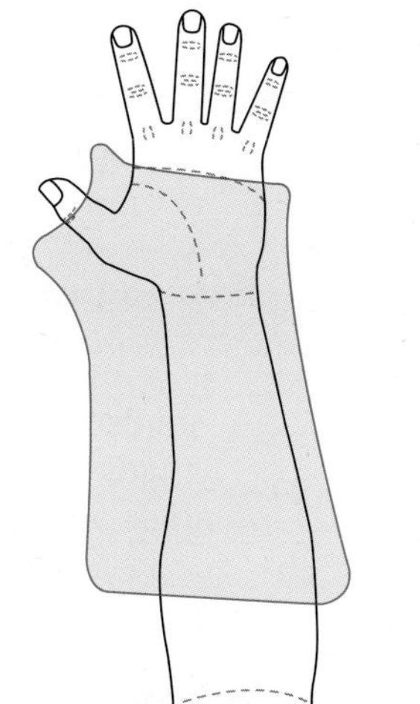

Figure 7–32

- Remember that elastic materials tend to shrink around proximal phalanx; do not remove until splint is completely set.
- Consider placing light layer of lotion on thumb before molding to ease removal of splint.
- Use coated material to allow material to pop apart once completely cooled. This forms trap door for easy donning and doffing of splint.
- Use 1/16" or 3/32" material for immobilizing patients with arthritis; this makes for lightweight splint with adequate rigidity.
- Consider perforated material when splint will be used during activity.

Cut and Heat

- Position patient with elbow resting on table and forearm slightly supinated for gravity-assisted molding.
- Position thumb per diagnosis. Commonly, position of function is gentle palmar abduction and opposition.
- If patient has difficulty supinating forearm (e.g., after cast immobilization), have patient flex elbow on table and adduct and externally rotate shoulder toward midline.

Evaluate Fit While Molding

- Lay warm material on towel, positioning thumb portion on correct side of material as if it were going to be placed on supinated forearm.
- Place thumb portion centrally over thumb and guide rest of material evenly along arm.
- Gently pull and overlap volar thumb material through web space to support proximal phalanx and lightly overlap onto dorsal piece. It is important for material to mold through web space to radial side of second metacarpal to provide adequate immobilization.
- Avoid direct pressure over radial styloid, STT joint, and dorsal MP joint.
- Do not grab proximal splint or try to secure with tight circumferential bandage. This may cause borders of splint to irritate skin. Instead, allow gravity to assist in forming forearm trough.
- While molding, place thumb joints in appropriate position.
- Carefully incorporate arches of hand by using smooth, even strokes and constantly redirecting material into arches.
- Make sure desired wrist position is maintained. Some patients tend to flex and deviate wrist while splint is being formed.
- Clear for radial and ulnar styloid, avoiding pressure over radial sensory nerve.
- Once material has cooled completely, pop apart overlapped thumb piece if concerned about doffing difficulty.

Strapping and Components

- Distal strap: 1" strap directed from radial dorsal web area to volar ulnar border. Use piece of adhesive foam under strap to further stabilize metacarpals.
- Middle strap: 2" strap just proximal to dorsal wrist crease; use piece of adhesive foam to further stabilize wrist in splint and prevent migration. Foam should lie directly over ulnar styloid and should not overlap splint edges.
- Proximal strap: depending on size of forearm, 1" or 2" strap may suffice; strap should have slight volar to dorsal angle.
- Apply small 1/2" strap across trap door.

Splint Finishing Touches

- Smooth and slightly flare all borders.
- Check for clearance of radial and ulnar styloids, elbow, thumb IP joint, and finger MP joints.
- Pay careful attention to IF MP, which frequently abuts radial portion of splint as it traverses through first web space. If splint is to be functional, check that patient can at least touch thumb to index fingertip.
- Make sure that patient does not experience pinching under overlapped thumb portion.

Dorsal Wrist/Hand (Optional Thumb) Immobilization Splint

(Fig. 7–33)

Common Names

- Dorsal protective splint
- Dorsal blocking splint
- Extension block splint
- Dorsal shell

Alternative Splint Options

- Cast

Primary Functions

- Immobilize wrist, MP, PIP, and DIP joints in flexion to allow healing of involved structures(s).

Additional Functions

- Promote early protected active and/or passive motion of repaired tendons to facilitate healing and prevent adherence to surrounding structures (mobilization or restriction splint).

Common Diagnoses and General Optimal Positions

- Optimal positions for tendon and nerve injuries depend on the severity of the injury, the integrity of repaired structures (tendon, nerve, vascular structures, pulleys, and bone), and the physician's rehabilitation protocol. Chapter 18 provides details.
- FDS or FDP tendon repair — Wr: 0 to 45° flex; MP: 30 to 60° flex; IP: 0 to 30° ext (depending on nerve status)
- FPL tendon repair — Wr: 0 to 45° flex; th CMC: 0 to 45° palm abd; MP: 20 to 40° flex; IP: 0 to 20°

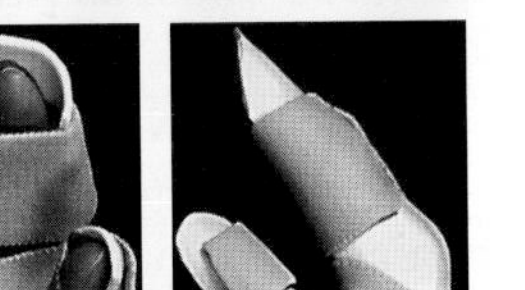
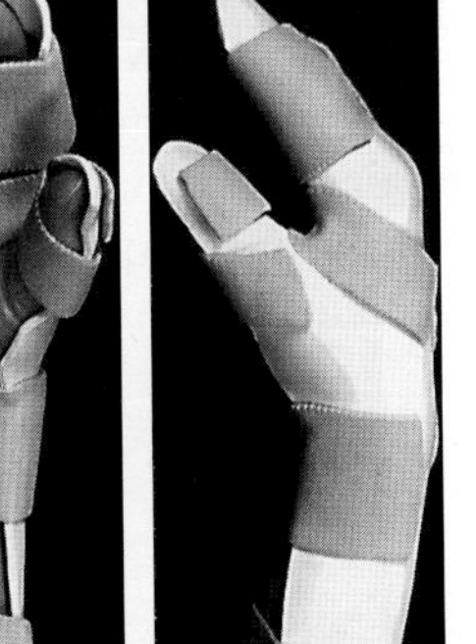
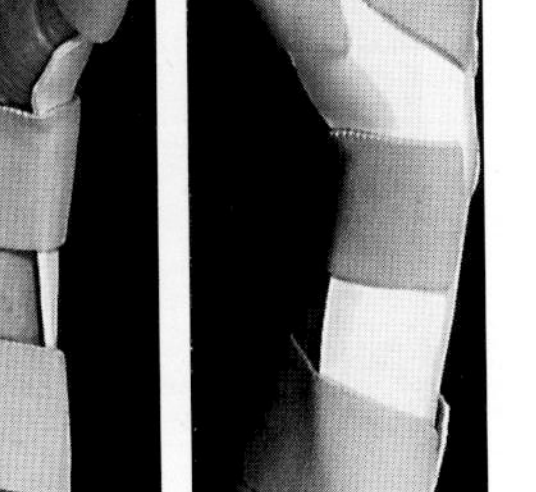

Figure 7–33

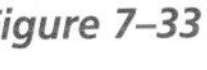
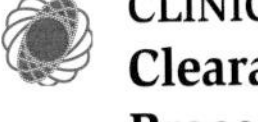

CLINICAL PEARL

Clearance of Radial and Ulnar Styloid Processes

Near the end of the molding process of a splint that includes the forearm, place the arm in both a pronated and supinated position to check for clearance of the styloid processes. Note that the forearm muscle bulk orientation changes as the forearm rotates. Using index fingers, gently reach under the slightly warm splint material and pull out or lift along the styloids. When using elastic materials, constant redirecting or reminding the material is necessary. For plastic materials, one gentle adjustment is all that is needed. For more rigid rubber materials, a stronger lift is necessary to achieve the desired clearance.

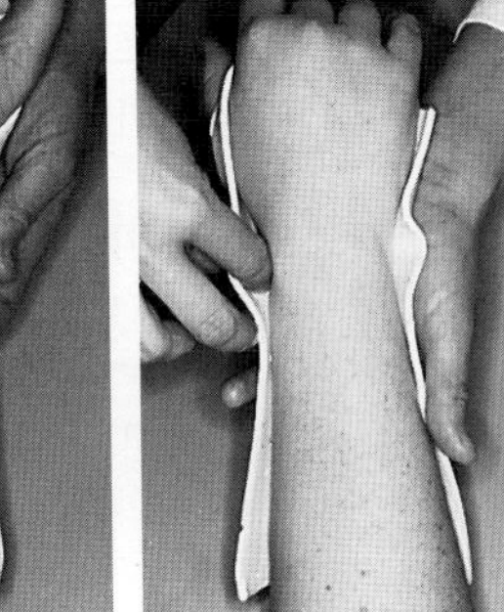
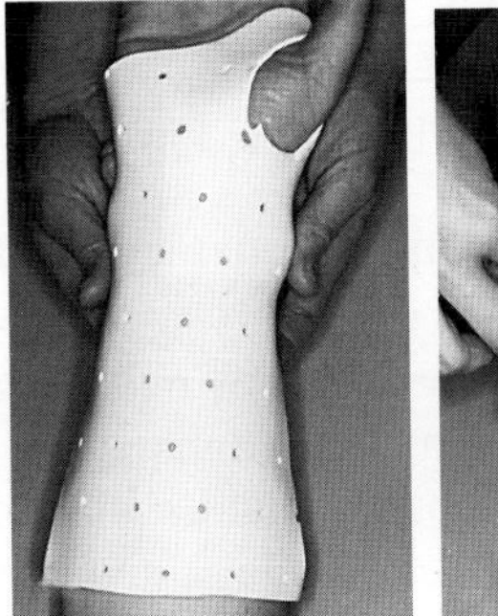

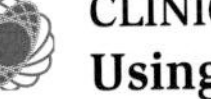

CLINICAL PEARL

Using Scrap Splint Material

Scrap pieces of splint material come in handy for many different situations. For example, material can be molded around a writing utensil to build up the handle. Also, scraps can be used for the fabrication of small digit splints and for securing mobilization components onto splint bases.

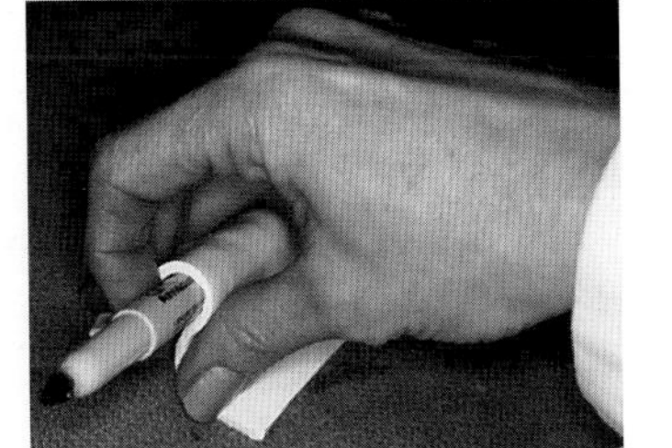

Fabrication Process

Pattern Creation (Fig. 7–34)

- Note: Because unimpeded active motion is contraindicated, draw pattern on uninjured hand, if possible.
- Mark for proximal border two thirds length of forearm.
- Mark distal border approximately 1" distal to fingertips; this additional material is necessary to compensate for flexed position of wrist and MP joints.
- If thumb is not involved, mark thumb clearance by making an arc from thumb MP to base of first STT joint (using thenar crease as landmark).
- If thumb is involved, mark 1" distally and allow enough material around borders to support thumb and allow for strap application (dotted line on pattern).

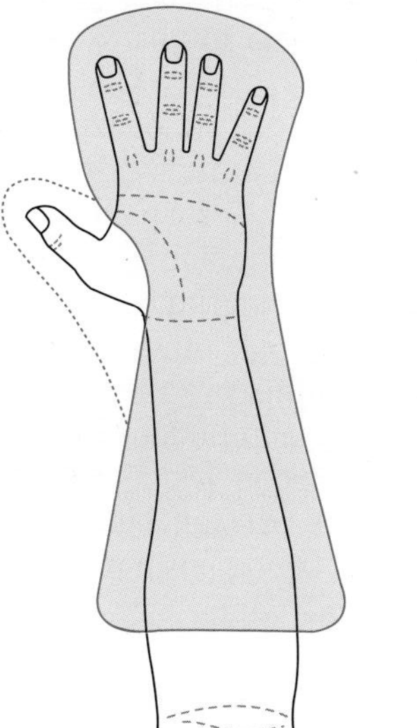

Figure 7–34

- Allow enough material to encompass half to two thirds circumference of forearm, remembering that forearm tapers distally.

Refine Pattern

- Proximal border should allow full elbow motion.
- Distal border should completely protect and cover fingertips (and thumb, if applicable).
- If thumb is not involved full mobility should be available.

Options for Materials

- Use $\frac{1}{8}$" thermoplastic material to provide needed rigidity to maintain joint positions.
- If patient has significant pain and swelling, splinting may be quite difficult. Consider uncoated materials or those that are slightly tacky and drapable to help prevent material from slipping and to make it easier to position patient and mold splint.
- Gel- or foam-lined materials help decrease sheer stress on ulnar styloid and metacarpal heads, decrease distal migration, and increase comfort.
- Materials that can be reheated and remolded several times are a good option if ongoing splint modifications become necessary to accommodate for fluctuations in edema or changes in desired joint position.
- Consider $\frac{1}{8}$" perforated material, because splint will likely be worn continuously for several weeks.

Cut and Heat

- Position patient with elbow resting on table and forearm pronated for gravity-assisted molding. If involved, position thumb in gentle palmar abduction and opposition.
- If wound dressings are necessary, they must be incorporated into splint. Place stockinette over dressing to prevent thermoplastic material from sticking. This can be easily cut away when molding process is complete.
- Consider using palmar support to rest hand on; this helps control of positioning wrist and MP joints during fabrication.
- Prepad ulnar styloid with adhesive foam or silicone gel.

Evaluate Fit While Molding

- Lay warm material on towel, positioning thumb cut out or thumb piece, if involved, on correct side of material as if it were going to be placed on pronated forearm.
- Position material on dorsum of involved hand, wrist, and forearm. Be sure to cover fingertips adequately. Allow gravity to aid in contouring about metacarpal heads and styloids.
- Depending on material chosen, splinting around IF and SF metacarpal borders may be difficult; buckling of material may occur.
- Do not grab proximal splint or try to secure with tight circumferential bandage. This may cause borders of splint to irritate skin. Instead, allow gravity to assist in forming forearm and hand trough.
- Digits often want to assume flexed posture secondary to edema, pain, and postsurgical complications, making molding of dorsal hood in 0° of IP extension a challenge. Gently lift material and approximate optimal position. Volarly applied soft strap progressively extends digits to reach dorsal hood.
- Make sure desired wrist and digit positions are maintained. It is crucial to use goniometer to ensure accurate positioning. Be careful of joint position during splint removal.

Dorsal Wrist/Hand (Optional Thumb) Immobilization Splint *(Continued)*

Strapping and Components

- Distal strap: 2" soft strap running slightly oblique from radial distal border to ulnar distal border. Strap should traverse and support all fingertips against dorsal hood. Use adhesive foam on straps to support digits in position.
- Volar MP strap: 1" to 2" (trimmed) strap provides support volarly to MP joints; use piece of adhesive foam to further stabilize wrist in splint and prevent migration. Foam should not overlap splint edges.
- Wrist strap: 2" soft strap with adhesive foam to further stabilize joints in splint and prevent migration.
- Proximal strap: 2" soft or elasticized strap.
- Thumb strap: 1" strap traversing on oblique angle to incorporate thumb IP and proximal phalanx.

Splint Finishing Touches

- Smooth and slightly flare all borders.
- Gently flare around dorsal thumb and lateral MP regions; do not roll, which makes future splint modifications difficult and unnecessarily bulky.
- Check clearance of elbow and thumb (if applicable).
- Check for compression stress at radial and ulnar styloid processes and over dorsal MP joints.
- Check for compression over radial and ulnar sensory nerves.

CLINICAL PEARL

Use of Hand Rest for Joint Positioning

A rest for the palmar surface of the hand can aid considerably when fabricating a dorsal wrist and hand immobilization splint. This device, consisting of a platform and rolled palmar support, can be constructed from thermoplastic material. The raised palmar support should be high enough to allow the fingers and thumb to drape over it without touching the table and keeping the wrist in the desired amount of flexion.

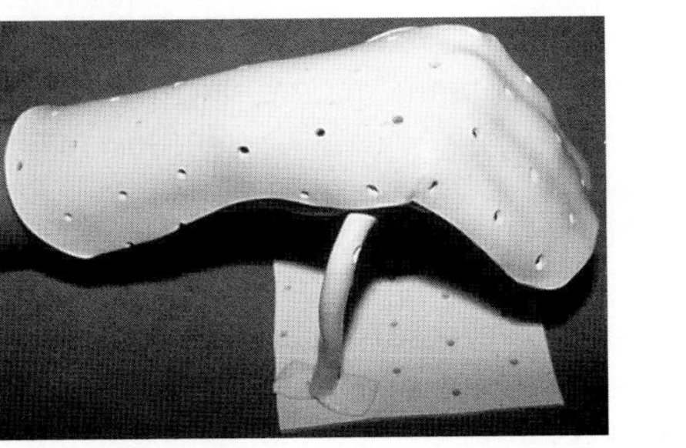

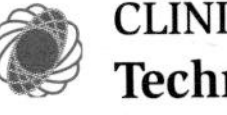

CLINICAL PEARL

Techniques for Accommodating MP Flexion Angle

When applying a dorsal splint over flexed MP joints, it can be challenging to accommodate for the flexion angle. Consider the following techniques (shown here from top to bottom): (1) Cut just enough material to support the area. With a small tug distally, the material will fall into place without overlapping. This is an advanced technique that takes much practice but provides the most cosmetically pleasing look. Be careful not to pull the material too much, or you will thin and weaken the area. (2) Dog ear the material by first snipping in approximately $1/2$" at the MP joints and then overlapping it. The material must be treated with solvent and heated with a heat gun to ensure a strong bond. This technique makes future modifications of the MP flexion angle difficult. (3) Gently stretch and overlap the material dorsally at the MP joints to take up the excess. Note that

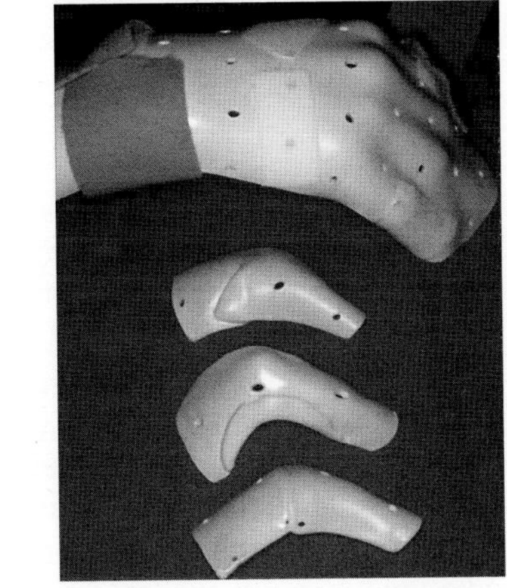

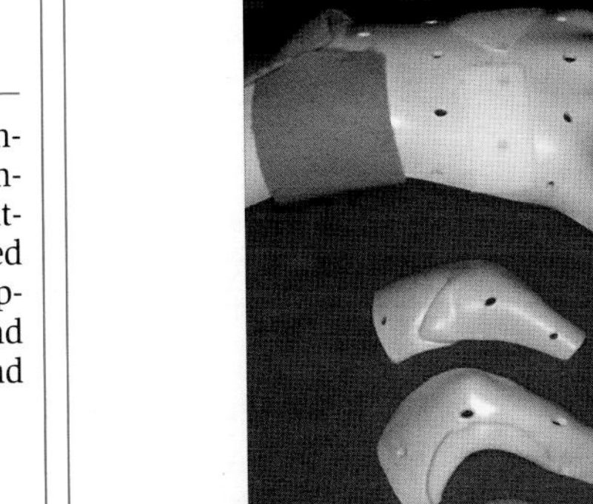

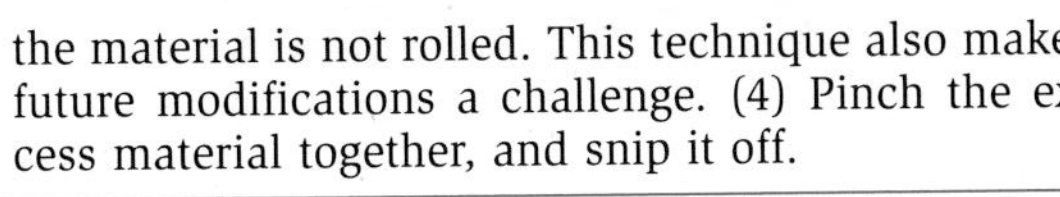

the material is not rolled. This technique also makes future modifications a challenge. (4) Pinch the excess material together, and snip it off.

CLINICAL PEARL

Wrist–Thenar Strapping Techniques to Prevent Migration

Splints may shift in position if not secured adequately. This can adversely alter joint angles and place the repaired or healing structures at risk. To help prevent this occurrence, the following strapping techniques can be employed. Apply an adhesive foam (such as T-Stick) to the 2" strap just proximal to the distal wrist crease (A). Trim the 2" strap in half at the thenar crease (B). Rivet an additional 1" strap to the MP joint strap at the midthenar crease to anchor the splint about the thumb (C). Mold a thermoplastic palmar bar from the radial dorsal aspect of the index finger MP area and guide a ulnar ward through the thumb web, along the palmar surface just proximal to the distal palmar crease, overlapping and securing on the distal ulnar small finger MP border (pull the material if needed for increased length) (D). Carefully incorporate the arches of the hand by using smooth, even strokes, constantly redirecting the material into the arches.

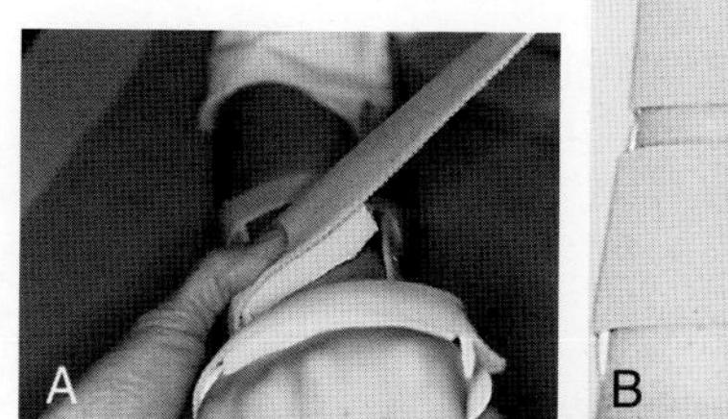
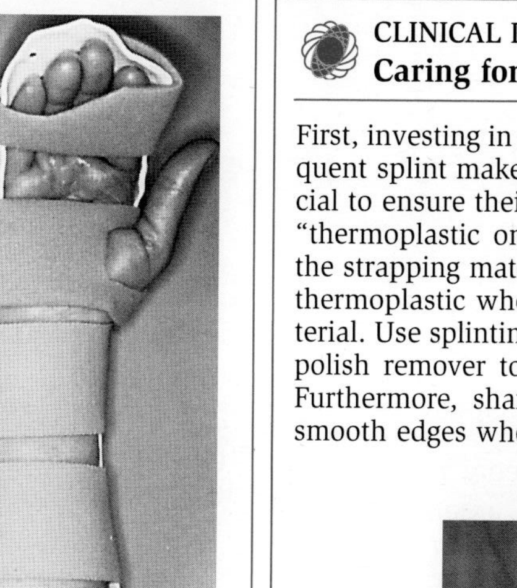
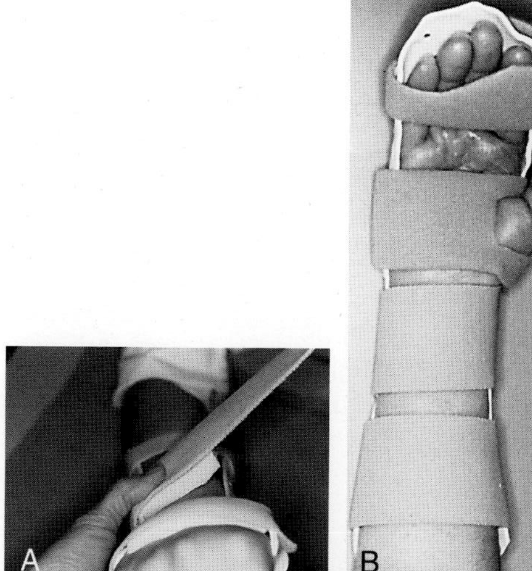
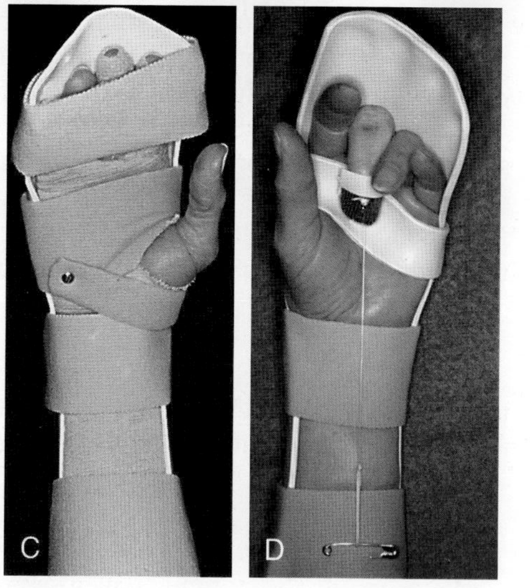

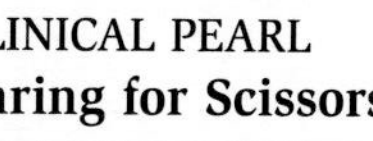

CLINICAL PEARL

Caring for Scissors

First, investing in quality scissors is a must for the frequent splint maker. Proper care of the scissors is crucial to ensure their effective use. Designating scissors "thermoplastic only" and "strapping only" prevents the strapping material's adhesive from sticking to the thermoplastic when cutting and trimming warm material. Use splinting solvent, adhesive remover, or nail polish remover to clean the adhesive from scissors. Furthermore, sharpen the scissors often to achieve smooth edges when fabricating splints.

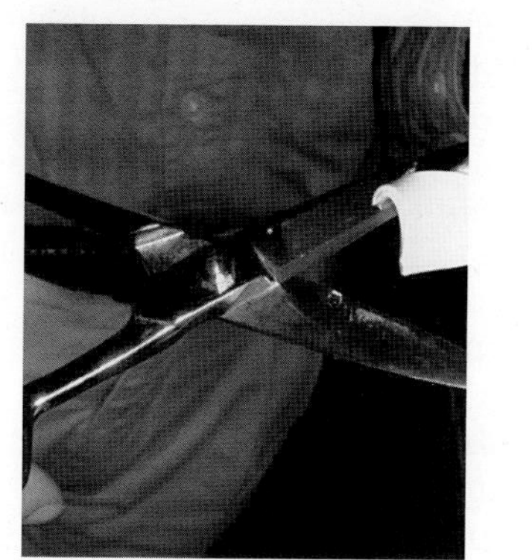

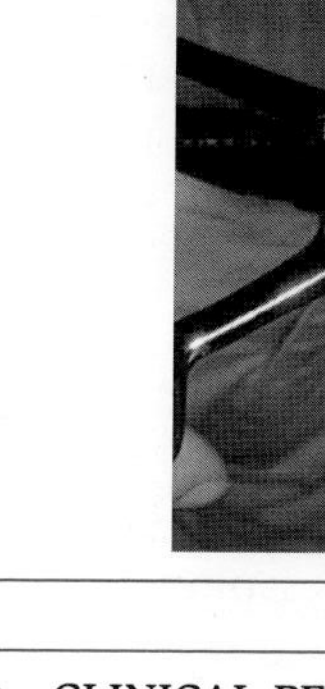

CLINICAL PEARL

Transferring Pattern to Material

There are many ways to transfer the paper towel pattern to the thermoplastic material. The main goal is to avoid an unsightly splint with markings along the edges. Here are some techniques: Allow the paper towel to adhere to the wet material during the cutting process (Left), use a wax pencil to outline the design (Right), or scratch the thermoplastic material with an awl to draw the pattern.

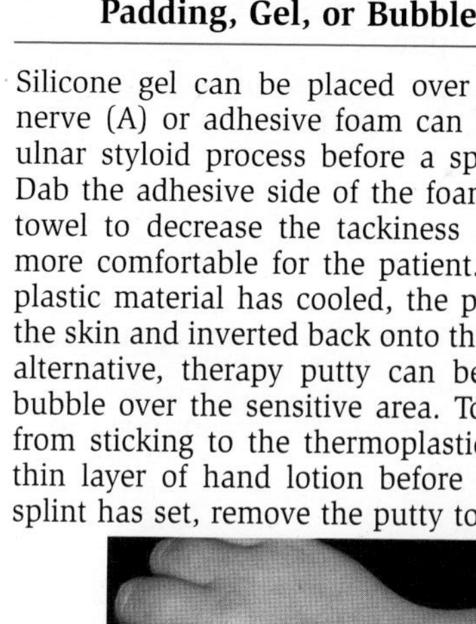

CLINICAL PEARL

Accommodating Sensitive Areas with Padding, Gel, or Bubble

Silicone gel can be placed over the radial sensory nerve (A) or adhesive foam can be used to pad the ulnar styloid process before a splint is applied (B). Dab the adhesive side of the foam a few times on a towel to decrease the tackiness and make removal more comfortable for the patient. Once the thermoplastic material has cooled, the padding is taken off the skin and inverted back onto the splint. As another alternative, therapy putty can be used to create a bubble over the sensitive area. To prevent the putty from sticking to the thermoplastic material, apply a thin layer of hand lotion before molding. After the splint has set, remove the putty to form the bubble.

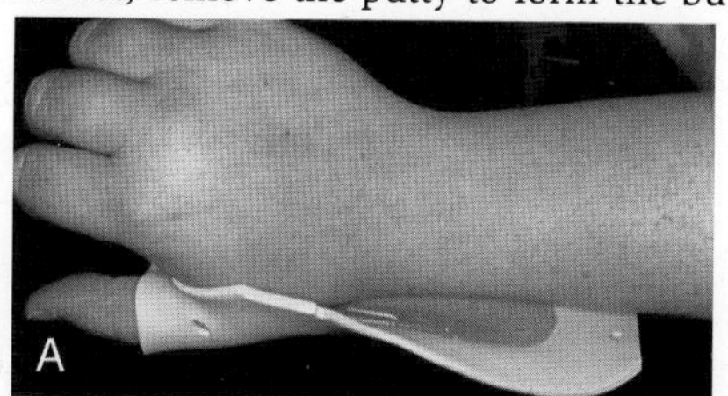
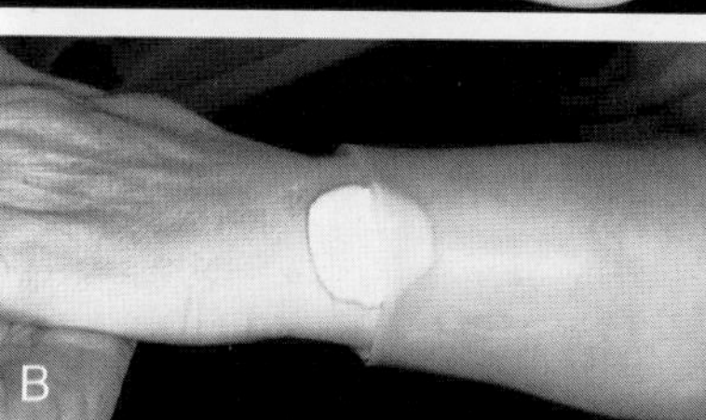

Volar Wrist/Hand (Optional Thumb) Immobilization Splint

(Fig. 7–35)

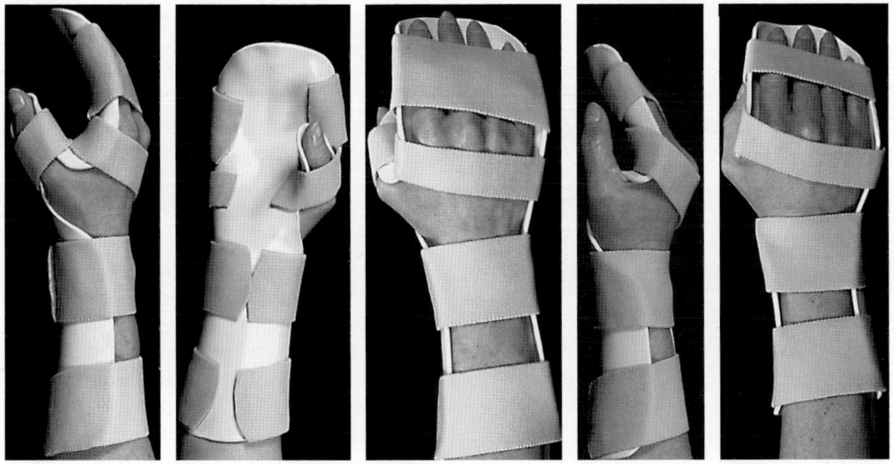

Common Names

- Resting hand splint
- Resting pan splint

Alternative Splint Options

- Prefabricated splint
- Cast

Primary Functions

- Immobilize wrist and hand (and thumb) joints to allow healing or rest of involved structures(s).

Additional Functions

- Statically position tight flexor tendons at maximum extension to facilitate lengthening of tissue (mobilization splint).
- Prevent or minimize joint contractures of wrist, fingers, and thumb.
- Prevent overstretching of weak or absent wrist and digit muscle–tendon units.
- Aid in reducing muscle tone in wrist and digits.

Common Diagnoses and General Optimal Positions

Diagnosis	Position
• Burn injury	Wr: 30° ext (volar or circumferential burns), 0° (dorsal burns); MP: 60 to 90° flex; IP 0°, th: between palm abd and th opp
• Rheumatoid arthritis	Wr: 30° ext; MP: slight flex; IP: comfortable flex; th: abd and th opp (Note: If patient has carpal tunnel symptoms, decrease wrist ext.)
• Crush injuries	Wr: 30° ext; MP: 60° flex; IP: 0°; th: palm abd
• Tendon transfers	Dictated by structures involved
• Extensor tendon repairs (zone V to VI)	Wr: 40 to 45° ext; MP: 0 to 20° flex; IP: 0°
• Radial nerve injury or repair	Wr: 30° ext; MP: 30 to 40° flex; PIP: 40° flex; DIP: 20° flex; th: rad abd
• Infection or cellulitis	Functional position or intrinsic plus position; include one jt higher than infection
• Replantation or transplantation	Dictated by structures involved
• MP capsulectomy	Wr: 10 to 30° ext; MP: 75 to 90° flex; IP: 0°
• Abnormal tone	Depends on therapist and physician rationale

Figure 7–35

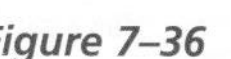

Fabrication Process

Pattern Creation (Fig. 7–36)

- Mark for proximal border two thirds length of forearm.
- Allow enough material to encompass half to two thirds circumference of forearm, remembering that forearm tapers distally.
- Mark width of hand plus 1/4" to 1/2" on each side to allow for hand trough.
- Mark distal border, approximately 1" distal to fingertips.
- Mark for thumb only if included in splint.
- Radial aspect of thumb: from distal border (approximately 1" radial to index fingertip), draw line through center of thumb IP joint proximally toward thumb MP joint, ending just proximal to CMC joint.
- Proximal and medial aspect: curve proximal and medial to CMC joint along palmar edge of thenar eminence. Curved thumb pattern should end at midthenar mass (along thenar crease), in line with third metacarpals.

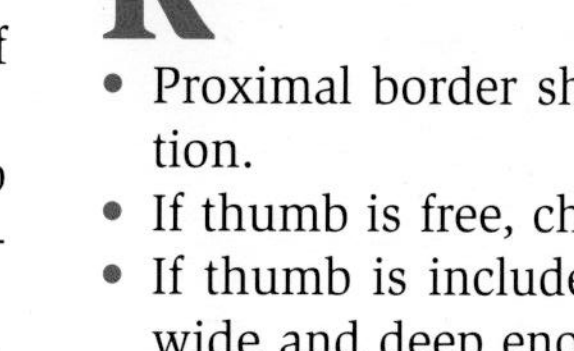

Figure 7–36

Refine Pattern

- Proximal border should allow full elbow motion.
- If thumb is free, check for nearly full motion.
- If thumb is included, thumb piece should be wide and deep enough to encompass thumb.

Options for Materials

- Material selection depends on requirements.
- Consider 1/8" thermoplastic material to provide needed rigidity to maintain stretch on tight tissue or support painful edematous hand.
- Materials with moderate stretch properties can be difficult to handle when fabricating this splint, especially if patient has increased tone.
- If patient has difficulty achieving supinated gravity assist position, consider uncoated materials or those that are slightly tacky to help prevent material from slipping and to make it easier to position patient and mold splint.
- Materials that can be reheated and remolded several times are a good option if ongoing splint modifications become necessary to accommodate for fluctuations in edema or changes in desired joint position.
- Gel- or foam-lined materials help provide volar wrist scar compression, decrease distal migration, and increase comfort.
- Consider perforated material when splint will worn continually or in conjunction with scar-management products such as Elastomer. Scar products seep through perforations, which helps anchor them into splint.

Cut and Heat

- Position patient with elbow resting on table with forearm supinated for gravity-assisted molding.
- Position thumb or leave free per diagnosis.
- If patient has difficulty supinating forearm (e.g., pain extremity), have patient flex elbow on table and adduct shoulder toward midline or lie supine with shoulder abducted and externally rotated 90° with elbow flexed.
- When cutting thumb area of splint, leave small space (make notch) between proximal thumb piece and radial forearm trough to keep material ends from touching and adhering during molding process.

Evaluate Fit While Molding

- Lay warm material on towel, positioning thumb piece on correct side of material as if it were going to be placed on supinated forearm.
- Position material on volar aspect of involved hand and wrist, with thumb component applied within index and thumb web space (commonly referred to as C-bar). Material must be stretched slightly to achieve even contouring along dorsal web and within palm.
- Lift thumb trough and place it centrally over thumb's medial/ulnar border. Once positioned, carefully stretch outer border to form C shape. Medial portion (snipped section) should adequately cover wrist and partially cover thenar eminence. Pay close attention to thumb joint positions.
- Use palmar aspect of hand to help support volar arches and first web space, simulating handshake hold.
- Position digits in slight abduction with MP, PIP, and DIP joints positioned per diagnosis.
- Guide rest of material evenly along arm.
- Borders of splint should be curved to from hand trough (1/4" to 1/2" at hand and thumb). These curved sides keep fingers from falling off splint's border.

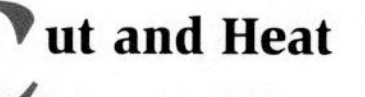

Volar Wrist/Hand (Optional Thumb) Immobilization Splint (Continued)

- Gravity tends to pull material away from thumb and toward IF continually reposition material as needed.
- Do not grab proximal splint or try to secure with tight circumferential bandage. This may cause borders of splint to irritate skin. Instead, allow gravity to assist in forming forearm trough.
- Check for pressure areas at ulnar aspect of thumb MP, and IF and SF MP joints.
- Check for compression of dorsal sensory branches of radial and ulnar nerves.
- Rotate forearm into pronated position at end of molding to check for clearance of ulnar and radial styloid processes; flare around styloids as necessary.
- Make sure desired wrist position is maintained. Some patients tend to flex and deviate wrist while splint is being formed. May use goniometer to ensure correct positioning; this is especially important for diagnoses requiring specific positioning (e.g., tendon repairs and transfers).
- Do not stress ulnar collateral ligament of thumb MP joint when attempting to palmarly abduct thumb.
- When splinting for increased tone or for use with serial static designs, it may be necessary to reinforce wrist portion with another strip of thermoplastic material, or consider different design, such as a dorsally based splint.

Strapping and Components

- Distal strap: 1" to 2" strap directed from radial border of proximal IF to ulnar border of proximal SF. Strip of adhesive foam can be used under strap to stabilize and contour about proximal phalanxes.
- Metacarpal strap: 1" strap directed from radial web space to midulnar border.
- Wrist strap: 2" strap just proximal to dorsal wrist crease; use piece of adhesive foam to further stabilize wrist in splint and prevent migration. Foam should lie directly over ulnar styloid and should not overlap splint edges.
- Proximal strap: depending on size of forearm, 1" or 2" strap may suffice; strap should have slight volar to dorsal angle.
- Thumb strap: 1" strap across proximal phalanx.
- In some cases (e.g., with severe edema), traditional strapping may not be appropriate; cotton wrap or elasticized bandage may be better option.
- Some conditions of arthritis may require straps or finger separators to aid in positioning deviating joints.
- Patients with an increase in tone may need additional straps to maintain joint position.

Splint Finishing Touches

- Smooth and slightly flare distal and proximal borders.
- Gently flare around thenar segment; avoid rolling, which makes future splint modifications difficult and leads to unnecessarily bulky splint.
- Check clearance of elbow, styloid processes, thumb, and IF to SF joints.

CLINICAL PEARL
Finger Separators

There are several creative ways to position deviating (or potentially deviating) joints of patients with rheumatoid arthritis. Finger spacers are often necessary for correct positioning and comfort. Thermoplastic separators can be formed using scissors, bandage applicator, or pencil (A). When designing the pattern, allow extra material at the hand width. While the material is still warm, gently take the edge of a pair of closed scissors (tip pointing into the web), or another similarly shaped object, and apply pressure volar to dorsal to create a trough for each digit that is approximately 1/2" deep. Lightly pinch together and move on to the next digit. Foam finger separators can be constructed using a adhesive-backed 3/8" foam, such as T-Stick (B). These do not need to extend completely into the web to provide slight abduction. Another option is to use Elastomer to create an insert for the hand to rest within (C). They are very comfortable and easy to apply. For patients with dense scar between the digits, a mold can be used to aid in remodeling (D). Fabricate soft strap separators from about 12" strip of 2" soft strapping (E). Apply adhesive hook to the volar portion of the splint, and form gullies or troughs with the soft strap. This technique works well for patients with arthritis or fragile skin.

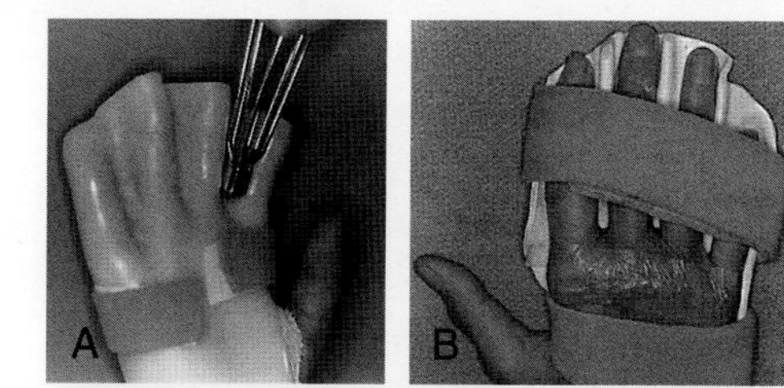

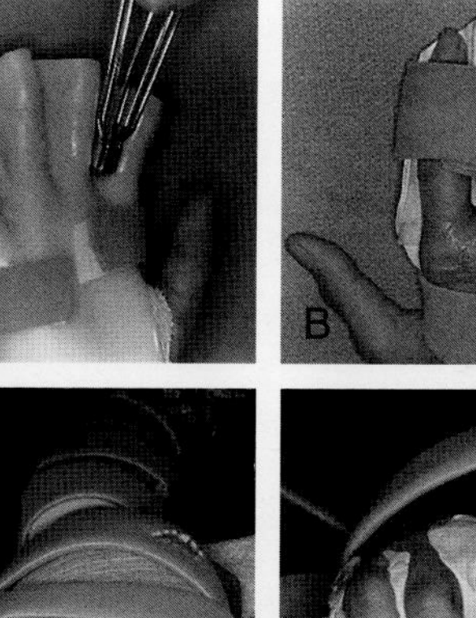

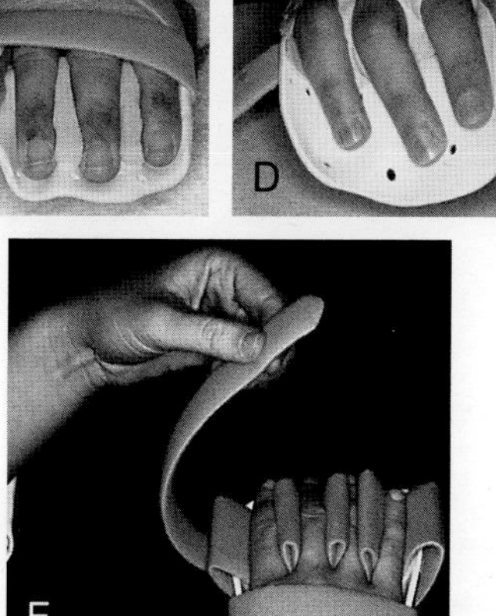

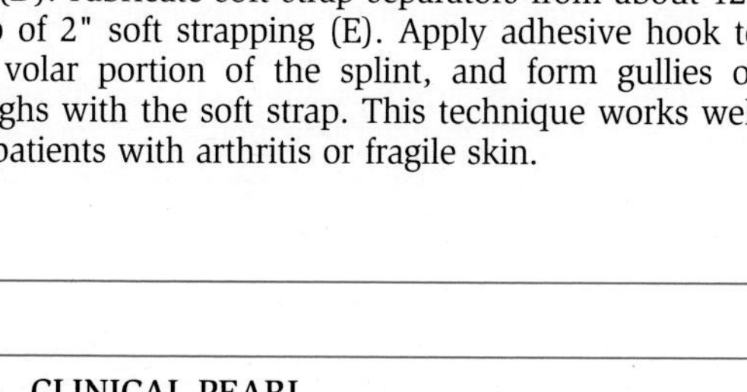

CLINICAL PEARL
Mitt-Style Wrist/Hand/Thumb Immobilization Splint

This pattern offers another way to immobilize the wrist, hand, and thumb. The appropriate diagnoses and optimal positions are the same as described for the wrist/hand/thumb immobilization splint. This particular splint can be easier to construct and may allow more latitude for altering the thumb position. However, it may not provide as secure positioning of the first web space as the other design.

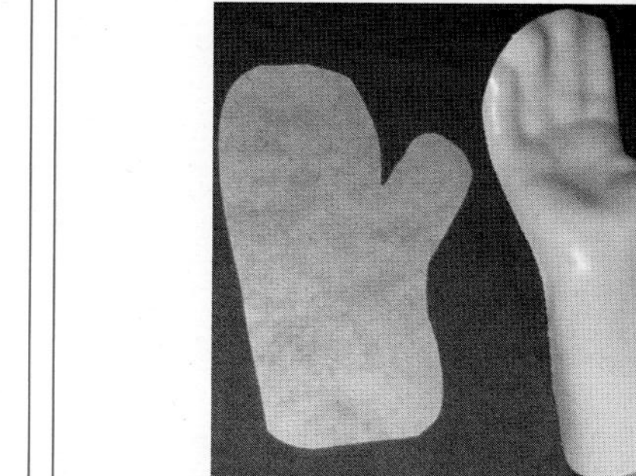

CLINICAL PEARL
Hints for Molding the First Web Space

The handshake hold technique helps control the thermoplastic material while maintaining the first web space. Use a light grasp distally while working proximally. Stretch and contour the material between the IF and thumb to create a C (similar to a thumb abduction splint) for the thumb and IF to rest in. Be careful not to dig the fingertips into warm material, creating potential pressure areas.

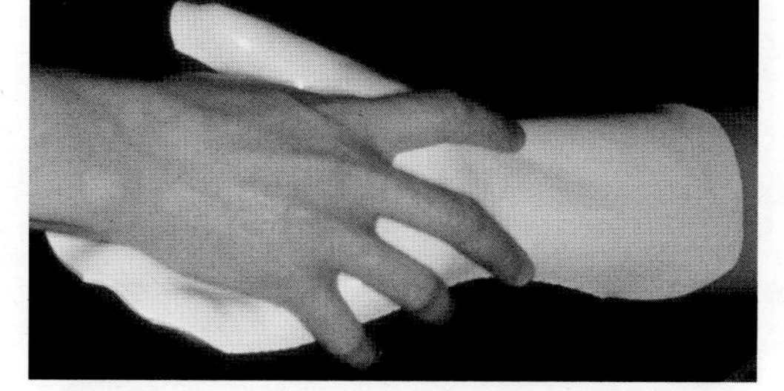

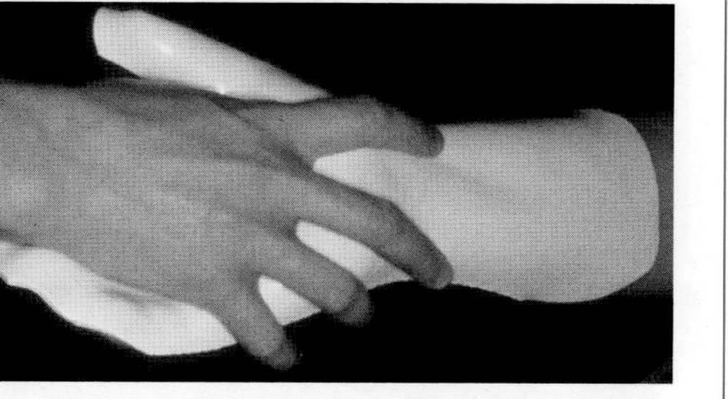

Volar Wrist/Hand (Optional Thumb) Immobilization Splint (Continued)

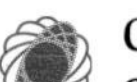

CLINICAL PEARL

Strap Placement to Facilitate Joint Alignment

Strapping can be the key to improving positioning of the distal joints. Here are some techniques. Riveting the radial end of the MP strap within the splint can help guide the IF metacarpal head ulnarward, while the distal straps can be directed radially (A). The placement of the distal strap can aid in aligning the proximal structures as well (B). Post extensor tendon realignment, the distally placed straps help prevent recurrent ulnar deviation and maintain neutral alignment of the digits (C). Weaving techniques work well to encourage proper digit alignment (D & E). Soft straps can be incorporated into a night resting splint for maintaining and correcting the digit position for diagnoses such as rheumatoid arthritis and Dupuytren's release. The slots can be made with a hole punch, drill, or heated awl. Adhesive hook is applied to the surface of the splint material corresponding to each involved digit. The loop material for each finger attaches first to the hook and then is directed about the digit and through the appropriate web space slot, terminating back on the hook.

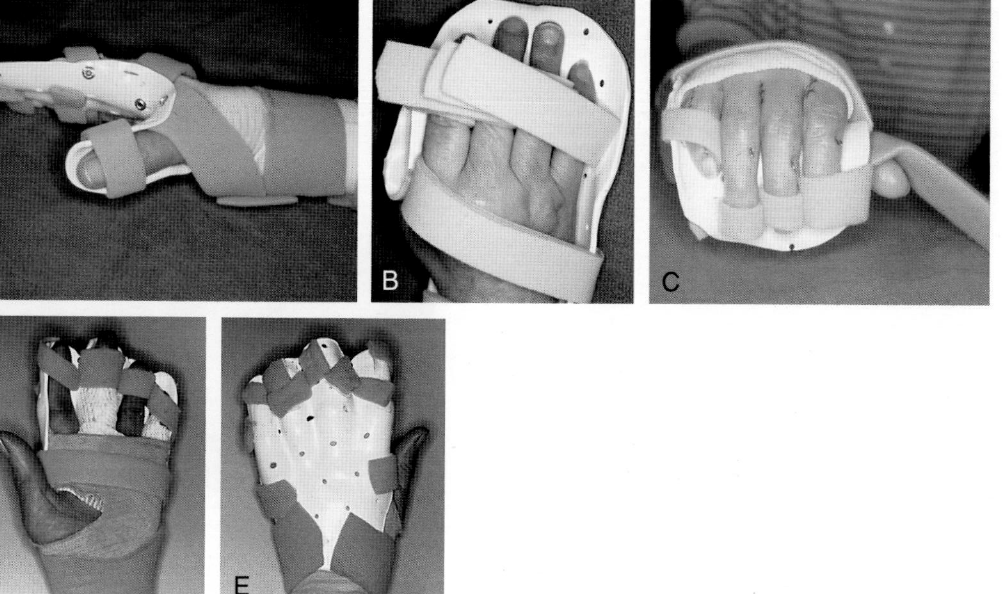

CLINICAL PEARL

Dacron Batting to Absorb Perspiration

Patients that have to wear splints for extended periods of time (e.g., after surgery), especially in warmer months, tend to perspire within the splint, which may lead to skin maceration and an unpleasant odor. Polyester batting, applied between the digits and lightly about the hand and forearm, wicks away moisture from the skin. The batting, readily available at most fabric stores, should be changed daily. Note the bias cut material used to securing the splint to the extremity. This nonelastic wrap applies gentle circumferential pressure to aid in reducing edema. It is applied with gentle tension in much the same manner as an elasticized Ace wrap.

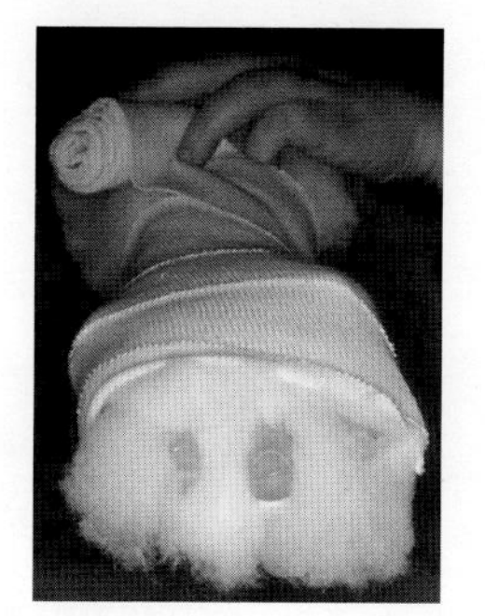

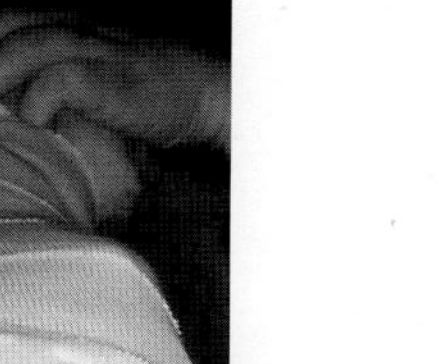

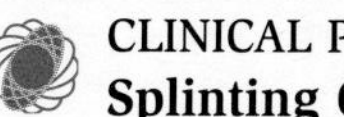

CLINICAL PEARL

Splinting Over Wound Dressings

During splint fabrication, the thermoplastic material can adhere to the wound dressing. Thus the dressing can be pulled. To avoid that risk, place a piece of stockinette over the dressing before molding the splint to the area. Once the splint is completely set, simply cut off the stockinette and remove the splint.

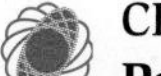

CLINICAL PEARL

Position of Function

In general, the position of function includes some degree of flexion at the MP, PIP, and DIP joints (shown here), whereas the antideformity position includes MP flexion with IP extension.

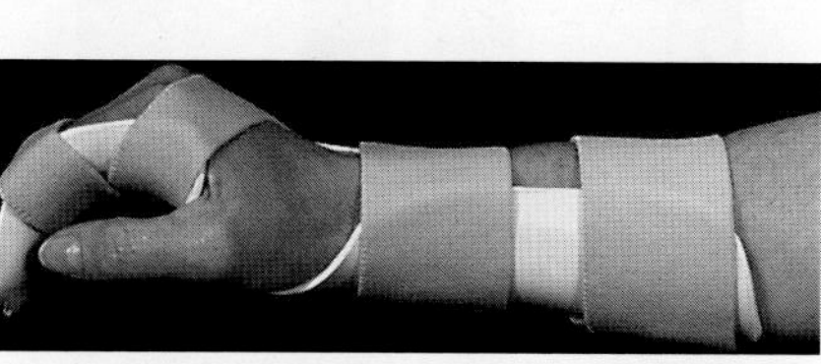

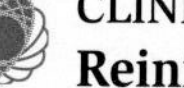

CLINICAL PEARL

Reinforcing Volar Portion of Splint

A strip of thermoplastic material can be used to reinforce potential areas of weakness within a splint. To reinforce a splint fabricated with a coated thermoplastic material, the therapist must first remove the coating with splint solvent or by vigorously scratching the surface.

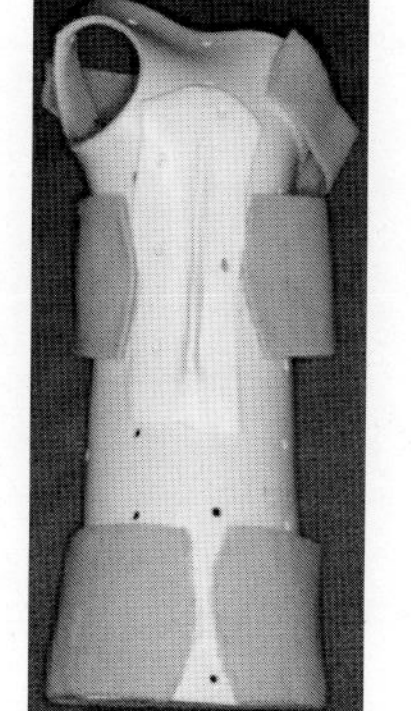

Volar-Dorsal Wrist/Hand Immobilization Splint (Fig. 7–37)

Common Names

- Antispasticity splint
- Bisurfaced forearm-based static wrist hand orthosis
- Dorsal platform splint
- Dorsal resting splint

Alternative Splint Options

- Cast
- Prefabricated antispasticity splint

Primary Functions

- Immobilize wrist and hand joints to allow healing, rest, or proper positioning of involved structures(s).

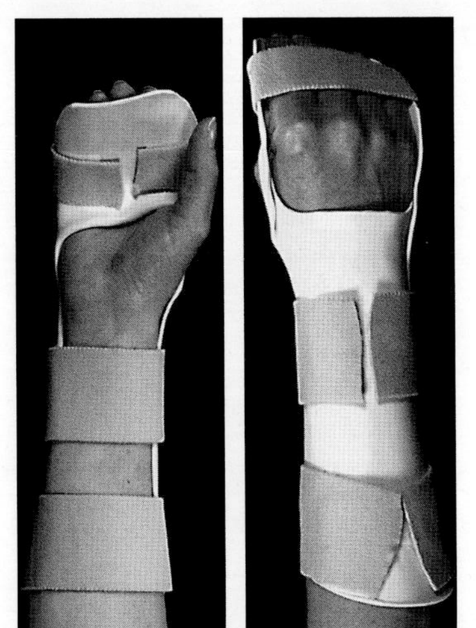
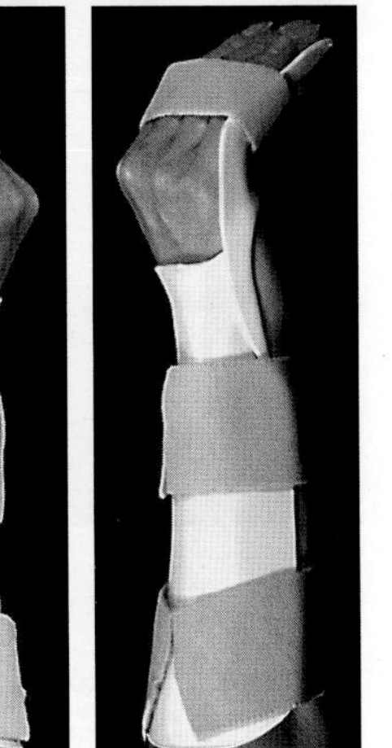
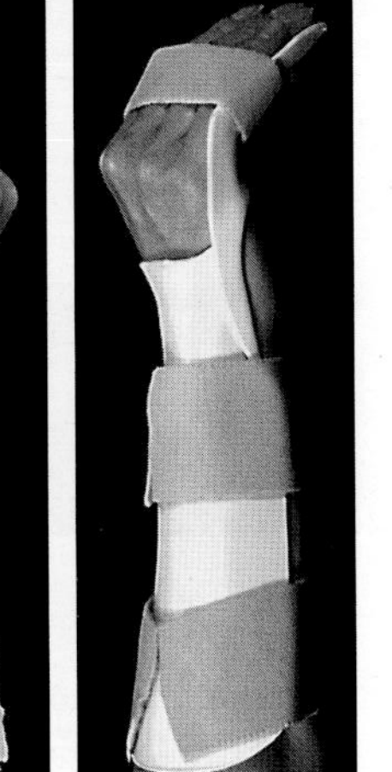
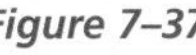

Figure 7–37

Additional Functions

- Statically position tight flexor tendons at maximum extension to facilitate lengthening of tissue and lessen joint contractures (mobilization splint).
- Aid in reducing muscle tone in wrist and digits.

Common Diagnoses and General Optimal Positions

• General hand trauma	Wr: 30° ext; MP: 60° flex; IP: 0°
• Burn injuries	Wr: 30° ext; MP: 60 to 90° flex; IP: 0°
• Rheumatoid arthritis	Wr: 30° ext; MP: slight flex; IP: comfortable flex; (Note: If patient has carpal tunnel symptoms, decrease wr ext.)
• Abnormal tone	Depends on therapist and physician rationale

Fabrication Process

Pattern Creation (Fig. 7–38)

- Can be an alternative pattern to volar or dorsal wrist and hand immobilization splint; may be used when it is necessary to avoid splinting over fragile or grafted dorsal or volar surfaces (burns, skin grafts, pins, open wounds)
- Positions depend on injury and structures involved.
- Mark for proximal border two thirds length of forearm.
- Allow enough material to encompass half to two thirds circumference of forearm, remembering that forearm tapers distally.
- Mark distal border approximately 1" distal to fingertips; this additional material may be necessary to compensate for material consumed by positions of joints.
- Mark thumb clearance by making an arc from thumb MP to base of first CMC joint.
- Opening for digits should be marked at mid-IF MP joint and run slightly oblique to SF MP joint.

Refine Pattern

- Proximal border should allow full elbow motion.
- Distal border should protect fingertips.
- Make sure that opening for digits is wide enough to accommodate width of MPs, allowing approximately $\frac{1}{2}$" material on sides.
- To aid in tone inhibition, incorporate finger separators into volar pan.

Options for Materials

- Use $\frac{1}{8}$" material because strength and rigidity are important characteristics for this splint, especially because of potentially weak and narrow area at junction of MPs.
- Materials with high resistance to stretch may offer more control for therapist; highly conforming materials may be difficult to control against gravity.
- Increase strength at borders of slotted piece by overlapping edges.
- If patient has significant pain and swelling, splinting with this design may be quite awkward and difficult; consider materials that are slightly tacky and drapable to help prevent material from slipping and to make it easier to position patient and mold splint.

Cut and Heat

- Before fabrication, use a technique to reduce tone in extremity if needed (see Chapter 21).
- Ideally, position forearm and hand in pronation; forearm can rest on elevated platform with MPs over edge.
- Prepad ulnar styloid with adhesive foam or silicone gel.

Evaluate Fit While Molding

- Lay warm material on towel and position MP slot on correct side of material as if it were going to be placed on pronated forearm. (The MP slot should be more distal on radial side.)
- Slide digits through slot; then carefully lay proximal portion on dorsal forearm and allow gravity to assist.
- One hand should simultaneously support volar piece at MPs and digits, incorporating arches.
- Fold MP flaps over onto material and flatten out to add strength to this potentially weak section.
- Do not grab proximal splint or try to secure with tight circumferential bandage. This may cause borders of splint to irritate skin. Instead, allow gravity to assist in forming forearm trough.
- Make sure desired wrist and digit positions are maintained.

Strapping and Components

- If splint is to be used for burn injury management, consider circumferential bandages to avoid localized pressure caused by straps on fragile healing skin or grafts.
- Distal strap: 1" or 2" strap to traverse across PIP joints. May use foam to improve extension positioning of digits.
- Wrist and proximal strap: 2" strap of soft, elasticized, or traditional loop.
- If adhesive foam is used to pad ulnar styloid during fabrication, carefully lift it off patient's skin and place it back into splint.

Splint Finishing Touches

- Check that opening for digits is wide enough for easy donning and doffing of splint.
- Make sure that sides of IF and SF MPs are strong enough to support weight of digits. If not, an additional strip of thermoplastic material may be added for support.
- May need to apply piece of thermoplastic material volarly to reinforce wrist position.

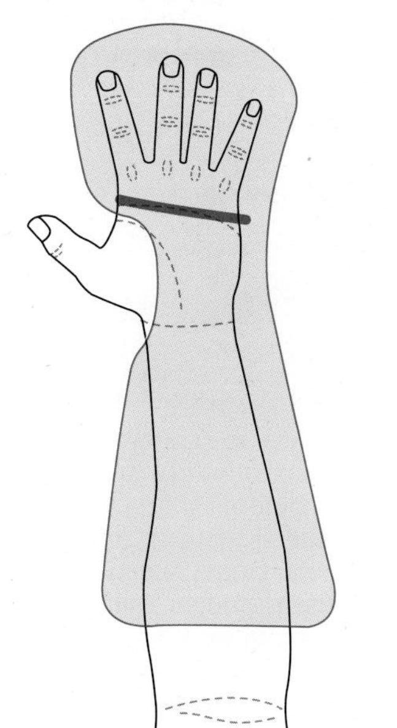

Figure 7–38

Antispasticity Cone Splint

(Fig. 7–39)

Common Names

- Antispasticity splint
- Forearm-based ulnar cone-style splint

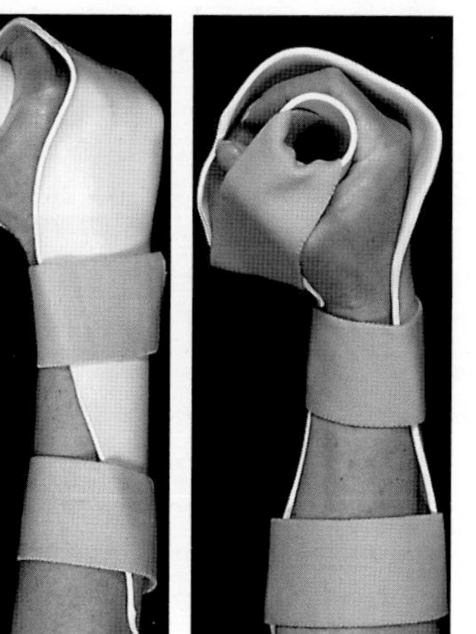

Figure 7–39

Alternative Splint Options

- Cast
- Prefabricated antispasticity splint

Primary Functions

- Immobilize wrist, digits, and thumb for individuals with moderate to severe spasticity.
- Help decrease tone and reduce risk of joint and soft tissue contracture.

Additional Functions

- Statically position tight flexor tendons at maximum extension to facilitate lengthening of tissue and reduce or prevent contractures (mobilization splint).

Common Diagnoses and General Optimal Positions

• Abnormal tone	Depends on therapist and physician rationale
• Jt contractures and muscle shortening	Functional position

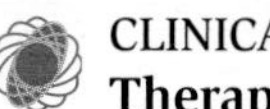

CLINICAL PEARL

Therapy Cone to Aid Fabrication of Antispasticity Splint

Using a cone when fabricating the central portion of this splint can extremely helpful. If an appropriately sized cone is not available, fabricate one out of scrap thermoplastic material. If there is any question that the materials may stick to each other during the fabrication process, simply wrap the cone with a wet paper towel, layer with lotion, or cover with a stockinette.

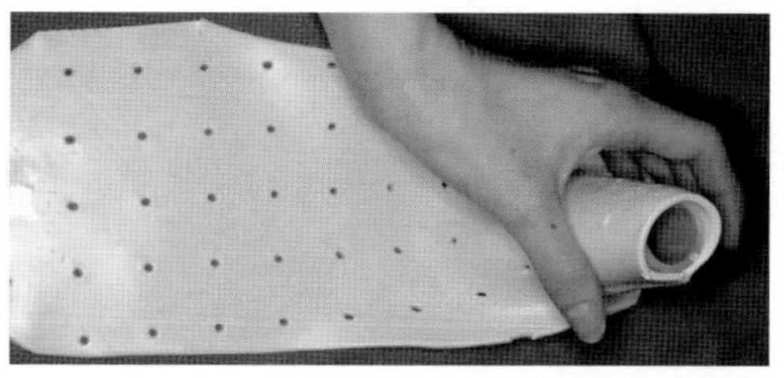

Fabrication Process

Pattern Creation (Fig. 7–40)

- Note: Because of increased tone, positioning extremity for creating this pattern may be quite difficult; draw pattern on contralateral extremity or estimate size.
- Mark for proximal border two thirds length of forearm.
- Allow enough material to encompass half to two thirds circumference of forearm, remembering that forearm tapers distally.
- Mark distal border using pattern illustration for an example. Material distally follows contour of digits.
- From MF distal phalanx tip radially, pattern extends beyond thumb approximately 2".
- Pattern follows contour of thumb proximally, leaving 1½" to 2" border radially. At this point, pattern comes in toward proximal thumb MP 1"; then continues proximally.

Refine Pattern

- Proximal border should allow full elbow motion.
- Distal border should protect digits.
- To prevent adherence, line cone (fabricated from thermoplastic or commercial) with light layer of lotion before placing on material.
- Make sure that pattern material for cone portion is generous and wide enough to accommodate hand size. Patients with tight, contracted hands may need to start with smaller cone that can be progressively enlarged as tissue elongates.

Options for Materials

- Use ⅛" material because strength and rigidity are important characteristics for this splint.
- Consider perforated materials, which allow air exchange between skin and splint, especially for patients who are cognitively impaired or who lack full sensation.
- Skin breakdown and maceration can become problem under these splints. Do not line splint with moleskin or similar padding, because they tend to absorb moisture and are difficult to clean. Closed cell foam that can be readily washed may work well.
- If patient has significant tone, splinting with this design may be quite awkward and difficult. Consider materials that are less conforming and more rigid to make it easier to position patient and mold splint.

Cut and Heat

- Before fabrication, use a technique to reduce tone in extremity (see Chapter 21.
- While material is heating, prepad ulnar styloid using self-adhesive padding or silicone gel.
- Ideally, position extremity with shoulder and elbow flexed and forearm neutral to achieve gravity-assist position.
- Make sure desired position is maintained.

Evaluate Fit While Molding

- Lay warm material on towel, positioning large radial section on correct side of material as if it were going to be placed on extremity.
- Place warm material on proximal forearm and allow gravity to hold it in place.
- Working distally, lay material into palm and place cone on material. Wide end of cone is on ulnar border pointing through web space.
- Wrap thumb portion over cone; then bring distal straight border over this material to forming cone. (While this occurs, ulnar aspect of splint should form an ulnar trough for digits to rest in.)
- Keep redirecting wrist into appropriate position. If there is considerable tone in hand, then splint can be made in sections. After molding forearm and wrist portions, cone section can be made while splint is off patient.
- Do not grab proximal splint or try to secure with tight circumferential bandage. This may cause borders of splint to irritate skin. Instead, allow gravity to assist in forming forearm trough.

Strapping and Components

- Digits: often not necessary.
- Cone straps: straps originating from top of cone can be quite effective for keeping hand correctly positioned. Soft 1" straps traversing just proximal to MP, PIP, DIP, thumb MP, and IP joint(s) are appropriate.
- Wrist and proximal strap: 2" strap of soft, elasticized, or traditional loop.
- If ⅜" adhesive foam or silicone was used to pad ulna styloid during fabrication, carefully lift it off patient's skin and place it back into splint to cushion styloid.

Splint Finishing Touches

- Smooth and slightly flare splint borders.
- Check that cone is of adequate width to position digits properly.
- Check clearance of elbow.

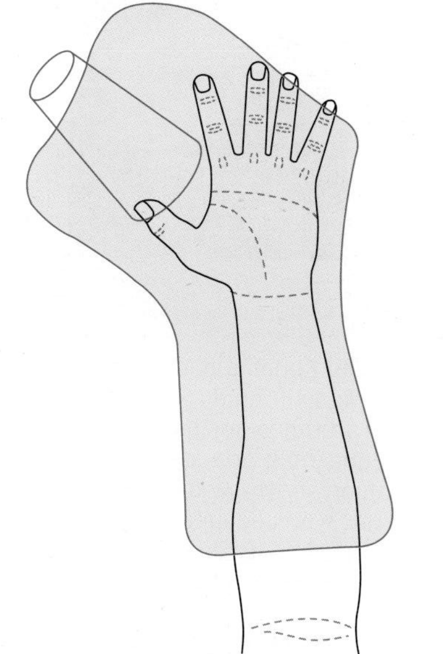

Figure 7–40

Antispasticity Ball Splint

(Fig. 7–41)

Common Names

- Antispasticity splint

Alternative Splint Options

- Prefabricated antispasticity splint

Primary Functions

- Immobilize wrist, digits, and thumb for individuals with moderate to severe spasticity.
- Aid in decreasing tone and reducing risk of tissue contracture.

Additional Functions

- Statically position tight flexor tendons at maximum extension to facilitate lengthening of tissue and to reduce or prevent contractures (mobilization splint).

Common Diagnoses and General Optimal Positions

• Abnormal tone	Depends on therapist and physician rationale
• Jt contractures and muscle shortening	Functional position

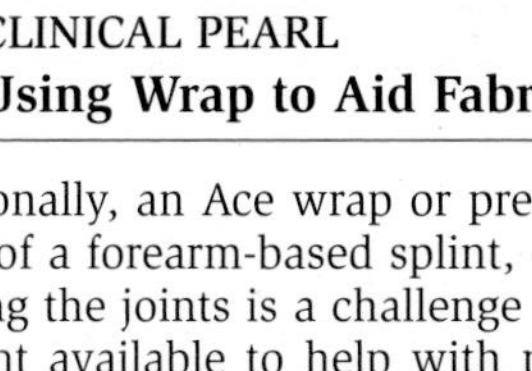

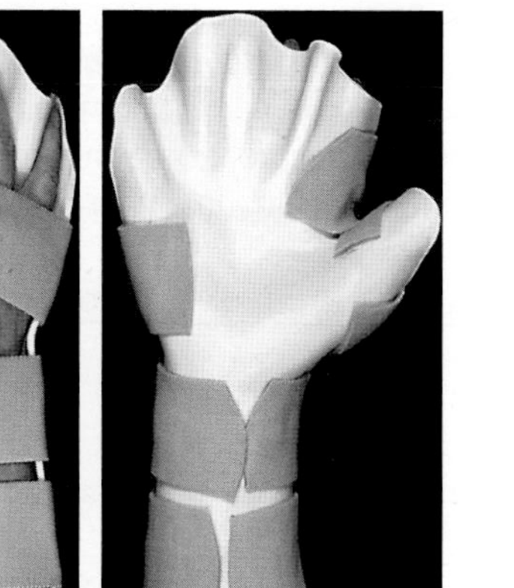

Figure 7–41

CLINICAL PEARL

Lining Perforated Splint with $^{1}/_{16}$" Material

Use $^{1}/_{16}$" material to line a splint's border. This works particularly well with perforated material, because its edges can irritate the skin. Cut $^{1}/_{16}$" material in $1^{1}/_{2}$" to 2" wide strips by what ever length is required to go around the periphery of splint. Once the material is thoroughly heated, gently stretch it (to disrupt the coating) and quickly place it along the splint's border. The material must be gently stretched and pinched over the edges. This application must be done quickly and accurately because thin materials set readily.

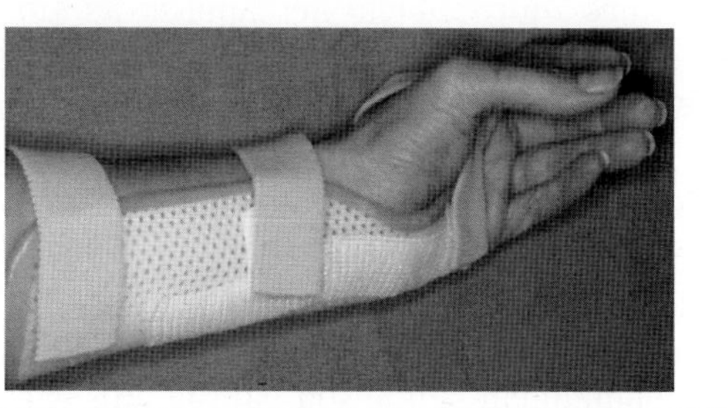

CLINICAL PEARL

Hand-Based Antispasticity Splints

This splint pattern can be easily modified into a hand-based design (A). The smaller version can be used for patients who have minimal wrist involvement. This design is especially useful for treating the pediatric population. An alternative is this preformed neutral position splint (B).

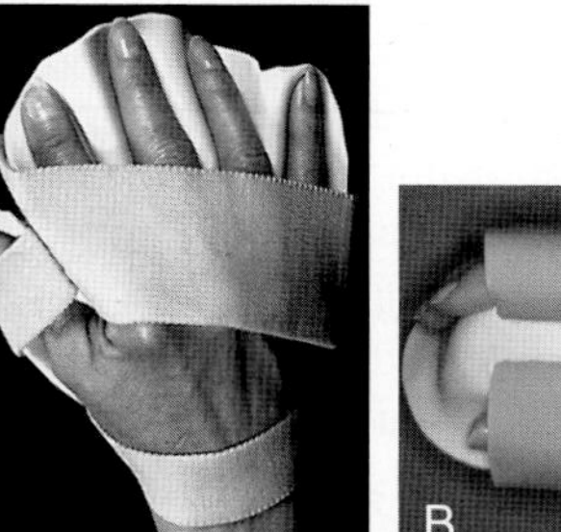

A

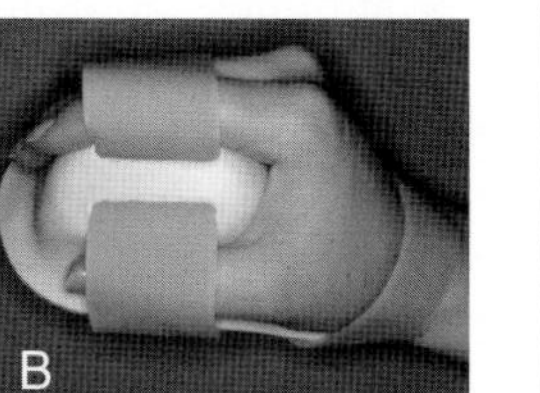

B

CLINICAL PEARL

Using Wrap to Aid Fabrication

Occasionally, an Ace wrap or prewrap aids the fabrication of a forearm-based splint, especially when positioning the joints is a challenge or when there is no assistant available to help with positioning. Use the wrap proximally to allow for hands-on positioning distally. Be sure to watch for compression forces at the forearm borders of the splint; just before the splint sets up, remove the wrap and gently flare the borders away from the skin.

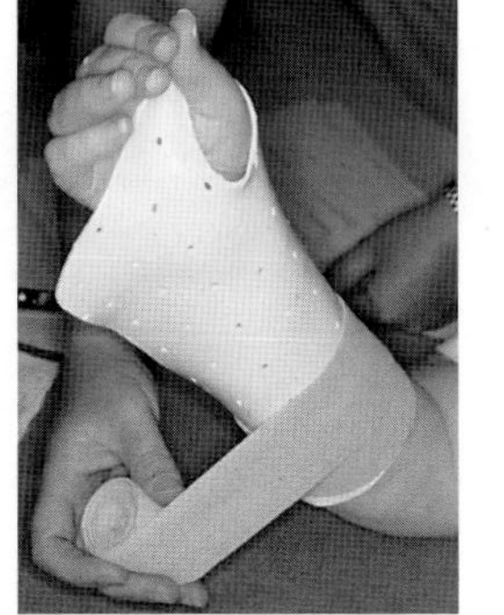

Fabrication Process

Pattern Creation (Fig. 7–42)

- Note: Because of increased tone, positioning extremity for creating this pattern may be quite difficult; draw pattern on contralateral extremity or estimate size.
- Mark for proximal border two thirds length of forearm.
- Allow enough material to encompass half to two thirds circumference of forearm, remembering that forearm tapers distally.
- Mark distal border, approximately 1" beyond fingertips, using pattern illustration for an example.
- Radially, follow contour of first web space along distal and radial thumb borders, meeting at thumb base. Allow ½" distally and 1" radially for sufficient troughing and strap application.

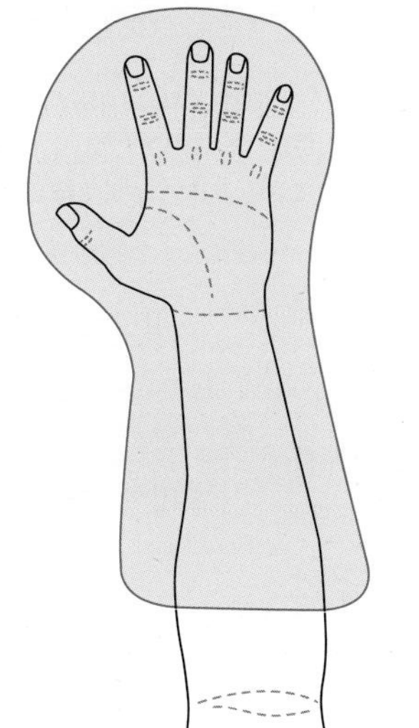

Figure 7–42

Refine Pattern

- Proximal border should allow full elbow motion.
- Distal border should extend just distal to fingertips.
- Make sure that digit and thumb material is generous and wide enough to accommodate web spacers.

Options for Materials

- Use ⅛" material because strength and rigidity are important characteristics for this splint.
- Consider perforated materials, which allow air exchange between skin and splint, especially for patients who are cognitively impaired or who lack full sensation.
- Skin breakdown and maceration can become problem under these splints. Do not line splint with moleskin or similar padding, because they tend to absorb moisture and are difficult to clean.
- Consider material with no memory, since maintenance of web spacers after material has been stretched is key to this splint design.
- If patient has significant tone, splinting with this design may be quite awkward and difficult. Consider materials that are less conforming and more rigid to make it easier to position patient and mold splint.

Cut and Heat

- Before fabrication, use a technique to reduce tone in extremity (see Chapter 21 for specific information).
- Consider placing light layer of lotion on ball before molding to prevent thermoplastic from adhering.
- Consider fabricating forearm trough first, and then making hand component as described below. This will allow more control over an already hard-to-control extremity.
- Prepare to pronate hand on medium-size ball (large enough to encompass entire hand).

Evaluate Fit While Molding

- To simplify fabrication process, warm forearm section first and carefully mold achieve good fit.
- Next, place warmed distal section on ball and rest patient's hand over it.
- Make sure that digits and thumb are fully abducted.
- Use pair of closed scissors, small dowel, or bandage applicator to pull material up between fingers and thumb.
- During this process, it helps to have an assistant maintain wrist and forearm position.

Strapping and Components

- Digits and thumb: 2" soft strap just distal to MP joints is sufficient. Some patients with severe flexor tone need straps threaded over proximal and distal phalanges.
- To prevent digits from lifting off palmar piece, 1" soft foam strap can be woven through web spacers.
- Wrist and proximal strap: 2" strap of soft, elasticized, or traditional hook can be used.

Splint Finishing Touches

- Smooth and slightly flare splint borders.
- Check that palmar section is of adequate width to properly position digits and allow easy donning and doffing of splint.
- Check clearance of elbow.

4 • Arm-Based Splints

Posterior Elbow Immobilization Splint (Fig. 7–43)

Common Names

- Posterior elbow splint

Alternative Splint Options

- Cast
- Prefabricated splint

Primary Functions

- Immobilize elbow joint and surrounding soft tissues to allow healing, rest, and/or protection of involved structures(s).

Additional Functions

- Limit or prevent forearm rotation.
- Statically position an elbow extension contracture at maximum flexion to facilitate lengthening of tissue (mobilization splint).
- Restrict specific degree of elbow extension (restriction splint).

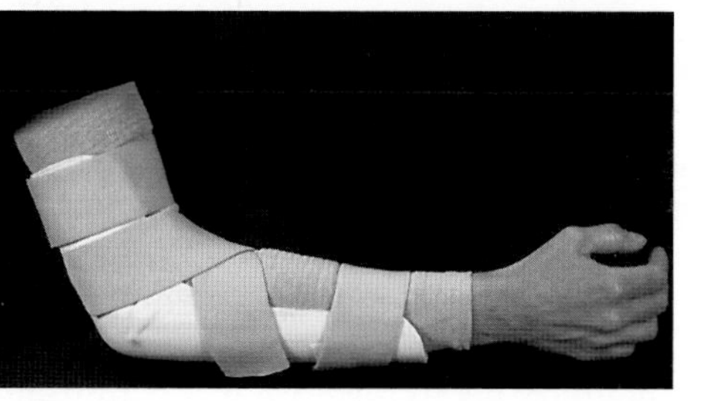

Figure 7–43

Common Diagnoses and General Optimal Positions

Diagnosis	Position
• Rheumatoid arthritis	Position of comfort
• Elb arthroplasty	Dictated by structures involved
• Ulnar nerve compression at cubital tunnel	Elb: 30 to 45° flex; FArm: neutral
• Ulnar nerve transposition:	Elb: 70 to 90° flex; FArm: neutral to 30° pro; wr: 0°
• Nerve repairs (high lesions)	Elb: 30 to 45° flex (depends on repair), FArm: neutral; wr: 0° to slight ext; digits free
• Tendon transfers for wr and digit extensors	Elb: 90°; FArm: pro; wr: 30 to 45° ext; MP and th: ext
• Biceps tendon repair	Depends on physician and status of tendon repair; generally start elb 45° active ext to 90° passive flex
• Posterior or anterior dislocation	Elb: 90°; FArm: neutral
• Collateral ligament repair (medial or lateral)	Elb: 90°; FArm: sup with 10° deviation to side of repair
• Proximal radius dislocation	Elb: 90°; FArm: sup
• Medial epicondyle fracture	Elb: 90 to 110°; FArm: pro
• Lateral epicondyle fracture	Elb: 90 to 110°; FArm: sup
• Olecranon fracture	Elb: 20 to 35° flex; FArm: neutral
• Acute lateral epicondylitis	Elb: 90°; FArm: neutral; wr: 30 to 45° ext
• Acute medial epicondylitis	Elb: 90°; FArm: neutral; wr: 0°

CLINICAL PEARL

Padding for the Olecranon Process

With a posterior elbow splint design, the olecranon process may rub against the splint. To prevent this, apply a small adhesive donut-shaped pad directly over the bony prominence. This helps keep pressure off the olecranon and onto the surrounding tissue. Once the splint is set, the pad can be removed from the skin and inverted back onto the splint.

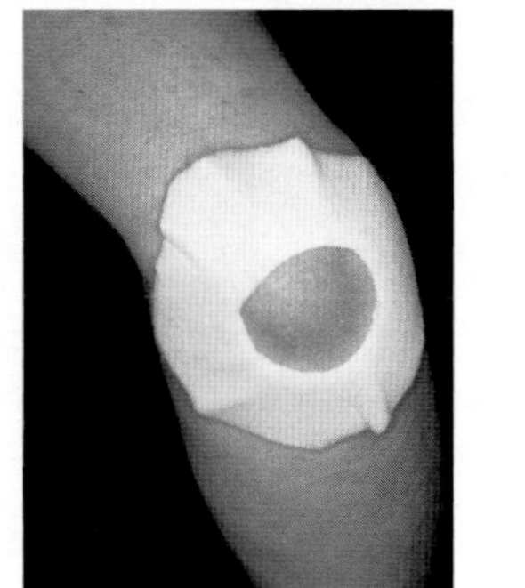

Fabrication Process

Pattern Creation (Fig. 7–44)

- Posterior design is better for positioning elbow at greater than 45° of flexion. Volar design is more appropriate for positioning elbow at less than 45°.
- Mark for proximal border $^2/_3$ length of humerus.
- Mark for distal border just proximal to ulnar styloid.
- Allow enough material to encompass half to two thirds circumference of upper arm and forearm.
- Remember that the longer and wider the splint, the more comfortable it is to wear.

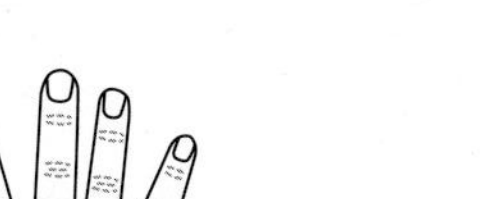
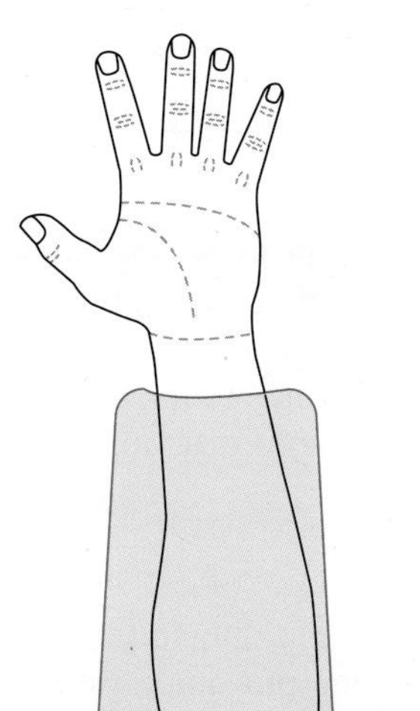

Figure 7–44

Refine Pattern

- Proximal border should allow unimpeded shoulder motion and not irritate axillary region with arm positioned at side of body.
- Distal border should allow full wrist motion.
- Note that pattern should be wider proximally because circumference of upper arm is greater than that of forearm.
- Make sure there is enough material to encompass elbow posteriorly. Insufficient material in this area requires stretching of material, which weakens splint's support.

Options for Materials

- Use $^1/_8$" material because strength is necessary for this splint.
- Consider rubber-based material, to have more control and to minimize stretching.
- Gel- or foam-lined materials help provide scar compression, decrease distal migration, and increase comfort.
- Consider perforated thermoplastics for patients who require full-time splint use.

Cut and Heat

- While material is heating, consider prepadding medial and lateral epicondyles and olecranon process.
- Position patient to allow for gravity-assisted molding: prone with shoulder neutral; supine with shoulder flexed 90°; or standing while leaning on table, forward flexed at waist and shoulder extended (upper arm parallel to floor).
- If possible, have an assistant help support proper elbow and forearm positions.

Evaluate Fit While Molding

- Drape warm material centrally over posterior aspect of upper arm and forearm, allowing gravity to assist. Be sure to position material proximal enough to support upper arm.
- Gently stretch and flare material around epicondyles and distal and proximal borders.
- Depending on desired degree of elbow flexion, excess material at elbow flexion crease may require attention.
- Do not grab splint or try to secure with tight circumferential bandage. This may cause borders of splint to irritate skin. Instead, allow gravity to assist in forming upper arm and forearm troughs.
- Check for clearance of ulnar styloid distally.
- Make sure desired elbow flexion and forearm rotation positions are maintained. Some patients tend to flex their elbows excessively while splint is being formed.

Strapping and Components

- Use stockinette or elasticized sleeve (if edema is present) to eliminate pinching of skin against splint borders once straps are applied.
- Proximal strap: 2" soft strap applied at most proximal portion of splint to anchor splint adequately to upper arm.
- Middle straps: crisscross design directly over anterior elbow to maintain elbow position.
- Distal strap: 1" or 2" soft strap.
- Consider securing splint with elasticized wrap if edema is problematic.

Splint Finishing Touches

- Smooth and slightly flare all distal and proximal borders.
- Check for clearance and/or irritation at axilla, ulnar styloid, epicondyles, and olecranon process.
- Check for compression of ulnar nerve at cubital tunnel area and of superficial sensory branch of radial nerve.

Anterior Elbow Immobilization Splint (Fig. 7–45)

Common Names

- Anterior elbow splint

Alternative Splint Options

- Cast
- Prefabricated splint

Primary Functions

- Immobilize elbow joint and surrounding soft tissues to allow healing of involved structures(s).

Additional Functions

- Limit or prevent forearm rotation.
- Statically position elbow flexion contracture at maximum extension to facilitate lengthening of tissue (mobilization splint).
- Restrict specific degree of elbow flexion (restriction splint).

Common Diagnoses and General Optimal Positions

Diagnosis	Position
• Rheumatoid arthritis	Position of comfort
• Ulnar nerve compression at cubital tunnel	Elb: 30 to 45° flex; FArm: neutral
• Nerve repairs (high lesions)	Elb: 30 to 45° flex (depends on repair); FArm: neutral; wr: 0° to slight ext; digits free
• Olecranon fracture	Elb 20 to 35° flex; FArm: neutral

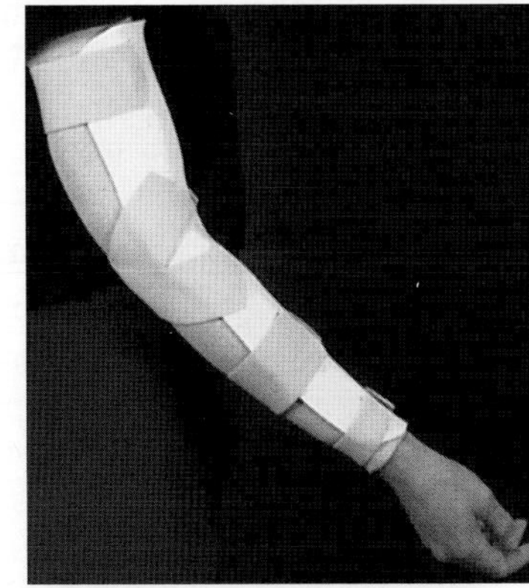

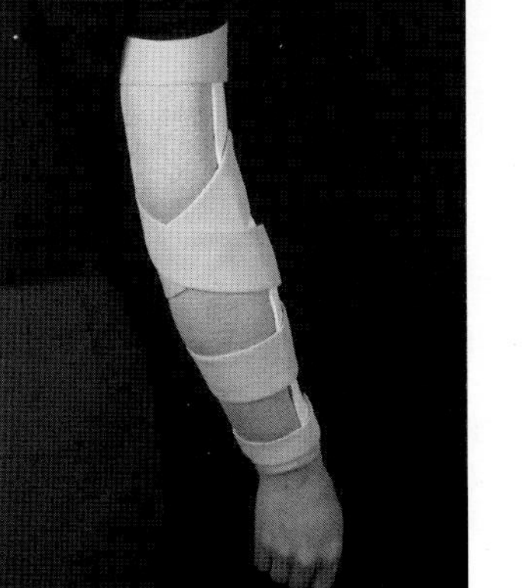

Figure 7–45

CLINICAL PEARL

Stretch, Pinch, and Pop Technique for Elbow Splints

Use 1/8" or 3/32" coated elastic material (Aquaplast). When the material is stretched, the coating is disrupted enough to produce a temporary bond when pieces are gently pinched together. Position the patient sitting, with the elbow flexed and forearm rotated in the desired position. The material can be applied to the volar or dorsal surfaces and stretched in the desired direction. As shown here, the material is placed on the anterior surface of the elbow and then quickly stretched and pinched segmentally along the posterior surface (A). Be sure to maintain the desired elbow and forearm positions while the material cools. Once the splint is completely set, pop the seams apart. Neatly trim and smooth any rough edges (B).

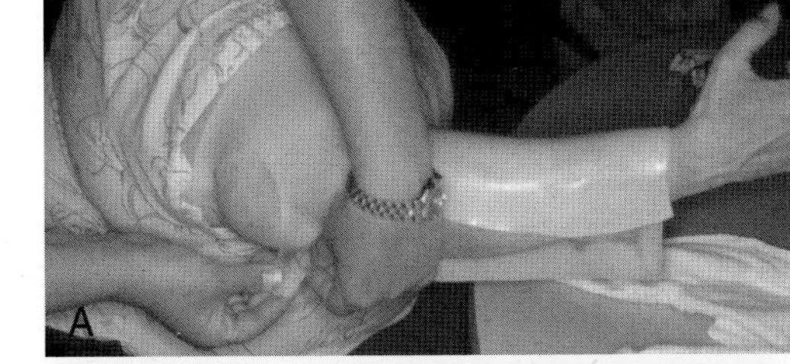

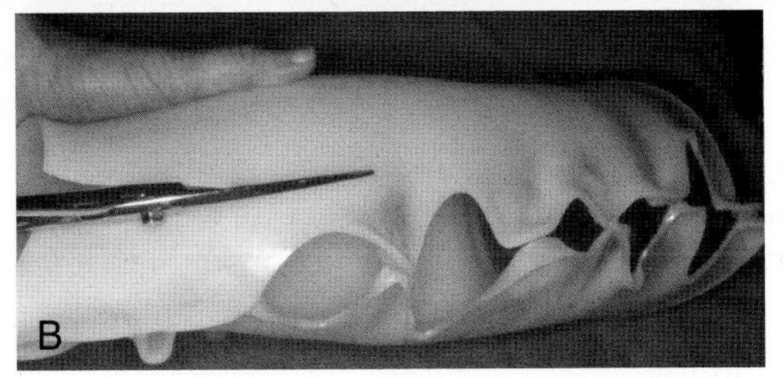

Fabrication Process

Pattern Creation (Fig. 7–46)

- Anterior design is best used for positioning elbow in less than 45° of flexion. Posterior design is more appropriate for positioning elbow greater than 45°.
- Mark for proximal border $2/3$ length of humerus.
- Mark for distal border just proximal to ulnar styloid.
- Allow enough material to encompass $1/2$ to $2/3$ circumference of upper arm and lower forearm.

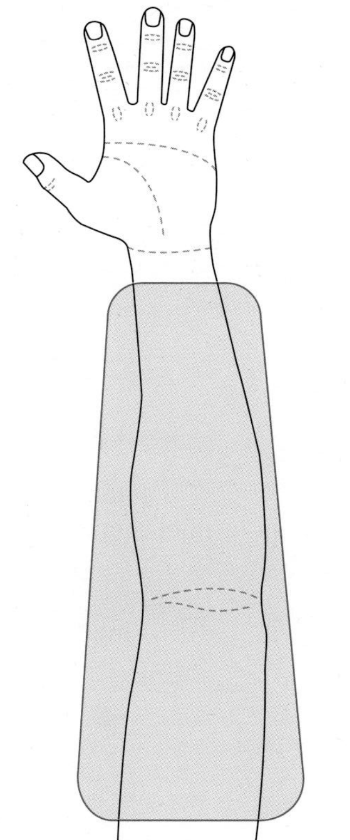

Figure 7–46

- Remember that the longer and wider the splint, the more comfortable it is to wear.

Refine Pattern

- Proximal border should allow unimpeded shoulder motion and not irritate axillary region with arm positioned at side of body.
- Distal border should allow full wrist motion.
- Note that pattern should be wider proximally because circumference of upper arm is greater than that of forearm.
- Make sure there is enough material to encompass elbow posteriorly. Insufficient material in this area requires stretching of material, which weakens splint's support.

Options for Materials

- Use either $3/32$" or $1/8$" thermoplastic material, depending on patient's arm size and desired splint strength.
- Gel- or foam-lined materials help provide scar compression, decrease distal migration, and increase comfort.
- Consider perforated thermoplastics for patients who require full-time splint use and when air exchange is necessary.

Cut and Heat

- While material is heating, consider prepadding medial and lateral epicondyles, if needed; remember that a well-formed splint does not require padding.
- Position patient to allow for gravity-assisted molding: supine with shoulder neutral or seated with elbow resting on table.

Evaluate Fit While Molding

- Drape warm material centrally over volar aspect of upper arm and forearm, allowing gravity to assist. Be sure to position material proximal enough to support upper arm.
- Gently flare material around epicondyles, distal, and proximal borders.
- Do not grab splint or try to secure with tight circumferential bandage. This may cause borders of splint to irritate skin. Instead, allow gravity to assist in forming upper arm and forearm troughs.
- Check for clearance of wrist distally.
- Make sure desired elbow extension and forearm rotation positions are maintained. Some patients tend to flex their elbows excessively while splint is being formed. Gently support patient's arm in correct position by supporting at wrist.

Strapping and Components

- Use stockinette or elasticized sleeve if edema is present to eliminate pinching of skin against splint's borders once straps are applied.
- Proximal strap: 2" soft strap applied at most proximal portion of splint to anchor splint adequately to upper arm and to prevent rocking.
- Middle straps: 2" straps to hold elbow adequately in splint.
- Distal strap: 1" or 2" soft strap.
- Consider securing splint with elasticized wrap if edema is problematic.

Splint Finishing Touches

- Smooth and slightly flare all distal and proximal borders.
- Check for clearance and/or irritation at axilla and epicondyles.
- Check for compression of ulnar nerve at cubital tunnel area and of superficial sensory branch of radial nerve.

Shoulder Abduction (or Adduction) Immobilization Splint (Fig. 7–47)

Common Names

- Gunslinger splint
- Airplane splint

Alternative Splint Options

- Prefabricated splint

Primary Functions

- Immobilize shoulder joint to allow healing of involved structure(s).

Common Diagnoses and Optimal Positions

Diagnosis	Position
• Brachial plexus injury	Sh: 30° abd, 30 to 45° flex, slight ER; elb: 90° flex; FArm: neutral rotation
• Tendon transfers for plexus injury	Sh: add, 30 to 45° flex, slight ER; elb: 90° flex; FArm: neutral rotation
• Sh and humeral arthroplasty	Sh: 30° abd and flex; 15° ER; elb: 90°, FArm: neutral rotation

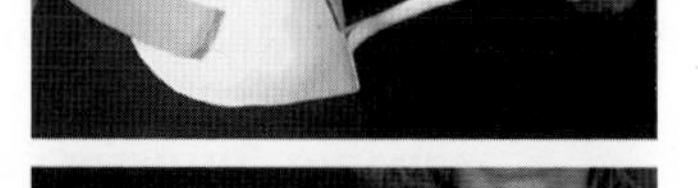
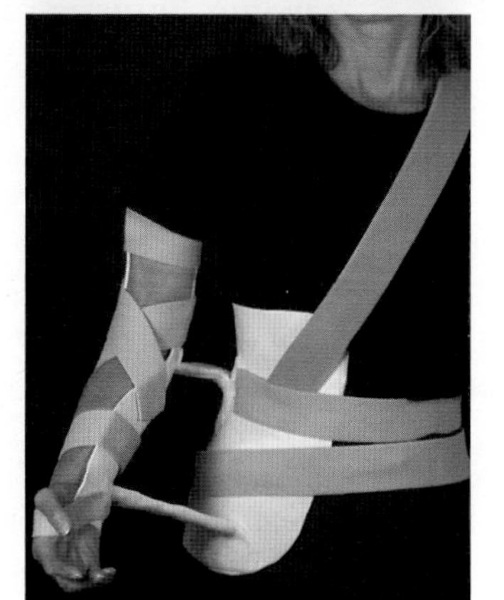

Figure 7–47

Fabrication Process

Pattern Creation (Fig. 7–48)

- Correct positions of shoulder and elbow depend on injury and/or surgical procedure. Communication with physician before splint application.
- Pattern should be made with patient's clothing on. If possible, fabricate trunk splint before surgical procedure; posterior elbow splint may also be fabricated before surgery. But remember that postoperative edema may alter fit, and accommodation may be needed.
- Posterior elbow component
  - Follow directions for posterior elbow immobilization splint, making certain that there is adequate troughing to accommodate connector bars.
- Trunk component
  - Take measurements on affected side with patient standing.
  - Mark distal border from midsternum to vertebral border dorsally.
  - Mark proximal border from naval to vertebral border dorsally.
  - Connect to form lateral borders (should somewhat rectangular).
- Connector component
  - Length of connector bars determined by desired shoulder position: the more elevation, the longer the bars.
  - Measure $1\frac{1}{2}$" to 2" for width. This material will be rolled onto itself for added strength.
  - Four 2" in diameter disks of thermoplastic material help secure connector bars onto trunk and elbow portions.

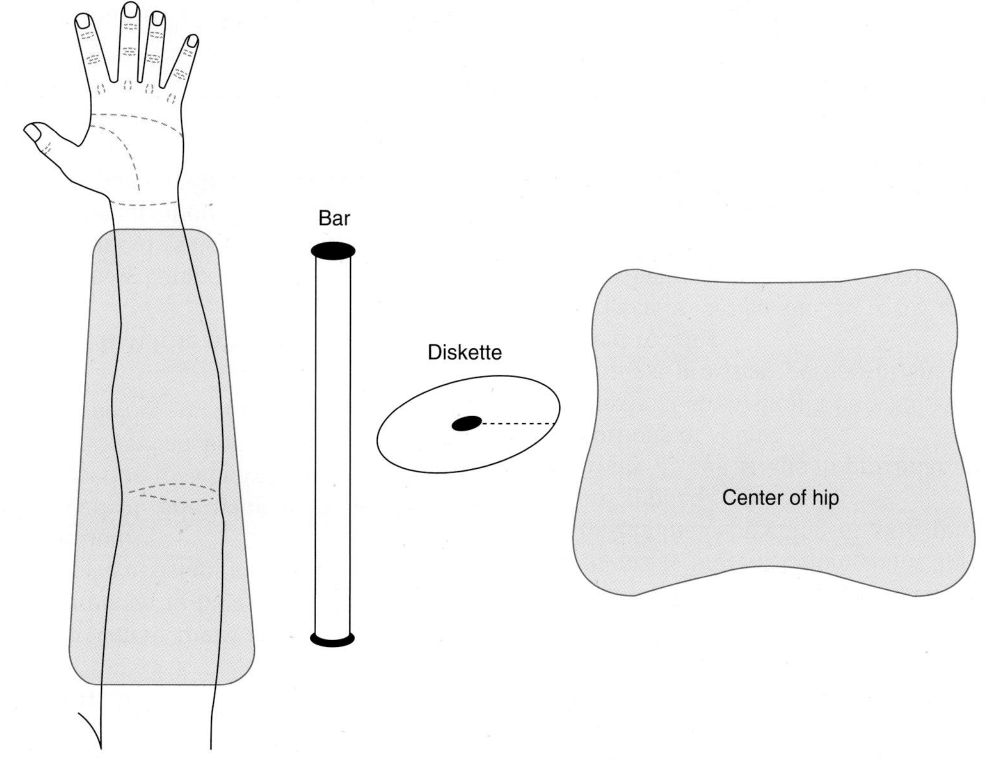

Figure 7–48

Refine Pattern

- Wrist inclusion is optional, depending on diagnosis and patient comfort.
- After determining length of connector bars, allow extra 1" on each end for application onto trunk splint.
- To provide added strength, include $\frac{3}{32}$" aluminum wire within thermoplastic roll. This is especially helpful for maintaining shoulder elevation, owing to potential high force delivered to connector bars.

Options for Materials

- Use uncoated splinting material to aid in bonding of connector bars. If uncoated materials are not available, then disrupt coating on all connected surfaces before adhering.
- Posterior elbow component: use $\frac{1}{8}$" uncoated perforated plastic or elastic-based material. Choose elastic material if patient has pain and/or cannot assist in shoulder positioning, because tackiness may aid during molding process.
- Trunk component: consider $\frac{1}{8}$" solid, rubber-based, uncoated material for its strength and stability.
- Connector component: use $\frac{1}{8}$" solid, rubber-based, uncoated material for bars and disks.

Shoulder Abduction (or Adduction) Immobilization Splint (Continued)

Cut and Heat

- Use plinth where there is full access to involved extremity, to increase ease of molding process. Have assistant support arm in appropriate position.
- Position patient side lying with affected extremity superior, to achieve gravity assistance.
- If necessary, prepad bony prominences: iliac crest, epicondyles, olecranon process, and ulnar styloid.

Evaluate Fit While Molding

- Posterior elbow component
  - Carefully mold as described for posterior elbow immobilization splint.
  - Allow enough material for connector bar application.
- Trunk component
  - Remove warm material from heating pan and support with both hands. Carefully place along trunk, as shown.
  - Mold well about waist and over iliac crest to prevent splint from sliding off hip.
- Connector component
  - Remove warm material, place on flat surface. Position wire in center of material and roll onto itself, forming thick bar. Repeat process for other bar.
  - Apply strapping before adhering components together.

Strapping and Components

- Posterior elbow component
  - Use stockinette or elasticized sleeve if edema is present before splint application, to eliminate pinching of skin once straps are applied.
  - Apply 2" soft straps to proximal and distal portions of splint.
  - Proximal strap should be wide and applied at most proximal portion of splint, to prevent rocking.
  - Crisscross design directly over anterior elbow helps maintain elbow securely in splint.
  - Consider using an Ace wrap or 3" Coban to secure, if edema is an issue.
- Trunk component
  - Apply one 3" to 6" soft strap or two 2" straps with D-ring closure about waist (width and number of straps depend on patient's trunk size).
  - Apply 2" soft strap directed from sternum, across uninvolved shoulder, to posterior vertebral border. D-ring attachment is recommended for ease of adjustment.
  - Pad portion of strap that traverses opposite shoulder to maximize comfort.
- Connector components
  - Disks act as reinforcements and should be applied once bars are attached.
  - While an assistant maintains desired position of shoulder, apply trunk and elbow splint.
  - Mark for upper and lower bar placements on both splint components.
  - Prepare all surfaces for bonding.
  - Heat 1" of both ends of two connector bars and secure to premarked areas.
  - Throughout process, check that correct shoulder position is maintained; making adjustments can be difficult.
  - Heat disk thoroughly; make slit halfway through disk; open; and wrap about bar and splint base, molding firmly into place.

Splint Finishing Touches

- Trunk splint can be lined with Microfoam tape or padding material (gel or foam) to help prevent migration and rotation.
- Smooth and slightly flare all distal and proximal borders.
- Check for clearance and/or irritation of trunk, axilla, ulnar styloid, epicondyles, and olecranon process (thumb and MP joints, if wrist included).
- Check for compression of ulnar nerve at cubital tunnel area and of superficial sensory branch of radial nerve.

CLINICAL PEARL

Techniques to Accommodate Elbow Flexion Angle

A common problem occurs when splinting the elbow in a flexed position (similar to splinting the MP joints in flexion): managing the excess material at the elbow flexion crease. There are several techniques that can be used to accommodate for this angle.

- Carefully take up material medially and laterally, and then overlap it onto itself, as shown (A). Make sure not to inadvertently apply excess pressure onto the bony areas. This technique adds strength and support to the curved area of the splint. However, making adjustments to the splint is difficult.
- Gently stretch and contour the material to provide a seamless, streamlined trough (B). This can be challenging for less experienced therapists and works best for angles of flexion that are less than 90°, as shown.
- The excess material can be pinched together rather aggressively (to ensure the material coating has been disrupted) and then cut to form a seam. This technique is the most cosmetically appealing and readily allows for splint adjustments. However, the splint is less stable and more susceptible to breaking at the seam point. Use solvent, and heat the area with a heat gun to create a strong seam.
- Take the excess material, pinch it, and then overlap it onto itself. This method is simple, but can be bulky and future modifications are difficult.
- Make small transverse snips medially and laterally, and dog ear the material onto itself. Use solvent and a heat gun to create a strong bond between the two surfaces. This method make future splint adjustments difficult, and the splint may look bulky and thick.

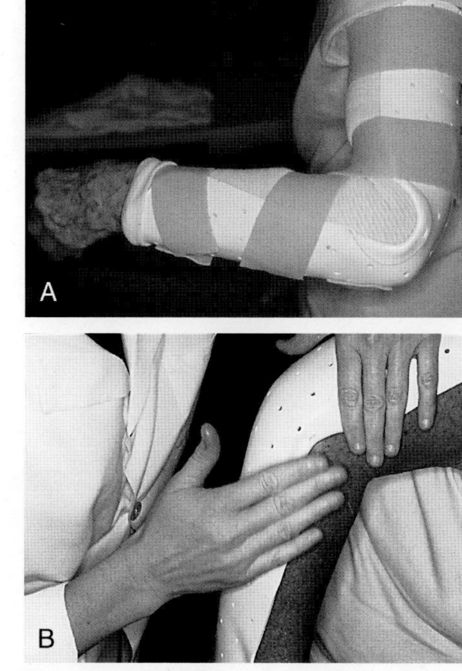

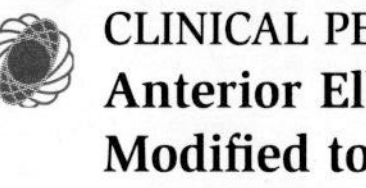

CLINICAL PEARL

Anterior Elbow Immobilization Modified to Include Wrist

The volar elbow immobilization splint can be easily modified to include the wrist, if required (A). Adjust the pattern by marking for the distal border at the distal palmar crease, incorporating the oblique angle that traverses from the IF to SF metacarpal heads. When molding, be sure to place the forearm in the desired amount of rotation. Note that this design it is easiest to splint with the forearm in neutral to full supination, allowing the splint to resemble a volar wrist immobilization splint distally. Make sure the material lies along the volar forearm and hand and extends to the distal palmar crease (B). A spiral design to reduce contact of material on the medial surface of the elbow can be extremely helpful when splinting to accommodate sensitive scars (C).

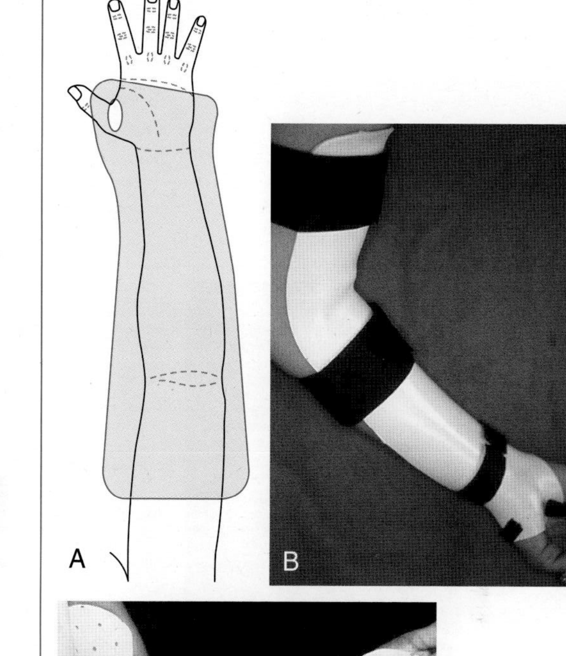

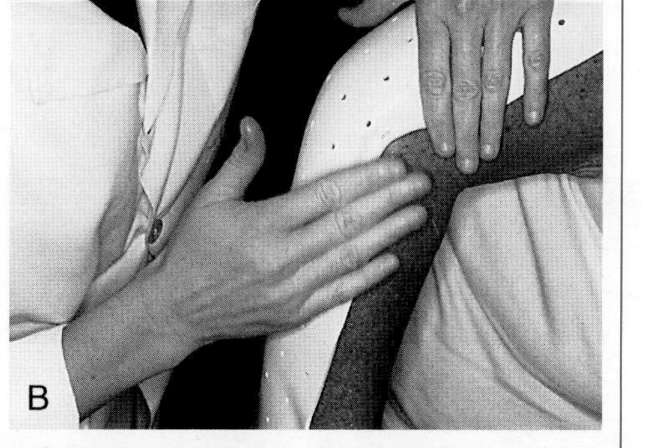

Chapter 8: Mobilization Splints

1 • Digit- and Thumb-Based Splints

Distal Interphalangeal (DIP) Flexion Mobilization Splint

(Fig. 8–1)

Common Names

- Dynamic DIP flexion splint

Alternative Splint Options

- Prefabricated
- Casting (serial static flexion)

Primary Functions

- Provide low-load, prolonged flexion mobilization force to DIP joint to facilitate lengthening of tissues.

Common Diagnoses and General Optimal Positions

• DIP jt ext contracture	Proximal interphalangeal (PIP) 0°; DIP: terminal flexion

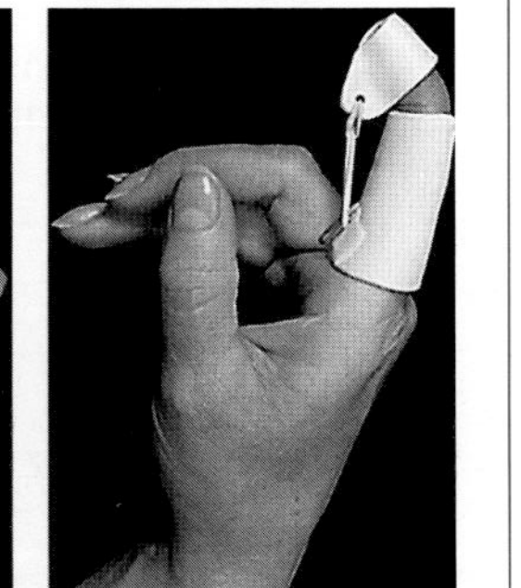

Figure 8–1

CLINICAL PEARL

Including Metacarpophalangeal (MP) Joint to Increase Effectiveness of DIP Stretch

To better secure the PIP joint, consider including the MP joint in the splint. The additional length allows for a longer line of pull, which can increase the effectiveness of this type of splint. This is especially helpful when splinting a small hand.

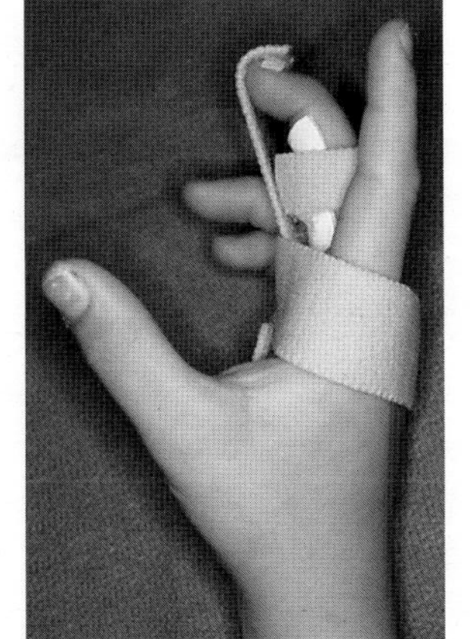

Fabrication Process

Pattern Creation (Fig. 8–2)

- For individuals with short digits, splint may need to include metacarpophalangeal (MP) joint to better stabilize PIP joint for optimal force application distally.
- For proximal attachment device prepare one scrap (1/2" by 1") of thermoplastic material.

Refine Pattern

- Make sure that digital web spaces are cleared and that PIP joint is held in 0° extension.
- DIP flexion crease should be cleared proximally.

Options for Materials

- Use nonperforated 1/16", 1/32", or 1/8" material.
- Plastic materials conform well to contours of digit.

Cut and Heat

- Position patient with hand supinated, digits slightly abducted, resting over platform.
- Warm material.
- Prepare mobilization components: sling, line, rubber band, and proximal attachment device.

Evaluate Fit While Molding

- Fabricate PIP splint.
- Clear distally to allow unimpeded DIP flexion.

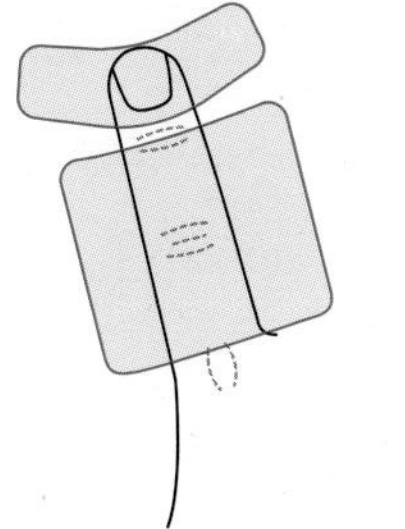

Figure 8–2

Strapping and Components

- Circumferential design does not require straps.
- Sling must be wide enough to distribute pressure over dorsum of DIP joint and short enough to prevent interference with line guide, if used.
- Secure proximal attachment device at most proximal border of splint, along longitudinal axis of proximal phalanx.
- Connect rubber band to sling and loop at proximal device.

Splint Finishing Touches

- Adjust tension per patient and/or tissue tolerance; goal is low-load stretch over prolonged period of time.

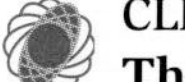

CLINICAL PEARL

Thermoplastic Distal Phalanx Caps

Slings used to stretch DIP joint extension contractures frequently slip during use. One solution is to fabricate a circumferential cap from 1/16" material to form a joined volar tab for the line attachment. Heat the material, and place it dorsally over the distal phalanx, quickly stretching to form a small volar tab. Pinch both ends to seal. Once set, punch a hole through the tab to serve as the attachment for the monofilament line.

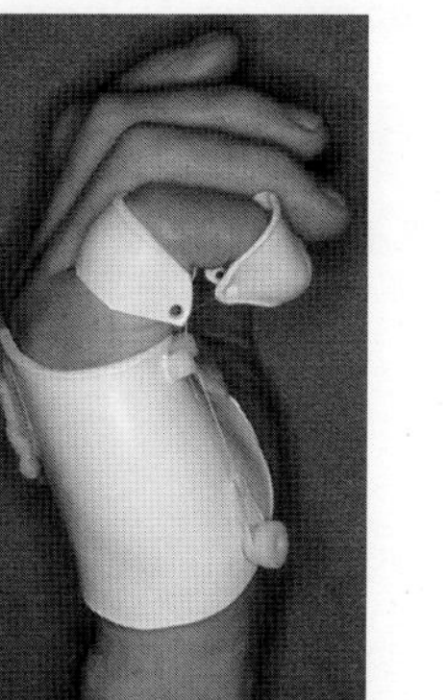

CLINICAL PEARL

Splints and Modalities

Splints can be used to enhance the use of therapeutic modalities. For example, a static progressive index finger (IF) MP flexion mobilization splint can be applied while ultrasound is used on the adherent extensor tendons over the dorsum of the IF. Another example is stabilizing the wrist (blocking the wrist flexors and extensors) with a wrist immobilization splint while applying neuromuscular stimulation to the extrinsic digital flexors and/or extensors to facilitate tendon glide. Splints can be worn directly over electrodes as long as the patient is instructed in proper electrode application and maintenance.

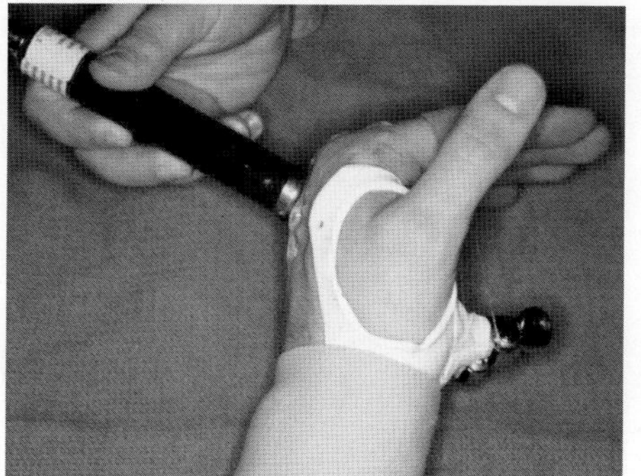

PIP/DIP Mobilization Splint
(Fig. 8–3)

Common Names

- PIP/DIP strap
- Interphalangeal (IP) flexion strap

Alternative Splint Options

- Taping in flexion
- Elasticized wrap
- Flexion glove
- Prefabricated straps

Primary Functions

- Provide low-load, prolonged flexion mobilization force to DIP and PIP joints to facilitate lengthening of tissues.

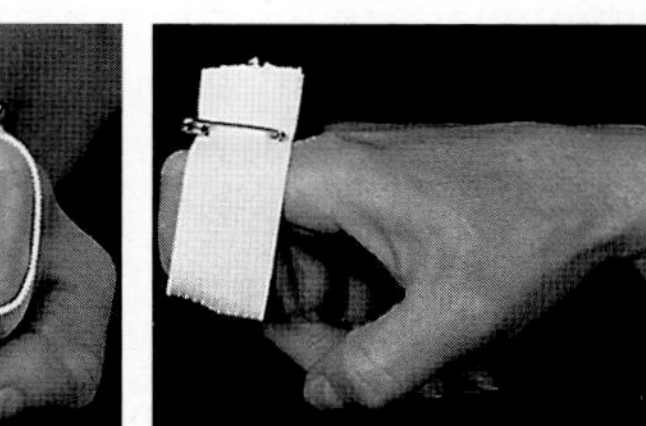

Figure 8–3

Additional Functions

- Facilitate extensor digitorum communis (EDC) function and glide during exercise.

Common Diagnoses and General Optimal Positions

• Intrinsic tightness	PIP/DIP terminal flex
• PIP and DIP jt tightness	PIP/DIP terminal flex
• Ext contracture	PIP/DIP terminal flex

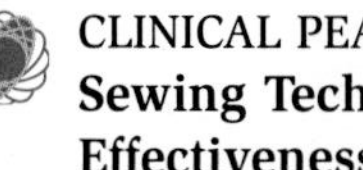

CLINICAL PEARL

Sewing Technique for Increasing Strap Effectiveness

When DIP joint flexion is extremely limited, applying a PIP/DIP strap can be challenging. One way to help keep the strap in place and provide a more effective stretch at the DIP joint is to sew the distal end of the strap diagonally to form a pocket for fingertip.

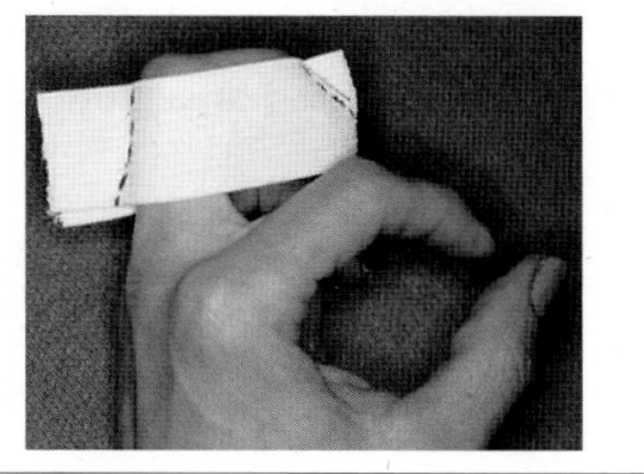

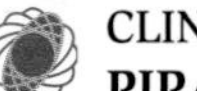

CLINICAL PEARL

PIP/DIP Strap for Increasing EDC Glide

PIP/DIP straps can be used to position the joints in flexion during exercises to increase the glide of the EDC tendons. Here, safety pins were used to secure the straps.

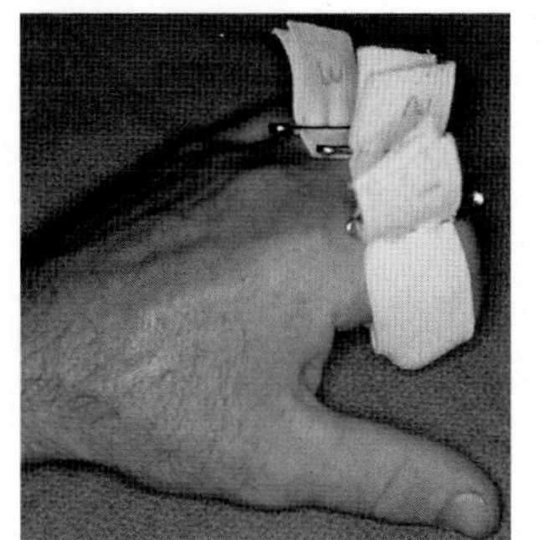

Fabrication Process

Pattern Creation (Fig. 8–4)

- Cut strip of 3/4" elastic strapping (pajama elastic) to approximately 1 1/2 times length of digit.

Refine Pattern

- Be sure width of elastic is adequate for size of digit.

Options for Materials

- 3/4" elastic strap is generally appropriate for adult digits, 1/2" for children.

Cut and Heat

- Be sure length is adequate to secure around digit.

Evaluate Fit While Molding

- While placing center of strip along dorsal distal phalanx have patient flex PIP and DIP joints of affected digit (claw position).
- Stretch strap ends to meet across dorsum of proximal phalanx, hold together, and adjust tension to tolerance.
- Mark both pieces of elastic and remove slowly from digit.

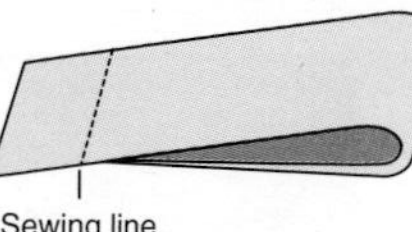

Figure 8–4

Strapping and Components

- Sew straps together on sewing machine, if available.
- Use safety pin or staples for simple, quick closure technique.
- May add a piece of soft foam under portion of straps that comes in contact with nail to soften contour of elastic over this sometimes sensitive area.

Splint Finishing Touches

- As range of motion (ROM) increases, tension in strap must be adjusted accordingly.
- Periodically check elasticity of strap; may need to be replaced with prolonged use.
- When fabricating straps for more than one digit, label them to ensure correct strap is placed on each digit.
- Adjust tension per patient and/or tissue tolerance; goal is low-load stretch over prolonged period of time.

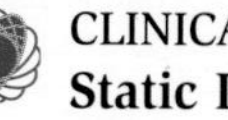

CLINICAL PEARL

Static Progressive PIP/DIP Mobilization Straps

Sometimes, using a static progressive approach for mobilizing stiff joints may yield better results. This technique may be helpful for patients who have difficulty donning the elastic PIP/DIP straps or who require frequent tension adjustments. Here are two ways to achieve this type of stretch.

Soft strap method (A). This works best with less severe contractures, because the foam strapping does not contour as well as the elastic strapping and may cause tissue irritation. Use soft 1/2" nonelastic foam strapping material. The severity of passive limitation determines the exact amount of strapping needed (i.e., the greater the contracture, the more material required). Use approximately two times the length of the digit. The fabrication method is the same as described for the PIP/DIP strap, except for the closure technique. A small strip of double-sided hook (adhesive hook folded onto itself) is placed on one end of the strap. Gentle tension is applied and then secured into place.

Thermoplastics and straps (B). For this method, fabricate a thermoplastic thimble over the distal phalanx and a thermoplastic sling on the proximal phalanx. Then apply a strip of adhesive hook on the lateral aspect of each thermoplastic piece. Connect the two segments with a 1/4" strip of nonelastic loop strapping material.

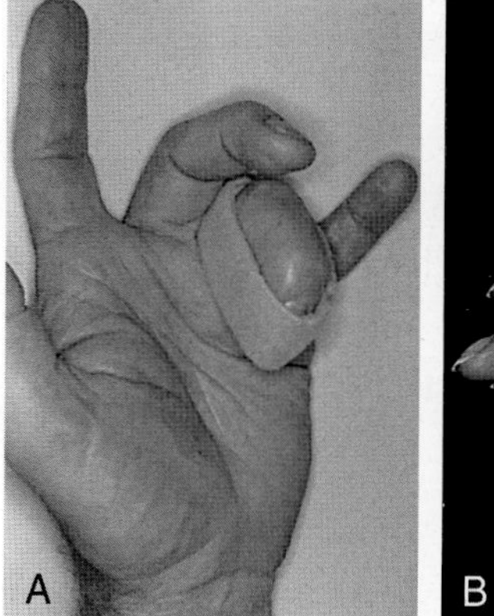

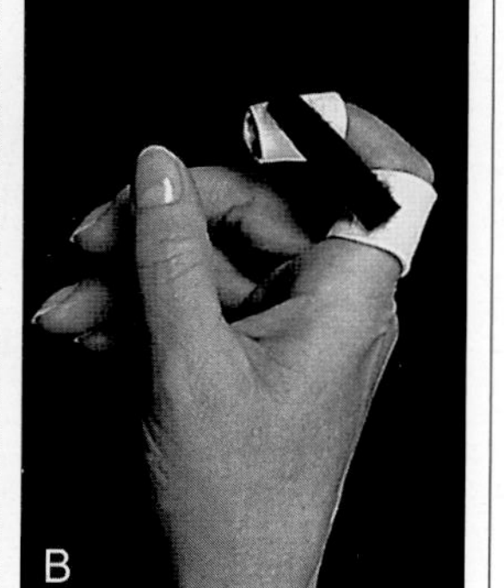

2 • Hand-Based Splints

PIP Extension Mobilization Splint (Fig. 8–5)

Common Names

- Dynamic PIP extension splint

Alternative Splint Options

- Cast (serial static)
- Prefabricated splint

Primary Functions

- Provide low-load, prolonged extension mobilization force to PIP joint to facilitate lengthening of tissues.

Additional Functions

- Facilitate extensor tendon function and glide during exercise.

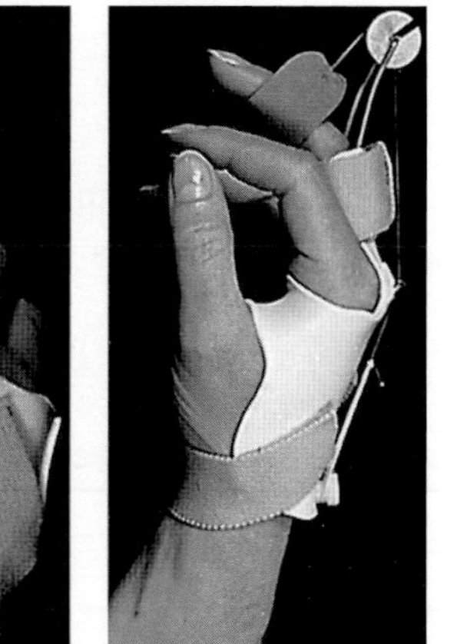

Figure 8–5

Common Diagnoses and General Optimal Positions

• PIP flex contracture	MP: 60°; PIP: terminal ext
• Zone III or IV ext tendon repair (for complex injury)	MP: 0°ext; PIP: 0°ext

CLINICAL PEARL

PIP Extension Mobilization Splint Using Rolyan Adjustable Outrigger

As an alternative, the Rolyan adjustable outrigger can be used to fabricate a PIP extension mobilization splint using the same pattern described for the Phoenix outrigger. Follow the manufacture's instructions for specific outrigger application.

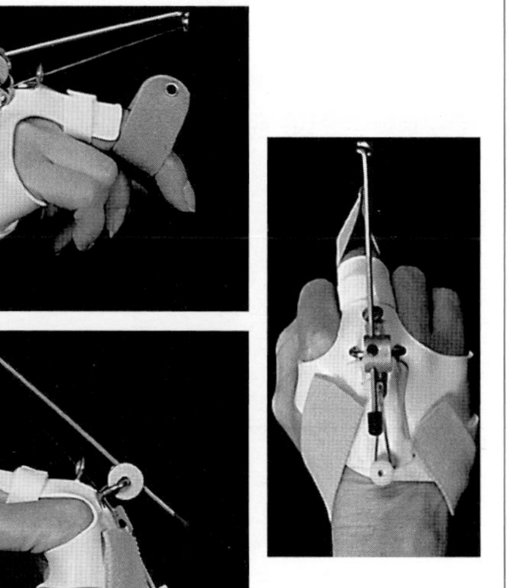

CLINICAL PEARL

Digit Extension Mobilization Splint Using Aquatube

Aquatube can be molded to form an outrigger. Here, the elastic is attached directly to the tube, providing the extension force.

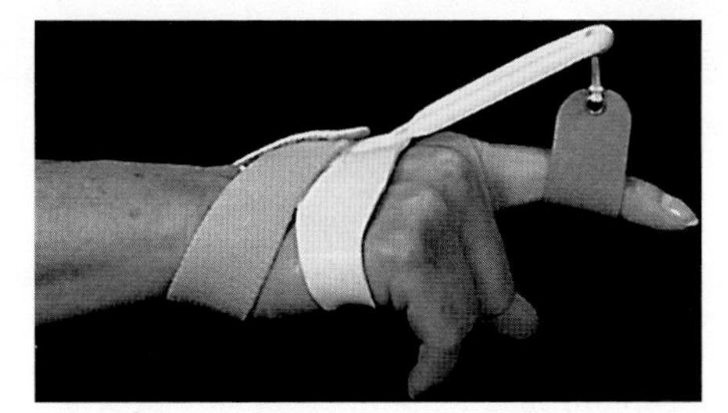

Fabrication Process (Using Phoenix Outrigger)

Pattern Creation (Fig. 8–6)

- Mark proximal border at wrist crease.
- If holding MP joint at 0°, mark distal border only to mid-PIP crease. If holding MP in flexion, mark distal border beyond PIP joint. Note: Additional material is needed to accommodate for flexion angle at MP joint.

Refine Pattern

- Proximal border should allow wrist motion.
- Lateral borders of PIP extension bar should trough proximal phalanx, encompassing half to two thirds of this segment.
- Ulnar aspect of hand splint should support hypothenar eminence.
- Make radial bar long enough to attach to volar ulnar border.

Options for Materials

- Use solid $^3/_{32}$" material, which is lightweight, yet strong enough to support MP joint in flexion while accepting extension force.
- Plastic materials contour well, with minimal handling into arches and digital web spaces.

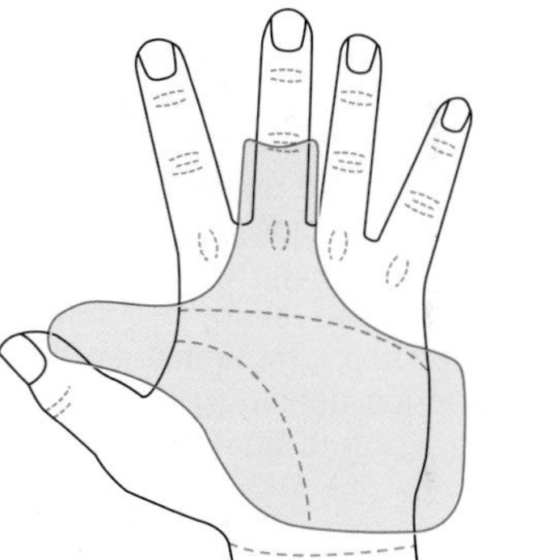

Figure 8–6

- If radial bar is intended to pop apart, coated material is necessary.
- If IF and/or small finger (SF) MPs are enlarged or if there is degree of thenar or hypothenar atrophy, the union must be popped open to ease donning and doffing.
- Use components of choice, following manufacturer's directions for correct application.

Cut and Heat

- Position patient with hand over platform, digits slightly abducted, and MP joint positioned per diagnosis.
- Heat two additional pieces of material (1" by 1") for securing outrigger and safety pin.

Evaluate Fit While Molding

- Dry and apply warm material onto hand, making sure to clear all creases, trough around involved proximal phalanx, and encompass ulnar border of hand.
- Gently pull radial bar through thumb web space and across volar MPs to meet with ulnar segment. Pinch and seal lightly.
- Make sure radial bar crosses proximal to MP joints and incorporates arches to help maintain proper splint position.
- Maintain MP joint position.

Strapping and Components

- Use $^1/_2$" to 1" strap at proximal phalanx.
- Attach 1" strap at ulnar–radial segment interface.
- Place an elasticized or soft foam strap at wrist to prevent splint migration.
- Mark desired outrigger attachment; position outrigger to extend distally over midportion of middle phalanx, extending it high enough so volar sling attached to line will clear pulley.
- Remove splint from patient and heat outrigger's proximal ends with heat gun. Press lightly to embed outrigger into marked area.
- Use extreme care when applying heated metal onto thermoplastic material. Metal may pierce through splint. Always perform this process off patient.
- Treat surfaces to be bonded with splint solvent. Place strip of heated thermoplastic material over outrigger and adhere to splint base.
- With flat-nose pliers, bend clasp part of safety pin at 90° angle. Heat same end over heat gun and embed into splint base over MP joint.
- Position eye of safety pin along longitudinal axis of involved digit; secure with thermoplastic material scrap.
- Attach Phoenix wheel to outrigger using appropriately sized Allen wrench.
- Affix proximal attachment device for rubber band at most proximal border.
- Attach line on both sides of sling and apply sling to middle phalanx.
- Thread line through pulley and safety pin.
- Loop appropriate rubber band onto end of line and connect to proximal attachment device.

Splint Finishing Touches

- Check for clearance of thumb, wrist, and uninvolved digits.
- Material should be flared about digital web spaces to avoid irritation.
- Check for equal traction on both sides of digit and for any possible rotational force.
- Adjust angles of pull by simply loosening pulley and rotating. Securely tighten in desired position with Allen wrench.
- Align pulley with longitudinal axis of proximal phalanx. Adjust by loosening pulley and sliding it transversely along width of outrigger. Securely tighten in desired position with Allen wrench.
- Adjust tension per patient and/or tissue tolerance; goal is low-load stretch over prolonged period of time.

CLINICAL PEARL

Forearm-Based PIP Extension Mobilization Splint

When splinting a patient with multiple PIP joint flexion contractures, or a PIP flexion contracture that is greater than approximately 60°, consider a forearm-based splint design. The longer design may also work well when addressing both MP and PIP joint contractures within one splint. The splint pattern is similar to the hand-based PIP extension mobilization splint but includes the wrist. Shown is a ring finger (RF) to SF PIP extension mobilization splint. The patient had significant, long-standing PIP flexion contractures secondary to an ulnar nerve injury. She presented with a 75° flexion contracture on the RF and a 45° flexion contracture on the SF. Note the length of the outrigger on the RF to achieve a 90° line of pull. The outrigger platform for the wheel had to be custom-made to incorporate the height and achieve the optimal angle of force application. The detachable extension outrigger can be positioned higher or lower, moved proximally or distally, and (to a lesser degree) slide radially and ulnarly. The more severe the contracture, the more distal and higher the rod will need to be. As the contracture resolves, the rod is retracted proximally and tightened back into place with the appropriate Allen wrench. The component shown here is the Rolyan adjustable outrigger, which can be adjusted to hold single or multiple rod extenders.

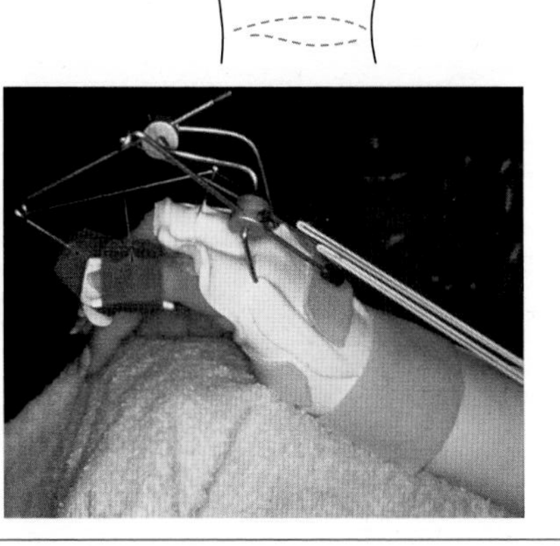

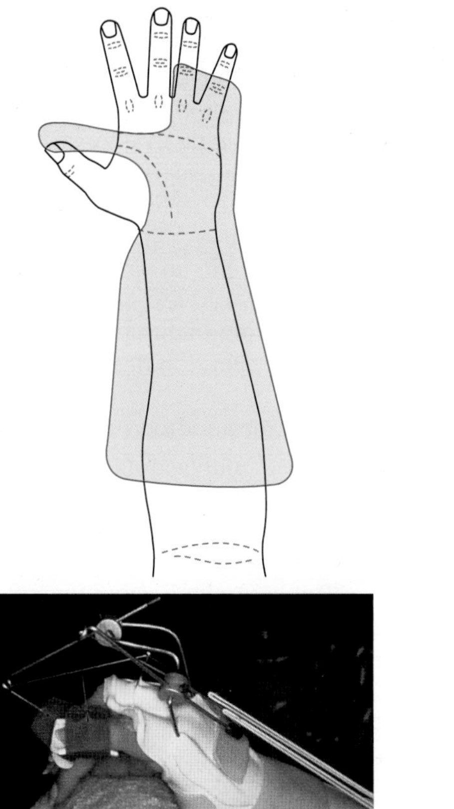

CLINICAL PEARL

Forearm-Based PIP and PIP/DIP Flexion Mobilization Splint

This splint pattern is similar to the hand-based PIP flexion mobilization splint, but the wrist is included (A). Be careful to accommodate for the differing heights of the PIP flexion creases to ensure adequate clearance for each individual digit (B). The dorsal design uses a static progressive approach to mobilization. Note the foam-lined slings, which improve patient comfort (C and D).

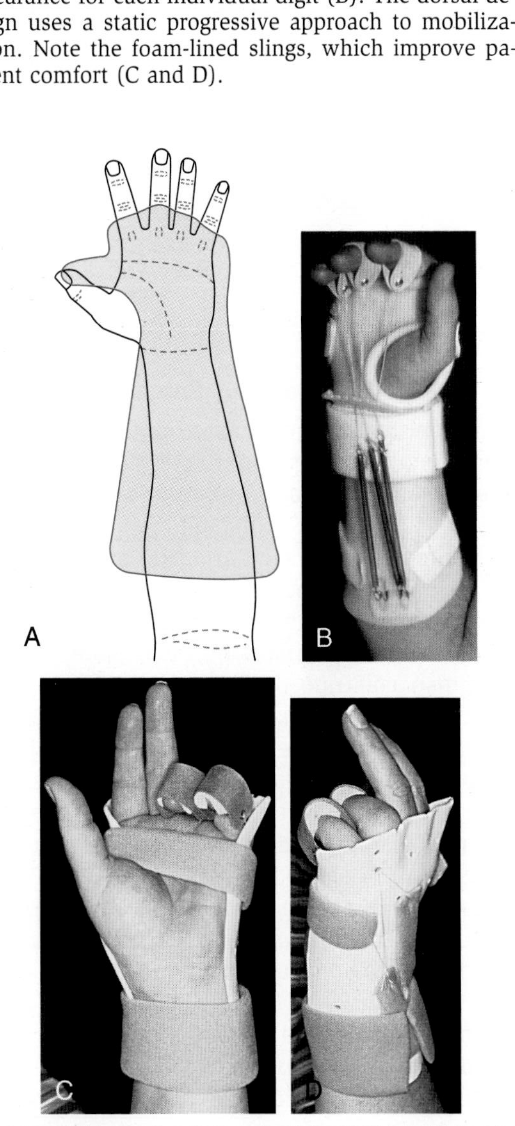

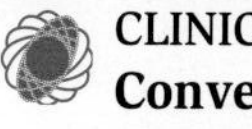

CLINICAL PEARL

Convert Dynamic Splint to Static Progressive Splint Using MERiT Component

These composite digit flexion splints have a similar design, except for the mobilization component. The composite SF flexion splint using a dynamic approach employs rubber band traction and homemade line guides (Aquatube) to increase SF MP, PIP, and DIP flexion (A). The composite middle finger (MF) flexion splint using a static progressive approach includes safety pins as line guides and a MERiT component to provide the static progressive force (B). The turn screw is gradually tightened to increase the tension applied to the MF.

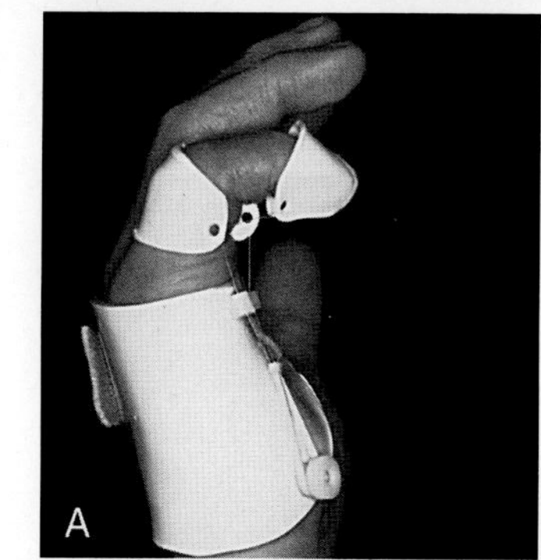

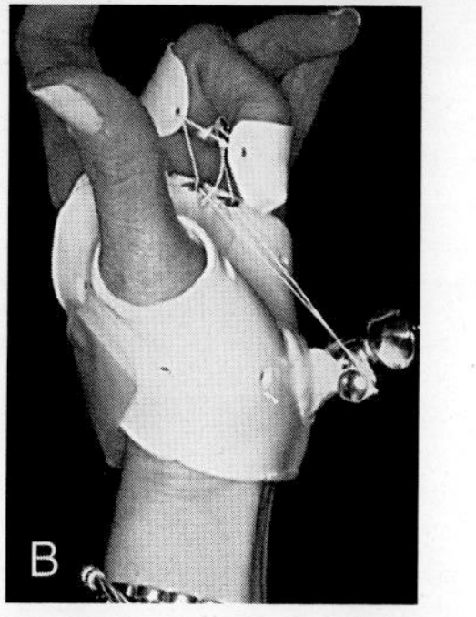

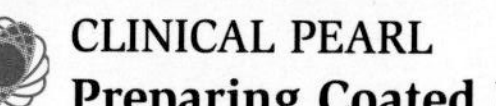

CLINICAL PEARL

Preparing Coated Materials for Bonding

When using thermoplastic material with a protective coating, the surfaces must be prepared if bonding of two pieces is necessary. To prepare the surfaces, use solvent to eliminate the coating on the material's surface or scratch and score the material's surface to disrupt the coating. To ensure a strong bond, press the materials firmly together. Use a heat gun to hyperheat the material, which helps make it tacky and more likely to adhere.

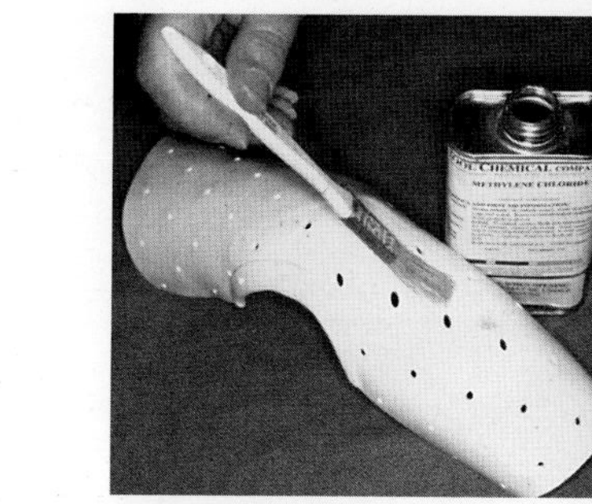

PIP Flexion Mobilization Splint (Fig. 8-7)

Common Names

- Dynamic PIP flexion splint

Alternative Splint Options

- Elastic wraps
- Flexion glove
- Prefabricated splints

Primary Functions

- Provide low-load, prolonged flexion mobilization force to PIP joint to facilitate lengthening of tissues.

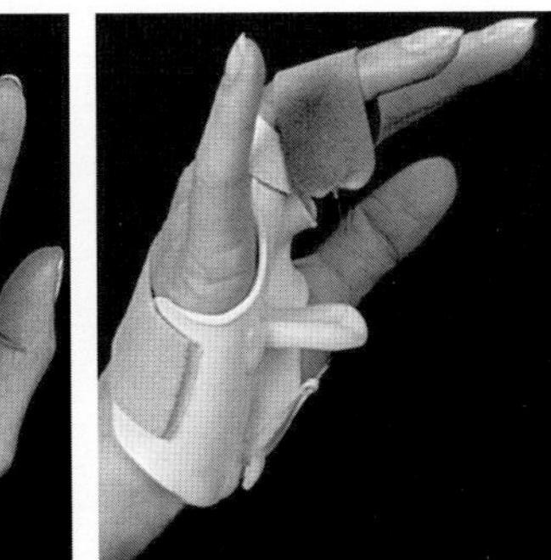
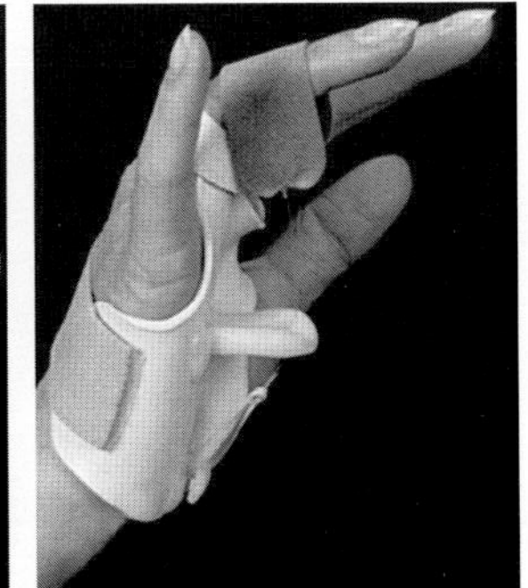
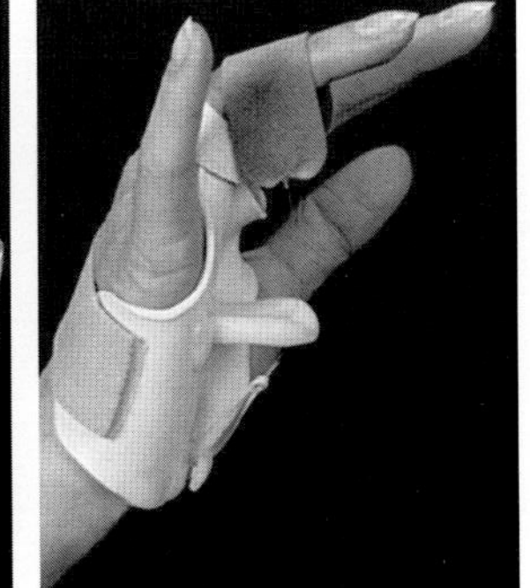
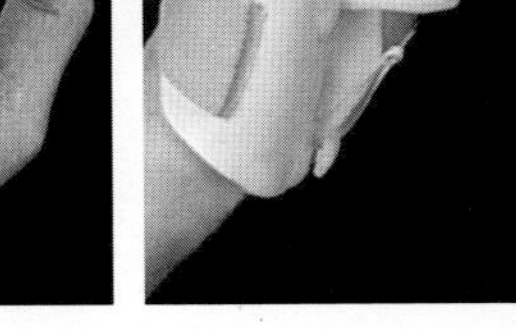

Figure 8–7

Common Diagnoses and General Optimal Positions

• PIP ext contracture	MP: 0°; PIP: terminal flex

CLINICAL PEARL

PIP Flexion Mobilization Splint Using Phoenix Outrigger

As an alternative, the Phoenix outrigger can be used to fabricate a PIP flexion mobilization splint using the same pattern described for the custom outrigger. Follow the manufacturer's instructions for specific outrigger application.

CLINICAL PEARL

PIP Flexion Mobilization Strap

An elastic or nonelastic strap can be used to effectively mobilize an isolated stiff PIP joint. The strap is directed from the middle phalanx of the involved digit, through the thenar web space, and across the ulnar border of the hand to terminate on the dorsum of the hand. Note the use of a thermoplastic cuff over the middle phalanx for optimal pressure distribution. The tension should be gentle and adjusted appropriately to maintain the correct stretch on the joint. When splinting a patient with both PIP and distal interphalangeal (DIP) tightness, it may help first to stretch the patient in this strap to address the PIP joint in isolation, and then apply the PIP/DIP strap.

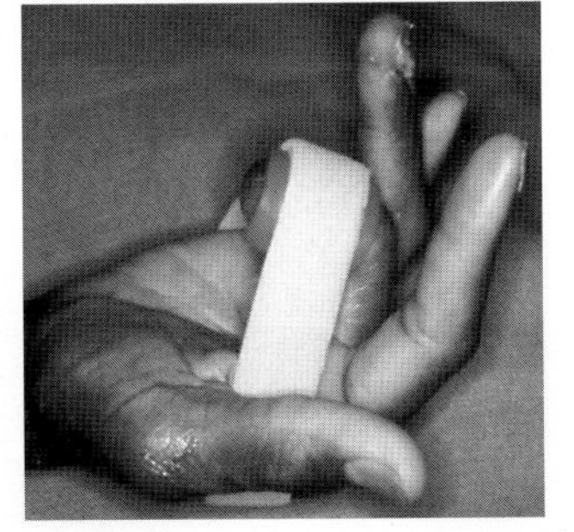

Fabrication Process

Pattern Creation (Fig. 8–8)

- Severity of contracture and number of joints involved determine whether splint is forearm or hand-based.
- This hand-based pattern can easily be modified to include wrist.
- Mark proximal border at distal wrist crease.
- Mark distal border at proximal PIP crease.

Refine Pattern

- Lateral borders should encompass half to two thirds of circumference of proximal phalanx (flush with dorsal surface).
- Borders should clear uninvolved MP joint creases and encompass hypothenar eminence.
- When splinting IF and middle finger (MF), there should be enough material molded around thenar eminence to allow for line guide attachment.
- Radial bar should traverse through thumb web space, across dorsum of hand, and attach to ulnar border.

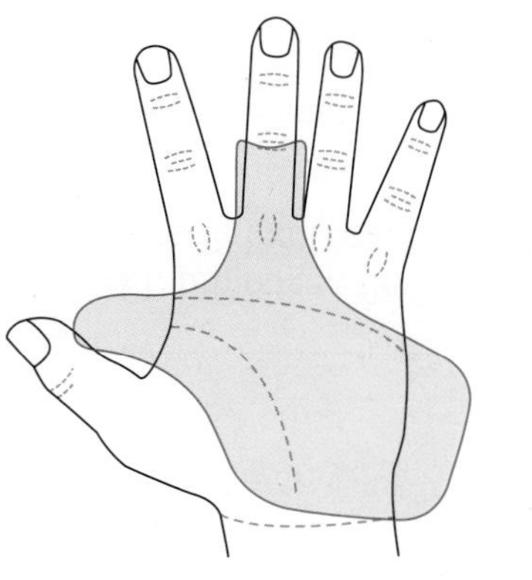

Figure 8–8

Options for Materials

- Use solid, coated $^3/_{32}$" material (elastic or plastic) for this splint; this makes for lightweight splint with adequate strength to support MP joint in extension while accepting flexion force.
- Elastic materials allow excellent visualization of creases during molding.
- Plastic materials tend to contour well, with minimal handling, into arches and about digital web spaces.
- To seal off circumference of splint, choose an uncoated material; however, if dorsal segment is intended to pop apart then coated material is recommended.
- Use components of choice (custom-fabricated line guide is shown).

Cut and Heat

- Position patient with hand supinated resting over platform, digits slightly abducted, and MP joint extended.

Evaluate Fit While Molding

- Dry and apply warm material onto hand, making sure to clear all creases; trough about involved proximal phalanx; and encompass ulnar border.
- Gently pull radial bar through thumb web space and across dorsum to meet with ulnar segment. Pinch and seal lightly, and return focus to volar aspect.
- Make sure arches are incorporated into the splint to maintain splint position properly on hand.
- MP joint should be positioned as close to 0° as possible.

Strapping and Components

- Use $^1/_2$" to 1" across proximal phalanx.
- If necessary, attach 1" strap dorsally at ulnar and radial segments. This area may be permanently sealed; however, if IF and SF MPs are enlarged or if there is some degree of thenar or hypothenar atrophy, it will be difficult to doff splint without popping it open.
- Place elasticized or soft foam strap at wrist to prevent migration (if needed).
- Position sling over middle phalanx.
- Apply line guide at level of distal palmar crease, making sure it is extended far enough to create 90° angle of pull when force is applied to middle phalanx.
- Proximal attachment device should be attached at most proximal border of splint.

Splint Finishing Touches

- Connect line to rubber band and loop about proximal device.
- Check for equal traction of both sides of digit and for any possible rotational force. Correct, if necessary, by adjusting monofilament line.
- Material should be flared, trimmed, and smoothed around digital web spaces to avoid irritation.
- Check that volar splint borders do not irritate uninvolved MPs.
- Adjust tension per patient and/or tissue tolerance; goal is low-load stretch over prolonged period of time.

Thumb IP Flexion Mobilization Splint (Fig. 8–9)

Common Names

- IP flexion splint

Alternative Splint Options

- Elastic wraps

Primary Functions

- Provide low-load, prolonged flexion mobilization force to thumb IP joint to facilitate lengthening of tissues.

Common Diagnoses and General Optimal Positions

• Th IP jt ext contracture	MP: 0°; (CMC): midpalmar–rad abd; IP: terminal flex

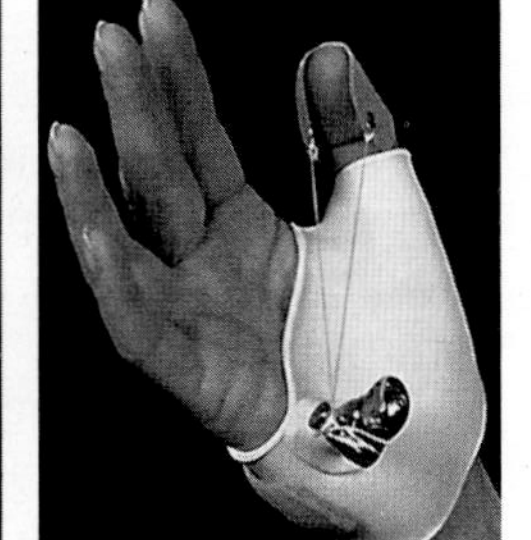
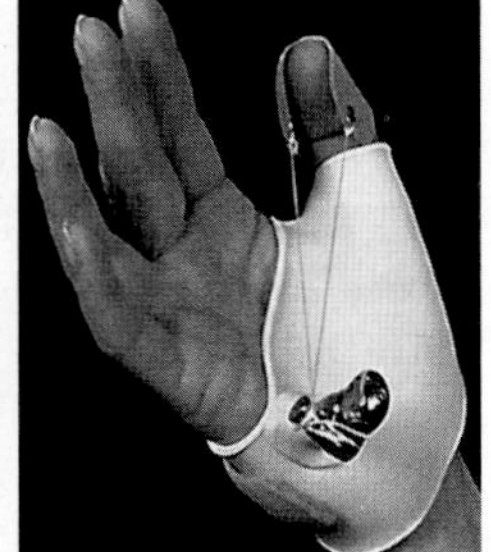

Figure 8–9

CLINICAL PEARL

Thumb MP/IP Flexion Mobilization Splint

Often after injury to the thumb, both the MP and IP joints can be stiff, requiring mobilization splinting. Stiffness may present after cast immobilization of the ulnar collateral ligament (UCL) or radial collateral ligament (RCL) sprain or repair, scaphoid fracture, scaphotrapeziotrapezoid (STT) fusion, carpometacarpal (CMC) joint arthroplasty, or other thumb injuries. To provide flexion forces to the MP and IP joints simultaneously, fabricate a splint similar to the thumb IP flexion mobilization splint but with the thumb portion extended only as far as the MP joint flexion crease (A). This allows adequate stabilization of the first metacarpal while forces are directed to the MP and IP joints. For a dynamic approach, use rubber band traction (B). A small piece of hook is adhered to the nail to allow for loop attachment. For a static progressive approach, use adhesive hook and loop strapping for the proximal attachment device (C). The adhesive hook is diagonally placed at the proximal border of the splint base, and the loop strapping is then directed to the hook and attached. This provides a gentle stretch that should be adjusted as patient tolerance permits.

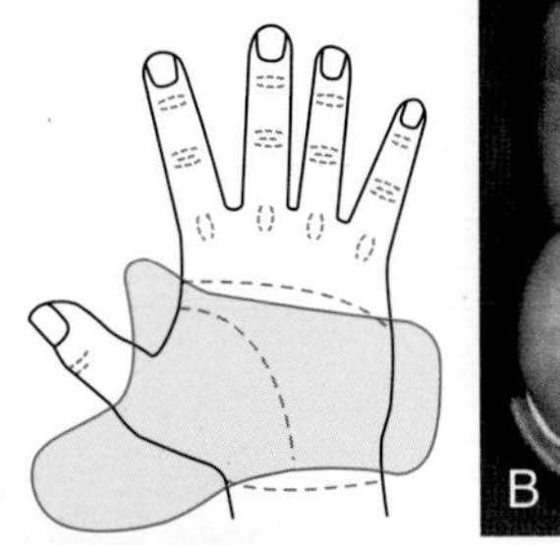

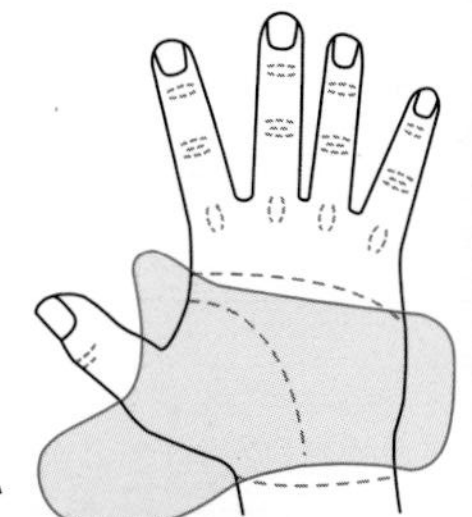

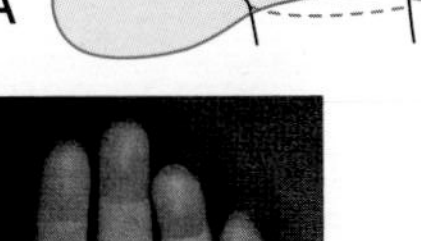
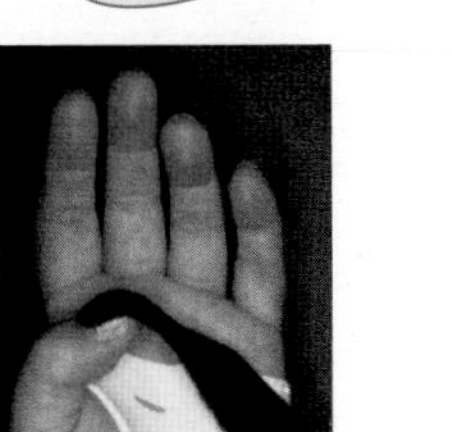

Fabrication Process (Using Splint Tuner Static Progressive Tension Adjuster)

Pattern Creation (Fig. 8–10)

- Mark proximal border at wrist crease.
- Mark distal border proximal to thumb IP flexion crease and distal palmar crease.

Refine Pattern

- Proximal border should allow full wrist motion.
- Distal border should allow unimpeded motion of digit MP and thumb IP flexion.
- Provide appropriate amount of material within and dorsal to web space to support thumb CMC and MP position adequately and provide surface area for strap application dorsally.

Options for Materials

- Use solid, coated, $1/16$" or $3/32$" material; this makes for lightweight splint with adequate strength to support CMC and MP joints while accepting flexion force to IP joint.
- Elastic materials allow excellent visualization of creases during molding.

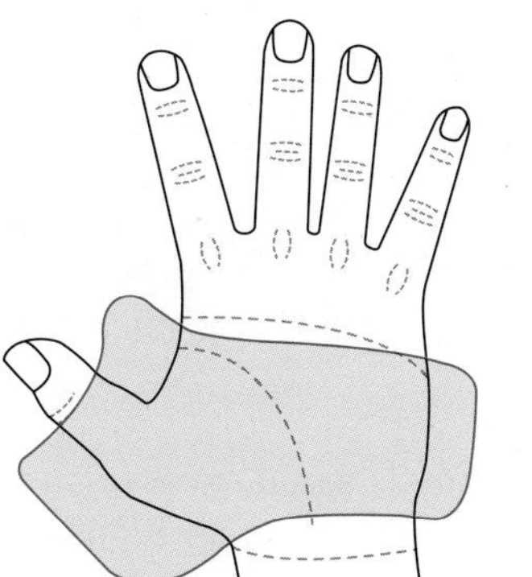

Figure 8–10

- Plastic material contours well, with minimal handling into arches and thumb web space.
- Use components of choice (Splint Tuner is shown).

Cut and Heat

- Position hand supinated over an armrest, with thumb in midpalmar and radial abduction.
- Heat an additional piece of material (1" by 1") to secure Splint Tuner component.

Evaluate Fit While Molding

- Lay warm material on towel, positioning thumb portion on correct side of material to place it on supinated hand.
- Place thumb section centrally over thumb proximal phalanx and guide rest of material evenly along palm.
- Take dorsal section of thumb material (between IF and thumb) and carefully contour through web space.
- Gently pull proximal volar thumb material and lightly overlap onto dorsal piece.
- While molding, avoid direct pressure over CMC joint and dorsal MP joint. Be sure to maintain thumb CMC and MP joints in appropriate positions.
- Carefully incorporate arches of hand by using smooth, even strokes and constantly redirecting material.
- Once material has cooled completely, pop apart overlapped pieces, if necessary; otherwise carefully remove splint.

Strapping and Components

- If necessary, attach $1/2$" strap dorsally at overlapped web space area.
- Attach 1" strap dorsally at ulnar and radial segments.
- To attach Splint Tuner component, first treat surfaces to be bonded with splint solvent (splint base and small thermoplastic piece).
- Heat small piece of material and wrap around component stem to form cylinder.
- Reheat material over heat gun; then set at predetermined site on splint base.
- Firmly press component into splint base and gently rotate cylinder to achieve an intimate fit about grooves of stem onto splint base.
- Position Splint Tuner component so axis of rotating cylinder is perpendicular to line.
- Apply sling to distal phalanx, then attach static splint line allowing enough so that splint can be easily donned and doffed but not so much that it is cumbersome to tighten up each time it is loosened.
- Thread line through hole in Splint Tuner component and tie line back onto itself.

Splint Finishing Touches

- Check for clearance of wrist, especially around radial and ulnar styloids.
- Smooth and slightly flare all borders and around thumb IP opening.
- Pay careful attention to IF MP, which frequently abuts radial portion of splint as it traverses through first web space.
- Make sure web tissue is not pinched under overlapped pieces.
- Adjust tension by rotating turn screw per patient and/or tissue tolerance; goal is low-load stretch over prolonged period of time.

MP Extension Mobilization Splint (Fig. 8–11)

Common Names

- Zero profile splint[1]
- Posterior interosseous nerve splint

Alternative Splint Options

- Dynamic MP extension splint
- Prefabricated splint

Primary Functions

- Dynamically support MP joints in extension while allowing active digit (and thumb) flexion.

Common Diagnoses and General Optimal Positions

• Returning radial nerve function	MP: 0°; PIP: free
• Posterior interosseous nerve injury	MP: 0°; PIP: free
• Weak extrinsic extensor function	MP: 0°; PIP: free

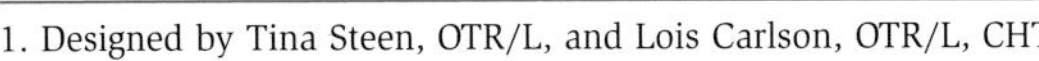

1. Designed by Tina Steen, OTR/L, and Lois Carlson, OTR/L, CHT.

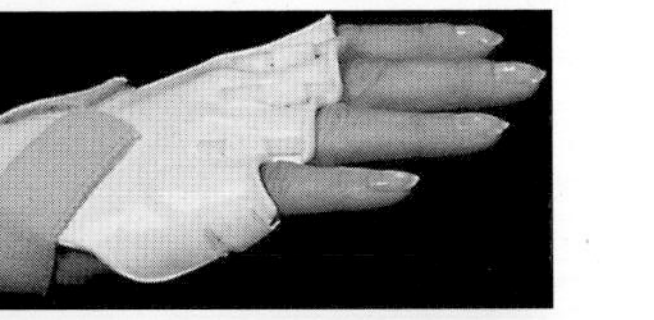

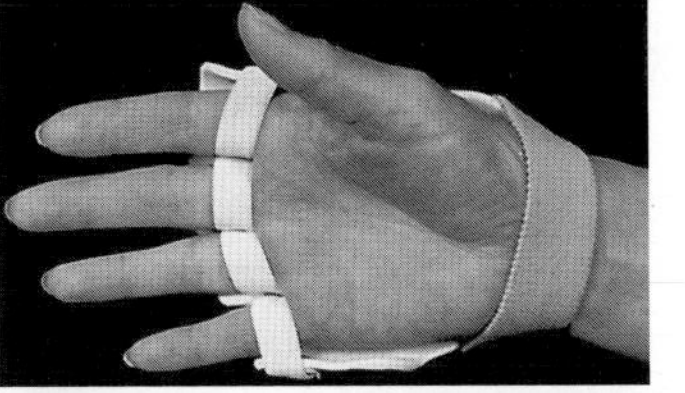

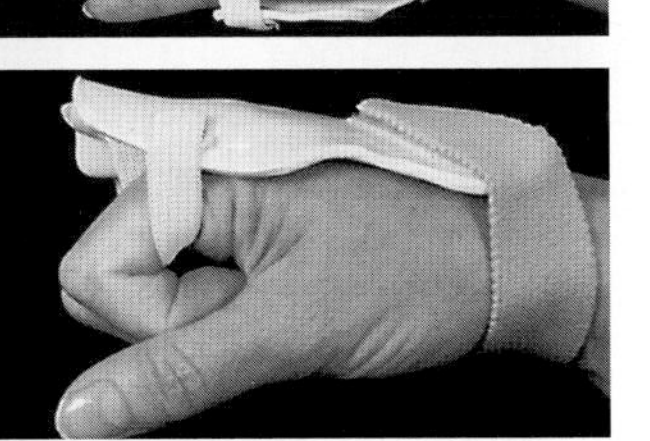

Figure 8–11

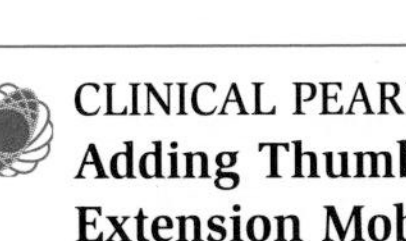

CLINICAL PEARL
Adding Thumb to Hand-Based MP Extension Mobilization Splint

Loss of thumb extension is commonly seen after radial nerve injury and can impair functional use of the hand. To better position the thumb (from a flexed and adducted posture) while awaiting reinnervation consider adding a dynamic thumb MP extension assist to the MP extension mobilization splint. The basic pattern does not change. A Phoenix or other similar outrigger works well to support the thumb passively in extension while allowing active thumb flexion.

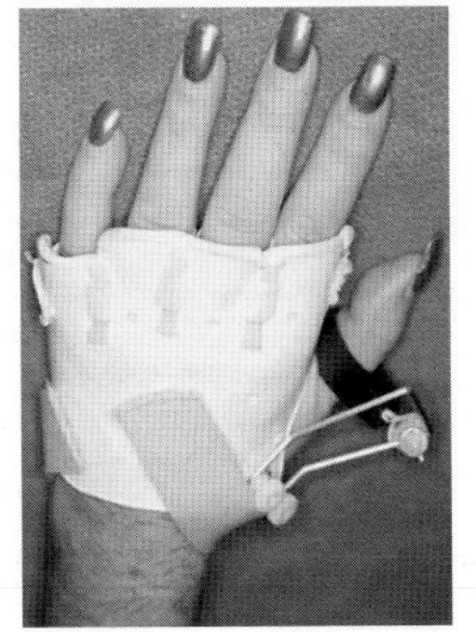

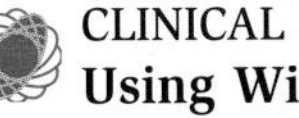

CLINICAL PEARL
Using Wider Elastic

Because of the difference in length of the proximal phalanges (adult male versus a young child), a wider elastic may be used to better support the digits in extension. On the bordering digits, the elastic may be folded over to provide better clearance at the PIP joint creases.

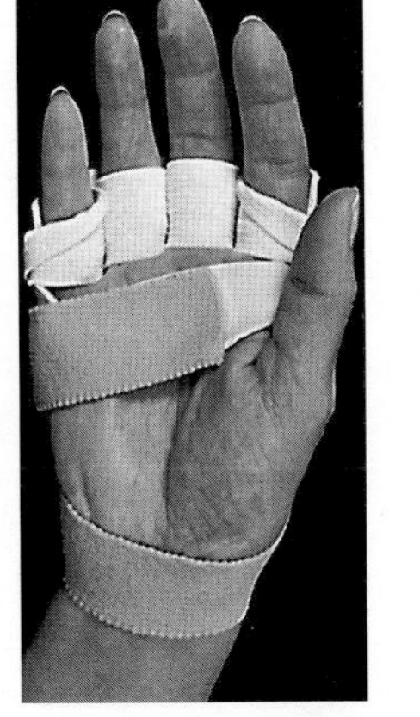

Fabrication Process

Pattern Creation (Fig. 8–12)

- Mark proximal border at wrist crease.
- Mark distal borders at middorsal PIP creases.
- Note small slits at digit web spaces for elastic to pass through.

Refine Pattern

- Radial aspect should extend enough to trough radial index and partially trough web space (just beyond proximal palmar crease); the trough should lie flush to volar surface and not interfere with digit flexion.
- Ulnar border should encompass hypothenar eminence but not interfere with MP flexion.

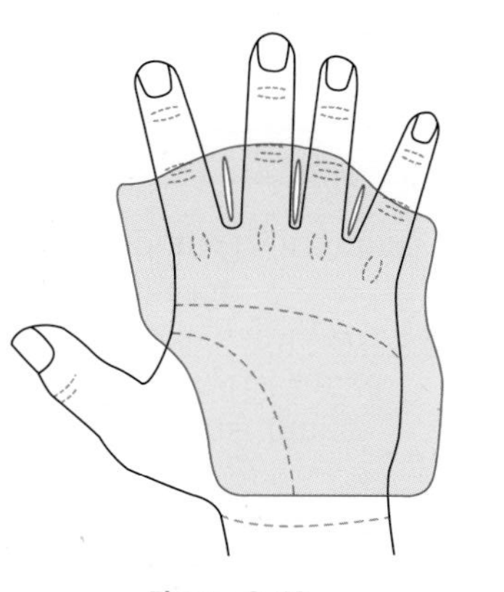

Figure 8–12

Options for Materials

- Use solid $^3/_{32}$" plastic material; this makes for lightweight splint with adequate strength to support MP joints in extension while accepting flexion forces.
- Plastic material contours well, with minimal handling about metacarpal heads and between digital web spaces.
- Cut $^1/_4$" to $^1/_2$" elastic strapping (pajama elastic), depending on size of hand, twice width of hand (at MP joint level); elastic should cover approximately two thirds length of proximal phalanxes.
- Use three small pieces of scrap thermoplastic material (or Aquatube) to secure elastic loops dorsally.

Cut and Heat

- Heat thermoplastics, including small pieces.
- Position hand, pronated with digits slightly abducted; MP joints should be positioned and held in extension. (Patient may need to support digits in extension with unaffected hand.)

Evaluate Fit While Molding

- Heat and apply material to dorsum of hand, carefully making sure that MPs are extended and proximal phalanxes are precisely contoured, forming small troughs.
- Mold with care over metacarpal heads to avoid pressure areas.
- Wrap about hypothenar border volarly along fifth metacarpal to add stability to splint.
- Radial border should be molded along radial aspect of IF and lay flush to its volar surface.

Strapping and Components

- Once set, use hole punch or hand drill to form slits that start approximately $^1/_2$" from distal splint border between the IF and MF, the MF and RF, and the RF and SF.
- Weave elastic through slits to support each proximal phalanx.
- Tension of elastic strap should be just enough to hold proximal phalanx in extension; excessive tension can lead to neurovascular compromise.
- Prepare surface of dorsal loop areas with splint solvent for adhering rods.
- Placed small pieces of warm thermoplastic material (rolled into rods) underneath each dorsal loop. Press rods into place, sealing elastic loop against splint base.
- Consider using rivets to secure radial and ulnar extensions of elastic.
- Use soft or elasticized 1" strap through palm and at wrist crease to secure splint on hand.

Splint Finishing Touches

- Check for pressure areas at dorsum of MP joints during active flexion.
- Check tension on each proximal phalanx support, monitoring for signs of neurovascular compromise.

3 • Forearm-Based Splints

Wrist Extension Mobilization Splint (Fig. 8-13)

Common Names

- Dynamic wrist extension splint
- Wrist mobilization splint

Alternative Splint Options

- Casting (serial static)
- Rolyan adjustable wrist hinge
- Rolyan incremental wrist hinge
- Rolyan preformed dynamic wrist splint
- MERiT wrist splint kit
- Orthotics (JAS splint, Dynasplint)

Primary Functions

- Provide low-load, prolonged extension mobilization force to wrist joint to facilitate lengthening of tissue

Alternative Functions

- Restrict specific degree of motion by blocking movement through hinge device (restriction splint).

Common Diagnoses and General Optimal Positions

• Wr flex contracture	FArm: pronated; wr: terminal ext

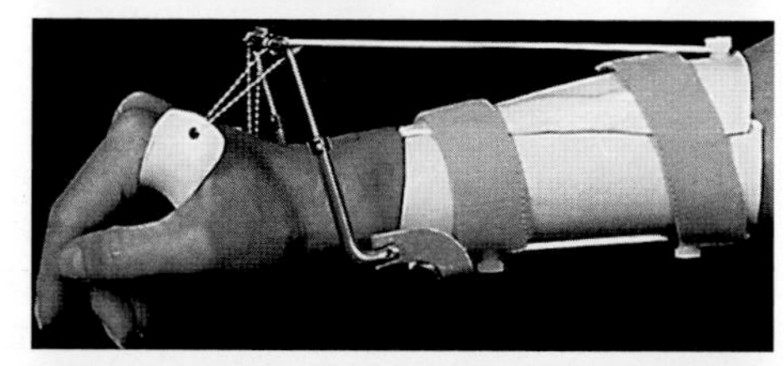

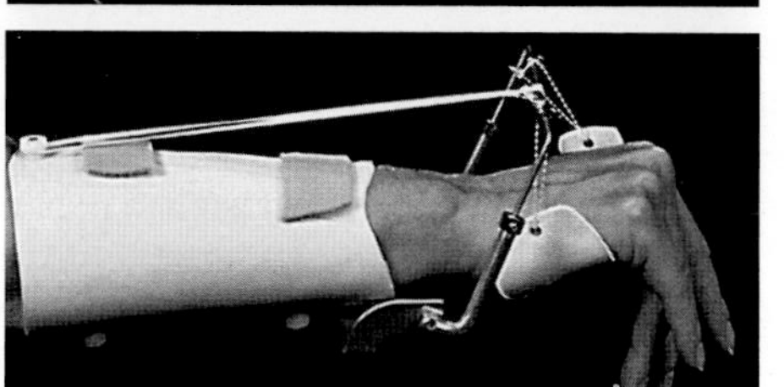

Figure 8–13

Fabrication Process (Using Phoenix Wrist Hinge)

Pattern Creation (Fig. 8–14)

- Forearm splint
  * Length of splint should be at least 5" to allow adequate attachment of outrigger.
- Hand splint
  * Width should be approximately $1\frac{1}{2}$ times width of hand (at distal palmar crease).
  * Length should extend ulnarly from distal palmar crease to hamate bone, and radially allow enough material to contour through first web space.

Refine Pattern

- Allow adequate clearance for unimpeded wrist motion.

Options for Materials

- Use $\frac{1}{16}$" or $\frac{3}{32}$" material for both splint pieces; the thinness allows for easy removal and application.
- Use components of choice (Phoenix wrist hinge is shown).

Cut and Heat

- Heat and fabricate each piece separately.
- For forearm splint, position forearm in neutral rotation.
- For hand splint, position forearm supinated.

Evaluate Fit While Molding

- Forearm splint
  * Prepad ulnar styloid process.
  * After heating material, place material on volar surface of forearm and gently wrap around onto itself.
  * Opening must be either on radial or ulnar aspect of forearm; volar or dorsal opening will impede outrigger placement.
  * If using coated material, lightly overlap so it will adhere to itself; if using uncoated material, place wet paper towel between overlapped layers.
  * Allow splint to set and then snap apart.
- Hand splint
  * Place material on volar hand and mold it around to dorsal surface.
  * Flare edges to clear thenar eminence and distal palmar crease.
  * Mark palmar splint for trimming just above ulnar and radial borders on dorsal surface.
  * Mark hole along ulnar and radial borders of hand splint for attaching nylon fasteners.
  * Remove splint, trim as needed, and smooth edges.

Strapping and Components

- Add straps once wrist hinge placement is determined.

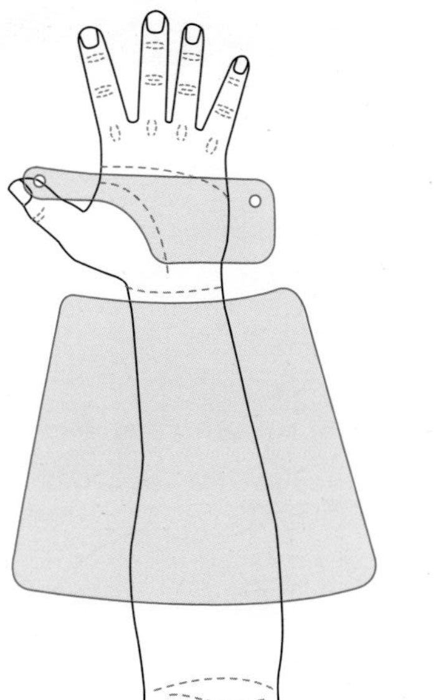

Figure 8–14

- Forearm splint
  * With forearm splint on patient, position wrist hinge volarly.
  * Align long arm of wrist hinge with axis of motion.
  * Mark two holes on volar splint to match up with holes on long arm of wrist hinge.
  * Remove splint and punch out holes.
  * Attach hinge with rubber band posts (included with Phoenix wrist hinge).
  * Affix rubber band post to proximal dorsal border for attachment of mobilization component.
  * Apply forearm splint to hand.
  * Set screws on lateral bars allow proximal and distal height adjustment of $1\frac{1}{2}$". Loosen set screws with Allen wrench and adjust distal bar to accommodate appropriate position; tighten screws.
  * Make necessary lateral adjustments for extreme radial or ulnar deviation by using screw on T-bar. Loosen with screwdriver and slide hinge radially or ulnarly to desired position.
- Hand splint
  * Punch holes on dorsal pieces.
  * Thread nylon fastener through dorsal holes on hand splint.
  * Apply hand splint.
  * Loop nylon fasteners around outrigger bar within movable collars of wrist hinge and adjoin fasteners.
  * Place wrist in maximum extension while adjusting fasteners to achieve 90° angle of pull with metacarpal bones.
  * Position two movable collars on distal bar of wrist hinge so they prevent nylon loops from slipping laterally.
  * Attach appropriate rubber band to distal bar, directing it to proximal attachment device.

Wrist Extension Mobilization Splint *(Continued)*

Splint Finishing Touches

- Add 1" to 2" strip of thin adhesive back padding (e.g., Moleskin) along length of inside border to prevent skin from being pinched when splint is overlapped and secured. Moleskin is doubled over (with thermoplastic edge in between adhesive sides of padding) and acts as flap.
- Line length of forearm splint and proximal and distal borders with nonskid material to decrease splint migration greatly. May use Microfoam tape, adhesive Dycem, or adhesive silicone gel sheets.
- Check for accomodation of ulnar styloid and full elbow range of motion.
- Adjust tension per patient and/or tissue tolerance; goal is low-load stretch over prolonged period of time.

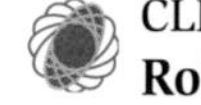

CLINICAL PEARL

Rolyan Incremental Wrist Hinge

As an alternative, the Rolyan Incremental Wrist Hinge can be used to fabricate a wrist mobilization splint. The pattern differs from the Phoenix wrist hinge, as shown. The hinge can be locked in position for serial static positioning, and components can be added to provide the mobilization forces. Follow the manufacturer's instructions for specific outrigger application.

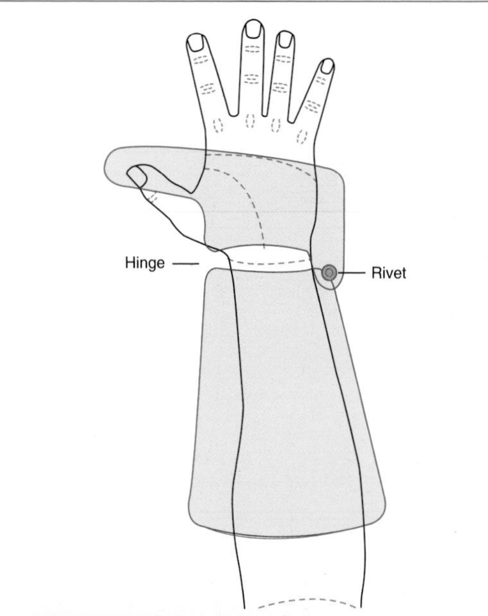

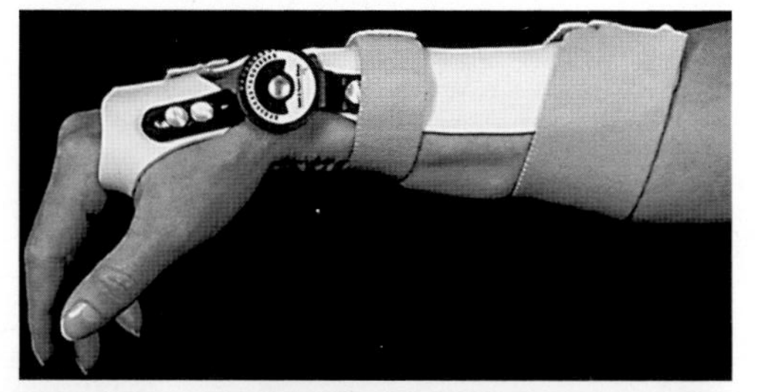

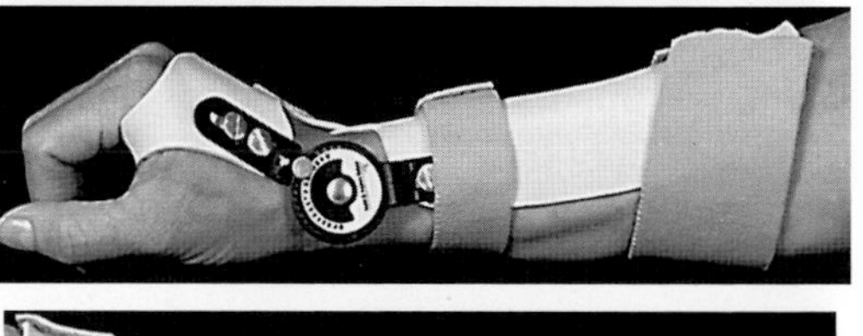

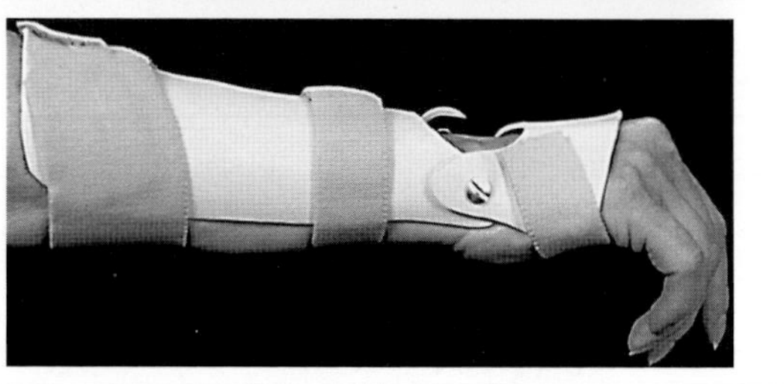

CLINICAL PEARL

Wrist Flexion and Combined Flexion/Extension Mobilization Splint

The pattern and instructions for the wrist extension mobilization splint (forearm splint and hinge) can be used with minor changes. The material for the forearm splint is applied to the volar surface. Place a rectangular piece of warm material on the dorsal surface of the hand and mold it well over the bony areas. Once set, pad the inner surface of the splint to prevent migration and improve comfort. The Splint Tuner, shown here, is used to provide the wrist flexion mobilization force (A).

Fabricating a wrist mobilization splint to address both extension and flexion limitations is a cost-effective way to address multidirectional wrist stiffness, which is common after cast immobilization. The hinge can be effective in both directions, as described for the wrist extension mobilization splint. When the patient has finished using the extension component, the hand is taken out of the palmar cuff and the hinge is left to drop volarly. The dorsal cuff is then applied and directed to a volar proximal attachment device (B). The patient can alternate use of wrist extension and flexion per therapist recommendations (C).

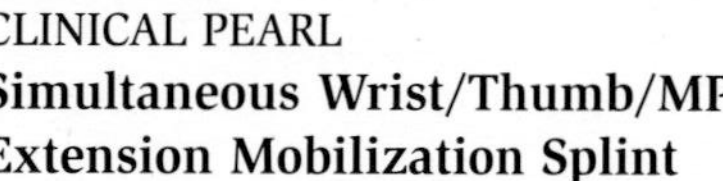

CLINICAL PEARL

Simultaneous Wrist/Thumb/MP/IP Extension Mobilization Splint

Patients who have sustained severe wrist fractures or extrinsic flexor tendon repairs, occasionally present with significant limitations in passive wrist extension and/or extrinsic flexor tendon adherence. A wrist extension mobilization splint can be converted to mobilize wrist extension and extrinsic flexor tendons simultaneously. The distal palmar bar of a wrist extension mobilization splint is replaced with a hand immobilization splint. To help achieve an intimate molding of the hand splint, make sure the wrist is flexed to place the extrinsic flexors on slack and allow optimal positioning of the digits in maximal extension during molding. If the thumb is included, the first web space should be positioned in maximal palmar abduction and opposition. Once set, punch holes at the level of the small finger and index finger MP joints. The nylon fasteners are attached at this level and directed to the distal bar of the hinge. The mobilization force is then connected and terminated on the proximal attachment device (A).

Note that if the contracture is severe, the distal bar (the side arms) may be too short to create an accurate 90° line of pull. A custom extended outrigger, fabricated from $^{3}/_{32}$" aluminum wire, can be fit in the side bar of the hinge. Several nylon fasteners may need to be linked together to accommodate the outrigger's extra length.

A serial static approach can address this same problem. Consider using QuickCast for digit and thumb IP extension splints and a volar thermoplastic base (made of elastic or rubber material to allow for frequent remolding as mobility increases) to serially elongate the extrinsic flexor tendons and increase the passive wrist motion.

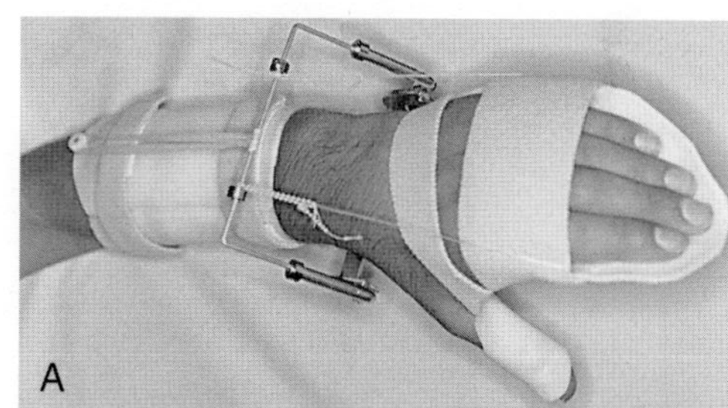
A

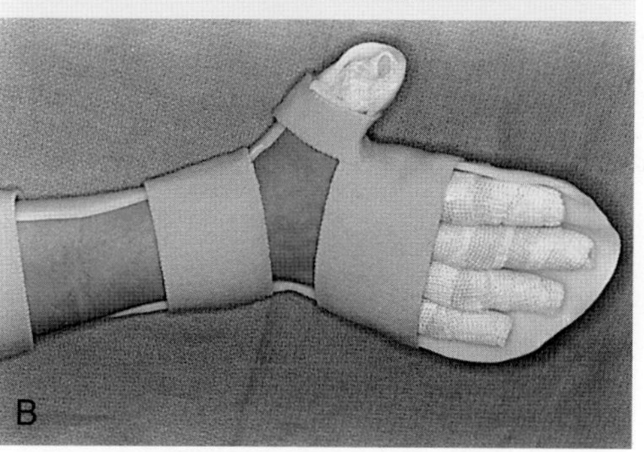
B

Wrist Extension, MP Flexion/Wrist Flexion, MP Extension Mobilization Splint (Fig. 8–15)[2]

Common Names

- Radial nerve palsy splint
- Tenodesis splint

Alternative Splint Options

- Phoenix extended outrigger kit
- Rolyan static radial nerve splint
- Wrist extension immobilization splint

Primary Functions

- Provide passive wrist and MP extension, allowing finger flexion, active wrist flexion, and digit and thumb extension. (Grasp and release through natural tenodesis action.)

Common Diagnoses and General Optimal Positions

- Radial nerve palsy
- Posterior interosseous nerve palsy

2. Designed by Judy C. Colditz, OTR/CHT.

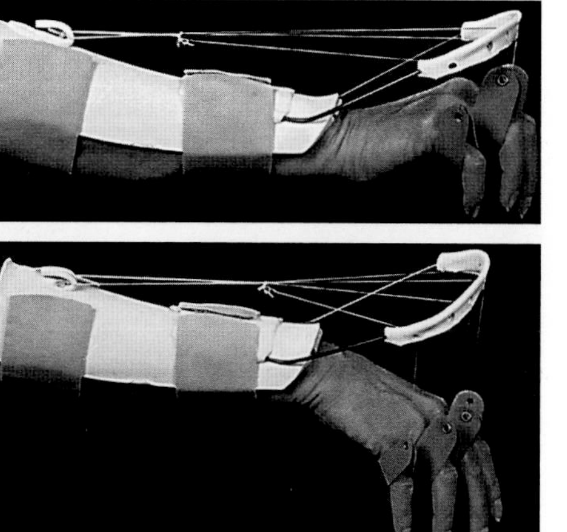

Figure 8–15

CLINICAL PEARL
Wrist Extension, MP Flexion/Wrist Flexion, MP Extension Mobilization Splint Using Phoenix Extended Outrigger

As an alternative, the Phoenix extended outrigger can be used to fabricate a wrist extension, MP flexion/wrist flexion, MP extension mobilization splint. This time-saving component is simple to apply. The rubber band posts secure the outrigger onto the splint base. Follow the manufacturer's instructions for specific outrigger application.

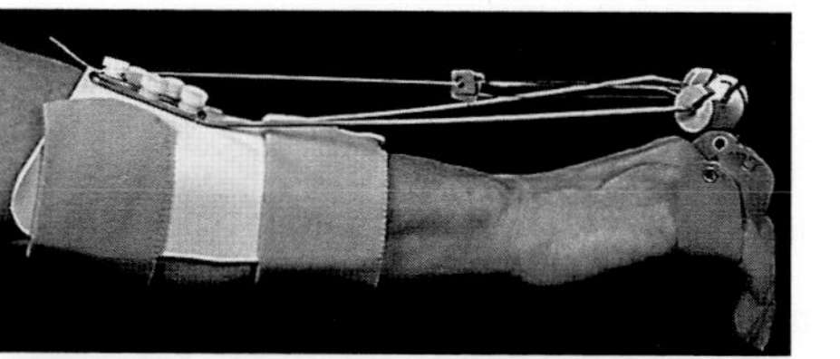

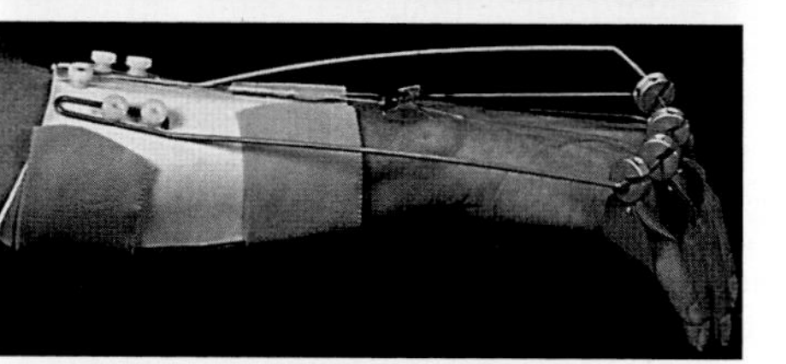

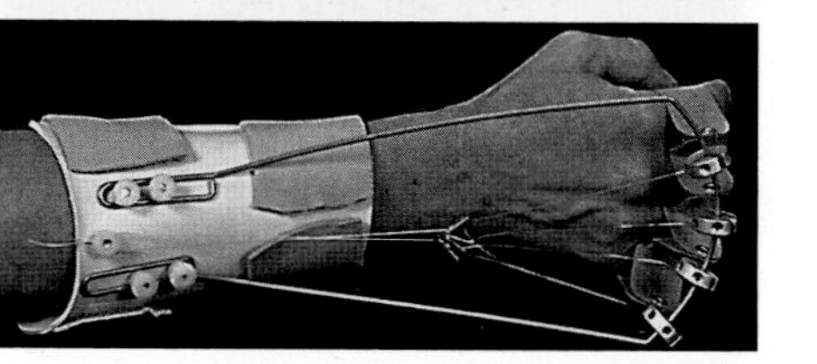

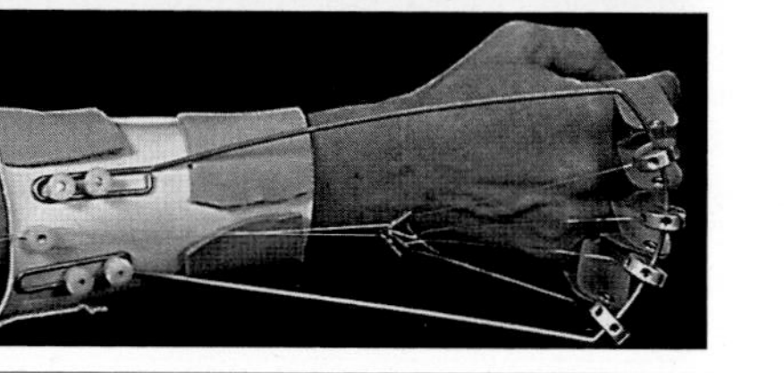

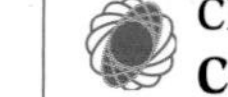

CLINICAL PEARL
Commercially Available Digit Slings

Several styles of slings are commercially available. Care should be taken with slings that converge into one line (also known as a loop). This design allows little accommodation for fluctuations in edema, potentially causing compressive forces about the lateral aspects of the digit, which may lead to neurovascular compromise.

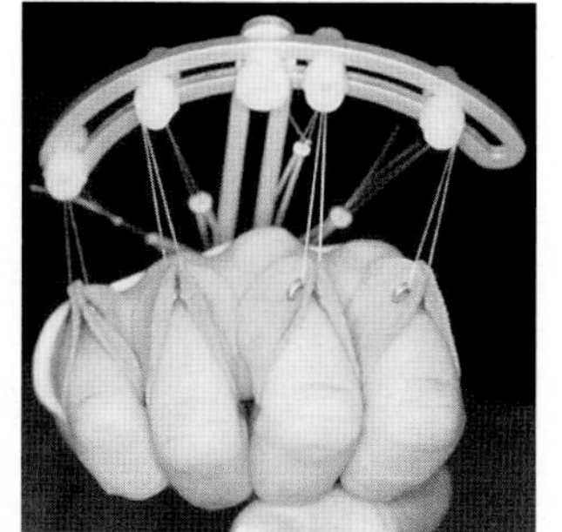

Fabrication Process

Pattern Creation (Fig. 8–16)

- Mark for dorsal forearm piece; proximal to wrist joint, and 1" to $1\frac{1}{2}$" in. distal to elbow crease.
- Circumference is half to two thirds of forearm.

Refine Pattern

- Adjust length and width appropriately.

Options for Materials

- Use $\frac{1}{8}$" thermoplastic material for splint base.
- Consider foam- or gel-lined materials to decrease distal splint migration.
- Cut two extra pieces of thermoplastic material (preferably noncoated): One to adhere outrigger onto splint base (2" by 2"), and one to form pulleys over distal outrigger wire (4" by 3") for individual proximal phalanx slings.

Cut and Heat

- Heat forearm piece while arm is resting pronated on table.

Evaluate Fit While Molding

- Apply heated material to forearm.
- Mold radial and ulnar aspects of forearm piece so they cup slightly.

Strapping and Components

- Apply distal and proximal strap to secure forearm splint. Elastic-based or D-ring-type straps may help prevent distal splint migration.
- Per pattern, bend an outrigger of $\frac{3}{32}$" wire into desired shape.
- Bend outrigger at level of wrist joint at approximately 40° of wrist extension.
- Off patient, heat proximal end of outrigger and apply it to splint. When placed on patient's hand, outrigger should rest at middle of each proximal phalanx with fist position.
- Check location of outrigger; if correct, apply solvent to splint surface around outrigger.
- Adhere warm piece of thermoplastic material intimately about outrigger (use solvent before heating) to form sturdy attachment, remembering that this area must accept weight of hand.
- Heat remaining strip of splinting material and apply to distal width of outrigger end, draping it over onto itself. Immediately trim to $\frac{1}{2}$" to $\frac{3}{4}$" width.

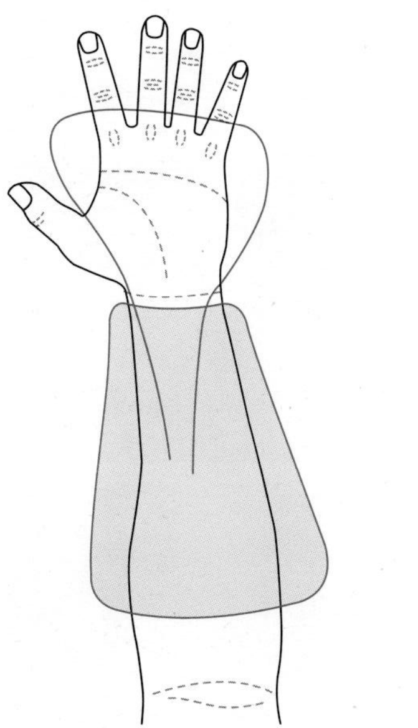

Figure 8–16

- When cool, mark and punch hole over middle of each proximal phalanx.
- Apply slings to cover two thirds length of proximal phalanxes. Premade leather slings work well, because they are soft, comfortable, and not bulky.
- Tie long piece of nylon line to each sling.
- Place sling under each proximal phalanx and direct cord through hole punched in splinting material on distal outrigger.
- Hold cords while patient lifts arm off of tabletop and passively opens and closes fist.
- Adjust tension on nylon lines so that MP joints are in 0° extension with neutral wrist, and wrist is in 20 to 30° extension with full finger flexion. Adjustment process may be easier with help of assistant.
- If dorsum of patient's hand touches outrigger during finger flexion, bend outrigger into greater extension.
- Once correct line tension has been determined, ask patient to again rest full fist on tabletop, so weight of hand is not on lines.
- Tie cords with firm knot and apply glue to secure it.

Splint Finishing Touches

- Flare distal edge and make sure that there is no abutment or irritation at ulnar styloid.
- If unlined material was used, consider lining splint with adhesive Dycem, gel, or Microfoam tape.

Thumb CMC Palmar/Radial Abduction Mobilization Splint

(Fig. 8–17)

Common Names

- CMC abduction splint
- Palmar abduction splint
- Thumb abduction splint

Alternative Splint Options

- Hand-based CMC abduction splint (serial static)
- Hand cones
- Air splints

Primary Functions

- Provide low-load, prolonged abduction mobilization force to first CMC joint to facilitate lengthening of tissue.

Common Diagnoses and General Optimal Positions

• Th CMC add contracture	Wr: 10 to 20° ext; CMC: terminal midpalmar and rad abd

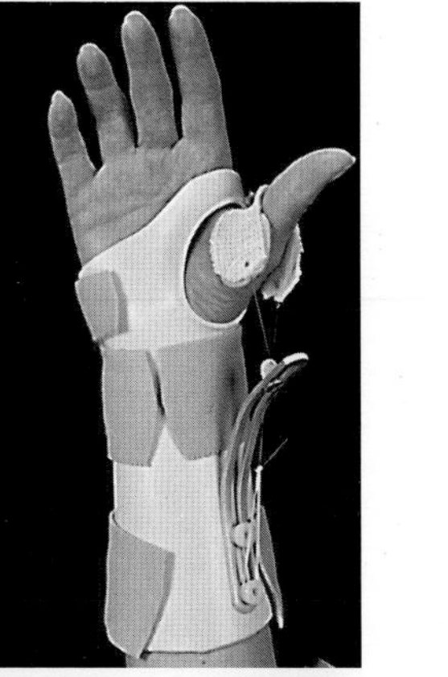

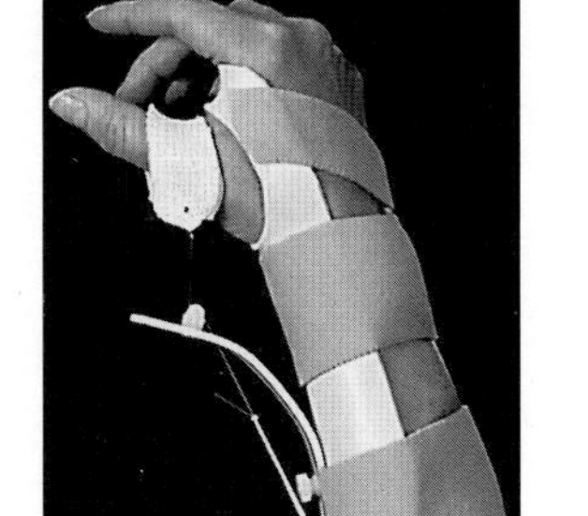

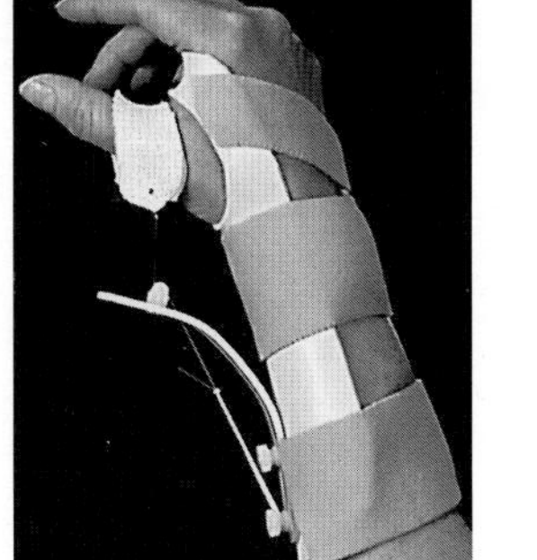

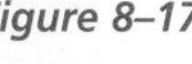

Figure 8–17

CLINICAL PEARL

Thumb CMC Radial Abduction, MP/IP Extension Mobilization Splint

Thumb flexion and adduction contractures can sometimes develop after flexor pollicis longus (FPL) repair or thumb fracture immobilization. Mobilization splinting can be a way to stretch the volar and ulnar soft tissue structures of the thumb. The dorsal wrist immobilization splint pattern is used for the splint base. The outrigger is aligned with the dorsal longitudinal axis of the thumb column and secured to the splint (a DigiTech outrigger is shown). A thermoplastic sling is molded to the volar thumb surface, supporting the proximal and distal phalanxes. Monofilament line is attached, threaded through the line guide on the outrigger, and attached proximally. Tension is adjusted per patient tolerance.

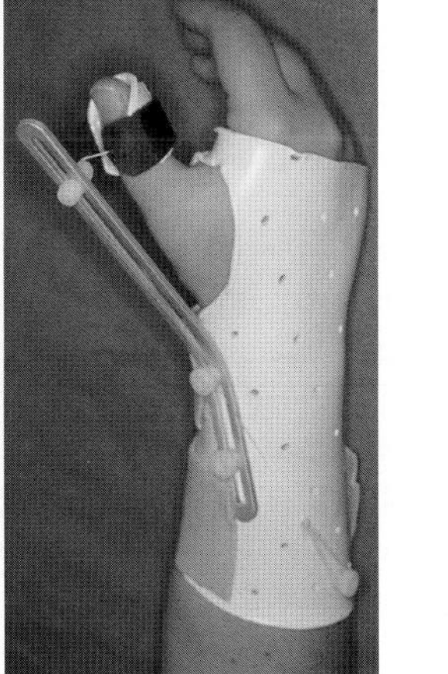

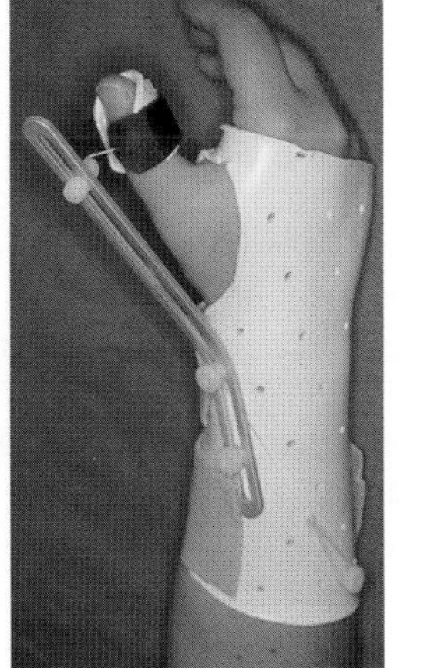

CLINICAL PEARL

Multipurpose Splint

Creating a splint that incorporates two functions—such as PIP flexion and PIP extension mobilization—can be a cost-saving measure and convenient for the patient. This splint addresses a stiff PIP joint with a custom outrigger for flexion mobilization and Phoenix outrigger for extension mobilization. The patient is effectively able to alternate between flexion and extension throughout the day using just one splint.

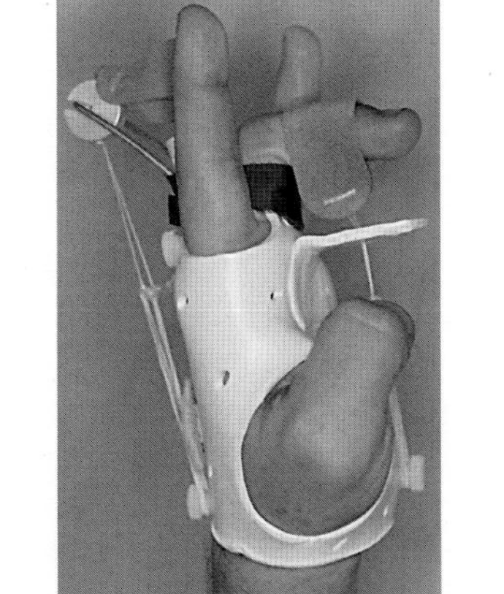

Fabrication Process (Using DigiTech System)

Pattern Creation (Fig. 8–18)

- Mark proximal border two thirds length of forearm.
- Mark distal border at distal palmar crease.
- Mark for thumbhole in distal central portion of pattern, approximately 1" down and in.
- Allow enough material to encompass half to two thirds circumference of forearm, remembering that forearm tapers distally.

Refine Pattern

- Proximal border should allow full elbow motion.
- Distal border should allow unimpeded motion of IF to MF MP joints and full thumb mobility.
- For average adult, thumbhole should be about size of elongated half dollar.

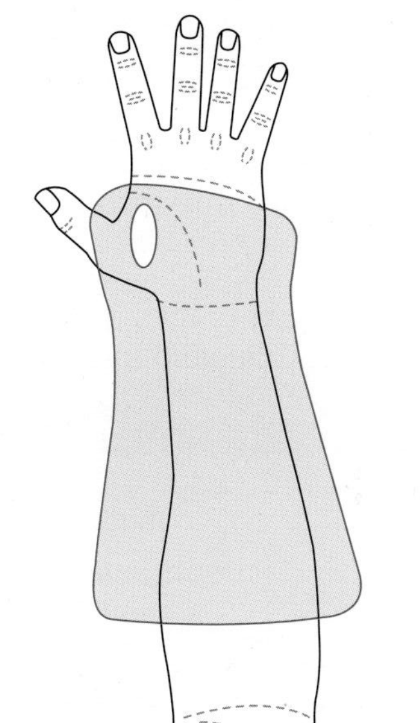

Figure 8–18

Options for Materials

- Consider 1/8" thermoplastic material to provide needed rigidity to withstand mobilization forces.
- Gel- or foam-lined materials may help decrease distal migration and increase comfort.
- Use components of choice (DigiTech outrigger system shown).

Cut and Heat

- Position patient with elbow resting on table and forearm supination for gravity-assisted molding; thumb should be held in gentle palmar abduction while molding.
- Cut out thumbhole in material either by making series of holes with hole punch before heating or by carefully piercing the slightly warm material with sharp scissors.

Evaluate Fit While Molding

- Lay warm material on towel, positioning thumbhole on correct side of material to be placed on forearm.
- Using index fingers, gently open hole, making it slightly larger and more elongated (egg shaped).
- Place thumbhole over thumb and guide rest of material evenly along volar wrist and forearm.
- Carefully incorporate arches of hand by using smooth, even strokes and constantly redirecting material into arches.
- Allow for clearance at base of CMC joint; as thumb abducts in splint, base of thumbhole may need to be adjusted.
- Rotate forearm at end of molding to check for possible abutment of ulnar and radial styloid processes, and flare as necessary.

Strapping and Components

- Distal strap: 1" strap directed from volar to dorsal border.
- Middle strap: 2" strap applied proximal to dorsal wrist crease; use piece of adhesive foam to further stabilize wrist in splint and prevent migration. Foam should not overlap splint edges.
- Proximal strap: depending on size of forearm, 1" or 2" strap.
- Position DigiTech outrigger along radial volar aspect of splint base.
- Position soft sling (sling made of QuickCast shown) in web space proximal to ulnar side of thumb MP (around metacarpal head). Positioning sling in this way directs forces to CMC joint, not MP joint ulnar collateral ligament.
- Check that sling and monofilament line are directed at 90° angle from first metacarpal; attachment on outrigger may appear more proximal than anticipated.
- Next, thread monofilament line to line guide on outrigger, attach mobilization force and secure to proximal attachment device.

Splint Finishing Touches

- Make sure sling does not irritate web space. Fabricating wider sling may assist in distributing pressure and increasing comfort.
- Adhesive-backed Dycem or silicone gel sheet may help sling stay in place.
- Smooth and slightly flare distal and proximal borders.
- Gently flare around thenar hole, especially at base; avoid rolling, which can make future splint modifications difficult and can lead to an unnecessarily bulky splint.
- Check clearance of elbow, irritation at radial and ulnar styloid processes, and digital MP motion.
- Adjust tension per patient and/or tissue tolerance; goal is low-load stretch over prolonged period of time.

MP Flexion Mobilization Splint

(Fig. 8-19)

Common Names

- Dynamic MP flexion splint

Alternative Splint Options

- Prefabricated splint
- Flexion glove

Primary Functions

- Provide low-load, prolonged flexion mobilization force to MP joint to facilitate lengthening of tissue.

Common Diagnoses and General Optimal Positions

• MP ext contracture	Wr: 10 to 20° ext; MP: terminal flexion

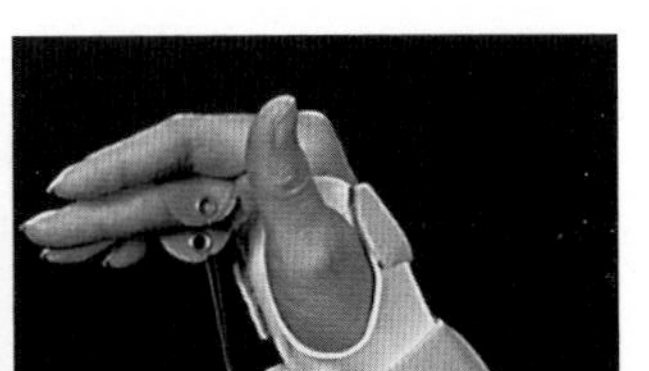
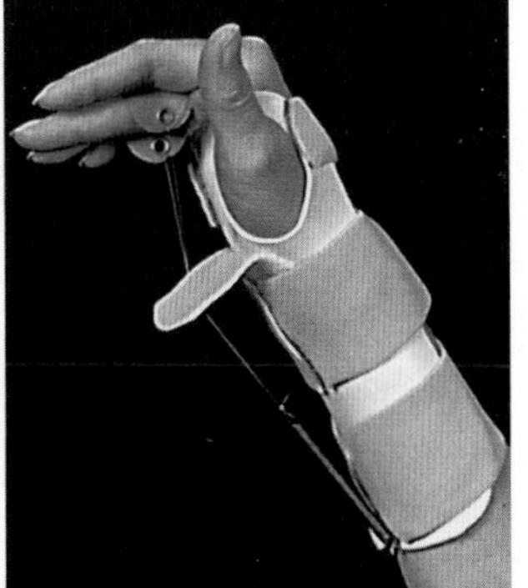

Figure 8–19

CLINICAL PEARL

MP Flexion Mobilization Splint Using Base2 Outrigger System

As an alternative, the Base2 outrigger system can be used to fabricate a MP flexion mobilization splint. Note the use of a MERiT component to provide a static progressive approach to mobilization. Follow the manufacturer's instructions for specific outrigger application.

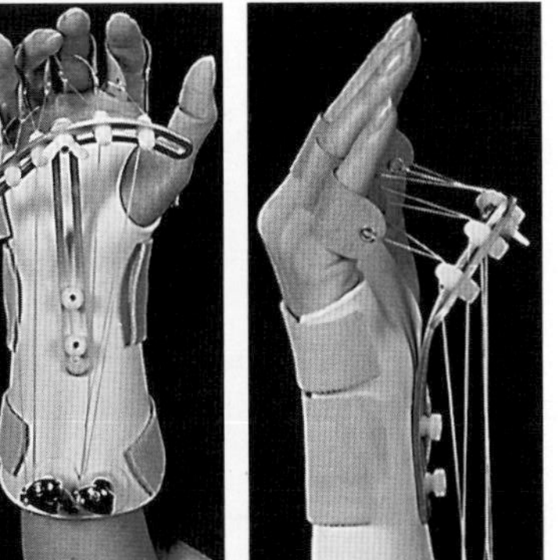
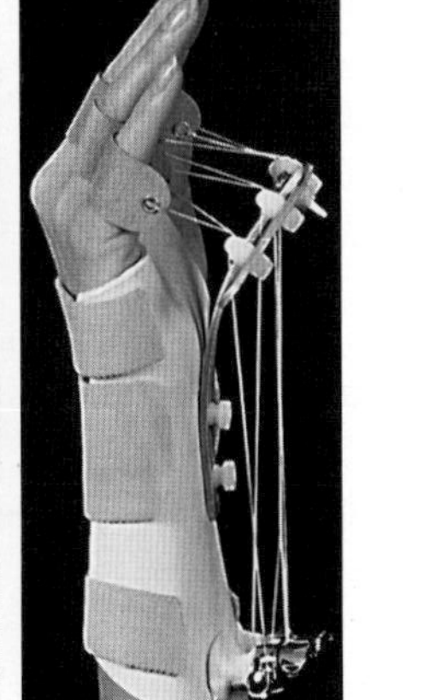
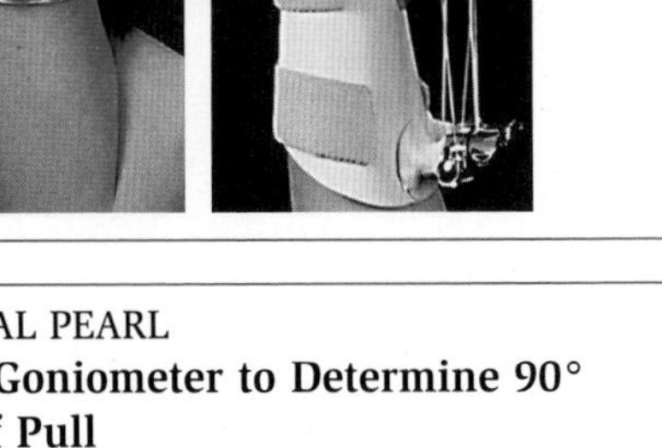
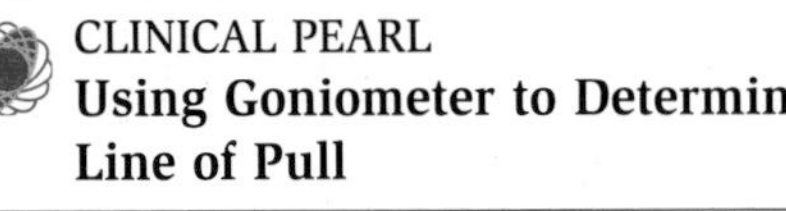

CLINICAL PEARL

Using Goniometer to Determine 90° Line of Pull

A goniometer ensures that a 90° line of pull has been achieved. This maximizes the effectiveness of the force application. Splints may need to be readjusted frequently, depending on the responsiveness of the tissue to the mobilization force.

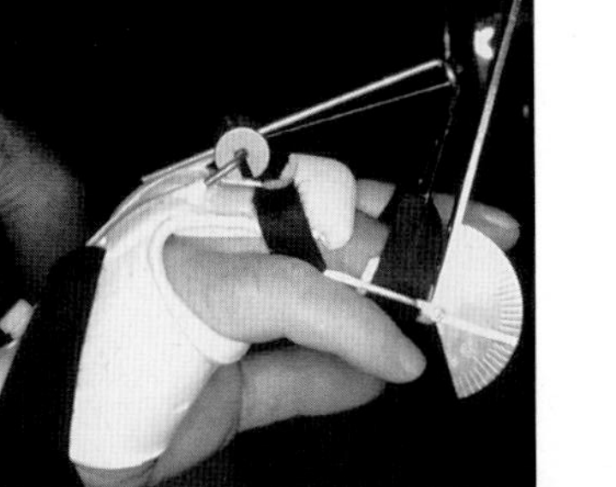

CLINICAL PEARL

Finger Sling Combined with Thermoplastic Material

Mold $^1/_{16}$" material to the volar (A) or dorsal (B) aspect of a digit to function as a sling. The material should extend the full length of the segment being mobilized (clearing the creases) and encompass half to two thirds the circumference of the segment. The thermoplastic sling maximally distributes pressure and prevents excessive compressive forces, which are sometimes caused by constrictive soft slings. A small strip of adhesive hook is placed on the mid-dorsal or volar portion of the sling. The midpoint of a 1" by 3" strip of loop material is placed over the adhesive hook. One hole is punched on both distal ends of the loop material. Monofilament line or elastic force is then attached at both ends of the loop and fed through the line guide and pulley to the proximal attachment device. A thin layer of foam can be added beneath the thermoplastic sling to increase comfort, if necessary.

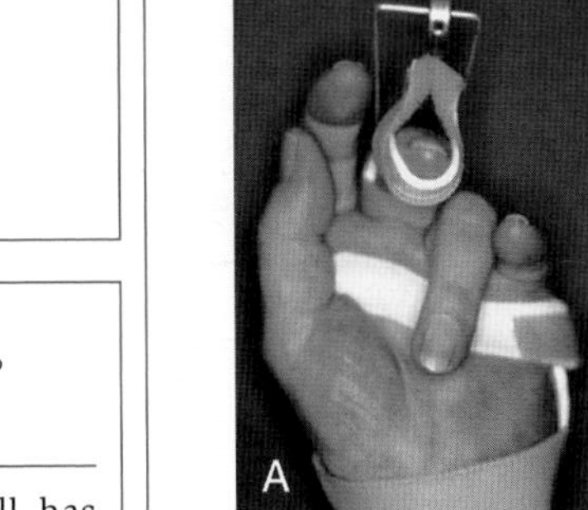

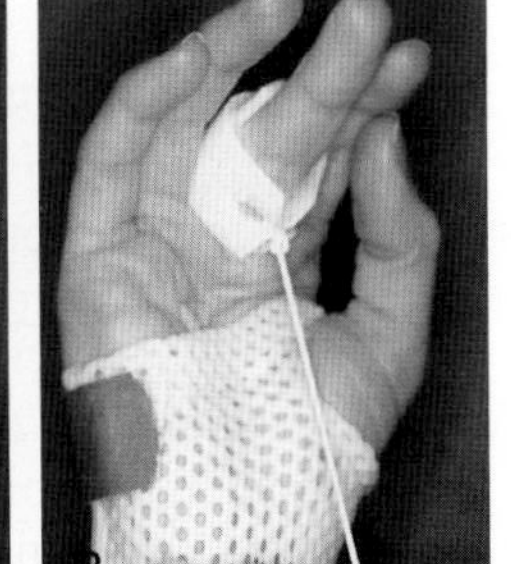

Fabrication Process

Pattern Creation (Fig. 8–20)

- Mark proximal border two thirds length of forearm.
- Mark distal border at distal palmar crease.
- Mark for thumbhole in distal central portion of pattern, approximately 1" down and in.
- Allow enough material to encompass half to two thirds circumference of forearm.

Refine Pattern

- Proximal border should allow elbow motion.
- Distal border should allow unimpeded motion of IF to MF MP joints and full thumb mobility.
- For average adult, thumbhole should be about size of elongated half dollar.
- Distal portion of splint should clear proximal palmar crease to allow MP flexion.

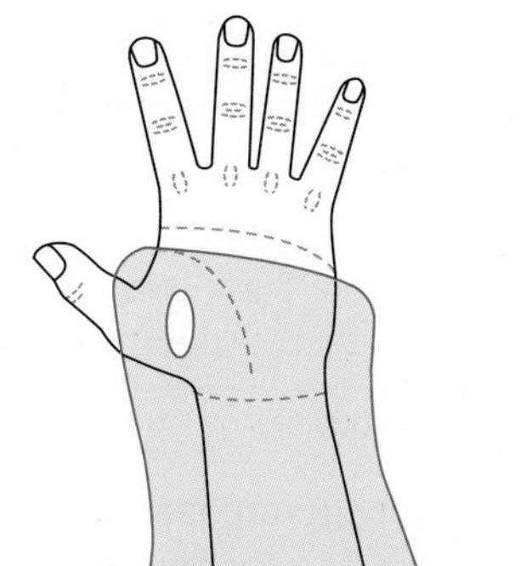

Figure 8–20

Options for Materials

- Use 1/8" material to provide needed rigidity to withstand mobilization forces.
- Gel- or foam-lined materials may help decrease distal migration and increase comfort.
- Custom-fabricated outrigger, made from 1/8" perforated material, acts as line guide. Solid thermoplastics can be used; however, smooth holes should be made using quality hole punch.

Cut and Heat

- Position patient with elbow resting on table and forearm supination for gravity-assisted molding.
- Cut out thumbhole in material either by making series of holes with hole punch before heating or by carefully piercing the slightly warm material with sharp scissors.
- Determine where outrigger should be positioned to achieve 90° angle of pull; it is generally placed at or about wrist crease and should be long enough to address degree of MP extension contracture.
- Prepare surface with solvent and heat thermoplastic outrigger.

Evaluate Fit While Molding

- Lay warm material on towel, positioning thumbhole on correct side of material to be placed on forearm.
- Using index fingers, gently open hole making it slightly larger and more elongated.
- Place thumbhole over thumb and guide rest of material evenly along volar wrist and forearm.
- Carefully incorporate arches of hand by using smooth, even strokes and constantly redirecting material into arches.
- Allow for clearance at base of CMC joint. As thumb abducts in splint, base of thumbhole may need to be adjusted.
- Rotate forearm to check for possible abutment of ulnar and radial styloid processes, and flare as necessary.

Strapping and Components

- Distal strap: 1" strap directed from volar to dorsal border.
- Middle strap: 2" strap applied proximal to dorsal wrist crease; use piece of adhesive foam to further stabilize wrist in splint and prevent migration. Foam should not overlap splint edges.
- Proximal strap: depending on size of forearm, 1" or 2" strap.
- Affix outrigger at correct angle on base.
- Mark holes on outrigger where monofilament will be threaded to apply correct angle of pull.
- Affix proximal attachment device; several are needed if multiple digits are involved.
- Affix individual slings to proximal phalanxes, thread monofilament through predetermined holes, attach mobilization force and attach to proximal attachment devices.
- Line of pull should be directed toward scaphoid bone, which follows natural cascade of digits.

Splint Finishing Touches

- Make sure that sling does not irritate web space. Fabricating wider slings may assist in distributing pressure and increasing comfort.
- Adhesive-backed Dycem or silicone gel sheet may help sling stay in place.
- Smooth and slightly flare distal and proximal borders.
- Gently flare around thenar hole, especially at base; avoid rolling, which can make future splint modifications difficult and can lead to an unnecessarily bulky splint.
- Check clearance of elbow, irritation at radial and ulnar styloid processes, and digital MP motion.

MP Flexion Mobilization Splint *(Continued)*

- As MP flexion gains are made, line of pull (changing hole in outrigger) must be adjusted and outrigger can be cut down.
- Adjust tension per patient and/or tissue tolerance; goal is low-load stretch over prolonged period of time.

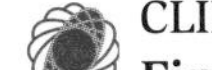

CLINICAL PEARL

Fingernail Attachment: Hook Material

Hook material (A). As an alternative to nail hooks, a small piece of hook strapping material (size should accommodate the length and width of the nail) can be glued to the fingernail using a gel-based glue. Once set, a strip of 1/2" loop (preferably soft material such as Velfoam or Betapile) can be added to the hook with the line attached and pulling proximally. This technique may work well for patients who have a large nail surface area.

Dress hook (B). A dress hook can be glued to the nail using a gel-based glue. Bend the hook slightly to provide optimal contour with the nail (contoured hooks can be purchased). Take care to place the hook as proximal on the nail as possible. If the hook is placed too far distally, the force may apply undue pressure on the nail bed. The line is either applied directly to the hook or attached first to a small piece of loop that has been attached to the dress hook. Some clinicians prefer this loop method, since it prevents the line from digging into the skin as it traverses over the fingertip.

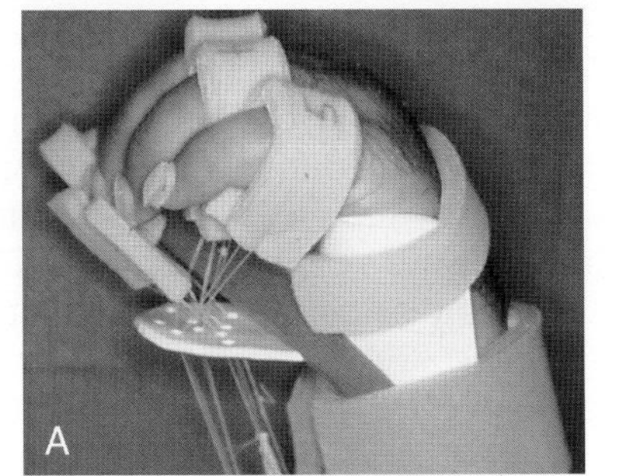
A

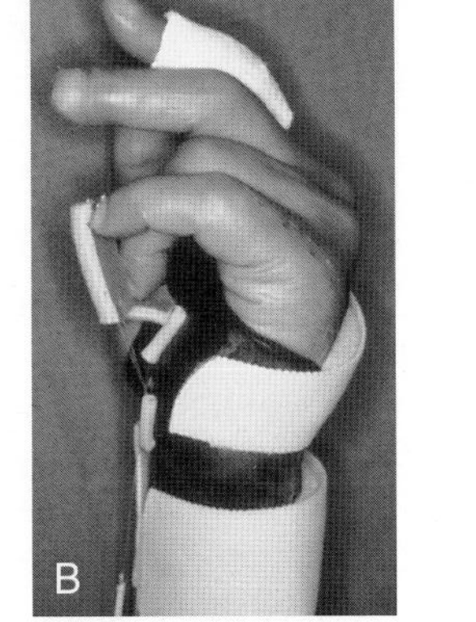
B

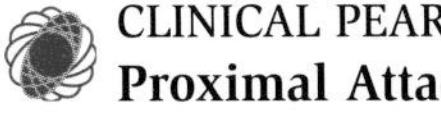

CLINICAL PEARL

Proximal Attachment Devices

A shows a splint being used as a mobilization device during the scar-remodeling phase of wound healing for a patient who sustained a severe crush injury. Rehabilitation focused on increasing digit ROM. Note the creative use of applying mobilization forces to the tissue. Static progressive stretch is applied to the MF via thin strapping material attached by hook on the nail and to the splint base proximally. The RF and SF are placed in PIP/DIP flexion mobilization straps. The SF has an additional sling that applies flexion force to the MP joint, creating a composite stretch to that digit. Note the Aquatube used as the custom-made proximal attachment device.

Paper clips and dress hooks can be bent, heated, and applied to the thermoplastic material. (B–far right) Rubber band posts and thumb nuts are also easy devices to apply to a splint for attaching mobilization components (B–middle). Another technique is to heat the small section where the proximal attachment device should be placed; then pierce through the material with scissors, lifting up from the splint base with a pencil (or similar object) to form an elongated hole that is approximately 4/5" This forms a raised area where rubber bands can be attached (B–far left).

Finally, commercially available devices provide a quick-and-easy way to attach mobilization components. They can be easily reused and/or adjusted. The splint shown has several holes for the rubber band post to allow for quick adjustment as ROM improves (C). Note that more than one device may be needed, depending on the number of rubber bands to be attached.

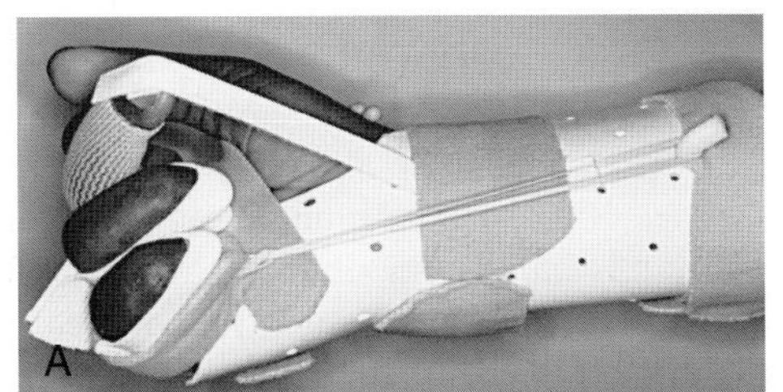
A

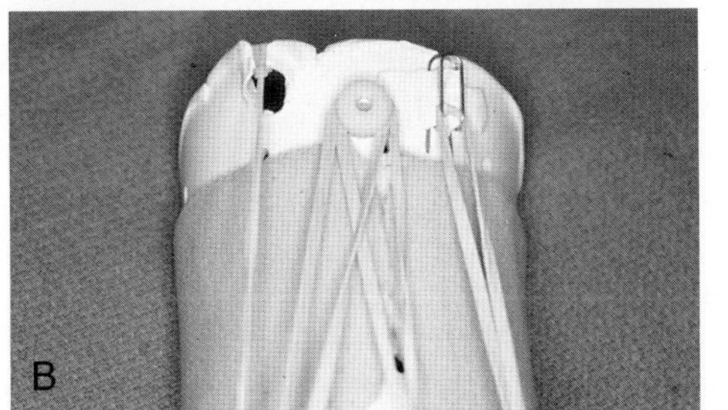
B

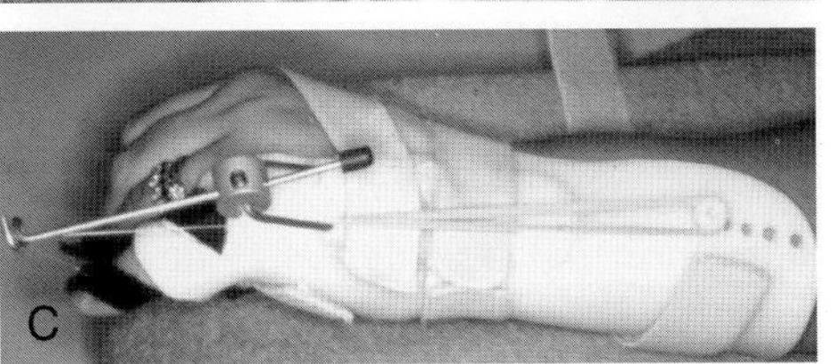
C

CLINICAL PEARL

Line Guides

Safety pin (A). A safety pin is a cost-effective way to provide a smooth and simple guide to a monofilament line. Shown is a combination PIP extension (dynamic) and PIP flexion (static progressive) mobilization splint. Note how the placement of the safety pin lifts the splint line off the dorsum of the MP joint, preventing the line from dragging across the splint base. To apply, bend and flatten the wide end of the safety pin. Heat this end with a heat gun and embed it into the desired area of the splint. This step should be completed with the splint off the patient's hand. Secure the safety pin by adding a scrap piece of thermoplastic material over the union. Allow the area to set before feeding the line through the hole.

Thermoplastic. A scrap piece of thermoplastic material can be used to create a line guide for an MP flexion mobilization splint (B). The length and width of the line guide depends on the location and severity of the contracture(s). Secure the line guide to the splint base while forming and maintaining a 90° angle with the segment that is to be mobilized (in this case the proximal phalanxes). Once set, use a hole punch to create holes at the appropriate area to form a 90° angle of force application. As ROM increases, create a new hole to maintain the desired angle of pull; the material can also be cut down. Highly perforated material provides many holes to choose from, eliminating the need for a hole punch.

An outrigger can be created by bending $^{3}/_{32}$" aluminum wire to form a dorsal segment (C). Cover it with heavily perforated material, slightly overlap the material at the wire's edge, then pinch and seal it. The slings are placed on the digits, and the line is threaded through the appropriate hole in the thermoplastic material to produce a 90° angle of pull. The rubber band or spring is then attached to the line and directed to the proximal attachment device.

Commercial. (D) Commercially available guides are simple to attach, remove, and reuse. However, some of these devices do not provide the extended length many splints require to obtain the desired 90°angle of force application. If the angle is not close to 90°, the line may drag through an edge of the line guide, creating increased frictional force.

Aquatube. Used as line guides, Aquatubes can prevent the lines from getting caught on an adjacent digit's line or on clothing and bed linens. Cut the Aquatube into $^{1}/_{4}$" disks, spot heat, and attach to a thermoplastic outrigger to create a line guide (E). Or cut it into small tubes (1" to 2") and use the pieces on the volar or dorsal surfaces to create a low-profile design (F).

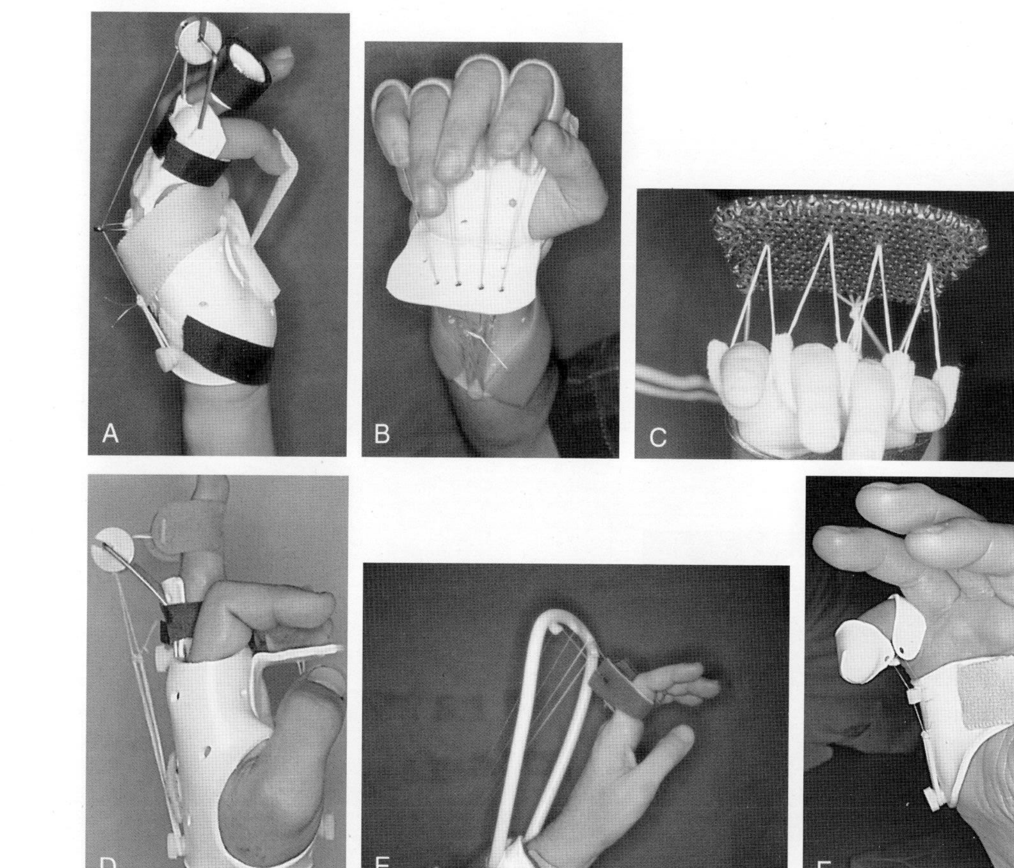

MP/PIP/DIP Flexion Mobilization Splint (Fig. 8-21)

Common Names

- Final finger flexion splint
- Composite flexion splint

Alternative Splint Options

- Finger flexion glove
- Phase II composite finger flexion loop attachments
- Prefabricated splints
- Splint Tuner final finger flexion kit
- Rolyan Biodynamic flexion system

Primary Functions

- Provide low-load, prolonged flexion mobilization force to MP, PIP, and DIP joints to facilitate lengthening of tissue.

Common Diagnoses and General Optimal Positions

- Extrinsic extensor tightness — Wr: 10 to 20° ext; MP/PIP/DIP: terminal flex
- MP, PIP, or DIP ext contractures — Wr: 10 to 20° ext; MP/PIP/DIP: terminal flex

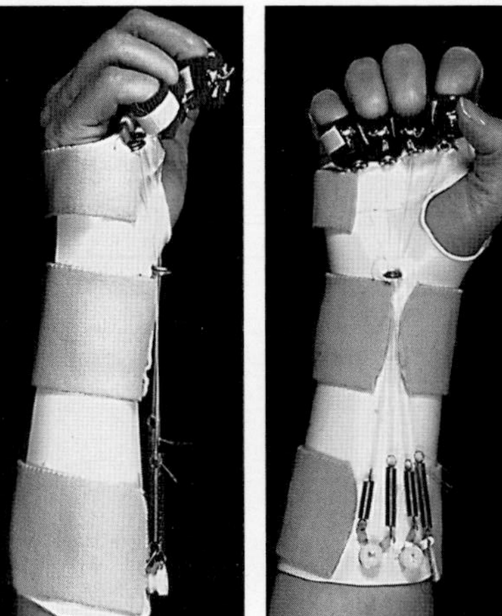

Figure 8–21

CLINICAL PEARL
Hand-Based Digit Composite Flexion Mobilization Splint

As an alternative when splinting a single digit, consider using a hand-based design ($^1/_{16}$" thermoplastic slings are shown).

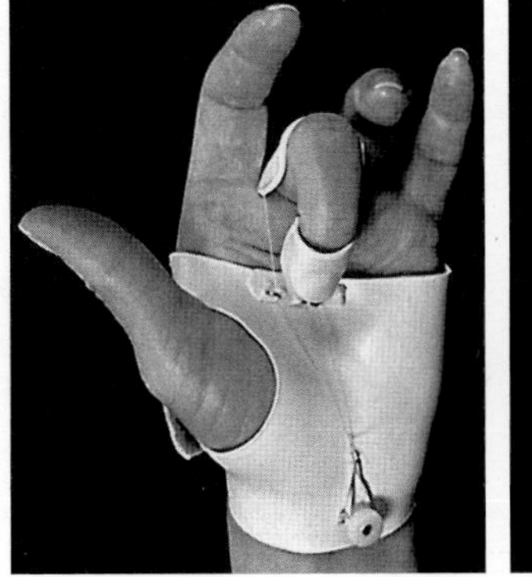
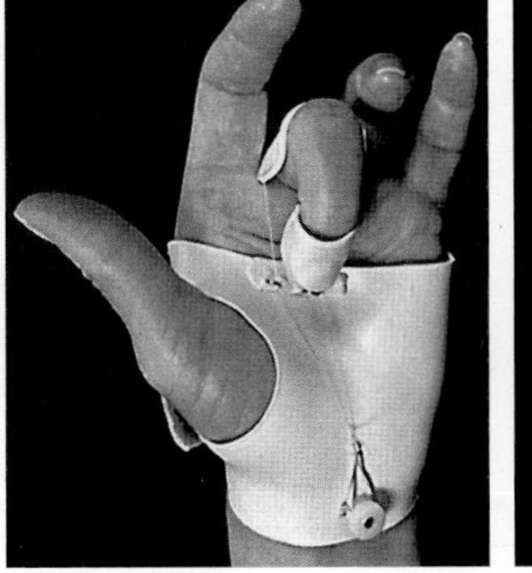

Fabrication Process

Pattern Creation (Fig. 8–22)

- Splint is most effective when MP and PIP joints have approximately 50% passive range of motion (PROM).
- Mark proximal border two thirds length of forearm.
- Mark distal border at distal palmar crease.
- Mark for thumbhole in distal central portion of pattern, approximately 1" down and in.
- Allow enough material to encompass half to two thirds circumference of forearm, remembering that forearm tapers distally.

Refine Pattern

- Proximal border should allow full elbow motion.
- Distal border should allow unimpeded motion of IF to MF MP joints and full thumb mobility.

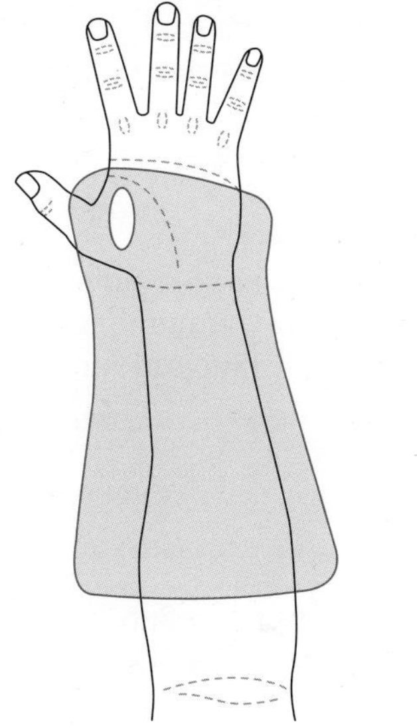

Figure 8–22

- For average adult, thumbhole should be about size of elongated half dollar.
- Distal volar portion of splint should clear proximal palmar crease to allow unimpeded MP flexion.

Options for Materials

- Consider 1/8" thermoplastic material to provide needed rigidity to withstand mobilization forces.
- Gel- or foam-lined materials may help decrease distal migration and increase comfort.

Cut and Heat

- Position patient with elbow resting on table and forearm supination for gravity-assisted molding. Thumb should be held in gentle palmar abduction while molding.
- Cut out thumb hole in material either by making series of holes with hole punch before heating or by carefully piercing the slightly warm material with sharp scissors.

Evaluate Fit While Molding

- Lay warm material on towel, positioning thumbhole on correct side of material to be placed on forearm.
- Using index fingers, gently open hole making it slightly larger and more elongated (egg shaped).
- Place thumbhole over thumb and guide rest of material evenly along volar wrist and forearm.
- Carefully incorporate arches of hand by using smooth, even strokes and constantly redirecting material into arches.
- Allow for clearance at base of first CMC joint. As thumb abducts in splint, base of thumbhole may need to be adjusted.
- Rotate forearm to check for possible abutment of ulnar and radial styloid processes, and flare as necessary.

Strapping and Components

- Distal strap: 1" strap directed from volar to dorsal border.
- Middle strap: 2" strap applied proximal to dorsal wrist crease; use piece of adhesive foam to further stabilize wrist in splint and prevent migration. Foam should not overlap splint edges.
- Proximal strap: depending on size of forearm, 1" or 2" strap.
- Apply line guides 1" to 3" from distal border of splint (approximately where digits would rest if composite fist were possible).
- Rolyan wrap-on finger hooks, used as distal attachment device, are shown.
- One or two lines guides per digit can be used. If using one line guide per digit, place in alignment with longitudinal axis of involved digit(s). If using two line guides, place in alignment with web spaces of involved digit(s).
- Line of pull should be directed toward scaphoid bone, which follows natural cascade of digits.
- Static line should be approximately triple length of hand; fold in half and guide from sling through line guides.
- Proximally, line is attached to rubber band post via springs.

Splint Finishing Touches

- Smooth and slightly flare distal and proximal borders.
- Gently flare around thenar hole, especially at base; avoid rolling, which can make future splint modifications difficult and can lead to an unnecessarily bulky splint.
- Check clearance of elbow, irritation at radial and ulnar styloid processes, and digital MP motion.
- Adjust tension per patient and/or tissue tolerance; goal is low-load stretch over prolonged period of time.

Thumb MP and IP Extension Mobilization Splint (Fig. 8–23)

Common Names

- Dynamic thumb extension splint
- Extensor pollicis longus (EPL) splint

Alternative Splint Options

- Casting (serial static)

Primary Functions

- Provide low-load, prolonged extension mobilization force to thumb MP and IP joints to facilitate lengthening of tissue.

Alternative Functions

- Maintain thumb MP and IP joints in extension, allowing restricted flexion within predetermined range, to facilitate tendon healing, tendon glide, and prevent tendon adherence (restriction splint).

Common Diagnoses and General Optimal Positions

• IP and MP flex contracture	Wr: 20 to 30° ext; CMC: mid rad/palmer abd; MP/IP: terminal ext

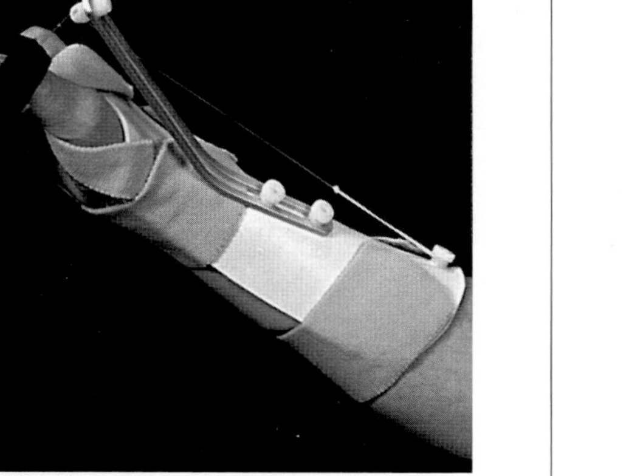

Figure 8–23

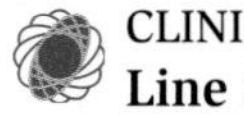

CLINICAL PEARL
Line Stops

Line stops provide the ability to limit a particular degree of motion. The device shown here requires pliers to press the stop in place. Stops are particularly helpful for treating extensor tendon injuries, for which limiting full ROM is needed to protect a healing repair.

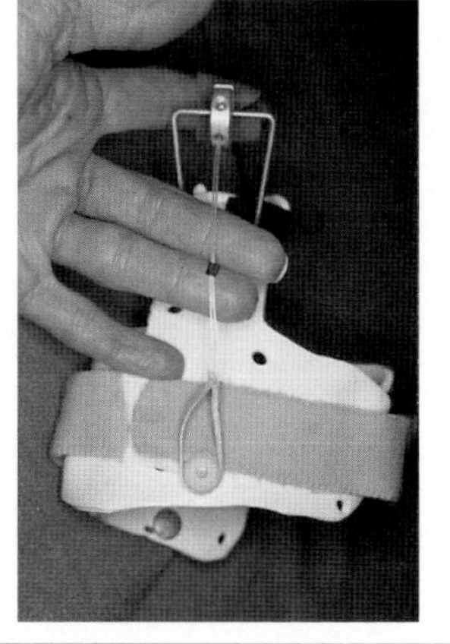

Fabrication Process (Using Base2 Outrigger System)

Pattern Creation (Fig. 8–24)

- Mark for proximal border two thirds length of forearm.
- Mark distal border, just proximal to dorsal digit and thumb MP joint skinfolds.
- Allow enough material to encompass half to two thirds circumference of forearm, remembering that forearm tapers distally.

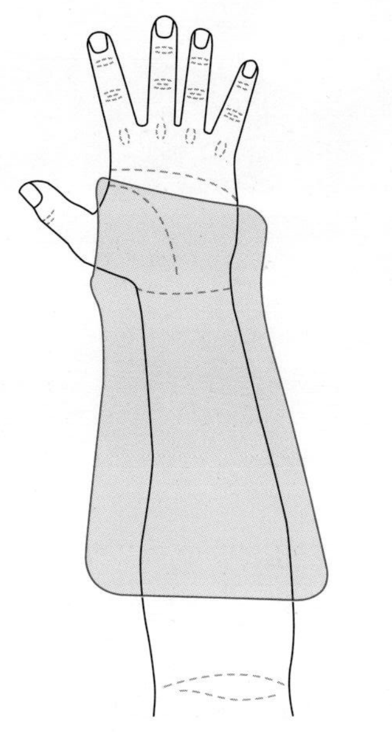

Figure 8–24

Refine Pattern

- Proximal border should allow full elbow motion.
- Distal border should allow unimpeded motion of digital MP and thumb MP and IP joints.
- Allow appropriate amount of material radially to provide surface area for component application.

Options for Materials

- Use 1/8" material to provide needed rigidity to maintain wrist joint position and accept extension mobilization force.
- Use components of choice (Base2 outrigger system show).

Cut and Heat

- Position patient with elbow resting on table and forearm pronated for gravity-assisted molding. Position thumb in abduction and opposition.
- Prepad ulnar styloid with adhesive-backed foam, putty, cotton ball, or silicone gel.

Evaluate Fit While Molding

- Position material on dorsum of involved hand and wrist just proximal to MP joints.
- Make sure desired wrist position is maintained. Some patients tend to flex and deviate wrist while splint is being formed.

Strapping and Components

- Thumb strap: apply volarly, allowing MP motion.
- Distal strap: 1" strap connecting distal radial and distal ulnar borders.
- Middle strap: 2" strap just proximal to dorsal wrist crease; use piece of adhesive foam to further stabilize wrist in splint and prevent migration. Foam should not overlap splint edges.
- Proximal strap: 2" soft or elasticized strap is good choice.
- Attach Base2 outrigger to splint base using rubber band posts. Be sure outrigger aligns with thumb column and extends distally entire length of thumb.
- Apply sling to distal phalanx thread monofilament line through line guide on outrigger, and secure mobilization component to proximal attachment device.

Splint Finishing Touches

- Smooth and slightly flare distal and proximal borders.
- Gently flare around dorsal thumb region; avoid rolling, which can make future splint modifications difficult and can lead to an unnecessarily bulky splint.
- Check clearance of elbow, radial and ulnar styloid processes, thumb, and MP joints.
- Adjust tension per patient and/or tissue tolerance; goal is low-load stretch over prolonged period of time.

MP Extension Mobilization Splint (Fig. 8–25)

Common Names

- Dynamic MP extension splint

Alternative Splint Options

- Rolyan preformed adjustable outrigger
- Prefabricated splint

Primary Functions

- Provide low-load, prolonged extension mobilization force to MP joints to facilitate lengthening of tissue.
- Passively support MP joints in extension while allowing active digital flexion.

Common Diagnoses and General Optimal Positions

Diagnosis	Position
• MP jt arthroplasty:	Wr: 30 to 45° ext; MP: 0 to 10° flex and slight RD
• Extensor tendon repair (zones V to VII)	Wr: 30 to 45° ext; MP: 0 to 10° flex (th zones IV to V) (if th involved: CMC ext and 45° rad abd)
• Radial or posterior interosseous nerve injury	Wr: 30 to 45° ext, MP: 0°
• Extrinsic flexor tightness	Wr: 45+°, IP: 0°, MP: terminal ext

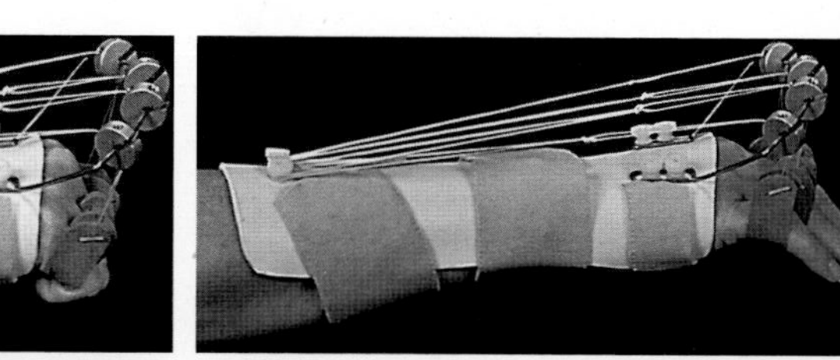
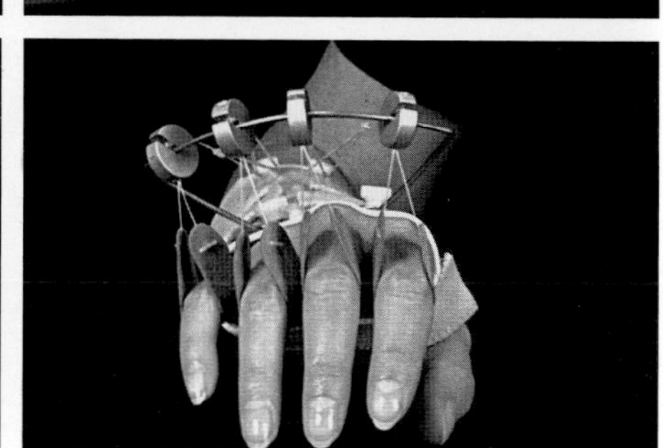
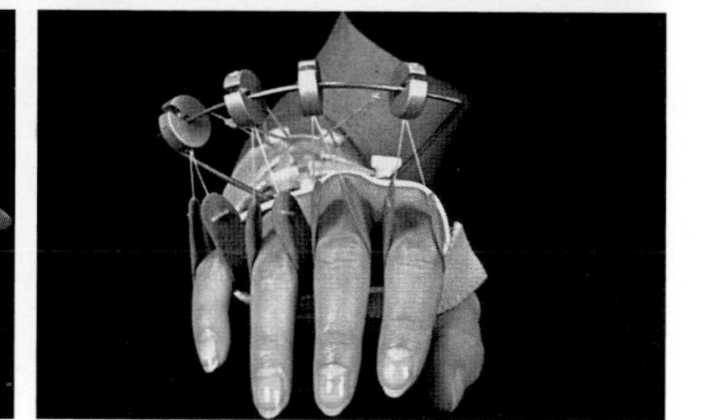

Figure 8–25

CLINICAL PEARL

PIP/DIP Extension Splints with MP Extension Mobilization Splint

A PIP/DIP extension mobilization splint or cast can be slipped under the slings of a MP extension mobilization splint to prevent or address concurrent PIP flexion contractures. These splints can be worn periodically throughout the day as an exercise tool to stretch tight PIP joints or to isolate or facilitate MP flexion with exercise.

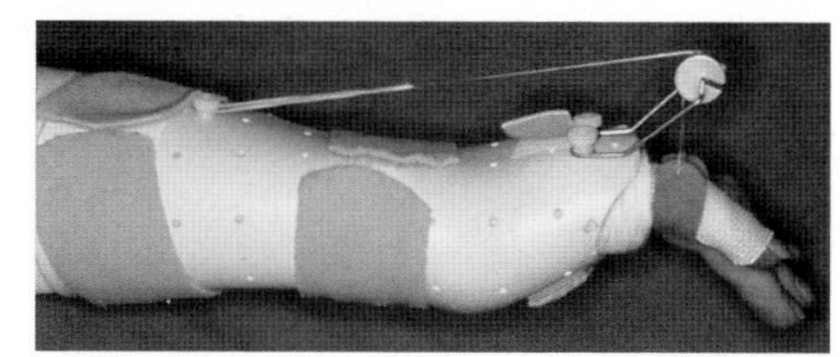

Fabrication Process (Using Phoenix Outrigger System)

Pattern Creation (Fig. 8–26)

- Mark for proximal border two thirds length of forearm.
- Mark distal border, just distal to dorsal digit MP joint skinfolds.
- Make radial tab (palmar bar) long enough (approximately 3") to traverse through palm and secure on distal ulnar border.
- Allow enough material to encompass half to two thirds circumference of forearm, remembering that forearm tapers distally.

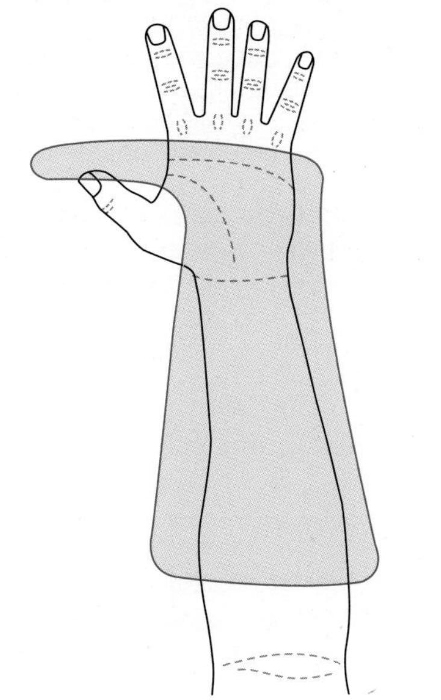

Figure 8–26

Refine Pattern

- Proximal border should allow full elbow motion.
- Extend distal portion of splint to MP head level.

Options for Materials

- Consider $1/8$" thermoplastic material to provide needed rigidity to maintain wrist joint position and accept extension mobilization force.
- Use components of choice (Phoenix outrigger system shown).

Cut and Heat

- Position patient with elbow resting on table and forearm pronated for gravity-assisted molding.
- Prepad ulnar styloid using adhesive-backed foam, putty, cotton ball, or silicone gel.

Evaluate Fit While Molding

- Position material on dorsum of involved hand and wrist just distal to MP joints.
- Gently pull radial bar through thumb web space and across volar MPs to meet ulnar segment. Pinch and seal lightly, and return focus to molding dorsum.
- Make sure desired wrist position is maintained. Some patients tend to flex and deviate wrist while splint is being formed.

Strapping and Components

- Distal strap: 1" strap connecting distal radial and distal ulnar borders (if needed).
- Middle strap: 2" strap just proximal to wrist crease; use piece of adhesive foam to further stabilize wrist in splint and prevent migration. Foam should not overlap splint edges.
- Proximal strap: 2" soft or elasticized strap.
- Mark desired outrigger attachment, positioning to extend distally over distal portion of proximal phalanx just proximal to PIP joints and extending high enough that, when volar sling is attached to monofilament line, it clears pulley.
- Use rubber band posts to secure outrigger on splint.
- Attach Phoenix wheels to outrigger using Allen wrench.
- Attach line on both sides of sling, apply sling to middle phalanx, and thread line through Phoenix wheels.
- Loop appropriate rubber band onto end of monofilament line, and connect to proximal attachment device.

Splint Finishing Touches

- Material should be flared distally to prevent irritation of MP heads during flexion exercises; if necessary, use layer of thin padding to increase patient comfort.

MP Extension Mobilization Splint *(Continued)*

- Check that mobilization force is strong enough to support and return MP joints to desired position after active digital flexion.
- Check that mobilization force is not too strong, impeding patient's ability to flex digits desired amount.
- Instruct patient to monitor for signs of increased pressure over ulnar styloid and radial and ulnar sensory nerve branches.

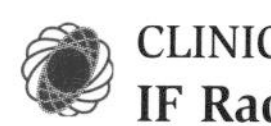

CLINICAL PEARL

IF Radial Outrigger to Prevent Pronation and Ulnar Deviation

An IF outrigger attachment is most often found in combination with an MP extension mobilization splint for patients who have undergone MP joint arthroplasty involving reconstruction of the IF radial collateral ligament. Consider applying an ulnarly positioned dress hook (with gel-based glue) or a piece of hook material to the fingernail. If using the dress hook, attach a thin strip of loop material (via a hole) directed ulnarly, crossing the volar aspect of the fingertip. Fasten a thin rubber band to the other end and attach it to the radial outrigger. If using adhesive hook material glued to the nail, place a thin strip of loop, directed as described for the dress hook. This should provide a gentle radial deviation and supination force to the IF. Note: If pronation is not an issue, a sling can be applied to the digit, directed radially.

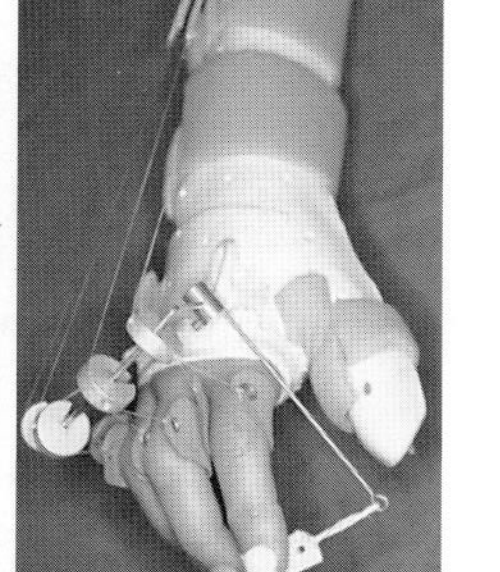

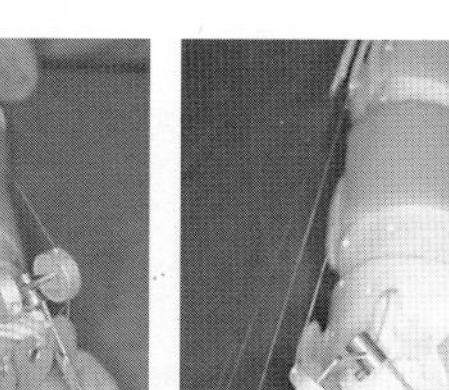

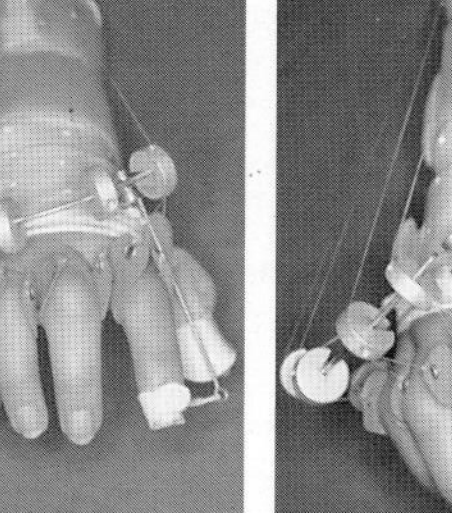

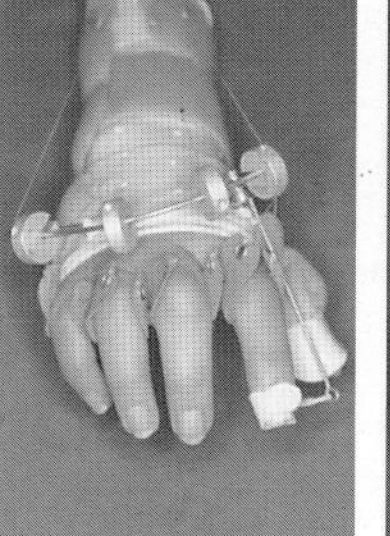

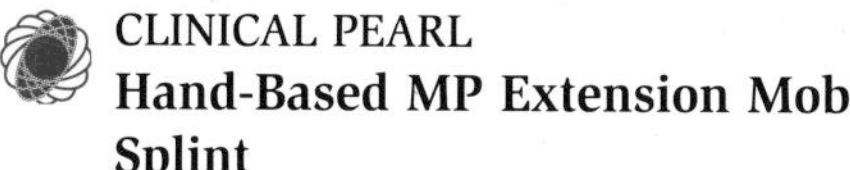

CLINICAL PEARL

Hand-Based MP Extension Mobilization Splint

The MP extension mobilization splint can be modified to a hand-based design. Shown here is the Rolyan adjustable outrigger system. Follow the manufacturer's instructions for specific outrigger application.

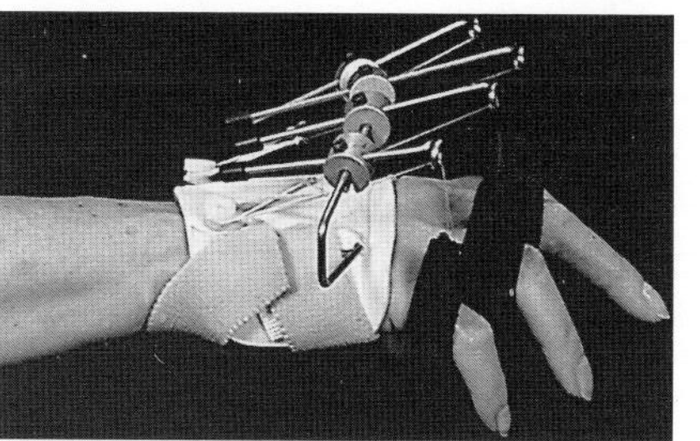

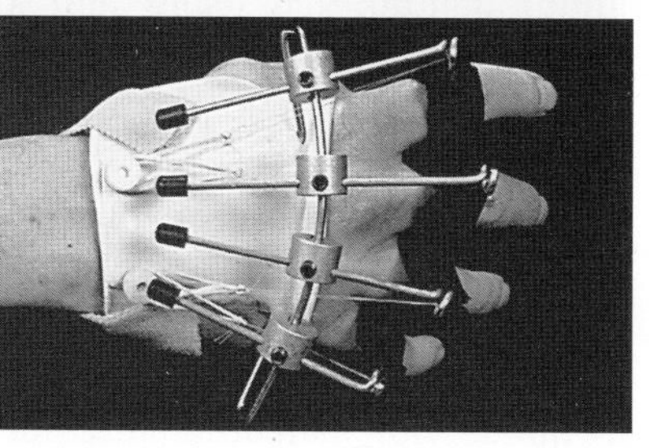

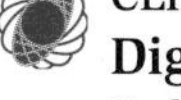

CLINICAL PEARL

DigiTech MP Extension Mobilization Splint

As an alternative, the DigiTech system can be used to fabricate a MP extension mobilization splint. Follow the manufacturer's instructions for specific outrigger application.

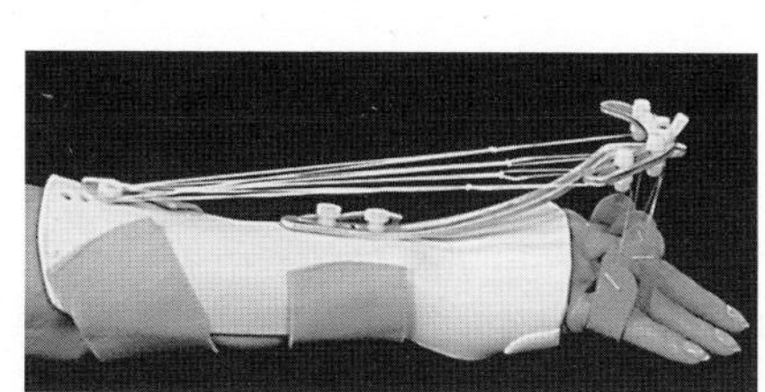

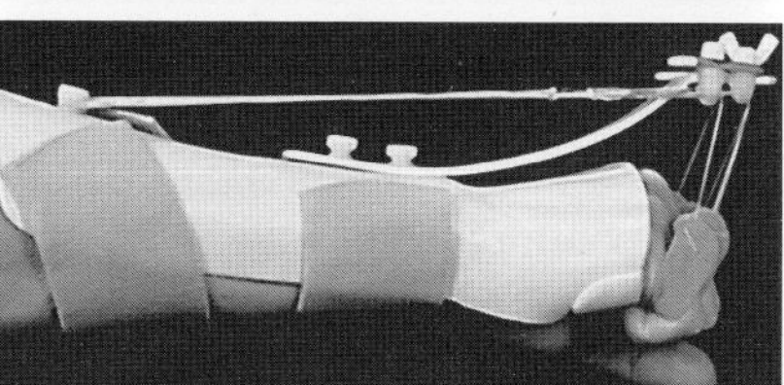

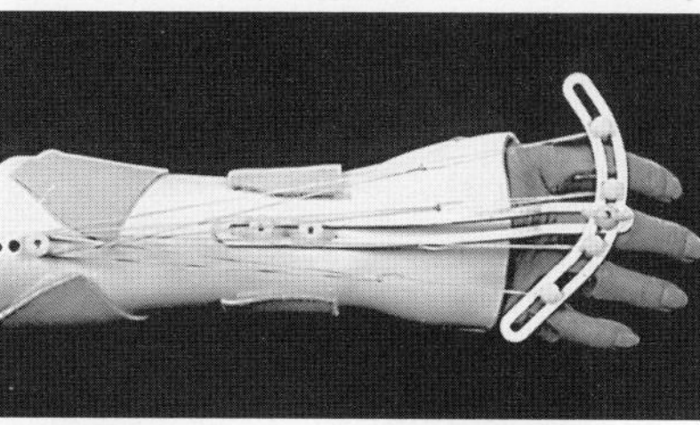

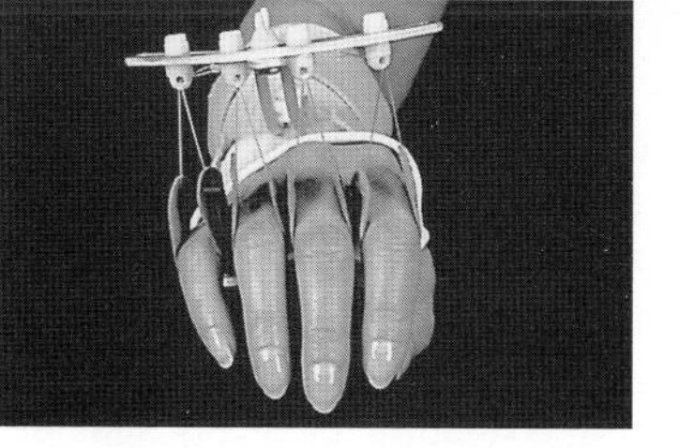

CLINICAL PEARL
Mobilization Forces

Elastic cord (A). Wrapped elastic cord is a quick and commonly used method for providing a mobilization force for dynamic splints. The wrapped elastic can be directly fastened from the sling to the proximal attachment device. Be aware that if the cord traverses through line guides, the friction (or drag) may alter the force placed on the intended structures. Because the elastic cord is wrapped with cotton it is less elastic and forgiving than rubber bands and should not be treated in the same way. Doubling the resting length of the cord will generate a much greater tension than doubling the length of a rubber band. This combination custom MP flexion mobilization splint includes a Phoenix outrigger for PIP extension mobilization.

Rubber bands (B). Rubber bands are the most commonly used component for generating tension in mobilization splints. They are readily available, inexpensive, easy to apply and adjust, and come in a variety of lengths and widths. Be aware that the tension generated is directly related to the rubber band's length and width. Thinner rubber bands provide less tension and are more susceptible to fatigue and breaking, thus they need to be replaced more often. The splint shown is a custom PIP flexion mobilization splint.

Spring coils (C). Graded spring coils offer a consistent way to control force accurately in a dynamic splint. Springs generate a given force based on their overall length and width, coil tightness, and the distance they have to travel from the proximal to distal attachment. Springs have been shown to be more durable and to last longer than rubber bands. However, they are more expensive than rubber bands and elastic cord. A clinic should have a variety of springs on hand to address a potential range of needs, although this may not always be feasible. The PIP joint fracture distraction splint shown includes a Base2 outrigger.

TheraBands (D). TheraBands work especially well with forearm-based designs such as wrist extension mobilization and forearm rotation mobilization splints. The force delivered to the tissue depends on the tension property of the band. A custom wrist and digit extension mobilization splint is shown.

Tape (E). Microfoam tape can be used to quickly fabricate a mobilization splint. The tape can be adjusted easily and can be effectively reused several times. A custom PIP flexion mobilization splint is shown.

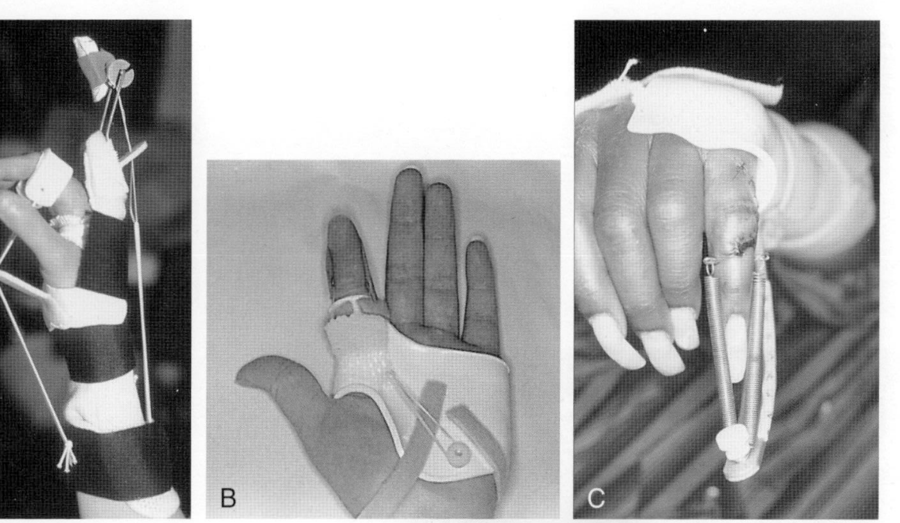

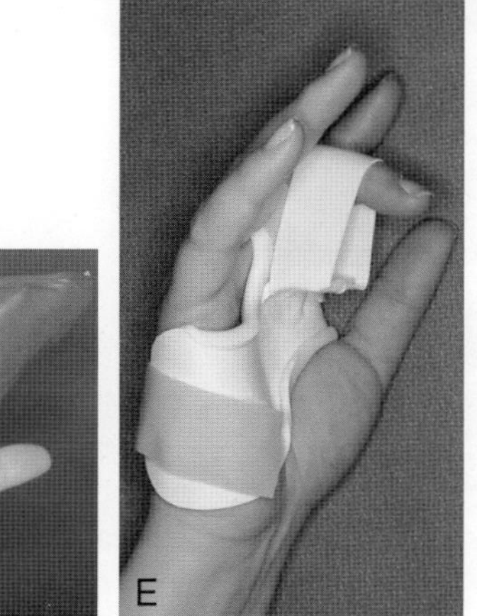

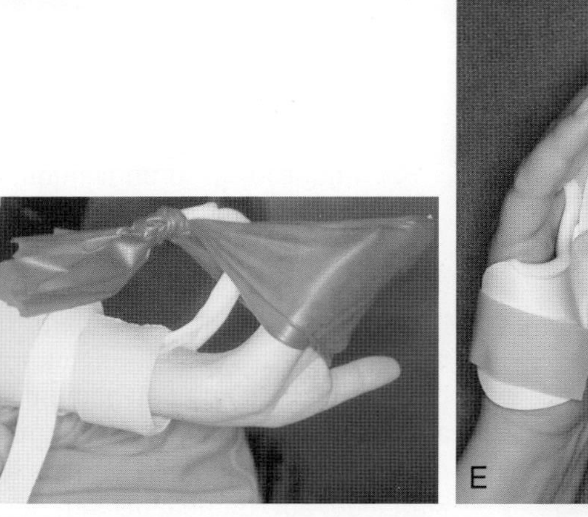

PIP Intra-Articular Mobilization Splint (Fig. 8–27)[3]

Common Names

- Dynamic traction splint
- Schenck splint

Primary Functions

- Provide gentle, controlled distal distraction to involved PIP joint to reduce articular fragments and realign joint surfaces.

3. Developed by Robert Schenck, MD, Laura Kearney, OTR/L, CHT, Krista Brown, OTR/L, CHT.

Common Diagnoses and General Optimal Positions

Note: Direction of distal traction, tension on rubber band, and passive arc of flexion and extension are set by the surgeon in the operating room. Any alteration to these placements should be discussed with the surgeon. This splint can be modified to accommodate intra-articular MP and thumb MP/IP joint injuries (Kearney & Brown 1994, Schenck, 1986, 1994).

- Pilon fracture of PIP
- Fracture dislocation of PIP
- Severe fracture of grade 3 or 4; grade 2 if combined with subluxation or dislocation
- Condylar fracture
- Oblique or spiral phalangeal shaft fracture

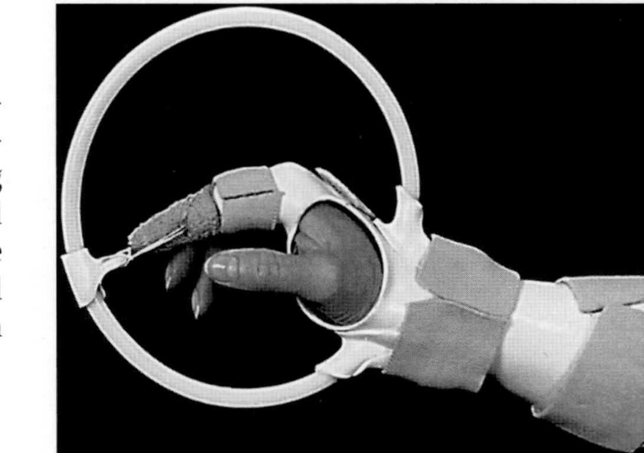

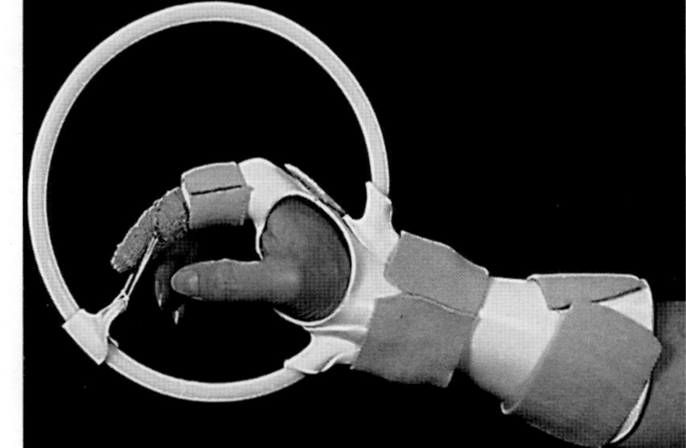

Figure 8–27

Fabrication Process

Pattern Creation (Fig. 8–28)

- Splint should be fabricated preoperatively or in operating room as physician places wire.
- Choose appropriate base pattern for digit.
  - * IF or MF (A): Radial wrist extension and MP flexion immobilization splint
  - * RF or SF (B): Ulnar wrist extension and MP flexion immobilization splint
  - * Thumb: Wrist and thumb MP immobilization splint or wrist immobilization splint.
- Fabricate 6" hoop or partial hoop.

Refine Pattern

- Make sure wrist is extended approximately 30° and MP joints flexed to approximately 60°.
- Splint can encompass bordering digit for maximal splint stabilization if necessary. Do not interfere with motion of uninvolved digits.
- Clear PIP flexion crease proximally.

Options for Materials

- Use $^{3}/_{32}$" or $^{1}/_{8}$" material.
- Hoop can be made from rolled thermoplastic material or wide Aquatubes.

Cut and Heat

- Prepare hoop by warming material around 6" cylindrical form (e.g., 5-lb therapy putty container) leaving about 1" extension on each end for attachment onto splint base.
- Position patient with forearm in neutral and digits slightly abducted.

Evaluate Fit While Molding

- Fabricate appropriate ulnar or radial wrist extension and MP flexion immobilization splint.
- Clear distally to allow unimpeded PIP flexion.

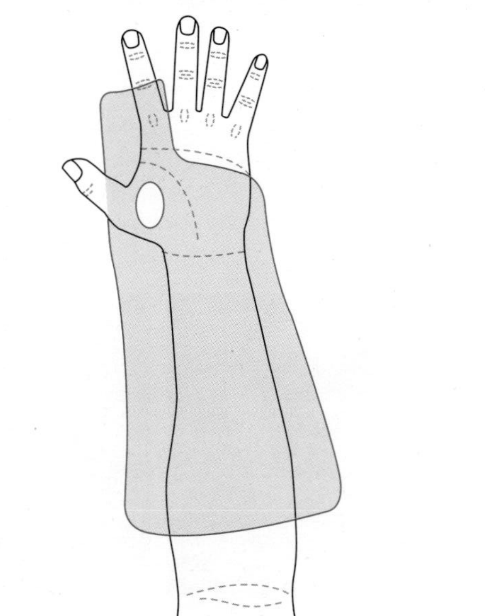

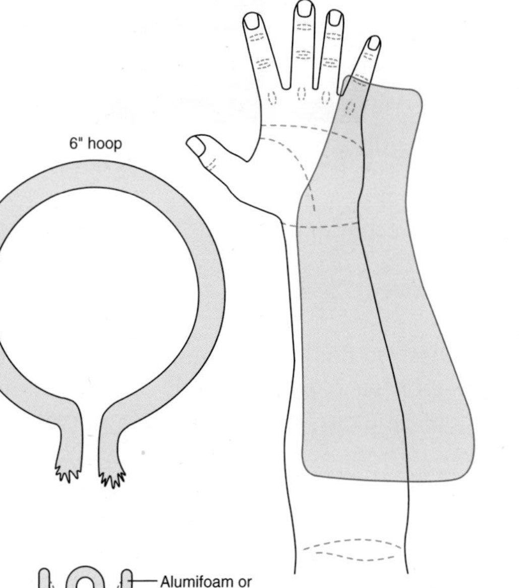

Figure 8–28

Strapping and Components

- Attach hoop to splint so involved joint is equidistant from hoop, align longitudinally with involved digit.
- Fabricate moveable component with either splinting material or AlumaFoam (see pattern).
- Apply rubber band traction (no. 19) or spring coils to interosseous wire and measure tension so it applies approximately 300 g of force.
- Mark flexion and extension limits (as set by physician) on hoop with tape or marker.
- Strap splint base at splint's distal border, wrist crease, and proximal splint border.
- Apply $^{1}/_{2}$" strap about proximal phalanx.

Splint Finishing Touches

- Carefully instruct patient on use of splint. Generally, patients should alternate between positions of flexion and extension. Beginning on first day of splint application patient should change positions every 10 min while awake. When sleeping, rubber bands should be placed midway between flexion and extension. Splint should be worn for 6 to 8 weeks (Schenck, 1994).

REFERENCES

Kearney, L. M., & Brown, K. K. (1994). The therapist's management of intra-articular fractures. *Hand Clinics, 10,* 199–209.

Schenck, R. R. (1986). Dynamic traction and early passive movement for fractures of the proximal interphalangeal joint. *Journal of Hand Surgery (American), 11,* 850–858.

Schenck, R. R. (1994). The dynamic traction method. Combining movement and traction for intra-articular fractures of the phalanges. *Hand Clinics, 10,* 187–197.

4 • Arm-Based Splints

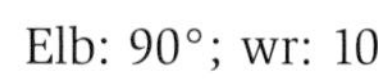

Supination and Pronation Mobilization Splint (Fig. 8–29)[4]

Common Names

- Forearm rotation splint
- Static progressive or dynamic supination/pronation splint
- Tone and positioning (TAP) splint
- MERiT SPS forearm rotation kit
- Dynamic/static progressive orthotic

Alternative Splint Options

- Dynamic supination–pronation splint[4]
- Cast (serial static)

Primary Functions

- Provide low-load, prolonged rotation mobilization force to proximal and distal radioulnar joints to facilitate lengthening of tissue.

Common Diagnoses and Optimal Positions

- Sup or pro contracture — Elb: 90°; wr: 10°

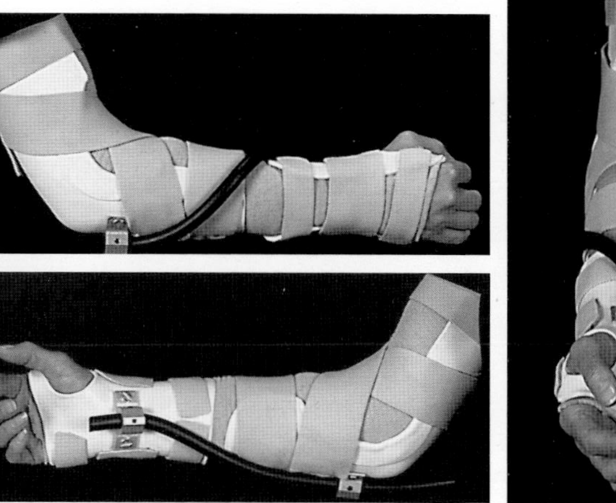

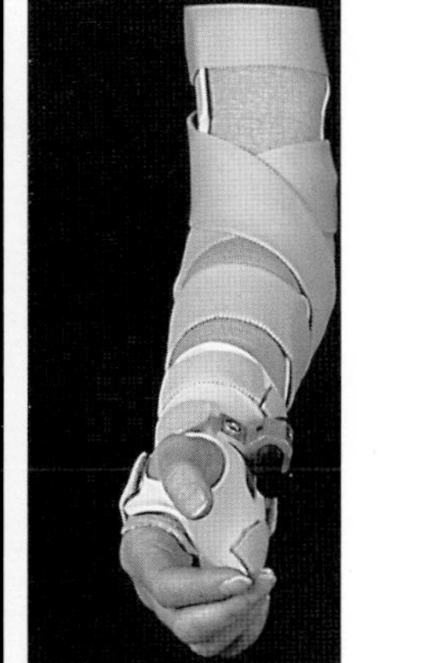

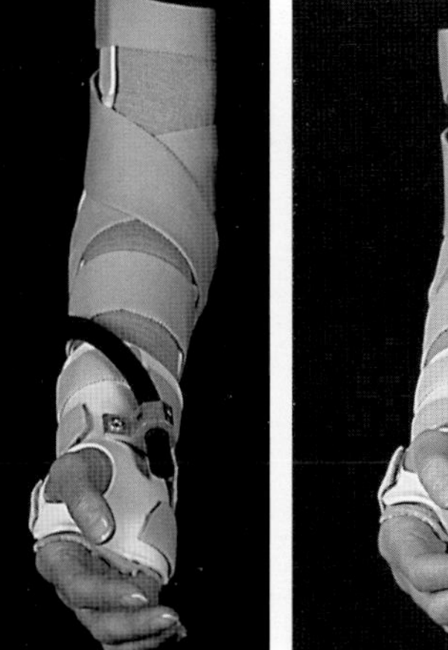

Figure 8–29

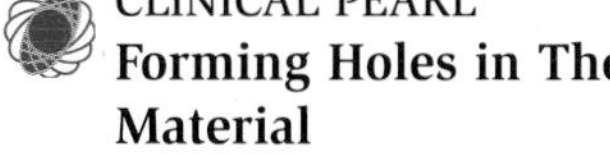

CLINICAL PEARL

Forming Holes in Thermoplastic Material

To form holes in thermoplastic material in regions where a hole punch cannot reach, heat a 3/32" piece of wire over a heat gun, using flat-nose pliers. Pierce the hot end of the wire onto the premarked area. Move the heated wire around, forming a small hole and immediately position the rubber band post or rivet in place. As an alternative, heat the end of an Allen wrench or awl instead of a wire. Note that this procedure should always be done with the splint off the patient. A small hand drill (such as a Dremmel) can be a handy tool to keep in a clinic, because it provides a quick-and-easy way to make holes in difficult to reach areas.

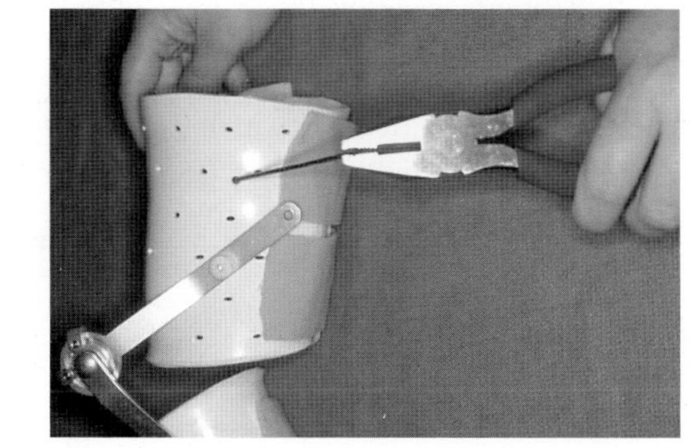

4. Designed by Kay Colello-Abraham.

Fabrication Process (Using Rolyan Pronation-Supination Kit)

Pattern Creation (Fig. 8–30)

- Proximal splint
  * Fabricate splint per posterior elbow immobilization splint design.
  * Splint should extend distally approximately 5" along ulnar border.

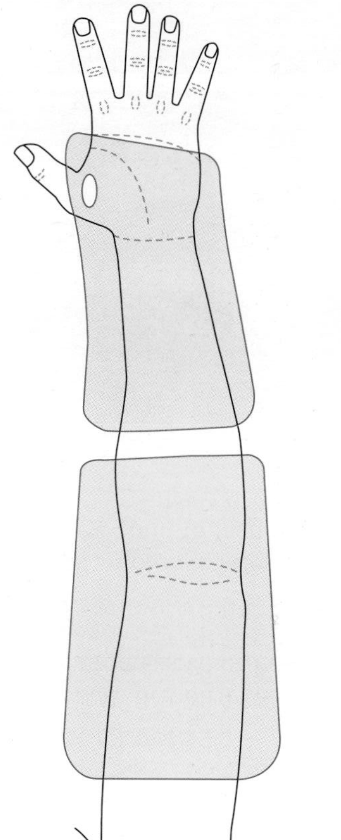

Figure 8–30

- Distal splint
  * Fabricate splint per volar wrist immobilization splint design.
  * Splint should extend proximally, leaving approximately 1" of space between proximal and distal splints, which should not overlap.

Refine Pattern

- Be sure to allow for clearance of MPs and thumb.
- Proximal splint border should allow full shoulder movement.

Options for Materials

- Use either perforated or nonperforated $^1/_8$" materials.
- Lightweight materials may not provide rigid support necessary for length and width of this splint.

Cut and Heat

- Position each splint as described for the individual splint.
- Heat and cut materials accordingly.

Evaluate Fit While Molding

- Mold dorsal elbow splint in 90° of elbow flexion and as close to neutral forearm rotation as possible.
- Check for clearance of medial and lateral epicondyles.
- Fabricate volar wrist immobilization splint, making sure to clear ulnar and radial styloids.

Strapping and Components

- Mark for housing units as described here; then apply straps so they do not interfere with cable.
- Using screws, apply two metal housing components, oriented transversely, on mid-portion of posterior elbow splint (just below olecranon) and on mid-portion of wrist splint.
- Large cable is set into proximal and distal housing units; distal end of tube is set in with Allen wrench and secured.
- For supination, cable is run from volar aspect of wrist around radial border to lateral elbow area and terminates in proximal housing unit on elbow splint (A and B).
- For pronation, cable is run from volar wrist around ulnar aspect of forearm to medial aspect of elbow and terminates on proximal housing unit of elbow splint (C and D).
- Twisting cable in opposite direction of desired motion controls force.
- Cut excess cable.
- Instruct patient in wearing schedule, donning and doffing techniques, and self-adjustments.
- Adjust tension as tissue accommodates.

Splint Finishing Touches

- Line length of proximal and distal splint as well as proximal and distal borders with nonskid material; this greatly decreases splint migration. Consider Microfoam tape, adhesive Dycem, or adhesive silicone gel sheets.
- Check for clearance of ulnar styloid, and epicondyles.
- Check for pressure on radial sensory nerve with supination design; cable may apply pressure directly over this area.

Elbow Flexion Mobilization Splint (Fig. 8–31)

Common Names

- Dynamic elbow flexion splint
- Static progressive elbow splint

Alternative Splint Options

- Prefabricated elbow flexion/extension kits
- Dynamic/static progressive orthotic

Primary Functions

- Provide low-load, prolonged flexion mobilization force to elbow joint to facilitate lengthening of tissue.

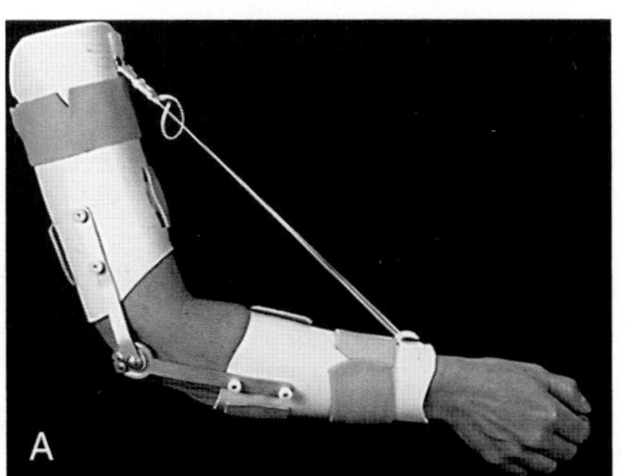

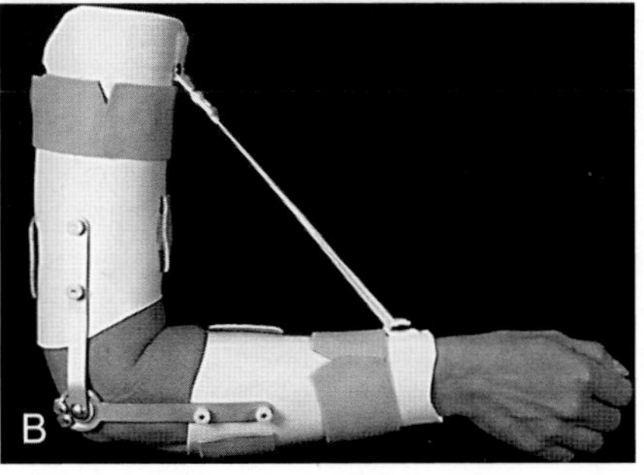

Figure 8–31

Alternative Functions

- Restrict full elbow extension or flexion.
- Restrict or prevent forearm rotation.
- Minimize medial or lateral stress at elbow.

Common Diagnoses and General Optimal Positions

- Elb ext contracture — Terminal elb ext

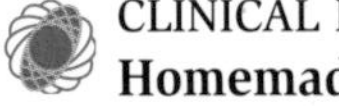

CLINICAL PEARL
Homemade D-ring Straps

Homemade D-rings can easily be fabricated out of thermoplastic material to accommodate the standard 1" and 2" straps as well as wider strapping material. (Commercially available D-rings come in a variety of sizes, commonly 1", 1.5", and 2") Use a scrap piece of thermoplastic material cut into a strip approximately ½" wide. The length depends on how big the D-ring has to be. Heat the material, roll it onto itself for rigidity, overlap the ends, and pinch together firmly. Use your index fingers to maintain the shape until the material is set. Be sure to prepare the surfaces of the material for bonding to ensure a strong attachment.

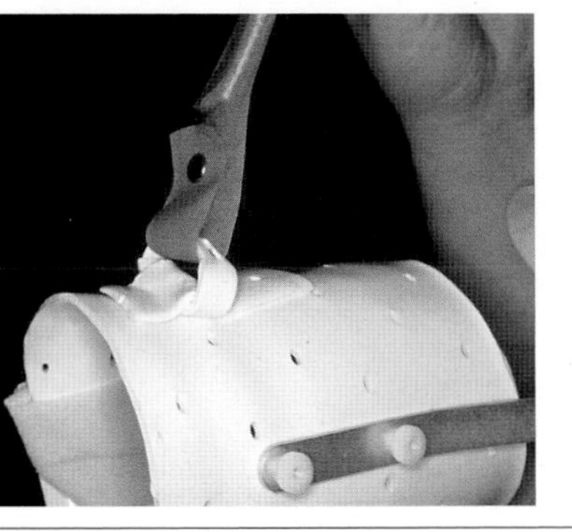

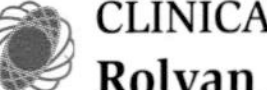

CLINICAL PEARL
Rolyan Adjustable Elbow Hinge

The Rolyan adjustable hinge device is designed to position the elbow statically in any degree of flexion or extension, to restrict motion, or to permit free elbow motion. The hinge's design (with set screws) allows it to be a versatile option for restriction and/or mobilization splinting approaches. Follow the manufacturer's instructions for specific outrigger application.

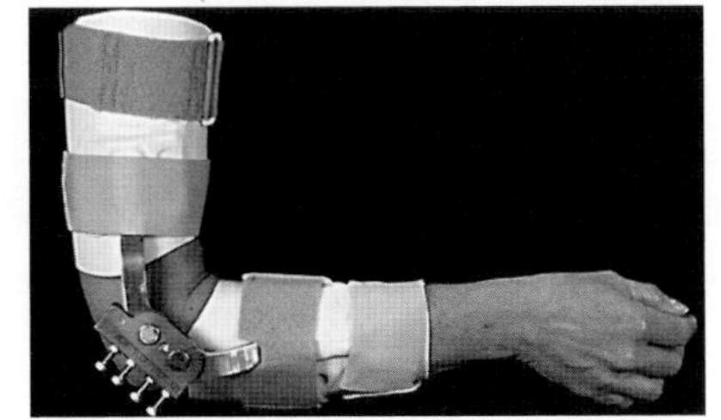

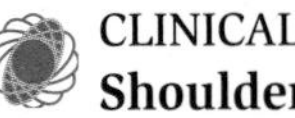

CLINICAL PEARL
Shoulder Harness to Secure Arm Splint

A shoulder harness can be fabricated from 2" soft strapping material (Betapile or Velfoam). The harness, which helps prevent distal migration of large arm splints, can be fabricated in a variety of ways. The strapping is initiated on the posterior border of the splint and directed across the back and toward the opposite shoulder. It then passes across chest to attach to the anterior splint. An additional strap is initiated on the anterior aspect of the splint and traverses posteriorly to attach to the other strap. The straps can be riveted together.

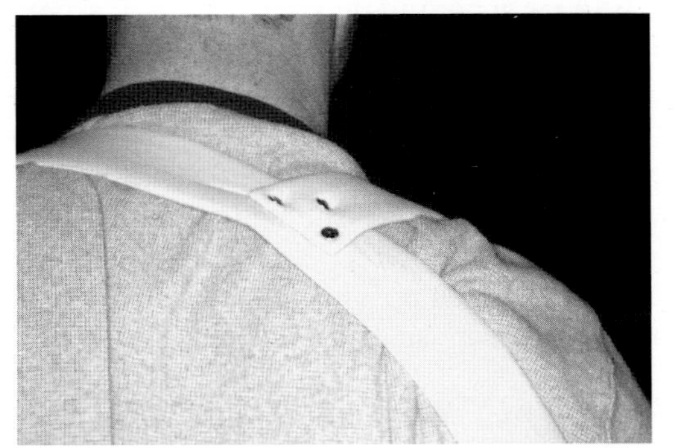

Fabrication Process (Using Phoenix Elbow Hinge)

Pattern Creation (Fig. 8–32)

- Proximal splint
  - * Fabricate nonarticular humerus splint.
- Distal splint
  - * Fabricate nonarticular forearm splint.
  - * If hand is extremely edematous, painful, arthritic, or weak, consider incorporating wrist in forearm splint.

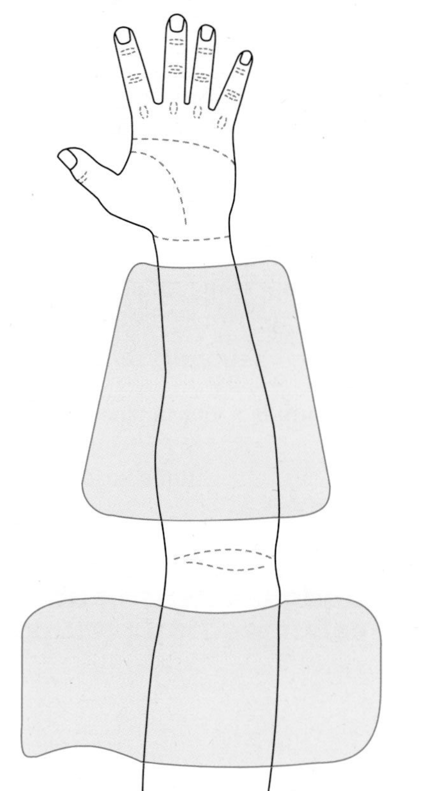

Figure 8–32

Refine Pattern

- Proximal splint borders should allow full shoulder motion and unimpeded elbow motion.
- Distal splint borders should allow unimpeded elbow and wrist motion.
- Check for irritation at epicondyles, olecranon, axilla, ulnar nerve (cubital tunnel), median nerve (wrist), ulnar styloid, and radial sensory nerve.

Options for Materials

- Use coated material so circumferential overlapped section can be popped open without permanent sealing.
- Remember that elastic materials tend to shrink around splinted part; do not remove until splint is completely set.
- Use material that has some degree of flexibility when set (slightly perforated $^1/_8$" and $^3/_{32}$" materials); important because splints need to give slightly to when removed for hygiene and guarded exercise (if appropriate).

Cut and Heat

- When molding distal splint, make certain forearm is in desired amount of forearm rotation.

Evaluate Fit While Molding

- Once both splints are formed, mark for hinge placement; align center (axis) of hinge with axis of rotation at elbow joint.
- Line inside of splint opening with Moleskin as described in splint pattern; consider using lining over border of axilla region for comfort.

Strapping and Components

- Plan and attach hinge before securing straps.
- D-ring straps work well because of ease of application.
- Direct straps so they secure on medial aspect of arm; may be applied over hinge arms.
- With both splints on and forearm in desired amount of rotation and elbow in flexion, line up axis of hinge with elbow joint and mark specific placement of hinge arms.
- Remove splints and attach hinge to proximal and distal splints using rubberband posts.
- Form hook with scrap material and attach to distal third of distal splint.
- Attach D-ring to proximal third of proximal splint.
- Apply elastic cord to attachment devices.

Splint Finishing Touches

- Consider a trial use in clinic because adjustments are frequently necessary.
- Make certain that lines of pull are appropriate for diagnosis (e.g., supination and flexion common for biceps repair, not pronation and flexion).
- Check for unwanted stress on collateral ligaments of elbow.
- Make sure splint allows clearance at elbow; there may be potential for abutment of distal and proximal splint segments as flexion increases, causing compression of skin in flexion crease and possible pressure areas. May need to trim distal border of proximal splint as flexion increases.
- Proximal portion of splint may migrate distally as tension is applied. Consider lining splint with adhesive Dycem, adhesive silicone gel, Microfoam tape, or foam. If this does not help, application of shoulder harness may be necessary.
- Adjust tension per patient and/or tissue tolerance; goal is low-load stretch over prolonged period of time.

Chapter 9: Restriction Splints

1 • Digit- and Thumb-Based Splints

Proximal Interphalangeal (PIP) Extension Restriction Splint

(Fig. 9–1)

Common Names

- Anti-swan-neck splint
- Figure-8 splint
- PIP hyperextension block splint

Alternative Splint Options

- Buttonhole splint
- Prefabricated splint: Silver Ring, 3-Point, Murphy ring
- Taping

Primary Functions

- Maximize functional use of digit by preventing PIP joint hyperextension while allowing PIP flexion.

Common Diagnoses and Optimal Positions

- Swan-neck deformity — PIP: slight flex
- PIP volar plate injury — PIP: 10 to 20° flex
- PIP dorsal dislocation — PIP: 15 to 30° flex (depends on severity)

CLINICAL PEARL

Buttonhole PIP Extension Restriction Splint

The buttonhole design is another option for the PIP extension restriction splint. This design can be more challenging to fabricate than the Figure-8 design. Remember that the degree of restriction for PIP extension depends on the diagnosis.

Use thin ($^{3}/_{32}$" or $^{1}/_{16}$") elastic material because its memory characteristic allows for a contoured intimate fit. Cut out the pattern on scrap piece of thermoplastic material (approximately 2" by 1" piece). Make the holes with the widest setting on a hole punch. Being careful not to overstretch the warmed material, gently feed the finger through both holes, orienting the proximal splint border on the dorsum of the proximal phalanx, the middle section volar, and the distal splint border on the dorsal surface of the middle phalanx.

Position the PIP joint in the desired amount of flexion and fold the lateral splint pieces onto themselves to minimize bulk in this area. Overlap any excess volar material on to the volar PIP piece to allow PIP joint flexion. Finally, remove the splint from the finger and smooth the edges, especially at the volar portion of the splint.

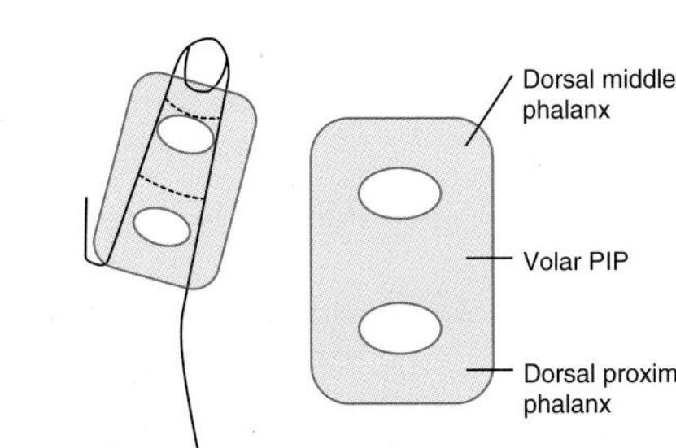

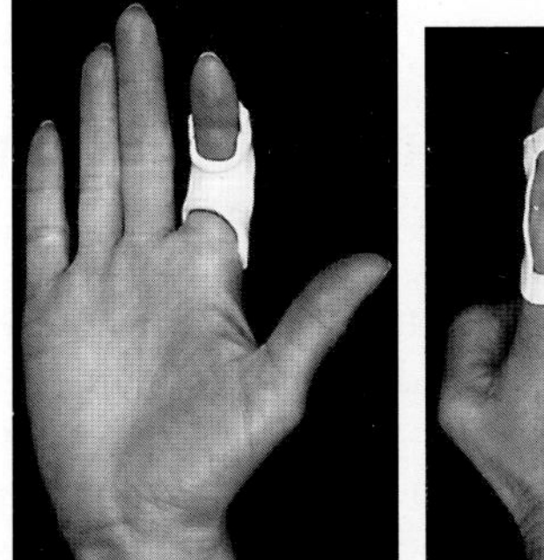

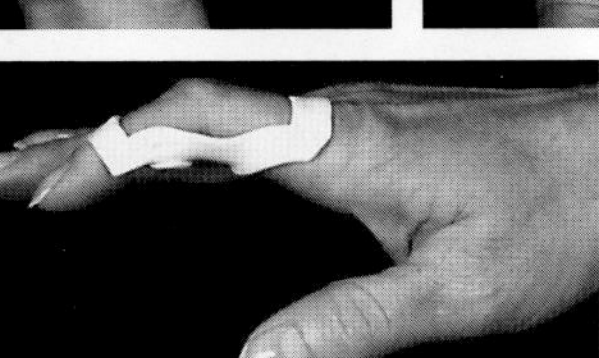

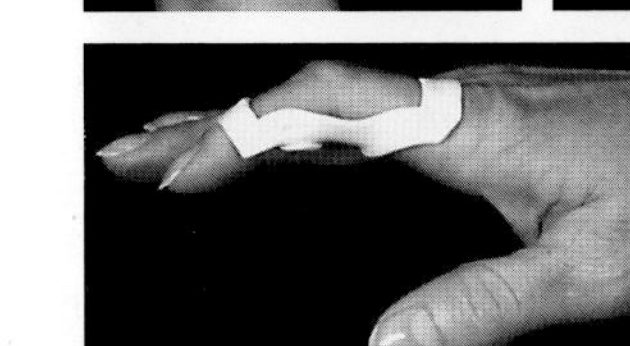

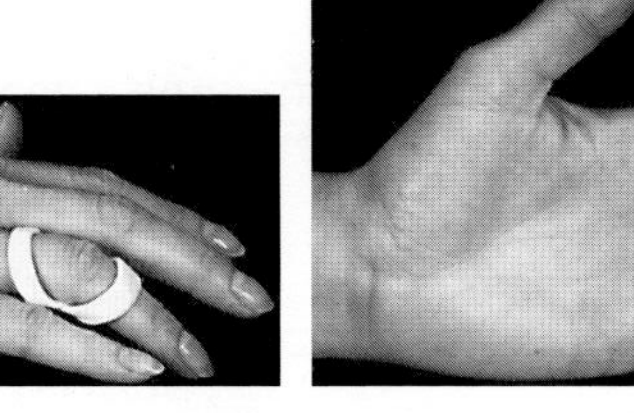

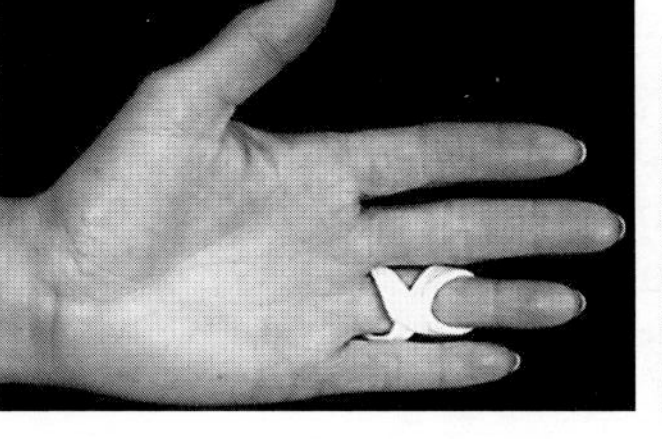

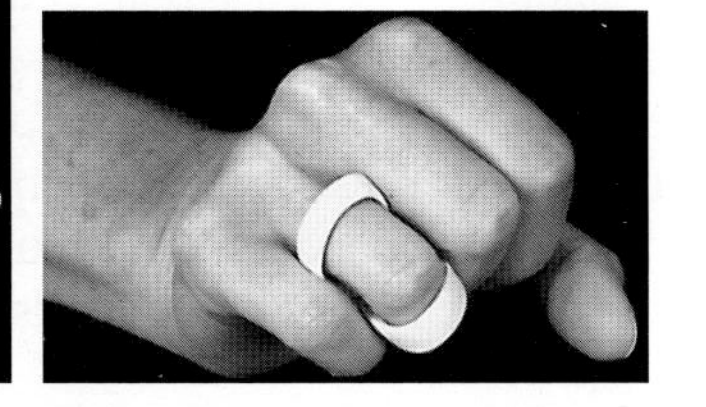

Figure 9–1

Fabrication Process

Pattern Creation (Fig. 9–2)

- Thermoplastic material for this splint should be approximately 4" long and 1/4" to 1/2" wide.

Refine Pattern

- Width of material depends on size of digit to be splinted; the larger the digit, the wider the strip of material.

Options for Materials

- Use thin (3/32" or 1/16") elastic material; memory characteristic allows for excellent contouring and intimate fit.
- Plan to overlap and/or roll material to increase strength.
- Medium to thin Aquatubes provide another option; size depends on strength required and size of digit.

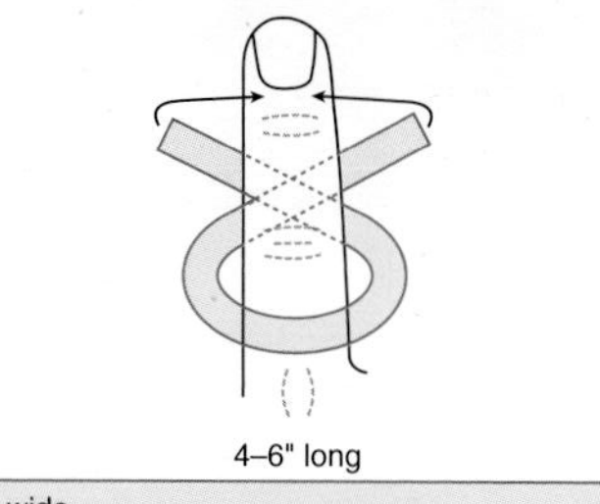

Figure 9–2

- The wider the dorsal segment, the more evenly distributed the pressure and the more comfortable the fit.

Cut and Heat

- Consider placing light layer of lotion on digit before molding to ease removal of splint.

Evaluate Fit While Molding

- Center strip on middle of proximal phalanx dorsally.
- Wrap both ends volarly around to PIP joint crease, dorsally on middle phalanx, ending dorsally.
- Cut and pinch ends so they overlap; smooth.
- While material is setting, position PIP joint in desired amount of flexion by gently providing pressure over volar crossed segment; make sure two dorsal ring pieces are contoured well around phalanges.
- Position dorsal segments close to metacarpophalangeal (MP) and distal interphalangeal (DIP) joints to maximize leverage and improve splint effectiveness.

Strapping and Components

- No strapping required.

Splint Finishing Touches

- Remove splint from patient and prepare overlapped pieces with splint solvent, spot heat and bend.
- Carefully spot heat volar crossed segment with heat gun to secure adherence and smooth edges.
- If DIP or PIP joints are enlarged owing to trauma or arthritis, gently flare rings laterally to allow extra space for removal.

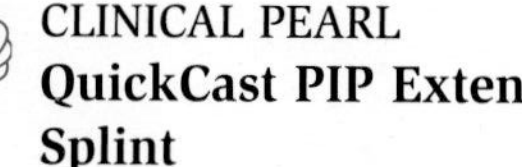

CLINICAL PEARL

QuickCast PIP Extension Restriction Splint

As an alternative, consider using QuickCast to fabricate a PIP extension restriction splint. This material can be easily trimmed to fit the dimensions of the digit and contours extremely well (see Chapter 12 for additional information).

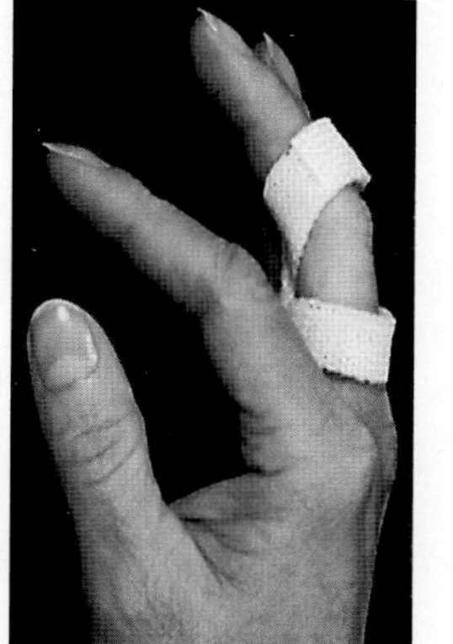

2 • Hand-Based Splints

MP Extension Restriction Splint

(Fig. 9–3)

Common Names

- Lumbrical blocking splint
- Anticlaw splint
- Ulnar nerve splint
- MP blocking splint
- Figure-8 MP blocking splint

Alternative Splint Options

- Prefabricated splints: spring coil, LMB, 3-Point
- Dynamic MP flexion splint
- Immobilization splint

Primary Functions

- Maximize functional use of hand by preventing MP joint hyperextension while allowing MP flexion for grasp.

Additional Functions

- Prevent MP collateral ligament tightness.
- Facilitate PIP extension.

Common Diagnoses and Optimal Positions

• Low-lesion ulnar nerve injury	RF and SF MPs: 45 to 75°flex
• Combined ulnar and median nerve lesion	IF to SF MPs: 45 to 75°flex

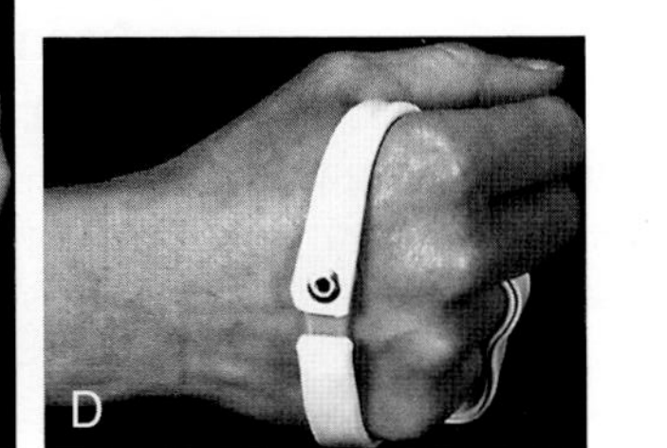
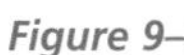
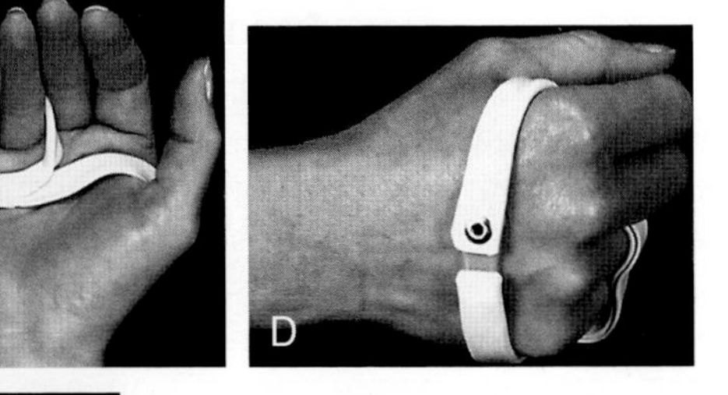

Figure 9–3

Fabrication Process

Pattern Creation (Fig. 9–4)

- Depending on combination of nerve injury, fabricate splint to include two to four MP joints (ulnar nerve: RF and SF; median and ulnar nerves: IF to SF).
- Thermoplastic material should be 8" to 12" long and 1" to $1^1/_2$" wide.

Refine Pattern

- Width of material depends on size of hand to be splinted.

Options for Materials

- Use thin ($^3/_{32}$" or $^1/_{16}$") elastic materials; memory characteristic allows for excellent contouring and intimate fit.

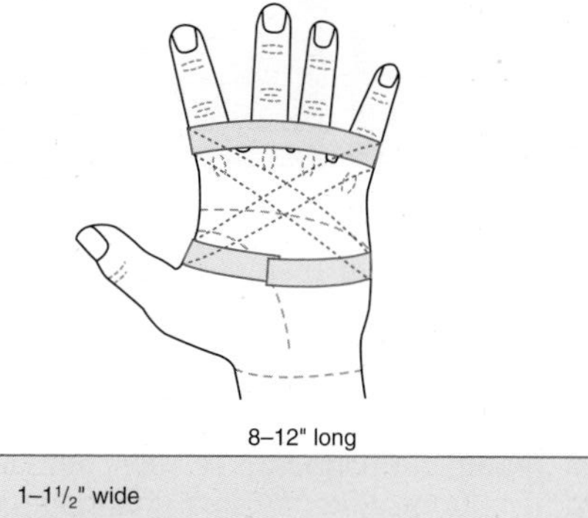

Figure 9–4

- When using elastic materials, constantly mold and redirect material over dorsum of metacarpal heads and proximal phalanges until material sets.
- If experienced splinter, may use plastic materials; allows effective use of gravity to contour between digits, forming comfortable troughs over proximal phalanges.
- Rolled thermoplastic or Aquatubes are not recommended; surface area in contact with skin is not wide enough to provide well-molded splint with adequate pressure distribution in most cases.
- Allow enough material to encompass minimum of one third length of proximal phalanxes; the wider the dorsal segments, the more evenly distributed the pressure and the more comfortable the fit.

Cut and Heat

- Position patient with elbow resting on table, wrist extended, in an intrinsic plus position: MPs flexed, IPs extended (patient may need to help position using unaffected hand).
- Warm material thoroughly.

Evaluate Fit While Molding

- Be sure to accommodate for natural descent of MPs; in fist, SF MP is lower than RF MP, which is lower than MF MP.
- Drape material centrally over middle of proximal phalanges, gently contouring material between digits; there should be an equal length of material draped on each side.
- Cross two draping pieces over each other on volar surface at distal palmar crease level.
- Press and flatten out intersection of two crossed pieces, forming less bulky bar. Constantly work material in palm to provide needed volar support for arches.
- Position remainder of pieces: one through radial web space and other over midulnar border; pinch together dorsally.
- While material is still warm, pull down and overlap excess material on ulnar SF MP and radial RF (or IF MP) areas to allow unimpeded MP flexion.

Strapping and Components

- None, unless there is significant atrophy.
- Many patients with long-standing ulnar nerve injury have significant atrophy of first web space and hypothenar eminence, which may make it difficult to remove the splint. Pop open splint dorsally and apply straps to ease donning and doffing. (Splint shown has riveted strap.)

Splint Finishing Touches

- Cut pinched dorsal piece, prepare surfaces with splint solvent, and spot heat to form permanent seal.
- If necessary, prepare surfaces and spot heat volar overlapped portion to adhere pieces together securely.
- May line dorsal bars with very thin adhesive silicone gel or wrap with Coban to help prevent splint migration during functional use and improve comfort.

MP Extension Restriction Splint *(Continued)*

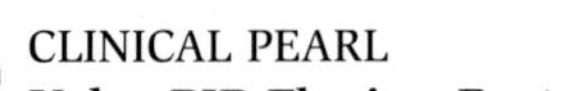

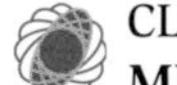

CLINICAL PEARL

MP Extension Restriction Splint with Thumb Included

With combined median and ulnar nerve injuries, the thumb is unable to abduct out of the palm, causing interference with functional use. A simple thumb abduction component can be incorporated into the MP extension restriction splint to position the thumb in palmar abduction and midopposition. The pattern is basically the same as described for the MP extension restriction splint.

Heat a 12" by 1" piece of thermoplastic material. Place the thumb in the desired position (patient may need to position using unaffected hand). Drape the material over the proximal phalanxes as described, except provide the ulnar portion with 3" to 4" of additional material.

Working quickly, cross the ulnar strip radially across the palm; then guide it dorsally around the thumb MP joint, traversing back through the first web space onto the dorsum of the hand. Next, pull the radial strip ulnarward across the palm to join the strip on the ulnar dorsum of the hand. Finish as described for the MP extension restriction splint. Hook and loop can be used to secure the closure and allow for easy donning and doffing. Note that the overlapped areas may need to be warmed with a heat gun to maximize adherence and minimize splint bulk within the first web space.

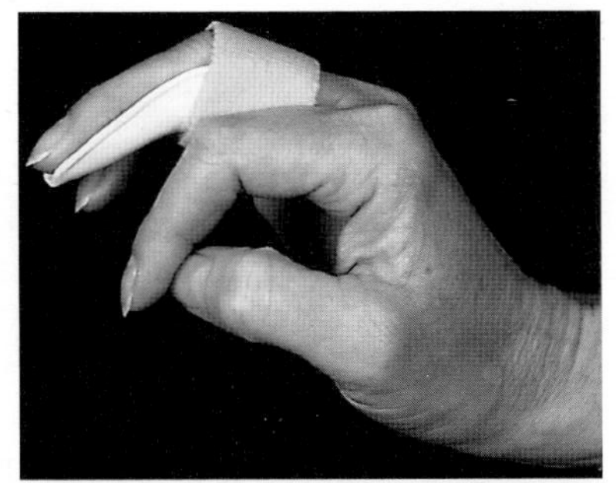

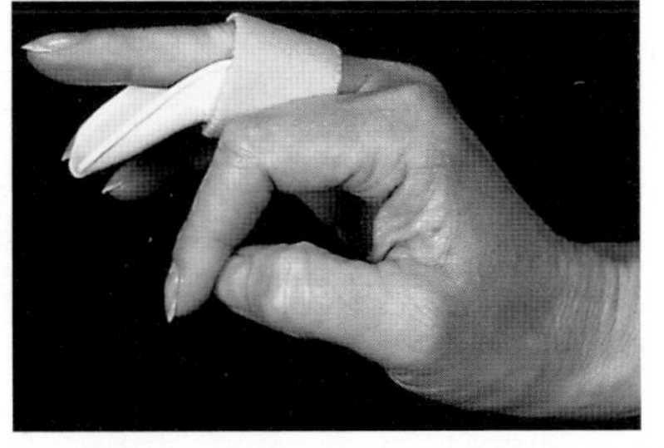

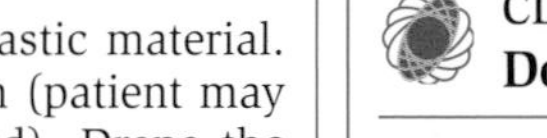

CLINICAL PEARL

Dorsal PIP Extension Restriction Splint

Restriction of full PIP joint extension may be required to allow adequate healing of structures such as the volar plate. The dorsal splint is fabricated in much the same way as the dorsal PIP immobilization splint (see Chapter 7), except for positioning the PIP joint in the desired amount of flexion. Once the proximal strap is secured, the distal strap can be periodically removed to allow active restricted (to the limit of the dorsal block) flexion and extension exercises of the PIP joint. Early motion can help prevent capsular tightness and allow tendon gliding.

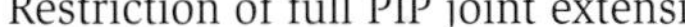

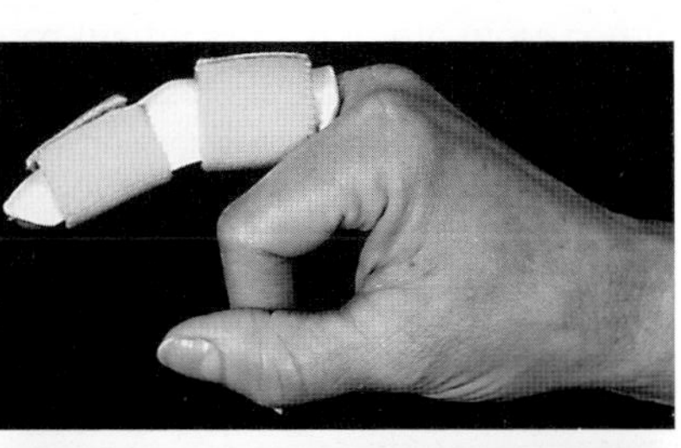

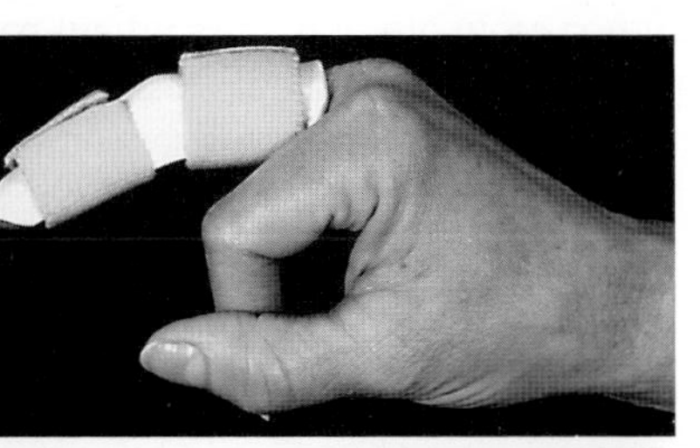

CLINICAL PEARL

Volar PIP Flexion Restriction Splint

The volar splint can be used as part of a specific extensor tendon protocol to limit a particular range of PIP joint flexion when treating zone II to IV injuries. The splint allows early protected motion to promote gliding of the injured or repaired extensor mechanism. The volar splint is fabricated in the same way as a volar PIP immobilization splint, except for positioning the PIP joint in the desired amount of maximum flexion (see Chapter 7). The splint is secured with a single proximal strap, because it is generally used only for exercise sessions. The patient may flex the PIP joint to the limits of the volar block and actively extend to neutral. The splint can be modified weekly as the healing progresses (see Chapter 18 for further details). Note: This protocol requires specific patient selection and physician approval; the therapist must have a full understanding of the theoretical basis behind any particular protocol before implementing it.

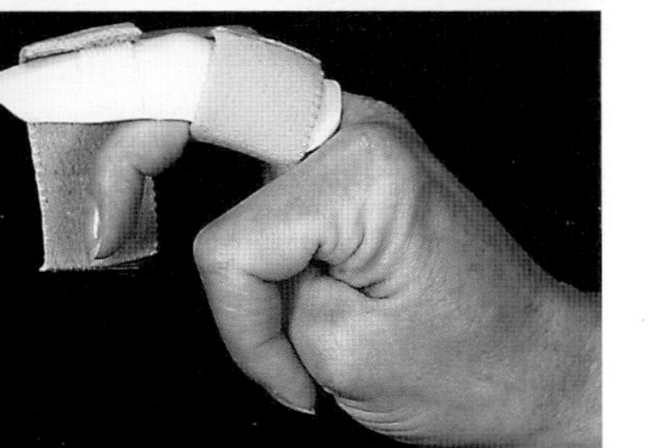

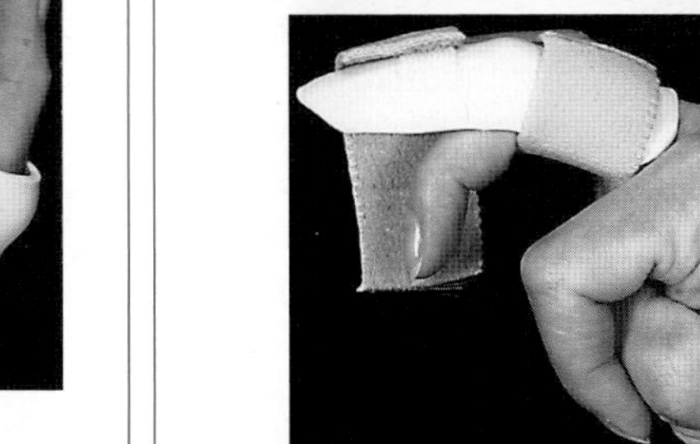

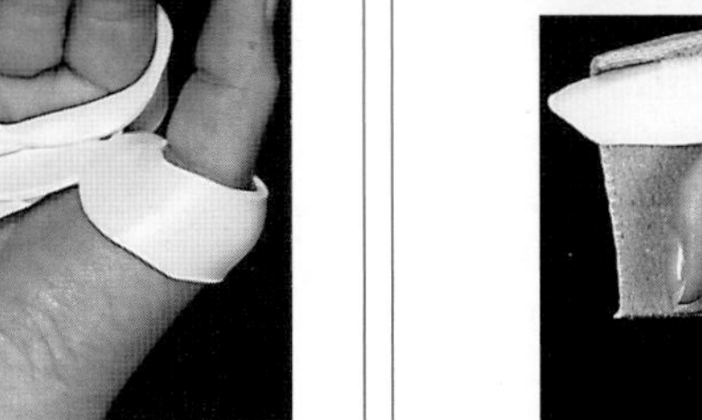

CLINICAL PEARL
Dorsal MP Extension Restriction Splint

This dorsal design provides a wider surface area of coverage. For some patients who have increased digital extensor tone or severe MP extension deformity, this may be the splint of choice. The additional material provides better pressure distribution, and the open volar aspect allows digital flexion. The thumb can easily be incorporated, if desired.

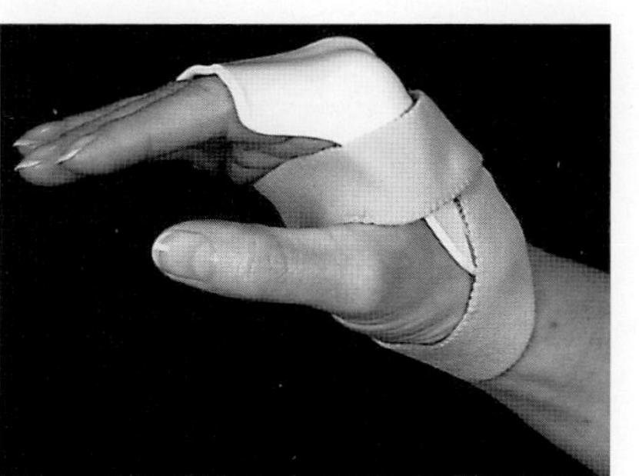

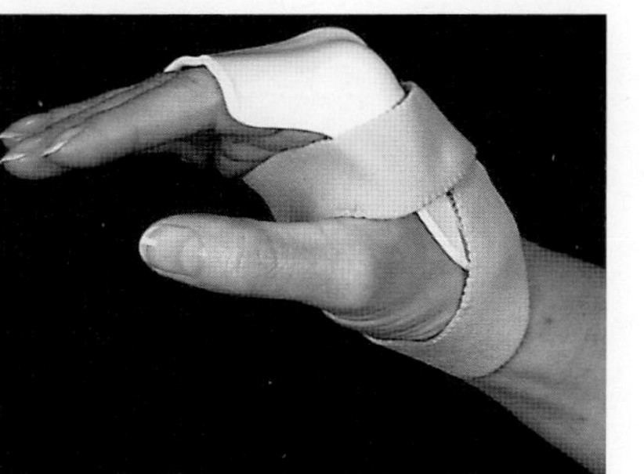

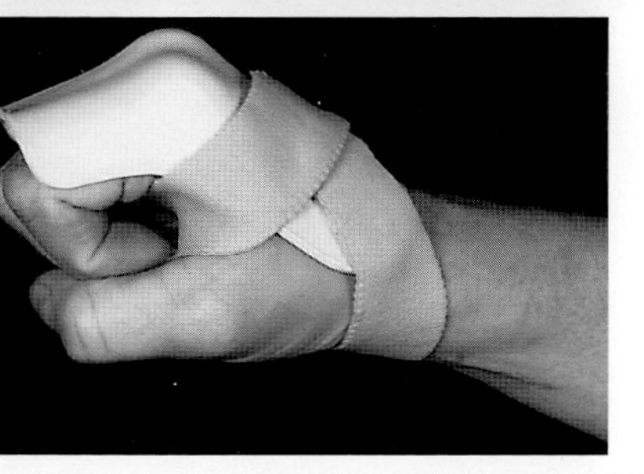

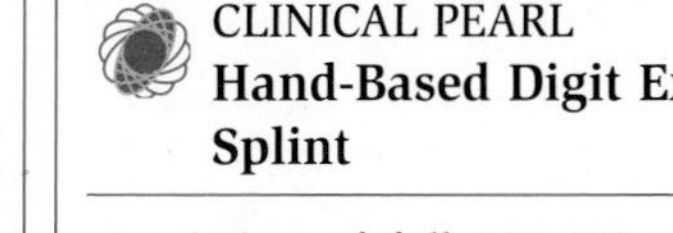

CLINICAL PEARL
Hand-Based Digit Extension Restriction Splint

Restriction of full MP, PIP, and DIP joint extension may be required to allow adequate healing of structures such as repaired digital nerves. This hand-based splint is fabricated in much the same way as the dorsal hand immobilization splint, except for positioning the MP, PIP, and DIP joints in the desired amount of flexion (see Chapter 7). Once the proximal strap is secured, the distal straps can be periodically removed to allow active restricted (to the limit of the dorsal block) flexion and extension exercises of the MP, PIP, and DIP joints. Early motion can help prevent capsular tightness and allow tendon and/or nerve gliding.

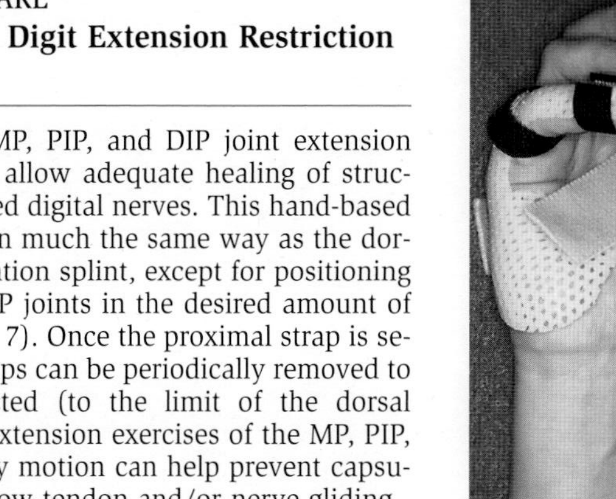

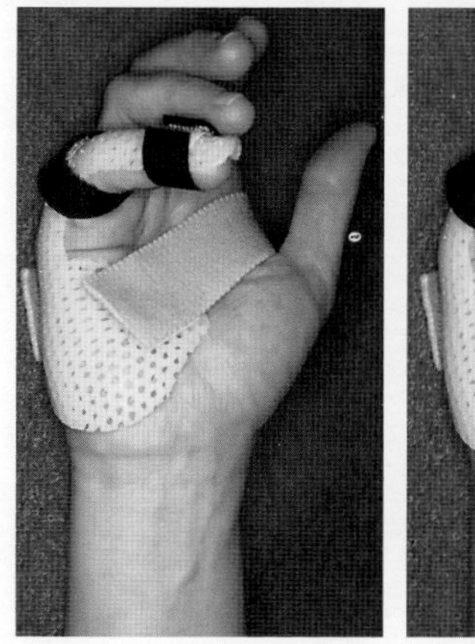

MP Deviation Restriction Splint (Fig. 9–5)

Common Names

- Ulnar deviation splint
- Protective MP splint
- Palmar MP stabilization splint

Alternative Splint Options

- Prefabricated Splints

Primary Functions

- Maintain MP joints in alignment to protect from ulnar deviating or volar subluxating forces.

Common Diagnoses and Optimal Positions

- Arthritis of MP jts — MP: 0 to 25° flex with slight RD

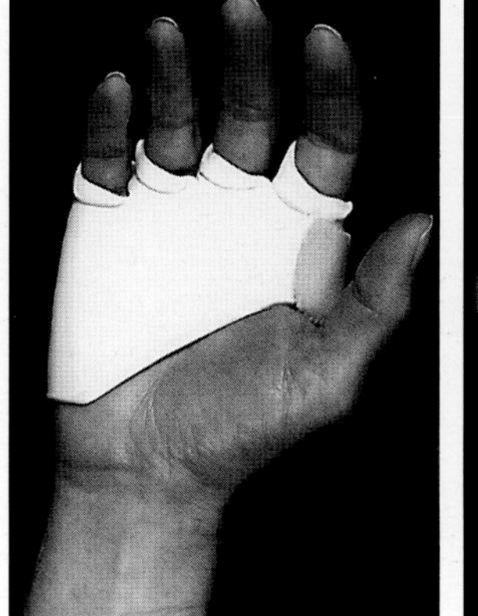

Figure 9–5

Fabrication Process

Pattern Creation (Fig. 9–6)

- Mark just distal to each PIP joint, appreciating the difference in their heights.
- Allow approximately 1" additional material on ulnar border.
- Allow enough material radially to traverse through thumb web, contouring pattern to allow thumb mobility.
- Mark just distal to wrist crease, allowing unimpeded wrist mobility.

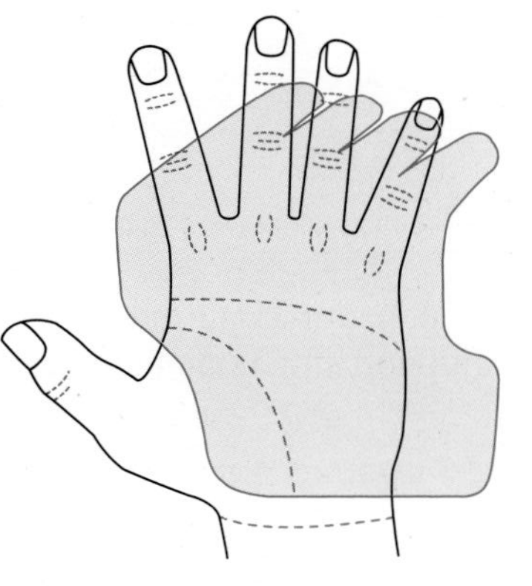

Figure 9–6

Refine Pattern

- Mark pattern from distal border to each digital web space, between IF and MF, MF and RF, and RF and SF.

Options for Materials

- Use thin ($^3/_{32}$" or $^1/_{16}$") elastic material; memory characteristic allows for excellent contouring and intimate fit.
- Consider $^1/_8$" plastic material; thinner plastics may become weak as material is gently stretched about proximal phalanxes.

Cut and Heat

- Position patient with forearm supinated on table and digits slightly abducted. Digits may need to be supported in position by assistant, especially if joints are significantly deviated and/or subluxed.
- Warm material thoroughly.

Evaluate Fit While Molding

- Dry material quickly, and cut slits marked between digits; separate into four tabs. Each tab should be wide enough (approximately $^1/_2$") to encompass proximal phalanx comfortably. Do not make this wrapped portion too narrow.
- Place material on volar aspect of hand. Working quickly, pull each tab around ulnar aspect of each proximal phalanx (onto dorsum).
- Overlap tabs onto themselves (for quick closure) or trim to form separate small cuffs.
- Constantly work material in palm to provide needed volar support for arches.
- MPs should be supported volarly and should rest in near neutral alignment.
- Check that material traversing between digits is not thick and is free of sharp edges.

Strapping and Components

- One strap to join radial and ulnar border.
- Consider riveted strap to allow for easy donning and doffing.

Splint Finishing Touches

- Smooth edges and between digits.
- Be sure MP joints are supported in optimal alignment.

Wrist and IF/MF Extension Restriction Splint (Fig. 9–7)[1]

Common Names

- Tenodesis splint
- RIC splint

Primary Function

- Maximize available grasp and release action of digits by redirecting portion of power generated during wrist extension into functional flexion arc of IF and MF against thumb (tenodesis).

Common Diagnosis and General Optimal Position

- Must have radial nerve function intact; loss of median and ulnar nerve function

1. Designed at the Rehabilitation Institute of Chicago.

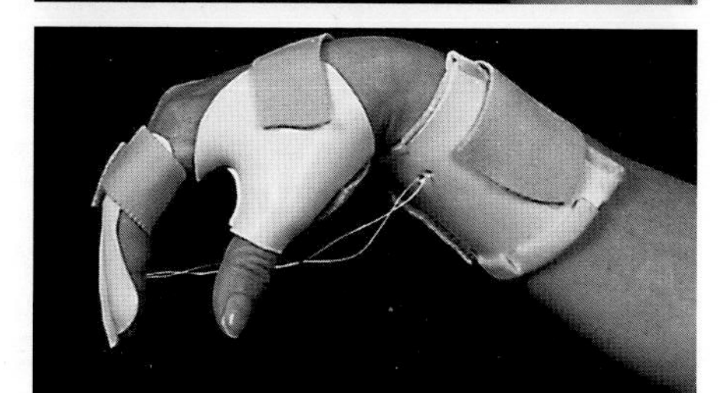

Figure 9–7

Fabrication Process

Pattern Creation (Fig. 9–8)

- There are three separate sections of this splint.
- Dorsal cap for IF/MF: Splint should encompass both proximal phalanges and terminate at tip.
- Thumb MP splint: Splint should stabilize thumb in midpalmar abduction and opposition; thumb MP joint should be held in slight flexion.
- Thermoplastic wristband: Splint is fabricated to surround two thirds circumference of wrist and is approximately $3^1/_2$" wide.

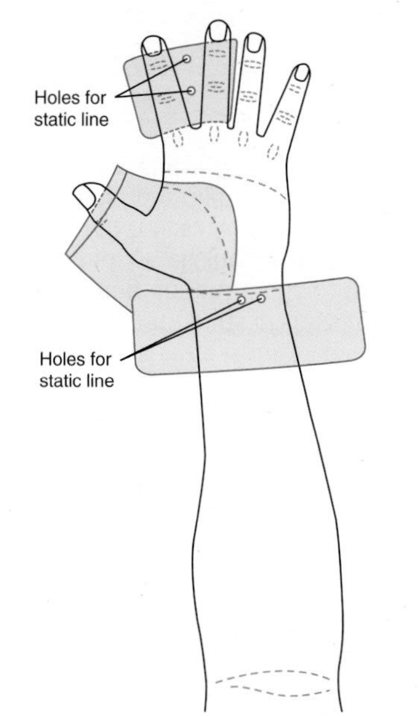

Figure 9–8

Refine Pattern

- Check that lateral borders of IF and MF dorsal splint do not irritate radial border of RF.

Options for Materials

- Use $^3/_{32}$" or $^1/_{16}$" material.

Cut and Heat

- Position patient with elbow resting on table, wrist extended and MPs flexed (tenodesis position).
- Warm material one section at a time.

Evaluate Fit While Molding

- Dorsal cap for IF/MF
  * Rest warm material over dorsum of IF and MF, making sure that PIPs are flexed to approximately 20°. There should be contouring between digits, distinguishing each one.
  * Proximal border of splint should extend just distal to MPs.
- Thumb MP splint
  * This splint is fabricated per instructions for thumb carpometacarpal (CMC) immobilization splint.
  * Position thumb in midpalmar/radial abduction and opposition; opposition should be to middle of IF and MF. MP joint should be slightly flexed.
- Thermoplastic wristband
  * This splint is fabricated proximal to wrist, allowing full passive wrist flexion and active extension.
  * Place material centrally over volar wrist, and wrap about radial and ulnar wrist borders. Material should terminate flush with dorsal skin.

Strapping and Components

- Thin strap of loop material secures dorsal splint onto digits and should be placed at proximal phalanx level.
- If needed, place optional strap distal, at middle phalanx level.
- Strap thumb splint from volar to dorsal.
- Wrist requires 2" strap across dorsum of wrist, connecting radial and ulnar borders.
- To connect dorsal IF/MF splint and wristband, punch two holes along indentation of IF/MF proximal phalanx crease; punch two more holes at middle of wristband at distal border.
- Place double length of static line through holes onto dorsum of splint, tie securely, and feed between phalanges. Place wrist in extension and feed line through wristband holes.
- Line should have enough tension to pull MP joints (along with dorsal splint) into flexion just to allow IF/MF tips to oppose thumb tip. Once proper tension is achieved, tie line through wristband holes.

Splint Finishing Touches

- To obtain maximum benefits from this splint, it is crucial to achieve appropriate amount of tension.
- Line dorsal splint and wristband with very thin adhesive silicone gel or wrap digits and wrist with thin layer of Coban (or similar material) to help prevent splint migration during functional use and improve comfort.

Wrist Extension, IF/MF/Wrist Flexion, IF/MF Extension Restriction Splint *(Continued)*

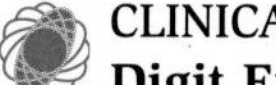

CLINICAL PEARL

Digit Extension Restriction Strap

Some flexor tendon protocols call for the use of a restriction strap to protect the healing repairs once the dorsal splint has been discontinued (at 4 to 5 weeks). This strap protects the repaired structures from simultaneous wrist and digit extension. It also prevents excessive and forceful wrist extension (see Chapter 18 for details).

For the wrist strap component, use a 8"-long, 2"-wide soft strap material (Betapile or Velfoam). Secure it about the wrist with a 3" piece of adhesive hook (folded onto itself), placing the strap so that the closure is on the dorsum of the hand. Then punch a hole on the volar surface of the 2" strap. Remember that the line of pull is always converging toward the scaphoid bone. Make a sling from 1" by 4" soft strap, and punch a hole on both ends of the sling. The overall length of the sling should be $1\frac{1}{2}$" to 2". Finally, thread rubber band or elastic cord through the MP sling and wrist strap holes. Adjust the tension so that as the wrist extends, the digit flexes and as the wrist flexes, the digits extend. Watch for neurovascular compromise.

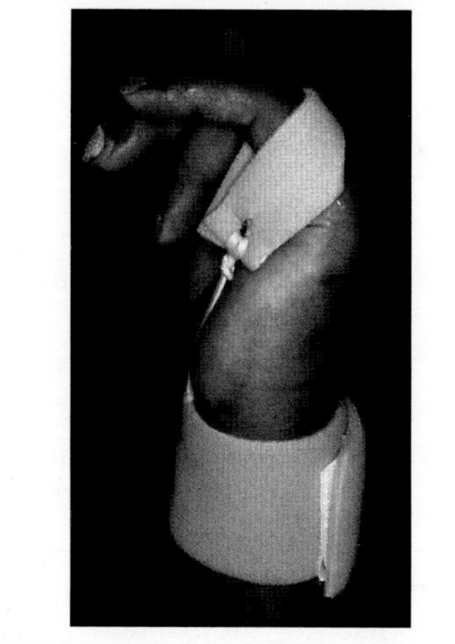

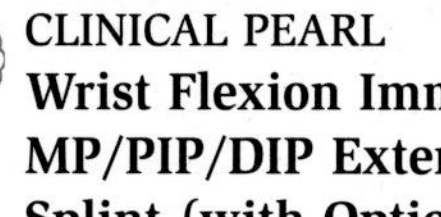

CLINICAL PEARL

Wrist Flexion Immobilization, MP/PIP/DIP Extension Restriction Splint (with Optional Thumb)

The intent of this splint design is to minimize tension on repaired structures during healing and to allow some degree of guarded motion to minimize adhesion formation. The healing structures may include one or all of the following: flexor tendons of the wrist, digits, and thumb; median and ulnar nerves; and vascular structures. The dorsal hand portion of the splint provides a block to full digit and thumb extension, which is required for most flexor tendon protocols (see Chapter 18 for further information). If only the flexor pollicis longus is involved, then the splint needs to protect just the wrist and thumb (the digits can be left free); see Chapter 7 for fabrication instructions.

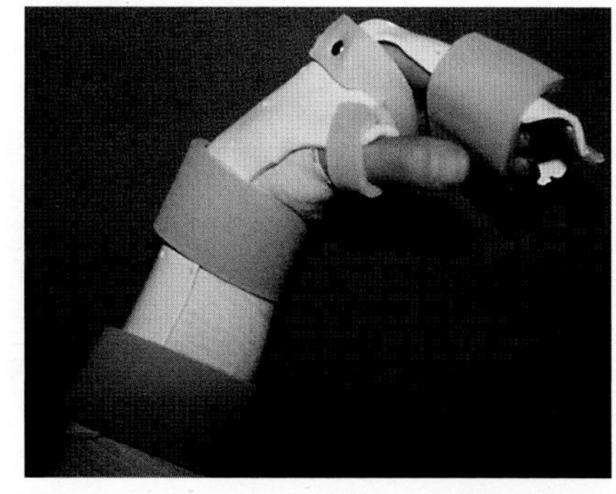

CLINICAL PEARL

Wrist Extension Immobilization, MP Flexion Restriction Splint

A & B) After operative repair of the extensor tendons (including the thumb), gentle and restricted gliding of the involved structures may facilitate tendon healing and minimize adhesion formation (see Chapter 18 for additional information). A volar thermoplastic block can be added to the splint to allow a restricted degree of MP flexion as per physician protocol. The patient can flex the MP joints actively to the volar block, and the dynamic component passively brings the digits back into extension. The volar block can be attached to the dorsal splint via loop and hook.

C) As an alternative to the volar block, a line stop can be placed on the line to limit motion, as required with some zone V extensor tendon and early mobilization protocols. This provides the therapist a way to restrict MP joint flexion to a specific degree. The patient is allowed to flex the MP joints actively within the range permitted by the stop bead; the dynamic component passively brings the digits back into extension. Stop beads (or line stops) can be purchased commercially or simply fabricated by using tape (although not as aesthetically pleasing). Commercial line stops are applied by placing the stop bead in the desired location and compressing it with pliers. Stops can be repositioned to allow for a progressive increase in motion as healing allows.

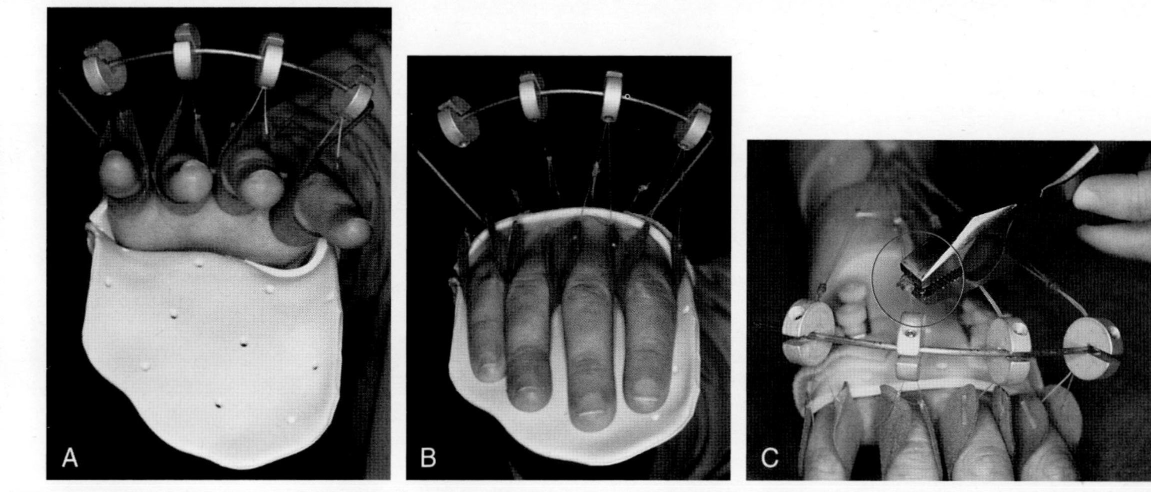

4 • Arm-Based Splints

Anterior/Posterior Elbow Extension or Flexion Restriction Splint

(Fig. 9–9)

Common Names

- Anterior/posterior elbow splint
- Bisurfaced static elbow orthosis
- Elbow extension-blocking splint
- Elbow flexion-blocking splint

Alternative Splint Options

- Prefabricated splint
- Hinged elbow splint

Primary Functions

- Restrict specific degree of elbow extension or flexion while allowing motion in opposite direction.

Additional Functions

- Limit or prevent forearm rotation.
- Statically position elbow flexion or extension contracture at maximum length to facilitate lengthening of tissue (serial static splint).

Common Diagnoses and General Optimal Positions

Diagnosis	Position
• Rheumatoid arthritis	Position of comfort and support
• Ulnar nerve compression at cubital tunnel	Elb: 30 to 45°flex; FArm neutral
• Posterior/anterior dislocation	Elb: 90°; FArm: neutral
• Dislocation proximal radius	Elb: 90°; FArm: sup
• Medial epicondyle fracture	Elb: 90 to 110°; FArm: pro
• Lateral epicondyle fracture	Elb: 90 to 110°; FArm: sup
• Olecranon fracture	Elb: 20 to 35° flex; FArm: neutral
• Acute lateral epicondylitis	Elb: 90°; FArm: neutral; Wr: 30 to 45° ext
• Acute medial epicondylitis	Elb: 90°; FArm: neutral; Wr: 0°
• Elb ext contracture	Terminal flex
• Elb flex contracture	Terminal ext

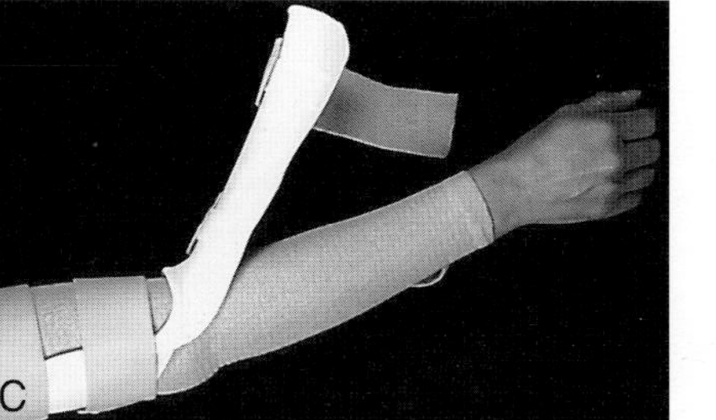

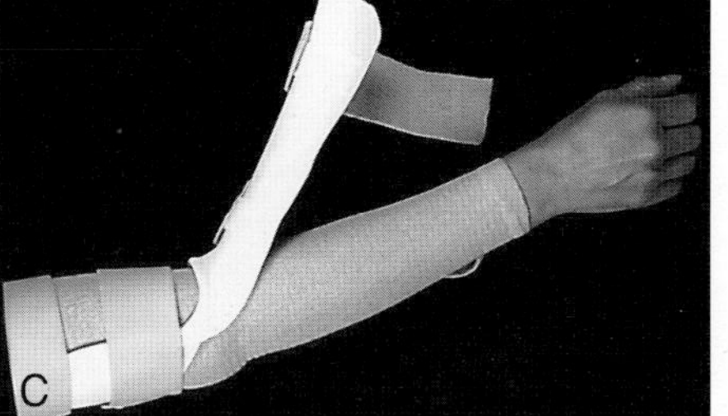

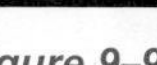

Figure 9–9

Fabrication Process

Pattern Creation (Fig. 9–10)

- This pattern may be alternative to anterior or posterior elbow immobilization splint design; consider when specific amount of flexion or extension must be restricted or when there are skin integrity issues(e.g., healing wounds or grafts).
- To restrict elbow extension: apply splint posteriorly on upper arm and anteriorly on forearm.
- To restrict elbow flexion: apply splint anteriorly on upper arm and posteriorly on forearm.

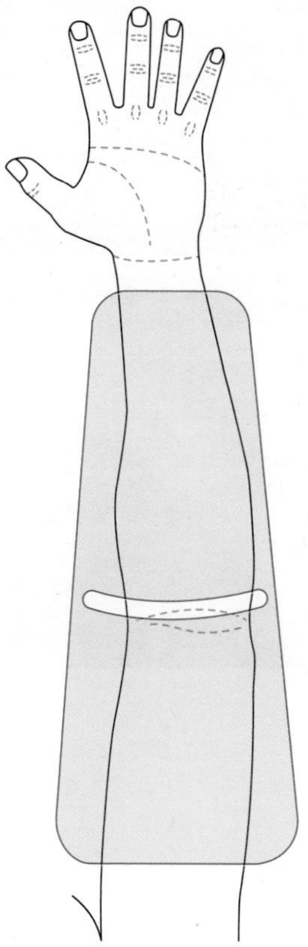

Figure 9–10

- Mark for proximal border two thirds length of humerus.
- Mark for distal border just proximal to ulnar styloid.
- Allow enough material to encompass half to two thirds circumference of upper arm and lower forearm, remembering that forearm tapers distally.
- Mark slit for elbow at elbow flexion crease.

Refine Pattern

- Proximal border should allow unimpeded shoulder motion and not irritate axilla region when arm is positioned at side.
- Distal border should allow full wrist motion.
- Note that pattern is wider proximally because circumference of upper arm is greater than that of forearm.
- Make sure that opening for elbow is wide enough to allow forearm and hand to pass through.

Options for Materials

- Use $1/8$" material because strength is important characteristic for this splint.
- Materials with high resistance to stretch (rubber) may offer more control for therapist.
- Consider material that has some degree of memory; material may stretch out as wrist and forearm pass through slotted piece.
- If patient has significant pain and swelling, consider uncoated materials or those that are slightly tacky to help prevent material from slipping making it easier to position patient and mold splint.

Cut and Heat

- Position patient seated to allow for gravity-assisted molding.
- Gravity can assist with molding only one portion of splint, rest of splint must be attended to by therapist.
- Have an assistant help support proper elbow and forearm positions if possible.

Evaluate Fit While Molding

- Before molding splint, decide on which surface to apply material.
- Drape proximal piece either anterior or posterior on upper arm, simultaneously sliding elbow carefully through slot; then place forearm portion either anterior or posterior.
- As one hand supports non-gravity-assisted piece, fold elbow flaps onto themselves to reinforce this potentially weak section.
- Do not grab proximal or distal splint segments or try to secure with tight circumferential bandage. This may cause borders of splint to dig in. Instead, allow gravity to assist in forming one trough while gently supporting the other segment.
- Check for clearance of wrist distally.

Strapping and Components

- Stockinette or elasticized sleeve (if edema is present) is recommended before splint application to help eliminate pinching of skin once straps are applied.
- 2" soft straps are recommended at most proximal and distal portions of splint.
- When used to restrict only one direction of elbow motion, forearm strap may be eliminated or released periodically to allow for exercise.

Splint Finishing Touches

- Smooth and slightly flare all borders.
- Check for clearance and/or irritation of axilla, ulnar styloid, and epicondyles.
- Check for compression of ulnar nerve at cubital tunnel area as well as sensory branch of radial nerve.

Forearm Rotation/Elbow Extension Restriction Splint

(Fig. 9–11)

Common Names

- Muenster splint
- Sarmiento elbow brace

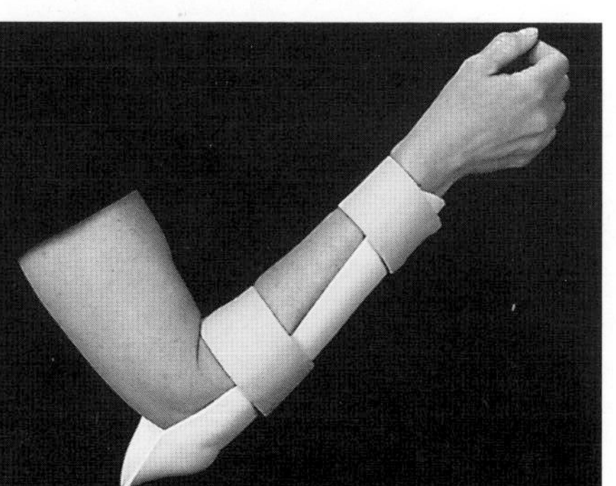

Figure 9–11

Alternative Splint Options

- Sugar tong splint
- Cast

Primary Functions

- Restrict elbow extension and provide full flexion to allow healing of involved structure(s).

Additional Functions

- Restrict some degree of forearm rotation.
- With wrist included, restricts forearm rotation and elbow extension.

Common Diagnoses and General Optimal Positions

Diagnosis	Position
• Proximal or distal radioulnar jt injury	FArm: neutral rotation
• Interosseous membrane injury	FArm: neutral rotation
• Proximal radius and ulna fracture	FArm: neutral rotation; Elb: restricted in ext (per physician's orders)
• Elb dislocation	Depends on structures involved

CLINICAL PEARL

Elbow Flexion Mobilization, Extension Restriction Splint

This dynamic elbow flexion splint with restricted elbow extension shown here is an example of the combined use of a mobilization splint with a restrictive component (see Chapter 8); it was designed for a patient who was referred 3 weeks after a biceps tendon repair. The splint bases were fabricated following instructions for the circumferential humerus and forearm splints. A hinge connects the splints, with the axis positioned at the elbow joint. Rubber band traction passively positions the elbow in flexion, and the hinge is set to restrict a specific amount of elbow extension. (Similar to distal flexor tendon injuries.) The patient periodically exercises within the splint limits (restricted active elbow extension with passive elbow flexion via the rubber band). Note that the hinge not only acts as an anchor for the rubber bands and a blocking mechanism to elbow extension but also prevents the proximal and distal splint segments from migrating toward each other when under tension from the rubber band. A static component can be added to immobilize the elbow between exercise sessions. The splint can be further secured to the shoulder girdle via a Figure-8-type strap. Note: This protocol must be reviewed by the referring physician before implementation.

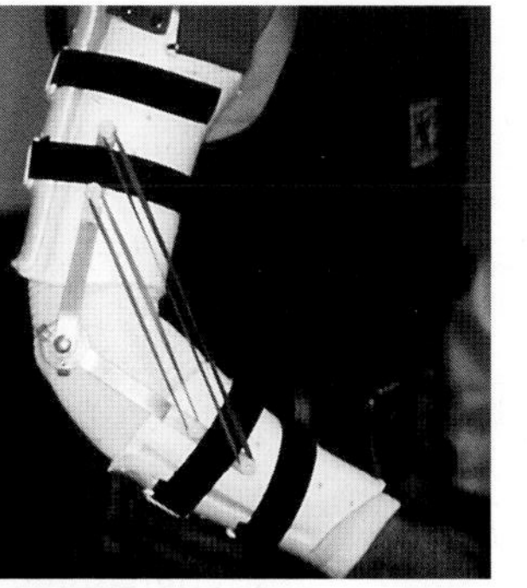

Fabrication Process

Pattern Creation (Fig. 9–12)

- Mark for proximal border approximately 2" above olecranon process.
- Mark for distal borders just proximal to wrist.
- Allow enough material to encompass half to two thirds circumference of forearm, remembering that forearm tapers distally.

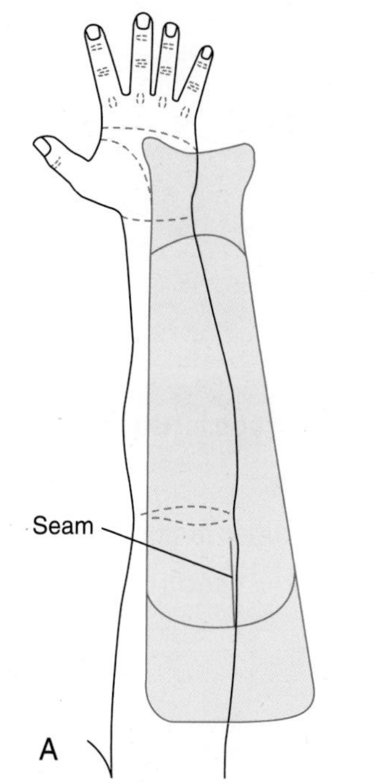

Figure 9–12

Refine Pattern

- Proximal border should allow limited elbow extension and unimpeded elbow flexion without irritating epicondyles or ulnar nerve.
- Distal border should allow full wrist and hand motion.

Options for Materials

- Use rubber materials (perforated or nonperforated).
- Consider elastic materials that are slightly tacky to help prevent material from slipping making it easier to position patient and mold splint.

Cut and Heat

- Have patient lying supine with shoulder flexed or prone with shoulder extended to achieve gravity-assist position. Place forearm in neutral and elbow in desired position.
- Have patient (or assistant) maintain this position during fabrication.
- While material is heating, prepad olecranon process and epicondyles with self-adhesive padding or silicone gel if desired.

Evaluate Fit While Molding

- While supporting entire piece of warm material, place centrally along ulnar border of forearm and distal humerus.
- Proximally, bring ends together and either cut warm material to form seam or overlap material ends. This seam can be reinforced with an additional piece of material later, if necessary.
- Make sure desired elbow and forearm positions are maintained. Some patients may tend to flex their elbows excessively while splint is being formed.
- When almost set, check for clearance of ulnar styloid and epicondyles. If patient complains of abutment, simply push material out.

Strapping and Components

- Distal strap: 2" elasticized strap just proximal to wrist crease; use piece of adhesive foam to further stabilize forearm in splint and prevent migration. Foam should not overlap splint edges; avoid excessive compression over radial sensory nerve.
- Proximal strap: 2" elasticized strap placed just distal to elbow crease.
- Note there is no strap proximal to elbow crease—this permits elbow flexion.

Splint Finishing Touches

- Smooth and slightly flare all edges.
- Check for complete clearance of wrist and desired elbow motion.

Chapter 10: Nonarticular Splints

1 • Digit- and Thumb-Based Splints

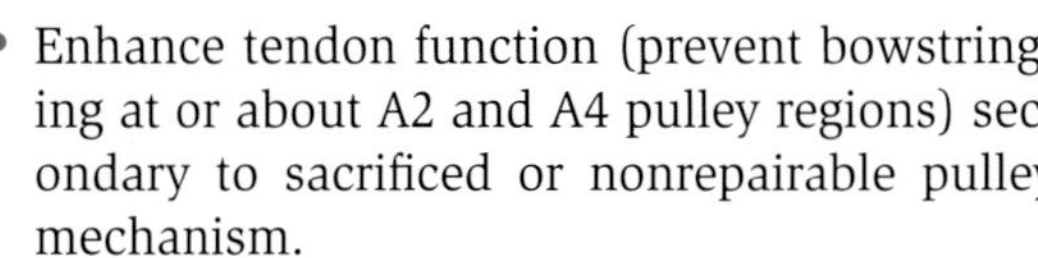

Proximal or Middle Phalanx Splint (Fig. 10–1)

Common Names

- Pulley ring

Alternative Splint Options

- Circumferential taping or strapping

Primary Functions

- Protect pulley reconstruction.

Additional Functions

- Enhance tendon function (prevent bowstringing at or about A2 and A4 pulley regions) secondary to sacrificed or nonrepairable pulley mechanism.

Common Diagnoses and General Optimal Positions

- Flexor tendon injury with pulley reconstruction (zones I and II)
- Iatrogenic injury to pulley secondary to flexor tendon repair or tenolysis

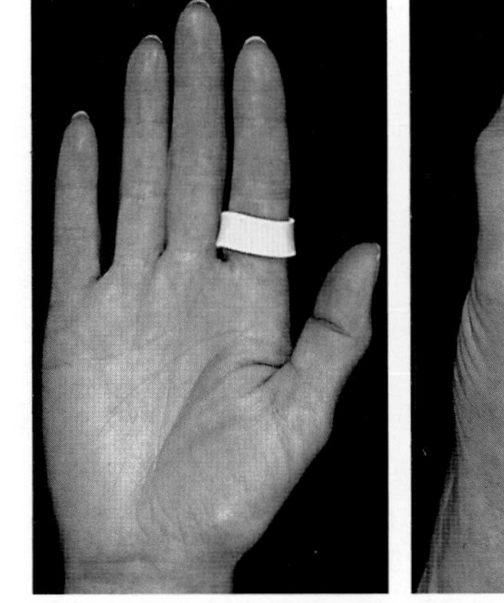

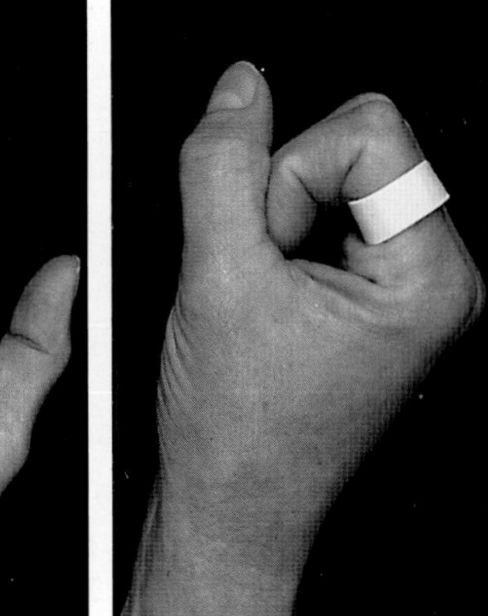

Figure 10–1

Fabrication Process

Pattern Creation (Fig. 10–2)

- Measure circumference of digit segment involved (e.g., proximal or middle phalanx).
- Measure width of segment involved; corresponding width of splint should be approximately $1/2$ to $1/3$ that of segment.

Refine Pattern

- Accommodate for use of circumferential wrappings (Coban) or wound dressings beneath splint.
- Splint should allow unimpeded flexion of metacarpophalangeal (MP), proximal interphalangeal (PIP), and/or distal interphalangeal (DIP) joints.

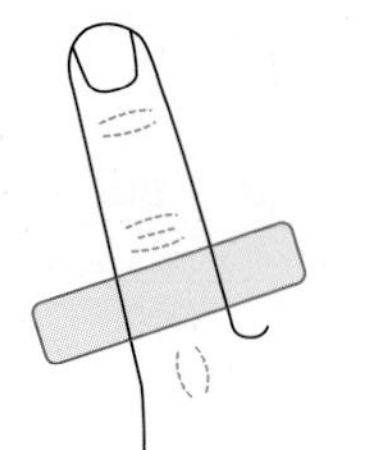

Figure 10–2

Options for Materials

- Use $1/16$" material, which provides adequate support.
- If strapping is used across dorsum of segment, consider thin strapping material.

Cut and Heat

- While material is heating, position patient with forearm supinated and digits slightly abducted.
- Protect patient with recent flexor tendon repair in wrist/hand extension restriction splint (dorsal blocking splint) during fabrication process.

Evaluate Fit While Molding

- Mold warm material around proximal or middle phalanx.
- For patient with no edema or with no wraps/dressings, consider circumferential design in which ring is overlapped and/or sealed circumferentially. Otherwise, leave gap over dorsum of phalanx for splint removal; small strap can be applied to join ends of splint.
- For patients with enlarged PIP or DIP joints, be sure to leave gap over dorsum for splint removal.
- Allow material to completely set before removing.

Strapping and Components

- If strap is necessary, it should be approximately same width as splint dorsally.
- Small metal rivet can be used to secure one end of strap.

Splint Finishing Touches

- Smooth borders and round strap ends.
- Check for unimpeded joint motion.
- Remember that splint will need to be modified as edema or wound dressings worn beneath splint change.

Proximal and/or Middle Phalanx Straps (Fig. 10–3)

Common Names

- Buddy straps
- Buddy splints
- Buddy taping

Alternative Splint Options

- Prefabricated
- Silver Ring splints
- Taping
- Thermoplastic material

Primary Functions

- Adjoin affected digit to border unaffected digit, minimizing lateral stress and allowing range of motion (ROM) and some function.

Additional Functions

- Facilitate passive and active ROM of affected digit via active motion of adjacent digit.
- Use in combination with hand-based splint to prevent rotation of digit.

Common Diagnoses and General Optimal Positions

- PIP collateral ligament injury
- PIP dislocation
- Volar plate injury
- Stiff digit
- Sagittal band injury

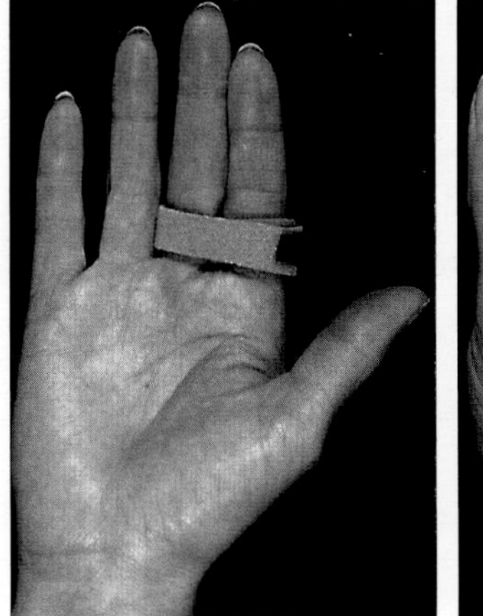

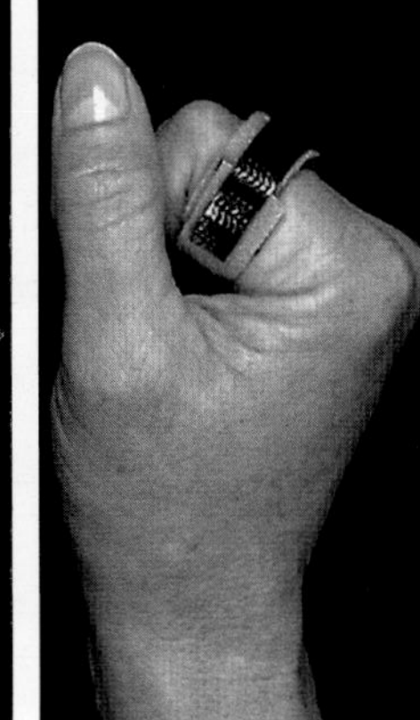

Figure 10–3

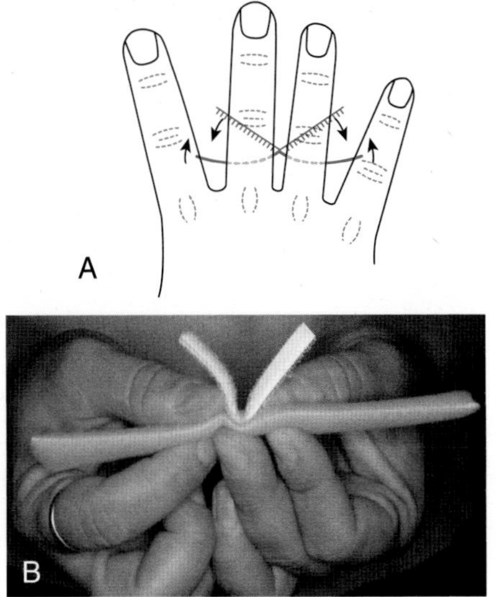

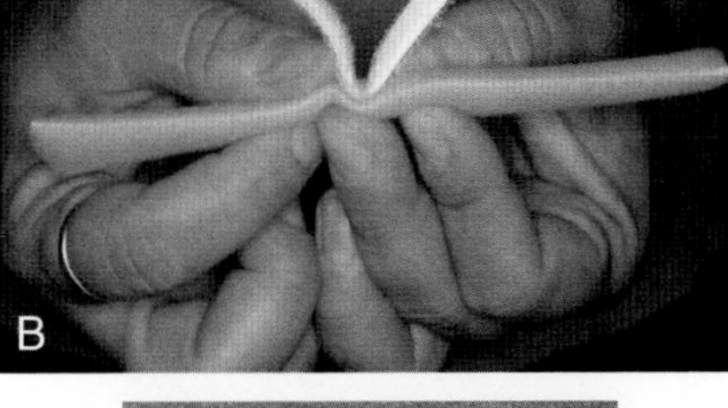

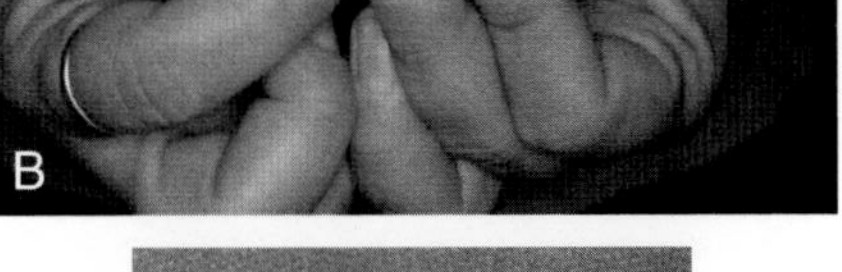

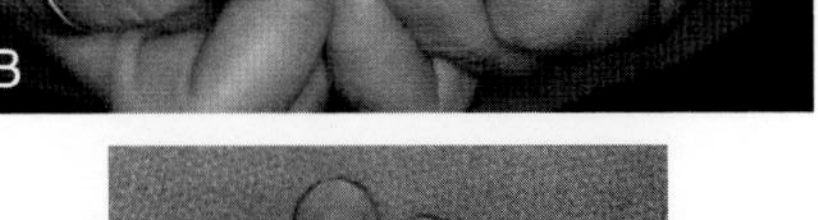

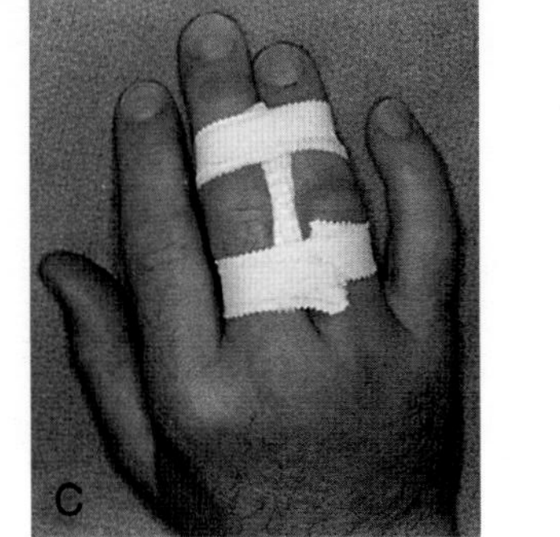

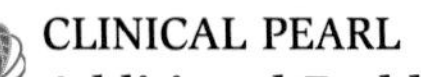

CLINICAL PEARL
Additional Buddy Strapping Techniques

Sewing method (A & B). Lay soft strap on a flat surface, and place the center of the hook strap in the middle of the soft strap. Stitch the strap onto the hook material at the center point. Loop each side of the soft strap material completely around the digit and back to the center, completely covering the hook material. With this design, dorsal closure leaves the soft strap on the volar surface to allow for unimpeded flexion of the digits.

Tape (C). Use $^1/_2$" athletic tape to secure the digits together. Note the use of gauze between the fingers to prevent maceration.

Fabrication Process

Pattern Creation (Fig. 10–4)

- Measure approximately 6" of 1/2" soft strapping material.
- Measure 1" to 1 1/2" nonadhesive hook.

Refine Pattern

- Measure width of segment involved; corresponding width of splint should be one half to one third that of segment.
- Consider additional strap at middle phalanx for added support, depending on size of digit.

Options for Materials

- Soft strapping material (Velfoam, Betapile, Neoprene) works best because they are nonelastic yet soft (Neoprene shown on previous page).
- Nonadhesive hook material to attach strap together.

Cut and Heat

- Trim both hook and soft strap according to digit size.

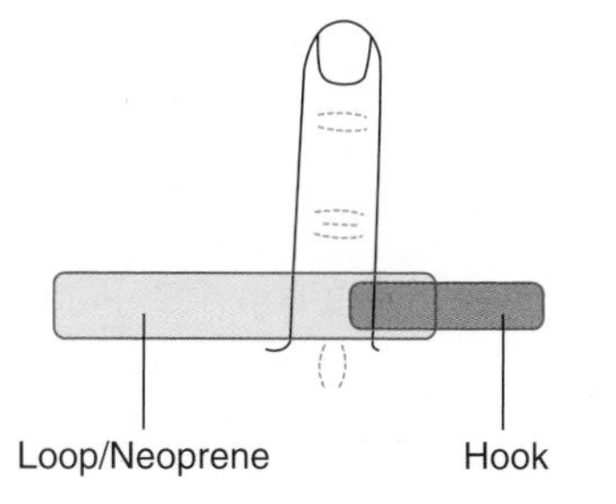

Figure 10–4

Evaluate Fit While Molding

- Position digits slightly abducted so there is adequate working room.

Strapping and Components

- From volar approach, place one end of soft strap between digits so that end is flush with dorsum of proximal phalanx.
- Wrap other end volar to dorsal and again volar to dorsal, attaching to hook.

Splint Finishing Touches

- Trim excess length and about digital web spaces if necessary.
- Consider use of gauze or polyester batting between fingers to reduce effects of perspiration.

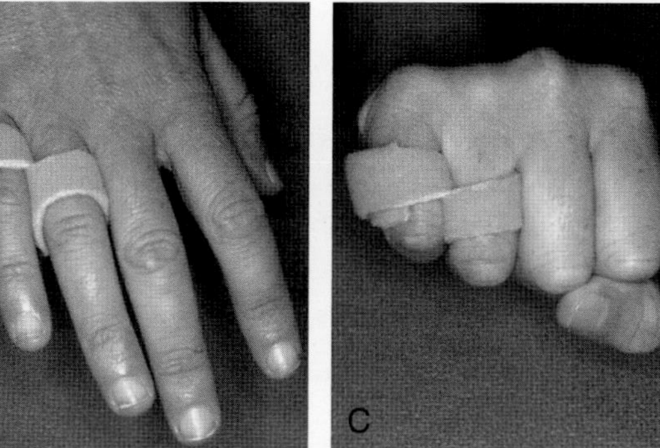

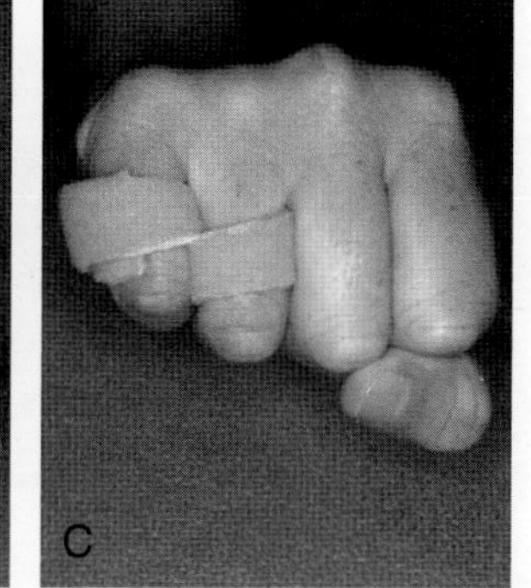

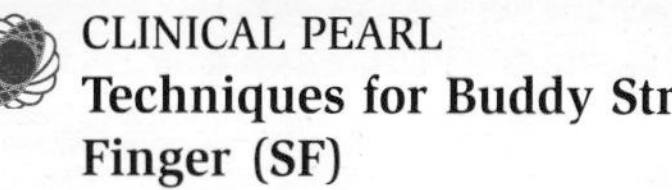

CLINICAL PEARL

Techniques for Buddy Strapping Small Finger (SF)

Buddy strapping the SF may pose a problem because it is much shorter than the RF, and the flexion creases of the fingers do not line up closely. To buddy strap these fingers effectively, consider the following techniques.

No-sew method (A–C). Zigzag or step-cut a piece of soft strap. Use hook to attach the loop together. The center portion of the strap should be quite narrow, to decrease bulk in this area. Make sure full motion is available.

Sewing method (D & E). Fabricate two separate loops and stitch them together, off center, to the degree necessary to accommodate the digit length differential. This technique allows for a good custom fit.

Proximal or Middle Phalanx Circumferential Splint (Fig. 10–5)[1]

Common Names

- Proximal phalanx fracture brace
- Middle phalanx fracture base

Alternative Splint Options

- Cast
- Digit immobilization splint

Primary Functions

- Support and protect proximal or middle phalanx during healing while allowing motion of proximal and distal joints.

Common Diagnoses and General Optimal Positions

- Stable proximal phalanx fractures (not requiring internal fixation)
- Unstable fractures requiring surgical fixation: pinning at 1 to 2 weeks postsurgery, depending on fracture stability; screw fixation 3 to 5 days postsurgery, depending on fracture stability

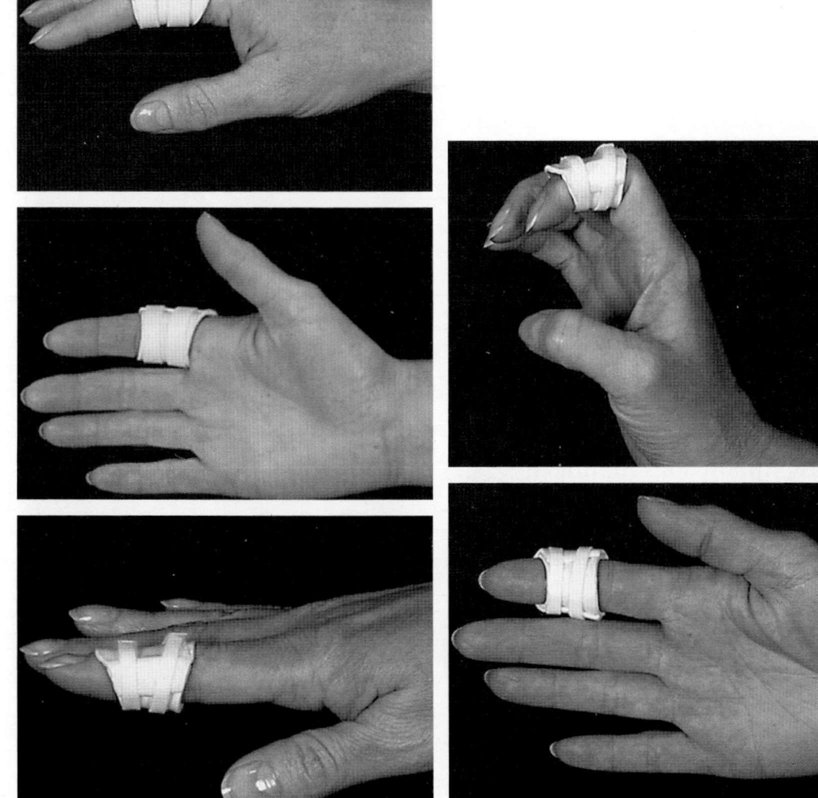

Figure 10–5

1. Described by Kim Oxford, MOT, OTR, CHT, and David H. Hildreth, MD, University of Texas Health Science Center.

Fabrication Process

Pattern Creation (Fig. 10–6)

- Mark pattern as close to digit length and circumference as possible.
- If patient cannot fully extend the involved PIP joint or is in pain, consider measuring unaffected digit.
- For more distal fractures, extend lateral supports to distal end of PIP joint.
- For more proximal fractures, extend material volarly and dorsally on MP joint.

Refine Pattern

- Remember to accommodate for use of circumferential wrapping (Coban) or wound dressing beneath splint.
- Splint should allow unimpeded flexion of MP, PIP, and DIP joints.

Options for Materials

- Use coated, elastic or plastic $^{1}/_{16}$" material.

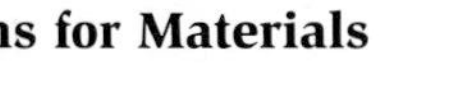

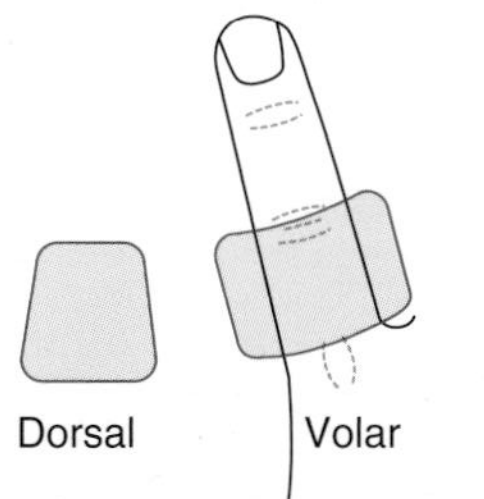

Figure 10–6

Cut and Heat

- Cut volar and dorsal pieces of material and heat.
- Apply Coban or compression garments as necessary before splint application.
- Position digits slightly abducted so there is adequate working room.

Evaluate Fit While Molding

- Fabricate volar portion of splint and allow to set before applying dorsal piece.
- For dorsal piece, lay warmed material over proximal phalanx, slightly overlapping it onto volar piece.
- Once completely set, pop splint apart.

Strapping and Components

- Use one or two $^{1}/_{4}$" to $^{1}/_{2}$" straps for optimal closure. This allows application of gentle circumferential pressure.

Splint Finishing Touches

- Smooth borders, especially between digital web spaces.
- Check for irritation of adjacent digits and possible neurovascular compromise.

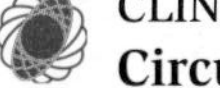

CLINICAL PEARL

Circumferential Phalanx Splints

Middle or proximal phalanx nondisplaced shaft fractures can also be managed with a circumferential splint design. Before application, examine the PIP for proximal phalanx injuries or the DIP for middle phalanx injuries to be sure that the joint is not enlarged, which would make this splint impossible to remove. Choose a $^{3}/_{32}$" or $^{1}/_{16}$" material that will readily adhere to itself once the coating has been disrupted. TailorSplint—which has a light coating but will form a smooth seam and strong bond when cut—was used for the splint shown.

Cut a strip of material the full length and approximately $^{1}/_{4}$" more than the circumference of the segment being splinted. Have the patient supinate the hand and slightly abduct the digits. Place the center of the warmed material over the volar proximal or middle phalanx and bring it around both the ulnar and the radial borders. Pinch the entire length of the ends together dorsally (this can also be done volarly). Carefully cut the excess material. Turn attention back to the volar aspect while still warm and check that the volar MP/PIP or PIP/DIP creases are cleared to allow motion.

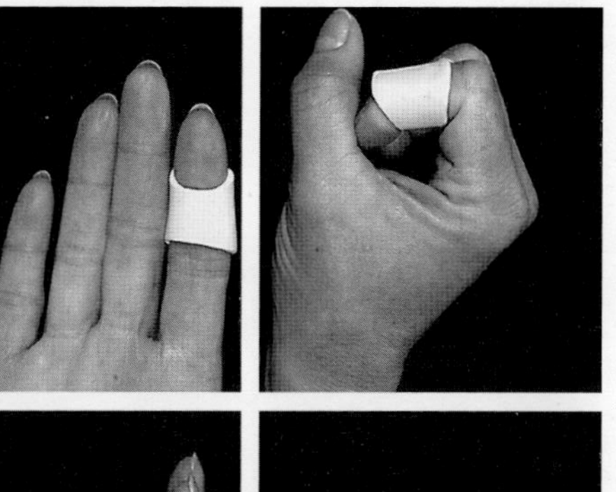
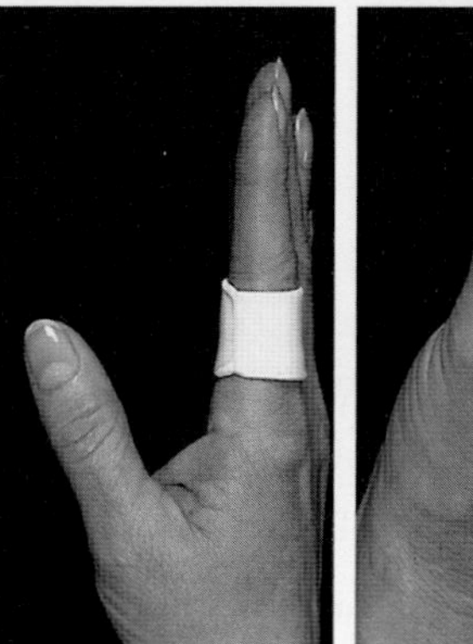
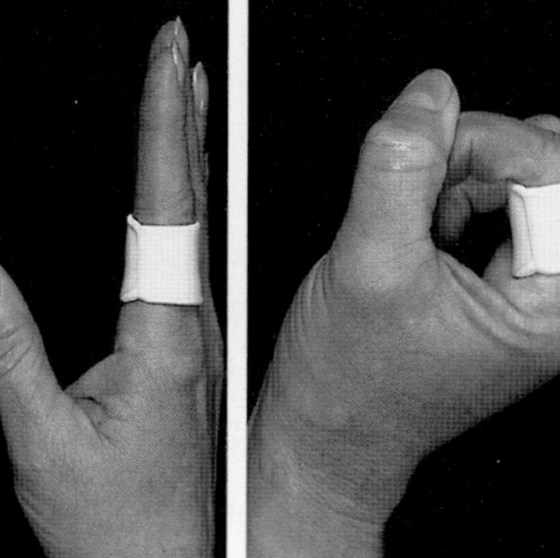
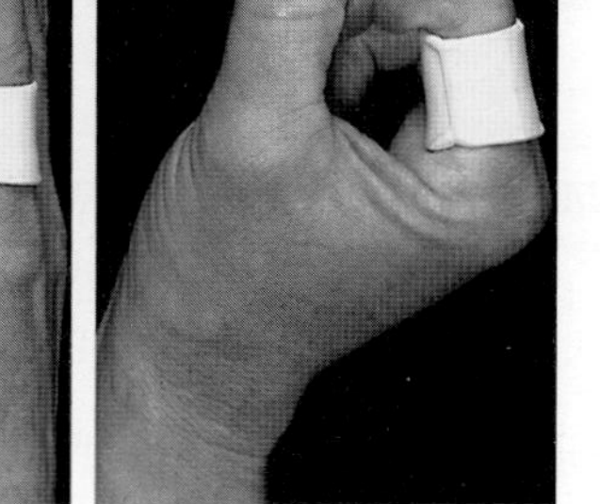

2 • Hand-Based Splints

Metacarpal Splint (Fig. 10–7)

Common Names

- Metacarpal fracture brace

Alternative Splint Options

- Cast
- Galvaston fracture brace
- Prefabricated

Primary Functions

- Stabilize and protect involved metacarpal during fracture healing.

Common Diagnoses and General Optimal Positions

- Stable/nondisplaced metacarpal fracture

CLINICAL PEARL

Splints to Facilitate Active PIP Joint Motion

Commonly, patients with stiff PIP joints compensate by hyperflexing at the MP joints when attempting to make a fist (A & B). Splinting can be an effective way to facilitate PIP joint flexion and minimize this abnormal movement pattern during functional use or exercise. This technique is most effective when addressing limitations of the MF or RF. Cut a 6" by ½" piece of thermoplastic material, heat, and place the central portion over the dorsum of the involved digit. The other two ends will wrap volar to dorsal about the adjacent digits, forming two rings. The MPs of the uninvolved digits are held in slight flexion while the involved digit is positioned in MP extension. Check that the splint borders do not interfere with active movement of the involved digit. Note that the splint must allow unimpeded MP and PIP motion. Placing a DIP immobilization splint can further isolate PIP flexion efforts.

Similarly, a splint fabricated for purpose of improving active PIP extension can be used (C & D). For this design, the middle portion of the splint is placed dorsally on the MF proximal phalanx to maximize PIP extension with active efforts.

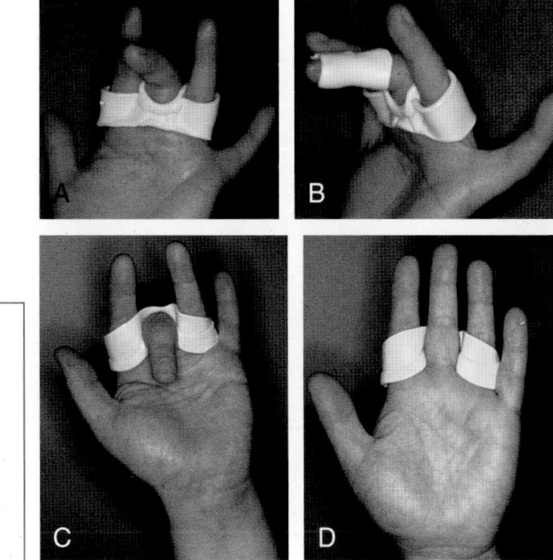

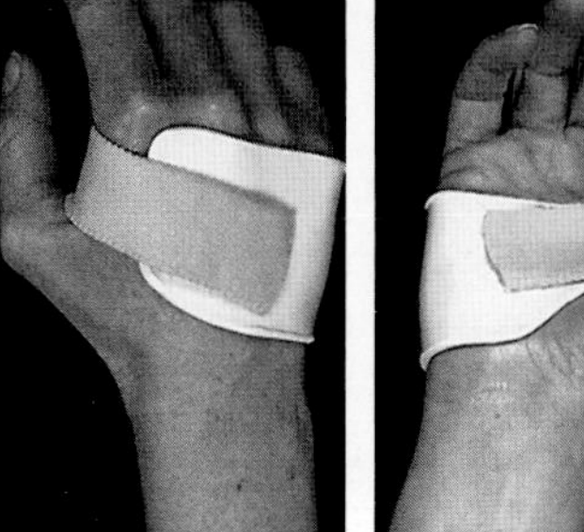
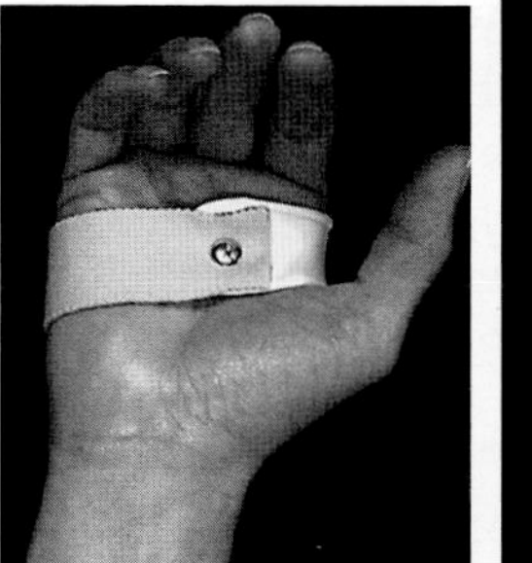
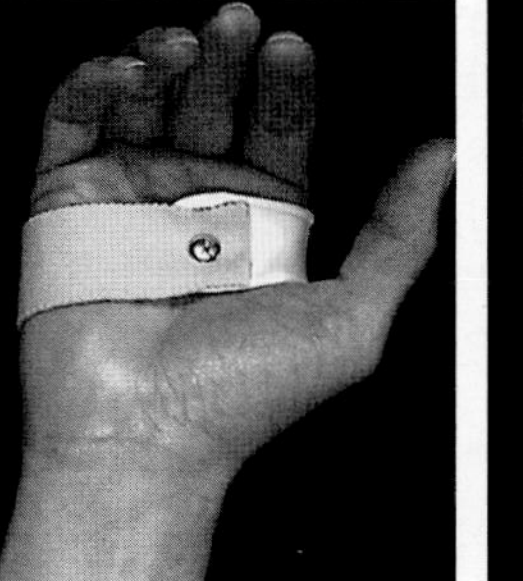
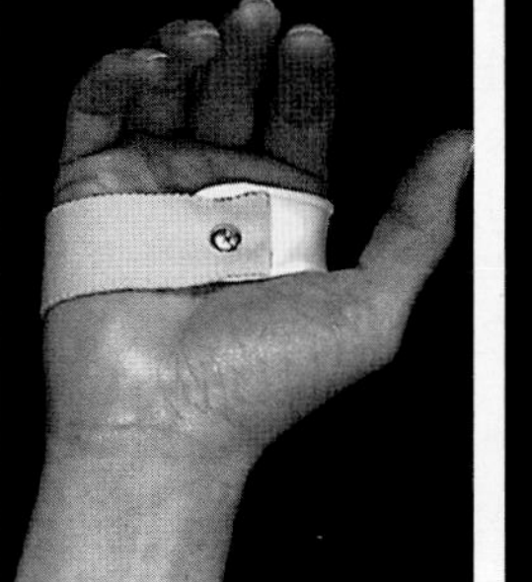
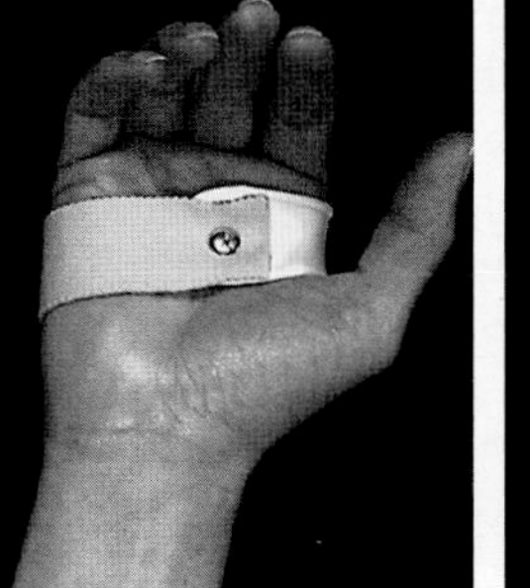
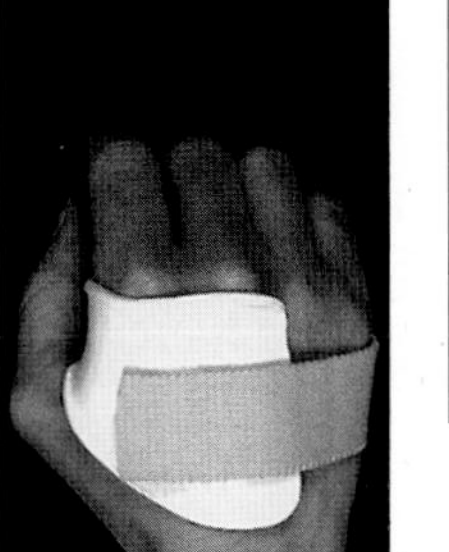
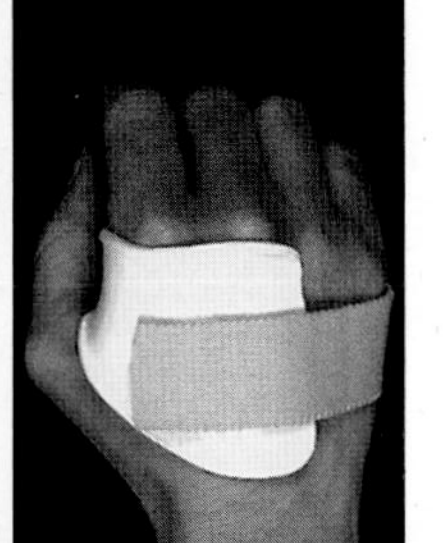
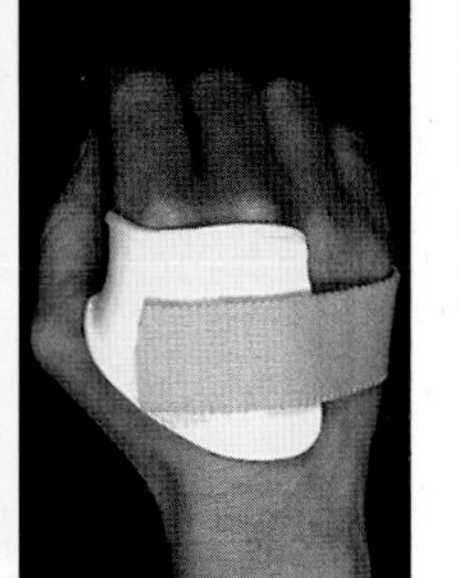
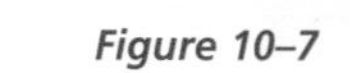

Figure 10–7

Fabrication Process

Pattern Creation (Fig. 10–8)

ULNAR DESIGN

- Mark proximal border at wrist crease.
- Mark just proximal to volar and dorsal borders of MF, RF, and SF MP joints.
- Volar surface should allow clearance of thenar muscles.

RADIAL DESIGN

- Mark proximal border at wrist crease.
- Mark just proximal to volar and dorsal borders of second and third metacarpals.
- Volar surface should allow for clearance of thenar muscles.

Refine Pattern

ULNAR DESIGN

- Proximal and distal borders should allow full wrist and MP joint motion, respectively.
- Thumb should have unimpeded motion.
- Make sure pattern encompasses third metacarpal for increased splint stability.

RADIAL DESIGN

- Proximal and distal borders should allow full wrist and MP joint motion, respectively.
- Thumb should have unimpeded motion.

Options for Materials

- Use lightly perforated material that retains some degree of flexibility when set. Splint must bend slightly to be removed for hygiene; perforations help prevent skin maceration.
- Material should provide intimate fit about metacarpals, provide stability and protection, and prevent splint migration.
- Materials that can be reheated and remolded several times are a good option if ongoing splint modifications become necessary to accommodate for fluctuations in edema.

Cut and Heat

- For ulnar design, position extremity with shoulder forward flexed and internally rotated, elbow flexed, and forearm pronated to achieve gravity-assist position (ulnar side of hand facing up).
- For radial design, position forearm in neutral rotation to achieve gravity-assist position.

Evaluate Fit While Molding

ULNAR DESIGN

- Place material centrally on ulnar aspect of hand just distal to wrist.
- On volar surface, material should rest just proximal to distal palmar crease and on dorsal surface, just proximal to MP joints.
- Allow gravity to assist while gently contouring and encompassing third to fifth metacarpals.

RADIAL DESIGN

- Place material centrally on radial aspect of hand just distal to wrist.
- On volar surface, material should rest just proximal to distal palmar crease and on dorsal surface, just proximal to MP joints.
- Allow gravity to assist while gently contouring and encompassing second to third metacarpals.

Strapping and Components

- Both ulnar and radial designs may need wrist strap to prevent migration; soft or elasticized strap works well.
- For ulnar design, use custom (trimmed) soft foam strap through first web space to maximize comfort and prevent skin irritation caused by friction (as sometimes seen with traditional loop material).
- For radial design, use elasticized strap on ulnar border to accommodate variations in muscle bulk during active hand use.

Splint Finishing Touches

- Smooth proximal and distal borders.
- Make sure there is no irritation from strap material in first web space with thumb motion.

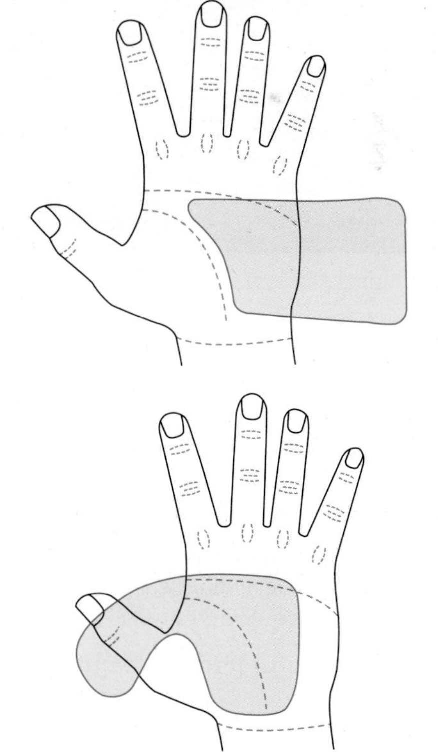

Figure 10–8

3 • Forearm-Based Splints

Forearm Splint (Fig. 10–9)

Common Names

- Forearm fracture brace

Alternative Splint Options

- Cast
- Prefabricated splint

Primary Functions

- Stabilize and protect radius and/or ulna during fracture healing by applying gentle, circumferential compression to surrounding soft tissues.

Additional Functions

- Can be used as transitional protective device for forearm fractures after healing has occurred, when patient must return to work and/or sports.

Common Diagnoses and General Optimal Positions

- Radius and ulna shaft fractures

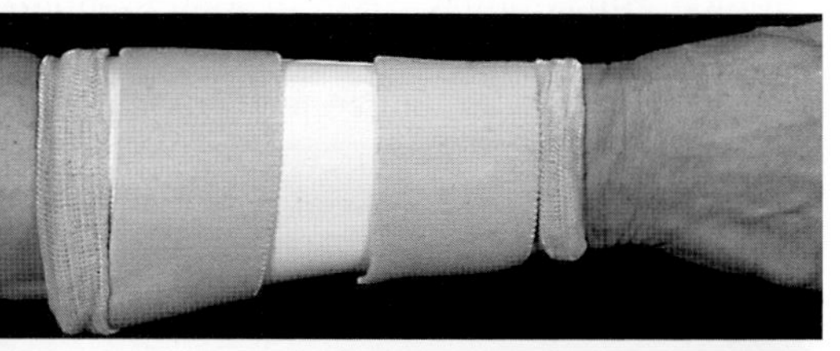

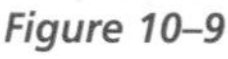

Figure 10–9

CLINICAL PEARL

Preventing Material from Adherence

There are a number of techniques for preventing the thermoplastic material from adhering to itself. When there is no choice but to use uncoated material, try one of these techniques. (1) Do not overstretch the splint material. (2) Do not be too aggressive when pressing the pieces together. (3) Place a wet paper towel between the pieces just before overlapping. (4) Apply a wet Ace wrap to the bottom piece (with an extra inch overlap directly onto the skin) and then wrap around gently over the entire splint. (5) Apply a thin layer of hand lotion on the warmed material's surface just before overlapping.

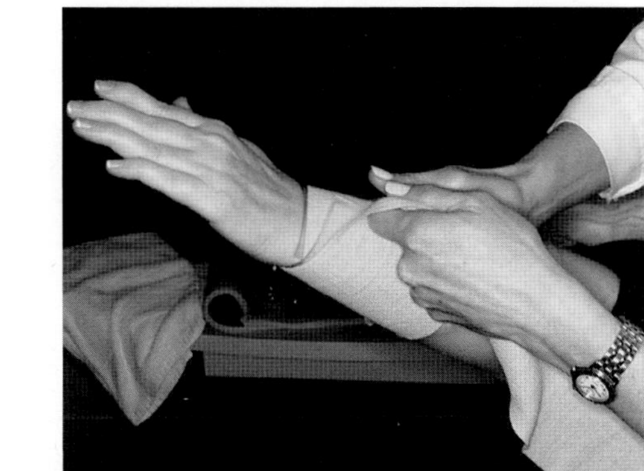

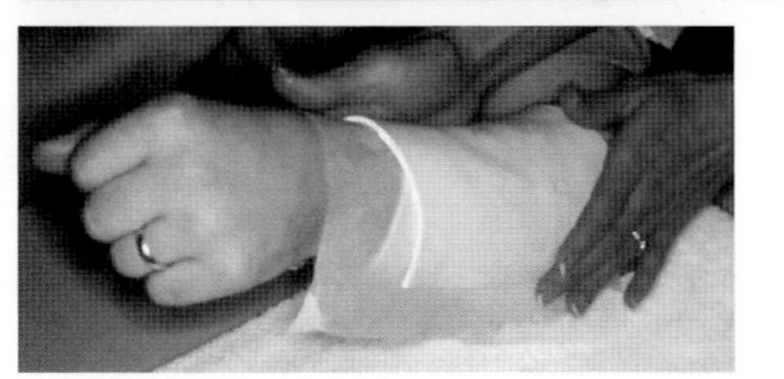

Fabrication Process

Pattern Creation (Fig. 10–10)

- Measure circumference of proximal border just distal to elbow flexion crease and add 1 in.
- Measure circumference of distal border just proximal to ulnar styloid, and add 1 in.
- Connect proximal to distal borders to account for length of splint.

Refine Pattern

- Be sure to allow enough material for approximately 1" overlap.
- In general, patients may find it easier to pull straps toward them rather than away; thus overlap material on ulnar forearm from volar to dorsal.

Options for Materials

- Use coated material to avoid permanent bonding of overlapped section and to allow splint to pop apart.
- For adults, $^3/_{32}$" material is adequate to stabilize forearm.
- For young children, $^1/_{16}$" material can be used.
- Lightly perforated material with some degree of memory may help provide intimate fit about forearm yet allow some flexibility for ease of removal and to increase air exchange.

Cut and Heat

- Position forearm in neutral rotation to achieve gravity-assist position.

Evaluate Fit While Molding

- Place warm material on towel, position so that wide section is applied proximally and narrow applied distally.
- Gently apply to forearm, keeping in mind desired overlap area.
- Begin evenly and lightly stretching material around forearm and overlapping it onto itself.

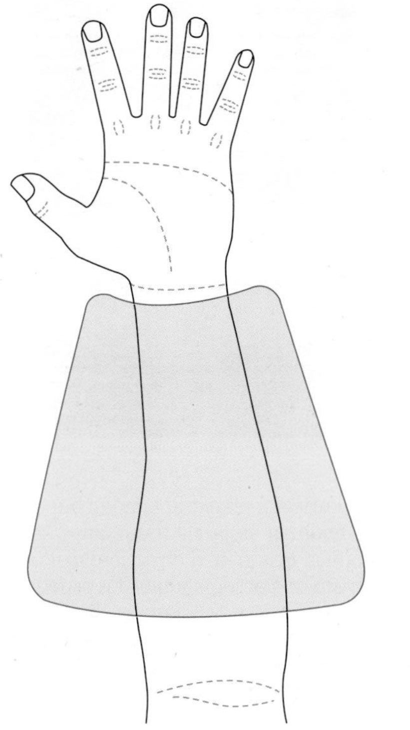

Figure 10–10

- Do not overstretch material, which may disrupt material's protective coating, causing inadvertent adherence.
- Once overlapped, apply constant moving pressure along length of splint until material is set.
- Remove splint when completely set, pop apart overlapped section, and remove from patient.

Strapping and Components

- Consider use of 1" or 2" self-adhesive D-ring straps, because they allow firm and easy closure.
- Attach D-rings so patient can tighten splint by directing pull of straps toward body.
- Alternatively, 2" elasticized straps allow patient to control compression placed on arm.
- Line entire length of inside seam with Moleskin or other thin liner. Overlap liner onto itself by approximately 1" to minimize potential of pinching forearm skin between splint pieces.
- Consider lining proximal and distal borders with soft liner, such as Moleskin or Microfoam tape to reduce migration.

Splint Finishing Touches

- Stockinette or Tubigrip under splint can provide comfort, aid with edema, and minimize splint irritation.
- Check for possible bony irritation and/or neurovascular compromise.
- Instruct patient to remove splint for hygiene only and to follow physician's protocol.

Proximal Forearm Splint

(Fig. 10–11)

Common Names

- Tennis elbow strap
- Tennis elbow cuff
- Golfer's elbow strap
- Lateral epicondylitis strap
- Medial epicondylitis strap
- Counterforce brace

Alternative Splint Options

- Prefabricated splints
- Taping

Primary Functions

- Decrease stress at proximal attachment of wrist extensors or flexors during functional use by providing counterforce and dispersing pressure about muscle bellies.

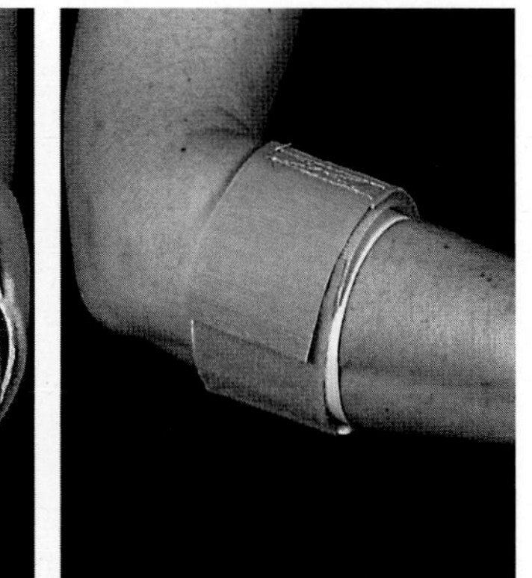

Figure 10–11

Common Diagnoses and General Optimal Positions

- Lateral epicondylitis (tennis elbow)
- Medial epicondylitis (golfer's elbow)

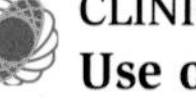

CLINICAL PEARL

Use of Elasticized Sleeve to Help Molding Process

An elasticized sleeve can be used to secure circumferential splints such as a proximal forearm splint. This technique allows for even pressure distribution while the material is setting. Do not use a size that is too tight, which may cause the splint's borders to dig in, possibly causing skin irritation. The patient can gently open and close the fist while the material is hardening, allowing the design to incorporate proximal forearm musculature.

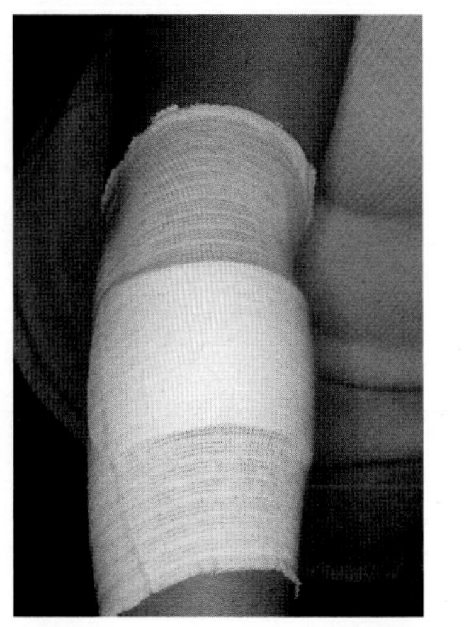

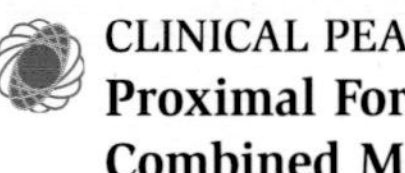

CLINICAL PEARL

Proximal Forearm Splint to Address Combined Medial and Lateral Epicondylitis

Two pieces of silicone gel or $^{3}/_{8}$" foam (2" by 2") can be added to a circumferential design to place pressure simultaneously over the proximal extensor and flexor muscle bellies. Occasionally, some patients with lateral epicondylitis, for example, may also have tenderness over the medial epicondyle secondary to overcompensation.

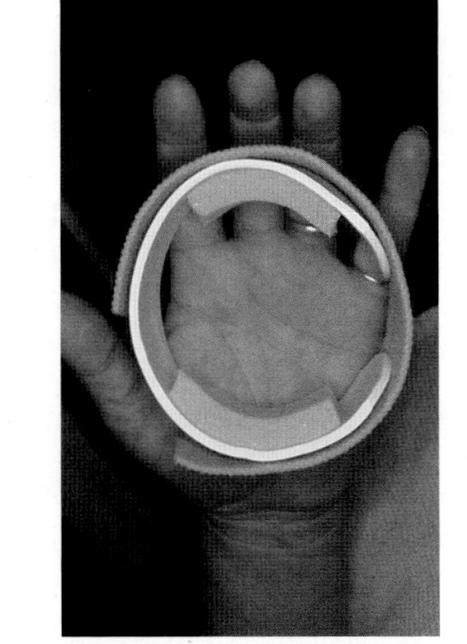

Fabrication Process

Pattern Creation (Fig. 10–12)

- Measure circumference of proximal forearm, 1" to $1\frac{1}{2}$" below epicondyles; subtract 1" to obtain circumference of splint.
- Width of splint should be approximately $2\frac{1}{2}$ in.

Refine Pattern

- Check length and width.

Options for Materials

- Use $\frac{1}{16}$" or $\frac{3}{32}$" material.
- Gel- or foam-lined thermoplastic materials eliminate added step of lining material over muscle bellies.
- When using traditional material, adhesive-backed foam or gel can be applied to molded thermoplastic in area over muscle bellies to disperse pressure.

Cut and Heat

- Position patient with elbow gently flexed, forearm neutral to slight pronation for lateral epicondylitis or neutral with slight supination for medial epicondylitis.
- Heat thermoplastic material.
- Note that some gel- and foam-lined materials can be heated in sealed plastic bag to prevent water from saturating lining (refer to manufacturer's instructions for details).

Evaluate Fit While Molding

LATERAL EPICONDYLITIS

- Rest warm material over proximal extensor muscle bellies, approximately two finger-breadths distal to lateral epicondyle.
- Wrap material from ulnar aspect of arm to radial volar aspect, leaving slight opening along ulnar border. Stockinette can be used to allow material to set with even pressure distribution.
- Once material is secured on proximal forearm, have patient lightly open and close fist to get contouring about muscle bellies.

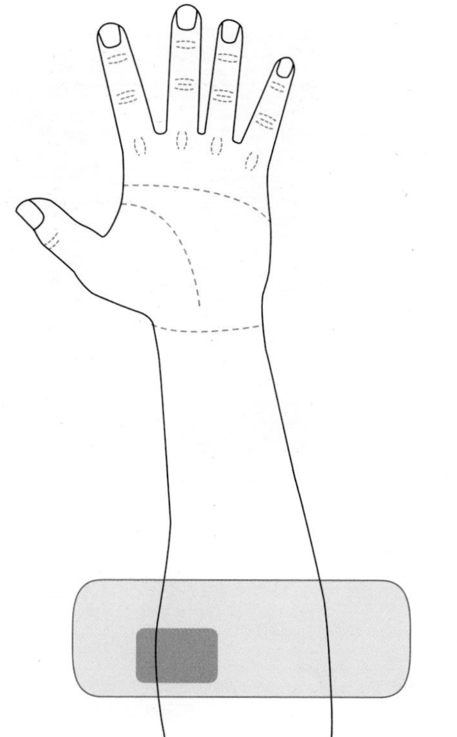

Figure 10–12

MEDIAL EPICONDYLITIS

- Rest warm material over proximal flexor muscle bellies approximately two finger-breadths distal to medial epicondyle.
- Once material is secured on proximal forearm, have patient lightly open and close fist to get contouring about muscle bellies.

Strapping and Components

- After material has set, apply adhesive foam or gel on portion of splint that will be resting over flexor and/or extensor muscle bellies.
- Adhesive hook is applied to nearly full circumference of splint to provide even pressure distribution throughout splint.
- Consider use of 2" elasticized strap to allow splint to accommodate for forearm musculature is contracting and relaxing.
- Apply strap with even tension across entire circumference of splint.
- D-ring strap also works well for this type of splint.
- Direction of strap application should provide for easy donning and doffing.

Splint Finishing Touches

- Smooth borders of splint's edges.
- Instruct patient in appropriate strap tightness and caution regarding signs of neurovascular compromise.
- Mark proximal and distal ends of splint and review proper splint placement.

4 • Arm-Based Splints

Humerus Splint (Fig. 10–13)

Common Names

- Humeral fracture brace
- Sarmiento humerus brace

Alternative Splint Options

- Cast
- Prefabricated splint
- Sling
- Orthotic

Primary Functions

- Stabilize and protect humerus during fracture healing by applying gentle, circumferential compression to surrounding soft tissues.

Additional Functions

- None.

Common Diagnoses and General Optimal Positions

- Humeral shaft fracture

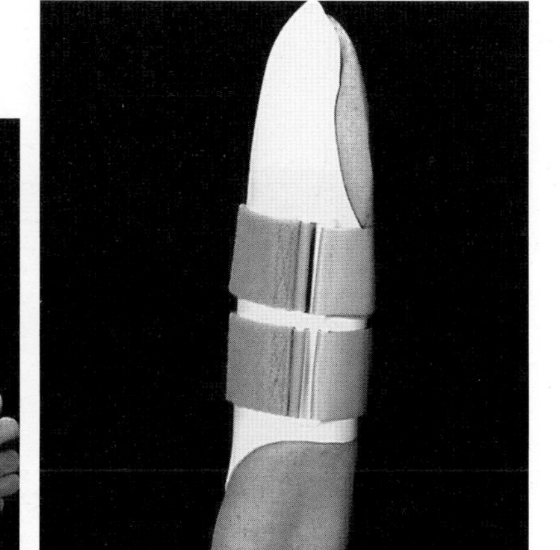

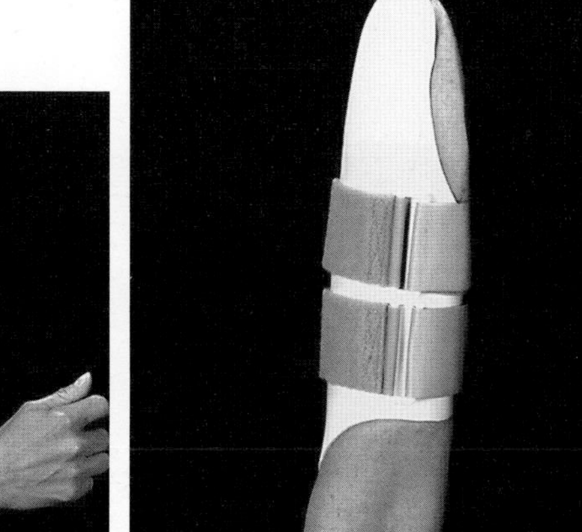

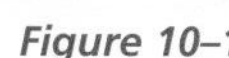

Figure 10–13

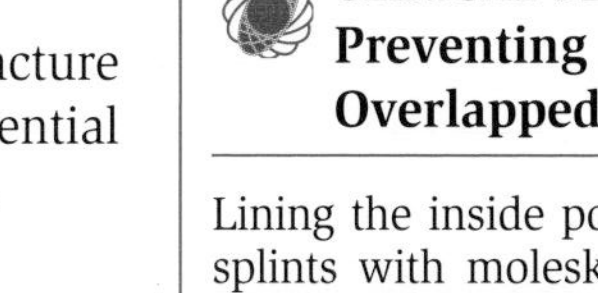

CLINICAL PEARL

Preventing Skin Irritation from Overlapped Segments

Lining the inside portion of circumferentially designed splints with moleskin (or a similar material) may reduce the potential for irritation at the splint/skin interface. The key is to overlap the lining onto itself to form an extra 1" to 2" soft flap on the inside of the splint. This technique can be used for most circumferential splint designs.

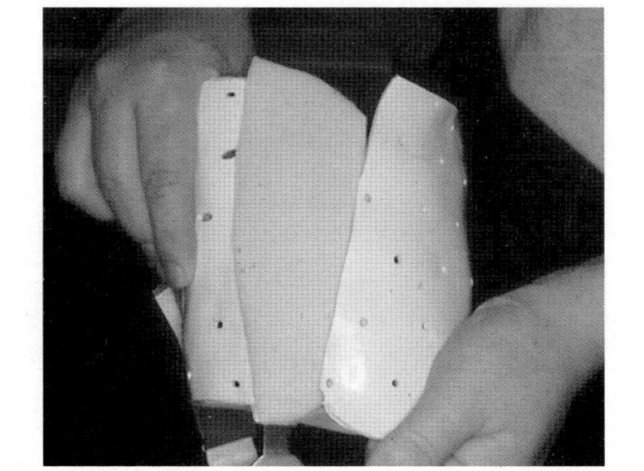

Fabrication Process

Pattern Creation (Fig. 10–14)

- Location of fracture along shaft dictates length of splint.
- For proximal shaft fractures, splint pattern should extend to proximal edge of acromion process and distal edge can terminate just above elbow crease.
- For distal shaft fractures, splint pattern should extend just distal to acromion process and distal edge can terminate over epicondyles medially and laterally.
- Both designs should support medial arm to axilla.

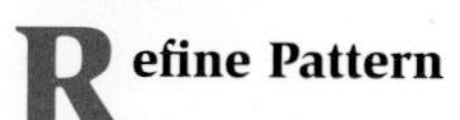

Refine Pattern

- Proximal border should allow nearly full shoulder motion.
- Distal border should allow unimpeded elbow motion.
- Check that there is enough material to encompass humerus circumferentially and add 1" to $1\frac{1}{2}$" extra for overlap.
- Avoid irritation to epicondyles, olecranon, axilla, and ulnar nerve at cubital tunnel.

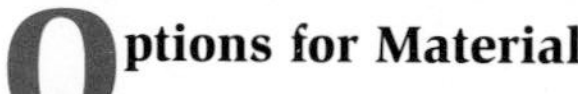

Options for Materials

- Use coated material so overlapped section can be popped open.
- For larger arms, $\frac{1}{8}$" or $\frac{3}{32}$" materials provide needed support.
- For smaller arms, $\frac{3}{32}$" or $\frac{1}{16}$" materials provide adequate support.
- Remember that elastic materials tend to shrink around splinted part; do not remove until splint is completely set.
- Use lightly perforated material that retains some degree of flexibility when set. Splint must bend slightly to be removed for hygiene; perforations help prevent skin maceration.

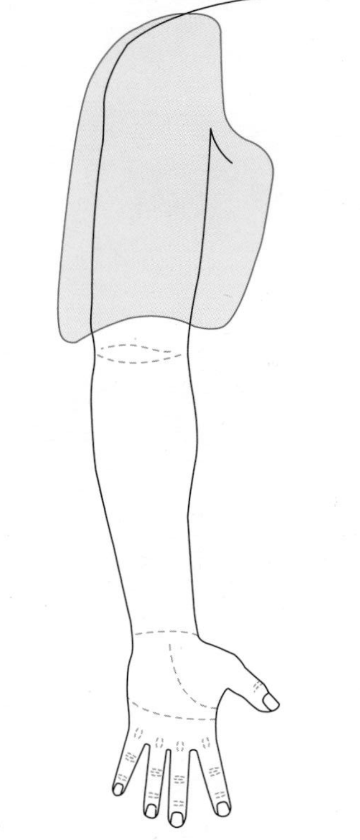

Figure 10–14

Cut and Heat

- Position patient seated with shoulder supported in slight abduction, it may help to have assistant position extremity during fabrication process to minimize patient discomfort.
- While material is heating, prepad medial and lateral epicondyles using self-adhesive padding or silicone gel, if necessary.
- Carefully cut pattern from material. Pattern has many curves; try to be accurate in pattern design and transfer onto material.

Evaluate Fit While Molding

- Supporting entire piece of warm material, place along anterior humerus, aligning cut out for axilla and anterior elbow appropriately; open section is positioned along posterior humerus.
- If splinting for proximal shaft fracture, simultaneously extend warm material over humeral head to acromion process.
- If splinting for distal shaft fracture, extend material distally over epicondyles making sure not to interfere with elbow mobility.
- Using both hands, carefully and gently stretch material anterior to posterior, under axilla, and over onto itself.
- Do not overstretch material, which may disrupt material's protective coating, causing inadvertent adherence.
- Gently flare material around proximal segment with careful attention to axilla (do not overlap material, which tends to irritate this sensitive region) and along distal borders.

Strapping and Components

- Use 2" self-adhesive D-ring straps, because they allow firm and easy closure; patient can make adjustments according to comfort
- Attach D-rings so patient can tighten splint by directing pull of straps toward body.
- Line inside of splint with Moleskin or other thin liner. Overlap liner onto itself by approximately 1" to minimize potential of pinching forearm skin between splint pieces.
- Line proximal and distal borders with Microfoam tape or self-adhesive gel liners to decrease distal migration.

Splint Finishing Touches

- Some patients may benefit from wearing stockinette or Tubigrip beneath splint to minimize splint irritation and aid with controlling perspiration.
- Check for migration and possible bony irritation or neurovascular compromise.
- Instruct patient to remove for hygiene only and to follow physician's protocol.

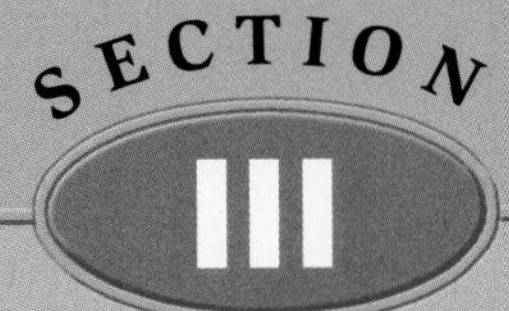

Optional Methods

CHAPTER 11

Prefabricated Splints

Janet Cope, MS, CAS, OTR/L

INTRODUCTION

Something that is designed to fit everyone fits no one well (Malick 1982). One size fits none. As therapists, we are by nature, skeptical of easy solutions to rehabilitation problems; and as hand therapists, we strive to design and create a comfortable and effective solution for the patient. It is the challenge of creating a well-fitting, purposeful splint for the patient that provides many therapists with joy in their work. However, owing to time constraints, monetary issues, and/or perhaps the lack of product availability, it is not always practical or appropriate to make a splint from thermoplastic, plaster, fiberglass, and soft splinting materials. Therefore, prefabricated splints offer an alternative treatment option and play an important role in the practice of upper extremity therapy.

This chapter outlines the considerations related to the use of **prefabricated splints** and includes information on how to become an educated consumer on the availability and application of these splints. Some of the commonly used and currently available splints are reviewed as well. Prefabricated splints can sometimes be used creatively for purposes other than what they were originally intended for; suggestions for these alternative uses are provided.

Splinting Considerations

There are a number of issues to consider before choosing either a custom-made or a prefabricated splint. The skill of the therapist is sometimes a determining factor for using prefabricated devices. That is, some therapists make splints only occasionally; therefore, they either do not have the skills to make the required custom splint or it would not be an efficient use of their time to do so. Adapting prefabricated splints may be helpful in these circumstances. Similarly, the setting in which a therapist works might dictate the choice of splints; those in home-health-care settings without the necessary equipment for custom fabrication may find that prefabricated splints are appropriate for some clients. In addition, one or any combination of the following factors may affect the selection of an appropriate splint for a particular patient:

- Specifics of the diagnosis.
- Patient needs.
- Time constraints.
- Appropriateness of the material.
- Ease of application.
- Cost effectiveness.

Specifics of the Diagnosis

In assessing the patient's needs, one must consider what is the best solution for the immediate situation. The therapist must clearly understand the patient's diagnosis and current status. Does the patient have a fracture with open wounds and a painful edematous hand? Perhaps a preformed resting splint will save fabrication time and assist in immobilizing the upper extremity more quickly and with less molding and fitting requirements than a custom splint. Does the patient have an external fixator, pins, or other hardware? These devices require customized splint fabrication. Does the patient require rigid immobilization or would a soft support suffice? For example, a patient with rheumatoid arthritis may use a prefabricated Neoprene ulnar deviation splint during the day and a custom thermoplastic resting splint at night (Dell & Dell, 1996).

Patient Needs

The therapist and patient need to negotiate a safe and reasonable splinting regime for home use. Patient education and involvement in the plan of treatment generally increase the likelihood of consistent implementation of the splinting schedule. When selecting a splint designed to increase function, "fit, comfort, and effectiveness through a range of functional activities" (Melvin, 1995) should be evaluated before dispensing the device to the patient.

The therapist must carefully consider the needs of the patients. Can the patient wait for the prefabricated splint to be ordered? Does insurance allow the patient the additional visit that is required to properly fit the splint that has been ordered? The patient's needs in both the home and the work setting should be considered. For example, someone who is a heavy laborer may require a rigid splint for work but may be more comfortable in a fabric-based prefabricated splint for home.

Time Constraints

Time can be a major factor in a for-profit organization. Today's demand for increased patient caseloads influences how much time the therapist has with each patient. The therapist must evaluate the need and weigh the benefits of a custom-made splint versus a prefabricated product. There are also preformed splints available that can save the therapist time. Specific splint patterns, or splint blanks, come ready to heat and apply to the patient. This saves a great deal of time in pattern development and cutting. Is it more appropriate to use a prefabricated or preformed elbow mobilization splint and to spend the patient's treatment time performing hands-on intervention or to fabricate a custom elbow splint? The therapist must decide what is the best use of the available treatment time.

Appropriateness of the Material

The type of prefabricated splint selected or the material used to fabricate a custom-made splint can have an effect on patient comfort, tissue healing, and position options. Patients who are slender and have prominent bony structures may be more comfortable in a splint that is fabricated out of Neoprene or another forgiving material. Thermoplastic is rigid and can be uncomfortable when constant use is required. Comfort is an important issue and is directly related to consistent wearing patterns (Rossi, 1988).

Thermoplastic material may be the most appropriate material to use if the patient is required to have his or her hands in water or heavy soil for any reason during the day. Thermoplastic material is easy to clean and tolerates moisture better than most fabric-based splints. However, there are patients who perspire and are thus prone to tissue maceration when solid thermoplastic materials are used; a light fabric-based splint should be considered for these patients.

Adjustments can be simple to make on soft splints with flexible metal inserts. No equipment is necessary, and the splints can be modified at the patient's bedside or in the home. A thermoplastic volar wrist support requires a heating source and patient compliance in upper extremity positioning while the material is molded and setting. This may not always be possible. Thermoplastic material may be the wisest and most appropriate choice when, for example, treating a patient with a flexor tendon injury that requires exact joint positions.

Ease of Application

Ease of application by the patient in the work or home setting is an important factor to consider when developing a splinting plan. The therapist must determine the simplest solution for the patient's requirements. A prefabricated digit extension mobilization splint may be easier for a patient to apply than a custom hand-based digit extension mobilization splint. Serial static casting might be the simplest solution for some patients.

If the patient has a number of issues (e.g., multiple joint contractures) that need to be addressed with splinting, they must be prioritized. The therapist must determine the feasibility of the splinting plan for the patient in the home setting; an individual who lives alone must be able to don and doff the device independently. Immobilization of healing structures may be the most important problem to be addressed, but increasing function may be deemed most important by the patient.

Cost Effectiveness

When evaluating the patient's needs, the therapist must consider all of the cost-effective variables. Is the splint going to be worn for a short period of time or will it be required on a more permanent basis? Will the patient's insurance pay for a prefabricated or custom-molded splint? The insurance carrier may or may not cover either type of splint. In some situations, the prefabricated splint may be more affordable to the patient without compromising the quality of treatment. It is appropriate to educate the patient regarding the options and to include him or her in the decision making. In some cases, the patient may require a number of splints, worn alternately throughout the day and night. Some of these splints may be custom-made and others prefabricated.

Educated Decision Making

An educated decision must be made each time a splint is selected for a patient. There is a wide variety of splinting materials, components, and prefabricated splints available for almost every splinting situation. It is challenging to keep abreast of all of the prefabricated splinting options, but there are many ways to stay informed.

To keep up with new splinting trends, therapists can attend upper extremity courses, including lectures and hands-on laboratories on successful splinting interventions. Conferences frequently feature vendor booths that allow therapists to investigate new materials and prefabricated splints. Therapists can try splints and equipment on and request further information. Vendors are eager to provide in-service training and information sessions at facilities, offer material or splint samples, and help with specific patient problem solving. Company representatives are often therapists who have decided to enter the equipment provision aspect of the business; they are integral to the development of new product lines and improvements of existing ones. In working with therapists all over the country, they collect valuable information on trends and helpful hints and are willing to share the tips they have learned.

Catalogs provide an expansive amount of information regarding splinting and therapy intervention. Updated yearly, they enable the therapist to stay abreast of therapy trends. See Appendix A for a list of vendors and rehabilitation companies along with contact information.

Therapists can also review articles in therapy and surgery publications to gain a better understanding of the theoretical basis behind the splinting decisions colleagues are making to solve splinting problems. There are many methods for solving every splinting situation. A custom-made splint might meet the biomechanical issues but may cause problems for the patient in the areas of maintaining skin integrity or comfort (Rossi, 1988). Solutions to many splinting problems can be found by reviewing current literature.

Prefabricated Splints for the Upper Extremity

This section, which presents a review of prefabricated splints, is organized according to where on the upper extremity the splint is to be applied. For each upper extremity part, a variety of prefabricated splints are discussed and comparisons are made to highlight specific splinting issues. This discussion is not meant to be inclusive of all available prefabricated splints; each manufacturer has versions of the commonly used prefabricated splints and available products are too numerous to mention all. Although **continuous passive motion (CPM) machines** can be considered treatment modalities, here they are referred to as an additional prefabricated splinting intervention.

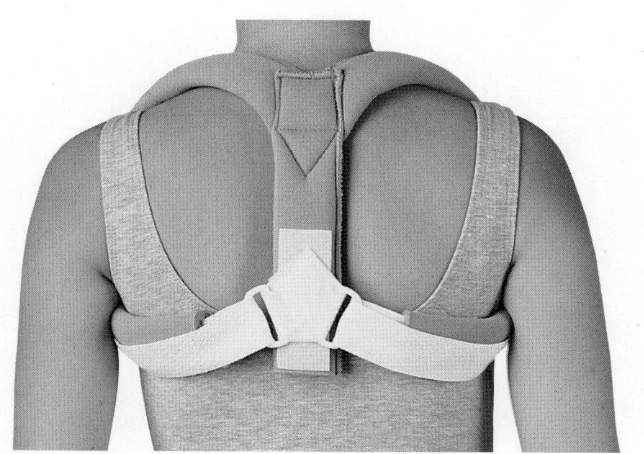

Figure 11–1 A Clavicle Posture Support. Observe the patient for 20 min after applying a clavicle brace to ensure proper fit. Check for any signs of neurovascular compression—numbness, tingling, coolness, or pain in the extremity—and readjust as needed. Photo courtesy of Rehabilitation Division of Smith+Nephew (Germantown, WI).

Shoulder and Upper Arm Splints

The diagnoses commonly treated with prefabricated splints at the shoulder and upper arm are clavicle, scapula, and humerus fractures; humeral head dislocation or subluxation; and rotator cuff injuries and surgical repairs. The types of prefabricated splints used to treat these conditions include clavicle braces, slings, functional fracture braces, and shoulder immobilization splints.

Clavicle Brace

Clavicle braces are available in a limited variety from most of the major rehabilitation suppliers (Fig. 11–1). Some providers also stock pediatric sizes. When fitting a patient with a clavicle brace, a key point to evaluate is an appropriate fit through the axilla. The strap system should not be too tight through this area, because it can create increased pressure on the brachial artery and brachial plexus, which innervates the arm. A loose fit may encourage a flexed cervical posture and is also not appropriate for proper clavicular stabilization. The patient should be able to relax the shoulders while good cervical and thoracic posture is sustained.

Sling

There is a wide array of **slings** available that stabilize healing structures about the shoulder (e.g, rotator cuff, capsule, ligaments, bone, or neurovascular) and provide support and properly position the hemiplegic shoulder (Fig. 11–2). Hemiplegic arm slings are recommended for patients who have hemiplegia or a subluxating humeral head. The therapist must carefully monitor patients who are using slings to ensure that they are removing the sling and exercising the injured extremity as recommended, to prevent complications of stiffness and distal edema.

There are a multitude of slings worn on the shoulder to provide support to an injured forearm, wrist, and/or hand. Selection of an appropriate sling is contingent on the patient's diagnosis. Shoulder immobilizers are recommended for patients with a humeral fracture or a humeral head dislocation. Patients with a stable humeral fracture may wear a sling for support and comfort; it should be removed regularly throughout the day for appropriate exercise (Colditz, 1995).

Humeral Fracture Brace

A prefabricated **humeral fracture brace** can be used for splinting a humeral fracture. A nonarticular design, which permits elbow motion, may be chosen for midshaft fractures (Fig. 11–3). For more distal humeral fractures, splints may be applied circumferentially to the

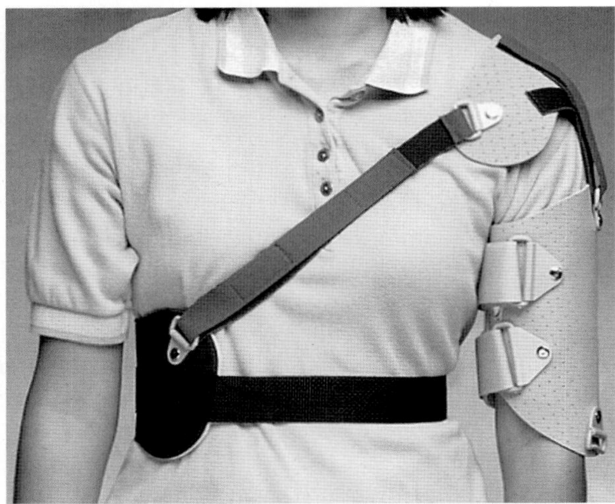

Figure 11–2 *Hemiplegic slings—designed to support the head of the humerus in the glenoid fossa—are commonly recommended for patients who have had a stroke. Slings should be judiciously used to protect the extremity of patients with complex forearm and hand injuries, owing to the possibility of stiffness and edema. The North Coast Hemiplegic Sling provides three points of pressure for optimal positioning and comfort. Photo courtesy of North Coast Medical (Morgan Hill, CA).*

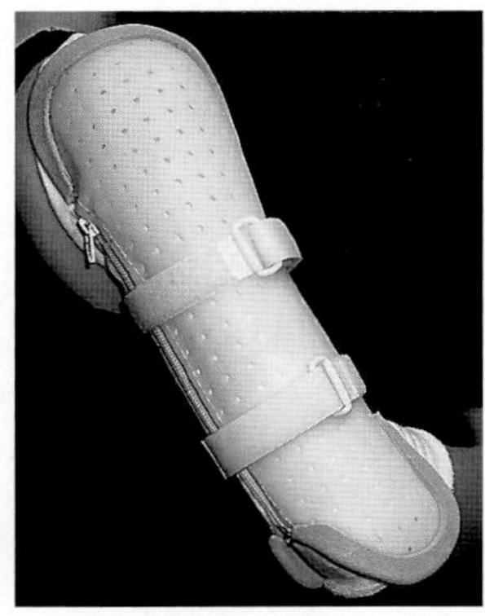

Figure 11–3 *This circumferential brace (Roylan AquaForm) allows elbow and forearm motion while providing good immobilization and support to the healing fracture. Photo courtesy of Rehabilitation Division of Smith+Nephew (Germantown, WI).*

humerus and the forearm with an elbow hinge connecting the components (Colditz, 1995).

Shoulder Immobilization Splint

A **shoulder immobilization splint** may be required for a fracture of the scapula or an injury of the rotator cuff. This splint immobilizes the humerus in the glenoid fossa and the scapula against the thoracic wall (Fig. 11–4).

CPM Machine

A **shoulder CPM machine** can be used for treating postoperative shoulders to prevent joint and soft tissue contractures. The Kinetic 7081 Shoulder CPM Machine (Smith+Nephew, Germantown, WI) is one example; it can be used with the patient in bed or in a chair.

Elbow and Forearm Splints

The elbow is a complex and challenging joint to splint, because it is made up of bony prominences and superficial nerves and is surrounded by forceful muscles. Some of the prefabricated splints that are used to treat the elbow are elbow protectors, Neoprene compression sleeves, proximal forearm splints (counterforce braces), elbow mobilization splints, and CPM machines.

Elbow Protector

Elbow protectors can be used before and after surgery for patients with cubital tunnel syndrome (ulnar neuropathy). The pad should be "worn over the posterior medial aspect of the elbow to protect the ulnar nerve from direct pressure or trauma" (Sailer, 1996). Available options incorporate a silicone gel pad insert to help reduce shock and vibration and to apply light compression to a postoperative scar in the region of the ulnar nerve (Fig. 11–5).

Neoprene Compression Sleeve

Neoprene compression sleeves may be used to treat ulnar neuropathies and muscle strains about the elbow (Fig. 11–6). They offer gentle compression, warmth, and support to surrounding tissues as well as provide gentle feedback to the patient to restrict elbow flexion. The sleeve should fit snugly but not tightly enough to increase or induce any neurologic symptoms (tingling, pain, or numbness).

Proximal Forearm Splint (Counterforce Brace)

Lateral and medial epicondylitis straps come with a wide variety of options (Fig. 11–7). Some have cushions

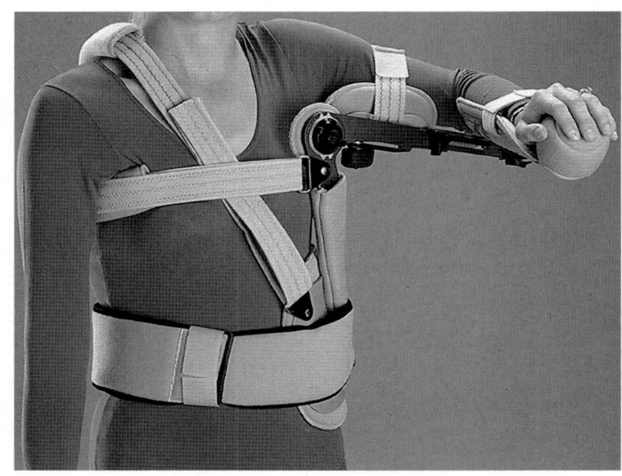

Figure 11–4 *This shoulder immobilization splint (Roylan Shoulder Brace) can be adjusted to place the humerus in a specific position of abduction and internal rotation. The elbow and forearm can be positioned by degree of flexion or extension and supination or pronation. Note that the wrist and hand are fully supported. Photo courtesy of Rehabilitation Division of Smith+Nephew (Germantown, WI).*

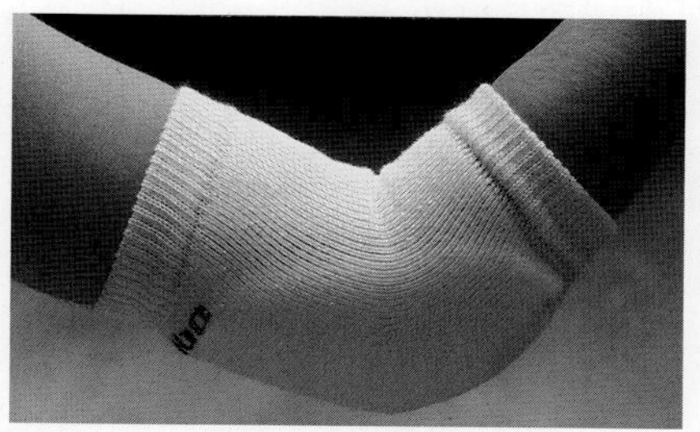

Figure 11–5 When fitting a patient with an elbow protector (Heelbo splint shown), measure the distance circumferentially around the patient's elbow flexion crease, keeping in mind that the protector is intended to fit snugly. Photo courtesy of North Coast Medical (Morgan Hill, CA).

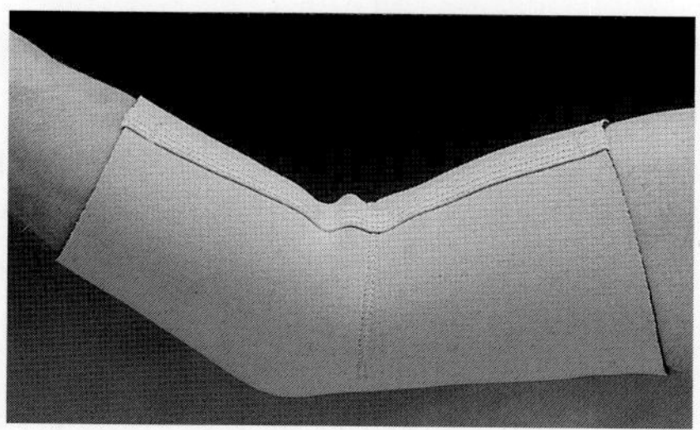

Figure 11–6 After applying a Neoprene Elbow Sleeve, monitor the patient for a short time, watching for any signs of neurologic symptoms. Photo courtesy of North Coast Medical (Morgan Hill, CA).

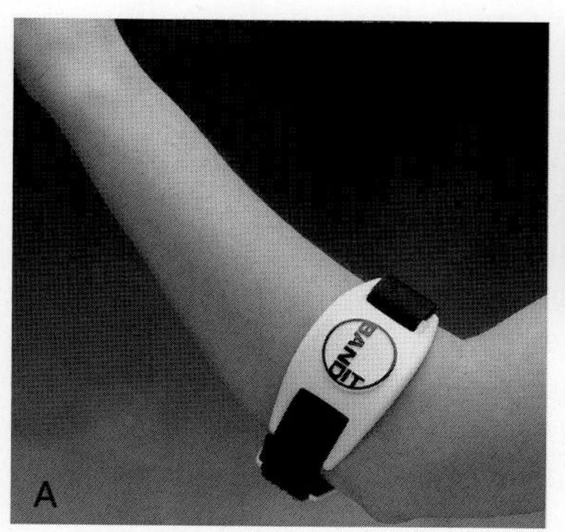

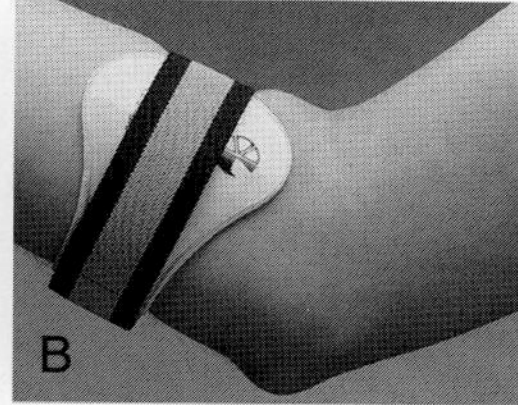

*Figure 11–7 An epicondylitis strap should reduce the patient's pain; reposition the strap distally or proximally as needed to increase patient comfort. **A,** The Band-It Therapeutic Elbow Band (used for patients with lateral and medial symptoms). **B,** The Tennis Elbow Epicondylitis Clasp with a wool-lined plastic device. Photo courtesy of North Coast Medical (Morgan Hill, CA).*

that apply a gentle compressive force to the forearm extensors in an effort to change the fulcrum from the epicondyle to the muscle bellies; they also help reduce the intensity of the muscle contraction. When treating a patient with lateral epicondylitis, apply the strap to the forearm extensors just distal to the lateral epicondyle; tighten the strap firmly. Then have the patient make a fist, extend the wrist, and flex the elbow to check for comfort. Caution the patient not to secure the strap too tightly, because the radial nerve is vulnerable to compression in this region (Aulicino, 1995; Kleinert & Mehta, 1996).

Many of the straps designed for the treatment of lateral epicondylitis can also be used in the treatment of medial epicondylitis by rotating the straps to apply pressure to the medial forearm flexors. There is a multipurpose strap called Band-It (North Coast Medical, Morgan Hill, CA) that can be used to treat patients who are diagnosed with both medial and lateral epicondylitis. This strapping system is designed to apply compression to both the extensor and the flexor muscle groups at the same time.

Elbow Mobilization Splints

Stiffness secondary to fractures and dislocations at the elbow can be treated with a variety of prefabricated **elbow mobilization splints** that provide a corrective force to the tissue. Splints like the Dynasplint (EMPI, St. Paul, MN) and Progress Elbow Hinge Splint (North Coast Medical) have Neoprene or foam cuffs with flexible metal attachments both proximal and distal to the elbow. These splints are flexible and comfortable for the patient and can be easily adjusted when there is a decrease in bandages or edema. Patients can wear this type of a splint with the load adjusted to provide a gentle stretch for sleep or intermittent daytime use. To maintain the gains in range of motion (ROM), the splint can be locked out at a specific degree, if desired. Both EMPI and North Coast Medical offer these splints in pediatric as well as adult sizes.

A static progressive stretch orthotic developed by Joint Active Systems (Effingham, IL) can be used to treat elbow flexion and extension contractures (Fig. 11–8). The application of a gentle stretch over a long period of time improves tissue extensibility and yields permanent tissue lengthening (Bonutti, Windau, Ables, & Miller, 1994). The device has proximal and distal cuffs, which can be adjusted to fit a variety of limb length, and a load-adjustable hinge centered at the olecranon. Patients with spinal cord injuries at C5-6 frequently develop elbow flexion contractures; these are treated with elbow extension mobilization splints. Splints designed to treat

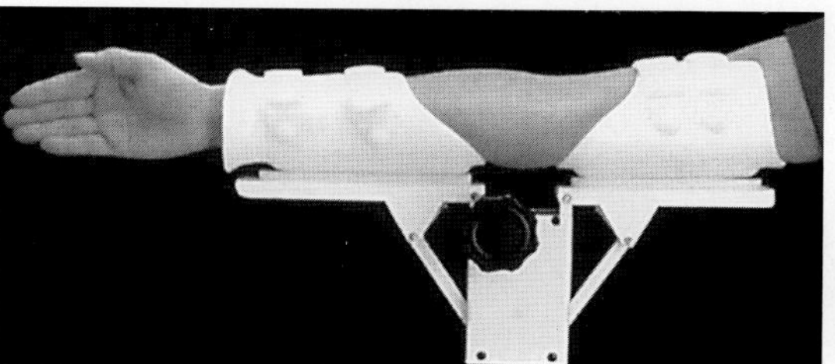

Figure 11–8 The JAS elbow system can be used to treat either flexion or extension contractures at the elbow. The patient can easily don this splint and adjust the tension until a mild stretch is felt. Photo courtesy of Joint Active Systems (Effingham, IL).

flexion contractures at the elbow work only at increasing the patient's ROM (Wierzbicka & Wiegner 1996).

Hinged splints can also be used as restriction splints, limiting ROM in one direction while allowing unrestricted motion in the other direction (Fig. 11–9). For example, when treating patients with a biceps tendon repair, the brace can be locked out to restrict full elbow extension, thereby preventing tension on the repaired tendon while allowing passive flexion and active extension exercises. As healing progresses, the extension restriction can be modified to increase ROM appropriately.

CPM Machine

An **elbow CPM machine** may be used to increase ROM. These are typically tabletop devices that can be set up to address limitations in flexion and extension at the elbow and supination and pronation of the forearm.

Wrist Splints

The wrist is made up several joints that allow multidirectional movement, which can be complicated to splint. When immobilization is the goal of splinting, it is essential to provide adequate support to the wrist in all planes of motion. When mobilization is the goal, it is essential to facilitate intended movement patterns. Some prefabricated splints used for treating diagnoses at the wrist are wrist immobilization splints, wrist/hand immobilization splints, supination/pronation mobilization splints, CPM machines, and wrist mobilization splints.

Wrist Immobilization Splint

"Commercially available wrist supports do not fit most distal radius fracture patients comfortably and can block full finger and thumb ROM" (Laseter & Carter, 1996). There are a number of issues to consider when fitting a patient with a prefabricated **wrist immobilization splint,** including clearance of the distal palmar crease, thenar eminence, and first web space and proximal fit at the forearm to reduce splint migration and ensure appropriate wrist position.

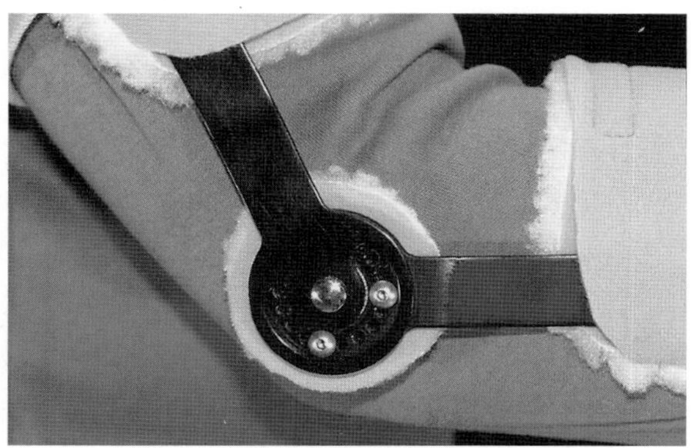

Figure 11–9 This brace (ROM Elbow Orthosis) has aluminum cuffs to provide a custom fit. The hinge can be adjusted to allow a specific restricted ROM. Photo courtesy of AliMed (Dedham, MA).

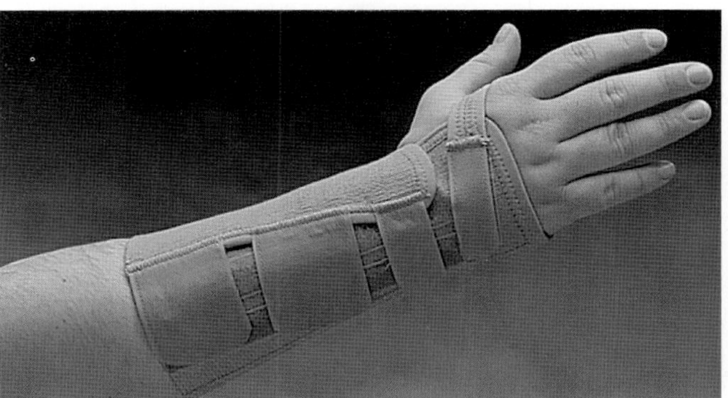

Figure 11–10 This wrist splint (Liberty Flare Splint) is a valuable option for patients with large forearms compared to wrist size. Photo courtesy of North Coast Medical (Morgan Hill, CA).

Adequate distal clearance is necessary for unrestricted grasp and pinch activities. The patient should be able to flex all fingers fully and comfortably with little or no interference from the distal portion of the wrist support, especially the radial portion. Patients with large forearms and narrow wrists have inherent problems with distal migration of wrist splints. The Liberty Flare (North Coast Medical) is a prefabricated splint that is designed specifically to accommodate this population (Fig. 11–10). If a prefabricated splint is unable to provide the patient with adequate use of the digits or a comfortable fit proximally, a custom-fabricated splint may offer a better option.

The actual position of the wrist should be measured while the prefabricated splint is on the patient and adjusted appropriately as per the specific diagnosis. For example, a patient with a wrist sprain is usually positioned for comfort, whereas an individual with a distal radius fracture is ideally positioned in 20 to 30° wrist extension after cast removal. If the patient is unable to obtain the desired range of extension, a prefabricated splint with a flexible metal or thermoplastic insert can be molded to the current wrist extension and later modified. The TECHlite Wrist Support (UE Tech, Edwards, CO) has a thermoplastic insert that can be heated and shaped to conform to the patient (Fig. 11–11) (Schultz-Johnson, 1996).

CARPAL TUNNEL SYNDROME

Prefabricated volar wrist supports are commonly prescribed to patients with carpal tunnel syndrome both before and after surgery. Gelberman, Hergenroeder, Hargens, Lundburg, and Akeson (1981) found that wrist flexion and extension increase the pressure in the carpal tunnel and compression of the median nerve. It is recommended that patients with carpal tunnel syndrome be splinted in a neutral to slightly extended position to provide maximum space at the carpal tunnel and reduce compression on the median nerve (Fig. 11–12). Splinting is frequently prescribed as the initial treatment of patients diagnosed with this syndrome (Kruger, Kraft, Deitz, Ameis, & Polissar, 1991).

The Rolyan Gel Shell Splint (Smith+Nephew) has a gel cushion along the volar surface to provide gentle, conforming compression to the incision site after carpal tunnel surgery (Fig. 11–13). This elastic canvas wrist wrap provides protection to the incision site and gives gentle feedback to the patient to avoid extreme positions of wrist flexion and extension postsurgery. A Neoprene Wrist Wrap is a nice transitional splint for a patient who is weaning off long-term use of a volar wrist support.

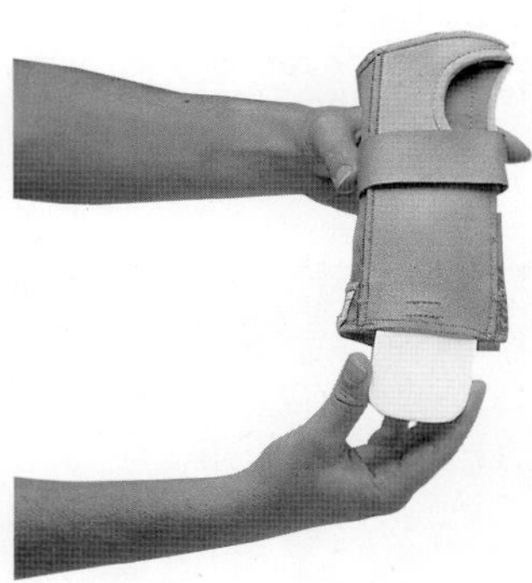

Figure 11–11 The TECHlite Wrist Support features a thermoplastic insert that can be heated and molded. The insert allows the therapist to adjust the rigidity of the splint and position the body part according to the patient's needs. Photo courtesy of UE Tech (Edwards, CO).

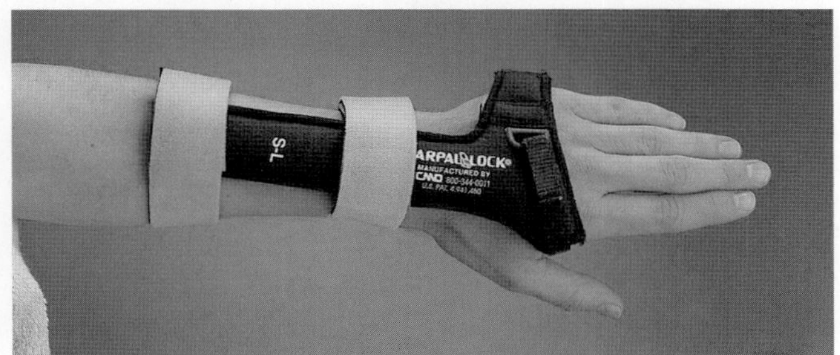

Figure 11–12 This dorsal-based wrist splint (Carpal Lock Wrist Splint) positions the wrist in neutral, allowing unrestricted digital motion. Photo courtesy of Sammons Preston (Bolingbrook, IL).

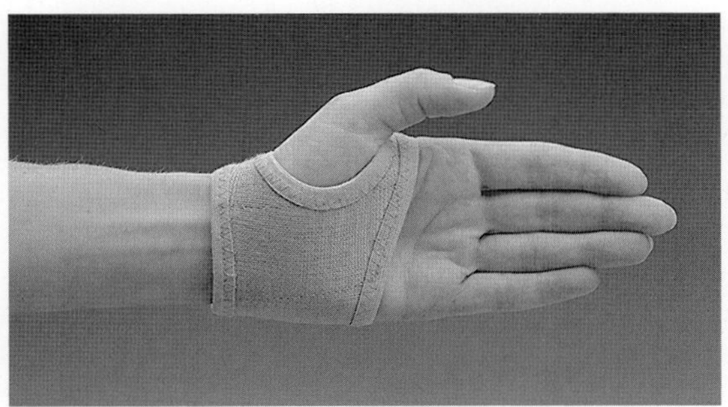

Figure 11–13 Replacement gel pads are available for the Rolyan Gel Shell Splint to provide scar management. Photo courtesy of Rehabilitation Division of Smith+Nephew (Germantown, WI).

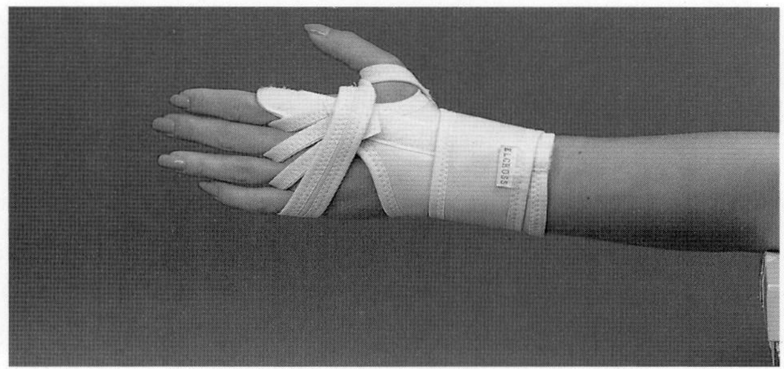

Figure 11–14 This ulnar deviation splint (Elcross) can enhance the function of patients who have rheumatoid arthritis affecting the wrist and MP joints. Photo courtesy of Sammons Preston (Bolingbrook, IL).

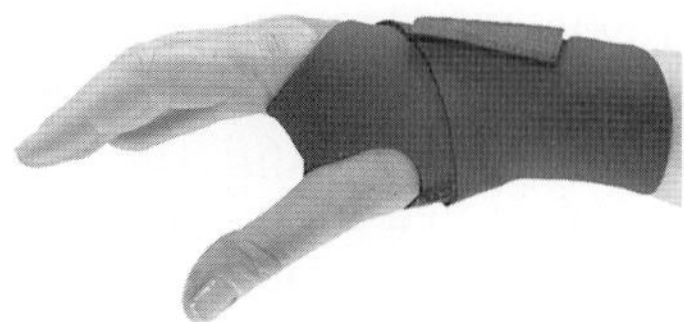

Figure 11–15 The thumbhole of this Neoprene Wrist Wrap can easily be modified by simply trimming with scissors. Photo courtesy of AliMed (Dedham, MA).

ARTHRITIS

Volar wrist supports afford mobility at the hand and digits and are frequently prescribed for people with arthritis as a means to rest the affected wrist joint. When patients with rheumatoid arthritis wear a volar wrist splint, they note improved muscle strength, functional abilities, and reduced pain (Jaffe, Chidgey, & LaStayo, 1996; Kjeken, Moller, & Kvien, 1995). Although wrist supports are beneficial, patient compliance for wearing them is relatively low (Tijhuis, Vliet Vlieland, Zwinderman, & Hazes, 1998). Patient concerns regarding wrist supports (whether prefabricated or custom made) include comfort of fit, interference with activities, appearance, cost, and reduced freedom of movement.

There are a wide variety of wrist supports designed specifically to meet the needs of patients with arthritis. Most suppliers have wrist supports, which provide metacarpophalangeal (MP) and/or thumb positioning (Fig. 11–14). These supports are available in Neoprene, breathable nylon fabrics, and preformed lined Aquaplast (Smith+Nephew). Neoprene Wrist Wraps are comfortable and warm but provide less support than their foam and fabric-based counterparts (Fig. 11–15).

When treating patients with arthritis, the therapist needs to clearly define all relevant issues and splinting goals to help determine which splinting regime best suits the needs of the patient. Some patients have problems with hyperhidrosis and prefer a light, breathable fabric splint, whereas others find warm splints to be helpful. Patients who are working or who are physically active tend to prefer the least restrictive splint. Patients may not tolerate MP support during the day but will use a wrist/hand immobilization splint to comfortably position the hand while sleeping.

Wrist/Hand Immobilization Splint

Individuals with a wide variety of diagnoses may require a **wrist/hand immobilization splint** for day and/or night use. There are a number of designs available for the treatment of patients with such diagnoses as arthritis, burns, crush injuries, and spasticity, and the splints come in volar- and dorsal-based and circumferential designs. There are soft splints that provide a gentle continuous stretch to spastic muscles and more rigid plastic splints that provide immobilization to healing structures (Wallen & O'Flaherty, 1990). Progress splints (North Coast Medical) come in several designs to provide a static progressive stretch to tissue (Fig. 11–16). These splints are machine washable, fabricated from soft foam to maximize comfort, and allow for easy adjustment.

Supination/Pronation Mobilization Splint

A tone and positioning (TAP) splint is a simple and comfortable alternative to a custom-molded **supination/pronation mobilization splint.** The Comfort Cool Spiral Arm Splint (North Coast Medical) provides a gentle, low-load supination or pronation stretch to aid in increasing functional hand position (Fig. 11–17). This device, although originally developed for neurologic patients, can be beneficial in facilitating supination or pronation ROM if the tissue at the forearm and wrist is not too dense (soft end feel). This splint is not capable of delivering the torque required for patients with hard end feel or long-standing limitations in ROM.

CPM Machine

Wrist CPM machines are frequently used to aid in increasing ROM at the radiocarpal joint. The Kinetec 8080 Hand and Wrist Machine (Smith+Nephew) is a tabletop wrist CPM unit that can produce flexion and extension and radial and ulnar deviation at the wrist joint (Fig. 11–18). Portable wrist machines include the Jace wrist W550 (Therakinetics, Cherry Hill, NJ) and the Kinetec 8091 (Smith+Nephew). These CPM machines provide adequate force throughout the ROM for patients with a soft end range. The Kinetec 8080 is most appropriate when more force is required.

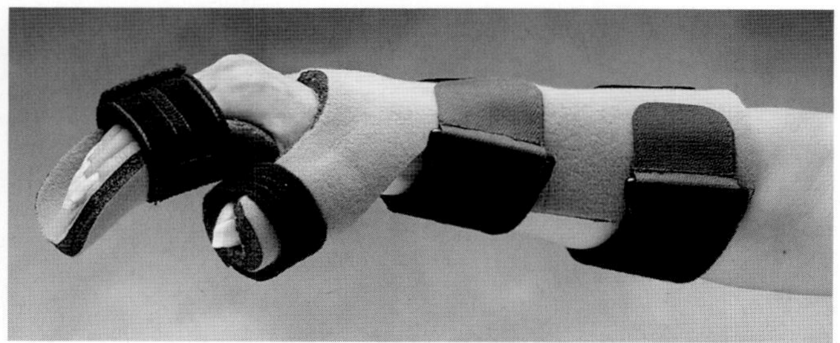

Figure 11–16 This wrist/hand immobilization splint (Progress Dorsal Antispasticity Splint) is recommended for patients with neurologic conditions such as spasticity. The metal frame can be repositioned progressively to obtain optimal positioning. The materials and specific positioning of the wrist, digits, and thumb depend on the diagnoses and splinting goals. Photo courtesy of North Coast Medical (Morgan Hill, CA).

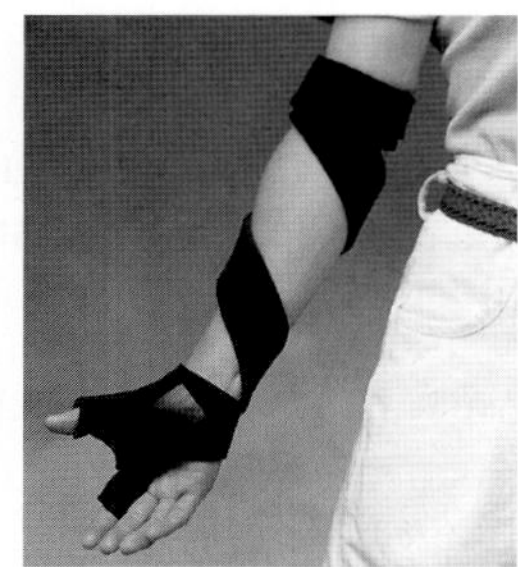

Figure 11–17 The Comfort Cool Spiral Arm Splint is made of Neoprene and is easily fitted, in either supination or pronation, to patients of all age groups. The Neoprene strap can be used with the included glove component or can be used with a custom-made thermoplastic volar wrist support. Photo courtesy of North Coast Medical (Morgan Hill, CA).

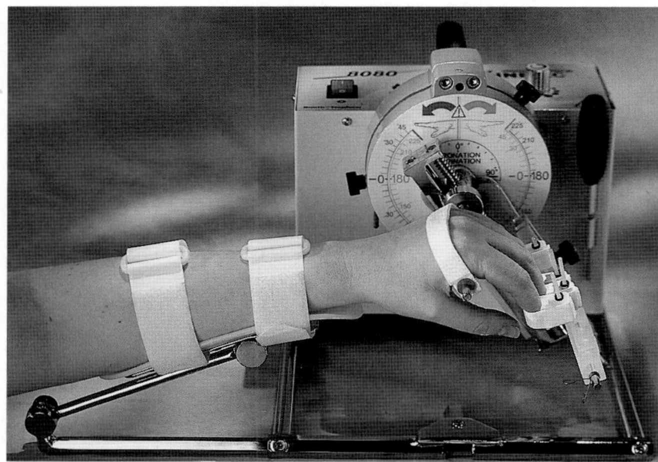

Figure 11–18 The Kinetec 8080 hand and wrist CPM machine can be set up to produce forearm supination and pronation as well as digit flexion and extension. Photo courtesy of Rehabilitation Division of Smith+Nephew (Germantown, WI).

Wrist Mobilization Splint

Prefabricated **wrist mobilization splints** using a static progressive and dynamic approach are commonly prescribed to increase wrist ROM. The JAS Progressive Splint (Joint Active Systems) is designed to increase wrist flexion and extension. The SP ROM Wrist Orthoses (DeRoyal/LMB, Powell, TN) provides an alternative for wrist flexion and extension mobilization (Fig. 11–19). The Ultraflex Dynamic Wrist Splint (Biotec, Malvern, PA) provides maximum ROM into wrist flexion and extension, is available in both adult and pediatric models, and is extremely comfortable for long-term use. The forearm component of this wrist splint is custom fabricated, which may assist in increasing the patient's comfort; but may take more time to fit, which may lead to an increase in the overall cost (Thompson & Wehbe, 1996).

Hand Splints

Because the hand is unique, the therapist is faced with many challenges in balancing the medically necessary restrictions with the patient's need for functional use. Some of the prefabricated splints used for treating the hand are CPM machines, composite digit mobilization splints, ulnar deviation splints, gloves, proximal interphalangeal (PIP) joint mobilization splints, distal interphalangeal (DIP) joint immobilization splints, boutonniere deformity splints, and swan-neck deformity splints.

CPM Machine

Hand CPM machines can be used to treat patients with severe burns (Fig. 11–20). Early goals for rehabilitation of patients with burn injuries to their hands include restored soft tissue coverage and "rapid advancement of active range of motion" at the MP joints (Barillo, Harvey, Hobbs, Mozingo, Cioffi, & Pruitt, 1997). Patients with burns who are unable to flex the MP joints to at least 70° and those who are unable to flex the digits actively secondary to the side effects of medication may use a CPM for 4 to 8 hr during the day and possibly while they sleep.

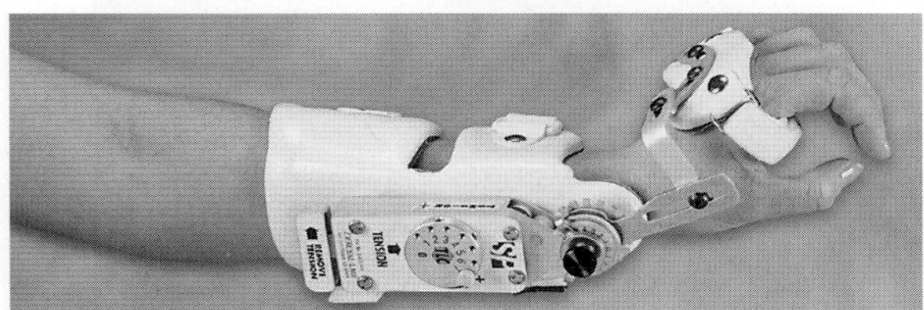

Figure 11–19 *The SP ROM Wrist Orthosis is easily adjusted to accommodate different sized wrists. The force application can be blocked to limit end ROM, if needed. This particular model can be used on either the right or the left hand in the direction of flexion or extension. Photo courtesy of DeRoyal (Powell, TN).*

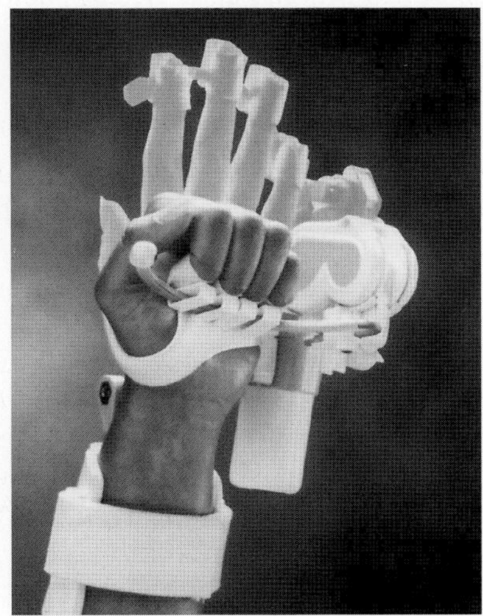

Figure 11–20 *The Jace Hand CPM is used in the early treatment of patients with severe burn injuries. This system can also be used to assist patients in obtaining a composite fist. Note that the force applied promotes maximal DIP flexion. Photo courtesy of Jace Systems (Cherry Hill, NJ).*

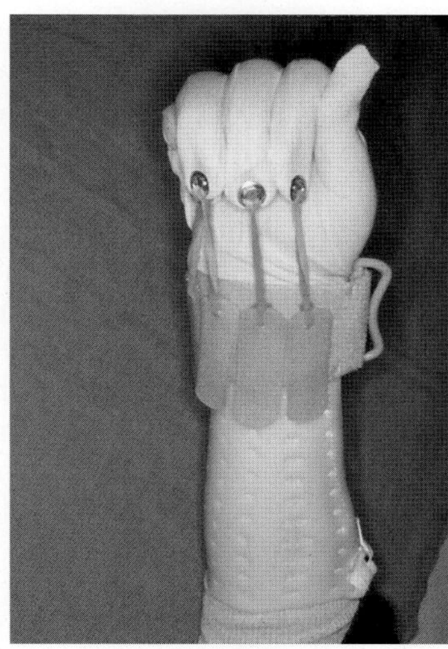

Figure 11–21 *A flexion glove with a circumferential wrist splint. The wrist splint is worn to prevent compensatory wrist flexion when force is applied to the digits.*

CPM machines are more commonly used to treat patients with stiff edematous fingers, a common complication of many injuries of the upper extremity. The CPM can be used to facilitate gentle ROM throughout the fingers or can be used to achieve increased motion at a specific joint. Note that obtaining full DIP flexion is a challenge when applying these devices. Furthermore, the unaffected joints often compensate by maximally flexing, thus decreasing the force aimed at the target joints. For example, when addressing tight PIP joints, the MP joints may hyperflex, thus prohibiting optimal stretch at the PIP joints. The therapist should carefully monitor the patient's use of a CPM machine and the settings should be checked frequently.

Digit Mobilization

A variety of prefabricated **digit mobilization splints** is available to address stiffness. The flexion glove is a staple found in most hand therapy clinics (Fig. 11–21). It can be used alone or in conjunction with a volar wrist support to apply a passive flexion stretch to the MP and interphalangeal (IP) joints as well as the extrinsic extensors. The wrist may need to be immobilized, because patients may collapse into compensatory wrist flexion when a flexion force is applied to their tight fingers. The patients can easily apply the glove and adjust it to a comfortable level of stretch.

Elasticized wraps—such as Coban (Smith+Nephew) and Coflex (AliMed, Dedham, MA)—can be used to treat limited flexion of the fingers. This reusable wrap is self-adherent, making it easy to apply and hold in place. The 2- to 4-in. rolls are useful for wrapping all fingers into flexion, if limited motion is consistent across the digits. The 1-in. rolls are best used when the fingers require individual levels of stretch. Many manufacturers have a version of this elastic wrap. The thinner wraps are useful for applying a stretch wrap to the digits and then dipping in paraffin, as the wax can seep into contact with the fingers fairly readily. The thicker wraps are best for gentle edema wrapping, because they provide support to a swollen, painful finger.

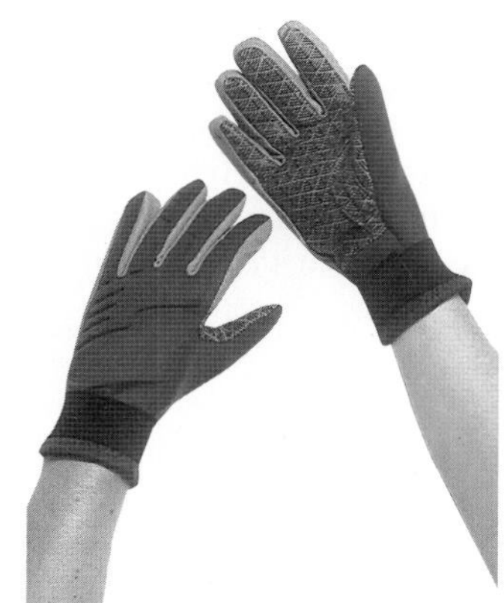

Figure 11–23 *Performance Gloves come in a variety of sizes and help patients who work in wet or cold environments. Photo courtesy of UE Tech (Edwards, CO).*

Ulnar Deviation Splint

The therapist should closely follow patients who have rheumatoid arthritis and are using supportive splinting to slow the progression of carpal collapse and the resulting ulnar deviation at the MP joints (Dell & Dell, 1996). Patients with ulnar drift may benefit from being splinted with soft **ulnar deviation splints** (Fig. 11–22). Hand-based splints and other suggested prefabricated splints for this population are reviewed in Chapter 17.

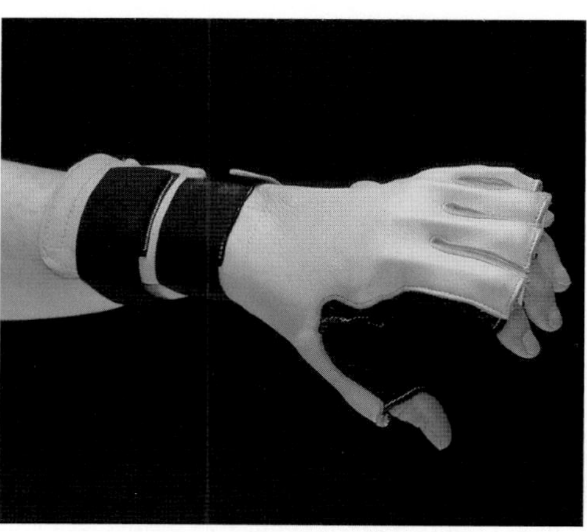

Figure 11–24 *The Robinson Peripheral Nerve Splint provides a low-profile and inexpensive alternative. This splint is available in hand- and forearm-based designs. A variety of peripheral nerve injuries can be addressed with this glove system. Photo courtesy of AliMed (Dedham, MA).*

Gloves

Various types of **gloves** are available—including short-fingered work gloves, bicycle gloves, and weight-training gloves—that are used to protect the hand from vibration, cold, or repetitive work activities. People who use wheelchairs frequently wear palmar-padded gloves to increase their ability to grasp and decrease the wear and tear on their hands.

Neoprene Performance Gloves (UE Tech) are specifically designed for patients with cold intolerance (Fig. 11–23). These durable work gloves also have some antivibration and antishock qualities. For patients with peripheral nerve injury, the Robinson InRigger Gloves (AliMed) provide digit extension dorsally while allowing full finger flexion. A variety of "in-rigger" systems are available to meet the needs of different patients (Fig. 11–24). Patients are fitted with a glove, and components are added to accommodate for losses secondary to the specific nerve injury.

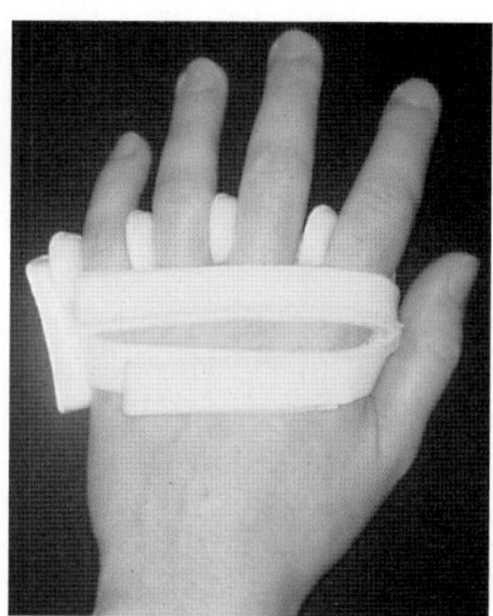

Figure 11–22 *A Soft-core Ulnar Deviation Splint (DeRoyal, Powell, TN) is worn to support the MP joints in extension and prevent radial deviation and enable the patient to better perform functional grasp activities.*

For patients with significant scarring to either the dorsal or the volar surface of the hand, the Bio-Form Pressure Glove (North Coast Medical) can help control edema and hypertrophic scarring (Fig. 11–25). This glove has open fingertips, which provide opportunity for vascular monitoring and sensory input. For scar management alone, fully lined silicone gloves are available.

The Electrode Glove (Sterling Medical Technologies, Plano, TX) can be used in conjunction with galvanic or electrical-stimulation units. This full glove electrode is especially helpful for edema reduction, pain management, and facilitating gross grasp stimulation of the digits.

The Ice-Aid Glove (AliMed) is made of Lycra and provides gentle compression to the hands and wrists. There is a pocket on the volar wrist and palm for a removable ice pack. This type of glove may prove beneficial to patients with carpal tunnel syndrome or who have undergone a surgical release.

PIP Mobilization Splint

Full ROM at the PIP joints is imperative for hand function; therefore, **PIP mobilization splints** are commonly used in the clinic. A loss of extension at this joint can limit a person's ability to grasp large objects or collect change with an open palm. A loss of flexion at this joint can severely limit the ability to grasp objects or even shake hands (Prosser, 1996).

EXTENSION MOBILIZATION

There are a wide variety of digit-based spring-loaded PIP extension splints for the treatment of PIP joint flexion contractures. The amount of padding, the length, and the ability to alter force depend on the design. The LMB Digit Extension Splint (DeRoyal/LMB) is one example of this common splint (Fig. 11–26).

Digit extension Neoprene sleeves, such as the Dynamic Digit Extensor Tube Splint (AliMed) can also be used to treat patients with PIP joint flexion contractures (Fig. 11–27). Patients may tolerate wearing this splint longer because the heat generated by wearing a Neoprene sleeve on the injured finger may increase tissue extensibility and blood flow while decreasing joint stiffness, pain, and muscle spasms (Michlovitz, 1990). Patients should be instructed in tissue monitoring, because maceration of the skin can occur owing to excessive perspiration (Clark, 1997).

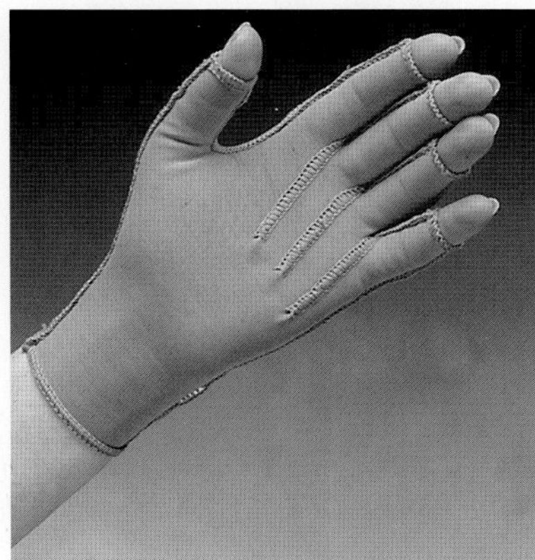

Figure 11–25 The Bio-Form Pressure Glove helps reduce edema, provides compression to scar tissue, and allows monitoring of vascularity. Photo courtesy of North Coast Medical (Morgan Hill, CA).

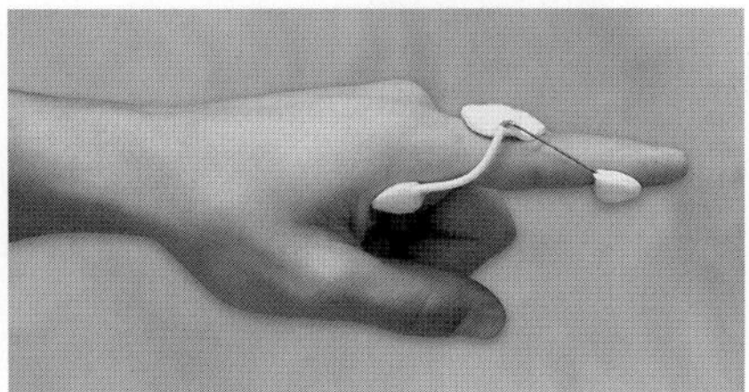

Figure 11–26 The DeRoyal/LMB Spring Finger Extension Assist Splint can be adjusted to provide more (straightening the splint out) or less (squeezing the proximal and distal pads together) force to the patient's finger. The lateral wires can also be pulled out a little to accommodate edema. Photo courtesy of DeRoyal (Powell, TN).

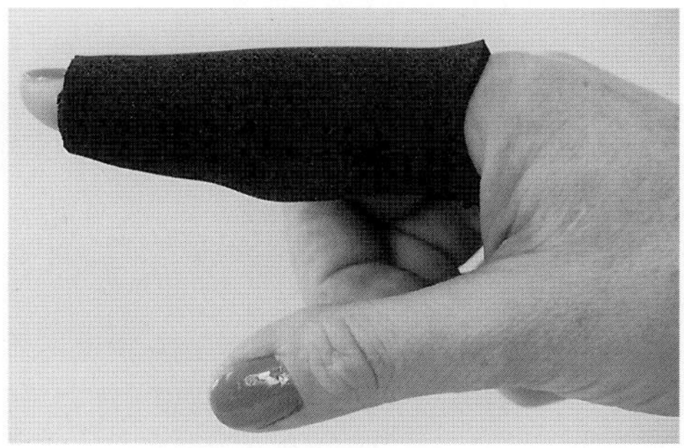

Figure 11–27 The Dynamic Digit Extension Tube is made of Neoprene and applies a low-tension load. This banana-shaped device is comfortable to wear and comes in a variety of sizes. Photo courtesy of AliMed (Dedham, MA).

Other PIP joint mobilization splints include the Joint-Jack (Joint-Jack Company, East Hartford, CT), Reverse Knuckle Bender (Sammons Preston, Bolingbrook, IL), and variations of the Safety Pin Splint (Sammons Preston). The Joint-Jack and Safety Pin Splints provide a static progressive (nonelastic) extension force to the PIP joints. Reverse knuckle benders have a somewhat higher profile (bulkier) with rubber bands that are applied to wire loops dorsally. The resistance can be easily adjusted via the rubber bands (Figs 11–28).

The Capener Splint (AliMed) is commonly used in the treatment of boutonniere injuries postoperatively and PIP joint flexion contractures (Fig. 11–29) (Capener, 1967; Colditz, 1990; Iselin, 1997; Prosser, 1996). In an investigation by Prosser (1996), patients reported that the low-profile (streamlined) Capener Splint was easy to wear during the workday. Patients are more likely to use a comfortable, low-profile splint, thus spending more time in the splint. Time spent at total end range is a significant factor; the greater the wearing time, the greater gains made in treating a PIP flexion contracture (Flowers & LaStayo, 1994; Prosser, 1996).

FLEXION MOBILIZATION

PIP/DIP straps are fabricated and sold by many companies to provide an flexion stretch to the PIP and DIP joints. However, the therapist can easily fabricate this simple splint by sewing 3/4" pajama elastic together to form a loop. Patients can readily increase the tension by sewing, stapling, or securing a safety pin to make the loop tighter. A Joint-Cinch Splint (Joint-Jack Company) can be used for individual fingers that require increased flexion at the PIP and MP joints (Fig. 11–30).

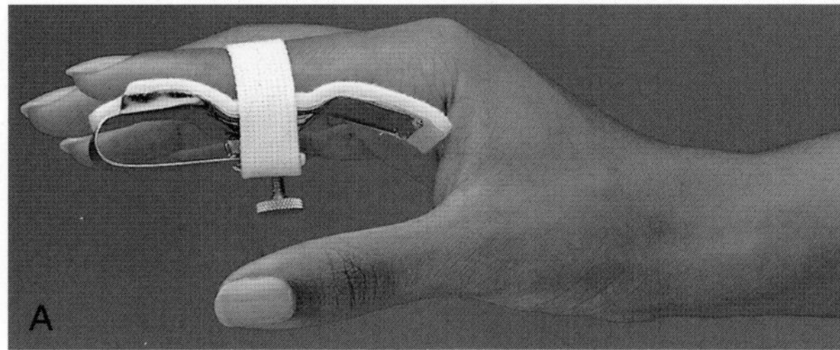

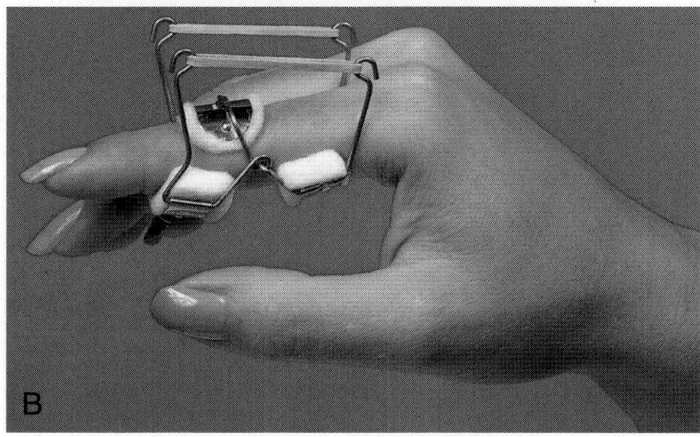

*Figure 11–28 The Joint Jack (**A**) and Reverse Knuckle Bender (**B**) may be most effective on joint contractures that are less than 30°. Photos courtesy of Sammons Preston (Bolingbrook, IL).*

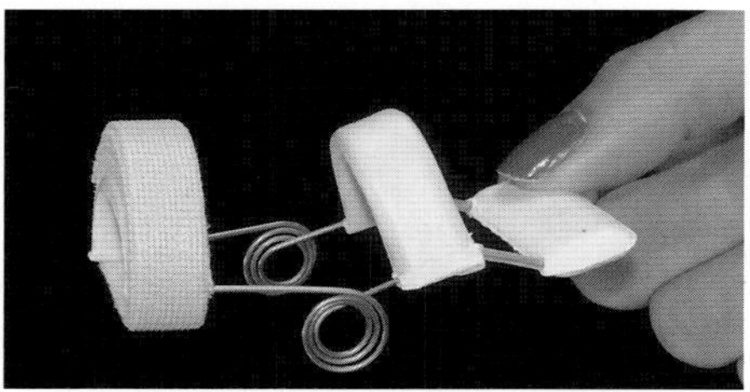

Figure 11–29 The Spring Coil Extension Assist Splint (Capener or Wynn Parry Splint) is a comfortable low-profile splint commonly used to treat boutonniere injuries. Photo courtesy of AliMed (Dedham, MA).

Buddy straps are used to treat many finger injuries, including amputation, fractures, dislocations, sprains, and extensor tendon injuries (Fig. 11–31) (Alexy & De Carlo, 1988). These straps are comfortable, minimize tissue damage, and are easily adjusted to fit to swollen or slender fingers. There are elastic double-digit finger sleeves (MBM, Pelham Manor, NY) are comfortable, flexible, and provide some compression while splinting two fingers together.

DIP Immobilization Splint

DIP immobilization splints, including aluminum padded splints and Stax Splints (North Coast Medical), are commonly used in the treatment of a mallet finger injury, which is the disruption of the terminal tendon at its attachment on the distal phalanx (Fig. 11–32). The goal of treatment is to immobilize the terminal tendon so that it may scar down during an uninterrupted period of 6 to 8 weeks (Alexy & De Carlo, 1988). One concern for the treating therapist and physician is maintaining tissue integrity on the dorsum of the DIP joint during the splinting. A benefit of the

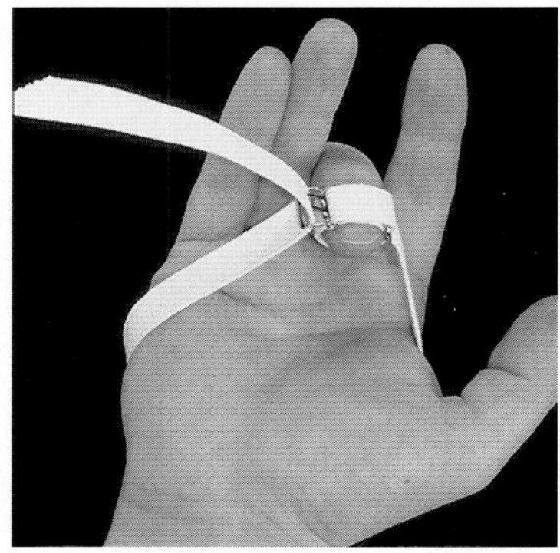

Figure 11–30 The Joint-Cinch Splint provides a nonelastic flexion force (static progressive). Photo courtesy of AliMed (Dedham, MA).

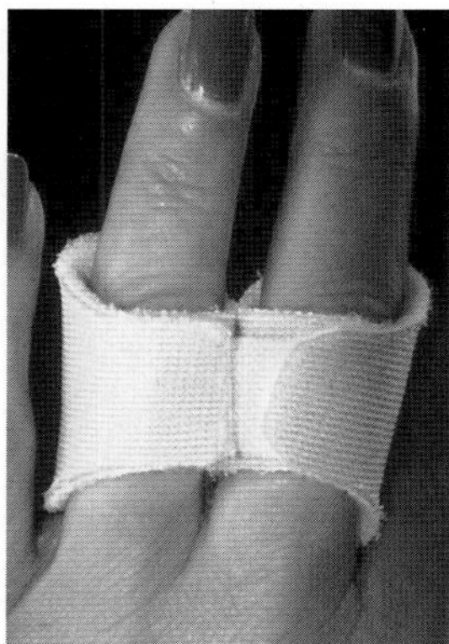

Figure 11–31 Soft Buddy Strap Splints are commonly used to ease the transition out of an immobilization splint. Photo courtesy of North Coast Medical, Inc. (Morgan Hill, CA).

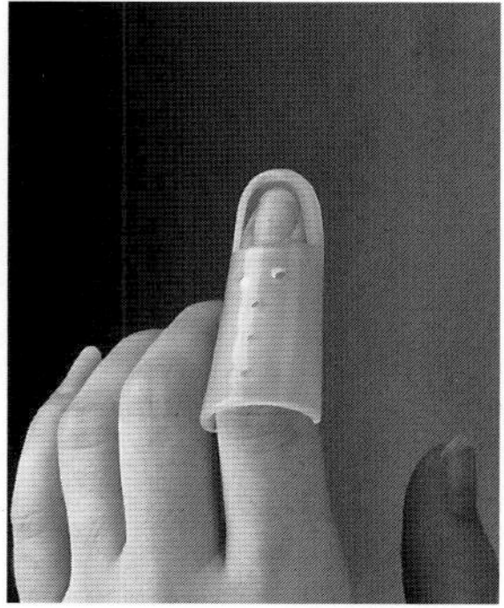

Figure 11–32 The Open-Air Stax Finger Splint is perforated, allowing air circulation and decreasing the likelihood of tissue maceration. Photo courtesy of North Coast Medical, Inc. (Morgan Hill, CA).

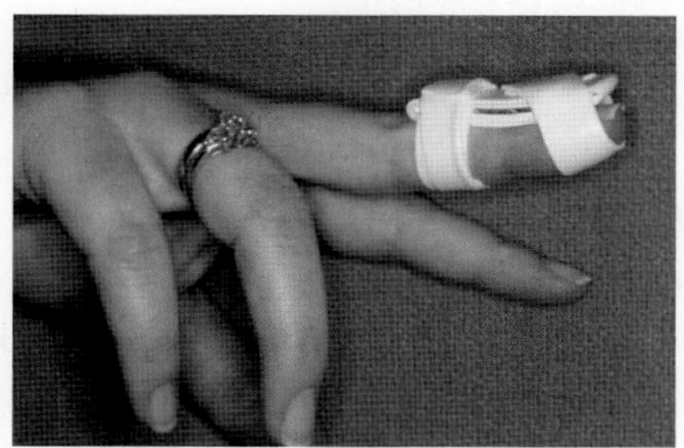

Figure 11–33 An aluminum splint secured with Microfoam tape. Applying the tape obliquely to the volar fingertip and then crossing it over the splint on the dorsal splint provides maximum distribution of force and secures the distal phalanx in good extension while the terminal tendon is healing (E. Rosenthal, personal communication, 1997).

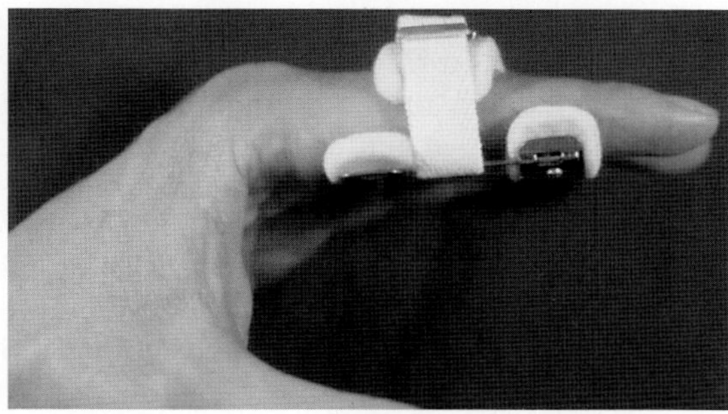

Figure 11–34 Note that the DIP joint is free to flex (Bunnell Mini, Modified Safety Pin Splint from North Coast Medical, Morgan Hill, CA).

clear plastic Stax splint is that it affords visualization of the tissue.

Aluminum splints are easily fitted to any digit and can be bent to increase extension at the DIP joint. To increase the stability of the splint (beneficial for maintaining dorsal tissue integrity), trim the foam to a thickness of 1/8" and then cover the device with silk tape. Aluminum splints can be held in place with 1/2" tape (Fig. 11–33). Garberman, Diao, and Peimer (1994) report that as long as the injured digit is continuously splinted for 6 to 10 weeks, the type of splint used is insignificant in the successful outcome of mallet finger deformity.

Boutonniere Deformity Splint

Boutonniere deformity, or the disruption of the central slip of the extensor tendon mechanism as it inserts onto the base of the middle phalanx, is acutely treated with splinting (Palchik, Mitchell, Gilbert, Schultz, Dedrick, & Palella, 1990). Aronowitz and Leddy (1998) treat all patients with acute boutonniere deformities with a Safety Pin Splint (Smith+Nephew) to position the PIP in extension, leaving the DIP free to move actively or to be moved passively (Fig. 11–34). Active and passive ROM at the DIP joint, while extension is passively maintained at the PIP joint, facilitates good anatomic positioning of the lateral bands.

Swan-Neck Deformity Splint

Swan-neck deformity—hyperextension of the PIP joint and flexion of the DIP joint—is commonly seen in patients who have rheumatoid arthritis or chronic volar plate injuries. The Silver Ring Splint (Silver Ring Splint Company, Charlottesville, VA) and splints such as the 3-Point Finger Splint (3-Point Products, Annapolis, MD) offer a low-profile, attractive, and extremely effective option to maximize function of the digit. When this type of splinting is required long term, patients tend to prefer the Silver Ring Splints because they are more attractive and often more comfortable and durable than thermoplastic splints (Fig. 11–35).

Thumb Splints

The thumb is responsible for approximately 40% of hand function (Swanson, de Groot, & Swanson, 1990). When splinting a patient's thumb, the therapist must consider that the thumb is involved in all tasks requiring grasping, pinching, or stabilizing an object or requiring sensory information to operate (King, 1992). It can be extremely challenging for the therapist and patient to find a splint, prefabricated or custom made, which is comfortable and functional while providing the proper support and positioning for the thumb. A painful carpometacarpal (CMC) joint can limit pinch or grip and severely impair hand function. An ideal splint for osteoarthritis at the CMC joint is one that stabilizes the joint in abduction, blocks adduction, and allows for full flexion at the IP joint (Fig. 11–36) (Melvin, 1995).

Neoprene Splint

Neoprene wrist and thumb splints (either prefabricated or custom) can provide warmth and support to the

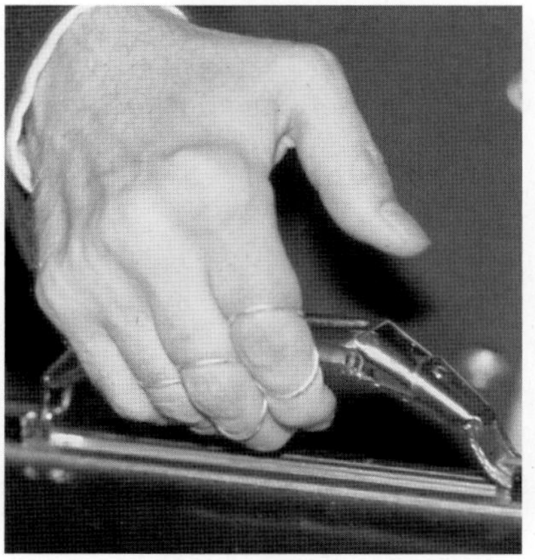

Figure 11–35 Silver Ring Splints are both functional and attractive. Photo courtesy of Silver Ring Splint Company (Charlottesville, VA).

thumb and wrist (see Chapter 14 for details). Custom-made thermoplastic splints for CMC arthritis are quite effective in immobilizing the thumb joint in a position of rest. Unfortunately, this immobilization can significantly hinder normal hand function. Patients often complain that the splints are uncomfortable and interfere with their daily routines. The Comfort Cool Thumb CMC Restriction Splint (North Coast Medical) is designed to stabilize the CMC joint while allowing some mobility (Fig. 11–37). Similar types of splints are available through different vendors and are made in a variety of Neoprene materials to provide joint warmth, gentle support, and protection around the CMC joint.

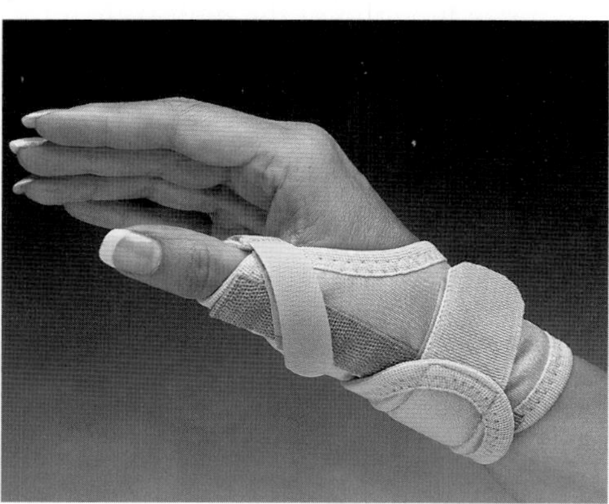

Figure 11–36 *The Otto Block Rheuma Thumb Support Splint allows unrestricted movement of the IP joint, while providing support to the MP and CMC joints. Photo courtesy of North Coast Medical (Morgan Hill, CA).*

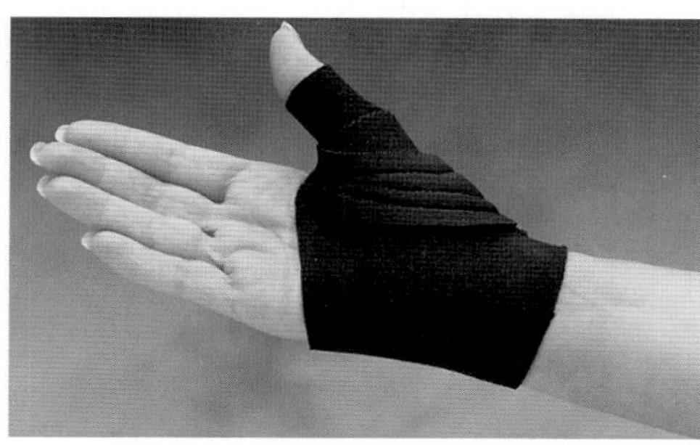

Figure 11–37 *The unique strap design of this Comfort Cool Thumb Restriction Splint provides support to the CMC joint. Photo courtesy of North Coast Medical (Morgan Hill, CA).*

Thumb Immobilization Splint

At times it is necessary to fully immobilize the patient's thumb. This means that the wrist should be included to stabilize the thumb's CMC joint. There are a wide variety of forearm-based prefabricated and preformed **thumb immobilization splints** available from almost every manufacturer.

It is imperative that the therapist pay close attention to proper biomechanical fit and comfort when splinting a patient's thumb. The requirements for positioning of the thumb depend on the specific diagnosis. Sometime the thumb CMC joint should be palmarly abducted and gently flexed at the MP joint, and other times the CMC joint must be placed in radial abduction with no flexion at the MP. Preformed thumb immobilization splints—available from many manufacturers—can provide the necessary immobilization and allow a time-efficient fit to the patient (Fig. 11–38). When less rigidity is required, a prefabricated thumb splint may be more comfortable for the patient.

The Rolyan Gel Shell Thumb Spica Splint (Smith+Nephew) is designed to provide comfortable support to the MP and CMC joints of the thumb (Fig. 11–39). This type of canvas-based splint may be used once less support is required at the wrist joint after surgery for deQuervain's tenosynovitis.

Prefabricated Splint Adaptations

Keeping abreast of all of the information on available splinting materials, components, and prefabricated splint options is both challenging and interesting. The therapist must be able to use all available resources to best meet the needs of his or her patients. Sometimes this means adapting prefabricated splints for purposes other than what they were originally intended to do. Table 11–1 provides a few creative ways to use prefabricated splints.

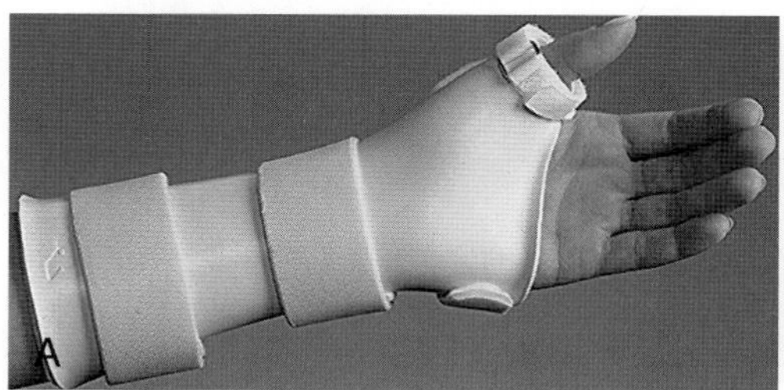

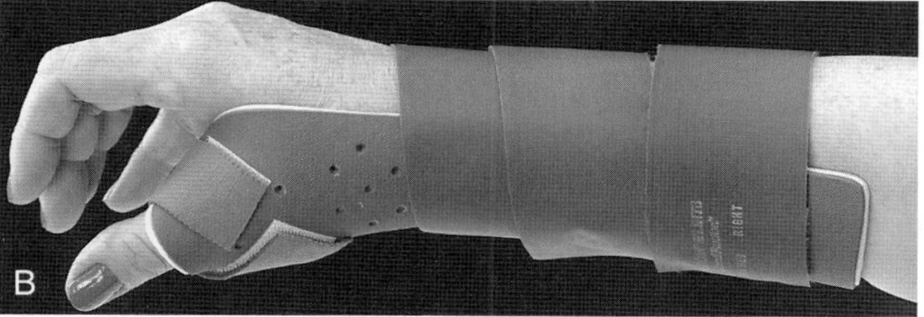

Figure 11–38 *Preformed thumb immobilization splints can save time and are easily altered to meet the positioning requirements of a variety of diagnoses.* ***A,*** *Rolyan Forearm-Based Thumb Spica Splint. Photo courtesy of Rehabilitation Division of Smith+Nephew (Germantown, WI).* ***B,*** *Freedom Memory Thumb Spica Deluxe. Photo courtesy of AliMed (Dedham, MA).*

TABLE 11–1 Created Uses of Prefabricated Splints

Prefabricated Splint	Intended Use	Expanded Use	Adaptations
Reverse knuckle bender	PIP extension	FDP or FPL exercise tool	Move splint to distal phalanx
LMB	PIP extension	Increase tissue extensibility	Use in combination with paraffin and hot packs
Digit extension tube	PIP extension	Increase PIP extension	Add 3/32" thermoplastic insert volarly
Padded palmar work gloves	Reduce shock and vibration in palm and digits	Reduce MP flexion in treating trigger finger	Patient wears glove to sleep or for day as needed
Isotoner glove	Edema reduction	As flexion glove in combination with volar wrist support	Punch holes at tips and run rubber bands to apply flexion force
Silipos Digicap	Scar management	Edema management	Wear for edema management
Digit cast	PIP extension	Isolated DIP flexion	Clear DIP proximally, use as exercise block
Coban	Edema control	Flexion wrap	Apply to individual digit or all digits in full-fist position

FDP, flexor digitorum profundus; FLP, flexor pollicis longus.

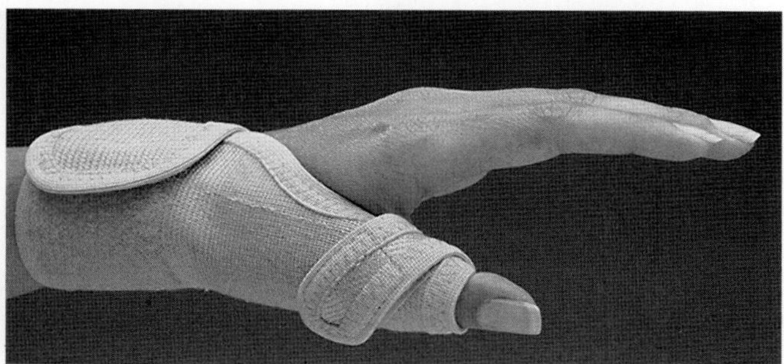

Figure 11–39 The Rolyan Gel Shell Thumb Spica Splint provides comfort and scar management to the incision site after surgery for deQuervain's tenosynovitis. Photo courtesy of Rehabilitation Division of Smith+Nephew (Germantown, WI).

CONCLUSION

Prefabricated splints play an integral part in the practice of upper extremity therapy. The therapist should carefully evaluate each patient and then determine which type of splint is most appropriate. When determining what splint to use, the therapist must consider the biomechanical goals, requirements for the treatment of a specific diagnosis, and most important, the patient's goals. Sometimes, a custom-made splint is more appropriate and at other times a prefabricated splint is the better choice.

REFERENCES

Alexy, C., & De Carlo, M. (1988). Rehabilitation and use of protective devices in hand and wrist injuries. *Clinics in Sports Medicine, 17,* 635–655.

Aronowitz, E. R., & Leddy J. P. (1998). Closed tendon injuries of the hand and wrist in athletes. *Clinics in Sports Medicine, 17,* 449–467.

Aulicino, P. L. (1995). Clinical examination of the hand. In J. M. Hunter, E. J. Mackin, & A. D. Callahan (Eds.). *Rehabilitation of the hand* (4th ed., pp. 53–75). St. Louis: Mosby Year Book.

Barillo, D. J., Harvey, K. D., Hobbs, C. L., Mozingo, D. W., Cioffi, W. G., & Pruitt, B. A. (1997). Prospective outcome analysis of a protocol for the surgical and rehabilitative management of burns to the hands. *Plastic and Reconstructive Surgery, 100,* 1442–1451.

Bonutti, P. M., Windau, J. E., Ables, B. A., & Miller, B. G. (1994). Static progressive stretch to reestablish elbow range of motion. *Clinical Orthopaedics and Related Research, 303,* 128–134.

Capener, N. (1967). Lively splint. *Physiotherapy,* 53, 371–374.

Clark, E. N. (1997). A preliminary investigation of the Neoprene tube finger extension splint. *Journal of Hand Therapy, 10,* 213–221.

Colditz, J. C. (1995). Functional fracture bracing. In J. M. Hunter, E. J. Mackin, & A. D. Callahan (Eds.). *Rehabilitation of the hand* (4th ed., pp. 395–406). St. Louis: Mosby Year Book.

Colditz, J. C. (1990). Spring-wire splinting of the proximal interphalangeal joint. In J. M. Hunter, L. H. Schneider, E. J. Mackin, & A. D. Callahan (Eds.). *Rehabilitation of the hand* (3rd ed., pp. 1109–1119). St. Louis: Mosby.

Dell, P. C., & Dell, R. B. (1996). Management of rheumatoid arthritis of the wrist. *Journal of Hand Therapy, 9,* 157–164.

Flowers, K., & LaStayo, P. (1994). Effect of total end range time on improving passive range of motion. *Journal of Hand Therapy, 7,* 150–157.

Garberman, S. F., Diao, E., & Peimer, C. A. (1994) Mallet finger: Results of early versus delayed closed treatment. *Journal of Hand Surgery [American], 19,* 850–852.

Gelberman, R. H., Hergenroeder, P. T., Hargens, A. R., Lundburg, G. N., & Ajesin, W. H. (1981). The carpal tunnel syndrome: A study of carpal canal pressures. *Journal of Bone and Joint Surgery (American volume), 63,* 380–383.

Iselin, F. (1997). Boutonniere deformity treatment: Immediate and delayed. In J. M. Hunter, L. H. Schneider, E. J. Mackin (Eds.). *Tendon and nerve surgery in the hand: A third decade* (pp. 580–583). St. Louis: Mosby.

Jaffe, R., Chidgey, L. K., & LaStayo, P. C. (1996). The distal radioulnar joint: Anatomy and management of disorders. *Journal of Hand Therapy, 9,* 129–138.

King, J. (1992). Traumatic injuries of the hand: Crush injuries and amputations. In B. G. Stanley & S. M. Tribuzi (Eds.). *Concepts in hand rehabilitation* (pp. 472–503). Philadelphia: Davis.

Kjeken, I., Moller, G., & Kvien, T. K. (1995). Use of commercially produced elastic wrist orthosis in chronic arthritis: A controlled study. *Arthritis Care and Research, 8,* 108–113.

Kleinert, J. M., & Mehta, S. (1996). Radial nerve entrapment. *Orthopedic Clinics of North America, 27,* 305–315.

Kruger, V. L., Kraft, G. H., Deitz, J. C., Ameis, A., & Polissar, L. (1991). Carpal tunnel syndrome: Objective measures and splint use. *Archives of Physical Medicine and Rehabilitation, 72,* 517–520.

Laseter, G. F., & Carter, P. R. (1996). Management of distal radius fractures. *Jouranl of Hand Therapy, 9,* 114–128.

Malick, M. (1982). *Manual on dynamic splinting with thermoplastic materials* (3rd. ed.). Pittsburgh: AREN.

Melvin, J. L. (1995). Orthotic treatment of the hand. What's new? *Bulletin on the Rheumatic Diseases, 44,* 5–8.

Michlovitz, S. (1990). Biophysical principles of heating and superficial heat agents. In S. Michlovitz (Ed.). *Thermal agents in rehabilitation* (2nd ed., pp. 88–108). Philadelphia: Davis.

Palchik, N. S., Mitchell, D. M., Gilbert, N. L., Schultz, A. J., Dedrick, R. F., & Palella, T, D. (1990). Nonsurgical management of the boutonniere deformity. *Arthritis Care and Research 3,* 227–232.

Prosser, R. (1996). Splinting in the management of proximal interphalangeal joint flexion contracture. *Journal of Hand Therapy, 9,* 378–386.

Rossi, J. (1988). Concepts and current trends in hand splinting. *Hand Rehabilitation in Occupational Therapy, ??,* 53–68.

Sailer, S. M. (1996). The role of splinting and rehabilitation in the treatment of carpal and cubital tunnel syndromes. *Hand Clinics, 12,* 223–241.

Schultz-Johnson, K. (1996). Splinting the wrist: Mobilization and protection. *Journal of Hand Therapy, 9,* 165–177.

Swanson, A., & de Groot Swanson. G. (1990). Evaluation of impairment of hand function. In J. M. Hunter, L. H. Schneider, E. J. Mackin, & A. D. Callahan (Eds.). *Rehabilitation of the hand* (3rd ed., pp. 1839–1986). St. Louis: Mosby.

Thompson, S. T., & Wehbe, M. A. (1996). Early motion after wrist surgery. *Hand Clinics, 12,* 87–96.

Tijhuis, G. J., Vliet Vlieland, T. P. M., Zwinderman, A. H., & Hazes, J. M. W. (1998). A comparison of the Futuro wrist orthosis with a synthetic thermolyn orthosis: Utility and clinical effectiveness. *Arthritis Care and Research, 11,* 217–222.

Wallen, M., & O'Flaherty, S. (1990). The use of the soft splint in the management of spasticity of the upper limb. *Australian Journal of Occupational Therapy, 38,* 227–231.

Wierzbicka, M. M., & Wiegner, A. W. (1996). Orthosis for improvement of arm function in C5/C6 tetraplegia. *Journal of Prosthetics and Orthotics, 8,* 86–92.

CHAPTER 12

Casting Techniques

Karen Schultz Johnson, MS, OTR/L, FAOTA, CHT

INTRODUCTION

Casting is the circumferential application of rigid material to a part of the body. The material can be a type of casting tape, **plaster of paris (POP), Softcast, fiberglass** (thermoplastic), or shrink-to-fit material such as **QuickCast.** Often the cast has no opening for removal, but it can be **univalved** or **bivalved** to allow the cast wearer to remove and replace it. **Serial stretchers,** often made of POP, incorporate half the extremity circumference (Tribuzi, 1990). A **drop-out cast** is circumferential on one side of a joint and incorporates half the extremity circumference on the other side. This design blocks joint motion in one direction but allows motion in another; thus the patient may use active motion to help resolve a passive limitation but cannot regress to a prior posture (Hill & Yasukawa, 1999). Although the cast, drop-out cast, and serial stretcher have no moving parts and are often considered static splints, they can provide or augment the functions of a mobilizing splint (Bell-Krotoski, 1987).

Indications for Use

Clinicians find casting to be a powerful weapon in their treatment arsenals. The casting technique helps solve several challenging problems that the therapist frequently identifies during the patient evaluation. Because casting provides optimal pressure distribution and because a cast usually remains on 24 hr per day, the patient population for casting includes those with sensory, motivation, and cognitive problems (Bell-Krotoski, 1987). Casting maintains the maximum tolerable end range position, and thus maximizes end range time. As described by Flowers and LaStayo (1994), the greater the end range time, the faster the contracted tissue lengthens and passive range of motion (PROM) increases.

Indications for casting include the following:

- Swollen, painful proximal interphalangeal (PIP) joints—common after joint dislocation and joint reconstruction (Bell-Krotoski, 1995).
- Acute, closed central slip avulsion without fracture (Coons & Green, 1995; Schneider & Smith, 1987).
- Acute, closed terminal extensor tendon rupture or avulsion (Brzezienski & Schneider, 1995).
- Extrinsic muscle/tendon unit tightness—a sequelae to protective positioning and common after many types of injuries, including extensive soft tissue injury to the hand or wrist, crush injury, tendon and nerve laceration, replantation, and fracture (Tribuzi, 1990).
- Hard end feel contractures of any joint—may be secondary to fracture; amputation; dislocation; tendon rupture, laceration, or repair; nerve repair, volar plate avulsion; and burn (Bell-Krotoski, 1995; Schultz Johnson, 1992; Tribuzi, 1990).
- Muscle-tendon unit imbalance at a joint—may be the result of ulnar nerve palsy, arthritis, tendon avulsion, or tendon laceration and repair (Bell-Krotoski, 1987).
- Proximal joint loss of PROM—improvement requires long lever arms via a mobilizing splint (Bell-Krotoski, 1987).
- Chronically stiff hand (Colditz, 2000a, 2000b).
- Compliance problems (Sailer & Salibury-Milan, 2000).
- Loss of PROM owing to spasticity (Goga-Eppenstein, Hill, Seifert, & Yasukawa, 1999).

Casts can be used for a variety of purposes, including the following:

- To rest and/or protect a joint, especially when edema needs to be controlled (Bell-Krotoski, 1995).
- To co-apt acutely ruptured tendons or bony avulsion and to immobilize the part to allow anatomic healing (Brzezienski & Schneider, 1995; Coons & Green, 1995; Schneider & Smith, 1987).

- To increase PROM by holding articular and periarticular structures at the maximum tolerable length for long periods of time, remodeling tissue (Flowers & LaStayo, 1994).
- To transfer a muscle-tendon unit force to adjacent joints (Bell-Krotoski, 1987).
- To rebalance flexor and extensor mechanisms at the PIP joint (Bell-Krotoski, 1987).
- To increase the effective lever arm and thus the force at a proximal joint when distal joints are casted (Bell-Krotoski, 1987).
- To act as a base for mobilizing splints when distributing pressure and minimizing migration are essential.
- To mobilize multiple joints by casting specific joints in positions of function and allowing self-mobilization of uncasted joints via active range of motion (AROM) (Colditz, 2000a, 2000b).
- To mobilize a joint by blocking motion in one direction and allowing motion in another (Goga-Eppenstein et al., 1999).
- To decrease tone and increase soft tissue length in spastic extremities.

Swollen, Painful PIP Joints

After joint dislocation and reconstruction, the PIP joint may require rest in the maximum available extension. This position reduces the incidence of PIP flexion contractures and places the joint structures in the optimal position to regain function. Dorsal dislocations or fracture dislocations are exceptions and require extension block splinting to protect the healing volar structures (Lubahn, 1988). A cast reduces edema and provides excellent pressure distribution. The hard shell offers protection from external forces. However, the cast may stress the PIP joint during removal, even if it is soaked first to soften it. Thus for highly acute joint involvement that results in extreme tenderness, the therapist may need to choose another form of splinting other than casting.

Acute, Closed Central Slip Avulsion

Casting is one treatment method for acute, closed central slip avulsion (Evans, 1995). The sooner this injury is identified and treated the better. However, even weeks and months after injury, if the finger still appears to be inflamed, the tendon may still benefit from a period of undisturbed extension in a cast (Fig. 12–1). Positioning the finger with the PIP in neutral and the distal interphalangeal (DIP) left free, coapts the ends of the torn central slip and allows the rebalancing of the extensor mechanism at the DIP joint. It also helps elongate the oblique retinacular ligament (ORL) and improve DIP flexion. Evans (1995) adds a nail hook and rubber band to the cast with a proximal rubber band attachment on the volar side of the cast to increase DIP flexion in the finger with a tight ORL. When the tendon is allowed to rest in the stressless, shortened position, it may heal without surgical intervention.

Ideally, if the finger demonstrates full PIP extension, the cast is left in place for approximately 6 weeks. If the finger has developed a flexion contracture, then the PIP needs to be serially casted into full extension and then held in that position for approximately 6 weeks. Some clinicians recommend starting guarded active motion at 3 weeks; however, this must be done with great care and with a responsible patient (Evans, 1995). If the patient flexes the PIP abruptly during this time, the therapist can assume that the continuity of the central slip has been compromised and the 6 weeks of extension must begin again. Making this information clear to the patient facilitates compliance. At the 6-week point, the patient is gradually weaned from the cast and can begin wearing a removable splint. Discontinuing extension positioning abruptly can compromise the end result.

Extrinsic Muscle-Tendon Unit Tightness

Extrinsic muscle-tendon unit tightness occurs after many types of injuries, including extensive soft tissue injury to the hand or wrist, crush injury, tendon and nerve laceration, replantation, and fracture. It can also be a sequelae to protective positioning. The therapist has many treatment options for minimizing the muscle-tendon unit shortening, although the POP stretcher is one of the most effective (Fig. 12–2).

The advantage of plaster lies primarily in its extreme rigidity. The initial plaster costs little. However, if the patient requires many serial stretchers, the price of the material added to the cost of setup and cleanup may equal or even exceed the cost of thermoplastic material. The serial static splinting treatment process necessarily involves progression of the splint's shape to position the tissue at ever-greater lengths. Although plaster cannot be remolded the way thermoplastic can, it often gives superior results. The thermoplastic that can withstand frequent remolding is often not rigid enough to maintain the joint at end range. Highly rigid thermoplastics cannot tolerate frequent remolding and must be discarded for new material. Reinforcing the thermoplastic requires effort each time the splint is revised. With a minimum of

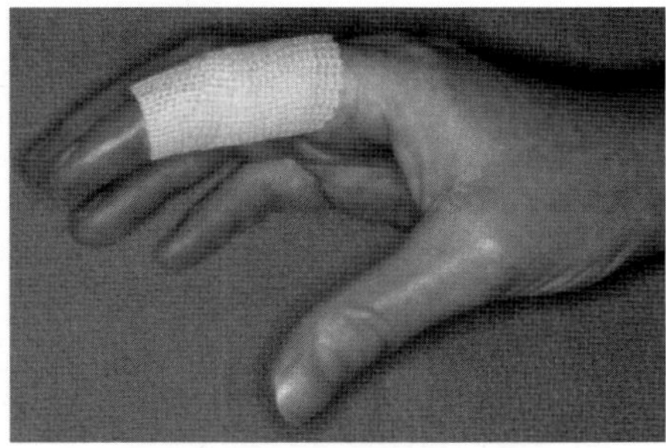

Figure 12–1 The PIP is cast in full extension, and the DIP is free to move.

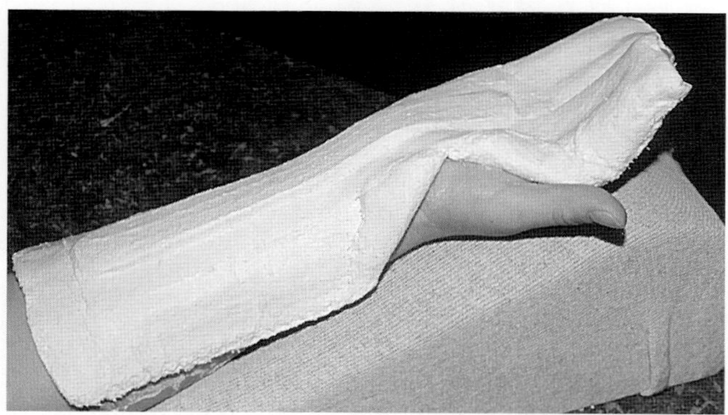

Figure 12–2 A POP stretcher is used to lengthen the muscle-tendon itself as well as any muscle-tendon unit adhesions.

practice, therapists can fabricate POP stretchers efficiently and cost effectively.

Another essential advantage is POP's superior drape and ability to distribute pressure. When pressure is distributed well along the skin surface, the patient can withstand higher forces (Brand, 1988). The limitations in the amount of force that can be generated in a splint are related to skin tolerance, because this is usually the weak link in force delivery. However, if the force is well distributed, the target tissue can often withstand higher loads (Brand, Hollister, Giurintano, & Thompson, 1999a). It is theorized that higher loads may have the potential to increase tissue length faster. Thus plaster provides the opportunity to increase PROM faster than materials that are less conforming and less efficient at distributing the load.

Hard End Feel Joint Contractures

Brand was the first clinician to use serial casting on hard end feel contractures of the PIP joints (see Chapter 15 for details). Since then, therapists all over the world have used this technique on PIPs and other joints of the upper extremity with great success (Fig. 12-1). Serial casting positions shortened tissue at maximum length but not beyond it, the way mobilizing splints with elastic traction tend to do. This positioning applies a mechanical stress to tissue, causing it to remodel in a longer form. Clinical experience has shown that almost any contracture involving live tissue, even one that is years old, will benefit from serial casting. Notable exceptions are Dupuytren's disease and contractures caused by fibrotic tissue (see Chapter 15 for details). Heterotopic ossification and exostosis do not respond to casting.

Tissue that has been overstretched will shorten when placed on slack for a significant duration in a cast. Clinical experience suggests that tissue remodeling to increase length occurs more rapidly than remodeling to shorten overstretched tissue. In the case of a PIP flexion contracture, the cast may reestablish enough length in the palmar tissues to allow full passive PIP extension. However, the overstretched dorsal hood extensor mechanism often will not be able to accomplish full active extension; thus surgery may be necessary. The surgical procedure creates an inflammatory response in the extensor hood. If immobilized long enough (usually 3 to 4 weeks) to allow collagen cross-linking to form and then mobilized at just the right speed, extension and flexion may be restored at 8 to 10 weeks postsurgery, without reproducing the previous extensor lag (R. Meals, personal communication, 1999). The patient will not be a candidate for the extensor procedure until the flexion contracture resolves.

Muscle-Tendon Unit Imbalance

Addressing the AROM and PROM limitations induced by nerve injury, Bell-Krotoski (1987) noted that casting can help "rebalance externally what has become imbalanced internally by a selective muscle loss." After paralysis of the hand's intrinsic muscles, an imbalance of the extensor mechanism—overpull of the proximal phalanx by the extensor digitorum communis (EDC) into extension and absent translational forces of the intrinsics on the dorsal hood—prevents the fingers from being fully extended at the interphalangeal (IP) joints (Fig. 12–3**A**). In addition,

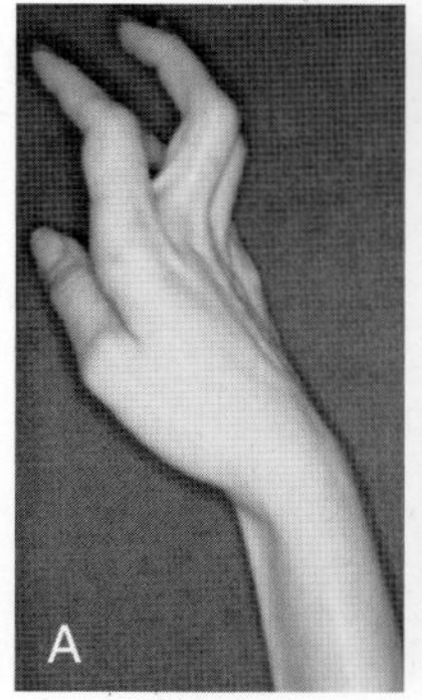

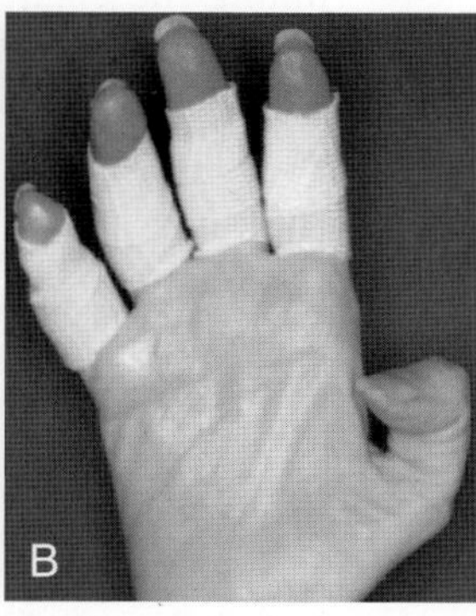

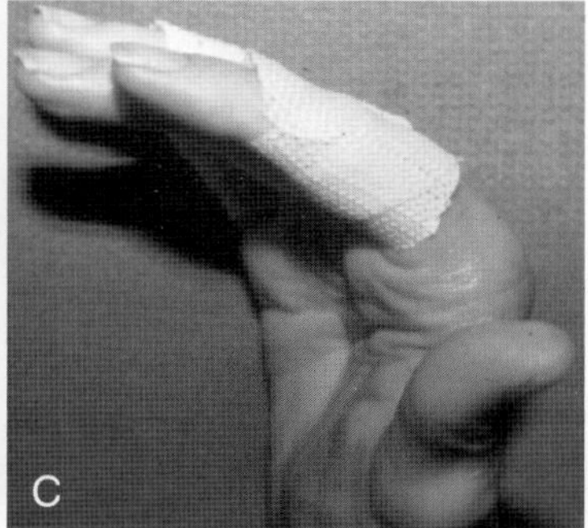

Figure 12–3 ***A,*** *Combined ulnar and medium nerve injury leading to intrinsic paralysis and an imbalance of the extensor mechanism prevents the fingers from being fully extended at the PIP joints. Casting of the PIP joints into extension allows the MP joints to be brought into full extension by the EDC (**B**) and full flexion by the FDS and FDP (**C**).*

the metacarpophalangeal (MP) joints lose their primary flexor, and these joints flex only after flexion of the IP joints by the flexor digitorum superficialis (FDS) and flexor digitorum profundus (FDP).

Bell-Krotoski (1987) explained that casting of the IP joints into extension allows the fingers to be brought into full extension by the EDC and into flexion at the MP joints by the FDS and FDP (Fig. 12–3**B,C**). Thus casting allows external rebalancing of the fingers and can be used temporarily before and after intrinsic replacement surgery in lieu of dynamic splinting. The hyperextension in the intrinsic minus hand commonly present at the MP joint does not usually continue after the casts are applied, because the primary flexion of the MP joint has been restored.

Lengthening Lever Arms

Occasionally, the therapist identifies a situation in which a contracture requires the use of higher force levels. In such cases, the physics of levers may help deliver the force. Casting is an excellent method for stabilizing a joint to increase mechanical advantage. As described in Chapter 4, the farther away the sling or loop is placed from the affected joint, the higher the force that the splint can generate (Bell-Krotoski, 1987). For example, when a splint is fabricated to increase MP joint flexion, the sling can be placed distal to the stabilized PIP to increase the force at the MP. Without PIP stabilization, the distally placed sling will instead act on both the PIP and the MP. This stabilizing technique is especially desirable for small fingers—the short proximal phalanxes result in a decreased mechanical advantage (Fig. 12–4). The therapist who uses long lever arms must first take note of joint stability and then closely listen to the patient for complaints of joint pain (Fig. 12–5) (Brand, Hollister, Giurintano, & Thompson, 1999b).

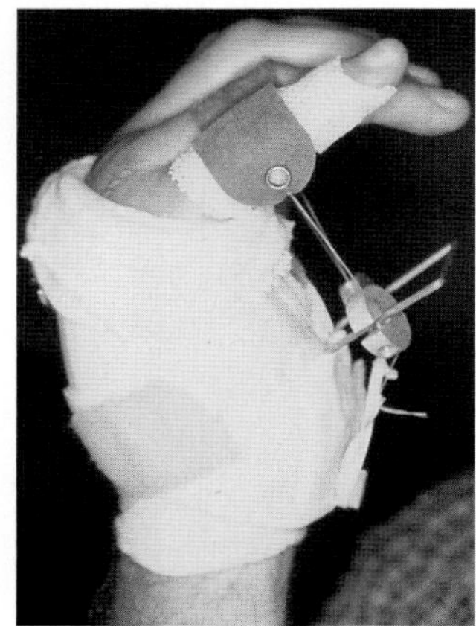

Figure 12–4 A PIP casting technique that is especially indicated when an MP extension contracture and a PIP flexion contracture co-exist.

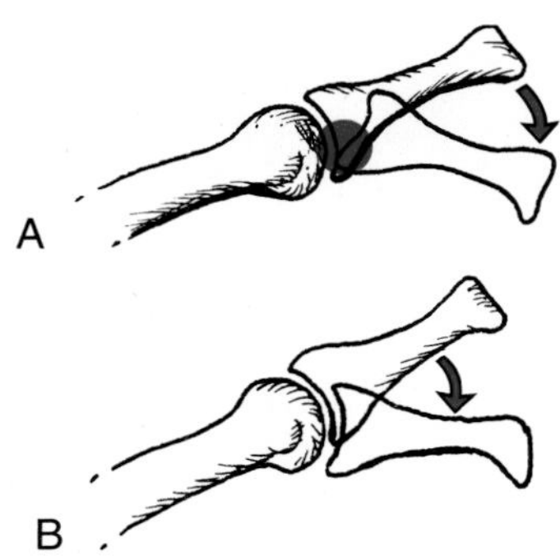

*Figure 12–5 Applying stress to a joint can result in undesirable tilting (**A**) or desirable gliding (**B**).*

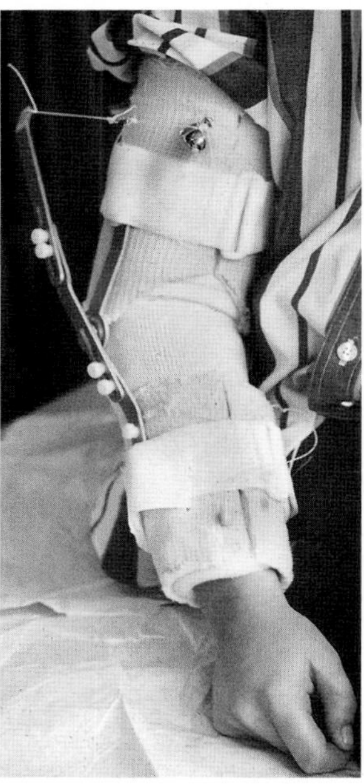

Figure 12–6 Using a circumferential splint as a base is one of the most effective means of maximizing stability and minimizing pressure problems.

Mobilizing Splint Base

Among the challenges that a therapist encounters when splinting the hand are splint stability and pressure distribution. With the addition of flexion or extension assists, the splint base tends to migrate or shift, and increasing the pressure at the splint edges (Fig. 12–6). A circumferential splint base minimizes migration and distributes pressure. A strategically positioned wrist or thumb can block the splint from migrating.

Chronically Stiff Hand

The management of a patient with chronic stiffness of multiple joints of the hand and upper extremity can seem overwhelming. The strategic casting of specific joints of the stiff hand and leaving other joints free for self-mobilization via AROM has proven effective when other approaches have failed (Colditz, 2000a, 2000b). Often the clinician notes chronic, unresponsive edema, stiff joints, and dysfunctional patterns of movement (e.g., wrist flexion with finger flexion rather than wrist extension with finger flexion). It is theorized that casting facilitates the lymphatic system, helps reeducate the patient to perform functional movement patterns, and allows the patient to focus on a few stiff joints at a time (Colditz, 2000a, 2000b). Although the casting of stiff joints such as the wrist and MPs in one position for a significant time may seem to contradict basic philosophies about how to mobilize joints, this approach has proven its effectiveness (Fig. 12–7).

Compliance Problems

Motivation, cognition, and maturity can each affect compliance. When compliance becomes a major concern in patient treatment, a circumferential, nonremovable cast offers the best opportunity for achieving treatment goals because it requires no judgment or cooperation. The patient need only keep the cast on and in good condition. If a caregiver is involved, then the clinician must instruct the caregiver to watch for signs of cast intolerance and how to remove the cast. The cast eliminates difficulties that result from donning and doffing the splint improperly and inconsistently.

Casting for Central Nervous System Disorders

Traumatic brain injury, stroke, and cerebral palsy commonly result in muscle tone and muscle synergy disorders that create joint contractures (see Chapter 21 for more information). Because patients with these disorders often lack the cognitive and sensory awareness to monitor their own status, their splints must distribute pressure optimally or harm to skin and joints can result. A frequently used splinting technique to increase PROM for central nervous system (CNS) disorders is serial casting (Goga-Eppenstein et al., 1999). The circumferential design provides even pressure distribution, edema control, and scar remodeling via pressure. Because the ROM problems confronting these patients is mostly owing to hypertonicity of muscle in consistent patterns, the clinician usually does not need to worry about losing motion in the opposite direction from the cast goal.

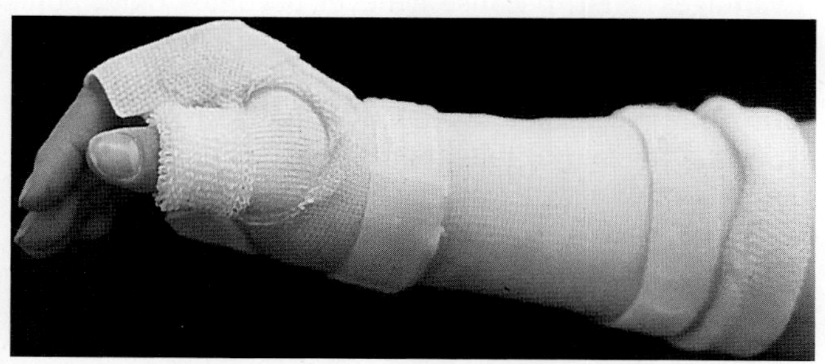

Figure 12–7 A QuickCast immobilization splint for the wrist and MP joints promotes active motion at the IP joints. The therapist must follow all the tenets of good splint and cast design and fabrication.

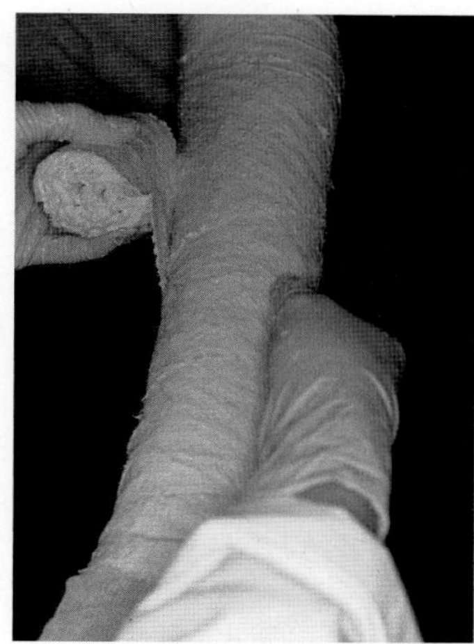

Figure 12–8 POP being used to fabricate an elbow cast to combat spasticity in a patient with a neurologically involved upper limb.

The therapist must carefully consider the number of joints incorporated into the cast, since hypertonicity controlled at one joint may increase tone at adjacent joints. For example, if an elbow cast does not control the wrist, flexor tone (now controlled at the elbow) may increase at the wrist, causing dramatic wrist flexion posture (T. Hackencamp, personal communication, 1999).

CNS Casting Materials

Many therapists use synthetic casting tape lined with cast padding to treat spasticity because it is strong, yet lightweight. Some therapists still favor plaster, especially for use around the fingers, thumb, and palm, because it conforms well and allows air exchange (Fig. 12–8). QuickCast, a product featuring shrink-to-fit technology, provides a means to achieve serial mobilization quickly. This product allows serial remolding at increased end range, because it can be gently heated while still on the patient. Like plaster, it allows air exchange.

Fabrication

For small patients, two people can fabricate the cast (T. Hackencamp, personal communication, 1999). One can position the patient's joint in a tolerable position—usually a submaximal position for the joint—while the other applies the casting material. Casting an adult, especially one in an agitated state, may require additional positioning assistance. All casting materials heat the extremity during fabrication, which can make the extremity more flexible. If the cast fabricator takes advantage of the increased PROM, the joint position obtained during casting may be too extreme for the patient to tolerate. As the joint position progresses, swelling may occur; should this happen, elevate the extremity.

Precautions

Casting for patients with CNS injuries has its own set of precautions and concerns (T. Hackencamp, personal communication, 1999). The clinician must frequently check for signs of cast intolerance by looking for color and temperature changes, swelling, and subtle signs of discomfort. To avoid the possibility of cast-caused trunk abrasions, the therapist may cover the cast with a soft material (Moleskin). The clinician must instruct the family and nursing staff to be sure that the patient does not put things into the cast. Taping the cast's edges prevents this possibility. All caregivers must remember to keep the cast dry.

CNS Cast Regimen

Do not initiate casting on a Friday if the patient cannot be checked over the weekend (T. Hackencamp, personal communication, 1999). If the setting permits, the therapist should check the first cast a patient receives several times a day. In an outpatient facility, the therapist must make sure that the patient and/or caregiver understand all precautions. If the patient does well, the cast can be left in place 3 to 5 days, after which it is removed. If it is clear that the patient has tolerated casting well, then the clinician may immediately replace the cast and leave it on for up to 2 weeks. Careful monitoring must continue.

Casting over a prolonged period will cause muscle atrophy. While considered a contraindication or negative side effect in the primarily orthopedic patient, in the patient with CNS dysfunction, this loss of muscle strength is considered a goal. The atrophy helps reduce flexion posture and subsequent joint contracture (see Chapter 12 for detailed information).

General Casting Materials and Equipment

Plaster of Paris

Traditionally, therapists used gauze impregnated with POP to cast finger contractures, especially PIP flexion contractures (Fig. 12–9). Plaster is the material first used by Brand for Hansen's disease patients in India and then in the United States (Wilson, 1965). Plaster has been the material of choice because it is readily available, inexpensive, breathable, friendly to skin and wounds, and meticulously conforming. Patient can be instructed in how to remove and apply plaster for use in a home program.

POP's primary disadvantage is that it is vulnerable to moisture. POP softens and loses its strength when exposed to water. Plaster is heavier and often thicker than thermoplastic. Although POP is messy to apply, the practiced therapist has developed a system to minimize cleanup. When POP and water mix, an exothermic chemical reaction takes place. Cases of burns caused by the application of POP have been reported; thus the therapist must observe the patient carefully for this possible complication (discussed in detail later in this chapter) (Becker, 1978; Grazer, 1979; Haasch, 1964; Kaplan, 1981; Schultze, 1967).

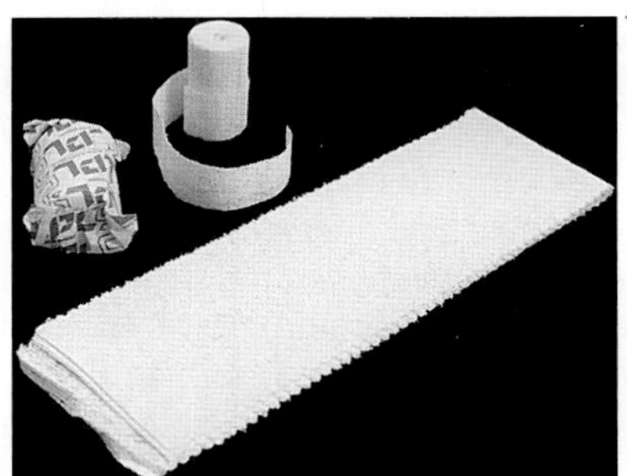

Figure 12–9 POP comes in rolls and sheets of various widths.

Fiberglass

With the advent of fiberglass casting materials (gauze impregnated with a water-activated resin), therapists have been able to take advantage of its lightweight quality to make larger casts. Fiberglass is rigid, durable, and lightweight, making it a good alternative for casting large joints. And it is available in bright colors. This material can be used for serial casting of wrists and elbows; however, it is not an option for casting fingers. Unfortunately, the skin does not tolerate the chemicals in the fiberglass and such casts require padding; thus finger casts are too bulky and nonconforming. Furthermore, fiberglass casts must be removed with a cast saw; thus it is unworkable for use in a home casting program. Fiberglass has a shorter shelf life than plaster.

Softcast

Softcast offers another alternative for casting. Unique in the world of casting materials, Softcast remains somewhat flexible and never sets rigidly, as does fiberglass and POP. In addition, while the material does adhere to itself, with a moderate pull, Softcast unwraps much like an Ace bandage. These characteristics offer two major advantages. First, because it never becomes rigid, Softcast can be used for patients who will benefit from slightly flexible immobilization. Second, Softcast does not require a cast saw for removal, so it can be used for patients who cannot tolerate a saw or who may need to remove the cast when away from the casting facility. It cannot be made into a bivalved cast.

Softcast can be applied directly to the skin, but some clinicians use it with a stockinette liner. The material has no shelf life once the package is opened. Any cast material not used must be discarded. The more layers of Softcast used, the more rigid the cast will be; however, this makes the cast heavier and bulkier. Placing a plaster splint underneath the Softcast increases overall rigidity.

QuickCast

In 1995, QuickCast (an elastic fiberglass mesh impregnated with heat-softened thermoplastic) entered the therapy market. QuickCast is available in 1-in. tape rolls; flat sheets; and cylindrical kits for the thumb, wrist, and elbow. The material shrinks when it is heated with a hairdryer. When the appropriately sized cylindrical kit is placed on an extremity and heated, it shrinks down to conform perfectly to the body part without any danger of constriction (Mahler & Pedowitz, 1996). QuickCast splint kits offer the therapist a means to make circumferential splints quickly and with excellent fit. By simply reheating the splint with a hairdryer, the therapist can easily reposition any joint included in a lined QuickCast cast (Fig. 12–10).

The flat sheets are intended for use as reinforcement and edging for the QuickCast kits. However, the cast maker can cut the sheets into strips and apply then in a similar fashion as conventional casting material. Once heated, the individual strips are placed either directly onto the skin or over some type of stockinette. Padding may also be added. When used in strips, the thick QuickCast stockinette liner does not need to be used, because the material is not heated directly on the skin as is a QuickCast cylinder kit.

The advent of QuickCast offered an important option in serial casting of fingers. For the first time, patients wearing finger serial casts could expose their hands to water. When used for serial casting, QuickCast can be laid directly against the skin or placed over a thin liner. (When a liner is used, the hand cannot get water.) QuickCast does contain live rubber (Latex); however, it is coated with thermoplastic. Because only one or two layers are required for a firm cast, QuickCast creates the thinnest finger cast yet available. Not only is this of great comfort to the patient but it allows the therapist to cast adjacent fingers without forcing them into extreme abduction. QuickCast sets up quickly—several minutes faster than plaster or fiberglass—making it a time-efficient material. The setup and cleanup for a QuickCast cast is minimal compared to plaster and fiberglass.

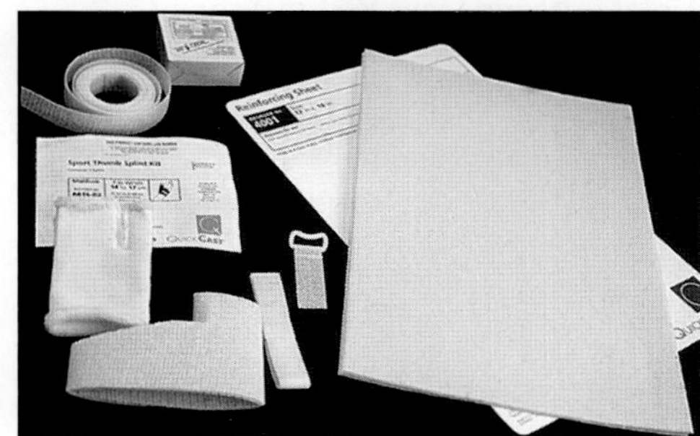

Figure 12–10 QuickCast is available in a variety of sizes and shapes. When heated, it conforms perfectly to the body part.

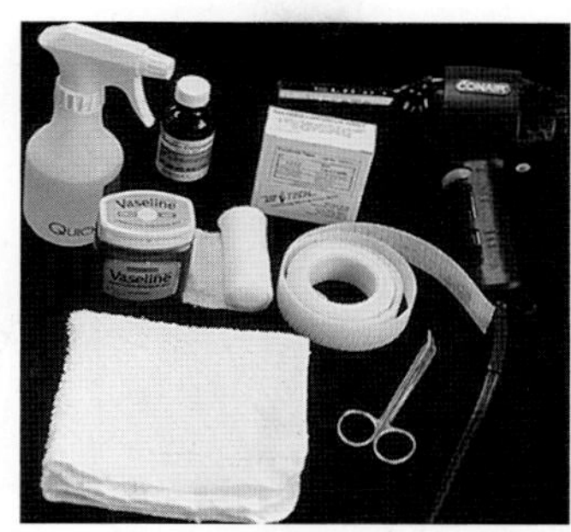

Figure 12–11 Materials and equipment needed to fabricate a QuickCast finger cast.

A QuickCast finger cast can be removed (discussed later in this chapter), reheated, and reused, as long as it does not have to be cut off the finger. In contrast, the therapist must discard other types of casting materials after removal. QuickCast conforms very well; the slight tackiness of the material also helps with serial cast application and conformity. The therapist can create univalve finger casts and QuickCast kits to make them removable with a special small scissors called a Splint/Cast Trimmer. The short blades are contoured for safety when cutting close to the skin, and the proportionally long handles provide excellent mechanical advantage.

Clinical Example: Serial Static PIP Extension Splint

Using QuickCast

Materials and Preparation

Making a QuickCast PIP extension cast requires the following materials (Fig. 12–11) (Schultz Johnson, 1999):

- QuickCast tape
- Hairdryer
- Splint/Cast Trimmers
- Towel
- Spray bottle with water (optional)
- Petroleum jelly (optional)
- Cast padding (optional)
- Tincture of benzoin (optional)

The hairdryer should be a long-nosed, 1600-W dryer with high airflow. This type of dryer heats the tape effectively and quickly. It is important that a long-nosed dryer will not shut off when hot air is funneled back into the end. Short-nosed dryers shut down when hot air returns into the nose, which often occurs when heating QuickCast. **Caution:** Do not use a heat gun with QuickCast.

To begin the cast fabrication process, cut the length of QuickCast needed for the finger. The length depends on the length and circumference of the finger and the number of joints being splinted (Fig. 12–12**A**). A QuickCast finger cast requires only a single layer of material with about 1/8" overlap.

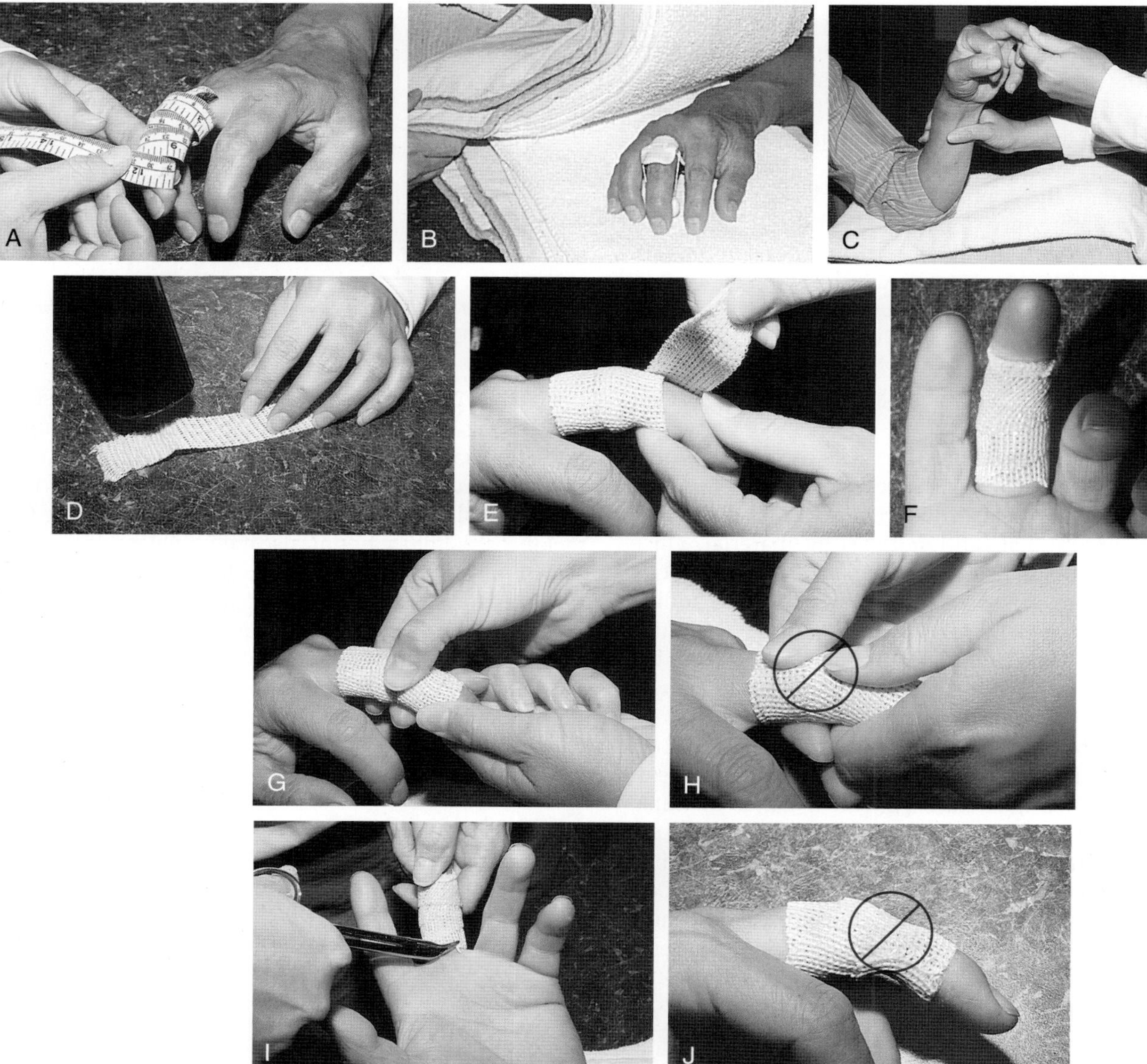

Figure 12–12 *Steps for fabricating a QuickCast finger cast.* ***A,*** *Estimate the amount of QuickCast tape needed by spiraling a cloth dressmaker's tape around the finger in the same configuration as the planned cast.* ***B,*** *Heat and a digit extension splint precondition the finger to gain maximum PROM just before casting.* ***C,*** *Extend the patient's PIP joint using axial traction.* ***D,*** *Hold the dryer above the tape, which will shrink as it becomes soft and hot. Keep the dryer steady; avoid moving it back and forth.* ***E,*** *Keeping the QuickCast tape stretched, wrap all the way around the proximal phalanx once; then begin to spiral distally, wrapping once for each layer and overlapping the previous layer.* ***F,*** *Wrap the finger so the DIP joint is free to move.* ***G,*** *Use a continuous rotary motion to conform the material closely to the finger and obtain an optimal fit.* ***H,*** *To avoid point pressure, do not poke at the cast with your fingertips; instead use the length of your fingers for maximal pressure distribution.* ***I,*** *Use the Splint/Cast Trimmers to contour and smooth the edges.* ***J,*** *If there are any indentations, the cast must be removed and remade.*

Method

PRECONDITIONING THE FINGER

Clinically, this author has found that the cast results are more rapidly achieved and of greater magnitude when the joint is preconditioned, or stretched out, just before casting. The therapist should use one of the following techniques to gain maximum PROM just before casting: compression and/or massage for edema reduction, heat and stretch, joint mobilization, active and passive exercise, and therapeutic activities (Fig. 12–12**B**).

POSITION AND TECHNIQUE

Before making the cast, decide on patient and finger positions. Practice with the patient. Be sure the patient understands the materials, technique, and rationale for cast application. Position the finger as follows:

1. Remove any rings from the finger to be casted.
2. Seat the patient, placing the elbow of the affected extremity on a firm but padded surface.
3. Have the patient (or an assistant) hold the finger to be casted at the distal phalanx, leaving the DIP crease free, and then pull the finger, using axial traction, while the patient (or an assistant) pulls the hand away from the traction force by extending the wrist or bending the elbow (Fig. 12–12**C**). The force must take the PIP joint to maximum available extension without causing pain.
4. Sustain the traction force until the cast is set.

Cut the QuickCast tape and place it flat on a towel. Set the hairdryer to the hottest setting and highest airflow. Hold the dryer directly above the tape, almost touching it (Fig. 12–12**D**). When all of the QuickCast is softened, pick it up and stretch it back to maximum length. (After the tape is applied on stretch to the finger, it will not shrink back down and overcompress the finger.) Because the tape will be tacky, the therapist should moisten his or her hands with water to prevent the QuickCast from sticking and make the material easier to work with.

Taking care to avoid the fragile skin of the finger web, place the tape as far proximally as possible on the proximal phalanx. Keeping the QuickCast tape stretched, wrap it all the way around the proximal phalanx; then begin to spiral distally, overlapping each wrap by about 1/8" over the previous wrap (Fig. 12–12**E**). If the DIP joint is to be left free to move, end approximately 1/16" proximal to the DIP joint flexion crease, but extend the cast fully to the DIP joint dorsally (Fig. 12–12**F**). Once the QuickCast has been applied to the entire finger, use a continuous rotary motion of the fingers to "screw" the material down onto the digit (Fig. 12–12**G**). **Caution:** Avoid point pressure against the QuickCast at all times (Fig. 12–12**H**).

Check and Revision

Inspect the palmar joint crease at the MP joint and be sure the patient can flex the MP without the proximal-palmar end of the cast pressing into the joint crease. If this occurs, use the Splint/Cast Trimmers to carve out some of the material and allow unimpeded movement (Fig. 12–12**I**). Next, check the DIP crease to be sure that the DIP joint can fully flex. Again, either push the material away from the crease or use the Splint/Cast Trimmers to trim the cast if needed. Finally, check the web spaces and contour or trim as needed. The Splint/Cast Trimmers present minimal risk to the patient's skin. All of the edges must be smooth to prevent skin irritation. Observe the cast closely for any signs of indentation along the substance of the cast. If any indentation is evident, remove the cast and start over (Fig. 12–12**J**).

If the cast appears unsatisfactory, simply unwind the material, even a few minutes after the cast is completed. After the QuickCast is off the finger, simply repeat the heating process and reapply the same material. Unwinding the material becomes quite difficult once the QuickCast is fully hardened. The cast will set up in 1 minute or less. Once the material has set, use the Splint/Cast Trimmer to cut the cast to remove it. **Caution:** Do not use the hairdryer to reheat the QuickCast when it is on the finger. The heat can cause great discomfort and may damage the tissue. The most commonly used finger casting technique lacks any insulating lining to protect the patient's skin.

Using POP

Materials and Preparation

Making a PIP extension cast from POP requires the following materials (Fig. 12–13):

- POP rolls cut into 2½-in. strips, folded in half
- Hot water
- Small clean bowl
- Plaster scissors
- Splint/Cast Trimmers
- Tissues
- Petroleum jelly
- Cast padding (optional)
- Drapes to protect work surfaces and patient's clothes

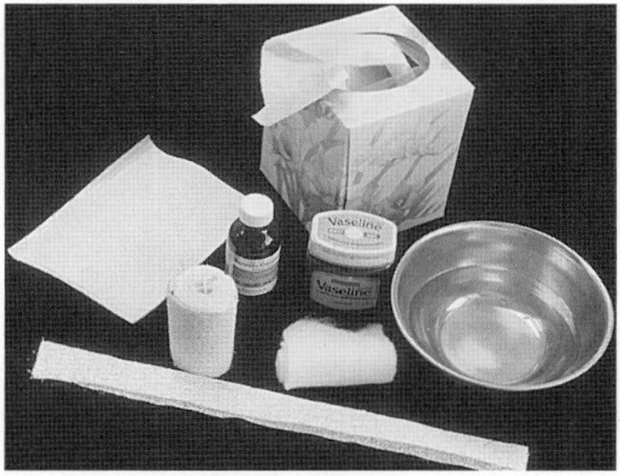

Figure 12–13 Materials and equipment needed to fabricate a POP finger cast.

This author prefers to use 3" wide POP folded in half and then trimmed to a 1¼" width. Choose the fastest-setting plaster obtainable. Gypsona (Smith+Nephew, Germantown, WI) is often the plaster of choice because of its fine texture that creates a smooth, strong cast that sets quickly.

Prepare the clinic for POP application and gather the required materials and equipment needed. To protect surfaces from plaster drippings, cover them with disposable waterproof covers. Place drapes over the patient's clothing. The therapist may wish to wear an apron. The therapist and patient may wish to remove watches and rings.

Fill a small clean bowl with hot water. The hotter the water, the faster the plaster will set. Cut the length of POP needed for the finger; the length depends on the length and circumference of the finger and the number of joints being splinted. Estimate the amount of POP needed by spiraling a cloth dressmaker's tape around the finger in the same configuration as planned to make the cast; then double the length (Fig. 12–12**A**). Remember that each layer of the cast requires two wraps of POP and each layer overlaps the preceding one by 50%, or ¾".

Method

Precondition the finger as described for making a QuickCast finger cast earlier in this chapter (Fig. 12–12**B**). Positioning for POP casting is virtually the same as that for QuickCast (Fig. 12–12**C**), with a few exceptions.

To begin the cast fabrication process, coat the finger with petroleum jelly (Fig. 12–14**A**), which protects against the drying effects of the plaster. Dip the length of plaster into the water; then run the POP between two fingers to remove excess water (Fig. 12–14**B**). Taking care to avoid the fragile skin of the finger web, place the tape as far proximally as possible on the proximal phalanx. Wrap all the way around the proximal phalanx twice and then begin to spiral distally, wrapping twice for each layer and overlapping the previous layer halfway, or by about ¾" (Fig. 12–14**C**). To allow the DIP joint to move freely, end approximately 1/16" proximal to the DIP joint flexion crease, but extend the cast fully to the DIP joint dorsally (Fig. 12–14**D**). Once the material is applied to the entire finger, use a continuous rotary motion of the fingers to coax the material down onto the finger (Fig. 12–14**E**). **Caution:** As for QuickCast, avoid point pressure against the material at all times (Fig. 12–14**F**).

Check and Revision

Once the POP has been applied and with traction sustained on the finger, check the cast. Inspect the palmar joint crease at the MP joint and be sure the patient can flex the MP without the proximal-palmar end of the cast pressing into the joint crease. If this occurs, push or roll the damp plaster back away from the crease or use the Splint/Cast Trimmers to carve out some of the material to allow unimpeded movement. Next, check the DIP crease to be sure that the DIP joint can fully flex. Again, either push or roll the damp plaster back away from the crease or use the trimmers to trim the cast if needed. Finally, check the web spaces and contour or trim as needed (Fig. 12–14**G**). The Splint/Cast Trimmers pose a minimal risk to the patient's skin. Of course, under optimal conditions, the cast will not need trimming. Observe the cast closely for any signs of indentation along the substance of the cast. If indentation is evident, remove the cast and start over (Fig. 12–14**H**).

If the cast appears unsatisfactory after making it, the therapist can remove the plaster and begin again with a clean bowl; clean water; and new plaster, petroleum jelly, and tissue. It may be possible to raise the end of the POP cast and unwind it. The patient may soak the POP cast off in very warm water. Alternatively, Splint/Cast Trimmers can be used to cut into the plaster either at the proximal or distal end to help remove it.

Helpful Techniques for Finger Casting

Cast Removal

Both the patient and the therapist must be familiar with techniques for cast removal. The patient should leave the clinic only after indicating a clear understanding of how to remove the cast. For the first few POP casts, mark the distal end of the POP with a pen; this will help with cast removal in an emergency and help assure the patient that they can unwind the cast (Fig. 12–15). The patient must be instructed that the cast cannot be removed with a cast saw, since there is no padding. However, after making hundreds of plaster casts, this author has had only two patients who needed to remove an initial POP cast before returning to the clinic. These patients had unusual psychological profiles and their need to remove the cast was owing to a sense of claustrophobia rather than any problem with edema or ischemia.

If the patient's contracture is approximately 30° or less, then the patient will most likely be able to pull the cast off. For patients with unstable MP joints (such as with rheumatic disease), the proximal phalanx will need to be stabilized before pulling off the cast. If the joint is too tender for this removal technique, if the joint is quite swollen, or if the contracture is more severe, then the cast removal is more involved.

SOAKING AND CUTTING

The patient can immerse the casted finger in the warmest tolerable water to soften the POP and unwind the cast (Fig. 12–16). This sometimes works for QuickCast as well, but the patient must be able to tolerate very warm water. The patient should soak the cast in the warmest water tolerable for 1 to 2 minutes for QuickCast and 5 minutes or longer for POP. Once the distal flap of the casting material is raised, it is possible to unwrap the cast. It may need to be resoaked several times before the

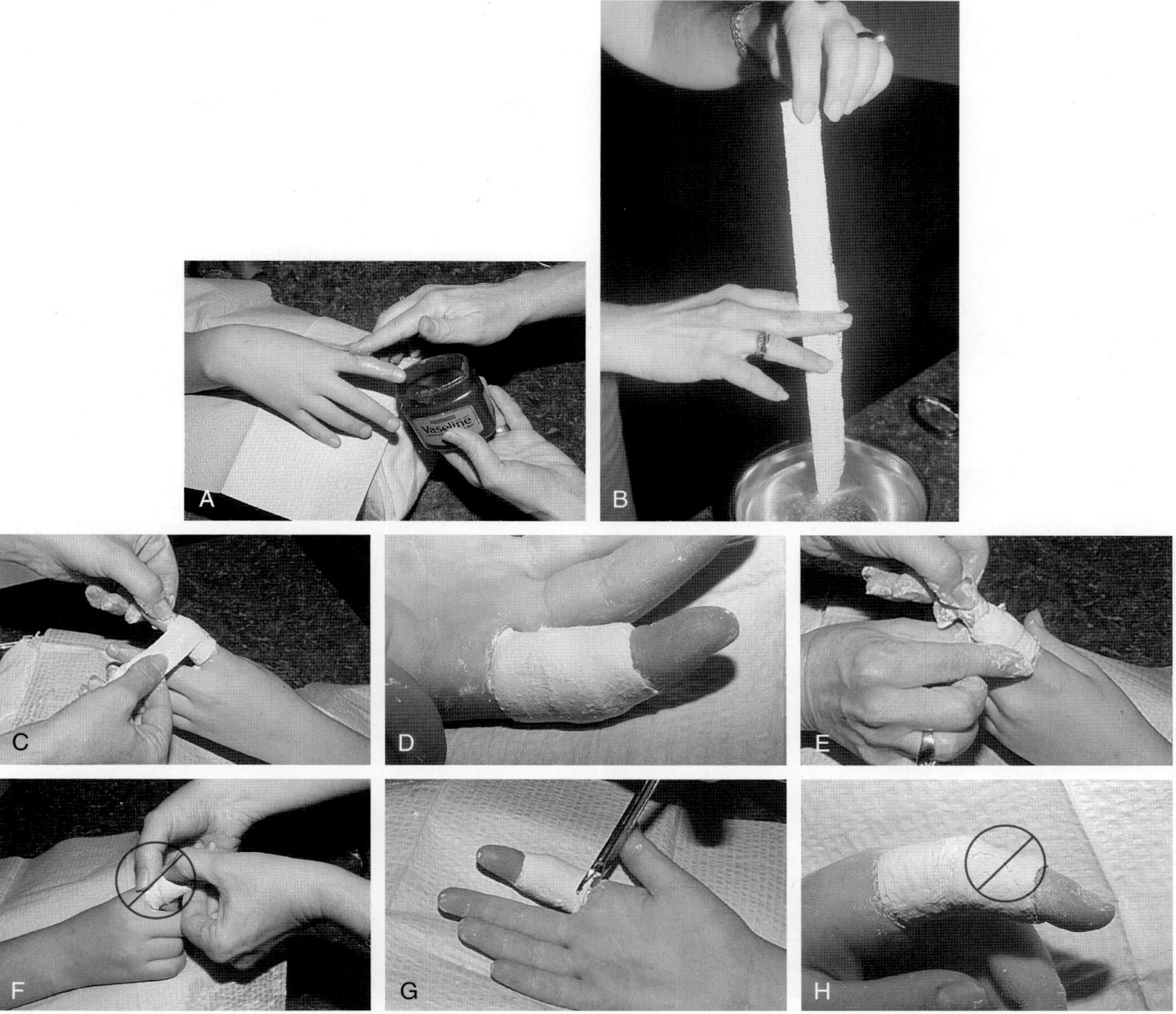

*Figure 12–14 Steps for fabricating a POP finger cast. **A,** The lubricating process helps protect the finger from the drying effects of the POP. **B,** Squeeze to remove excess water. **C,** Wrap all the way around the proximal phalanx twice; then spiral distally, wrapping twice for each layer and overlapping the previous layer. **D,** To allow the DIP joint to move freely, end just short of the DIP flexion crease. **E,** Use a continuous rotary motion to closely form the material to the finger and obtain optimal fit. **F,** To avoid point pressure, do not poke at the cast with your fingertips; instead use the length of your fingers for maximal pressure distribution. **G,** Use the Splint/Cast Trimmers to contour and smooth the edges. **H,** If there are any indentations, the cast must be removed and remade.*

cast can be removed. The therapist or patient can soak the cast to soften it partially and then use Splint/Cast Trimmers to cut it off.

Patients who cannot pull off a QuickCast cast can cut it off with Splint/Cast Trimmers. A pair of trimmers can be sent home with the patient. Cutting off a QuickCast cast does not require soaking, but a POP cast does.

The therapist may choose one of two approaches to cut the cast for removal. Bell-Krotoski (1987) described a window technique by which the dorsal aspect of the cast is cut out along the proximal phalanx. With this section of the cast removed, the patient can usually slip the cast off (Fig. 12–17**A**). The other option is to create a univalve in the cast with a longitudinal cut along either the radial/palmar or the ulnar/palmar border (Fig. 12–17**B**). The location for these cuts has two advantages. The palmar skin has more subcutaneous padding that the dorsal skin, and the volar approach avoids the PIP condyles. Cutting over a bony prominence usually creates discomfort for the patient. Either the window or the univalve approach can be used to make the cast removable for intermittent wear. However, in this author's experience, the removable cast is not as ef-

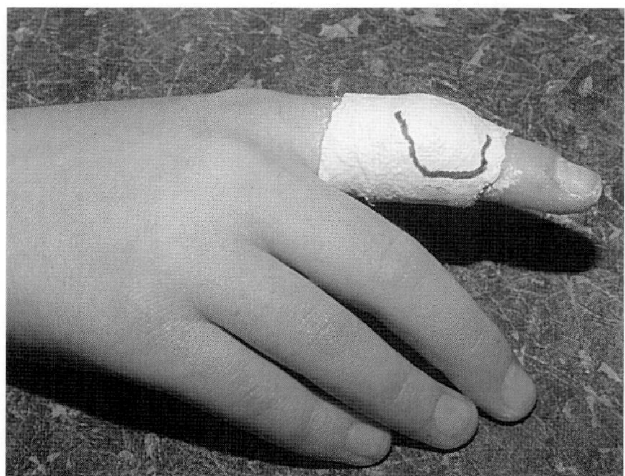

Figure 12–15 Mark the cast to ease removal.

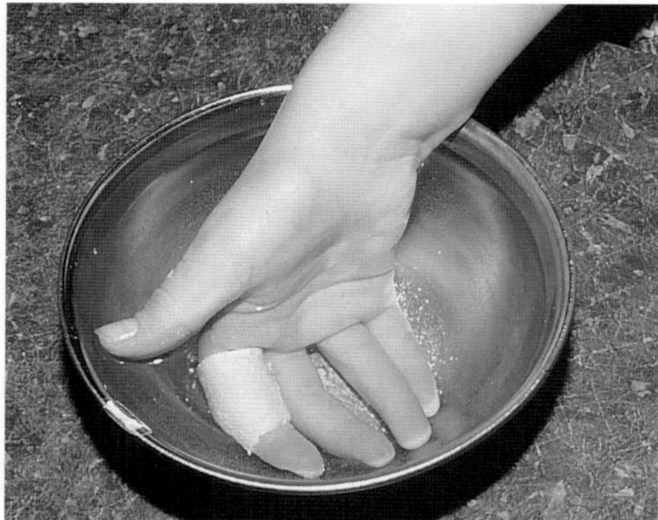

Figure 12–16 Remove a cast by soaking it in warm water.

fective as the nonremovable cast approach. As noted earlier, do not use a hairdryer to heat QuickCast when it is on the patient's finger.

Securing the Cast in Place

Occasionally, the patient will have trouble keeping the cast on. This occurs rarely, but is most frequently seen with very small fingers that are approaching full extension and fingers that were edematous when the cast was applied and have since lost volume. When presented with this problem, the cast maker must be certain that the cast was applied properly. For example, that the QuickCast was fully heated, fully stretched after being heated and shrunk, and applied firmly to the finger. This author has found three techniques helpful for maintaining cast position on the finger when the proper casting technique does not result in a secure cast:

1. **Nonadhesive wrap.** The patient can wrap the cast and adjacent skin with self-adherent nonadhesive wrap, such as Coban. The wrap can be applied around the cast and then through the palm (Fig. 12–18**A,B**).
2. **Additional material.** The therapist can cut an additional piece of material, laminate it to the proximal end of the cast, and continue wrapping through the first web space and around the palm (Fig. 12–18**C**).
3. **Tincture of Benzoin.** Also known as Tough Skin, this product is a alcohol-based liquid that creates a tacky surface on the skin. A tiny amount of this can be dabbed on the skin before applying the cast. The tincture can be removed with rubbing alcohol when desired.

Protecting Adjacent Fingers

Sometimes, the finger adjacent to the casted finger becomes irritated from rubbing against the cast. To prevent this or to relieve it once it occurs, the patient may cover the adjacent finger with Moleskin, a bandage (Band-Aid), or light Coban wrap.

Home Program

With the encouragement of Brand, this author began teaching patients and their caregivers or family to apply casts at home (Johnson and Johnson Orthopaedic Division, 1985). While most patients prefer the therapist to perform the casting, the complicating factors of geogra-

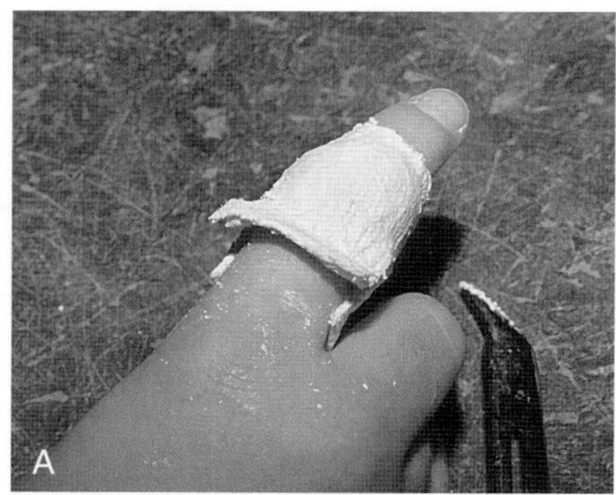

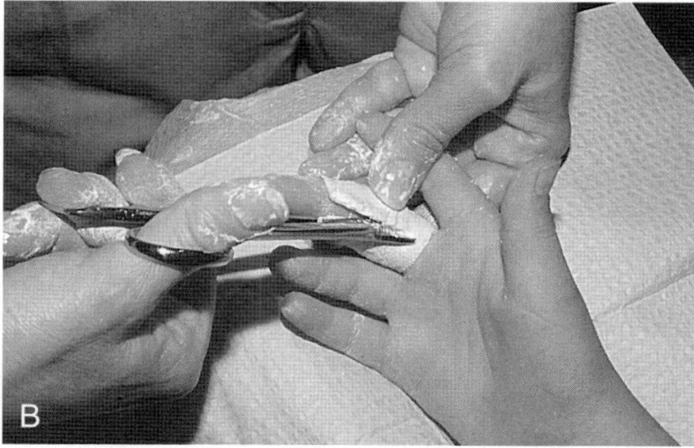

*Figure 12–17 Window (**A**) and univalve (**B**) cutting techniques for cast removal.*

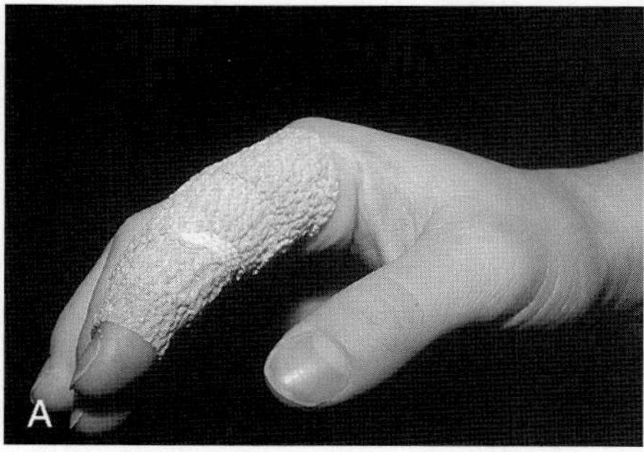

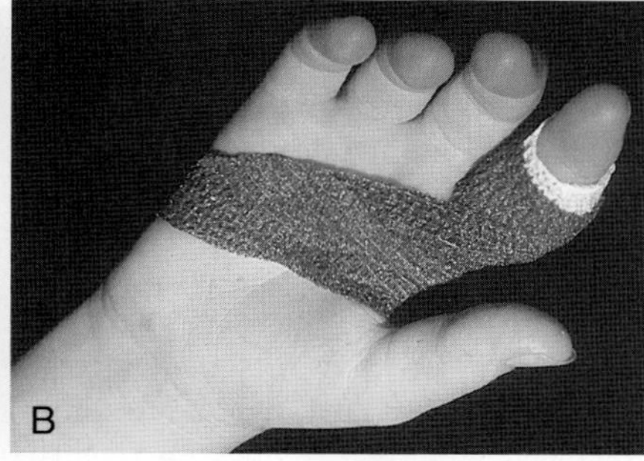

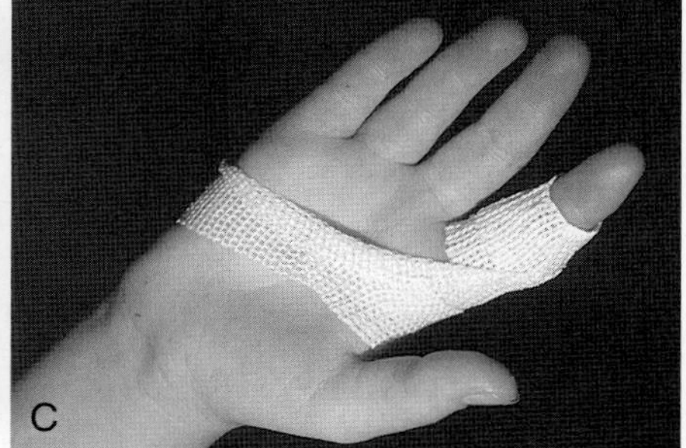

*Figure 12–18 Techniques for securing a finger cast include Coban (or similar material) wrapped around the cast and adjacent skin (**A**), Coban (or similar material) wrapped around the cast and through the palm (**B**), and additional material attached to the cast and wrapped through the web space and palm (**C**).*

phy (the patient lives too far away to come regularly) or finances (the patient cannot afford to have the therapist provide the care) sometimes make a home program desirable. The therapist must thoroughly instruct the patient and caregivers and must document this comprehensive instruction. The patient should be provided with written instructions, complete with precautions, as well as materials for casting. It is the responsibility of the therapist to screen patients for their ability to follow a home casting program. Patients and their caregivers must demonstrate excellent verbal comprehension, a high level of motivation, appreciation of precautions, and adequate skill in the clinic to be cleared for a home casting program.

Precautions for Finger Casting

Material Tolerance

If the patient does not tolerate the QuickCast directly against the skin (in this author's experience this problem is extremely rare) or if additional padding is desired, one or more layers of tubular finger bandage may be applied to the finger before making the cast. In the case of wounds or the use of padding, the patient must avoid getting the finger wet. Techniques for keeping the finger dry in a cast range from putting a plastic bag around the whole hand to cutting a finger from a surgical glove and placing it over the cast (Fig. 12–19).

Therapists' reports of POP intolerance are virtually nonexistent. In 22 years of clinical practice using POP, this author has seen one possible case of POP sensitivity. Bell-Krotoski (personal communication, 1999) notes that she has never seen a case of POP intolerance, despite many years of use. Tribuzi (1990) reported that contact sensitivity to POP is rare but noted two studies that describe this problem (Lovell & Staniforth, 1981; Staniforth, 1980).

Casting over Wounds

Each clinician must use personal judgment when the finger still has open wounds. POP casts can be applied over open wounds and over dressings. QuickCast can be applied over open wounds that are dressed (Brand & Yancey, 1997). The thinner the dressing the better. A layer or two of a petroleum gauze such as Xeroform may be all that is needed. The person applying the cast must take care to keep the dressing in place during cast application.

Indications for Cast Removal

The therapist must thoroughly instruct the patient in symptoms that signal an ill-fitting cast. A poorly made cast can compromise nerve, vascular structures, and/or skin. Vascular compromise, if not dealt with, can cause skin breakdown. Sharp cast edges—proximally or distally—can also compromise skin integrity. Point pressure directly against a digital nerve can cause a neuropraxia. The symptoms that signal vascular compromise are tingling, numbness, unusual pain, color change, unusual

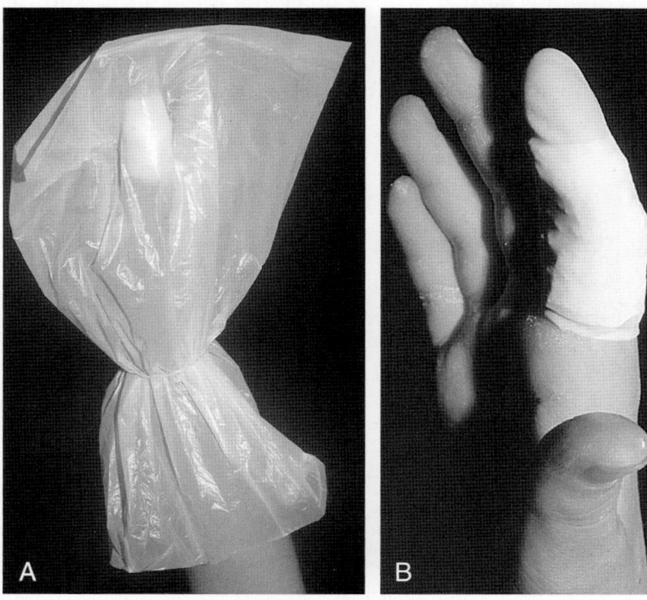

*Figure 12–19 To keep a finger cast dry, use a plastic bag (**A**) or surgical glove (**B**).*

coolness, and persistent throbbing. The symptoms that signal pressure on a nerve are tingling, numbness, and unusual pain. The symptoms that signal skin compromise from sharp edges are unusual pain and red skin just proximal or distal to the cast.

SENSORY COMPROMISE

Casting the patient with sensory compromise places an even greater responsibility on the therapist to make a well-fitting cast. The patient with numbness will not have the primary signal (pain) to warn that the cast is causing problems. However, it is helpful to know that Brand's initial casting population suffered extreme sensory compromise from Hansen's disease but did extremely well with POP casting. It is precisely the pressure-distributing nature of the circumferential cast that makes it appropriate for this at-risk population. Placing a 3-Point pressure splint on a numb part is often not an option that can be considered. Still, the therapist must strongly emphasize the potential risks to the patient and teach him or her to inspect the skin regularly to check for problems that the nervous system may miss.

VASCULARITY

When the cast is completed, the therapist must inspect the color of the fingertip. It may appear slightly darker red than the adjacent fingers or can change color so much as to appear purplish, which indicates difficulty with venous outflow. The finger may also become white or dusky, indicating difficulty with arterial inflow. The patient must remain in the clinic until the color of the finger normalizes. This usually happens within 5 to 10 minutes. However, this author had patients take more than 20 minutes before their vascular tone normalizes for vascular outflow difficulty. Usually, the discoloration occurs in a patient who is receiving a first cast, and the problem does not recur. The person applying the cast must use judgment to determine whether the color of the finger means that the cast should be left on or removed and redone. A sustained color change can signal that focused pressure against major arteries or veins exists and must be relieved.

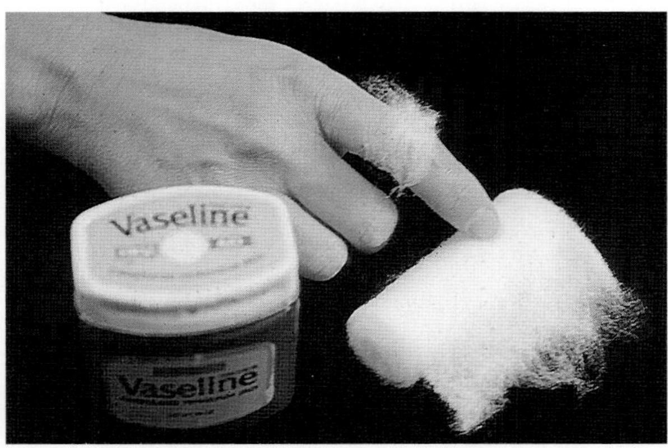

Figure 12–20 A minimalist approach to padding relieves pressure over the PIP in the cast. Petroleum jelly helps stabilize the wisp of padding.

PIP DORSAL SKIN TOLERANCE

If the patient presents initially with erythema of the dorsal aspect of the PIP joint or develops this over a period of time in the cast, casting does not have be discarded or discontinued. Bell-Krotoski (1987) described a technique using clouds, or wisps, of cast padding to protect vulnerable tissue (Fig. 12–20). To make the cloud, pull a small fluff of cast padding from the roll. Apply petroleum jelly over the area where the padding will go, to keep the cloud in place during cast fabrication. With the padding over the dorsum of the PIP, the normal casting procedure can begin. The therapist must be sure that the padding stays in place during cast fabrication. Bulkier approaches to padding the cast usually do not have a satisfactory result (Bell-Krotoski, 1987).

Skin Lubrication

The literature often mentions the application of petroleum jelly to the skin before POP cast application. As mentioned, petroleum jelly helps lubricate the skin under the moisture-robbing plaster. It also helps secure small amounts of padding. On one occasion, this author saw a finger—treated by another therapist—that had been dipped in paraffin before being casted in POP. The result was the loss of the superficial layers of the skin, extreme erythema, and pain. The nature of this reaction to paraffin is not known. The patient stated she had tolerated the paraffin application in the clinic, so it did not seem that she was generally allergic to the substance. Although I had never considered using paraffin under a cast, many therapists have reported doing so on a regular basis. However, because of the problems seen, this author believes that paraffin under a cast is risky.

Casting Regimen

Frequency of cast changes vary with the characteristics of the patient. Diagnosis, severity and duration of contracture, and wound and sensory status all help determine the number of times a week or month a patient will be seen for a cast change. In this author's experience, the issues of geography, financial status, patient schedule, and motivation usually have more impact on the regimen than the medical factors.

Some patients seem to benefit from less frequent cast changes, whereas others have the best results with frequent cast changes. Theoretically, the more frequent cast changes will have better results because a new end range is captured with each cast change, enhancing the mechanical signal to the tissue to remodel.[1]

1. This section has been adapted and reprinted with permission from Schultz Johnson, K. S. (1999). *PIP serial casting with QuickCast*, UE TECH, Edwards, CO.

Clinical Example: Forearm Splint as a Base for a Mobilization Splint (Using QuickCast)

Materials and Preparation

The following materials are needed for a QuickCast forearm splint (Fig. 12–21):

- QuickCast forearm kit
- QuickCast tape
- Hairdryer
- Splint/Cast Trimmers
- Bandage scissors
- Spray bottle of water (optional)
- A 3" cotton, polypropylene, or synthetic stockinette

The QuickCast kit contains a splint tube, a terry liner, two one-piece straps and one two-piece strap. The hairdryer requirements were discussed earlier in this chapter. The stockinette is required to make the terry cloth liner removable for cleaning.

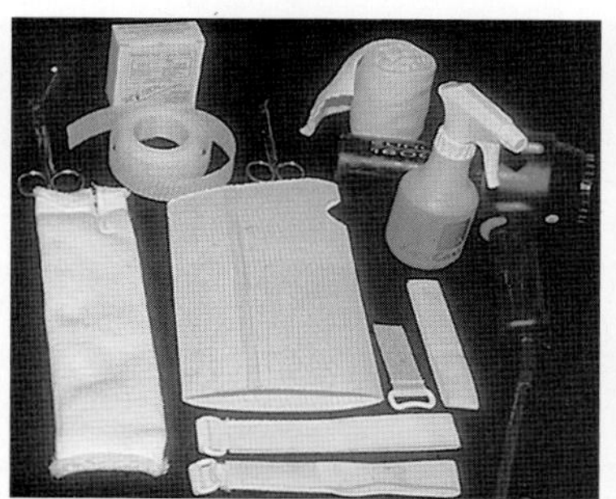

Figure 12–21 Materials and equipment needed to fabricate a QuickCast forearm splint.

Methods

Position and Technique

Before making the QuickCast forearm splint, decide on patient and wrist positions. Practice with the patient. Be sure the patient understands the materials, technique, and rationale for splint application. Position the patient as follows:

1. Remove any watches or bracelets from the arm to be splinted.
2. Make sure the forearm area is clean and dry.
3. Seat the patient, and place the elbow of the affected extremity on a firm but padded surface. Ideally, the forearm is held in neutral rotation during fabrication.
4. Have the patient place the wrist in a position of maximum tolerable extension to ensure that the splint will not migrate (wrist creates a mechanical block). Then have the patient abduct the fingers while the palm portion of the splint is fabricated to prevent metacarpal adduction when the heated material shrinks. If the patient is unable to participate, an assistant may help.

To determine proper size of the splint, measure the smallest circumference of wrist and follow the manufacturer's guidelines for sizing. Bunch up the terry cloth liner and slide it onto patient's arm. Ensure that the liner fits properly in the web space of the thumb and that no wrinkles are present before the application of the splint tube (Fig. 12–22**A**).

Apply the QuickCast tube over the arm and thumb. Check the length of the splint on the forearm. If it is more than two thirds the length of the forearm, remove the splint and trim it to the proper length (Fig. 22–22**B,C**). Preheat the edges of the thumbhole at the web space before reapplying the tube to the arm (Fig. 12–22**D**). Set the hairdryer on high airflow and high heat to heat the edges of the thumbhole. As noted earlier, do not use a heat gun on QuickCast.

Begin heating the splint in the palm area of the hand. Hold the hairdryer as close to the splint as possible (Fig. 12–22**E**). Be sure the nozzle of the hairdryer is not pointed at the patient's face. Keep the hairdryer slowly moving while heating. Maintain a steady and continuous motion. Avoid wiggling the hairdryer back and forth. Continue heating in a circumferential fashion and move from the palm to the proximal end of the splint. Note: The therapist must avoid point pressure at all times.

As the QuickCast softens and shrinks around the palm, it will tend to compress the metacarpals together. Finger abduction assists in maintaining adequate splint width across the palm (Fig. 22–22**F**). If the patient is unable to abduct the fingers, the therapist or assistant may need to spread the fingers and metacarpals passively. While the splint is still warm, mold the wrist and hand in the desired position, and allow the material to cool (Fig. 12–22**G**). QuickCast requires minimal molding, because it simply shrinks around the extremity and exactly mimics its shape. Positioning the wrist in maximum tolerable extension minimizes migration because of the mechanical block this wrist position creates.

To accelerate cooling, apply a vapocoolant spray, if the patient has no known respiratory conditions. Other options for facilitating material cooling and setup include applying cool air with the hairdryer set on cool and misting the splint with cool water.

With the splint fully heated, trim the liner at the proximal end to the desired length. Fold the liner back onto splint (Fig. 12–22**H,I**). The liner will adhere to the warm splint. If the splint has cooled, it may be necessary to reheat the edges of the splint before folding back the liner. Repeat this procedure for the distal end of splint. Cut the liner covering the thumb, if desired. Roll back and adhere the liner around the thumb portion of the splint.

The ideal time to create a univalve splint is when it has mostly set, but is still slightly warm. If the cut is made while the splint is still soft, the material will spring back and deform. The position for the cut can be any-

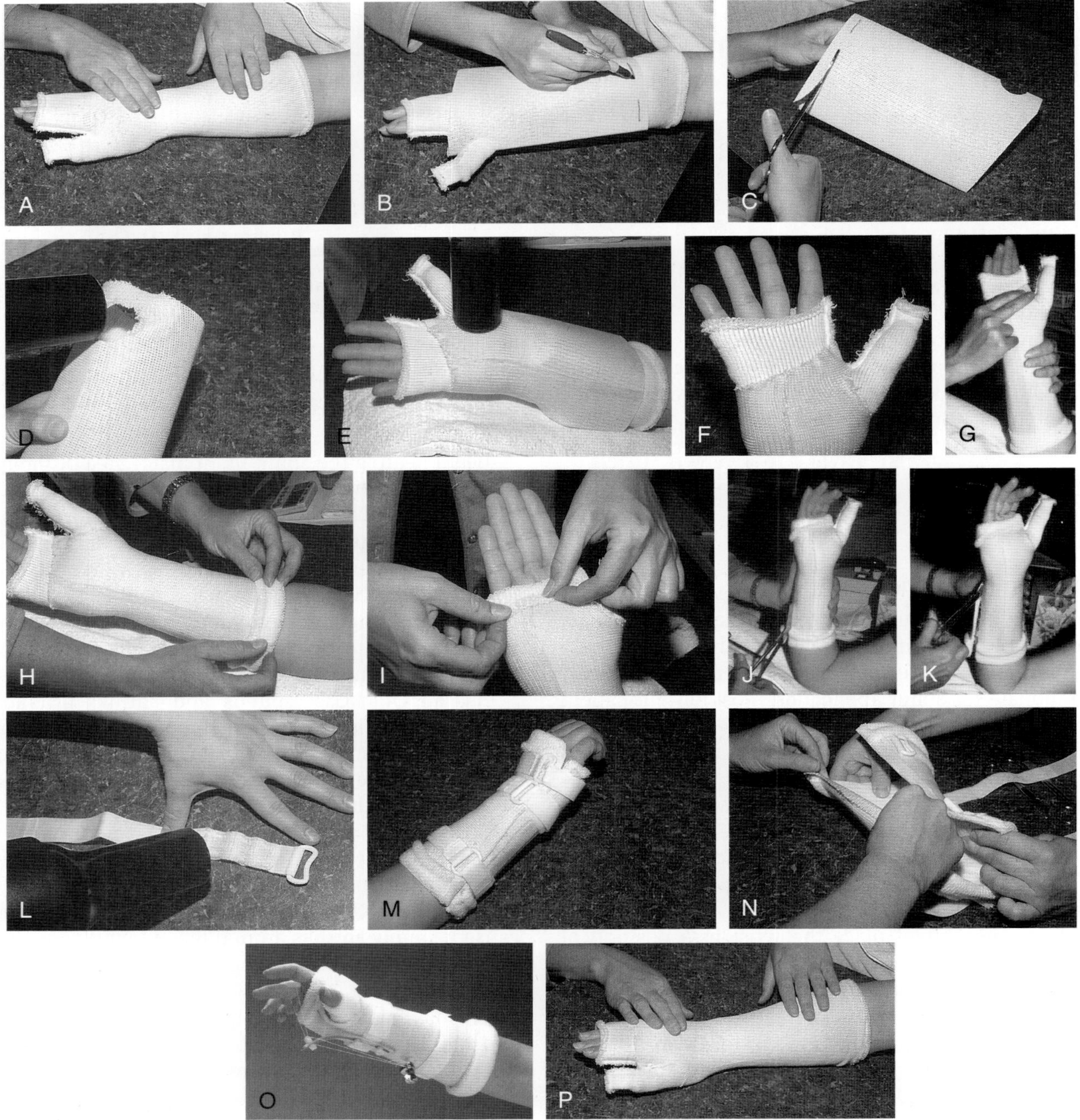

Figure 12–22 *Steps for applying a QuickCast forearm splint.* ***A,*** *Smooth out the wrinkles in the QuickCast liner to avoid adversely affecting the final fit.* ***B,*** *Mark the desired length of the cast.* ***C,*** *Trim the cast.* ***D,*** *Preheat the edges of the thumbhole at the web space.* ***E,*** *Holding the hair dryer as close to the cast as possible, heat the tube from distal to proximal.* ***F,*** *Abduct the fingers during cast fabrication to help maintain adequate cast width across the palm and avoid metacarpal compression.* ***G,*** *While the splint is still warm, mold the wrist and hand in the desired position and allow the material to cool.* ***H and I,*** *Fold the liner back onto the splint. The material must be heated to allow the liner to adhere correctly.* ***J and K,*** *Univalve the splint with bandage scissors and/or Splint/Cast Trimmers. First, cut proximal to distal until resistance is felt. Then cut from the distal end to the end of the first cut.* ***L,*** *To apply straps, heat the QuickCast material on the back of the straps and laminate it to the cast by rubbing with the fingers. Do not pull on the straps until the QuickCast material on the strap has completely cooled and set.* ***M,*** *The finished QuickCast forearm splint with straps.* ***N,*** *QuickCast finishing tape used to finish the edge.* ***O,*** *Splint components can be attached to a QuickCast splint in the same manner as they are attached to conventional low-temperature thermoplastic splints.* ***P,*** *Stockinette placed over the terry liner allows the liner to be interchangeable.*

where on the splint except on the seam where the material is laminated together. The therapist makes the choice for cut location with consideration for strap application, ease of splint application and removal, and position of hardware (force generators, hinges, outriggers). Common choices for cut location are either the dorsal or the ulnar aspect of the splint. Avoid making the cut directly over the distal ulna. Cutting in this location is difficult for the therapist and uncomfortable for the patient. Create a univalve splint with bandage scissors and/or Splint/Cast Trimmers (Fig. 12–22**J**,**K**).

Next, apply the straps. Heat the QuickCast material on the back of the one-piece D-ring strap (Fig. 12–22**L**). The material will begin to curl when sufficiently heated. Briefly warm the area of the splint to which strap will be applied. Place the strap on the proximal end of the splint with the D-ring just to one side of the cut, and laminate it to the splint by rubbing with your fingers. Using the same technique, affix the second one-piece strap at the wrist; this strap secures splint. Heat the D-ring portion of the two-piece strap. Using the same technique, attach the D-ring just to one side of the cut. Using the same heating technique, heat the other portion of the two piece strap. Place it on the splint so the loop portion of the strap is directly opposite the D-ring (Fig. 22–22**M**). The splint may now be removed from patient.

To finish edges, especially where the QuickCast was univalved and around the thumb hole, the clinician may wish to apply QuickCast tape (Fig. 12–22**N**). After measuring the length needed, heat the tape, stretch it out to maximum length, and lay it over the edges of the cast—half on the inside and half on the outside. Using firm pressure, burnish the finishing strap onto the cast.

The cast/splint is now ready for attachment of outriggers and force generators, such as static progressive components or springs. Splint components can be attached in the same manner that they are attached to conventional low-temperature thermoplastic splints (with thermoplastic, rivets, or screws). Any warm low-temperature thermoplastic will adhere to the QuickCast. Strips of QuickCast tape or QuickCast sheeting will also effectively secure components to the cast (Fig. 12–22**O**).

Using an Interchangeable Liner

The QuickCast kit was designed so that the terry liner adheres to the QuickCast shell. Some therapists prefer to make the terry liner removable and to have an additional liner so the patient can wash and change liners. To accomplish this, an additional terry liner and a thin stockinette (cotton, synthetic, or polypropylene) are required. The terry liner becomes removable because the QuickCast adheres to the thin stockinette.

To use the interchangeable liner technique, follow the instructions outlined earlier, except after placing the terry liner on the patient's arm, place the thin stockinette over the terry liner (Fig. 12–22**P**). Next, place the QuickCast tube over the thin stockinette. Be sure the stockinette covers all of the area under the QuickCast. Shrink the QuickCast; trim the stockinette, leaving at least 1 in. beyond the edge of the splint. Fold the thin stockinette over onto the outside of the QuickCast. If the QuickCast is warm, the stockinette will stick to it. Create a univalve splint, as described, being careful to cut only the thin stockinette, leaving the terry liner intact. This is easier to achieve when the terry liner is pulled taut from both the proximal and the distal ends.

Check and Revision

The therapist can easily adjust the QuickCast splint and reposition each joint incorporated in the splint over the course of treatment with the following technique. Be sure the splint is on the patient, because if it is heated off the patient it may shrink and will no longer fit. Stretching the splint out once it has shrunk is difficult.

Heat the area of the splint to be repositioned until soft. When heating the splint, soften it at least 2 in. proximal and 2 in. distal to the area to be repositioned. In addition, be careful when heating the cut edges of the splint. Overheating may cause the edges to deform. While the splint is soft, reposition the limb. Smooth out any wrinkles. Allow the splint to cool.

The terry liner provides excellent padding and is all that is required to protect the distal ulna. Be sure to check the radial aspect of the thumb carpometacarpal (CMC) for a pressure area. Ask the patient if the palmar aspect of the splint is comfortable.

Casting Precautions

The same precautions for splinting over wounds as discussed for finger casting apply to forearm casting. QuickCast splints should not be placed directly over wounds, but can be placed over a dressing. The patient must be instructed to beware of excessive moisture buildup under the splint.

Material tolerance was discussed earlier in this chapter. Unlike finger casts, forearm QuickCast splints include a thick terry liner, making it one of the best tolerated and comfortable splints available. The terry liner minimizes skin contact and risk of irritation, protects the skin from hairdryer heat, provides mechanical padding, and wicks moisture away from skin surface. Do not use QuickCast splints on any patient who has previously shown sensitivity to the material.

Heating QuickCast

Use a hairdryer to apply QuickCast splints. A heat gun is hazardous and may cause patient injury. QuickCast cast and splints kits are applied with heat while on the patient. Conventional hairdryers, if used too close to the skin or without sufficient motion, can generate enough heat to cause discomfort, pain, or even skin burns. Avoid applying excessive heat application to any area near bare skin. Cover any exposed skin with towels or padding. When working at the edges of the splint and around the thumb, place fingers on the exposed skin of the patient. This way, the therapist will know when the temperature becomes uncomfortable and will avoid causing the patient discomfort.

As with any low-temperature thermoplastic, excessive heat exposure (e.g., hot oven, fireplace, car dashboard, or furnace) may soften QuickCast splints to the point of compromising the splint structure. The patient should be instructed to avoid extended exposure to temperatures over 115°F (46°C). Should the splint deform as a result of accidental exposure to heat, the patient should be instructed to get away from the heat source and contact the responsible clinician as soon as possible.

Patients should be instructed to keep QuickCast splints clean and dry. Care must be taken to prevent excessive moisture buildup in the padding between the QuickCast and skin. As with any immobilization device, excessive moisture may cause dermal irritation or maceration. To wash the splint, submerge it in warm soapy water and allow to air dry.

Indications for Splint Removal

As noted earlier, the therapist must thoroughly instruct the patient in the symptoms that signal an ill-fitting cast. The signs of vascular compromise, pressure over a nerve, and skin compromise are same as those outlined for finger casts.

Splint Regimen

The frequency and duration of splint wear are similar to that which the therapist normally uses for a mobilizing splint. The excellent pressure distribution and stability of the splint or cast owing to its circumferential design may allow the patient to wear the splint longer. As with any removable splint, the patient should initially wear the splint for a trial period of 20 to 30 minutes to determine skin tolerance. Once tolerance is determined, the patient can gradually increase time in the splint. The clinician adjusts the tension and angle of pull in the same way as for splints with noncircumferential thermoplastic bases.

Clinical Example: Serial Static POP Stretcher for Modifying Scar Tissue

Materials and Preparation

The materials needed to make a POP stretcher are as follows (Fig. 22–23):

- Approximately 10 plies of POP cut from rolls or strips
- Stockinette
- Additional POP strips for finishing
- Hot water
- Clean bowl

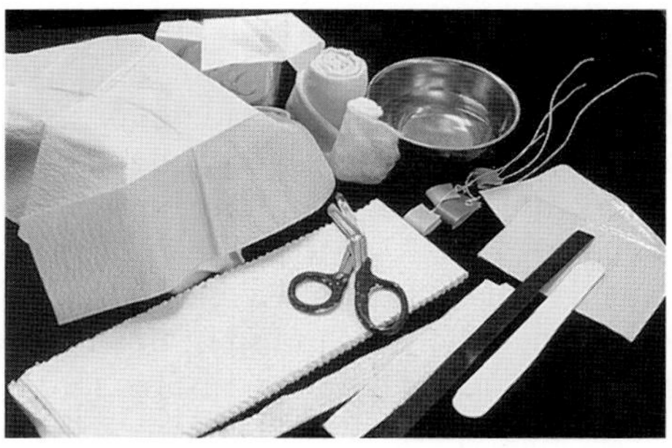

Figure 12–23 Materials and equipment needed to fabricate a POP stretcher.

- Plaster scissors
- Tissues
- Drapes to protect work surfaces and patient's clothes
- Finger loops of vinyl with line attached or flexible surgical drain tubing
- Cast padding (optional)
- Draped arm wedge (optional)
- Banding metal, thermoplastic strips, or additional POP strips for reinforcement (optional)

The number of initial POP strips depends on the size of the arm to be splinted. The hotter the water, the faster the plaster will set; but be careful not to burn the patient. Finger loops are especially necessary if flexor tightness differs significantly among the digits. The optional arm wedge may be foam or solid.

Prepare the clinic for POP application. Gather the required materials and equipment. To protect surfaces from plaster drippings, cover them with disposable, waterproof covers. Both the therapist and patient will want to protect their clothing with drapes or aprons and should remove watches and rings.

Determine the amount of POP required for the stretcher (Fig. 12–24**A,B**) by measuring the greatest width of the extremity, generally the palm or proximal forearm. Be sure to include the drape of the material halfway down the forearm or palm in the measurement. Measure length from longest fingertip to two thirds of the way up the forearm to determine POP strip length. Round the corners of the plaster. Lay the plaster down on the hand to determine the location of the thenar eminence (Fig. 22–24**C**). Cut a slit in the plaster at the midway point of the thenar eminence. This will be turned back to leave the thumb free, and the overlap will reinforce this thinner part of the splint (Fig. 12–24**D**). Finally, fill a large clean bowl with hot water.

Method

Tissue Preconditioning

As for finger casting, this author has found that gains in PROM of the forearm are more rapid and of a greater magnitude if the tissue is preconditioned or stretched out just before splinting. Methods of preconditioning were discussed earlier in this chapter. Note that patients with sensory compromise may not be candidates for tissue preconditioning.

Position and Technique

Before making the POP splint, decide on patient and joint positions. Practice with the patient. Be sure the patient understands the materials, technique, and rationale for cast application. Position the patient and prepare the tissue as follows:

1. Clean and dry the area of the arm to be covered.
2. Seat the patient and place the affected extremity on a firm but padded surface (a foam wedge is excellent) with the forearm supinated and position the joints as desired.

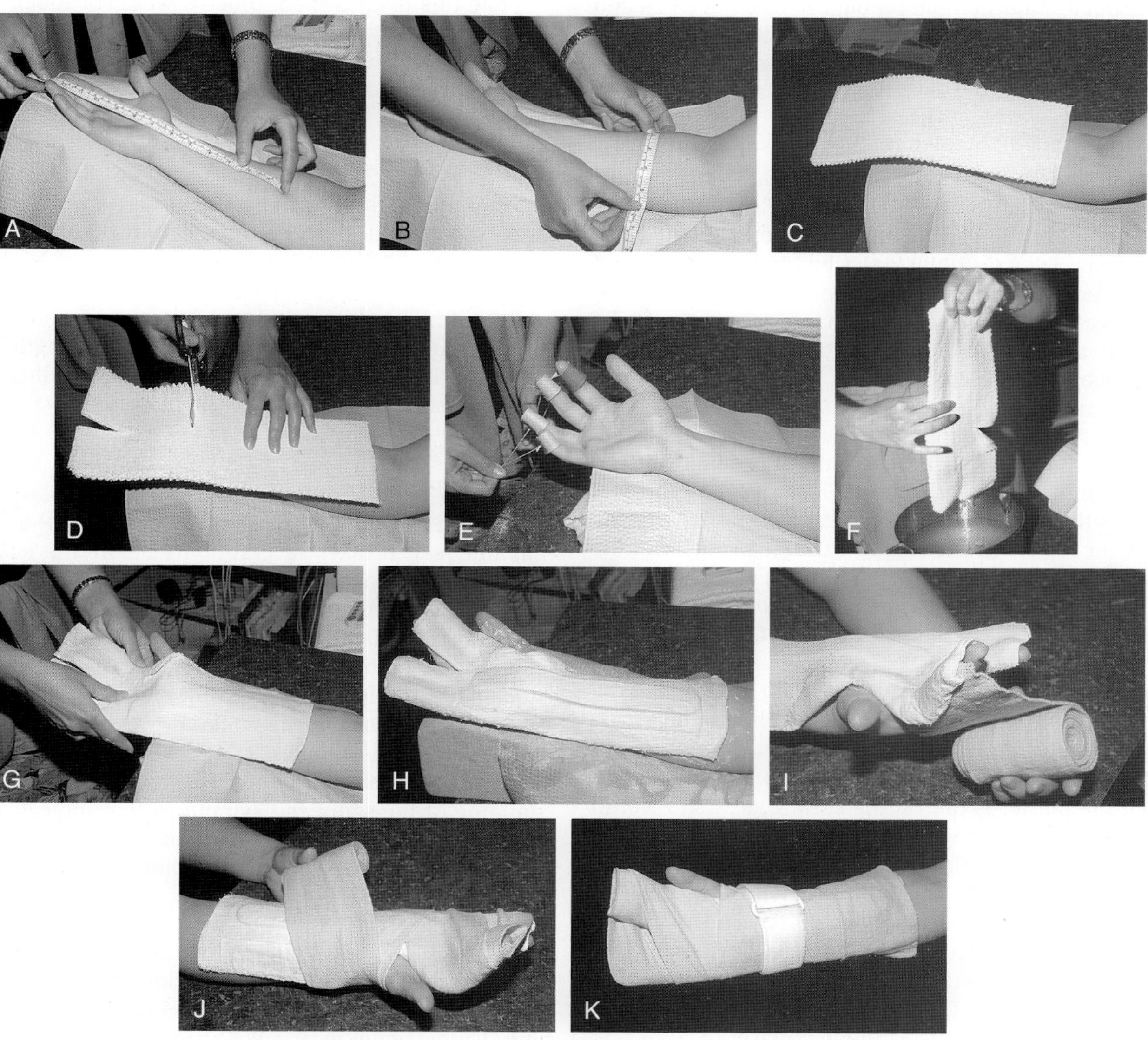

Figure 12–24 *Steps of applying a forearm POP stretcher.* ***A and B,*** *Determine the appropriate plaster dimensions by measuring the length and greatest width of the extremity.* ***C,*** *Check that the plaster is of the proper dimensions.* ***D,*** *Cut a slit in the plaster at the midway point of the thenar eminence. If the range of motion of the fingers differs significantly, cut the plaster longitudinally between the fingers to position the fingers at different angles.* ***E,*** *This traction maneuver maximizes the stretch on the affected tissue. The fingers may be stretched individually as well.* ***F,*** *Immerse the plaster in water for 5 to 10 sec, and remove any excess water.* ***G,*** *Gently mold the POP to the arm, avoiding point pressure.* ***H,*** *If reinforcement is desired, contour the plastic or metal to the stretcher and cover it with two or three layers of POP to secure it in place.* ***I and J,*** *Tuck the end of the wrap in between the index finger and POP stretcher and wrap proximally. The tips of the digits are left uncovered so a patient with diminished sensation can check color and temperature.* ***K,*** *D-ring hook-and-loop straps help secure the stretcher in position and distribute the pressure.*

3. Start with the wrist in neutral and place the MP and IP joints in maximum available extension; once the fingers demonstrate full passive extension, begin progressing the wrist into extension while maintaining digit extension until full composite extension is achieved.
4. To position the fingers, especially if the flexor tightness varies significantly between digits, place vinyl finger slings or loops with line attached or place flexible surgical drain tubing over the fingertips and have the patient or an assistant place the fingers under traction into maximum tolerable extension (Fig. 12–24**E**). **Caution:** Avoid point pressure at all times.

Applying the POP Stretcher

As the process begins, keep in mind that even with extra-fast-setting plaster, the therapist will have adequate time to contour the POP to the arm. The POP will set in 3 to 5 min. Tribuzi (1990) described the application of padding or stockinette before applying the POP. However, this author has never used an interface between the POP and the skin in the fabricating process, and has never encountered a complication.

Using care to fully saturate all of the POP, all the strips are immersed as a group into the water. Remove the POP as a unit and gently squeezes along the length of the strips to remove excess water (Fig. 12–24**F**). The wet plaster is then placed on the patient's arm and over the fingers (or fingers in the slings, if used). Using all of the POP layers as a single unit, mold the POP to the arm, carefully contouring the forearm, palm, fingers, and spaces between the fingers (Fig. 12–24**G**). No pressure need be applied to the POP. The person positioning the fingers controls the finger and wrist joint angles, and the person forming the stretcher simply follows the shape and position of the hand and arm.

When the POP is set, remove it from the arm. Although the plaster is dry on the surface, it is still wet in the deeper layers and will still be soft enough to smooth edges by hand or with a plaster scissors. At this point, the therapist may add any reinforcement desired to increase the rigidity of the splint. Thermoplastic and banding metal are both effective reinforcement materials. The reinforcement bar should extend over most of the length of the stretcher (Fig. 12–24**H**). Additional strips of POP secure the reinforcements to the POP base.

Securing the POP Stretcher

Once the final POP stretcher revisions are made, the patient puts it on and wraps it into place with an elasticized bandage (Ace wrap). The therapist must carefully instruct the patient in proper wrapping technique to avoid vascular compromise. To start the wrap, the patient tucks the end of the wrap in between the index finger and POP stretcher and then starts wrapping proximally in a Figure-8 or spiral fashion (Fig. 12–24**I,J**). D-ring hook-and-loop straps may be added to reinforce the wrist or finger position (Fig. 12–24**K**).

If the arm underwent preconditioning before stretcher fabrication, the therapist must instruct the patient in cast application when the lengthened tissue returns to its shorter length. When first applied, the arm will not fit perfectly into the stretcher. The wrap will have to be readjusted over time as the patient wears the stretcher and tissue once again lengthens. Some patients do not tolerate this readjustment process well. For them, avoid tissue preconditioning. Patients with sensory compromise are not candidates for the readjustment period because pressure distribution is poor and the risk of skin injury high.

Check and Revision

Check the stretcher for sharp edges, cracks, and pressure areas. Sharp edges can be rounded with the application of hot water. A pair of sharp plaster scissors is also effective. Should cracks appear in the plaster, apply warm water to the cracked area and add two or more strips of plaster. These strips do not need to be the length of the whole splint, but must be long enough to adhere well and give adequate reinforcement.

Casting Precautions for the POP Stretcher

Material Properties

Care must be taken to avoid stressing the POP before it has fully set. It takes several hours before the POP will have its full strength. After the initial exothermic heat reaction, the plaster will be quite cold for the next few hours until it fully dries. Some patients may find this uncomfortable. However, providing the patient with a stockinette (preferably polypropylene) may resolve this problem. Tolerance to the material was discussed in detail earlier in this chapter.

As always, the patient must have a thorough understanding of the signs and symptoms that indicate splint removal. Vascular, dermal, and neurologic symptoms were discussed earlier in this chapter.

Skin Lubrication

POP wicks moisture from the skin and can be very drying. Having the patient wear a stockinette as an interface between the arm and the POP can improve skin lubrication. Patients who wear a POP stretcher may need to apply a skin lubricant more frequently.

Pressure Areas

The patient must be instructed to check for the deep red marks in the skin that indicate pressure areas and to report these to the therapist. Teach the patient to attempt to resolve pressure areas with repositioning the stretcher, adjusting the wraps and straps, or inserting small temporary bits of tissue or cotton. Pressure problems that do not respond to these interventions indicate that the stretcher cannot be worn until the therapist can make the appropriate revisions.

Casting over Wounds

Casting over wounds was discussed in detail earlier in this chapter. Plastic wrap placed over a dressing protects the dressing during stretcher formation and will keep it free from POP and moisture. Clinical experience suggests that POP aids wound healing. Bell-Krotoski (personal communication, 1999) believes that the POP wicks away exudate when it is applied either directly to the wound or over a light dressing. She further comments that, although some clinicians may fear that the wound will stick to the plaster, the adherence aids in wound healing, since it prevents sheer stress (the greatest enemy to wound healing).

Thermal Effects of POP

When POP and water mix, an exothermic chemical reaction takes place. The literature does report cases of thermal burns with the application of POP bandages (Becker, 1978; Grazer, 1979; Haasch, 1964; Kaplan, 1981; Schultze, 1967). When working with plaster, therapists should keep this thermal effect in mind. Tribuzi (1990) noted that casts reach maximum temperature in 5 to 15 minutes after application. She listed several variables that may increase the temperature of the exothermic reaction, including high room temperature, high humidity, cast thickness of more than eight plies, undersaturation or oversaturation with water, use of fast-setting plaster, dipping temperature, and inadequate ventilation during the drying period. Inadequate ventilation can occur from overwrapping the freshly applied plaster with cotton or elastic bandages, covering the plaster with blankets, or placing the cast or splint near a pillow or mattress (Johnson and Johnson Orthopaedic Division, 1985; Kaplan, 1981; Lavalette, Pope, & Dickerson, 1982).

Bell-Krotoski (personal communication, 1999) postulates that these injuries may actually be caused by pressure from an improperly applied POP rather than from heat. In 22 years of practice, despite use of extra-fast-setting plaster, the hottest dipping temperature tolerable, and applying finger casts and POP stretchers directly against the skin, the author has never seen a burn complication from POP.

When working with plaster, the clinician must always use clean water, because the plaster residue left in the dipping container from previous casts is thought to act as an accelerator and increase the exothermic reaction. In addition, shards of set plaster can accidentally be incorporated into the splint and cause irritation and discomfort.

Although Tribuzi (1990) noted that POP should never be applied directly to the skin, Bell-Krotoski (personal communication, 1999), on the other hand, states that she is unaware of any contraindication to this practice (Brand & Yancey, 1997). Certainly, any time a clinician applies a circumferential plaster cast to an extremity, cast padding must be placed first. A cast saw cannot be used if there is no padding under the cast. The risk of burn may be increased with a circumferentially applied cast then with a half-shell stretcher.

Stretcher Regimen

Deciding when to fabricate a new stretcher is easier than deciding how frequently to change a serial cast, because the extremity demonstrates what it needs. When a patient is consistently able to lift out of the stretcher by 5° at the target joint(s), the time has come for a new stretcher.

It is the responsibility of the therapist to assess the characteristics of each patient to determine a safe and effective wearing schedule. As with any removable splint, the patient should initially wear the splint for a trial period of 20 to 30 min to determine skin tolerance. Once tolerance is established, the patient can gradually increase time in the splint. This author has worked with many patients who were able to wear the stretcher at night during sleep. This achieves 6 to 8 hours of end range positioning and then leaves the extremity free during the day for exercise. When the goal is stretcher wear during sleep, the therapist may want to decrease the amount of stretch placed on the tissue during stretcher fabrication or may avoid preconditioning before fabrication.

For the patient who cannot sleep while wearing the stretcher, the therapist must achieve a balance between stretcher wear, activities of daily living, and exercise. Remember that the more the patient wears the stretcher, the faster the patient will reach the therapeutic goals. A minimum amount of time in the stretcher (which depends on the individual patient) must occur for it to have any effect (see Chapter 15 for details) (Flowers & Michlovitz, 1988). The therapist may consider combining other splints or POP finger casts with stretchers. Applying the finger splint or casts before stretcher fabrication may help achieve optimal IP joint position.

CONCLUSION

Casting is a powerful treatment technique that has the ability to provide outcomes that no other splinting approach can offer. The circumferential approach to splinting has many benefits, including improved pressure distribution and minimized sheer and migration. Casting offers an efficient and effective means to decrease contractures, including those with a hard end feel. Even patients with cognitive and sensory impairment can benefit from casting.

As with any treatment approach, the therapist must carefully consider the nature of the problem before applying the cast. Patients with PROM limitations owing to soft tissue abnormalities that will not respond to low-load, prolonged stress should not receive a cast. Joint limitation caused by heterotopic ossification, exostosis, or loose body will also not benefit from casting. The circumferential design of the cast allows mobilization of a joint that might not be a candidate for conventional splinting, e.g., in the case of some forms of joint instability and acute inflammation. However, avascular necrosis, infection, unstable fracture, marked demineralization, myositis ossificans, and stress across healing structures without adequate blood supply or tensile strength to withstand tensile stress remain contraindications to cast application.

The family of casting products continues to increase, offering patients and clinicians more options. Familiarity with the characteristics of each product helps the therapist choose the material that best meets the patient's needs. Circumferential and noncircumferential casting techniques to serially increase PROM require skills that are unique to this modality. This chapter describes several of these. Continued innovation in the use of casting will benefit patients in new and effective ways.

ACKNOWLEDGMENTS

Many thanks to Trudy Hackencamp, OTR, CHT, for the information she provided regarding casting spasticity. Thanks also to Judy Bell-Krotoski for our many discussions over the years regarding the use of POP and serial casting of fingers. Finally, thanks to Jessica Hawkins, my patient of many years, who has worn more casts than anyone can count and has given me invaluable feedback.

REFERENCES

Becker, D. (1978). Danger of burns from fresh plaster splints surrounded by too much cotton. Plastic and Reconstructive Surgery, 62, 436–437.

Bell-Krotoski, J. A. (1987). Plaster casting for the remodeling of soft tissue. In E. E. Fess & C. Phillips (Eds.). Hand splinting: Principles and methods (2nd ed., pp. 449–466). St. Louis: Mosby.

Bell-Krotoski, J. A. (1995). Plaster cylinder casting for contractures of the interphalangeal joints. In J. M. Hunter, E. J. Mackin, & A. D. Callahan (Eds.). *Rehabilitation of the hand* (4th ed., pp. 1609–1616). St. Louis: Mosby Year Book.

Brand, P. W. (1988). Biomechanics of Deformity. Paper presented at the Insensitive Hand Seminar. Long Hansen's Disease Center, Baton Rouge, LA.

Brand, P. W., Hollister, A. M., Giurintano, D., & Thompson, D. E. (1999a). External stress: Effect at the surface. In P. W. Brand & A. M. Hollister (Eds.). *Clinical biomechanics of the hand* (3rd ed., pp. 215–232). St. Louis: Mosby.

Brand, P. W., Hollister, A. M., Giurintano, D., & Thompson, D. E. (1999b). External Stress: Forces that effect joint action. In P. W. Brand & A. M. Hollister (Eds.). *Clinical biomechanics of the hand* (3rd ed., pp. 233–246). St. Louis: Mosby.

Brand, P. W. & Yancey, P. (1997). *The gift of pain: Why we hurt and what we can do about it.* Grand Rapids, MI: Zondervan Publishing House.

Brzezienski, M. A., & Schneider, L. H. (1995). Extensor tendon injuries at the distal interphalangeal joint. *Hand Clinics of North America, 11,* 373–386.

Colditz, J. (2000a). Preliminary report on a new technique for casting motion to mobilize stiffness in the hand. *Journal of Hand Therapy, 13,* 68–73.

Colditz, J. (2000b). *Presentation outline: Therapist's management of the stiff hand.* Paper presented at the Surgery and Rehabilitation of the Hand Symposium, Philadelphia, PA.

Coons, M. S., & Green, S. M. (1995). Boutonniere deformity. *Hand Clinics of North America, 11,* 387–402.

Evans, R. B. (1995). An update on extensor tendon management. In J. M. Hunter, E. J. Mackin, & A. D. Callahan (Eds.). *Rehabilitation of the hand* (4th ed., pp. 565–606). St. Louis: Mosby Year Book.

Flowers, K. R., & LaStayo, P. (1994). Effect of total end range time on improving passive range of motion. *Journal of Hand Therapy, 7,* 150–157.

Flowers, K. R., & Michlovitz, S. L. (1988). Assessment and management of loss of motion in orthopedic dysfunction. In *Postgraduate Advances in Physical Therapy.* Alexandria, VA: APTA.

Goga-Eppenstein, P., Hill, J. P., Seifert, T. M., & Yasukawa, A. M. (1999). Theoretical background and rationale for cast intervention. In P. Goga-Eppenstein, J. P. Hill, P. A. Philip, A. Philip, T. M. Seifert, & A. M. Yasukawa (Eds.). *Casting protocols for the upper and lower extremities* (pp. 1–4). Gaithersburg, MD: Aspen.

Grazer. F. (1979). Danger of burns from fresh plaster splints surrounded by too much cotton. *Plastic and Reconstructive Surgery, 63,* 560.

Haasch, K. (1964). Verbrennungen unter dem Gispverband. *Hefte Unfallheilkd, 78,* 264.

Hill, J. P., & Yasukawa, A. M. (1999). Upper extremity casts: types and application descriptions. In P. Goga-Eppenstein, J. P. Hill, P. A. Philip, A. Philip, T. M. Seifert, & A. M. Yasukawa (Eds.). *Casting protocols for the upper and lower extremities* (pp. 23–66). Gaithersburg, MD: Aspen.

Johnson and Johnson Orthopaedic Division. (1985). *Fracture management orthopaedic learning system reference.* New Brunswick, NJ: Johnson & Johnson.

Kaplan, S. (1981). Burns following application of plaster dressing. *Journal of Bone and Joint Surgery (American volume), 63,* 670–672.

Lavalette, R., Pope, M., & Dickerson, H. (1982). Setting temperature of plaster casts: The influence of technical variables. *Journal of Bone and Joint Surgery (American volume), 64,* 907–911.

Lovell, C, & Staniforth, P. (1981). Contact allergy to benzalkonium chloride in plaster of Paris. *Contact Dermatitis, 7,* 343–344.

Lubahn, J. D. (1988). Dorsal fracture dislocations of the proximal interphalangeal joint. In R. I. Burton (Ed.). *Small joint injuries* (pp. 15–24). Philadelphia: Saunders.

Mahler, L. R., Pedowitz, R. A., Byrne, T. P., & Gershuni, D. H. (1996). Pressure generation beneath a new thermoplastic cast. *Clinical Orthopaedics and Related Research, 322,* 262–266.

Sailer, S. M., & Salibury-Milan, D. L. (2000). Hand therapy. In T. E. Trumble & S. M. Sailer (Eds.). *Hand surgery and therapy* (pp. 603–623). Philadelphia: Saunders.

Schneider, L. H., & Smith K. L. (1987). Boutonniere deformity. In J. M. Hunter, L. H. Schneider, & E. J. Mackin (Eds.). *Tendon surgery in the hand* (pp. 349–357). St Louis: Mosby.

Schultze, R. (1967). Verbrennungsschaden im Gipsverband. *Hefte Unfallheilkd, 9,* 236.

Schultz-Johnson, K. S. (1999). *PIP serial casting with QuickCast.* Edwards, CO: UE Tech.

Schultz-Johnson, K. S. (1992). Splinting: A problem solving approach. In B. G. Stanley & S. M. Tribuzi (Eds.). *Concepts in hand rehabilitation* (pp. 238–271). Philadelphia: Davis.

Staniforth, P. (1980). Allergy to benzalkonium chloride in plaster of paris after sensitization to centrimede. *Journal of Bone and Joint Surgery (British volume), 62,* 500–501.

Tribuzi, S. M. (1990. Serial plaster splinting. In J. M. Hunter, L. H. Schneider, E. J. Mackin, & A. D. Callahan (Eds.). *Rehabilitation of the hand* (3rd ed., pp. 1120–1127) St Louis: Mosby.

Wilson, D. C. (1965). *Ten fingers for God: The true story of a surgeon's quest for an end to the ravages of leprosy.* New York: McGraw-Hill.

CHAPTER 13

Taping Techniques

Ruth Coopee, OTR/L, CHT

INTRODUCTION

Research supports the theory of encouraging early motion to improve healing time and the quality of tissue repair (Cyr & Ross, 1998). Casting and immobilization in rigid splints, though beneficial at certain stages of healing, do not allow motion (Fess & McCollum, 1998). Hinged braces and splints are often cumbersome and not practical for performing activities of daily living (ADLs). Silicone and soft splints that offer semirigid support have been introduced to provide protected motion during return to activity and to prevent injury or reinjury of soft tissue (Birrer, 1994; Canelon, 1995; Henshaw, Satren, & Wrightsman, 1989). This type of splint fabrication is helpful but time-consuming and not always cost effective.

In sports medicine and athletic training, strapping and taping techniques have been used successfully for early, protected return to activity (Hilfrank, 1991). **Taping** is a cost-effective treatment alternative for many common injuries and overuse syndromes seen in the clinic and does not affect grip strength (Rettig, Stube, & Shelbourne, 1997). Taping is not applicable for conditions requiring the protection of rigid splinting, but it may be incorporated along the recovery continuum to allow for protected mobilization or to assist in neuromuscular retraining. A skilled and extensive evaluation to determine the appropriateness and the timing for proper implementation is necessary before incorporating taping. As with many such modalities, effective taping is employed as a complement to a comprehensive rehabilitation program.

This chapter provides a brief overview of three popular taping methods and techniques: **traditional athletic taping, McConnell taping,** and **Kinesio taping.** Table 13–1 compares the distinctly different taping methods and provides a summary of their features. Specialized training is recommended for each technique to provide proficiency and improve comprehension of the underlying mechanisms and associated therapeutic programs. Instruction is offered through a variety of venues; see Suggested Reading for the URLs to helpful Web sites. Accessibility to some training programs may be limited based on clinical training or expertise (e.g., training in spinal manipulation) and on the scope of practice laws in individual states.

The clinician must have an extensive clinical knowledge of anatomy, kinesiology, and the physiology of healing to determine if taping is indicated and, if so, to determine the best choice of technique and material. Note that each patient and injury is unique and requires a comprehensive evaluation by the physician and therapist before therapy intervention (Austin, Gwynn-Brett, & Marshall, 1994). The evaluation should include knowledge of the physical demands and requirements of the patient, the structure(s) involved, the degree of injury, and the stage of healing. Table 13–2 is a general guide to the application of taping based on the specific degree of injury.

Patients using taping techniques should be closely monitored. Frequent re-evaluation of the injured body part, healing process, tension, and tape placement as well as the taping materials themselves is essential to maximize the success of taping as a method of treatment. Inspection of the completed taping should be conducted to ensure proper support and proper taping application. Patients are at risk for significant harm if they return to activity with inadequate support or limitation of movement. Therefore, sound professional clinical judgment and proper diagnosis are imperative to ensure a positive outcome. Treatment may also include instruction of proper tape application and removal by the patient, family member, or other caregiver. It is important to educate the patient about the precautions and to stress the necessity of frequent monitoring of the body part for changes in skin integrity and neurovascular and lymphatic function.

TABLE 13–1 Comparison of Three Taping Techniques

Technique	Athletic	McConnell	Kinesio
Materials	Adhesive spray Undertape Prewrap Padding Adhesive tape	Undertape Brown adhesive tape	Kinesio Tex tape
Evaluation	Analysis of muscle, joint, and soft tissue integrity	Analysis of structural alignment and dysfunctional biomechanics	Analysis of muscle, soft tissue. and fascial dysfunction and its relationship to pathology
Indications	Joint injury Ligament injuries (grade 1–3) Muscle injury Rigid yet flexible protection	Postural re-education Muscle retraining Joint alignment	Scar and soft tissue modification Relieves myofascial pain Edema reduction Muscle support and re-education Joint support (correction) Postural re-education
Purpose	Provides progressive amount of support and immobilization to healing tissues and prevents reinjury while allowing continued participation in activity	Passively repositions soft tissue and holds bony structures in proper alignment to retrain and restore normal static and dynamic functional biomechanics	Specially developed elastic tape and application technique facilitates neurosensory and physiologic mechanisms of skin, lymphatics, and muscle and affects soft tissue, fascia, and muscle tension to modify functional biomechanics and reduce pain
Advantages	Maximum support to healing structures	Provides support to weak structures and allows full ROM	Gentle approach to treatment of myofascial pain and soft tissue injuries and allows full ROM
Disadvantages	Tape trauma Skin irritation Must be replaced and checked often for maximum support Patient dependency	Tape trauma Skin irritation Pulling of tape may be pain restrictive in exercise Not appropriate for grade 3 injuries	Complexity of technique Tape allergy Not appropriate for grade 2–3 injuries, though may be used in combination with athletic tape

ROM, range of motion.

TABLE 13–2 Injury Classification and Taping Recommendations

Type of Injury	Definition	Characteristics	Taping Duration
First-degree injury	Damage with little or no elongation of ligaments or soft tissue	No instability	3–10 days
Second-degree injury	Overstretch with partial tear and moderate ligament involvement	Some laxity to joint	4–6 weeks
Third-degree injury	Complete rupture with abnormal movement on stress testing	Major loss of joint ligament integrity and structural function, requiring probable surgical intervention	Minimum of 4 months, with close monitoring

TABLE 13–3 Commonly Used Materials

Material	Function and Use
Skin tougheners and adhesive sprays	Applied to skin in either pad or spray before taping Improves adhesion of tape to skin and decreases chemical tape irritations Tougheners have additional astringent to prepare skin These products can cause irritation if used for prolonged periods
Undertapes	Adhesive-backed, nonelastic material used as base to which sports tape is applied Serves as light padding to protect skin and bony areas and to prevent skin blisters and cuts
Prewraps	Similar to undertape but does not have an adhesive backing Composed of fine, porous polyester foam material that has light stretch to help conform to contours Provides increased padding to skin and bony areas but requires spray adherent to increase skin contact
Adhesive tapes	Rated by number of vertical fibers per inch, which relates to tensile strength and weight Available in ½", 1", 1½", and 2" widths Often referred to as white tape, zinc oxide tape, or linen tape Inelastic and provides a high degree of joint support and immobilization
Elastic tapes	Possess certain amount of recoil or stretch Percentage of stretch determines amount of controlled movement in a joint and functional muscle support

Taping Materials

There are many types of sports tape and products on the market, each with its own indications. Tape should not be confused with bandages or cohesive circumferential wraps that do not adhere directly to the skin. All tapes should be stored flat to maintain the roll shape and in a cool dry location to maintain its adhesive quality. Table 13–3 lists commonly used materials along with their functions (Arnheim & Prentice, 2000; Austin, et al. 1994).

Athletic Taping

General Principles

The main function of athletic taping is to restrict or immobilize specific joint structures while allowing for some degree of active movement (Arnheim & Prentice, 2000; Austin et al., 1994; Jim Wallis ATC, personal communication, 2000, 2001). Tape is applied across a joint in several layers and it is positioned to provide outside support and restrict forces that would apply stress to an injured part. Tape can also support and protect a weakened muscle by limiting tendon excursion. Depending on the technique of application, taping can provide minimal to moderate constraint of healing tissues while allowing joint motion for controlled protected healing. Encapsulating acutely injured joint structures assists in edema control via compression and active muscle pumping. To reduce edema associated with muscle contusion, an elastic tape is used to provide localized compression and allow supported contraction and relaxation. Tape also serves as an anchor for attaching tape strips. The goals of athletic taping are as follows:

- Support and protect weakened joint structures.
- Limit harmful movement and assist in planes of movement.
- Provide a progressive method for achieving pain-free functional movement.
- Allow for movement of an injured part to improve circulation and healing.
- Assist in controlling edema.
- Prevent worsening of injury and muscle atrophy.
- Improve kinesthetic awareness in an acutely injured joint.
- Allow early return to function.

Indications for Use

Athletic taping is most often used in the treatment of sprains, strains, subluxations, and dislocations with ligament tears or ruptures resulting in unidirectional or multidirectional instability. When a thorough medical evaluation determines it appropriate and if applied properly, taping creates a rigid support and provides for maximal soft tissue control. This technique is particularly effective in the conservative management of subacute second- and third-degree injuries. For grade 3 injuries or after repetitive injury, taping is combined with activity restriction to allow tissue healing.

Technique

Multiple layers of **nonelastic adhesive tape** are applied across the joint to provide rigid stability for ligament injuries. Elastic tapes are used for contractile tissue injuries (muscle and tendon) and to provide localized pressure. The manner in which the tape is applied determines the degree of mobility or immobility across a joint. Table 13–4 lists common techniques and methods used in athletic taping.

The skin overlying the area to be taped needs to be cleansed of all oils, perspiration, hair, and old adhesive before application of a **skin toughener** or **spray** adher-

TABLE 13–4 Techniques and Methods Used in Athletic Taping

Technique	Method of Application
Anchor	Circumferential pieces of tape placed proximal and distal to injury from base to attach tape strip ends May use elastic tape if room for muscle expansion needed
Stirrup	U-shaped loop of nonelastic tape used to create lateral stability
Vertical strips	Tension applied as tape is attached, moving from distal to proximal anchor Increased stability of affected joint is achieved through joint compression and fascial restriction
Butterfly or check reins	Multiple strips of tape applied at angles to each other with apex at joint to limit movement in unidirectional or multidirectional planes (X or star) Variation of technique to inhibit abduction in fingers is applied with anchors to adjacent digits; tape between anchors twisted onto itself to create rein that limits movement
Locks	Smooth roll application with increased tension at key points of support and reinforced joint stability Allows protected functional movement (Figure-8 with cross-point at support point)
Figure-8 or locking strip	Used to complete taping, covers open areas and tape strip ends while adding stability
Compression	Elastic adhesive tape stretched from center and applied directly down with pressure over muscle injury No tension is applied at ends to avoid vascular constriction Provides support to muscle and fascia while assisting in edema reduction
Closing up (in) and coverup	Strips of tape applied to cover all open areas and finish taping job Increases durability and provides consistent coverage to prevent blisters and constriction with focal edema
Strip	One strip of tape is placed in specific direction with highly controlled tension from one anchor to other
Smooth roll	Use of one single continuous uninterrupted piece of tape May begin and end at same anchor, as with joint locks

ent. This creates a microscopic layer to protect the skin from tape irritants and increase the adhesive quality of the tape. **Undertape** or **prewrap** is then applied to protect bony prominences, soft skin creases, or superficial arteries. In addition, prewrap may be used to hold additional padding in place. **Tape anchors** are applied proximal and distal to the joint being taped. The joint is placed in a well-supported unstressed position. Depending on the degree of injury, the target joint is taped in either an anatomic neutral position or placed in a slack position to restrict movement stress on healing structures. The person applying the tape should be in an efficient and comfortable position, to help proper application technique. The amount of support and joint restriction is dictated by the degree of injury and is achieved by the technique and tension applied during taping.

The joint should be evaluated on completion to determine if there is adequate restriction of motion to protect from re-injury. There should be no pain. Inspection must include evaluation for distal patency and surrounding tissue assessment to ensure there is no occlusion or impairment of circulatory or lymphatic function. Taping may be used for a particular event or may stay in place for several days. The taping becomes progressively looser with activity and should be checked regularly so the joint does not become vulnerable.

Tape removal should always be performed carefully so as not to damage or accidentally tear the skin. Blunt-ended bandage scissors are used on the opposite side of the injury to tunnel under the tape and slowly ease the tape off of the skin. Slowly cut and gently peel the tape away by pressing down on the exposed skin while drawing the tape parallel to the surface of the skin. Do not pull up on the tape, because this may tear the skin and cause subcutaneous hemorrhaging. Close inspection and evaluation of the skin are imperative for preventing breakdown from adhesives, chronic shearing forces, or tape irritation.

Precautions

The patient should be counseled against developing a false sense of security and/or dependency on taping. Examination of circulation and tape performance should be completed after application and throughout the day. Inspection of the skin for maceration or allergic reaction (blistering, rash) between tapings is necessary; taping should be suspended or discontinued if these signs are noticed. Do not tape over abrasions, blisters, lacerations, or cuts. Decreased sensibility from ice or edema may mask tissue response and sensation of pain during taping, resulting in injury. Do not use ice or heat before taping, particularly in the subacute phase. Reduction in interstitial tissue volume from the ice application may create a progressive tightening of the taping as the tissue warms up. Conversely, tissue volumes may decrease after heat application, resulting in reduction of support. It is important to note that improper application can aggravate an existing injury or create a new one.

Helpful Hints

- Place the joint in a position that stabilizes or protects it.
- Overlap at least half the width of the underlying tape strip to prevent separation.
- Avoid the continuous smooth roll method; apply only one turn around a joint then tear. Continuous wrapping increases tension and may become constrictive.
- Smooth and mold each strip as it is placed on the skin, allowing it to flow around the natural contours of body part. This is more difficult to achieve with heavier, stiffer tapes.
- A nonadhesive foam prewrap, in contrast to an adhesive-backed undertape, potentially decreases stability and support owing to the increased movement between skin and tape.
- Maximum control is achieved by the degree of skin adherence.
- Do not tape immediately after application of heat or cold; wait until the tissue returns to normal temperature.

McConnell Taping

General Principles

McConnell taping was developed in 1989 by McConnell, an Australian physical therapist, and was initially used for the conservative management of patellofemoral pain (J. McConnell, personal communication 2001; Murphy, 1996; Tremain, 1996). Later, McConnell successfully expanded her philosophy and treatment techniques to the spine and upper extremity. The McConnell technique involves not only the use of taping but also an extensive muscle evaluation and an analysis of individual biomechanics and posture. Treatment of structural misalignment in conjunction with poor movement patterns is addressed through a comprehensive rehabilitation program, and taping assists in the physical re-education of the body. McConnell method taping is employed to reduce pain and to improve muscle function and biomechanics. Other goals are as follows:

- Position a joint into more appropriate alignment.
- Increase stability of a joint (ligament support).
- Correct articular orientation by inhibiting short, tight muscles.
- Facilitate firing capacity of weak, lengthened, overstretched muscles.
- Enhance muscle retraining by balancing the tissue length/tension relationship.
- Assist in both static and dynamic neuromuscular re-education.

Besides taping, the McConnell program includes evaluation and mobilization of the spine to improve scapular and upper extremity alignment, stretching exercises, therapeutic exercise to improve motor control and coordination, and biofeedback.

Indications for use

Taping is used as a vehicle to directly control fascia and establish proper structural alignment for improved muscular recruitment and neuromuscular retraining. These techniques help reduce pain, which encourages compliance in an exercise program, usually designed to strengthen and lengthen the muscular structures involved in pathology. Proper analysis of the underlying pathology is essential to maximize the effectiveness of the method, which focuses on re-establishing a proper length/tension relationship and motor control. Subluxation, unidirectional or multidirectional instability, impingement, postinjury or postoperative retraining, overuse, and poor alignment respond well to McConnell taping.

Technique

A thorough evaluation is completed to determine the pathologic mechanisms involved and how best to correct them. Specific taping materials are used in this technique owing to their tensile strength and durability. First, a **white adhesive undertape** is applied to the skin without tension. This provides a protective bed for application of a heavyweight working **brown adhesive tape.** The undertape is extremely important, as it protects the skin from shearing forces and the strong holding adhesive of the brown tape. Taping with a vertical strip technique gains control of muscle tissue and fascia. If applied correctly, there should be an immediate reduction in pain and no restriction of normal movement. Taping should be completed before exercise to allow proper pain-free exercise performance.

To support joint alignment and ligaments, the working tape uses the surrounding fascia to hold the joint in a corrected, tension-free position. To treat shortened tissues or inhibit overactive muscles, the goal is to create a multidirectional stretching force to the muscle belly or shortened tissue. The working tape is applied with tension, perpendicular to the alignment of muscle fibers and with downward force to create both a lateral and compressive stretch to the muscle fibers and fascia. To treat lengthened or weak muscles, the working tape is used to draw the fascia or muscle proximally to passively shorten the fibers. This provides support through somatosensory feedback and prevents overstretch. To ensure proper joint and bone alignment during application of the working tape, the desired position is maintained manually by the nontaping hand or an assistant. The tape will then maintain the body in the proper position to assist in neuromuscular and postural re-education. Return to previous poor postural movement patterns are discouraged through sensory feedback.

The tape may remain in place for 1 to 3 days before replacement is necessary. Remove the tape as described earlier for athletic tape. The skin should be evaluated and cleansed thoroughly before re-application.

Precautions

Avoid taping patients with known allergies to tape. Do not apply to fragile, thin, or healing skin or tissue that is susceptible to stress injury. Skin integrity and examination for irritation or sensitivity should be continuously evaluated and taping should be discontinued as necessary. During application, care should be taken not to apply strong tension, as this can create shearing forces to adjacent as well as target tissues. When taping the shoulder, be careful not to compress the brachial plexus as it crosses the humerus. Remember that the patient should experience immediate improvement and reduction in pain; if the patient experiences an increase in pain, the tape should be removed immediately. This continued pain may be the result of improper evaluation of causal factors or improper taping procedure.

It is important to have received training by a certified instructor, which will improve effectiveness and proficiency in the technique. Taping is just one part of the McConnell multifaceted treatment approach to correcting structural dysfunction. Instruction in evaluation techniques to determine individual taping needs, and a comprehensive exercise program to retrain full-body maladaptive movement patterns, is important to the successful implementation of this technique.

Helpful Hints

- Using a skin toughener or adhesive spray may help reduce skin irritation.
- There should be at least a 50% reduction in symptoms.
- Tape must improve the symptoms immediately.
- Discontinue the technique if it is not effective.

Kinesio Taping

General Principles

Kinesio taping has been used extensively in Japan and was introduced to the United States in 1994 (K. Kase, personal communication, 2000, 2001; Kase, 1994; Kase, Hashimoto, & Okane, 1996). Both the method and special tape used for this technique were developed in 1973 by Kase, a Japanese chiropractor. After chiropractic training in the United States, he specialized in rehabilitation and therapeutic medicine. Intrigued with kinesiology and conservative ways of treating traumatized soft tissue, he used sports tape to assist in soft tissue control. Not satisfied with the stiff restriction of athletic tapes, he searched for a material that would work with the mechanisms of the body to facilitate healing. He developed **Kinesio Tex tape** to mimic the elastic properties of muscle, skin, and fascia.

Proper application of the tape does not restrict soft tissue movement, as do conventional adhesive tapes, but rather relies on the movement of skin for multilevel effects. The elastic recoil of the tape is used to provide support to weak muscle and encourage full joint movement. The movement of taped skin and soft tissue creates a massaging effect that promotes lymph and blood flow, decreasing pressure on mechanoreceptors, thus reducing pain and edema. Sensory receptors located in the skin also act on ascending and descending neurologic pathways to reduce pain and assist in control of muscle tension via Golgi tendon organ input. The application technique may specifically address sensory receptors in the skin, lymphatic movement for edema and circulation, muscle tension control, or joint support. The goals of Kinesio taping are as follows:

- Decrease pain and abnormal sensation in skin and muscle.
- Reduce edema and inflammation.
- Normalize muscle tone and abnormality of fascia involved in pathology.
- Support a weakened muscle in movement (expanding effects) by preventing overstretch and reducing fatigue.
- Reduce spasm or overcontraction of a shortened muscle.
- Improve range of motion (ROM).
- Provide muscle and proprioceptive re-education.
- Correct misalignment of a joint by re-establishing a muscular balance.
- Support normal joint alignment for rehabilitation.
- Prevent injuries in exercise or ADLs.
- Improve kinesthetic awareness of proper posture and structural alignment.

Indications for Use

Kinesio taping is used to address soft tissue pathology created by muscle imbalance and assists in removing chemical substances and edema while retraining the body in improved structural alignment. An indirect approach, it works on the neurologic, somatosensory, and physiologic processes of the body. The tape, in combination with the method, has multisystemic effects on vascular, lymphatic, soft tissue, joint, and muscular dysfunctions. A thorough and comprehensive understanding of pathology and its relationship to muscle physiology and kinesiology is essential to the success of this form of taping. An evaluation of muscle, fascia, soft tissue continuity, and structure is completed to determine the causal factors of the pathology.

Kinesio taping is used to complement a therapeutic program and can be easily taught to patients, family members, or other caregivers for continued application in chronic conditions for self-management. This technique is effective in treating many orthopedic and complex conditions such as subluxation, sprains, impingement syndromes, reflex sympathetic dystrophy, fibromyalgia, overuse, edema, adhesions and scars, muscle dysfunctions, and postural re-education.

Technique

Kinesio Tex tape was specifically developed to be used with this technique. The high elasticity qualities of the tape, combined with proper application, affects the superficial fascial structures in the skin and creates a lifting or ripple effect in resting tissue. These changes cause a reduction in subcutaneous interstitial pressure, improving lymphatic drainage of toxic chemicals and reducing edema. During normal movement, there is constant tactile stimuli to low-threshold cutaneous mechanoreceptors of the skin. This stimulates muscle, decreases pain, and enhances proprioception for neuromuscular re-education.

The high elastic recoil of the tape also provides support to weak muscles, reducing fatigue. The thickness and weight of the tape are approximately the same as skin, and when applied properly is rarely perceived by the patient. It stretches in the longitudinal axis only up to 40% of its resting length. The tape is made of a 100% woven cotton fabric and there is no Latex or medicinal properties in the tape. An acrylic, heat-activated adhesive forms a fingerprint glue pattern, with holes between to allow for passage of perspiration and air.

The tape is applied to a paper substrate with a 10% stretch that is available in 2" and 3" widths. It is also available in three colors and in a water-resistant variety for patients who perspire heavily or who are involved in water sports. The tape may be worn for up to 4 days, and the patient is able to shower with the tape in place. Care should be taken when drying the body part so as not to roll up the edges of the tape. A thorough evaluation is critical to obtain positive results, because taping must address both the pain and the cause of the pain to provide correction of the pathology.

The specific taping technique is determined by the target fascia and tissue to be treated, which also affects how the tape is cut. The most commonly used cuts are the Y- and I-shaped cuts from 2" wide Kinesio Tex tape. Table 13–5 lists techniques and methods used in Kinesio taping, and Table 13–6 defines appropriate tape tension.

To treat a tight, shortened muscle and decrease spasm, the tape is anchored on the insertion or moveable segment. Move the body so the muscle and skin are on stretch and apply the tape around the lateral and medial margins of the target muscle, ending at the origin or fixed aspect of the muscle (insertion to origin). To provide support to a weak muscle, anchor the tape at the origin or fixed part of the muscle. Move the body so the muscle and skin are on stretch and apply the tape around the lateral and medial margins of the target muscle, ending at the insertion or moveable aspect of the muscle (origin to insertion). When providing treatment to the cause of the disability, it is important to re-establish balance at the joint by addressing both the agonist and the antagonist (e.g., to effectively treat an overstretched upper trapezius, the shortened, tight pectoralis minor must also be addressed).

After application, lightly rub the tape to activate the heat-sensitive glue. The tape may be applied over fine hair, but more coarse hair should be clipped short with scissors or shaved. Once rubbed to activate the glue, the tape may not be reapplied. For best adherence it should be applied 20 to 30 min before activity so it can tolerate perspiration. It is not necessary to use an adhesive spray before application, except when applying the tape to moist tissue areas or when the patient's skin is sensitive to the adhesive.

To remove the tape, it is best to start at the proximal end and work distally, moving with the direction of hair growth. Brushing the tape briskly while rolling it onto itself is most effective for overstimulating sensory receptors and decreasing discomfort. The tape is easily removed during a shower or bath.

Precautions

Do not stretch the tape, unless using a correction technique. The elasticity of the tape provides the therapeutic effect, and if the tape is improperly applied, it will increase pain. If applied correctly, there should be immediate pain relief. Some patients have experienced sensitivity to the adhesive; application of a spray adherent may prevent irritation. Because the acrylic adhesive is heat activated, direct application of high heat such as hotpacks or fluidotherapy should be avoided, as this will make the tape difficult to remove. A hair dryer may be used on the no-heat setting to dry the tape after a shower or exposure to water.

The multiple effects of Kinesio taping often create an evolutionary process in symptom presentation; therefore tissue and muscle re-evaluation before each application is critical to the successful correction of the underlying problem. Alterations in taping are commonly required to address physical changes and individual needs of the patient. Owing to the complex nature of this taping method, formal training from an experienced and certified instructor is highly recommended.

Helpful Hints

- Complete a thorough evaluation for pain and the cause of pain.
- Move through a full ROM before applying the tape to maximize tissue movement.
- Clean the skin of oils; then dry.
- Use a spray adherent, if necessary.
- Cut the tape into the appropriate shape to address the target tissue or function (edema).
- Use water-resistant tape for application to the hand or if extended exposure to water is anticipated (aquatic therapy).
- Apply the anchor of the tape securely without tension while the body is in a neutral position.

TABLE 13–5 Techniques and Methods Used in Kinesio Taping

Technique	Method of Application
I or single strip cut	May be used on all muscles In correction technique Encourages rotation Applied along center of a muscle group (e.g., wrist flexors) 1" width is used for small muscles 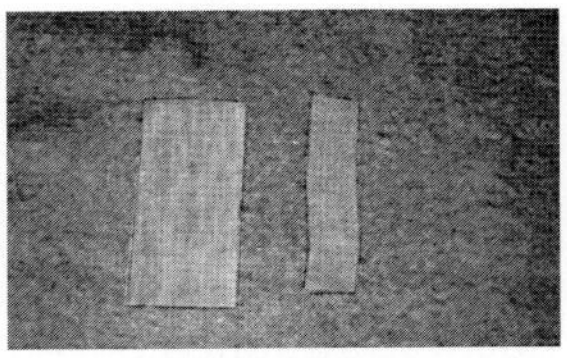
Y cut	Used to surround multiple or large muscle belly Base of Y is used as anchor Separation of ends or tails assists in changing tension of tissue between, lifting it to increase lymphatic flow 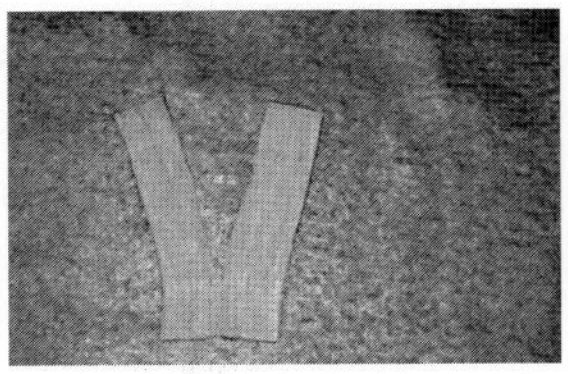
X cut	Used to stabilize at joint for treatment of rhomboidal-shaped muscle or in correction technique 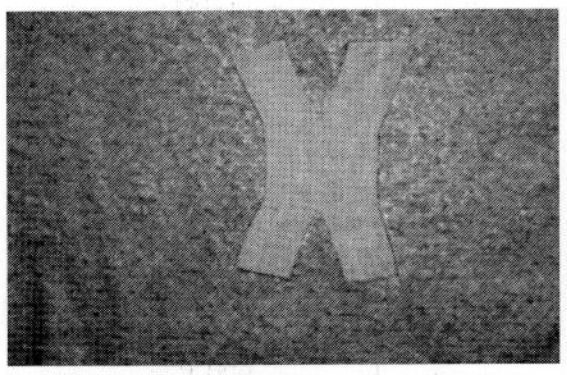
Fan cut	Used primarily for edema reduction Anchor serves as drawing point to which the lymph will drain 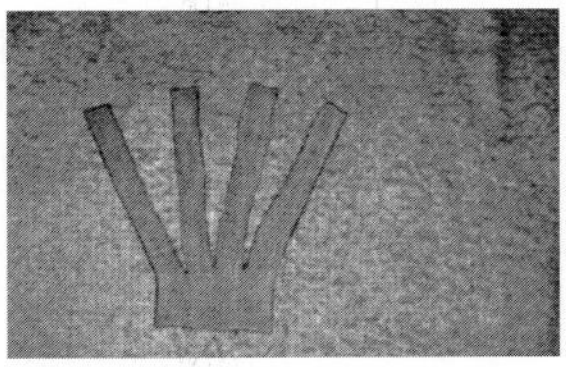
Buttonhole cut	Used as an anchor in forearm tapings to prevent rolling 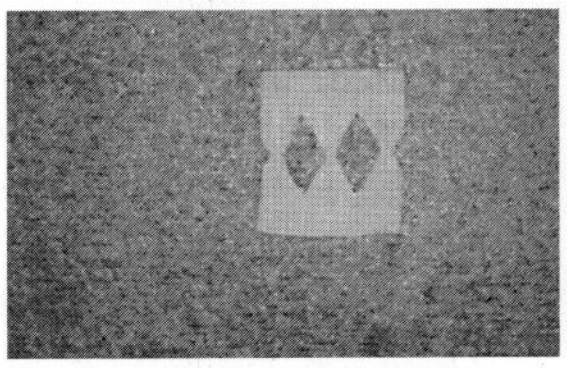

TABLE 13–6 Definitions of Kinesio Tape Tensions

Technique	Method of Application
No tension	No pull at anchor or end of tape
10 to 25%	Pull off paper stretch is most effective tension
50%	Tape may be slightly stretched if applied to nonstretched skin (e.g., joint contracture or contraindications to joint movement).
75 to 100%	Tape is applied with all elastic stretch taken out only when using a “correction” technique

- The target muscle and fascia are moved into maximal elongation (end ROM).
- Apply the tape off the paper backing at 25% stretch, unless used in the correction technique.
- Place the tape so it surrounds the muscle or as appropriate to the cut shape of the tape.
- Apply the tape without tension at the end attachment.
- Be sure of the placement before smoothing down the tape; work from the center outward to prevent rolling up of the ends.

Clinical Examples of Athletic Taping

Wrist Sprain and Instability

Application

When using athletic taping for the wrist, first shave the skin, if necessary, and apply a spray adherent to the areas to be taped (Fig. 13–1) (Arnheim & Prentice, 2000; Austin et al., 1994). The materials required are 1½" to 2" wide white adhesive or linen tape and underwrap. If additional support is needed, a dorsal X taping may be used before closing in. After taping, check for appropriate application and motion restriction.

General Considerations

The therapist must understand which structures require the most support to allow proper positioning of the wrist; if necessary, apply an additional tape strip for maximum protection. Tape strips are placed on tension to provide support but should not be so constrictive as to impinge on the skin or vascular structures.

The patient instructions should include periodic evaluations to ensure proper support and appropriate timing for replacement. If possible, teach the patient how to apply the tape. The wrist taping may stay in place for 2 to 4 days, depending on the degree of restriction and the activity level of the patient. Instruct the patient to remove the tape immediately if there is an increase in pain or adverse vascular signs. A backup splint may be necessary to protect the wrist between tapings or as needed.

Athletic taping achieves support and restriction through the quality of the material, the specific technique used, the tension applied by the tape, and the number of layers used to restrict movement. Keeping this in mind will assist in customization for individual needs and diagnosis.

Thumb Ulnar Collateral Ligament Injury

Application

Before using athletic taping for a thumb ulnar collateral ligament (UCL) injury, shave the area, if necessary, and apply adhesive spray (Fig. 13–2) (Arnheim & Prentice, 2000; Austin et al., 1994). The material required is 1", 1½", or 2" wide white adhesive tape. Because there is increased tension on the UCL, parallel ½" strips of tape may be placed from the interphalangeal (IP) anchor to the wrist for added support. After taping, check for appropriate application and motion restriction.

General Considerations

Avoid stress to the UCL during the taping procedure. Instruct the patient in self-evaluation of the taping. The patient should replace the tape if gapping or loosening is noted and should remove the tape immediately if pain, numbness, or vascular changes are noted. The tape should be replaced in 2 to 3 days, depending on the activity level of the patient.

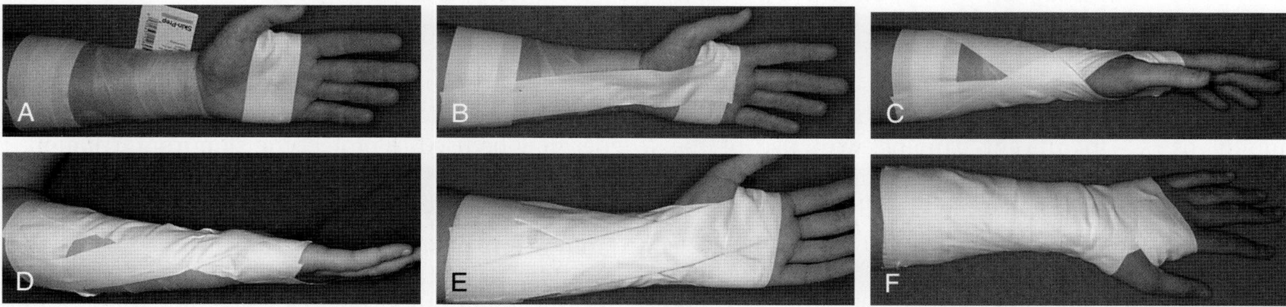

Figure 13–1 ***Athletic taping for a wrist sprain or instability. A,*** *Apply undertape or prewrap circumferentially to protect the forearm; place white tape anchors around the proximal forearm and at the metacarpals. The skin may be further protected with an adhesive spray or prep pad.* ***B,*** *Place the wrist in neutral (unless otherwise indicated), and apply a strip of white tape, with tension, from the distal anchor to the proximal anchor. To provide more support or restriction to extension, another strip may be placed, overlapping and parallel to the longitudinal piece along the ulnar aspect.* ***C,*** *Apply two strips, with tension, from the distal anchor (dorsal and volar), forming an X to support the radial aspect of the wrist.* ***D,*** *Repeat the X support on the ulnar aspect of the wrist.* ***E,*** *Form another X support on the volar aspect of the wrist to further restrict extension. Note the positions of the X supports. (Another X support may be placed dorsally to limit flexion, if necessary.)* ***F,*** *Complete the taping by applying a top anchor strip to secure the distal ends. Close in the forearm by applying overlapping circumferential strips, moving distal to proximal.*

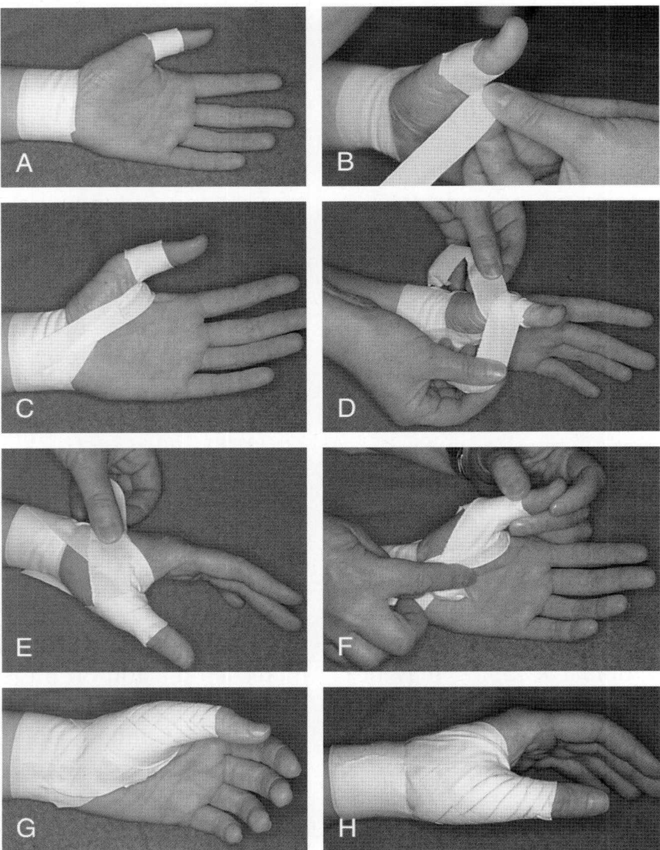

Figure 13–2 ***Athletic taping for a thumb UCL injury. A,*** *Apply circumferential anchors at the wrist (two 1½" to 2" wide strips with light tension) and distal proximal phalanx (1" wide strip).* ***B,*** *Form a diagonal anchor by attaching a 1½" wide strip to the distal anchor and pinching it in half at the first web space.* ***C,*** *Place the fold against the web space and reopen the tape for attachment at the base of the thumb.* ***D,*** *Use 1" wide tape in a Figure-8, with downward equal pull, to form the crosspiece.* ***E,*** *Anchor the dorsal attachment on the diagonal strip with pressure to adduct the thumb and restrict abduction.* ***F,*** *Secure the volar attachment to the diagonal strip at the base of the thumb.* ***G,*** *Continue the Figure-8 taping pattern proximally, overlapping the previous strip by ½", until the thumb is encapsulated.* ***H,*** *To close in, repeat the diagonal and circumferential wrist anchor strips to secure the Figure-8 strip ends.*

When placing the Figure-8 strips, be sure to overlap a minimum of ½" to prevent gapping with use of the hand. A check rein can be applied under this taping to provide more support: circumferentially anchor a ½" strip at the metacarpophalangeal (MP) joint, hold and twist the tape to form a string tether section, and then circumferentially anchor the tape to the proximal phalanx of the index finger (IF) close to the MP joint.

Clinical Examples of McConnell Taping

Postural Correction

Application

McConnell taping can be used for postural correction (Fig. 13–3) (C. Bailey, personal communication, 2001). The materials required are brown heavyweight adhesive tape and an undertape. A spray adherent or skin toughener may be used to protect the skin from irritation.

General Considerations

Taping for postural correction serves as a gentle reminder to the patient. Exercise caution when applying the longitudinal tape; do not upwardly compress the joint capsule, which can lead to shoulder impingement or bursitis. If the patient experiences paresthesias, increased pain, or discomfort, the tape should be removed. Taping should be combined with a comprehensive program to improve strength and proper muscular recruitment and coordination during active movement.

The therapist should place the extremity in the proper position. Do not overcorrect, which may be uncomfortable to the patient and inhibit normal use of the extremity.

Shoulder Subluxation

Application

When taping for a shoulder subluxation, use a spray adherent or skin toughener to protect the skin from irritation, if necessary (Fig. 13–4) (J. McConnell, personal communication, 2001). The materials required are brown heavyweight adhesive tape and an undertape.

General Considerations

McConnell taping for the shoulder may cause increased irritation, depending on the condition of the muscle carrying the weight of the arm. This taping does not address multidirectional instability, only the anterior subluxation commonly seen in patients who have undergone cerebrovascular accidents (CVAs). If the patient experiences increased pain or paresthesias, remove the tape immediately. This taping may stay in place for 3 to 4 days. Depending on the patient's age, overall medical condition, diagnosis, and skin condition, the technique shown here may not be appropriate.

Use caution with all shoulder tapings employing nonelastic tape. Excess force and pressure can have adverse effects on joint and soft tissue structures. This technique should be combined with a comprehensive strengthening program for the muscles affecting the joint, to provide extrinsic stability and prevent further damage or stretching of supporting ligaments and joint structures.

McConnell taping for shoulder subluxation also works well for treating anterior instability. When applying the working tape, avoid pulling straight up, which may create additional stress to the skin. Rather, move parallel to the skin and gently take up the slack, observing the skin on the edges for signs of excess tension. When taping a patient who has suffered a CVA or who has weakened deltoids, have respect for the increased loading of the skin.

Lateral Epicondylitis

Application

Lateral epicondylitis can be treated with McConnell taping. Use a spray adherent or skin toughener, if necessary, to protect the skin from irritation (Fig. 13–5) (C. Bailey, personal communication, 2001). The materials required are brown heavyweight adhesive tape and an undertape cut into 1-in. strips. The taping technique shown uses a diamond unloading pattern to shift the fascia and soft tissue restrictions away from the lateral epicondyle.

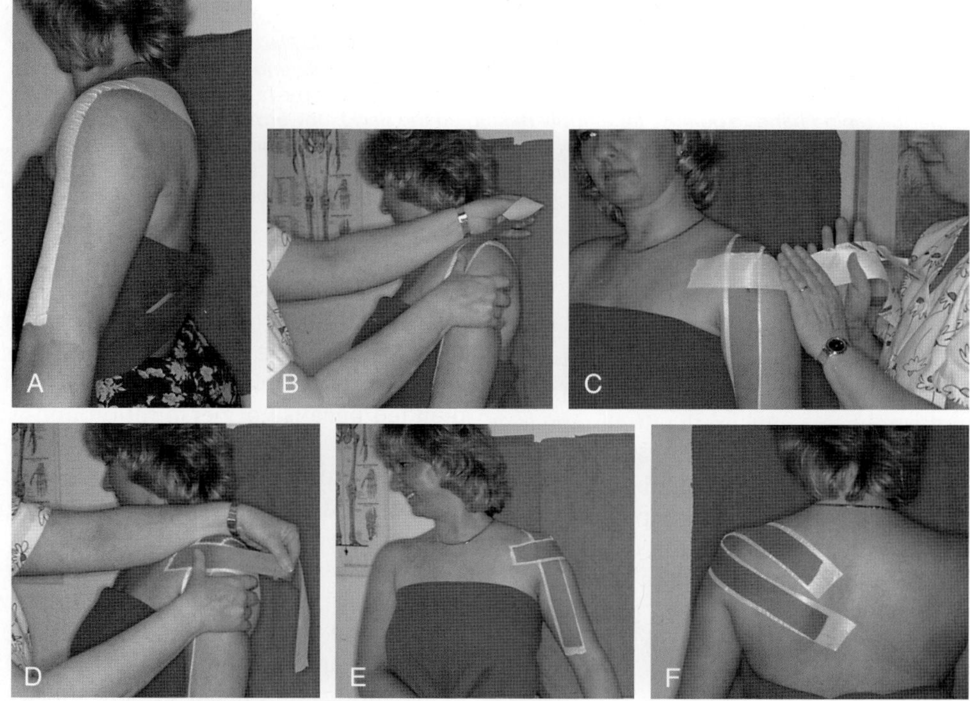

Figure 13–3 ***McConnell taping for postural correction.*** ***A,*** *Apply the undertape over the anterior surface of the upper arm, beginning at the elbow and ending just medial to the scapula.* ***B,*** *When applying the brown adhesive tape on top of the undertape, position the extremity in the proper desired posture of external rotation and humeral and scapular depression and retraction, ending at the scapula.* ***C,*** *Place the next undertape perpendicular to the first, for scapular retraction and external rotation of the humerus.* ***D,*** *Use the nonworking hand to position the patient properly.* ***E,*** *Position of anterior tapes at completion.* ***F,*** *Position of tapes across scapula when completed*

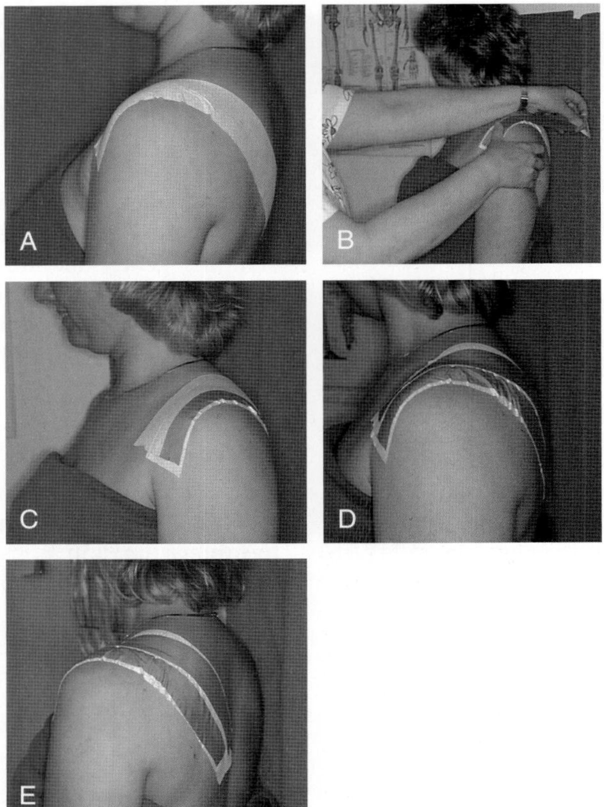

Figure 13–4 ***McConnell taping for anterior shoulder subluxation. A,*** *Place the undertape from the anterior aspect of the glenohumeral joint across the acromion process, ending at the medial inferior border of the scapula.* ***B,*** *Use the nonworking hand to lift the head of the humerus up and back while using the taping hand to pull the tape firmly (taking up the slack), upward and diagonally, to create uplift and external rotation of the humeral head. Secure the tape diagonally across the scapula.* ***C,*** *For additional support, repeat, positioning the second tape just medial to the first tape.* ***D,*** *Placement of anterolateral tape after completion.* ***E,*** *Placement of posterior tape after completion.*

General Considerations

The patient should experience immediate decrease or relief of symptoms after taping. The taping can remain in place for 2 to 3 days before needing to be replaced. Be careful to maintain the adhesive tape on the undertape to prevent skin contact and irritation on removal. The taping for lateral epicondylitis should be combined with a comprehensive stretching and strengthening program for the upper extremity, focusing on the forearm extensors.

Do not pull up on the tape, rather glide the fascia parallel to the skin. When the taping has been completed, there will be a puckering and lifting of the skin over the lateral epicondyle.

Clinical Examples of Kinesio Taping

Lateral Epicondylitis

Application

Kinesio taping for lateral epicondylitis addresses the tight forearm extensor muscles by applying the tape from insertion to origin and providing assistance to the overused supinator muscle (Fig. 13–6). The technique requires 2" wide combination buttonhole and Y-cut tape for the extensors. Water-resistant tape is recommended because of perspiration and water exposure of the hand.

The buttonhole technique is used to secure the tape on the hand and prevent removal during functional activities. Use a short, or half, version for this application, because the tape is applied to the dorsum of the arm only. A $1\frac{1}{2}$" to 2" end is needed to provide a secure anchor in the palm. The long end is then cut down the middle to approximately 4" (or two boxes, if using the demarcations on the back of the substrate) from the buttonhole.

General Considerations

If the patient has long or coarse forearm hair, it may need to be shaved to ensure adhesive contact. Shave the hair only where the tape is to be applied. A special cosmetic shaver with a 1" blade is available for creating a track for tape application. Apply tape with pull-off-paper tension. The patient should experience rapid relief of symptoms, unless he or she has a chronic condition. For chronic lateral epicondylitis, a few days are required to reduce the edema in the tissues and for the patient to experience relief. There should be no irritation from the tape, unless it was applied with too much tension or the patient is allergic.

Allergic responses to the adhesive are seen as a blister-type rash or hives. To ensure that the patient is not allergic to the acrylic adhesive, apply a small piece of tape—without tension—on an area of skin that does not pass across a joint. This will remove human error as the cause of any reaction.

Round the corners of the tape to prevent lifting of the anchor or ends. Anchors should be a minimum of 1". and secured by rubbing before moving the fascia into the taping position. The anchors and ends of the tape are secured while the patient is in a neutral position. The paper substrate may be torn through the cotton tape, but if

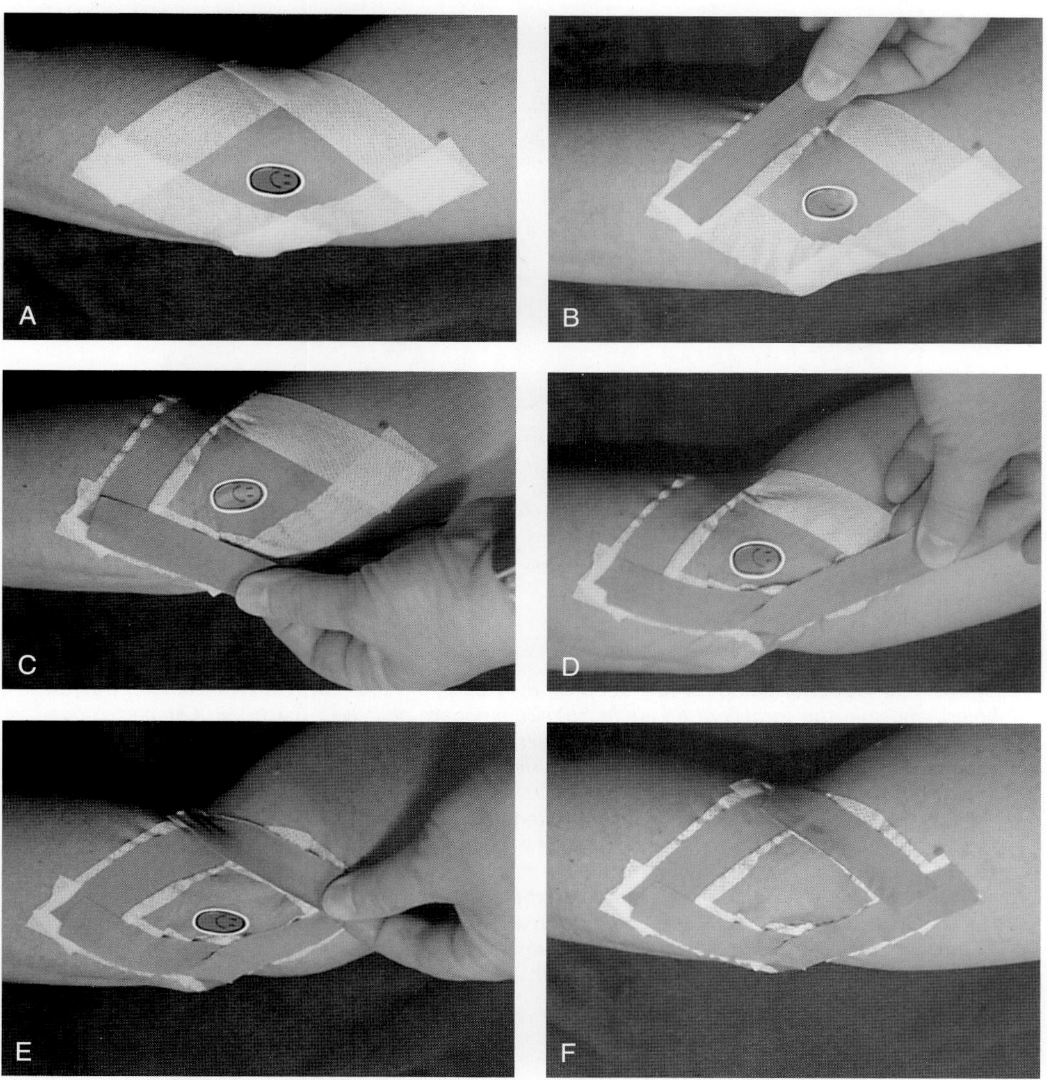

Figure 13–5 ***McConnell taping for lateral epicondylitis*** *(left elbow, lateral view).* ***A,*** *Place the undertape in a diamond configuration to surround the area of pain (noted with marker).* ***B,*** *Attach the brown tape at the inferior anterior section of the diamond, starting at the inferior apex. Stretch the fascia superior and anterior along the course of the undertape, and attach it at the anterior apex of the diamond.* ***C,*** *Repeat the process, placing the tape in the direction of the inferior posterior aspect of the diamond.* ***D,*** *Repeat, placing the tape at the posterior superior aspect of the diamond.* ***E,*** *Place the last tape at the anterior superior aspect to complete the diamond.* ***F,*** *Completed diamond deloading, without the pain marker.*

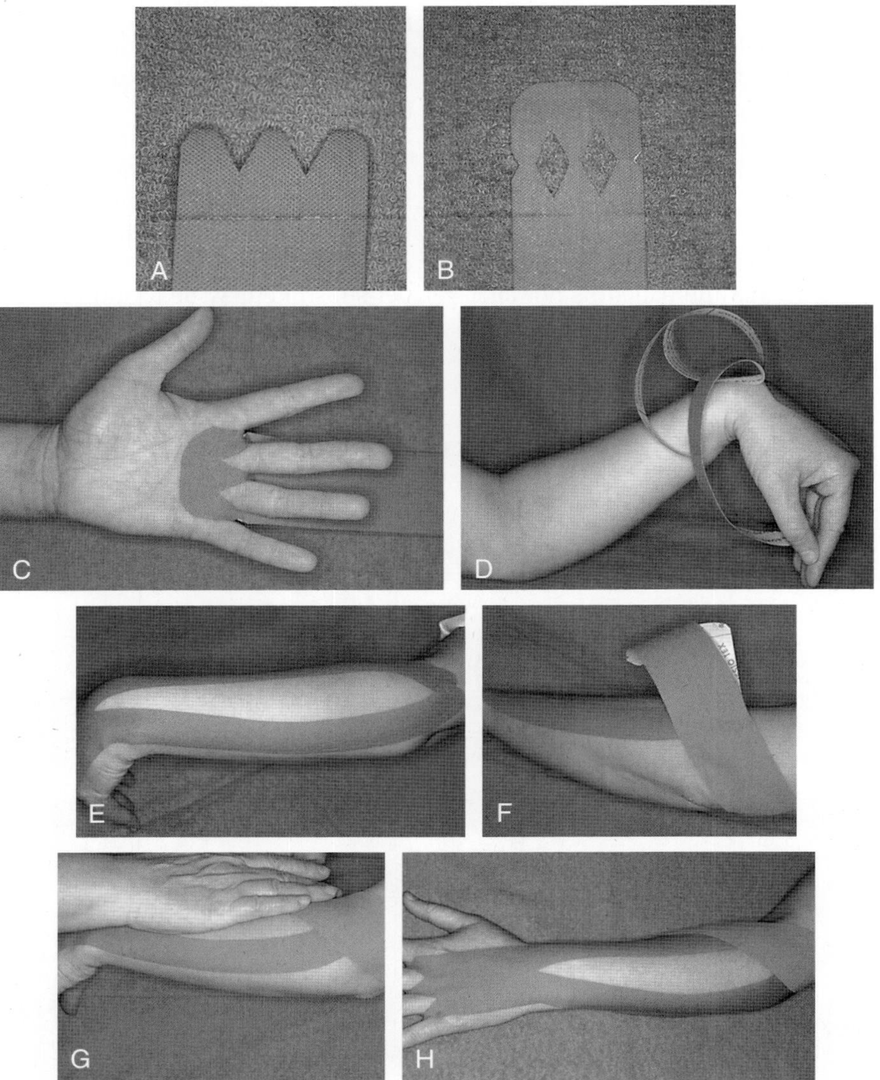

Figure 13–6 ***Kinesio taping for lateral epicondylitis. A,*** *Fold the tape, cut two triangles (fingerholes), and snip the corners at an angle (to accommodate digit web spaces).* ***B,*** *Completed buttonhole cut.* ***C,*** *Place the middle and ring fingers through openings and secure with a 1" to 2" volar anchor.* ***D,*** *Position the wrist in maximum flexion, and apply the tape over the dorsum of the hand to the wrist. The split should be located at the dorsum of the proximal wrist (over the muscle belly).* ***E,*** *Maintaining the wrist position, extend the elbow and apply the tape around the medial and lateral margins of the extensor muscle wad, ending at the lateral epicondyle.* ***F,*** *Apply an additional tape to help the supinator muscle relax, because it may put pressure on the radial nerve, creating similar symptoms. Apply the tape anchor just proximal to elbow, on an angle at the midline of the humerus.* ***G,*** *Position the forearm in pronation with the elbow in slight flexion to prevent compensatory movement of the humerus. Apply the tape over the lateral epicondyle and supinator, terminating on the medial ulnar side of the forearm.* ***H,*** *Completed taping.*

torn on the edge and pulled, it will tear across and not affect the elastic tape. To improve tension control, tear the paper substrate just after the anchor and fold back the edge of the paper to create a handle. Keeping the tape parallel and close to the skin, pull on this handle with one hand and follow behind with the IF of the opposite hand, smoothing the tape onto the skin while moving toward the end attachment site. Rub to create friction heat to secure.

The demarcations on the back of the substrate indicate the stretch direction (longitudinal marks) and 2" boxes. These can be used to help measure and cut the tape and when providing directions to the patient for self-application.

There may be some redness after removal, but it should resolve in about 30 min. To remove the glue from the skin, rub an oil or skin lotion (or cream) into the tape or use soap during bathing to decrease the removal trauma.

Carpal Tunnel Syndrome

Application

Kinesio taping for carpal tunnel syndrome uses a correction technique to lift the skin, creating a space in the area of inflammation or pain to improve lymph and vascular movement (Fig. 13–7). The target tissue is the retinacular ligament. The material required is a 2" wide I-cut tape.

General Considerations

The tape may be applied to either the volar or the dorsal aspect of the wrist, depending on the response of patient. The patient may experience changes over a 24-hr period and may benefit from the edema taping in combination with the correction technique. Do not apply tension to the ends of the tape from the midline of the wrist to the final attachment to the skin.

To best handle the tape for this technique, tear the edge of the substrate and pull, this will run the tear across the paper. Fold back the substrate to form two handles. Hold these in a lateral pinch fashion, and draw them apart directly over the area to be taped. Apply direct downward pressure; then smooth for good contact.

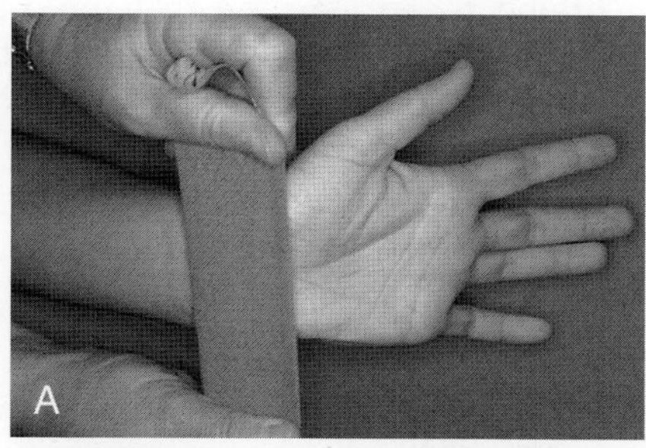

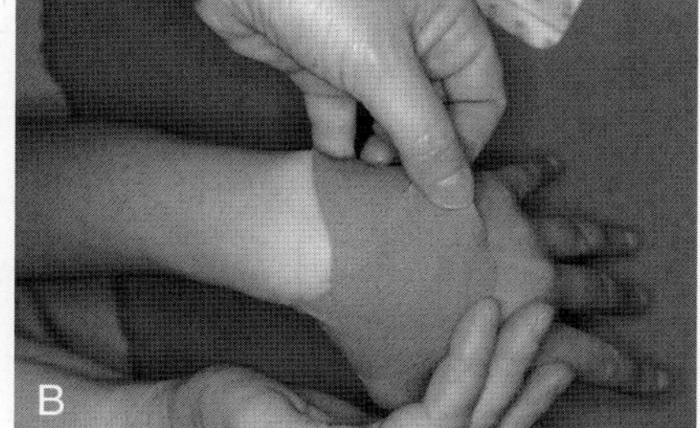

Figure 13–7 ***Kinesio taping for carpal tunnel syndrome.*** ***A,*** *Position the hand in tolerable active wrist extension. Apply correction tape (I-cut tape with all the stretch taken out of the center and applied directly down onto the area) over the transverse carpal ligament.* ***B,*** *move the wrist into relaxed flexion, and apply the ends without tension.*

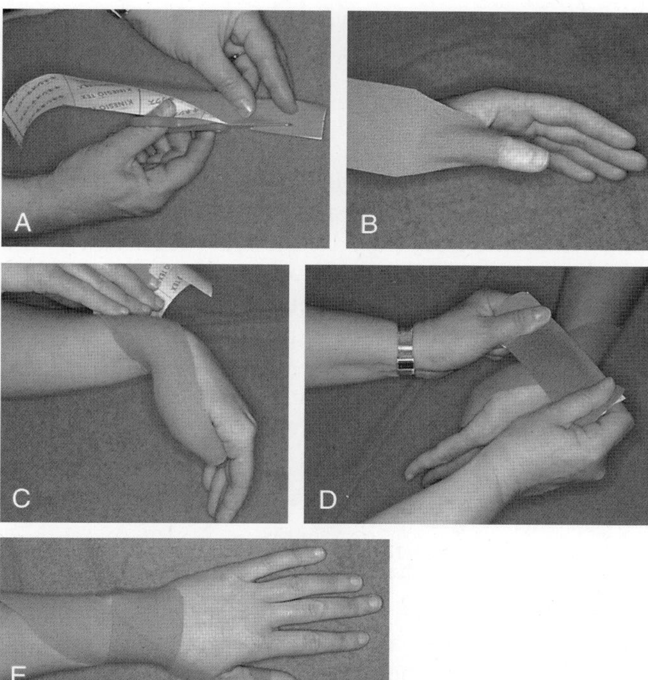

Figure 13–8 ***Kinesio taping for deQuervain's tenosynovitis.*** ***A,*** *Trim the end of the tape in a scallop or curved form to prevent circumferential restriction of the proximal phalanx.* ***B,*** *Place the anchor just proximal to thumb IP joint.* ***C,*** *With the elbow flexed, move the thumb into flexion and ulnarly deviate and flex the wrist as tolerated. Apply the tape along the radial aspect of the wrist and up onto the extensor surface, ending at the midforearm (origin of the abductor pollicis longus).* ***D,*** *Maintain the wrist position. A correction tape (all the stretch taken out) is placed over the retinacular ligament at the radial aspect of the wrist. Then apply the ends with no tension and the wrist relaxed in a neutral position.* ***E,*** *Circumferentially secure the distal thumb anchor with crosscut pieces of ½-in.-wide Kinesio Tex tape (inelastic).*

deQuervain's Tenosynovitis

Application

The target tissues for Kinesio taping for deQuervain's tenosynovitis are the inflamed extensor pollicis brevis and abductor pollicis longus; therefore, the tape is applied from insertion to origin (Fig. 13–8). Retinacular ligament taping uses a correction technique to lift the skin and fascia, reducing edema and improving vascular flow. The materials required are a 2" wide I-cut tape, 2" wide I-cut tape (as described earlier for carpal tunnel syndrome), and two ½" crosscut pieces of tape.

General Considerations

The ½" securing tapes for the anchor should be applied loosely, so as not to constrict, and may be applied after the muscle taping. This taping is also affective for relieving some forms of carpometacarpal (CMC) pain and edema. To increase the I tape conformity on the thumb and web space, fold the tape and scallop it slightly to create a 1" area of tape contact on the dorsal thumb, gradually increase to cover the thenar area of the thumb.

Edema and Scar Management

Application

The target tissue for Kinesio taping for edema and scar management is tight flexor and extensor muscles that inhibit lymphatic flow (Fig. 13–9). The movement of the fascia during normal activity also assists in lymph drainage. A correction technique is used at the wrist to lift the scar tissue in a second plane of motion, decreasing adhesions. This tape can be placed along the original taping at any point. The materials required are a 2" water-resistant tape, buttonhole cut (as described for lateral epicondylitis).

General Considerations

This technique is effective for treating postoperative pain and edema, but take care with acutely healing tissues. Taping may be placed on the dorsum, avoiding contact with surgical areas, and still be effective in reducing edema. The taping should be combined with active motion, as this creates movement and massaging of the skin to improve lymphatic return.

To assist in proper adherence in finger web spaces, gently pull the tape and then relax to allow it to settle and improve skin contact. Kinesio Tex tape has improved adherence when it is in contact with itself.

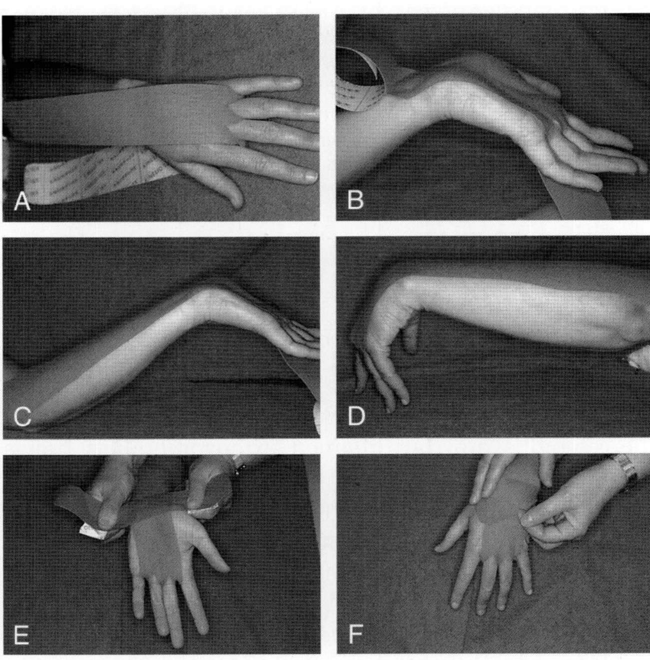

Figure 13–9 ***Kinesio taping for edema and scar management.*** ***A,*** *Place buttonhole-cut tape through the middle and ring fingers.* ***B,*** *With the wrist in maximum extension, apply the tape to the volar surface of the hand to the wrist.* ***C,*** *Apply the tape over the flexor muscle mass. ending at the medial epicondyle.* ***D,*** *Move the wrist into maximum flexion. Apply the tape over the dorsum of the hand, wrist, and extensor muscles, ending at lateral epicondyle.* ***E,*** *Place the scar (volar) on stretch, and apply a correction tape (all the stretch out) perpendicular to the first taping.* ***F,*** *Then move the wrist into flexion, and apply the tape without tension to the edge of the dorsal strip to prevent circumferential restriction.*

CONCLUSION

Taping is not for every patient or therapist and should be employed with caution and sound clinical judgment. In addition, taping should not be viewed as a replacement for traditional forms of splinting, because it holds a special place in upper extremity rehabilitation. The advantages of soft tissue support and increased joint mobility that taping provides place it in a class of its own. Athletic taping has had a longer history and is supported by more clinical research studies than the other taping methods. This is primarily the result of its popularity in sports medicine.

There is limited available research on McConnell or Kinesio taping. Unpublished anecdotal reports can be found on the World Wide Web, and clinical studies are in progress. Web sites also provide information on educational opportunities and links or resources for obtaining taping supplies. Some sites offer instructional vignettes to assist the novice.

The limitations of splinting may also be found with taping. For example, patients may not want to wear the tape in public or may object to wearing the tape for a prolonged period of time. Patients may become frustrated when learning to handle and manage the tape. Therapist may have difficulty finding clinical education. A strong educational base is important; but as with all new skills, it takes time and practice to develop proficiency.

REFERENCES

Arnheim, D., & Prentice, W. (2000). *Principles of athletic training* (10th ed.). New York: McGraw-Hill.

Austin, K., Gwynn-Brett, K., & Marshall, S. (1994). *Illustrated guide to taping techniques.* London: Mosby-Wolfe.

Birrer, R. B. (1994). *Sports medicine for the primary care physician* (2nd ed.). Boca Raton, FL: CRC Press.

Canelon, M. F. (1995). Silicone rubber splinting for athletic and wrist injuries. *Journal of Hand Therapy, 4,* 152–157.

Cyr, L. M., & Ross, R. G. (1998). How controlled stress affects healing tissues. *Journal of Hand Therapy, 2,* 125–130.

Fess, E. E., & McCollum, M. (1998). The influence of splinting on healing tissues. *Journal of Hand Therapy, 2,* 157–161.

Henshaw, J., Satren, J. W., & Wrightsman, J. A. (1989). The semi-flexible support: An alternative for the hand injured worker. *Journal of Hand Therapy, 1,* 35–40.

Hilfrank, B. C. (1991). Protecting the injured hand for sports. *Journal of Hand Therapy, 2,* 51–56.

Kase, K., Hashimotom, T., & Okane, T, (1996). *Kinesio taping perfect manual.* Albuquerque: Kinesio Taping Association.

Kase, K. (1994). *Illustrated Kinesio-taping* (1st ed.). Tokyo: Ken'iKar.

Murphy, J. (1996). A wrap-up on taping. *Advance for Physical Therapists, 7*.

Rettig, A. C., Stube, K. S., & Shelbourne, K. D. (1997). Effects of finger and wrist taping on grip strength. *American Journal of Sports Medicine, 1,* 96–98.

Tremain, L. (1996). Meeting the needs of managed care with McConnell method. *Advance Rehabilitation, 5,* 37–39.

SUGGESTED READING

Sports Medicine Council of British Columbia. (1995). *Manual of athletic taping* (3rd ed.). Philadelphia: Davis.

WORLD WIDE WEB RESOURCES

Kinesio Taping Web Site. www.kinesiotaping.com. Accessed Dec. 11, 2001.

McConnell Institute. www.mcconnell-institute.com. Accessed Dec. 11, 2001.

Nicholas Institute of Sports Medicine and Athletic Trauma. www.nismat.org. Accessed Dec. 11, 2001.

CHAPTER 14

Splinting with Neoprene

Nicole Jacobs, OTR/L, CHT, and Christy Halpin, OTR/L, CHT

INTRODUCTION

Neoprene (polychloroprene) is a synthetic Latex-free polymer. Neoprene was first used for making wetsuits because of its flexibility and insulation properties (Stern, Callinan, Mark, Schousboe, & Yutterberg, 1998). Therapists have come to use Neoprene as an option for splinting because of these same properties. The material is able to conform and drape, making it easy to work with. Neoprene is a unique splinting alternative as it can offer support to the incorporated joint(s) while still allowing for some motion (Colditz, 1999). Until recently, fabricating custom-made Neoprene splints required sewing, which was impractical for many therapists. Thus prefabricated Neoprene splints were the preferred option; however, proper fit can be a challenge and it is costly to maintain the necessary inventory. New custom Neoprene materials offer an alternative and an inexpensive way to fabricate these soft splints without the use of a sewing machine (Colditz, 1999).

Benefits of Neoprene

Why use Neoprene? Neoprene is an excellent insulator, protecting the involved area from at-risk situations such as water and cold temperatures. The compressive qualities help reduce edema while providing comfort and warmth. Neoprene is able to conform over bony prominences with minimal concern of creating localized areas of pressure. Although Neoprene is flexible, it also provides a gentle support. Thermoplastic reinforcement can be added to the Neoprene splint base, which increases the rigidity of the splint if more support is required. Finally, Neoprene can be washed and air-dried with ease.

Common Uses

Neoprene splinting may be an option for a variety of situations and diagnoses. These uses include arthritis, cold intolerance, repetitive strain injuries and occupational assists, pediatric disorders, neuromuscular problems, and sports injury protection.

Arthritis

Neoprene can be used for patients who have osteoarthritis, rheumatoid arthritis, or a related rheumatic disease. Neoprene has the ability to protect and support the involved joint(s) gently while providing warmth and gentle compression. For example, a soft hand-based thumb splint may be fabricated for an individual with symptoms of a first carpometacarpal (CMC) joint osteoarthritis (Fig. 14–1**A**,**B**). Neoprene may also reduce friction and irritation, prevent abutment of bony prominences (such as Bouchard nodes), and protect subcutaneous nodules from pressure irritation (Anderson, Hall, & Martin, 2000; Colditz, 1999; Melvin, 1995). Neoprene can be quickly and easily fabricated into a comfortable splint for combating ulnar drift (Fig. 14–1**C**,**D**).

Cold Intolerance and Hypersensitivity

Individuals with Raynaud's phenomenon or a crush injury with resultant sensory problems may benefit from the neutral warmth and gentle compression Neoprene materials can provide. These characteristics may promote blood flow and increase functional tolerance (Colditz, 1999; Melvin, 1995). For example, a digit cap or sleeve may be fabricated out of Neoprene to protect an individual with a healing digital nerve repair (Fig. 14–2). The cap may be small enough to fit under a work glove while allowing near full mobility. Neoprene splints may be an option in the workplace when symptoms are resolving and a rigid support is no longer necessary (Wright & Rettig, 1995). Such splints can offer protection

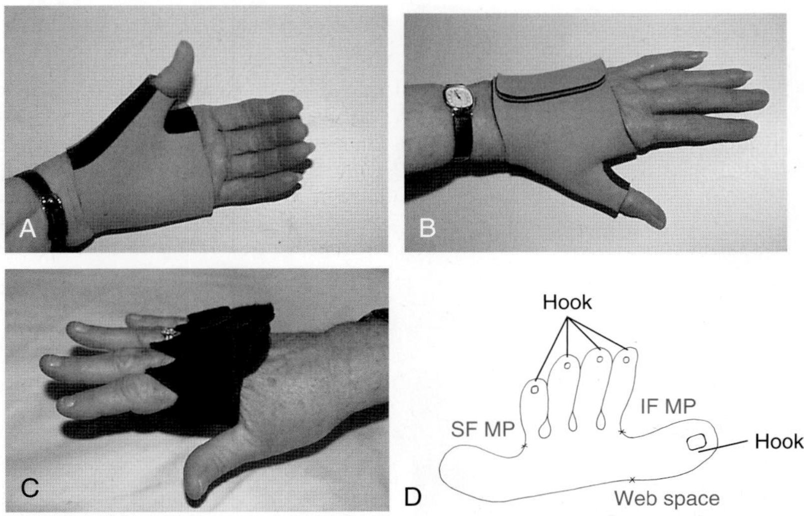

Figure 14–1 *Volar (**A**) and dorsal (**B**) views of a thumb splint for CMC joint osteoarthritis. An ulnar drift splint (**C**) and pattern (**D**) for rheumatoid arthritis at the MP joints. Mark for the first web space and small finger and index finger MP joints. Iron on the hook and trim as needed.*

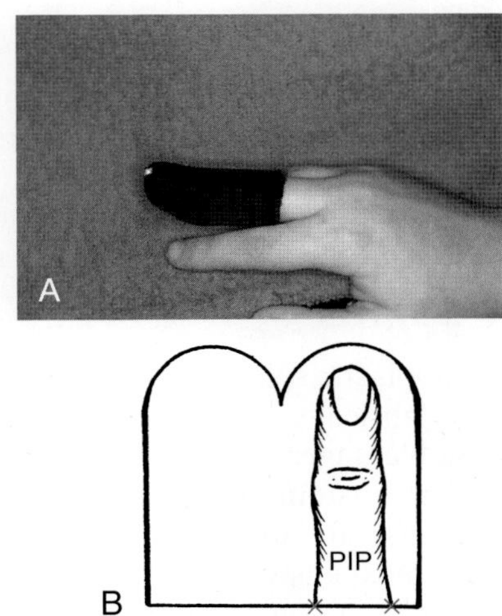

Figure 14–2 ***A,** A digit cap is commonly used to protect a hypersensitive digit during healing of a digital nerve repair. **B,** Use 3/32" or 1/16" material and allow for a 1/4" seam. Add tape, iron on for closure.*

to a vulnerable area from occupational hazards such as cold temperatures and/or vibration related to tool and machine use. For example, a thin circumferential Neoprene material may be used to protect and insulate a sensitive stump after an amputation at the distal interphalangeal (DIP) joint level while allowing the patient to return to work in a factory setting.

Repetitive Strain Injuries

Musculotendinous injuries such as deQuervain's tenosynovitis, wrist tendonitis, and lateral or medial epicondylitis may benefit from Neoprene's compression, light restriction, and warmth properties. A circumferential Neoprene wrap, with a foam or gel insert, serves as a proximal forearm splint (counterforce brace) for lateral or medial epicondylitis (Fig. 14–**3A**). Another example is a distal forearm-based wrist/thumb splint for a hairstylist who has intersection syndrome (tenosynovitis at the junction of the first and second dorsal compartments) and who is not able to wear a stiff thermoplastic splint because of the nature of his or her work (e.g., scissors use, blow drying) (Fig. 14–**3B,C**) (Leonard, 1995). Neoprene may be an alternative to rigid splinting for a worker that has carpal tunnel symptoms; the material may aid in reducing friction, absorbing shock and vibration, dispersing the impact area of vibratory tool use, and preventing extreme wrist positioning (Anderson et al., 2000).

Pediatric Patients

Thermoplastic splints can often aid in positioning the hands and limbs of young children; but, at the same time, they can significantly restrict function and inhibit sensation. Neoprene is an ideal choice for splinting when dynamic mobility is the goal. Splints made from Neoprene allow for functional use while maintaining optimal joint positioning (Casey & Kratz, 1988; Wilton, 1997). Neoprene can also be used to aid in managing tone and preventing joint contractures (see Chapters 21 and 22 for more information) (Lohman, 1996; McKee & Morgan, 1998). Small Neoprene splints are lightweight, stretchable, and easy for even children to apply. The color selection makes splint wearing fun for children and, it is hoped, increases compliance.

Neuromuscular Problems

Neoprene can be used as a functional transition splint (from a rigid thermoplastic splint to a soft splint) for a

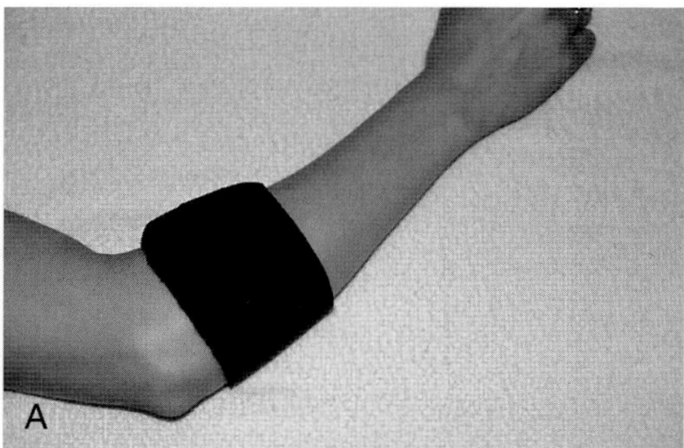

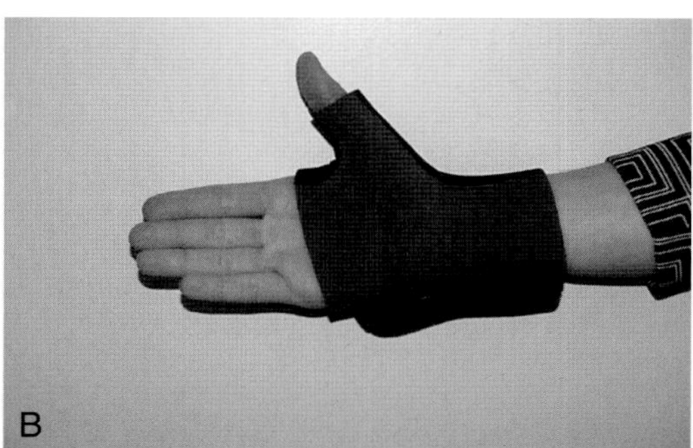

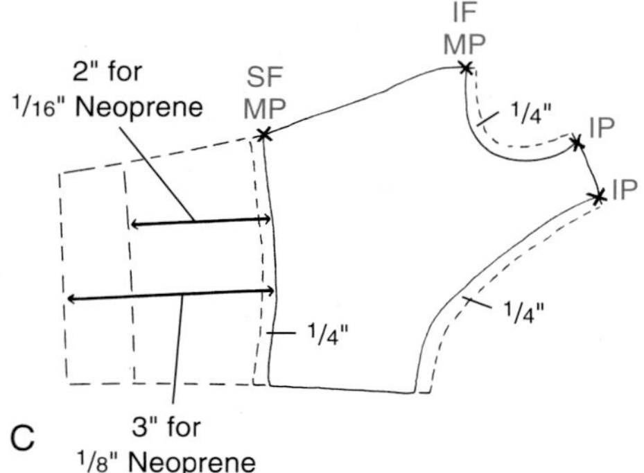

*Figure 14–3 Splints commonly used for repetitive strain injuries. **A,** proximal forearm splint for lateral or medial epicondylitis. **B,** Wrist/thumb splint for deQuervain's tenosynovitis. **C,** The final pattern for the wrist/thumb splint involves two pieces. Allow ¼" for the seam and 2" to 3" for the overlap depending on the material's thickness and stretch.*

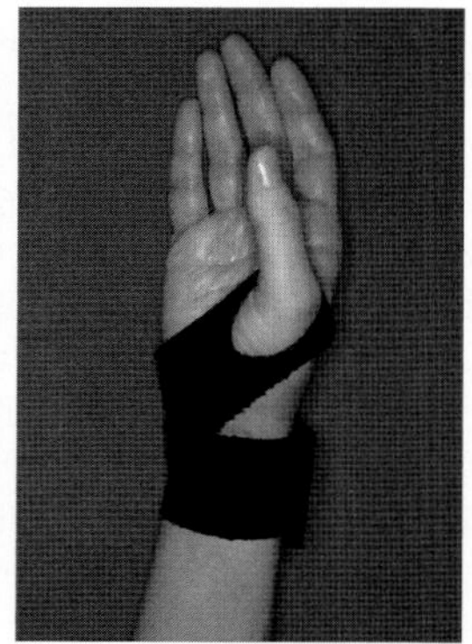

Figure 14–4 This thumb abduction/opposition strap is being used 6 weeks after median nerve repair.

variety of diagnoses (e.g., regenerating nerve), for protection after a tendon transfer, or to assist a weak muscle. Because of its light weight and elastic qualities, Neoprene can help with joint positioning while allowing some degree of mobility. For example, Neoprene can be used for a thumb abduction/opposition strap after median nerve laceration or repair (Fig. 14–4).

Sports Injury Protection

Various types of Neoprene sleeves can be custom fabricated to provide comfortable circumferential pressure and warmth as well as a light, nonrestrictive support for a chronic sports injury (Anderson et al., 2000). Examples include a wrist splint for a suspected distal ulna instability in a gymnast and an elbow splint for a baseball pitcher who is diagnosed with medial tension overload syndrome in the elbow (Fig. 14–5) (Anderson et al., 2000; Wright & Rettig, 1995).

Prefabricated Versus Custom Neoprene Splints

Similar to thermoplastic splinting, Neoprene splints are available in prefabricated designs. There are advantages and disadvantages to both the prefabricated splints and the custom-made ones. Prefabricated splints can be easy to apply and adjust. Generally, these splints are inexpensive, but the rehabilitation department must have a constant stock of several types and sizes, which may lead to an increase in the overall splint cost. Custom-designed Neoprene splints are relatively inexpensive to make and can be fit to the patient. The material is available with several different fabric liners and in a variety of colors. This makes the splint not only comfortable but also aesthetically pleasing.

Figure 14–5 Simple wrist wrap for a gymnast with distal ulna instability. This strap helps to decrease distal ulna mobility, thereby decreasing pain with forearm rotation.

These qualities may increase patient compliance in wearing the splint (Simin, 2000).

Characteristics of Neoprene

When considering the different types of Neoprene, one must understand the characteristics unique to this splinting material. Neoprene is a black rubber material, and it is covered by fabric when used for splinting. Companies and vendors who sell Neoprene may use their own terminology For example, North Coast Medical (Morgan Hill, CA) has its own line of Neoprene, which is called Neoloop and Comfortprene. These materials all stem from Neoprene and have similar qualities.

Elasticity

Neoprene is very elastic, enhancing its conformability about the intimate structures of the upper limb. Neoprene, when stretched, has 100% memory; however, with repeated stress and stretching, the material may lose 10 to 15% of its elasticity (Colditz, 1999). The outer covering that encases the core Neoprene can alter the material's ability to stretch. Such Neoprene liners are commonly made from **nylon, unbroken loop (UBL) cloth,** or **terry cloth** (Colditz, 1999; Simin, 2000). Material selection is key for diagnosis-specific splint fabrication. The characteristics of each fabric are as follows:

Nylon

- Adds no bulk to the Neoprene (is thin).
- Allows full stretch and drape.
- Provides moderate durability of exterior or interior linings.
- Takes time to add fasteners (needs iron-on hook and loop).
- Feels slick and cool against the skin.
- Bonds best with iron-on seam tape.

Unbroken loop

- Feels similar to loop strapping material.
- Adds bulk to the Neoprene (is thick).
- Reduces the amount of stretch and drape.
- Offers maximum durability for exterior or interior linings.
- Feels cushiony, fuzzy, and warm against the skin.
- Takes no time to add fasteners (use hook strap directly anywhere).
- Bonds well with iron-on seam tape.
- Allows quick application of supportive straps for any splint.

Terry cloth

- Adds no bulk to the Neoprene (is thin).
- Allows full stretch and drape.
- Provides maximum durability for interior linings (rarely used on exterior).
- Takes minimal time to add fasteners (use hook strap for short term, iron-on fasteners for permanent use).
- Feels soft and cool against the skin.
- Bonds well with iron-on seam tape.

Thickness

Neoprene comes in a variety of thicknesses. It is important to remember that the thickness measurement applies only to the black rubber core (Colditz, 1999). The thickness is increased when exterior or interior linings are adding (Simin, 2000). The range of available thicknesses allows for creativity in splint design. The clinical applications of different thicknesses of Neoprene are similar to those of thermoplastic materials. Larger body parts are best splinted with thicker materials, because they provide stronger support, protection, and compression but tend to be less conforming (Simin, 2000). Thinner materials may be the best option for smaller body parts, because they provide a lighter support, protection, and compression and tend to allow greater motion and functional use. Thinner materials also provide more conformability and drape (Simin, 2000). For example, a thin Neoprene core with a nylon covering can be used for a digit cap, and a thicker Neoprene core with a terry lining can be used for an elbow sleeve. The most common core thicknesses of Neoprene materials used in splinting are $\frac{1}{8}$" (5 mm), $\frac{3}{32}$" (2.5 mm), and $\frac{1}{16}$" (1.5 mm) (Colditz, 1999; Simin, 2000).

Insulation

The black rubber core of Neoprene is composed of closed cells. Because of this, Neoprene allows minimal air and water exchange and acts as an excellent insulator (Colditz, 1999). Some Neoprene materials are commercially available with **macroperforations** and **microperforations.** For example, North Coast Medical's Comfortprene is a perforated material. These perforations can affect Neoprene's insulating properties; the macroperforations allow good air exchange for keeping the skin dry and cool, which can be excellent choice for athletic use. The increase in perforations may make the splint lighter and less bulky with a greater degree of stretch about the body part it is applied. Because of the larger holes, smooth, neat edges may not always be possible (Simin, 2000). Microperforations allow less airflow to the skin. The weight, drape, and stretch properties of the perforated material are similar to those of solid Neoprene sheets (Simin, 2000). The characteristics of perforated Neoprene are as follows:

Macroperforated

- Provides maximum air exchange to keep the skin dry and cool.
- Decreases the weight of the splint.
- Moderately increases the drape and stretchability.
- Creates bumpy appearance and jagged cut edges

Microperforated

- Provides some air exchange to keep skin dry and cool.
- Slightly decreases weight of splint.

- Minimally increases drape and stretchability.
- Creates neat cut edges and a smooth surface finish.

Cushioning

Neoprene is an ideal cushion between two surfaces and over bony prominences because of its closed cellular makeup. This helps decrease sheer stress to the underlying tissue, which is sometimes caused with rigid splinting. Because of this quality, Neoprene does not sustain permanent changes with prolonged compression, making it a good option for padding (Colditz, 1999).

Colors

Neoprene is available in a variety of colors, depending on the vendor. Patients who are given the option to choose a color may demonstrate increased compliance with overall wear (Simin, 2000). For the athlete, colors can be combined (material, taping, and strapping) to match school colors or uniform clothing. For people with arthritis who are self-conscious about their hands, a neutral skin tone color may be the preferred choice.

Precautions

Although it is rare, there are reported cases of **allergic contact dermatitis (ACD)** and **prickly heat (miliaria rubra)** caused by Neoprene use (Colditz, 1999; Stern et al., 1998). When issuing a prefabricated or custom-designed Neoprene splint, it is important to instruct patients to monitor skin integrity frequently. The wonderfully warm compressive qualities of Neoprene may be very inviting to some patients; but for others, it may be intolerable. Caution should be used when dispensing these splints for use during strenuous exercise or heavy manual labor and for use in very warm climates. Skin breakdown and maceration may become problematic (Colditz, 1999).

To reduce the risk of skin irritation, the splint should be frequently hand washed with mild soapy water or machine washed in a gentle cycle with all hook and loop fastened. Neoprene splints should be thoroughly air dried before reapplication. Stockinette helps absorb sweat but does not act as a barrier to ACD (Stern et al., 1998). Neoprene is also available with perforations that may be useful in minimizing these issues.

General Guidelines for Neoprene Splinting

The guidelines of splinting with Neoprene are similar to splinting with thermoplastics. Make a paper pattern, taking into consideration the characteristics of the material. Fit the pattern to the patient and trim as needed. Once a pattern has been traced, the actual splint fabrication does not require the patient to be present. This is beneficial if time constraints are a factor. Transfer the pattern to the Neoprene with a vanishing-ink pen (so the lines do not show on the completed splint). Cut out the Neoprene, making sure to cut squarely so that the edges fit when making a seam.

Glue the core Neoprene material with cement made specifically for Neoprene. The glue will adhere immediately but requires approximately 24 hr to reach its maximum strength. Reinforce the seams with iron-on seam tape. Fit the splint to the patient, and trim as necessary (Colditz, 1999). If the patient is not present during splint fabrication, make final fitting adjustments at the follow-up visit. The specific materials required to get started and a step-by-step process are described below. The materials needed for fabricating a Neoprene splint are as follows (Fig. 14–6):

- Neoprene material.
- Iron-on seam tape.
- Iron-on hook-and-loop tape or strips.
- Iron.
- Seal cement.
- Disappearing-ink marking pen.
- Thenar web space thermoplastic form.
- Small dowel.

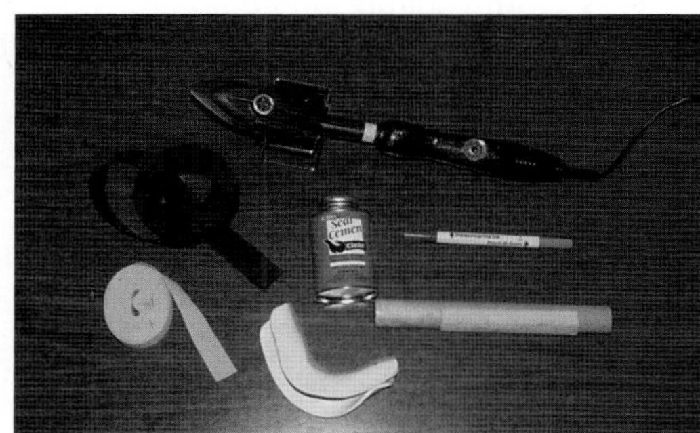

Figure 14–6 Equipment and materials needed to fabricate Neoprene splints.

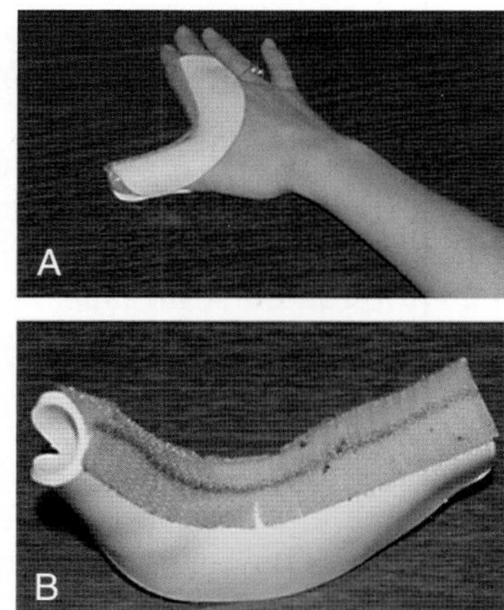

*Figure 14–7 Thumb web space form on **(A)** and off **(B)** the patient. Note that a marker was used as a guide to line up the two pieces of material during the gluing process.*

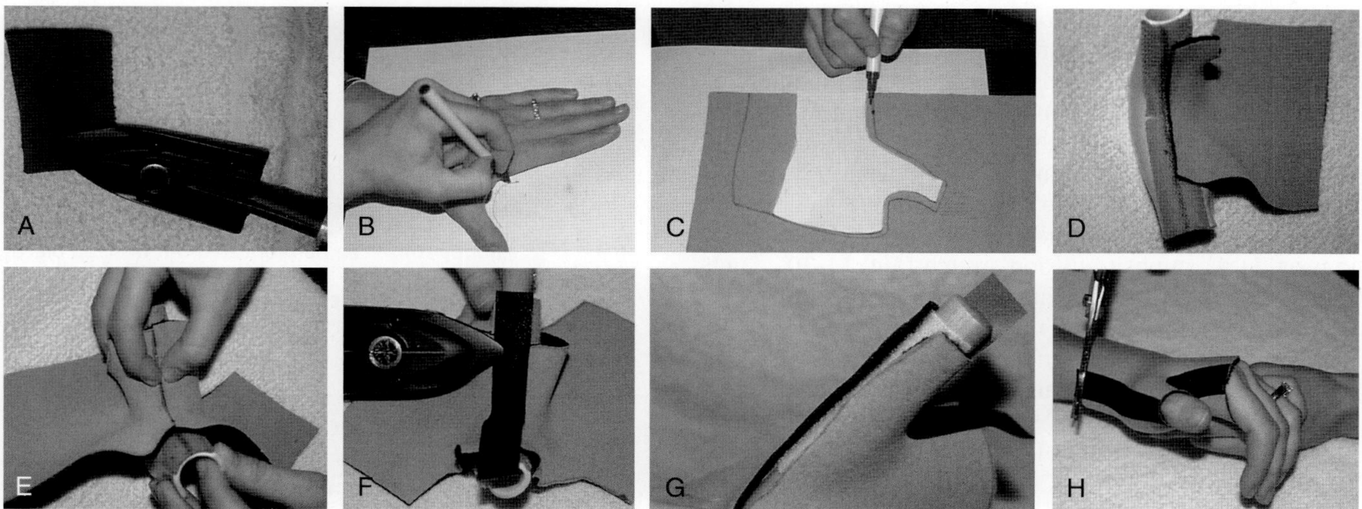

*Figure 14–8 Steps for fabricating a Neoprene thumb splint, **A,** Set the iron to the midrange on the dial, and let it heat; test a small area of the Neoprene and heat-sensitive seam tape. If the Neoprene and tape do not adhere within 15 sec, increase the temperature and test again. **B,** Trace the patient's hand on paper from the MP joints to the wrist, making sure the wrist is in neutral and not radially or ulnarly deviated. Trace the thumb in full radial abduction, paying special attention to tracing the thumb web space as precisely as possible. **C,** Place two pieces of Neoprene material, wrong sides facing, and use folded-over sticky backed hook between the layers to stabilize them. The piece of Neoprene that will be the dorsal piece should be 2" to 3" wider than the other. Trace the pattern onto the top (dorsal) piece of Neoprene material. Trace ¼" wider than the pattern along the radial side to allow for the seam. Add 2" to 3" of width to the top piece along the ulnar side. **D,** Cut out the pattern. Remember that the top piece is wider than the bottom (volar) piece. It is important for the two pieces to be attached with hook so they are cut exactly the same. Keep the scissors parallel to the Neoprene to maintain a flat edge, which is necessary for bonding of the radial-side seam. Take the volar piece of Neoprene and place the web space area from the Neoprene pattern onto the thermoplastic web space form. Match up the Neoprene with the line drawn down the middle of the piece of hook on the web space form. Lightly apply the seal cement (glue) to the black core material of Neoprene in the web space area of the dorsal piece. First, heat the seal cement with a heat gun until the cement has set up. Small bubbles will be seen in the seal cement when it is ready. **E,** Now attach the web spaces from both pieces together onto the web space form, using the line drawn onto the hook for alignment. Using your fingers, pinch the edges together, moving from distal to proximal. Allow a few moments for the seam to set up before moving on to the next step. **F,** Press the seam tape over the seam while it is still on the web space form. Apply the iron directly to the tape for 15 sec at a time. Look for melted glue to show along the edges of the tape. If the iron is held in one spot too long, the seam glue can come apart. **G,** Remove the splint from the web space form. Apply glue to the next seam, and use a dowel to align edges to form the thumbhole. Follow the same steps, substituting the dowel for the web space form. Remove the splint from the dowel. Attach the iron-on hook strip to the Neoprene by placing a piece of paper towel between the iron and the hook material. Apply the iron for 15 sec at a time, and look for the melted glue on the edges of the hook strip. Let the strip cool or at least 30 min before applying stress. **H,** Check the fit, and trim as necessary. Trim the seam tape.*

The particular type of Neoprene material used depends on the goals of the splint, as discussed earlier. A household iron can be used, or the therapist may use a small iron developed for splint fabrication (e.g., Handy Iron from North Coast Medical). Be sure to choose a cement that is specifically formulated to work with Neoprene. Simin (2000) suggests adding a piece of adhesive hook material to the thermoplastic web space form and drawing a line down the center of the hook material to aid in matching up the two halves of Neoprene during splint fabrication (Fig. 14–7). The steps for fabricating a Neoprene thumb splint are outlined in Figure 14–8).

Alternative Uses of Neoprene

As with thermoplastics, tapes, and other casting materials, the possibilities of therapeutic uses of Neoprene are endless. Neoprene makes an excellent strap choice when dealing with patients with skin integrity issues or when strapping over bony and/or easily irritated areas, such as the posterior elbow, volar wrist, and thenar web space (Fig. 14–9) (Colditz, 1999). Neoprene can be cut to any width, which is ideal for distributing forces over a larger area, as may be necessary with an edematous extremity or when splinting over a healed skin graft or burn site.

The length and shape can be contoured to accommodate challenging areas, such as the digital web spaces.

The Neoprene straps can be used in combination with a thermoplastic splint to provide a mobilization force to a tight joint. For example, with a splint base of a wrist extension/metacarpophalangeal (MP) flexion immobilization splint, a Neoprene strap can be applied to traverse the proximal interphalangeal (PIP) and DIP joints to provide a composite flexion stretch (Fig. 14–10). Such a splint/Neoprene combination is easy to fabricate and, when worn appropriately, may be quite effective. Small leftover scraps of Neoprene material can be used for padding around bony prominences, buddy strapping two digits, or strapping around small areas, such as the digital and thenar web spaces (Fig. 14–11).

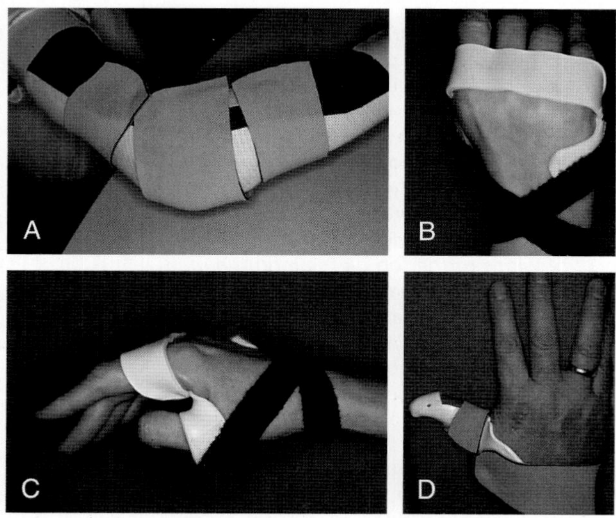

Figure 14–9 Using strapping with Neoprene splints. ***A,*** *Anterior elbow immobilization splint with wide conforming straps.* ***B and C,*** *Wraparound straps for an MP extension restriction splint can be challenging to secure when atrophy is present.* ***D,*** *Comfortable strapping about the wrist used with a thumb immobilization splint.*

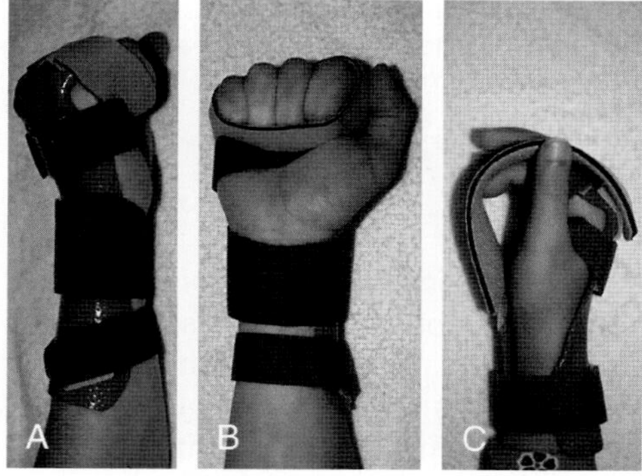

Figure 14–10 Composite flexion splints that use both Neoprene and thermoplastic materials. Ulnar ***(A)*** *and volar* ***(B)*** *views of a composite flexion splint.* ***C,*** *Index finger composite flexion splint that utilizes a dorsal strap application.*

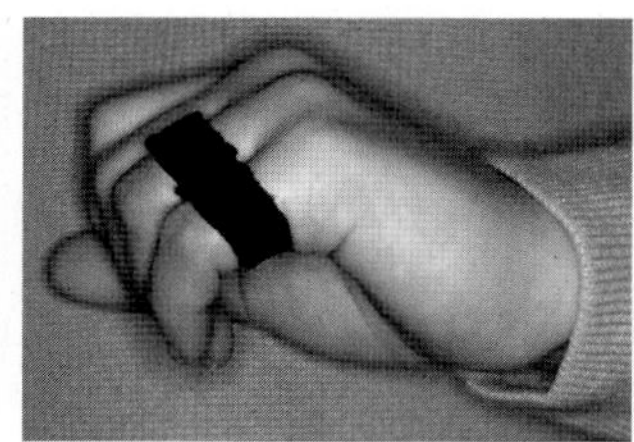

Figure 14–11 Buddy straps can be fabricated out of scrap pieces of Neoprene.

CONCLUSION

Neoprene is an excellent choice for splinting, based on its characteristics, ease of application, soft texture, and cosmesis. The new and easy approach for fabricating Neoprene splints without sewing makes it an excellent option for therapists. As with any therapeutic intervention, monitoring the tissue status is key to preventing progression of any adverse reactions to this unique material.

REFERENCES

Anderson, M. K., Hall, H. J., & Martin, M. (2000). *Sports injury management* (2nd ed.). Philadelphia: Lippincott Williams & Wilkins.

Casey, C. A., & Kratz, E. J. (1988). Soft splinting with Neoprene. The thumb abduction supinator splint. *American Journal of Occupational Therapy, 42,* 395–398.

Colditz, J. C. (1999). *Splinting with Neoprene.* Morgan Hill, CA: North Coast Medical.

Leonard, J. B (1995). Joint protection for inflammatory disorders. In J. M. Hunter, E. J. Mackin, & A. D. Callahan (Eds.). *Rehabilitation of the hand* (4th ed., pp. 1377–1383). St. Louis: Mosby Year Book.

Lohman, M. (1996). Antispasticity splinting. In B. M. Coppard & H. Lohman (Eds.). *Introduction to splinting: A critical-thinking and problem-solving approach* (pp. 194–224). St. Louis: Mosby Year Book.

McKee, P., & Morgan, L. (1998). *Orthotics in rehabilitation: Splinting the hand and body.* Philadelphia: Davis.

Melvin, J. L. (1995). Scleroderma (systemic sclerosis): Treatment of the hand. In J. M. Hunter, E. J. Mackin, & A. D. Callahan (Eds.). *Rehabilitation of the hand* (4th ed., pp. 1385–1397). St. Louis: Mosby Year Book.

Simin, H. (2000). *Splinting with Neoprene* [Course Syllabus]. Morgan Hill, CA: North Coast Medical.

Stern, E. B., Callinan, N. J., Mark, L. E., Schousboe, J. T., & Yutterberg, S. R. (1998). Neoprene splinting: Dermatological issues. *American Journal of Occupational Therapy, 52,* 573–578.

Wilton, J. C. (1997). Splinting and casting in the presence of neurological dysfunction. In J. C. Wilton (Ed.). *Hand splinting: Principles of design and fabrication* (168–197). Philadelphia: Saunders.

Wright, H. H., & Rettig, A. C. (1995). Management of common sports injuries. In J. M. Hunter, E. J. Mackin, & A. D. Callahan (Eds.). *Rehabilitation of the hand* (4th ed., pp. 1809–1838). St. Louis: Mosby Year Book.

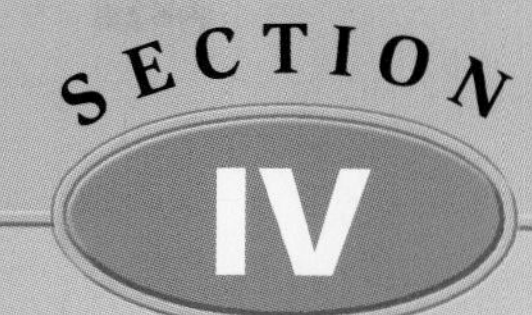

Splinting for Specific Diagnoses and Populations

CHAPTER

15

We should regard the hand as a mobile organ and never let it stiffen. It must move to survive.

—STERLING BUNNELL, 1947

Stiffness

Karen Schultz-Johnson, MS, OTR/L, FAOTA, CHT

INTRODUCTION

In the 1999 keynote address at the American Association of Hand Surgeons Seminar on Joint Stiffness, Hardy noted that, while the profession has made great strides in hand surgery and rehabilitation, joint stiffness continues to remain a challenge. **Stiffness,** the loss of normal passive range of motion (PROM) and active range of motion (AROM), remains one of the most common reasons for visiting an upper extremity therapy clinic (Copeland, 1997). Although the clinician has many weapons in the therapy armamentarium for improving PROM, splinting is the most powerful.

But how do clinicians know when to apply a splint and what type will offer the best outcome for the patient? To find the answer, therapists combine a thorough understanding of the diagnosis with a comprehensive evaluation. The clinician also needs the well-honed ability to see into the future. This does not suggest the ability to be clairvoyant but, rather, states the importance of knowing, according to the tissues affected, the predictable effects of position, the progression of wound healing (see Chapter 3 for more information), and the potential contractures.

This chapter describes how the therapist applies knowledge of wound healing and of the unique anatomy and mechanics of each joint to predict and avoid or to evaluate and treat joint stiffness. After reviewing the nature and cause of joint stiffness, the effect of splinting on tissue length is presented. The contribution of a variety of clinical entities to the loss of PROM is discussed along with a joint-by-joint review of the structures that, when wounded, adversely positioned, or affected by scar, lead to limited PROM. Table 15–1 summarizes the common contractures seen in the upper extremity.

PROM Loss

Trauma, especially in conjunction with immobilization, often results in decreased PROM (Akeson, Ameil, Avel, Garfin & Woo, 1987; Akeson, Ameil, & Woo, 1980; Akeson, Ameil, Mechanc, Woo, Harwood, & Hamer, 1977; Ameil, Woo, Harwood, & Akeson, 1982; Enneking & Horowitz, 1972). This loss of joint flexibility has two major sources: **scar formation** and **adaptive shortening** (Flowers & Michlovitz, 1988). Both create formidable barriers to motion.

Scar Formation

Formed to repair tissue defects, scar is deposited not only between discontinuous structures but also in noninjured tissues surrounding the wound. All wounded and some nonwounded structures become attached, resulting in the one wound/one scar phenomenon (Peacock, 1984). An **adhesion,** the pathologic attachment of one structure to another via scar, limits the excursion of articular and periarticular structures, restricting useful joint motion. As the scar matures over time, it

TABLE 15–1 Common Contractures of the Upper Extremity

Joint	Contracture(s)
DIP	Flexion or extension (decreased extension or flexion)
PIP	Flexion (decreased extension)
MP	Extension (decreased flexion)
Thumb MP	Flexion (decreased extension)
Thumb CMC	Adduction (decreased abduction)
Wrist	Flexion and ulnar deviation (decreased extension and radial deviation)
Forearm	Pronation (decreased supination)
Elbow	Flexion (decreased extension)
Shoulder	Decreased flexion, abduction, and external rotation

DIP, distal interphalangeal; *PIP*, proximal interphalangeal; *MP*, metacarpophalangeal; *CMC*, carpometacarpal.

contracts and becomes denser (Akeson et al., 1980; Frank, Ameil, Woo, & Akeson, 1985).

Adaptive Shortening

Inflamed tissue undergoes remodeling in a shortened form when it is immobilized in a slack position and deprived of constant stress in the form of motion (Brand, 1985). Brand (1985) theorized that this adaptive shortening occurs when lack of stress signals the body to reduce tissue constituents, creating structures with less length. Research has proven this true for the biceps muscle (Williams & Goldspink, 1978). Inadequate tissue length limits joint motion. Both scar and normal tissue may become adaptively shortened and contribute to loss of motion.

Stress and Restoration of PROM

To reverse the motion-robbing effects of scar and adaptive shortening, the clinician faces the challenge of changing the length and density of the adhesions and shortened tissue. To achieve the desired length change, the clinician controls the environmental demands on the tissue and applies the mechanical stimulus of **stress.** Living tissue, including scar, will reorganize and change in response to stress. The stress stimulus of tension triggers an increase in the length of the tissue (Arem & Madden, 1976).

The scientific community has not yet quantified the exact amount of stress required to stimulate change in tissue length. Clinically, it is apparent that the amount of stress required increases as the maturation of the scar progresses. Research supports the hypothesis that the longer tissue remains at maximum tolerable length, the more it will increase in length (Flowers & LaStayo, 1994). Typically, the clinician employs experience and data from repeated evaluation to determine optimal stress loads. In addition to intensity, the clinician must also consider the effect of the variables' duration and frequency, as they mediate total stress delivery (Flowers & Michlovitz, 1988).

Optimal Stress Application: Delivery Approach

Clinical experience, observation of some cultures' success at altering the body's configuration, and the orthodontic and orthopaedic literature support the use of **low-load, prolonged stress (LLPS)** over any other combination of load and stress for achieving permanent increase in tissue length and, therefore, in PROM (Arem & Madden, 1976; Flowers & LaStayo, 1994; Hotchkiss, 1995, n.d.; Light, Nuzik, Personius, & Barstrom, 1984). Clinically, low-load, brief stress (LLBS); high-load, brief stress; and high-load, prolonged stress have failed to demonstrate effectiveness in producing permanent length change. Although the mechanism of action is unknown, LLPS appears to work by providing a mechanical stimulus that causes scar to remodel biologically into a permanently lengthened form. Clinically, the most effective way to apply LLPS is initially to stress the tissue to maximum length with LLBS. Then the tissue is maintained in its lengthened state with light to moderate force for a prolonged period of time. Thus the key to reducing a PROM limitation is an extended time of low-load stress to position the shortened tissue at or near the end of its currently available length.

Low-Load, Prolonged Stress

The clinician has several options for applying LLPS to tissue. However, the most powerful LLPS technique of the longest duration is splinting. Splinting maintains the tissue elongation gained during therapy, a home program, and functional use of the hand. Using low tension, it maintains the newly gained length over long periods of time. Brand (1985) theorizes that the application of mechanical stress via splinting signals contracted tissue to grow or add cells while the body absorbs redundant tissue. In the clinic, therapists note that splinting at end range brings about increases in PROM much more quickly than LLBS and exercise. Sometimes splinting creates increases in PROM that were previously unavailable by any approach short of surgery.

Characteristics of Splint Approaches

When increasing PROM is the splint goal, the clinician may choose one of three splint approaches: **dynamic, serial static,** or **static progressive.** The American Society of Hand Therapists' splinting nomenclature classifies each of these three types of splints as a **mobilizing splint** when it is used to mobilize a joint. Clinicians often incorrectly describe splints designed to mobilize joints as dynamic (Cassanova, 1992) The following discussion shows that the term *dynamic* has a different, and specific, meaning.

Dynamic Splints

Dynamic splints have self-adjusting resilient or elastic components—such as spring wire, rubber bands, or springs—that create "a mobilizing force on a segment, resulting in passive or passive-assisted motion of a joint or successive joints" (Fess & Phillips, 1987). In addition, dynamic splints allow active-resisted motion in the direction opposite of their line of pull. The dynamic tension generated continues as long as the elastic component can contract, even when the shortened tissue reaches the end of its elastic limit (Fig. 15–1).

Static Progressive Splints

Static progressive splinting involves the use of inelastic components, such as hook-and-loop tapes, static lines, progressive hinges, turnbuckles, and screws. These components allow progressive changes in joint position as PROM changes without needing to change the structure of the splint. Only the line of pull must be changed as PROM progresses. A static progressive splint holds shortened tissue at its maximum length. Because the components lack the elasticity of those used in dynamic splinting, the appropriately set tension of the splint does not continue to stress tissue beyond its current maximum length limit (Fig. 15–2) (Schultz-Johnson, 1992).

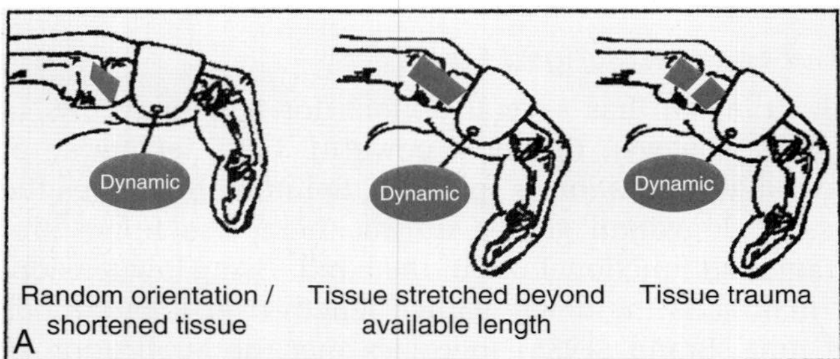

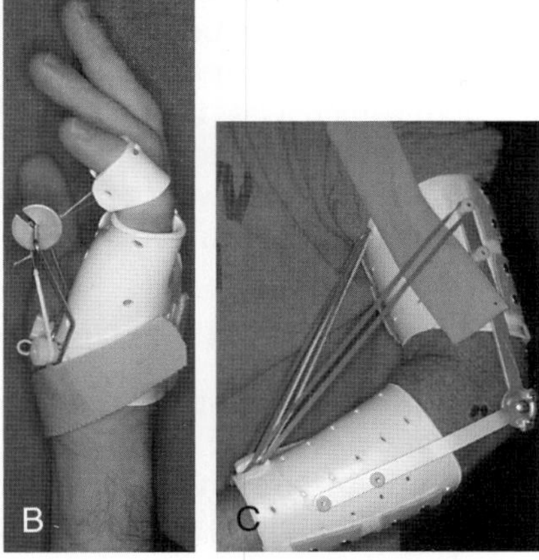

Figure 15–1 ***A,*** *A dynamic splint generates tension as long as the elastic component can contract, even when the shortened tissue reaches the end of its elastic limit; thus tissue trauma can result.* ***B,*** *A dynamic PIP flexion mobilization splint using a Phoenix outrigger.* ***C,*** *A dynamic elbow flexion mobilization splint utilizing a Phoenix elbow hinge.*

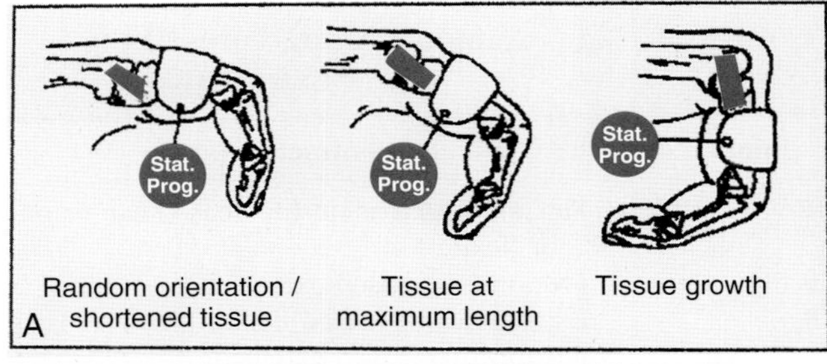

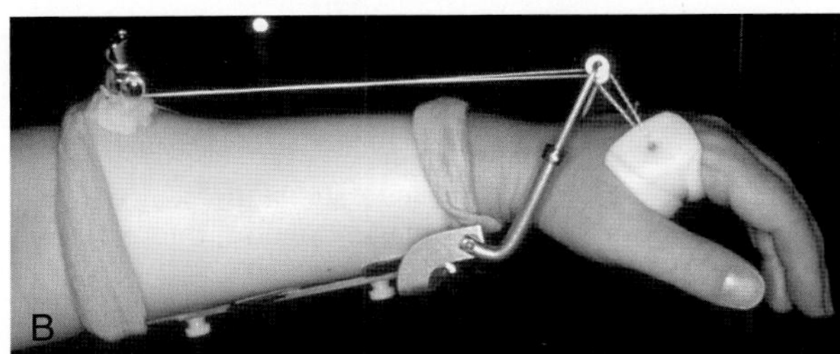

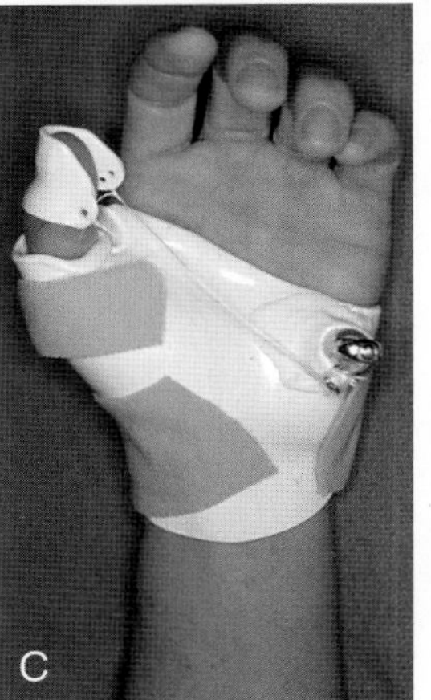

Figure 15–2 ***A,*** *Because static progressive components lack the elasticity of those used for dynamic splinting, the appropriately set tension of the splint does not stress tissue beyond its current maximum length limit. Tissue lengthening occurs without tissue trauma.* ***B,*** *A wrist extension mobilization splint using a Phoenix wrist hinge and MERiT component.* ***C,*** *A thumb IP flexion mobilization splint utilizing a MERiT component.*

Serial Static Splints

Serial static splinting differs from static-progressive splinting in that the clinician must remold the splint to accommodate increases in mobility. Proximal interphalangeal (PIP) serial casts and serial wrist extension splints exemplify this splinting approach. The clinician establishes the tension of the splint to maximum tolerable end range. Therefore, the splint does not continue to stress tissue beyond its current maximum length limit (Schultz-Johnson, 1992). No change in joint position occurs until the clinician modifies the splint (Fig. 15–3).

Indications for Splint Approach

Splint Algorithm

As a foundation for making the choice among the splinting approaches, clinicians have developed an algorithm that matches the type of splint with the phase of wound healing (Fig. 15–4). This algorithm serves as a guideline only. Therapists must choose the approach that best suits each patient's many characteristics.

Based on this algorithm, many clinicians have delayed using static progressive splinting until the later phases of wound healing because they consider it a high-load generator. This is a misconception. A static progressive force generator has a wide range of load application from extremely low to extremely high. Because the static progressive force generators are infinitely adjustable, the range of force is more diverse than that achievable from a rubber band or spring. Thus any tissue that can tolerate dynamic traction can tolerate static progressive traction. In addition, tissues that cannot tolerate dynamic splinting may tolerate static progressive traction. It is up to the clinician to establish the correct amount of tension or load for the given tissue and to set up the splint appropriately (Schultz-Johnson, 2000). Table 15-2 compares the approaches (Schultz-Johnson, 2000).

Torque-Angle Range of Motion

Assessment of **torque-angle range of motion (TAROM),** the quantification of the amount of torque force required to gain a certain amount of PROM at a joint, helps the therapist decide what type of splint will resolve the patient's PROM limitations (Roberson & Giurintano, 1995). If a joint requires a significant amount of torque to gain maximum PROM and the torque-angle curve has a rapidly rising slope, then the joint will have a **hard end feel** (Fig. 15–5**A**). Serial static or static progressive splinting is probably the only means to increase PROM. However, if a joint requires only a low amount of torque to gain maximum PROM and the torque-angle curve has a slowly rising slope, then the joint will have a **soft or springy end feel** (Fig. 15–5**B**). A soft end feel joint can benefit from serial static, static progressive or dynamic splinting. However, clinical experience has shown that the dynamic approach requires more time than the static approaches to produce the desired result (Schultz-Johnson, 1992).

A soft end feel joint indicates either relatively young scar tissue that has not yet formed significant cross-linking or transient physiologic changes, such as swelling or mal-

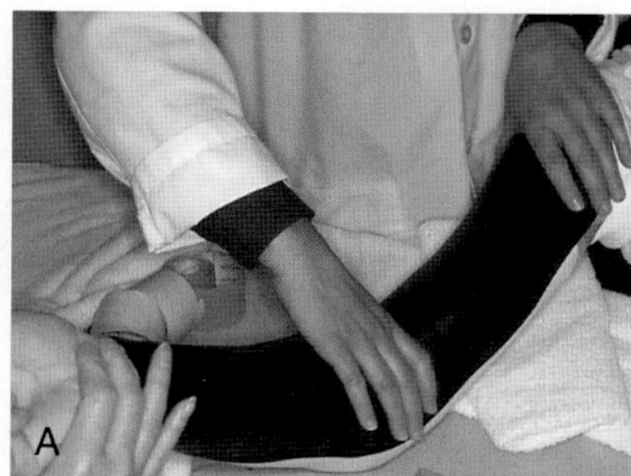

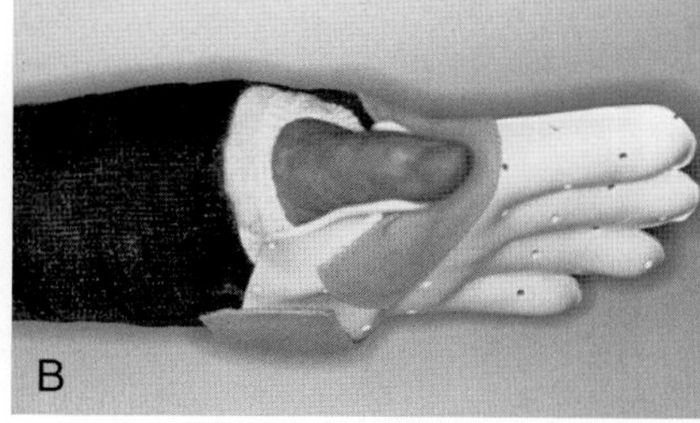

*Figure 15–3 Examples of serial static approach to gain elbow extension (**A**) and a serial static digit extension splint to increase length of tight extrinsic flexors (**B**).*

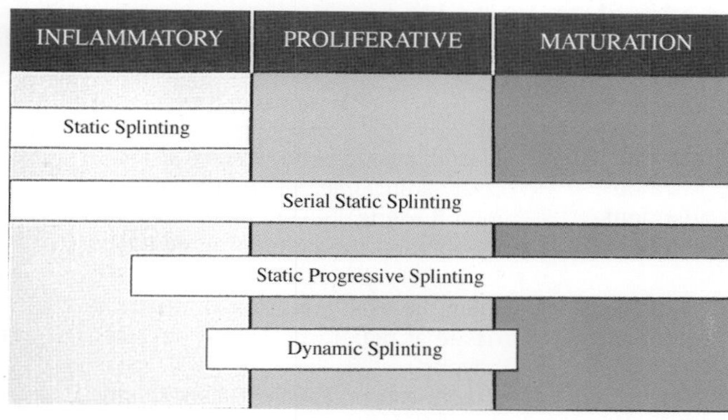

Figure 15–4 Algorithm for matching the type of splint with the phase of wound healing.

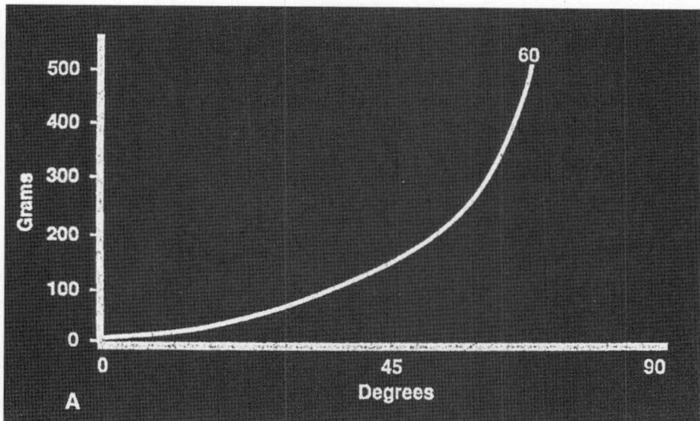

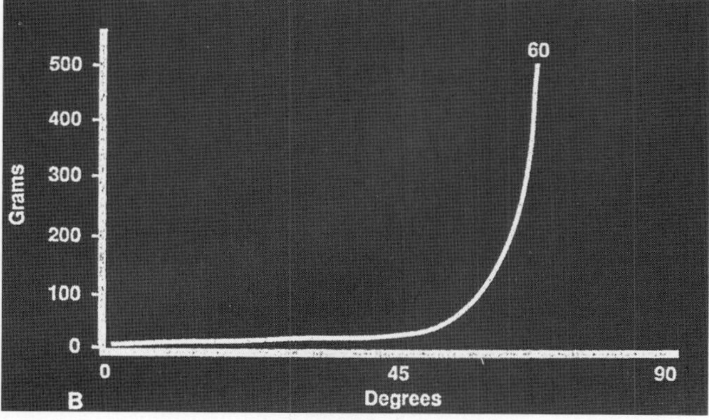

*Figure 15–5 **A,** A hard end feel joint requires a significant amount of torque to gain maximum PROM and has a torque-angle curve with a rapidly rising slope. **B,** A soft end feel joint requires only a low amount of torque to gain maximum PROM and has a torque-angle curve with a slowly rising slope.*

TABLE 15–2 Comparison of Mobilization Splint Approaches

Characteristic	Dynamic	Serial Static	Static Progressive
Force and ROM adjustment	• Elastic tension is not readily or precisely adjustable; when applied to a joint it exerts a given force and places the joint at a given point in its PROM • Extremely difficult to establish a tolerable elastic tension that places tissue at maximum length but not beyond • Patient can pull against the dynamic force, shortening the tissue on an intermittent basis, which thwarts the purpose of the splint (to hold the tissue at its maximum length for long periods of time)[a]	• Creates constant tension and joint positioning • End range position with tolerable tension is easily achieved • Patient cannot move from the end range established by the clinician; splint holds tissue at its current maximum length	• Static progressive tension and joint positioning are infinitely adjustable • Always possible to establish a static tension that places tissue at maximum length but not beyond it • As tissue remodels into a longer form, splint can immediately be adjusted to capture increased length and PROM • Patient remains at end range until splint is readjusted to optimize the combination of ROM and tension
Tension	• Dynamic component continues to shorten even when tissue has reached the end of its available length, which causes microtears and increased scar • Microtears, in turn, undergo the normal phases of wound healing • As the scar matures, it contracts and further limits PROM	• Holds the tissue at maximum length and does not stress beyond it	• Holds the tissue at maximum length and does not stress beyond it
Force control	• Springs and elastics deform over time • Neither clinician nor patient has control of forces	• Clinician has control over forces	• Clinician can maintain control over forces or instruct patient in proper use, so the patient has control
Splint tolerance and time dose	• Because dynamic component continues to shorten, it frequently stresses tissue beyond its available length, leading to poor splint tolerance and the inability to wear the splint for as many hours as required to achieve permanent length change[a]	• Appropriate stress fosters consistent splint wear, resulting in tissue growth and reorganization in a longer form and creating a permanent length change	• Appropriate stress fosters consistent splint wear, resulting in tissue growth and reorganization in a longer form and creating a permanent length change
Splint tolerance and sleep	• Because patient often cannot tolerate the splint during sleep, the splint must be worn during the day, which interferes with functional use of the hand • If the dynamic force is light enough to allow sleep, it probably is not taking the joint to end range	• Patient can tolerate the splint during sleep, minimizing need for daytime wear	• Patient can tolerate the splint during sleep, minimizing need for daytime wear
Joint end feel	• Improves PROM in joints with soft end feel but is ineffective for hard end feel joints	• Improves ROM of soft end feel joints faster than do dynamic splints • Improves PROM in joints with soft or hard end feel[a,b]	• Improves ROM of soft end feel joints faster than do dynamic splints • Improves PROM in joints with soft or hard end feel[a,b]
Efficiency	• Requires many more weeks or months in splint and in therapy than do static approaches	• Highly effective in increasing PROM, especially for patients with compliance and sensory problems	• Increases PROM faster than any other approach and, sometimes, when no other treatment approach is successful[c]

[a]Bell-Krotoski, J. A. (1987). Plaster casting for the remodeling of soft tissue. In E. E. Fess & C. Phillips (Eds.). *Hand splinting: Principles and methods* (2nd ed., pp. 453–454). St. Louis: Mosby.
[b]Fess, E. E. & Phillips, C. (Eds.). (1987). *Hand splinting: Principles and methods* (2nd ed). St. Louis: Mosby.
[c]Bonutti, P. M., Windau, J. E., Ables, B. A., & Miller, B. G. (1994). Static progressive stretch to re-establish elbow range of motion. *Clinical Orthopaedics and Related Research, 303,* 128–134.

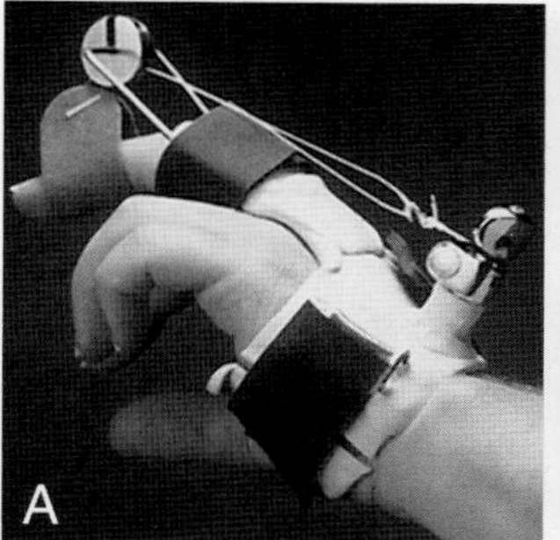

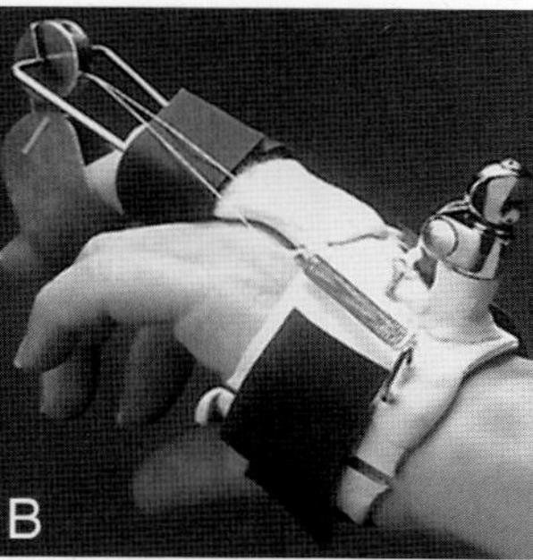

*Figure 15–6 This PIP extension mobilization splint incorporates both static progressive (**A**) and dynamic (**B**) approaches. The patient is able to alternate between the two approaches. Shown using Phoenix outrigger and MERiT component.*

nourished cartilage, that have produced a contracture and the body has not yet absorbed the cells required for normal range of motion (ROM) (Bell-Krotoski, 1987). A hard end feel joint indicates mature scar tissue with advanced cross-linking, the presence of a check rein, or the absorption of tissue required for normal passive motion (e.g., a PIP flexion contracture when the body absorbs volar skin and joint capsule) (Bell-Krotoski, 1987).

Clinical experience has shown that using static approaches to PROM limitations offers the fastest results without additional tissue trauma. However, when optimal results require tissue excursion and the joint limitation feels soft, dynamic splinting provides the best solution. The clinician can design a splint that incorporates both static progressive and dynamic approaches, so the splint wearer can alternate between the two (Fig. 15–6). The analysis of the duration and nature of the contracture, coupled with the information gained from TAROM measurements, helps the therapist select the appropriate splint.

TAROM can also help the therapist discover the quality of the stiffness. Sometimes, the pure AROM or PROM measurement does not change over time; however, the patient will note that the joint feels better. This description does not generally indicate a decrease in pain. Further assessment may reveal that the arc of motion is more easily available, which means that either the clinician does not have to push as hard during the PROM evaluation and/or the patient does not have to contract the muscle as hard to achieve the arc of motion. If the clinician had been performing TAROM evaluations all along, it would be obvious that the plotted slope of the torque-angle curve was becoming less steep. Thus the quantification of the degree of stiffness relative to both noninvolved joints and to previous evaluations of the joint in question is a valuable piece of information in the battle against stiffness. Such data can help the clinician in treatment planning and splint assessment.

Contraindications to Splinting

Just as it is important to know the indications for mobilizing splints and for splint approaches that match a given problem, it is important to know contraindications to splints that seek to mobilize joints. Common contraindications include the following:

- Joint instability.
- Avascular necrosis.
- Acute inflammation.
- Infection.
- Unstable fractures.
- Marked demineralization.
- Myositis ossificans.
- Heterotopic ossification.
- Exostosis formation.
- Loose body in joint.
- Stress across healing structures without adequate blood supply or tensile strength to withstand tensile stress.

In addition, three special diagnostic categories that are contraindications to mobilizing splints require special comment: Dupuytren's contracture, motion loss due to irradiation, and Ashworth's disease.

Dupuytren's contracture does not respond to low-load, prolonged stress (Abbott, Denney, Burke, & MGrouther, 1987; Sampson, Badalamente, Hurtst, Dowd, Sewell, Lehmann-Tprres. Ferraro, & Semon, 1992). Owing to its nature, Dupuytren's tissue, made up of myofibroblasts, does not remodel in the same way as normal tissue or scar. Only in the postoperative period will Dupuytren's contracture respond to splinting, because the surgery removes the unresponsive tissue and replaces some of it with scar.

Irradiated tissue does not usually respond to low-load, prolonged stress. The tissue is mostly fibrotic and does not possess the same viscoelastic properties as normal connective tissue. It lacks the live cells required to respond to the mechanical stimulus and to reorganize.

The last category, which this author calls Ashworth's disease, has no formal name in the literature. Hand surgeon Ashworth (personal communication, 19??) described the condition as nameless and extremely rare. Ashworth believes he has seen more of it than any other physician in the United States. Ashworth's disease is a congenital anomaly that causes its bearer to have supernumerary muscles. The condition may present in a limited manner in a part of the upper extremity or may involve the entire extremity, including the shoulder and neck. Before puberty, it causes no limitation and, in fact, can provide some cause for pride in patients who value extra muscle bulk and strength. However, at puberty the disease becomes active and causes the supernumerary muscles to fibrose and contract, often creating severe deformity. The contracting tissue is powerful enough to sublux joints. Clinical experience shows that this fibrotic tissue does not respond to splinting.

Whenever the clinician applies a splint—and especially when any doubt about splint appropriateness or tolerance exists—he or she must rigorously check for the following signs that indicate a problem with this splint:

- Pain (dolor).
- Heat (calor).
- Redness (rubor).
- Edema.
- Decreased ROM.
- Decreased strength.
- Decreased sensation.

If any of these symptoms and signs are seen, the therapist must thoroughly check the splint for fit and pressure distribution. It is important for the clinician to rethink the rationale for splint application to be certain of its appropriateness.

Causes of Joint Stiffness

When discussing joint stiffness, the nature of the limitation in joint PROM must be addressed. Changes in the soft tissue structures surrounding a joint, the peri-articular structures (e.g., ligament, joint capsule, volar plate, and sagittal bands) can cause such motion limitation. Changes in the structure of the articular surfaces of the bones forming the joint can also lead to loss of PROM. The relationship of adjacent bones to one another also affects arc and ease of motion.

Spasticity and congenital anomalies may cause joint stiffness (see Chapters 21 and 22 for further information). Although metastatic and primary bone tumors and Paget's disease can lead to stiffness, they will not be specifically addressed here (Copeland, 1997).

As noted, peri-articular structures may adaptively shorten when positioned on slack for a significant period of time; inflammation hastens this process. Madden described how peri-articular structures may fold on themselves, like an accordion, and become stuck in that position when scar forms between these folds (Fig. 15–7). Spot-welding of peri-articular structures may also occur during scar formation when the scar attaches the normally

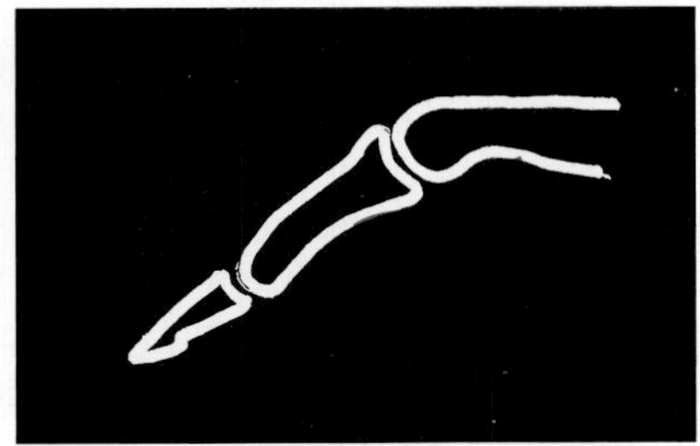

Figure 15–7 The accordion phenomenon is caused by scar formation between the folds, leading to decreased PROM.

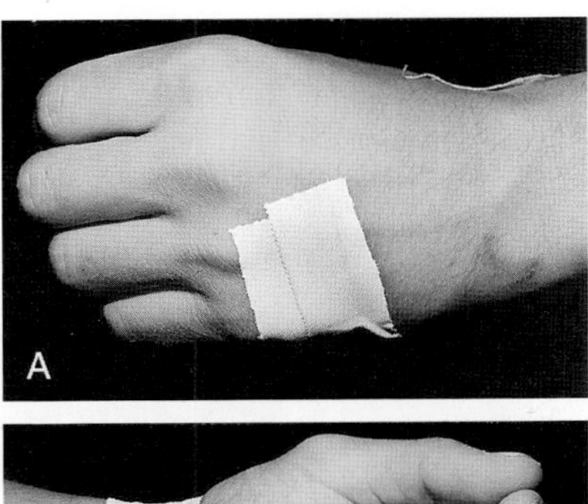

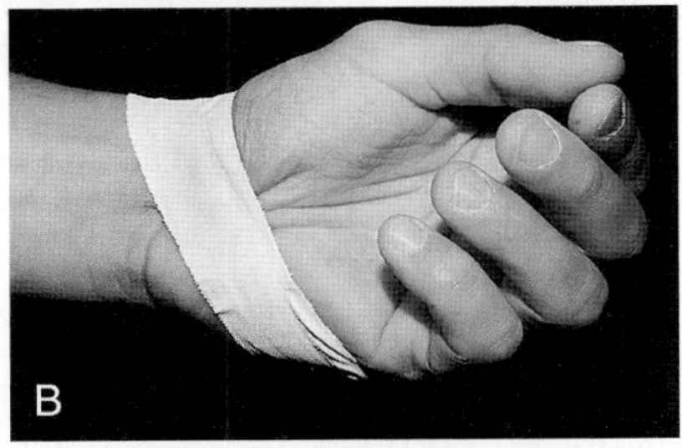

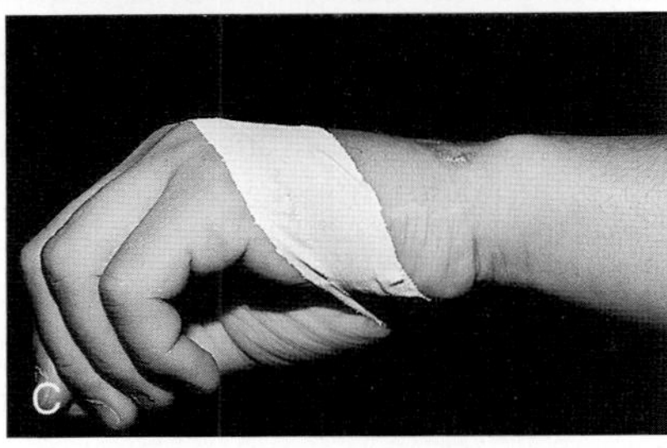

*Figure 15–8 Dorsal (**A**), volar (**B**), and ulnar (**C**) views of Mulligan taping, which mimics splinting. Splint/tape combinations can be used to augment this often effective technique.*

mobile tissue to less mobile tissue. This leads to a decrease in extensibility and glide (Flowers & Michlovitz, 1988).

The aforementioned changes in peri-articular tissue and the joint surface have long been part of the literature pertaining to joint stiffness. Mulligan (1999), a physiotherapist from New Zealand, described the newest theory in the search for understanding the cause of decreased motion. When he combined joint mobilization techniques with passive physiologic motion, Mulligan found he was able to restore normal, pain-free motion in many patients. This success was achieved even in many cases in which the loss of motion and pain had existed for years. Although Mulligan has spent years honing his techniques for restoring motion, he has not used the scientific method to examine why his techniques are so often effective. Mulligan postulates that the reason for many PROM limitations is a "positional fault" that "mobilization with movement" corrects. Once the correct joint relationship is restored, the joint moves normally and pain diminishes. Mulligan advocates the use of taping techniques to enhance his mobilization approach (Fig. 15–8).

Each joint possesses a unique anatomy that, when subjected to trauma or autoimmune processes and to inflammation, produces predictable patterns in the limitation of flexibility. When presented with the diagnosis and duration postinjury or since onset, the clinician uses knowledge of these patterns to plan treatment. Often, the treatment consists of splinting to prevent or decrease the effect of the pathology.

Precipitating Conditions for Stiffness

Edema

In the presence of diffuse edema, the hand assumes the position of ease: wrist flexed, MP joints extended, and interphalangeal (IP) joints flexed (Fig. 15–9) (Grigsby, deLinde & Miles, 1995). This position minimizes tension on the dorsal skin of the hand, on the ligaments, and on the peri-articular structures. When the edema remains and the hand is left untreated, the wrist loses extension, the MPs develop extension contractures, and the IPs develop flexion contractures. The clinician must immediately seek to control edema and position the hand appropriately. Splinting provides the desired extremity posture. Strategic application and design of splint strapping may assist in edema management. The position of choice for minimizing or preventing hand stiffness and deformity is called the antideformity position (Fig. 15–10): wrist in 20 to 25° extension, if available; maximum tolerated MP flexion; and maximum tolerated IP extension. Even if the PROM limitations do not permit the initial splint to secure the desired position, serial splint changes will generally accomplish the goal.

Paralysis

Paralysis of the primary IP extensor and MP flexor occurs with loss of ulnar or combined ulnar and median motor function. This leads to sustained flexion of the IP

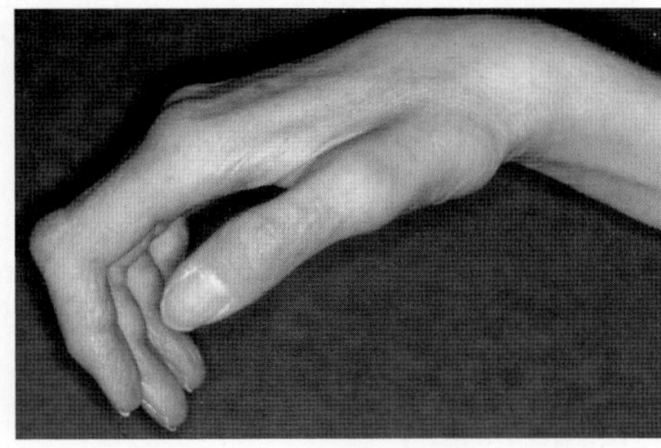

Figure 15–9 The position of ease with wrist flexed, MPs extended, and IPs flexed.

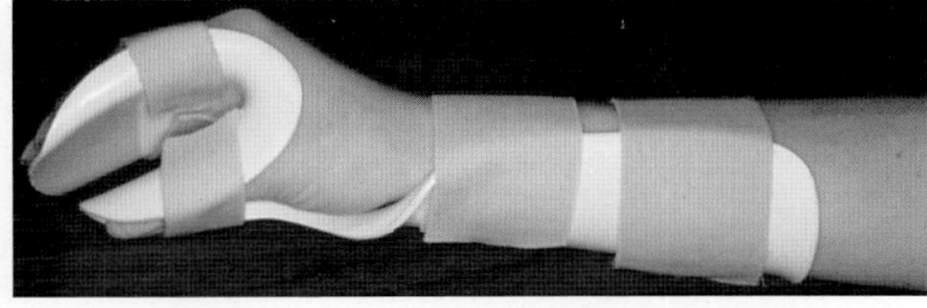

Figure 15–10 The antideformity position is the position of choice for minimizing or preventing hand stiffness and deformity.

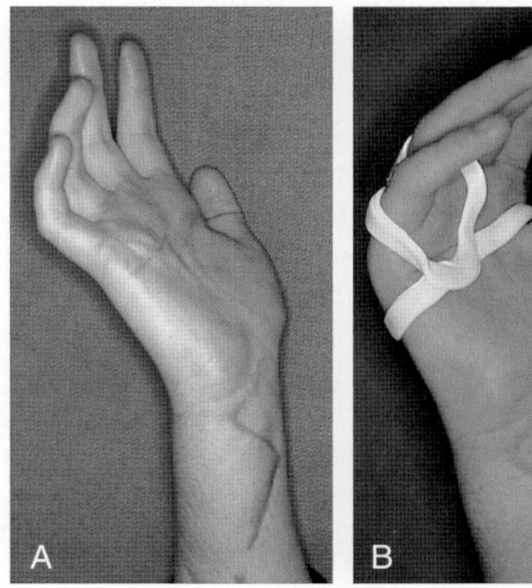

*Figure 15–11 **A,** Claw deformity is commonly seen with ulnar nerve injury. **B,** An MP extension restriction splint.*

joints and hyperextension of the MP joint as the patient attempts to straighten the fingers with only the extrinsic extensor digitorum communis (EDC) (Fig. 15–11) (Brand & Hollister, 1999). Over time, this unopposed flexion alone can produce IP flexion contractures owing to adaptive shortening. The hyperextension at the MP joint further facilitates the loss of IP flexion and subsequent contracture. Left to the whims of the extrinsic flexor, the MP joint flexes only after both IP joints have done so. The combination of MP hyperextension (when the patient attempts to open the palm for function) and lack of functional MP flexion facilitate the loss of MP flexion.

The presence of edema and/or of inflammation often hastens the contracture. When the therapist notes loss of ulnar or combined ulnar and median nerve function, the treatment plan must immediately include MP flexion splinting. With the MP joint flexed, the power of the EDC transfers to the IP joint and re-establishes active IP joint extension (Brandsma, 1993). Edema or inflammation indicates the need for a static IP extension splint to prevent contracture. Established IP flexion or MP extension contractures require a mobilizing splint to increase PROM (see Chapter 19 for details).

Loss of the ulnar innervated intrinsic muscles produces the loss of ulnar finger metacarpal rotation and results in the loss of the cupping function of the palm (Fig. 15–12). When the metacarpals remain immobile and the intrinsic muscles become fibrotic, the transverse metacarpal arch is lost. The palm assumes a narrow and flattened appearance, a sign of intermetacarpal contractures. Splints that incorporate the palm must be carefully contoured to preserve the metacarpal arch (Malick, 1972).

Intrinsic Tightness

Injury or disease can create spasm or scarring of the intrinsic hand muscles. Intrinsic tightness causes loss of simultaneous MP extension and IP flexion. When these movements are impaired, the clinician should perform a test of intrinsic length (Fig. 15–13) (Aulicino, 1995). If intrinsic tightness is noted, the therapist begins the appropriate splint and exercise regimen to increase composite MP extension and IP flexion. Intrinsic tightness can create an imbalance that results in swan-neck deformity at the PIP and distal interphalangeal (DIP) joints (Melvin, 1989). Loss of intrinsic function can result in loss of the intermetacarpal movement, as described earlier. When intrinsic muscles become fibrotic, they seem to be resistant to splinting and exercises geared to increase their length. It is possible that fibrotic tissue lacks an adequate number of living cells to respond to tension stimuli and to reorganize in a manner conducive to length increase.

Extrinsic Tightness

Injury and overuse are the primary culprits of extrinsic tightness (Lowe, 1992). Extrinsic tightness can occur in either the flexor/pronator or extensor forearm muscles. Extrinsic extensor tightness condition leads to the loss of composite finger flexion (MPs and IPs simultaneously) or the loss of composite finger flexion combined with wrist flexion (Fig. 15–14). Just the reverse is true for extrinsic flexor tightness; it creates the loss of composite finger extension (MPs and IPs simultaneously) or the loss of composite finger extension combined with wrist extension (Fig. 15-15). When the problem is the result of overuse, it usually disappears with proper stretching exercises. However, when scarring is the cause, composite extension or flexion splinting is often necessary to lengthen adhesions and increase motion.

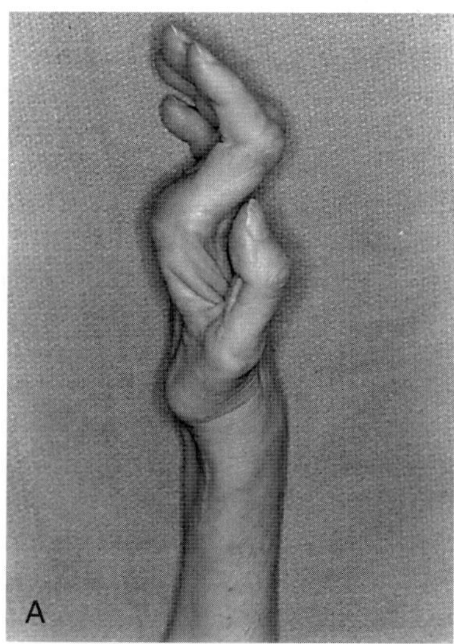

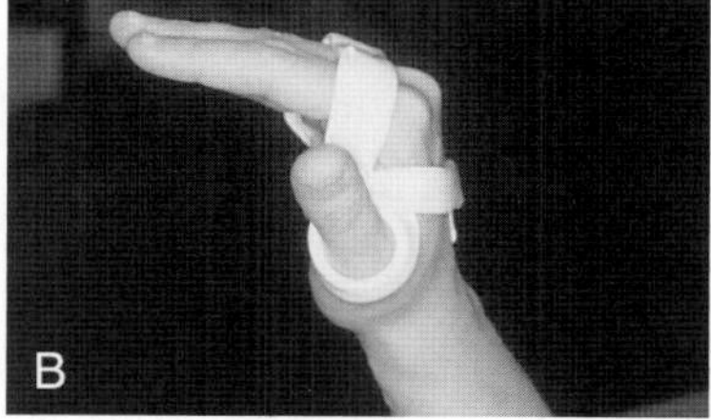

Figure 15–12 ***A,*** *With paralysis of the intrinsics post median and ulnar nerve injury, there is a loss of the arches in the hand.* ***B,*** *An MP extension restriction splint.*

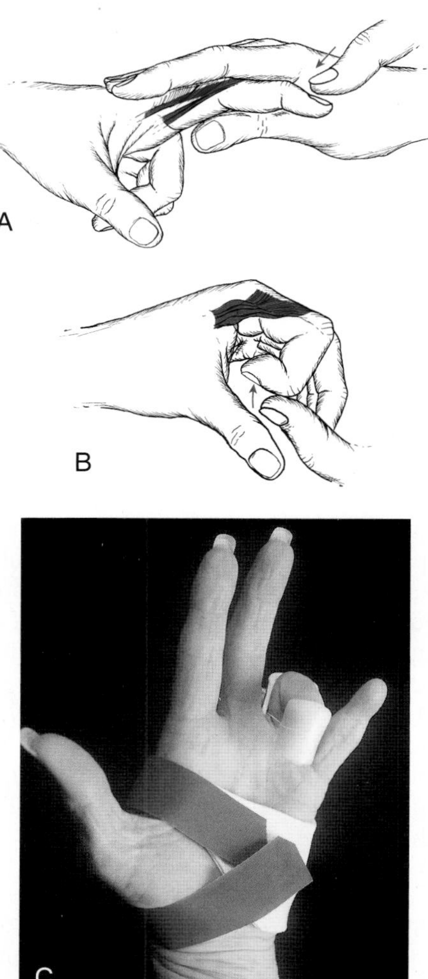

Figure 15–13 ***A and B,*** *The intrinsic tightness test. Note the loss of simultaneous MP extension and IP flexion.* ***C,*** *A PIP/DIP mobilization splint to stretch the tight intrinsics.*

Extensor Tendon Injury

Extensor tendon injury creates motion loss at different joints, depending on the level of injury. Zone I and II tendon disruptions cause loss of active DIP extension (Brzezienski & Schneider, 1995), which if left untreated leads to a DIP flexion contracture. Lack of treatment over many months creates an imbalance at the IP joints, resulting in overpull at the lateral bands, shifting them dorsally. Eventually, a swan-neck deformity, with PIP hyperextension and its concomitant loss of flexion at the PIP, occurs (Fig. 15–16). The adhesions caused from nonoperative or operative treatment can limit DIP flexion, leading to a DIP extension contracture (Fig. 15–17).

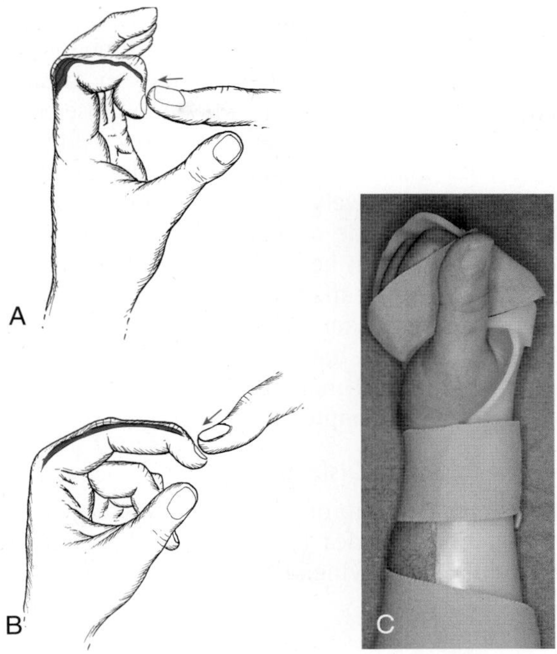

Figure 15–14 ***A and B,*** *The extrinsic tightness test. Note the loss of composite finger flexion.* ***C,*** *A composite digit flexion mobilization splint.*

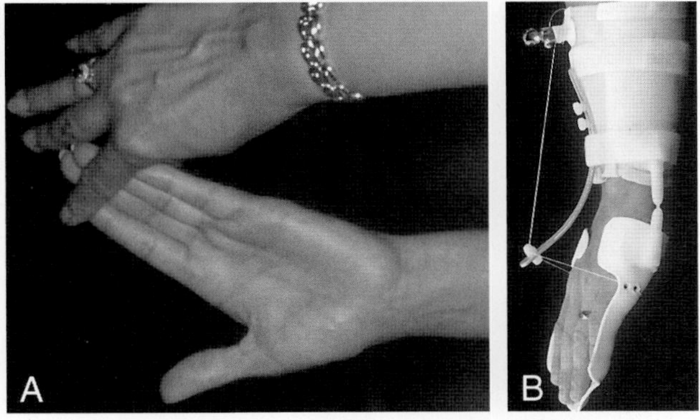

Figure 15–15 ***A,*** *Extrinsic flexor tightness leading to loss of combined wrist and digit extension.* ***B,*** *A wrist and digit extension mobilization splint.*

A Zone III or IV tendon disruption results in loss of active PIP extension (Coons & Green, 1995), causing loss of passive PIP extension. If left untreated, a PIP flexion contracture results. Lack of treatment over many months creates an imbalance at the IP joints, shifting the lateral bands volarly. This leads to a boutonniere deformity, with PIP flexion and its concomitant loss of flexion at the DIP (Fig. 15–18). When the oblique retinacular ligament (ORL) adaptively shortens, it creates a DIP hyperextension deformity and loss of flexion at the DIP (Fig. 15–19). The adhesions that result from nonoperative or operative treatment can limit PIP flexion, leading to a PIP extension contracture (see Chapter 18 for further information).

Flexor Tendon Injury

To repair a Zone II flexor tendon laceration, the surgeon must invade the flexor tendon sheath. The finger is then positioned in flexion for many hours a day owing to inflammation, edema, and scar synthesis. As described earlier, this combination creates the perfect situation for the formation of IP flexion contractures (Stewart & van Strien, 1995). Flexor tendon injury in other zones may also cause IP flexion contractures, owing to the flexion posture of the digit coupled with the generalized edema and inflammation that often involves much of the hand.

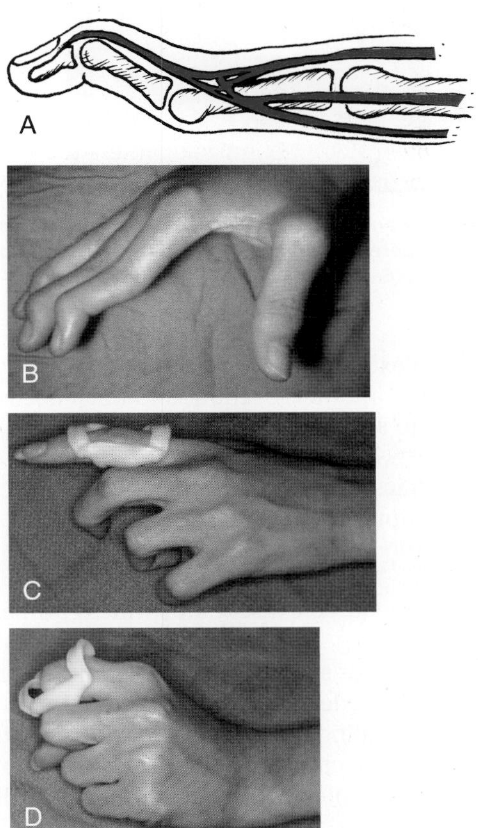

Figure 15–16 ***A and B,*** *Swan-neck deformity: note the PIP hyperextension and DIP flexion. A PIP extension restriction splint with extension (****C****) and flexion (****D****).*

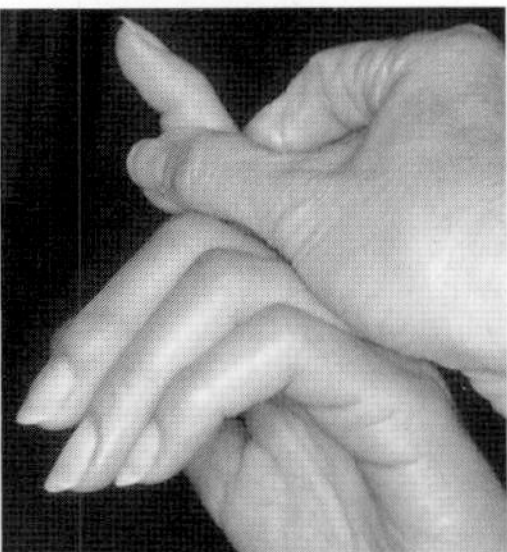

Figure 15–17 *Adhesions following Zone I extensor tendon injury limit active DIP flexion.*

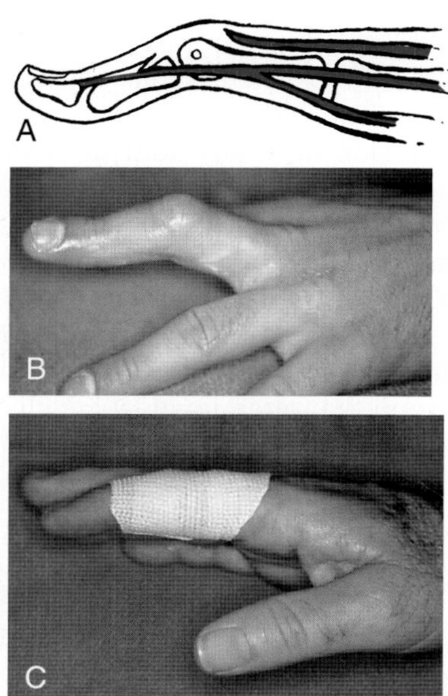

Figure 15–18 ***A and B,*** *Boutonniere deformity: note the PIP flexion and DIP hyperextension.* ***C,*** *A PIP extension immobilization splint using QuickCast.*

When the flexor digitorum sublimis (FDS) ruptures or is transferred to another location, an imbalance is set up that can lead to swan-neck deformity (Fig. 15-16) (Brand & Hollister, 1999). As noted, when left untreated, the faulty mechanics can lead to loss of motion at the IP joints (see Chapter 18).

Burn Injury

Partial-thickness burns cause joint stiffness primarily via adaptive shortening of peri-articular structures. Tight skin positions these structures on slack in the presence of inflammation, edema, and scar formation. Healing scar contracts, pulling the joint along with it. Skin damage across motion creases is the most likely to create joint stiffness (Chapter 23 provides details). Full-thickness burns can also damage tendon. The loss of active motion coupled with the adaptive shortening creates a powerful mechanism for joint stiffness. The clinician must be aware of the tendon's vulnerability to thermal injury. The splint should not only prevent primary joint contracture but also protect vulnerable tendon structures, such as the central slip of the extensor hood mechanism (dorsum of the PIP) (Grigsby et al., 1995).

Fracture

Fracture causes joint stiffness via several mechanisms. For example, edema and inflammation accompany most fractures. Cartilage defects also produce loss of PROM, which occurs in a predictable cascade of increased friction, leading to inflammation that in turn creates pain and edema. The normal reflex arc and the patient's normal response to pain limit active motion at the joint. When the joint fails to go through its full arc of motion, peri-articular structures shorten; and eventually, the joint will lose motion.

A fracture may produce loose bodies in an adjacent joint (Raney, Brashear, & Shands, 1971). A loose body limits joint motion mechanically. If the loose body persists and the joint limitation is sustained, the peri-articular structures may adaptively shorten, causing joint stiffness.

Structures that glide over bone may become trapped in the scar callus that heals the bone. This may lead to extrinsic tightness or may involve a prime joint mover, such as a wrist extensor. When this occurs, the muscle-tendon unit does not have adequate excursion, and the ability to restore and maintain joint motion is severely compromised (see Chapter 16 for details).

Ligament Injury or Dislocation

A sprain directly compromises structures supporting the joint. Ligament injuries tend to heal slowly owing to poor vascularity (Levine, 1992). They also tend to be

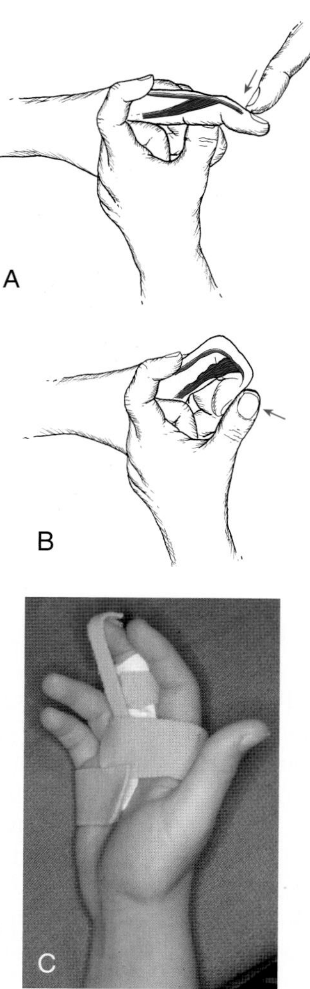

Figure 15–19 ***A and B,*** *The oblique retinacular ligament tightness test. Note the lack of isolated DIP flexion.* ***C,*** *A DIP flexion mobilization splint using loop snapping for a static progressive approach.*

painful for months and even years after they are healed. Clinical experience shows that edema after ligament injury of the small IP and MP joints tends to linger much longer than for other types of injuries (Mannarino, 1992). The edema and pain severely limit motion. The therapist must splint carefully to prevent joint contracture. Once a joint contracture establishes itself, the therapist must carefully note sprain classification, swelling, color, and temperature to avoid aggravating the joint while attempting to restore motion.

Infection

As part of the initial evaluation of a trauma patient with wounds or percutaneous pins, the therapist should obtain information about the patient's risk for infection. When risk factors are present, the therapist must be on constant alert for signs of infection. Infection causes an acute and severe inflammatory reaction. Edema always accompanies infection and is the primary reason that infection frequently results in stiffness. Some organisms not only trigger inflammatory reactions but also produce toxins that destroy tissue. Frequently, infection management involves immobilization of the involved part, which contributes to joint stiffness. Sepsis has the capacity to turn a good surgical result into a poor one because of its motion-robbing effects (Nathan & Taras, 1995).

Psychopathology

No discussion of stiffness is complete without addressing the contribution that psychopathology can make to PROM loss. The problems take many forms, including the following:

- Contribution to causing an accident (Hirschfeld & Behan, 1963).
- Self-inflicted wound (Wallace & Fitzmorris, 1978).
- Noncompliance with postinjury care.
- Refusal to move a joint via nonfunctional co-contraction (Simmons & Vasile, 1980).
- Refusal to move a joint for a significant period of time (Brand, 1988).

Improving PROM in a patient with these tendencies usually involves psychotherapy, since the stiffness serves the patient in some way (I. Schultz, personal communication, 2001). The patient perceives attempts to increase motion as undesirable and will resist.

Stiffness at Specific Joints

DIP Joint

The DIP joint is vulnerable to stiffness in both flexion and extension. The DIP presents a unique challenge in that once the joint becomes stiff, the short length of the distal phalanx offers little in terms of a lever arm to torque the joint into the desired ROM. The joint is unique in that the motor sensors surrounding the joint are singular and do not have the redundancy that is available at the other joints of the hand. Thus, if one of the motors becomes injured or ineffective, stiffness is likely to result.

The DIP has a dense volar plate that can become folded and adherent in scar in the presence of inflammation. The resultant flexion contracture often occurs with zone I or distal zone II flexor tendon injury, especially in the case of flexor digitorum profundus (FDP) advancement (Evans, 1990). With advancement, the flexed position of the DIP is encouraged with the introduction of a pull-out wire and button that introduce even more scar and inflammation. Although some loss of DIP extension might be considered desirable in the face of lost flexor excursion, the resulting extreme flexion contractures can be disfiguring and disabling. The therapist must respect the time for tendon healing, but should begin to extend the DIP as soon as the type of repair and the health and cooperation of the patient permit. Progressive isolated DIP extension splinting improves PROM and minimizes stress on the flexor tendon. However, even though such a splint attempts to extend only one joint in the series that the FDP affects, splinting so close to the repair can lead to attenuation or rupture.

When the extensor of the joint is avulsed from its insertion in the case of a mallet injury, the joint cannot actively extend. If left untreated, the volar structures undergo adaptive shortening, and a flexion contracture results. An untreated mallet injury can also lead to imbalance of the entire extensor mechanism of the finger and affect the PIP joint. The mallet injury must be immediately splinted in extension to co-apt the tendon ends and allow restoration of extension (Fig. 15–20). Clinical experience has shown that after days or even weeks have elapsed since the time of injury, if the dorsal aspect of the DIP remains reactive, it is possible that instituting extension splinting will restore tendon continuity.

With a diagnosis of a PIP central slip injury, the therapist must include a program of DIP flexion to prevent ORL tightness. If the injury is old and the DIP has already lost flexion, the clinician must progress the patient through a combination of PIP extension/DIP flexion splinting and exercise to restore normal PROM (Figs. 15–18 and 15–19) (Evans, 1995). As mentioned, scarring of zone I or II extensors can lead to loss of DIP extension. In addition, any dorsal scar in this location can create loss of DIP flexion.

PIP Joint

The PIP joint can become stiff in either flexion or extension. However, it is the PIP flexion contracture that is the most challenging to resolve, for the following reasons (Fig. 15–21) (Liuch, 1997; Sokolow, 1997):

- The tendency for the volar plate to shorten or fold on itself after trauma.
- The prevalence of a flexed finger posture in the position of ease and during function.

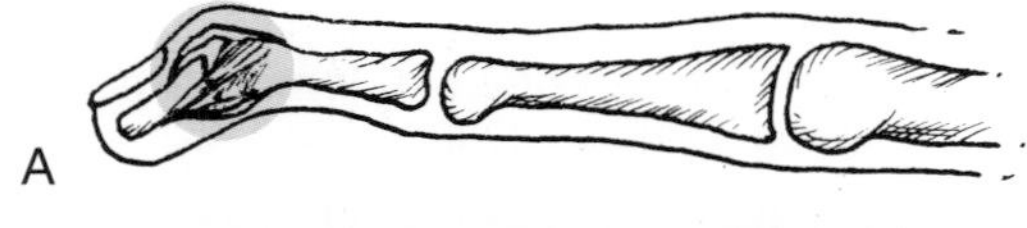

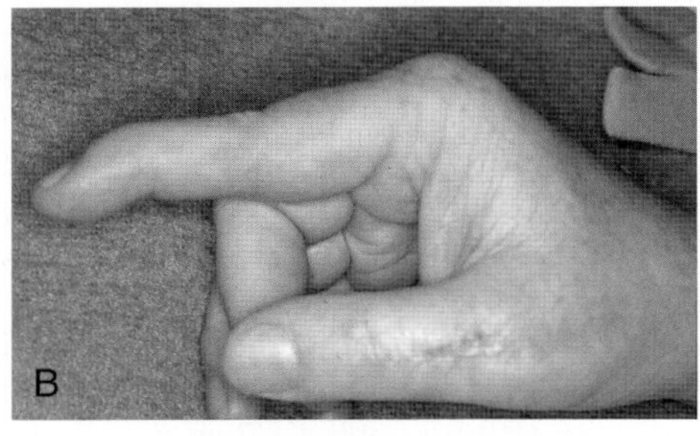

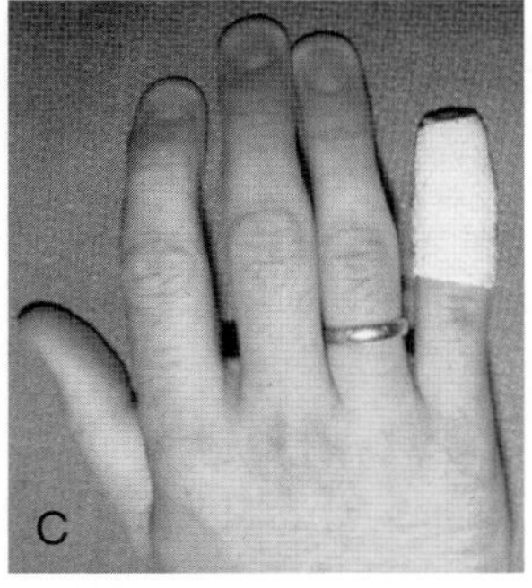

Figure 15–20 ***A and B,*** *IF DIP joint flexion contracture.* ***C,*** *SF DIP extension mobilization splint using QuickCast.*

- The vulnerability of the extensor mechanism (it is thin, superficial, and intimate with the underlying bone).
- Length loss caused by proximal phalanx fractures, leading to redundancy in extensor mechanism length and causing lack of full active extension.
- Extensor hood attenuation from prolonged positioning in flexion, rendering the mechanism too long to provide full extension even when the contracture has resolved (Brandsma, 1993).
- The density of the PIP volar plate, making it prone to adaptive shortening, and the thickness of the structure, making its lengthening difficult.

PIP joints are usually held in flexion, and hands are used in flexion. When a patient uses his or her hands for normal function during the day, the PIP joints are frequently in some degree of flexion. The position of comfort and rest is flexion. In the face of pain and edema, the PIPs are held in flexion to place the peri-articular structures on slack. During sleep, the PIP joints assume a flexed position.

Many types of trauma to the finger cause the extensor mechanism to become adherent to the bone and skin. This adhesion of the dorsal hood creates loss of excursion. Without full excursion, the PIP joint cannot actively assume full extension (Mannarino, 1992). If the patient fails to perform PROM consistently, the volar structures adaptively shorten, causing a flexion contracture.

Proximal phalanx fractures can result in shortening of the bone. However, the extensor hood length remains the same. This length redundancy makes complete active extension mechanically impossible. As for dorsal hood adhesions, with active extension lost, the volar structures adaptively shorten.

If the PIP flexion contracture remains for any significant period of time, the extensor hood becomes attenuated. The discrepancy in length between bone and tendon creates a mechanical deficit. The extensor mechanism cannot generate adequate tension to extend the joint fully. For this reason, even though many therapists argue for prioritizing PIP flexion to regain functional use of the hand, this author prioritizes PIP extension, especially in the face of an FDP with good excursion, evidenced by good DIP flexion. Hand surgeon Ashworth (personal communication, 1987) offers the following clinical gem. When the IP joints lack flexion, if the FDP has the ability to take the DIP through full available PROM, then the outcome for IP flexion is good. Over the years, Ashworth's indicator has proven itself to be consistently correct. Once the extensor hood length increases, the likelihood of its shrinking to normal proportions again is nil. Therefore, prevention of PIP contractures becomes of paramount importance. Even if splinting and therapy resolve the volar restrictions causing the contracture, the adverse dorsal mechanics of length or dorsal adhesion may prevent the maintenance of the improved extension.

Loss of PIP PROM in flexion can result from many of the factors described earlier. In the presence of a functioning

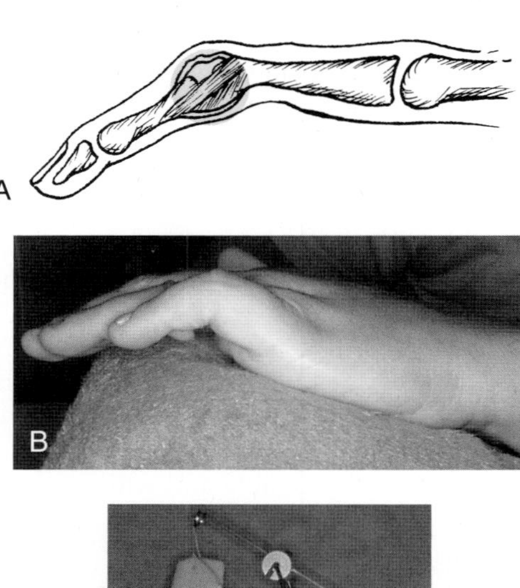

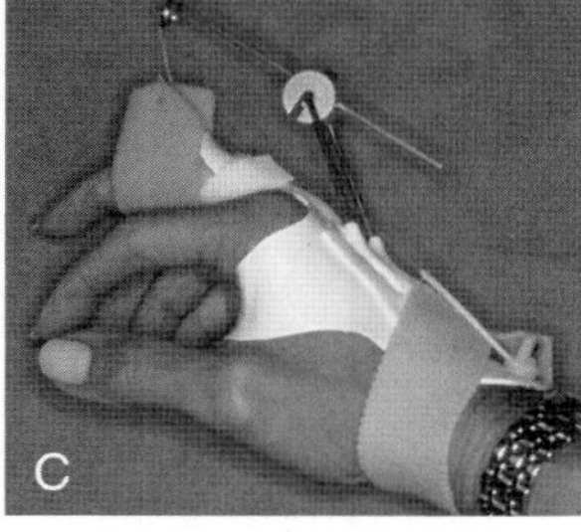

Figure 15–21 ***A and B,*** *SF PIP joint flexion contracture.* ***C,*** *A PIP extension mobilization splint utilizing Roylan outrigger.*

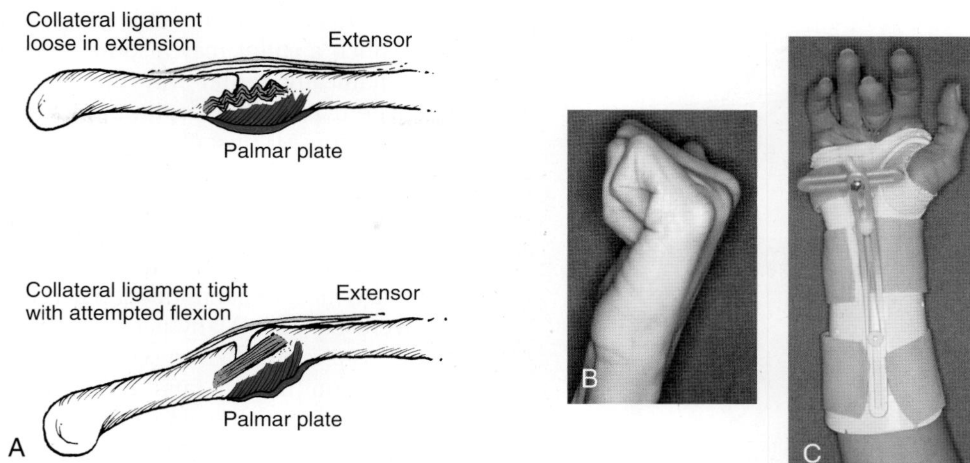

Figure 15–22 ***A and B,*** *SF MP joint extension contracture.* ***C,*** *MF MP flexion mobilization splint using Digitec outrigger.*

FDP, most PIPs eventually flex. One notable exception is a fracture or dislocation (especially one that is immobilized too long) that results in significant scarring at the joint. This extra tissue can create a physical block to motion that only surgical excision of the scar tissue can improve.

Finger MP joint

Problems at the finger MP joint rarely result in loss of extension. Even when the joint has been held in flexion for years by Dupuytren's fascial contracture, surgical release of the fascia readily returns the joint to extension. Injuries involving the soft tissue crossing the MP crease at a 90° angle or involving the majority of soft tissue in this location (e.g., burns, degloving injuries, and palmar skin graft) create loss of extension. However, restoration of soft tissue length restores normal motion. With rheumatic disease, the patient may lose passive MP extension owing to multiple factors, including loss of joint capsule and ligament integrity, intrinsic tightness, and ulnar subluxation of the EDC (Melvin, 1989).

The bane of the hand specialist's existence at the MP joint is the extension contracture (Fig. 15–22). Diagnoses associated with this problem are any injury causing generalized edema of the hand, intrinsic paralysis, crush injury, metacarpal and proximal phalanx fractures, dorsal or circumferential burns, and zone V extensor tendon injury that is not mobilized properly. Each of these injuries results in the sustained extension of the MP joint, often in the presence of edema, inflammation, and scar formation. The MP joint's unique anatomy predisposes it to the extension contracture.

The collateral ligaments of the MP joint are slack in extension and taut in flexion (Chase, 1989). When the ligaments are allowed to remain slack, especially in the presence of inflammation and scar formation, they can fall prey to the accordion phenomenon, adaptive shortening, or both. Like the volar plate of the PIP, these collateral ligaments are dense and recalcitrant to lengthening. A well-established MP extension contracture may require 23 to 24 hr a day of end range time to change length and increase PROM.

Thumb MP joint

Trauma to the thumb often causes stiffness at the MP joint. The diagnoses of fracture, collateral ligament injury, tendon, and nerve injury all frequently present with loss of MP flexion. The problem with restoring thumb MP flexion mirrors those of contracture at the finger but does not have the same primary cause. The collateral ligaments of the thumb have a different architecture than those of the finger MPs (Imaeda, An, & Cooney, 1992; Kapandji, 1982; Melone, Beldner, & Basuk, 2000). The loss of flexion seems to originate with joint swelling, which may be worsened by dorsal adhesions.

The thumb MP may lose extension with the loss of extensor pollicis brevis (EPB) continuity and a concomitant rent in the extensor expansion. This imbalance creates a dynamic similar to that of the finger boutonniere deformity. Left untreated, the IP joint of the thumb loses flexion and assumes a hyperextended position. Over time, a fixed deformity can result. A grade 3 tear of either the ulnar or the radial collateral ligament of the thumb MP can lead to MP joint instability with subsequent subluxation and the creation of a flexion contracture.

Rheumatic disease can create various thumb contractures (Melvin, 1989). Rheumatoid arthritis, lupus, and similar diseases can create the Nalebuff type 1 thumb, characterized by MP flexion and IP hyperextension (Fig. 15–23). The appearance is similar to the boutonniere deformity of the finger. This occurs as a result of chronic synovitis of the thumb MP joint, intrinsic muscle tightness, weakening or attenuation of the EPB, and ulnovolar displacement of the EPL (Melvin, 1989). Clinicians most commonly use splints to prevent this deformity.

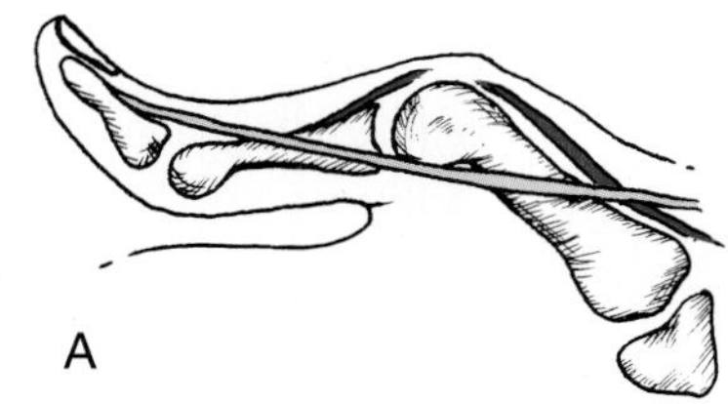

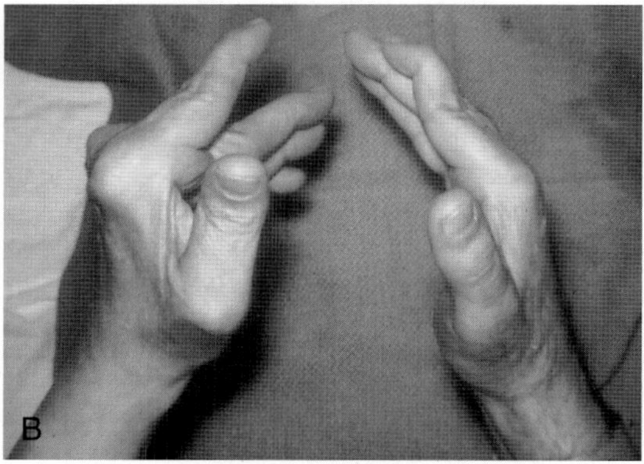

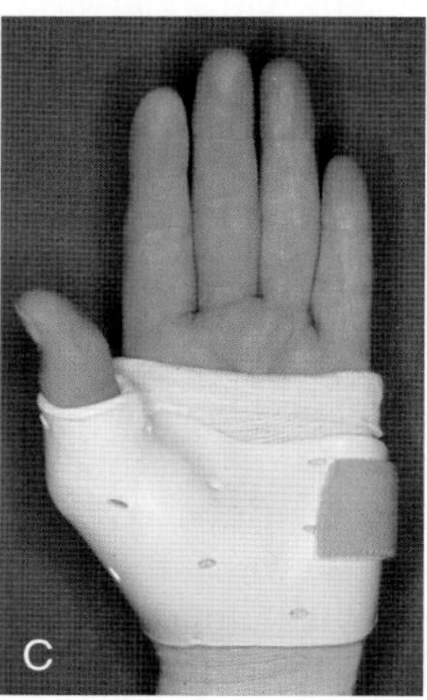

Figure 15–23 ***A and B,*** *The Nalebuff type 1 thumb: MP flexion and IP hyperextension on left hand.* ***C,*** *A thumb immobilization splint.*

However, aggressive disease or late treatment may present the clinician with the need to address this deformity. Goga-Eppenstein, Hill, Seifert, & Yasukawa, (1999) describe a casting technique used successfully for a patient with juvenile rheumatoid arthritis. The casting was followed-up with a program of static splinting and electrical stimulation to the thumb extrinsic extensors.

In contrast, the stiffness problem commonly associated with osteoarthritis is the Nalebuff type 2 thumb (Fig. 15–24). The condition associated with this classification is carpometacarpal (CMC) synovitis of the joint, which stretches the joint capsule and allows the joint to sublux or dislocate in adduction. This adducted posture results in shortening of the adductor pollicis muscles and web space. MP hyperextension develops with attempts to abduct the contracted first metacarpal (Melvin, 1989). Once this deformity exists, a splint will not improve it. A thumb MP extension restriction Silver Ring splint minimizes the hyperextension and may prevent it from getting worse. Such a splint may also help distribute forces in a biomechanically sound way that will unload the CMC joint. The main role for splinting for MP hyperextension secondary to CMC instability is prevention.

Thumb CMC joint

The CMC joint of the thumb has a unique saddle architecture that renders it highly mobile (Kapandji, 1982). The thumb is critical to hand function and is a frequently used and overused joint. Many people experience thumb CMC arthritis as a result of overuse, trauma, or a multijoint disease. Pelligrini, Olcott, and Hollenberg (1993) hypothesized that over time, overuse or trauma compromise the ligament system supporting the joint. This allows the joint surfaces to lose congruency, which leads to friction that wears away the cartilage, creating CMC arthritis. Clinical experience shows that osteoarthritis often first presents at the basal joint of the thumb. This disease has an insidious onset, and the cause and the cure are as yet unknown.

Joint incongruity, weakness, and pain all lead to loss of motion at the thumb CMC. As the cartilage loses integrity, the joint becomes painful and inflamed. The joint receptors send a signal to the spinal cord to inhibit efferent signals. The patient experiences loss of coordination and strength and has trouble performing activities of daily (ADLs). The condition leads to loss of motion, inflammation, and pain.

No matter the cause, at the end stage of thumb CMC arthritis (stage 4 disease), the metacarpal dislocates from the trapezium altogether (Fig. 15–24) (Eaton & Glickel, 1987). This dislocation usually occurs ulnarly. With such joint compromise, the thumb abductors are no longer able to function and the first metacarpal remains in an adducted position. Over time, the thumb adductor shortens. Even when the patient undergoes CMC arthroplasty to restore joint kinematics, the shortened adductor prevents normal thumb motion and function. Although splinting and exercise to restore the width of the first web

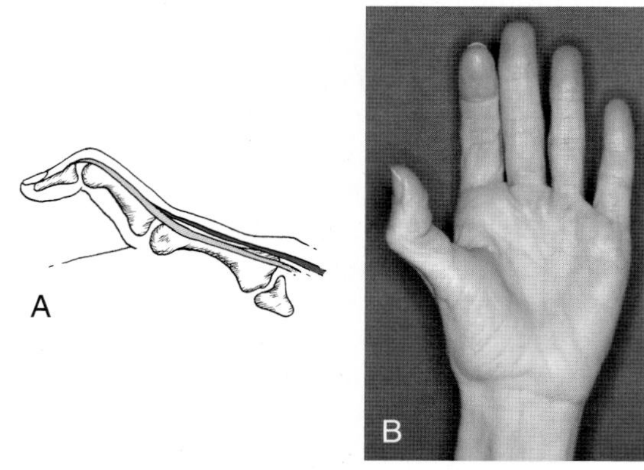

Figure 15–24 ***A and B,*** *The Nalebuff type 2 thumb: MP hyperextension and IP flexion.*

space can increase ROM, in my experience, it does not restore normal abduction. It is critical that the patient be aware of this and undergo a joint reconstruction before adduction contracture occurs. Splinting may be able to improve web space width or may stabilize the joint and improve comfort and function; however, the only real solution at the current level of technology is surgery.

With the loss of the median innervated thumb musculature, the thumb is unable to abduct in the palmar plane. Without the ability to lengthen the thumb adductor, the muscle shortens, producing a first web space contracture (Fig. 15–25). In the case of combined ulnar and median paralysis, the ulnar innervated thumb adductor ceases to function and often becomes fibrotic. This speeds up the formation of a first web space contracture. Clinicians use web space splinting to protect the length and width of this web space (Brandsma, 1993).

Wrist Joint

Unlike the joints discussed so far, the wrist is not generally predisposed to any particular patterns of motion loss. The wrist consists of a complex of joints and contains multiple articulations. As with other joints, stiffness here can arise from intra-articular or extra-articular pathology. Some causes of stiffness at this level are unique to this joint (Saffar, 1997):

- Certain types of idiopathic arthritis (gout).
- Avascular necrosis of the lunate.
- Volkmann ischemic contracture (produces wrist flexion).
- Ligamentous injury and carpal instability, including carpal collapse.
- Carpal non-union, especially of the scaphoid.

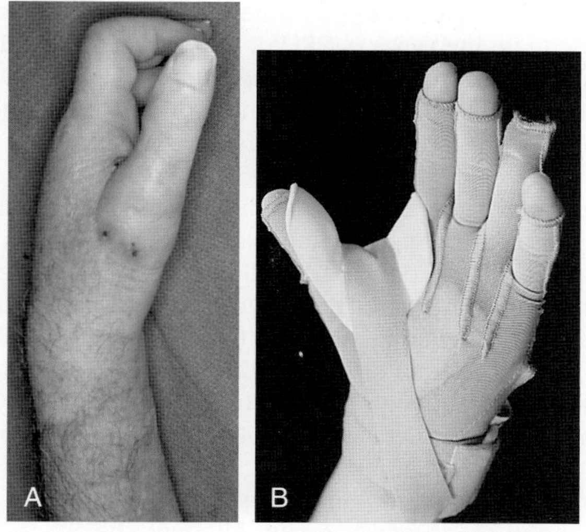

Figure 15–25 The thumb is unable to abduct with median innervated thumb musculature paralysis. ***A,*** *Without splinting, a first web space contracture will result.* ***B,*** *A thumb abduction mobilization splint using a serial static approach. Note use of compressive glove for edema.*

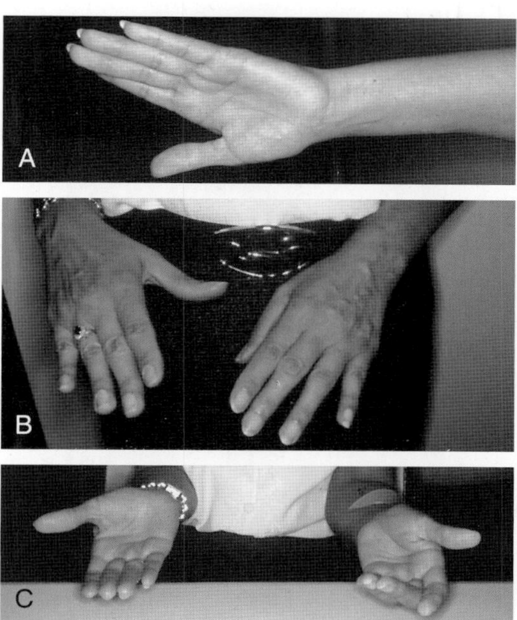

*Figure 15–26 Note the lack of motion on the patient's left side with wrist extension (**A**), radial deviation (**B**), and forearm supination (**C**).*

Trauma and its sequelae are the most commonly causes of lost wrist PROM. Saffar (1997) states that carpal instability causes 70% of chronic wrist stiffness. He describes post-traumatic osteoarthritis secondary to carpal joint injuries as a frequent cause of wrist stiffness. The position of the wrist during immobilization often predetermines the direction of stiffness.

The most common type of wrist fracture, the Colles, requires reduction of the wrist in a flexed, ulnarly deviated and pronated position to align the dorsally displaced distal fragment with the proximal radius (Frykman & Kropp, 1995). The patient remains in the cast for many weeks and often cannot attain a neutral wrist or forearm even after weeks out of the cast. The direction of wrist stiffness is always the opposite of the position in which the patient was casted. Thus for the common Colles fracture, the patient lacks extension, radial deviation, and supination (Fig. 15–26).

According to LaStayo (personal communication, 2000), the greater the distal radius malunion, the more opportunity exists for what appears to be an ulnar shift of the proximal row. This ulnar shift can occur if the radial inclination is lost and there is a distal radioulnar joint (DRUJ) disruption. The ulnar shift limits radial deviation; without radial deviation, normal wrist extension can never be achieved.

Soft tissue scarring in the forearm can also limit wrist PROM (Saffar, 1997). When extrinsic flexor and/or extensor muscle-tendon units become adherent to either bone or surrounding less mobile soft tissue, wrist PROM suffers (Fig. 15–27). In the case of predominantly dorsal extensor scarring, wrist flexion decreases. When volar

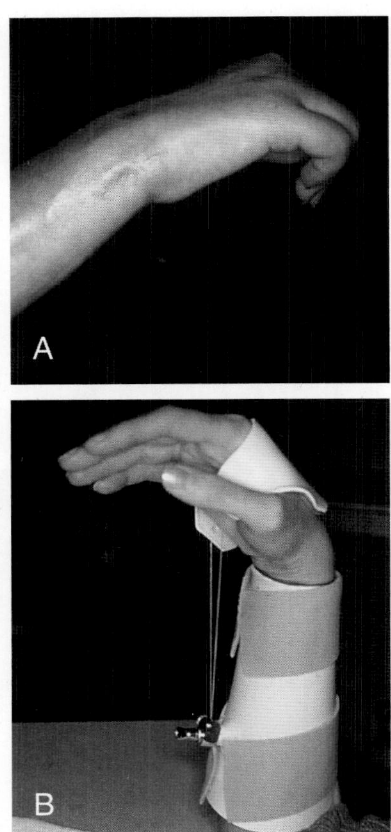

Figure 15–27 ***A,*** *Loss of wrist flexion.* ***B,*** *A wrist flexion mobilization splint using a static progressive stretch provided by a MERiT component.*

flexor scarring occurs, the wrist loses extension. It is important to note that if these extrinsic problems can be addressed early and if the wrist is spared involvement in inflammation and scar formation, then the wrist complex itself remains healthy and true stiffness of the joint will not result. However, in the case of long-standing extrinsic adhesions, especially if the inflammatory process of the injury involves the radiocarpal joint or the carpal complex, the wrist may become stiff.

Loss of wrist motion in rheumatoid arthritis has multifactorial origins (Garcia-Elias, 1997). The presence of significant synovitis alone can take up so much space that the wrist cannot achieve normal ROM. Loss of articular cartilage and supporting ligaments causes the wrist to shift in a characteristic manner. Usually, the adult with rheumatoid arthritis experiences carpal volar subluxation and an ulnar shift of the carpus rotating the hand radially on the forearm. With juvenile rheumatoid arthritis, volar subluxation of the carpus occurs; however, frequently, the carpus shifts radially, creating an ulnar deviation deformity at the wrist (Melvin, 1989). See Chapter 17 for more information.

Overt (visible and palpable) and occult (by MRI or differential diagnosis) ganglions can limit wrist ROM much in the same way that edema does (Angelide, 1988). The soft mass takes up space and limits normal tissue excursion and extensibility. When ganglions affect nerves, they cause pain, and the patient purposely restricts ROM. If the ganglion remains over a long period of time, wrist ROM can suffer, largely from adaptive shortening. More often, however, ganglion-related stiffness results from operative treatment.

Ganglions can present volarly or dorsally. In this author's experience, the dorsal ganglion is more common. When surgically excised, it frequently results in a loss of wrist flexion that is recalcitrant to active and passive exercise and scar-modification techniques. This scenario indicates the need for wrist flexion mobilization splinting (Fig. 15–27). Splinting the wrist in flexion is a foreign concept for many therapists. Most clinicians focus on wrist extension for function. Placing the wrist in a flexion splint for sustained periods leads to concerns about median nerve compression. Certainly, it is important to instruct the patient about monitoring for median nerve sensory status; however, this author has successfully used wrist flexion splinting after dorsal ganglion excision to restore normal PROM in flexion without median nerve compromise and without loss of wrist extension. Likewise, patients who have lost passive wrist extension after volar ganglion excision can benefit from a mobilizing splint for wrist extension (Fig. 15–2B).

The patient with carpal instability may undergo surgery—e.g., partial fusion, ligament repair, or wrist capsulodesis—to restore stability and decrease pain. In this case, wrist stiffness is iatrogenically introduced; the patient trades some motion to have a stable, pain-free wrist. However, these patients remain immobilized postoperatively for a long duration and frequently come out of the cast with little or no motion. When diligent therapy, including a thorough home program, fails to result in adequate increases in PROM, a dilemma arises. Opinions diverge about treatment indications (Levine, 1992).

Some clinicians believe that the stiffness will resolve somewhat over a very long period of time, perhaps of 1 year or more. They also believe that passive approaches to increasing motion are contraindicated, because these methods compromise the surgically induced stiffness and ultimately may produce instability and pain. Other clinicians introduce guarded passive exercise and carefully monitored mobilizing splinting to improve PROM. They use guidelines from several studies on cadavers that underwent partial fusion to limit the goals of motion (Gellman, Kauffman, Lenihan, & Botte, 1988; Ruby, Cooney, An, Linscheid, & Chao, 1988). These clinicians do not seek to restore full motion, the goal is the amount of motion the studies suggest as safe. Although the concerns of the more conservative clinicians warrant consideration, waiting a year or more to regain functional motion may not be an option for all patients. In addition, surgically induced stiffness can produce pain in and of itself. The careful and strategic application of passive treatment, including mobilizing splinting after surgery to restore carpal stability, can result in a more rapid return to motion and function that is both safe and comfortable.

Forearm

As for the wrist, a common cause of lost forearm PROM is trauma. And the position of the forearm in the cast usually dictates the direction of stiffness. Because wrist and forearm fractures are often reduced in pronation, loss of supination is more common than the loss of pronation (Fig. 15–26C). However, clinical experience shows that with severe forearm fractures and complex fractures of the DRUJ or the proximal radioulnar joint (PRUJ), the patient often loses rotation in both directions. Reduction of the radius that produces a less-than-optimum DRUJ relationship reliably decreases forearm rotation. Safar (1997) states that radiocarpal joint stiffness is associated with decreased pronosupination. The formation of exostosis is associated with forearm fractures. A bony bridge between the radius and ulna fuses the two bones together. Exostosis is easily diagnosed on radiographs and represents a contraindication to PROM exercise and mobilization splinting. Only surgical excision resolves the PROM loss (Raney, Brashear, & Shands, 1971).

Although fractures commonly cause loss of forearm motion, soft tissue injury (with or without fracture) can

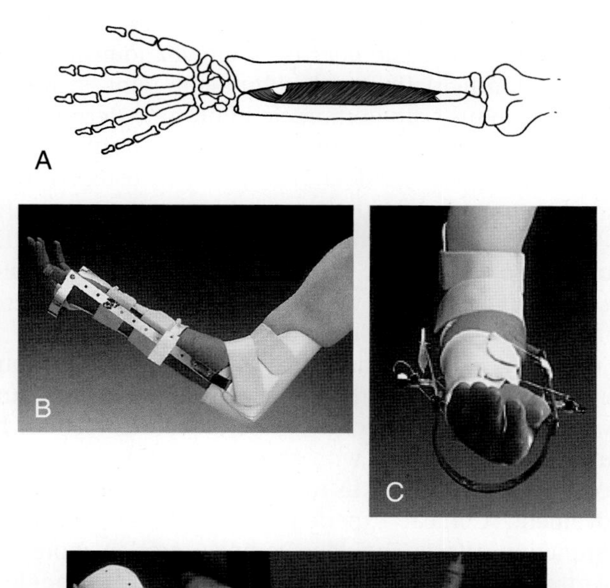

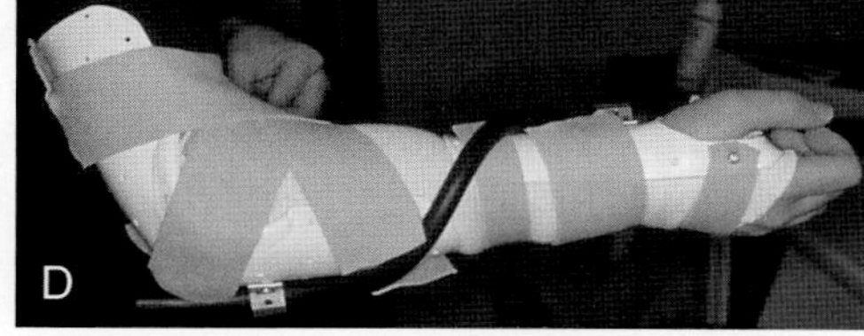

Figure 15–28 ***A,*** *The dense interosseus ligament joins and stabilizes the radius and ulna along their entire course.* ***B and C,*** *MERiT SPS Forearm Rotation Splint.* ***D,*** *Roylan Forearm Rotation Splint.*

also cause PROM limitation. Injury to the triangular fibrocartilage complex (TFCC) limits rotation and tends to affect supination more than pronation. Adaptive shortening or scarring of the interosseus ligament prevents the normal rotation of the radius (Fig. 15–28) (Stanley, 1997). Injury to other peri-articular soft tissues, such as the supinator muscle or either of the pronator muscles, can limit forearm rotation. In particular, the pronator quadratus has been implicated in restriction of supination (P. Dell, personal communication, 2000).

Rheumatoid arthritis affects both the DRUJ and the PRUJ. Bone and cartilage erosions, ligament instability, and joint effusions all contribute to forearm PROM loss.

Elbow Joint

Although fractures are the most common injuries that result in post-traumatic stiffness, other conditions such as central nervous system dysfunction, osteoarthrosis, burns, infection, and hemophilia can also lead to elbow contractures (Evans, Larson, & Yates, 1968; Figgie, Inglis, Mow, & Figgie, 1989; Josefsson, Gentz, Johnell, & Wendeberg, 1989; Jupiter, Neff, Holzach, & Allgower, 1985; Millard & Ortiz, 1965; Sherk, 1977). Many factors contribute to elbow stiffness after trauma (Hotchkiss, 1999). Delay in instituting active motion causes stiffness. Elbow stiffness also comes from mechanical causes. Galley, Richards, and O'Driscoll (1993) studied the effect of intra-articular effusions to explain the early development of flexion contracture from trauma. This condition causes the joint to assume a position of flexion to maximize capacity and minimize pressure. Hotchkiss describes how the uninjured elbow joint has a thin and usually transparent capsule that leaves adequate clearance for full flexion and extension. However, after trauma, the capsule thickens and limits both flexion and extension as a doorstop and a tether (Fig. 15–29). Loss of motion can also occur owing to a fracture that has fallen apart because of failed internal fixation or a persistently dislocated elbow (Jupiter et al., 1985).

Weiss and Sachar (1994) address a wide range of elbow PROM problems and describe a loss of terminal extension as a result of olecranon fracture and complete joint ankylosis as a result of high-energy injuries. They describe the unique way the soft tissue structure surrounding the elbow joint responds to trauma.

The medial and lateral collateral ligaments are often injured in elbow fractures and have a propensity toward calcification (Thompson & Garcia, 1967). The brachialis muscle is broad and lies directly on the capsule as it crosses the elbow joint. It is highly vascular, has no tendinous portion at this point, and thus bleeds in response to trauma. Hematoma has been implicated as an inciting cause of heterotopic ossification and subsequent capsular contracture (Glynn & Neibauer, 1976; Husband & Hastings, 1990; Urbaniak, Hansen, Beissinger, & Aitken, 1985). Both the anterior and the posterior cap-

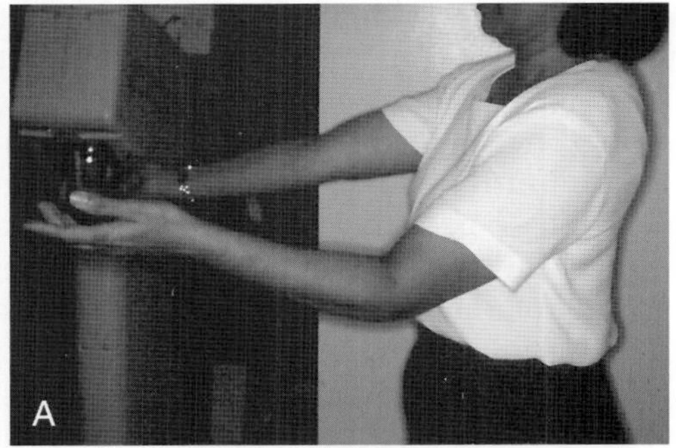
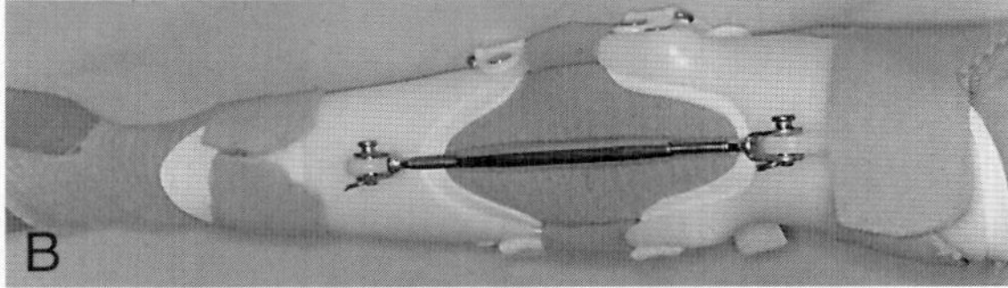
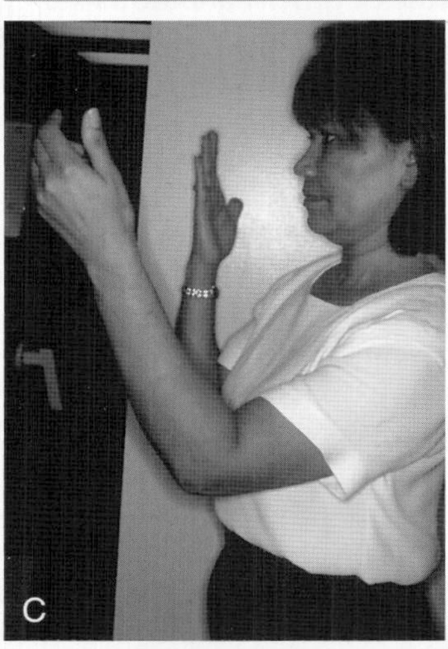
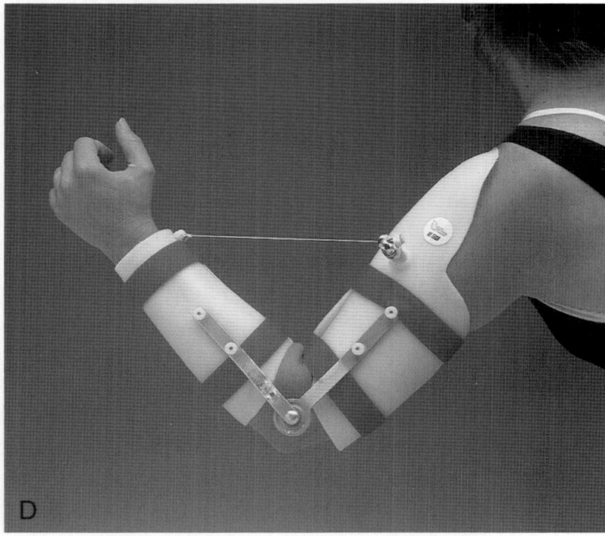

*Figure 15–29 After trauma, the elbow capsule thickens and limits both flexion and extension. **A,** note the elbow flexion contracture. **B,** An elbow extension mobilization splint using turnbuckle for static progressive positioning. **C,** Elbow extension contracture. **D,** An elbow flexion mobilization splint using the Phoenix elbow hinge and a MERiT component to exert a static progressive force.*

sule often contract. Heterotopic ossification is not amenable to splinting.

Ectopic ossification about the elbow can result from various local or systemic insults, including direct injury, neural axis trauma, burns, and genetic disorders (Viola & Hasting, 2000). The most common cause of elbow ectopic ossification is direct elbow trauma (Green & McCoy, 1979). Pathologic bone formation at the elbow level forms an unyielding block to motion and is generally not amenable to splinting and ROM treatment. As stated earlier, ectopic ossification is a contraindication for a mobilization splint.

Rheumatic disease at the elbow can affect the synovial lining at both the humeroradioulnar joint and the proximal radioulnar joint. Pain encourages the patient to position the arm in flexion and pronation, leading to contractures caused by prolonged positioning (Melvin, 1989). Static splinting at comfortable end range and soft splints that limit flexion during sleep may help minimize flexion contractures. Prevention of deformity provides the best results.

Morrey (1965) proposed a classification system for post-traumatic elbow stiffness that helps plan treatment and influences prognosis. Morrey categorizes stiffness as caused either by intrinsic factors (intra-articular adhesions) or extrinsic factors (capsular contractures). In addition, stiffness may have a mixed origin, which is associated with increased morbidity.

Shoulder Joint

Like the wrist, the shoulder is a complex joint made up of several articulations: glenohumeral joint, acromioclavicular joint, scapulothoracic joint, and sternoclavicular join. According to Copeland (1997), trauma is the primary cause of shoulder stiffness with osteoarthritis, and rheumatoid arthritis is a close second. Other rarer inflammatory arthropathies can contribute to shoulder motion problems. Soft tissue inflammation, especially rotator cuff tendonitis with impingement and subacromial bursitis, may result in permanent motion loss.

Common extrinsic factors related to regaining shoulder motion are the health and balance of the cervical and thoracic spine and rib cage; these complexes cannot be ignored when working with shoulder motion loss. Compromise of brachial plexus function often affects shoulder movement. Clinical experience shows that myofascial dysfunction affects shoulder complex motion more frequently than any other upper extremity joint. Shoulder stiffness has some causes unique to the glenohumeral complex. Primary frozen shoulder, or adhesive capsulitis, has no known cause. Copeland (1997) emphasizes the need for a general systemic assessment as part of the comprehensive shoulder stiffness examination to rule out contributions from remote sites, including Pancoast tumor, myocardial infarction, esophagitis, subphrenic abscess, cholecystitis, and gastric ulcer. Shoulder PROM loss may also result from shoulder immobilization. This immobilization may occur as treatment for primary shoulder pathology or may happen as the result of sling immobilization or self-treatment during recovery from injury to the distal joints. Copeland (1997) notes that of all the upper extremity joints, the shoulder most frequently responds to decreased movement with rapid onset of stiffness.

The shoulder demonstrates patterns of motion limitation. Impingement syndrome usually results in loss of elevation, abduction, and horizontal abduction. Cyriax (1978) described the capsular pattern, with loss of elevation and external rotation greater than internal rotation. The clinician frequently encounters this capsular pattern after sling immobilization (Fig. 15–30).

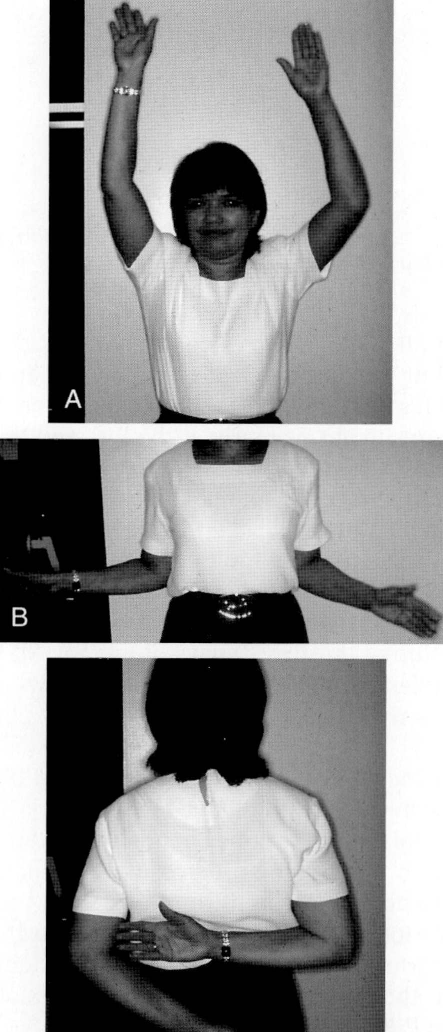

*Figure 15–30 Capsular pattern in the patient's left shoulder after sling immobilization with loss of elevation (**A**), external rotation (**B**), and internal rotation (**C**).*

Because shoulder splints are often bulky, heavy, and difficult to fabricate and fit, clinicians and patients rarely chose a shoulder splint as the first line of treatment. Because a large shoulder splint renders the entire extremity nonfunctional, compliance is predictably poor. The diagnosis of axillary burn and rotator cuff repair are notable exceptions, and the shoulder abduction splint or wedge is applied at the earliest possible moment. Compliance in such instances improves significantly because of the acuity of the problem and prophylactic nature of the device.

CASE STUDY SECTION

The case studies presented here are meant as teaching guidelines only. Treatment and splinting protocols vary greatly from surgeon to surgeon and from therapist to therapist. The therapist should check with the referring physicians and colleagues to define the preferred treatment and splinting methods.

CASE STUDY 1: **Hand Crush Injury**

MM is a 27-year-old right-dominant male baker who sustained a crush injury to his right hand when it went into a baguette-making machine. His index and middle fingers were crushed up to the proximal phalanx and his thumb was crushed up to the CMC joint. His ring and small fingers were generally unaffected. He had small superficial lacerations on the affected fingers and thumb that were healing well.

He was referred 10 days postinjury with a diagnosis of right crush injury with middle finger (MF) and thumb distal phalanx tuft fractures and a chip fracture of the MF middle phalanx. He presented with moderate edema and hematoma under the nails of the index finger (IF), MF, and thumb. He was generally hypersensitive and unwilling to move his hand, apparently owing to pain. His hand postured with his affected fingers in MP extension, PIP flexion, and DIP in neutral. His thumb MP postured in hyperflexion with the IP joint in slight hyperextension. This thumb posture suggested an undiagnosed soft tissue injury at his thumb MP joint that would affect active and passive MP extension. This concern was shared with the treating physician and patient. A subsequent radiograph revealed a mild subluxation of the thumb MP joint, confirming the diagnosis of a grade 2 to 3 sprain and extensor mechanism compromise.

The therapist discussed the treatment priorities with MM and the rationale for them. MM was told that most physicians and patients prioritize regaining finger IP flexion. However, the therapist's clinical experience supported prioritizing extension. The patient did demonstrate FDP function, and so prognosis for gaining flexion was excellent. MM learned that if the extensor mechanism was left attenuated over the flexed IP joint, it would almost certainly be permanently lengthened and would never be able to provide full extension again. This would sentence MM to lifelong PIP flexion contractures. MM agreed to the plan.

MM's initial splint focused on providing a safe position, with the finger MPs in maximum tolerable flexion and the IPs in maximum tolerable extension (Fig. 15–31). The thumb was placed in maximum tolerable abduction with the MP in maximum tolerable extension and the IP neutral. The patient received a custom, palmar, hand-based splint made of 1/8" combination rubber and plastic material. This type of thermoplastic provides a rigid splint owing to its plastic content while allowing for easier modification owing to the rubber content. In conjunction with his splinting program, the patient was provided with a comprehensive home program of edema control, gentle ROM to the fingers and thumb IP, and desensitization. The splint was progressed at each subsequent treatment session to achieve the goal of 75° finger MP flexion, 0° IP extension, 50° thumb abduction, and 0°thumb MP extension. He rapidly achieved his finger MP flexion and thumb abduction goals. He progressed in finger PIP and thumb MP extension.

Once the diagnosis of thumb soft tissue injury was confirmed, the patient was placed in a nonremovable, hand-based thumb cast made of 1" QuickCast tape without a liner, to allow MM to bathe and wash his hands (Fig. 15–32). When fabricating such a cast without a liner, extreme care must be taken to keep all parts of the cast smooth and all edges padded with small pieces of synthetic cast lining, trimmed or folded back on themselves. The patient was provided with a Splint/Cast Trimmer to trim the cast as needed as well as with additional cast padding to add or change padding as needed.

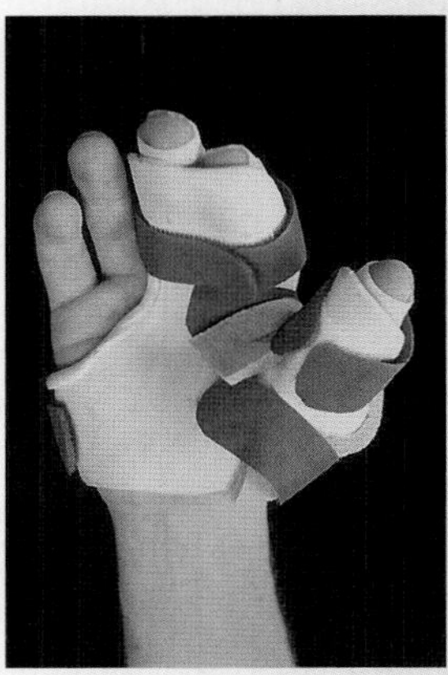

Figure 15–31 Hand-based IF, MF and thumb immobilization splint in the safe position.

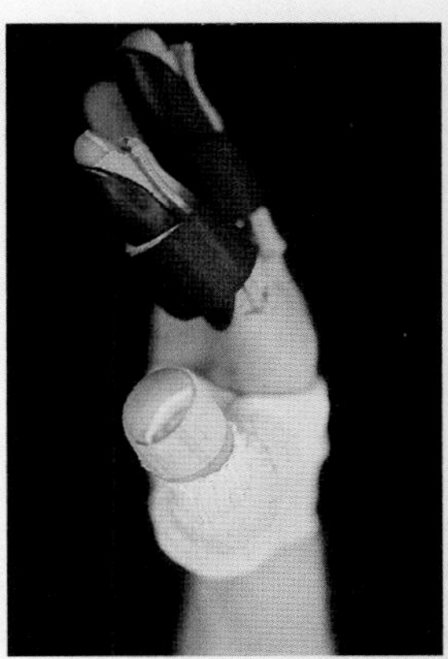

Figure 15–32 Hand-based QuickCast thumb cast and with custom gutter splints and 1-in. strap directly over the PIPs.

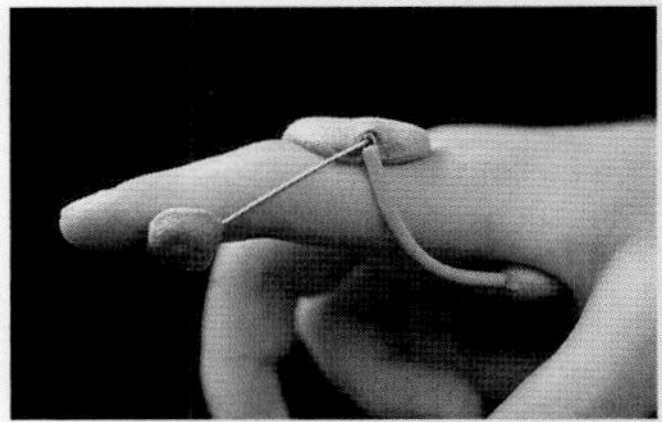

Figure 15–33 Prefabricated PIP extension mobilization splint. The patient was taught how to adjust the tension.

For the PIPs, the MM received custom gutter splints fabricated of 1/16" thermoplastic with a 1" strap directly over the PIPs (Fig. 15-32). The contours of the gutter splints were straight palmarly at the PIP, and the patient was instructed to tighten the loop strap gradually until the finger met the splint. The patient was also provided with a prefabricated PIP extension mobilization splint to be used intermittently as tolerated (Fig. 15–33). MM achieved neutral PIPs 1 week after receiving the new PIP splinting regimen. It is important to note that during the 7 to 10 days of therapy MM would not have tolerated the extension forces he was able to tolerate when switched to the gutter/spring splint combination.

After achieving neutral extension at the PIPs, the patient received a flexion glove (Fig. 15–34). The therapist replaced the rubber bands with static line to allow MM to use a static progressive approach to stretch composite flexion of the fingers. MM was instructed to focus on flexion but to return to the gutter splints intermittently if he began to lose extension; 2 days later, the patient had increased his flexion by 40° at the PIPs. He could still extend fully.

The thumb cast was changed every other day until the MP reached neutral, for a total of three casts. It should be noted that significant pressure had to be applied to achieve maximum thumb MP extension. Ini-

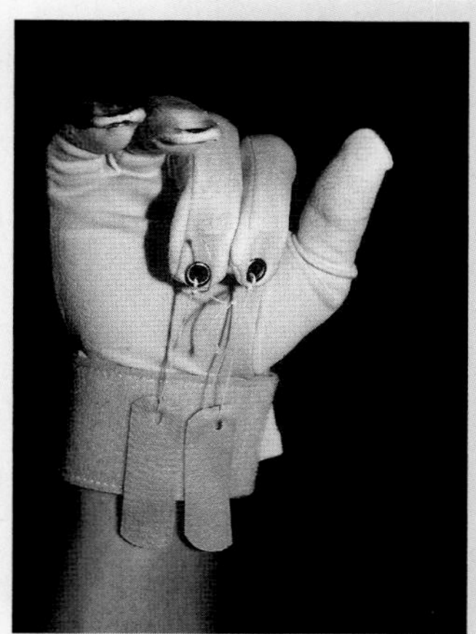

Figure 15–34 Static lines provide a static progressive approach to composite flexion of the fingers.

tially, the patient would not have tolerated this degree of force. It should also be noted that after application of each thumb cast, the thumb tip turned a deep red. The patient was asked to remain in the clinic until the color normalized, which it did for every cast.

MM was then placed in a final QuickCast thumb cast that included a rigid dorsal stay made of QuickCast; it positioned the thumb MP in anatomic neutral. This splint remained in place for 6 weeks, at which time the thumb extensor mechanism was evaluated for competence and a radiograph was taken to confirm anatomic alignment.

CASE STUDY 2: **Elbow Capsulotomy and Osteotomy**

LS is a 23-year-old, right-dominant, female graduate student who sustained a left intra-articular fracture of the humerus, ulna, and radius in a motor vehicle accident. She initially underwent an open reduction and internal fixation (ORIF) but did not have functional ROM after diligent therapy. She then underwent a subsequent manipulation under anesthesia (MUA). This too failed to yield functional motion. She then underwent two osteotomy and soft tissue releases with the most recent 2 days before presentation. She was referred for fabrication of a custom elbow splint to allow her to position herself alternately at maximum extension and maximum flexion.

LS presented with a minimal dressing and a compression sleeve. Her drain was discontinued the same day she arrived for therapy. She demonstrated 135° of flexion and 10° of extension. Her goal was to maintain this mobility, which proved difficult after the previous surgeries.

A static progressive elbow splint (MERiT SPS elbow extension kit) was chosen to meet the goals for this patient (Fig. 15–35). The splint was fabricated using a circumferential approach with 3/32" Aquaplast T for the humeral cuff and 1/16" Aquaplast T for the forearm cuff. The splint involved an elbow hinge and an extension outrigger adjusted to provide a 90° angle of pull. The MERiT kit, mounted to the forearm cuff, generated tension, which LS could control after receiving thorough instructions about use and precautions. The splint line was done in a three-part fashion, with one line attached to the MERiT component and a bra hook, one line attached to the extension outrigger and a bra loop, and the last line attached to the humeral cuff and a bra loop. This allowed the MERiT kit to attach alternately to the flexion or extension component.

LS immediately grasped the function and use of the splint and stated that she was pleased. She was instructed in precautions for skin pressure areas and was taught to monitor the sensation of the ulnar innervated digits while positioned in flexion. Her goal was to wear the splint for as many hours as possible during the day, alternating between flexion and extension.

Because LS lived a long distance from the clinic, she was referred to another rehabilitation facility for ongoing therapy. A 3-month follow-up visit revealed she had maintained her excellent ROM.

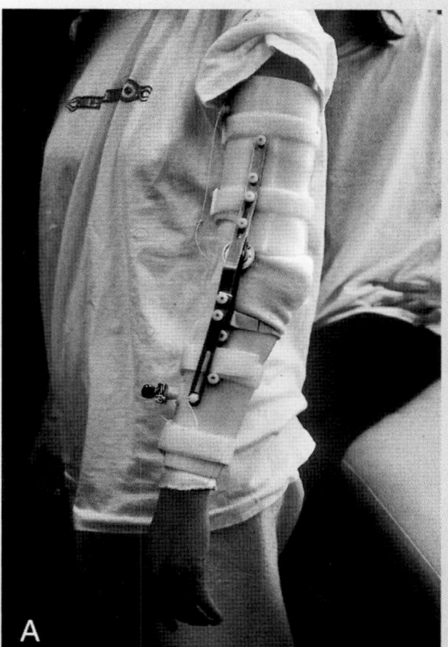

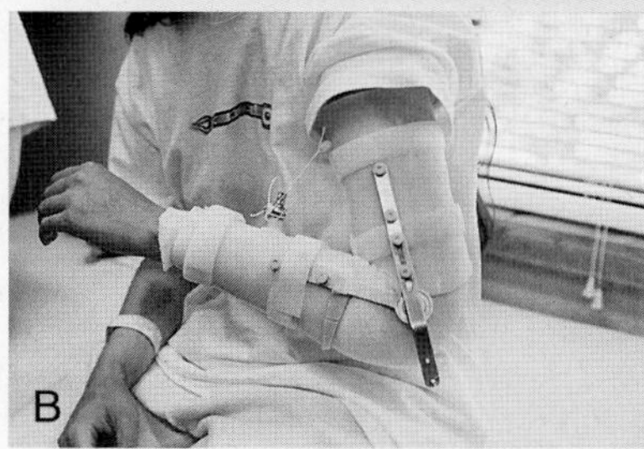

*Figure 15–35 A static progressive splint allows the patient to position herself at maximum extension (**A**) and maximum flexion (**B**). Shown is a MERiT SPS Elbow Extension Kit.*

CONCLUSION

The stiff joint continues to be one of the great challenges in hand surgery and rehabilitation. With unique anatomy, each joint presents its patterns of response to injury and disease. Understanding the tendencies for a joint to respond to trauma and disease in a certain way helps the therapist predict problems with stiffness and often provides the opportunity to prevent loss of motion. To work toward the goals of either preventing stiffness or minimizing the duration of stiffness, therapists must continue to study the nature of stiffness at the molecular, histologic, and joint complex levels.

REFERENCES

Abbott, K., Denney, J., Burke, F., & McGrouther, D. A. (1980). A review of attitudes to splintage in Dupuytren's contracture. *Journal of Hand Surgery (Edinburgh, Lotham), 12,* 326–328.

Akeson, W. H., Ameil, D., & Woo, SL.-Y. (1980). Immobility effects on synovial joints. The pathomechanics of joint contracture. *Biorheology, 17,* 95–110.

Akeson, W. H., Ameil, D., Avel, M., Garfin, S. R., & Woo, S. L. (1987). Effects of immobilization on joints. *Clinical Orthopaedics and Related Research, 219,* 28–37.

Akeson, W. H., Ameil, D., Woo, SL.-Y., Mechanc, G. L., Woo, S. L., Harwood, F. L., & Hamer, M. L. (1977). Collagen cross/linking alternations in joint contractures: Changes in the reducible crosslinks in periarticular connective tissue collagen after nine weeks of immobilization. *Connective Tissue Research, 5,* 15–19.

Ameil, K., Woo, SL.-Y., Harwood, F. L., & Akeson, W. H. (1982). The effect of immobilization on collagen turnover in connective tissue: A biochemical-biomechanical correlation. *Acta Orthopaedica Scandinavica, 53,* 325–332.

Angelides, A. C. (1988). Ganglions of the hand and wrist. In D. P. Green (Ed.). *Operative hand surgery* (2nd ed., pp. 2281–2289). New York: Churchill Livingstone.

Arem, A., & Madden, J. (1976). Effects of stress on healing wounds: Intermittent noncyclical tension. *Journal of Surgical Research, 20,* 93–102.

Aulicino, P. (1995). Clinical examination of the hand. In J. M. Hunter, E. J. Mackin, & A. D. Callahan (Eds.). *Rehabilitation of the hand* (4th ed., pp. 53–75). St. Louis: Mosby Year Book.

Bell-Krotoski, J. A. (1987). Plaster casting for the remodeling of soft tissue. In E. E. Fess & C. Phillips (Eds.). *Hand splinting: Principles and methods* (2nd ed., pp. 453–454). St. Louis: Mosby.

Bonutti, P. M., Windau, J. E., Ables, B. A., & Miller, B. G. (1994). Static progressive stretch to re-establish elbow range of motion. *Clinical Orthopedics and Related Research, 303,* 128–134.

Brand, P. W. (1985). *Clinical biomechanics of the hand.* St. Louis: Mosby.

Brand, P. W. (1988). The mind and spirit in hand therapy. *Journal of Hand Therapy, 1,* 145–148.

Brand, P. W. & Hollister, A. M. (1999). *Clinical biomechanics of the hand* (3rd ed.). St. Louis: Mosby.

Brandsma, J. W. (1993). *The intrinsic minus hand.* Doctoral thesis (Proefschrift). Rijksuniversititeit Utrecht, The Netherlands.

Brzezienski, M. A., & Schneider, L. H. (1995). Extensor tendon injuries at the distal interphalangeal joint. *Hand Clinics of North America, 11,* 373–386.

Cassanova, J. S. (1992). *ASHT Splint Classification System.* Chicago: American Society of Hand Therapists.

Chase, R. A. (1989). Anatomy and kinesiology of the hand. In J. M. Hunter, E. J. Mackin, & A. D. Callahan (Eds.). Rehabilitation of the hand: Surgery and therapy (4th ed., pp. 24–35). St Louis: Mosby.

Coons, M. S., & Green, S. M. Boutonniere deformity. *Hand Clinics of North America, 11,* 387–402.

Copeland, S. A. (1978). Shoulder stiffness: Introduction. In: Copeland S. A., Gschwend, N., Landi, A., & Saffar, P. (1997). *Joint Stiffness of the Upper Limb.* London: Dunitz.

Cyriax, J. (1978). *Textbook of orthopaedic medicine* (7th ed., vol. 1). London: Bailliere Tindall.

Eaton, R. G., & Glickel, S. Z. (1987). Trapeziometacarpal osteoarthritis: Staging as a rationale for treatment. *Hand Clinics, 3,* 455–469.

Enneking, W. F., & Horowitz, M. (1972). The intra-articular effects of immobilization on the human knee. *Journal of Bone Joint Surgery (American volume), 54,* 973–985.

Evans, R. B. (1990). A study of the zone I flexor tendon injury and implications for treatment. *Journal of Hand Therapy, 3,* 133–148.

Evans, R. B. (1995). An update on extensor tendon management. In J. M. Hunter, E. J. Mackin, & A. D. Callahan (Eds.). *Rehabilitation of the hand* (4th ed., pp. 565–606). St. Louis: Mosby Year Book.

Evans, E. B., Larson, D. L., & Yates, S. (1968). Preservation and restoration of joint function in patients with severe burns. *Journal of the American Medical Association, 204,* 91–96.

Fess, E. E., & Phillips, C. (1987). Hand splinting: Principles and methods (2nd ed.). St. Louis: Mosby.

Figgie, M. P., Inglis, A. E., Mow, C. S., Figgie, H. E. (1989). Total elbow arthroplasty for complete ankylosis of the elbow. *Journal of Bone and Joint Surgery (American volume), 71,* 513–520.

Flowers, K. R., & LaStayo, P. (1994). Effect of total end range time on improving passive range of motion. *Journal of Hand Therapy, 7,* 150–157.

Flowers, K. R., & Michlovitz, S. L. (1988). Assessment and management of loss of Motion in orthopedic dysfunction. *Postgraduate Advances in Physical Therapy,* (pp. 1–12). Alexandria, VA: APTA.

Frank, C., Ameil, D., Woo, SL.-Y., & Akeson, W. (1985). Normal ligament properties and ligament healing. *Clinical Orthopedics and Related Research, 196,* 15–24.

Frykman, G. K., & Kropp, W. E. (1995). Fractures and traumatic conditions of the wrist. In J. M. Hunter, E. J. Mackin, & A. D. Callahan (Eds.). *Rehabilitation of the hand* (4th ed., pp. 315–318). St. Louis: Mosby Year Book.

Galley, S. H., Richards, R. R., & O'Driscoll, S. W. (1993). Intraarticular capacity and compliance of stiff and normal elbows. *Arthroscopy 9,* 9–13.

Garcia-Elias, M. (1997). General causes of radiocarpal stiffness. In S. A. Copeland, N. Gschwend, A. Landi, & P. Saffar (Eds.). Joint stiffness of the upper limb (pp. 170–177). London: Dunitz.

Gellman, H., Kauffman, D., Lenihan, M., & Botte, M. J. (1988). An in vitro analysis of wrist motion: The effect of limited intercarpal arthrodesis and the contribution of the radiocarpal and midcarpal joints. *The Journal of Hand Surgery, 13,* 378–383.

Glynn, J. J., & Neibauer, J. J. (1976). Flexion and extension contractures of the elbow. Surgical management. *Clinical Oropaedics and Related Research, 117,* 89–291.

Goga-Eppenstein, P., Hill, J. P., Seifert, T. M., & Yasukawa, A. M. (1999). Considerations with specific diagnoses. In P. Goga-Eppenstein, J. P. Hill, P. A. Philip, A. Philip, T. M. Seifert, & A. M. Yasukawa (Eds.). *Casting protocols for the upper and lower extremities* (pp. 125–156). Gaithersburg, MD: Aspen.

Green, D. P., & McCoy H. (1979). Turnbuckle orthotic correction of elbow flexion contractures after acute injuries. *Journal of Bone and Joint Surgery (American volume), 61,* 1092–1095.

Grigsby deLinde, L., & Miles, W. K. (1995). Remodeling of scar tissue in the burned hand. In J. M. Hunter, E. J. Mackin, & A. D. Callahan (Eds.). *Rehabilitation of the hand* (4th ed., pp. 1267–1294). St. Louis: Mosby Year Book.

Hardy, M. (1999). Keynote address presented at the American Association of Hand Surgeons Seminar on Joint Stiffness.

Hirschfeld, A. H., & Behan, R. C. (1963). The accident process: Etiological considerations of industrial injuries. *Journal of the American Medical Association, 186,* 193–???.

Hotchkiss, R. M. (1995). *Application of hinged external fixator for elbow limitations.* Paper presented at the ASSH meeting, Snowmass, CO.

Hotchkiss, R. M. (n.d.). *Design rationale.* Literature accompanying elbow compass hinge.

Hotchkiss, R. N. (1999). Elbow contracture. In D. P. Green, R. N. Hotchkiss, & W. C. Pederson. (1999). *Green's operative hand surgery* (4th ed., 667–682). New York: Churchill Livingston.

Husband, J. B., & Hastings, H. I. (1990). The lateral approach for operative release of post-traumatic contracture of the elbow. *Journal of Bone Joint Surgery (American volume), 72,* 1353–1358.

Imaeda, T., An, K.-N., & Cooney, W. P. (1992). Functional anatomy and biomechanics of the thumb. *Hand Clinics, 8,* 9–15.

Josefsson, P. O., Gentz, C. F., Johnell, O., & Wendeberg, B. (1989). Dislocations of the elbow and intra-articular fractures. *Clinical Orthopaedic and Related Research, 246,* 126–130.

Jupiter, J. B., Neff, U., Holzach, P., & Allgower, M. Intercondylar fractures of the humerus: An operative approach. *Journal of Bone and Joint Surgery, 67,* 927–930.

Kapandji, I. A. (1982). *The physiology of the joints: Annotated diagrams of the mechanics of the human joints. Vol. 1: Upper Limb* (5th ed.). New York, Churchill Livingstone.

Levine, W. (1992). Rehabilitation techniques for ligament injuries of the wrist. *Hand Clinics, 8,* 669–681.

Light, K., Nuzik, S., Personius, W., & Barstrom, A. (1984). Low-load prolonged stretch versus high-load brief stretch in treating knee contractures. Physical Therapy, 64, 330–333.

Lluch, A. (1997). In S. A. Copeland, N. Gschwend, A. Landi, & P. Saffar (Eds.). *Joint stiffness of the upper limb* (pp. 259–264). London: Dunitz.

Lowe, C. (1992). Treatment of tendinitis, tenosynovitis, and other cumulative trauma disorders of musicians forearm, wrist and hands . . . restoring function with hand therapy. *Journal of Hand Therapy, 5,* 84–90.

Malick, M. H. (1972). Manual on static hand splinting (2nd ed.). Pittsburgh: Harmarville Rehabilitation Center.

Mannarino, S. L. (1992). Skeletal injuries. In B. G. Stanley & S. M. Tribuzi (Eds.). *Concepts in hand rehabilitation* (pp. 312–315). Philadelphia: Davis.

Melone, C. P., Beldner, S., & Basuk, R. S. (2000). Thumb collateral ligament injuries: an anatomic basis for treatment. In C. P. Melone (Ed.). *Update on management of sports injuries* (Vol. 16, pp. 345–357). Philadelphia: WB Saunders.

Melvin. J. L. (1989). *Rheumatic disease in the adult and child: Occupational therapy and rehabilitation* (3rd ed.). Philadelphia: Davis.

Millard, D. R., & Ortiz, A. C. (1965). Correction of severe elbow contractures. *Journal of Bone and Joint Surgery (American volume), 47,* 1347–1354.

Morrey, B. F. (1965). Post-traumatic contractures of the elbow: Operative treatment, including distraction arthroplasty. *Journal of Bone and Joint Surgery (American volume), 47,* 1347–1354.

Mulligan, B. R. (1999). *Manual therapy "NAGS", "SNAGS", "MWMS" etc.* Wellington, NZ: Plane View Services.

Nathan, R., & Taras, J. S. (1995). Common infections in the hand. In J. M. Hunter, E. J. Mackin, & A. D. Callahan (Eds.). *Rehabilitation of the hand* (4th ed., pp. 251–260). St. Louis: Mosby Year Book.

Peacock, E. E. (1984). *Wound repair* (3rd ed.). Philadelphia: Saunders.

Pelligrini, V. D., Olcott, C. W., & Hollenberg, G. (1993). Contact patterns in the trapeziometacarpal joint: The role of the palmar beak ligament. *The Journal of Hand Surgery, 18,* 238–244.

Raney, R. B., Brashear, H. R., & Shands, A. R. (1971). *Shand's handbook of orthopedic surgery.* St. Louis: Mosby.

Roberson, L. & Giurintano, D. J. (1995). Objective measures of joint stiffness. *Journal of Hand Therapy, 8,* 163–166.

Ruby, L. K., Cooney, W. P., An, K. N., Linscheid, R. L., & Chao, E. Y. S. (1988). Relative motion of selected carpal bones: A kinematic analysis of the normal wrist. *Journal of Hand Surgery, 13,* 1–10.

Saffar, P. (1997). Extrinsic and intrinsic causes of radiocarpal stiffness. In S. A. Copeland, N. Gschwend, A. Landi, & P. Saffar (Eds.). *Joint stiffness of the upper limb* (pp. 156–167). London: Dunitz.

Sampson, S. P., Badalamente, M. A., Hurtst, L. C., Dowd A., Sewell, C. S., Lehmann-Torres, J., Ferraro, M., & Semon, B. (1992). The use of a passive motion machine the postoperative rehabilitation of Dupuytren's disease. *Journal of Hand Surgery, 17,* 333–338.

Schultz-Johnson, K. S. (1992). Splinting: A problem solving approach. In B. G. Stanley & S. M. Tribuzi (Eds.). Concepts in hand rehabilitation (pp. 238–271). Philadelphia: Davis.

Schultz-Johnson, K. S. (2000). *Static-progressing splinting* (2nd ed.). Edwards, CO: UE Tech.

Sherk, H. H. (1977). Treatment of severe rigid contractures of cerebral palsied upper limbs. *Clinical Orthopaedics and Related Research, 125,* 151–155.

Simmons, B. P., & Vasile, R. G. (1980). The clenched fist syndrome. *Journal of Hand Surgery, 5,* 420–424.

Sokolow, C. (1997). Extrinsic causes of stiffness of the proximal interphalangeal joint. In S. A. Copeland, N. Gschwend, A. Landi, & P. Saffar (Eds.). *Joint stiffness of the upper limb* (251–258). London: Dunitz.

Stanley, J. (1997). Causes of stiffness of the distal radioulnar joint. In S. A. Copeland, N. Gschwend, A. Landi, & P. Saffar (Eds.). *Joint stiffness of the upper limb* (201–219). London: Dunitz.

Stewart, K. M., & van Strien, G. (1995). Postoperative management of flexor tendon injuries. In J. M. Hunter, E. J. Mackin, & A. D. Callahan (Eds.). *Rehabilitation of the hand* (4th ed., pp. 433–462). St. Louis: Mosby Year Book.

Thompson, H. C., & Garcia, A. (1967). Myositis ossificans: Aftermath of elbow injuries. *Clinical Orthopaedics and Related Research, 50,* 129–134.

Urbaniak, J. R., Hansen, P. E., Beissinger, S. F., & Aitken, M. S. (1985). Correction of post-traumatic flexion contracture of the elbow by anterior capsulotomy. *Journal of Bone and Joint Surgery (American volume), 67,* 1160–1164.

Viola, R. W. & Hasting, H. (2000). Treatment of ectopic ossification about the elbow. *Clinical Orthopaedics and Related Research, 370,* 65–86.

Wallace, P. F., & Fitzmorris, C. S. (1978). The S-H-A-F-T syndrome in the upper extremity. *Journal of Hand Surgery, 3,* 492–494.

Weiss, A. C., & Sachar, K. (1994). Soft tissue contractures about the elbow. *Hand Clinics, 10,* 439–451.

Williams, P & Goldspink, G (1978). Changes in sarcomere length and physiological properties in immobilized muscle. *Journal of Anatomy, 127,* 459–468.

SUGGESTED READINGS

Raphael, J., & Skirven, T. (2001). *Atlas of the hand clinics: Contractures and splinting.* Philadelphia: Saunders.

CHAPTER 16

Fractures

Kristina E. Manniello, MS, OTR/L, CHT

INTRODUCTION

Splinting after an acute fracture can play an important role in the care of these injuries. Splints not only are used occasionally to replace cast immobilization of a healing fracture but also are used after healing to address range of motion (ROM) limitations. The careful application of splints during the initial fracture healing phase can permit the fracture to mend while allowing at least partial mobility of adjacent structures. Unlike casts, splints are usually lighter in weight and can conform quite nicely around small areas of the upper extremity, such as the metacarpals. However, the therapist must always appreciate that prolonged immobilization may contribute to stiffness, especially in older patients.

This chapter reviews acute fractures and splinting intervention sequentially, from the shoulder complex to the distal phalanx. Tables present a quick reference for splinting management of the fractures discussed. The splint and positioning recommendations outlined in this chapter are meant as a general guideline only, because each fracture is unique and therapy intervention must be individualized to meet each patient's needs. This chapter does not discuss every possible fracture or dislocation that can occur in the upper extremity; instead it focuses on common injuries. Splinting to gain ROM is detailed in Chapter 15.

Fracture Classification and Treatment

Fractures are generally classified by the **anatomic location** (base, neck, or shaft) and the **direction of the break line** (longitudinal, transverse, or spiral) (Fig. 16–1). They are further categorized by whether they are **linear** (two fragments) or **comminuted** (several fragments) (Fig. 16–2) and **open** (tissue disrupted; fragment exposed to environment) or **closed** (soft tissue intact) (Harkess & Ramsey,1991).

The treatment of fractures includes a **closed, immobilization** approach, which involves manipulation to reduce the fracture and then casting, traction, or splinting to hold the bones in the corrected position. Traditional methods immobilize the joints proximal and distal to the fracture site. Functional splinting immobilizes the fracture site only. The physician almost always directs the type of immobilization method to be used. **Operative treatment** is performed when closed means are unsuccessful or may be the primary method of treatment for some types of fractures. Techniques for fracture management include external fixation, percutaneous pinning, and plate and screw fixation (Harkess & Ramsey, 1991). The mechanism and severity of the injury and the age of the patient dictate the type of resultant fracture. Table 16–1 highlights the most common types of fractures.

Scapula Fractures

The therapist does not often manage fractures of the shoulder girdle in the acute stage, unless there is some associated distal involvement, as often seen in multiple trauma cases (i.e., motor vehicle accidents). The associated injuries commonly include distal fractures of the extremity. There is a place, however, for educating patients regarding edema management, activity limitations, and instruction in appropriate home exercises of the uninvolved joints to decrease edema, prevent joint contractures and stiffness, and maximize function.

Scapula fractures occur infrequently (Butters, 1991), probably because it is protected by covering muscles and

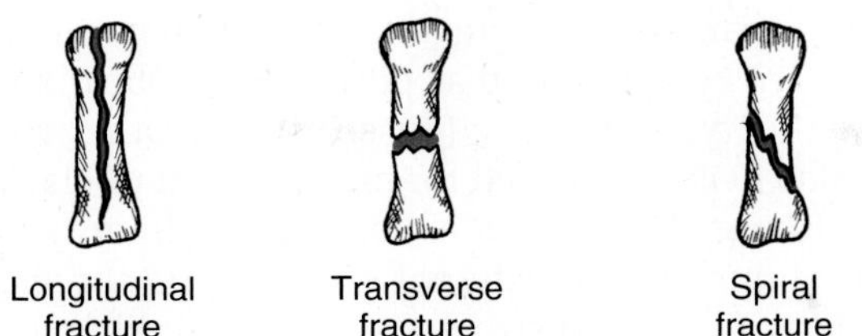

Figure 16–1 *Fractures can be classified by the direction of the fracture.*

Figure 16–2 *Linear fractures produce two fragments; comminuted fractures produce more than two fragments.*

TABLE 16–1 Common Upper Extremity Fractures

Fracture	Definition
Avulsion	Occurs when a bony attachment tears away
Complicated	May disrupt nerves, arteries, or viscera
Comminuted	More than two pieces or fragments
Compound	Associated with an open wound; susceptible to infection if not properly treated
Greenstick	Impacted or buckling from bony cortex; associated with the pediatric population
Osteochondral	Involves articular cartilage of bone

its close proximity to the rib cage (Fig. 16–3). The scapula, a broad bone that provides major support for the arm, is fractured mainly in cases of severe trauma. Acromion and coracoid fractures are usually isolated injuries, which can be caused by a direct blow to the area; but they may be found in combination with humerus fractures. They often heal without complication (Fig. 16–4) (Brown, 1983; Butters, 1991).

Splinting Options

The splinting or acute management options for nondisplaced scapula fractures include immobilization for 2 to 3 weeks with a broad arm sling (Fig. 16–5) (Brown, 1983). After this time, therapeutic exercises are started to prevent stiffness. If found in isolation, acromion and coracoid fractures may be treated with a sling, to provide symptomatic relief during the healing process.

Clavicle Fractures

The clavicle connects the arm to the shoulder girdle and trunk and protects the brachial plexus and subclavian vessels. The clavicle consists of three parts: distal third (lateral third), middle third (midshaft), and proximal third. This S-shaped bone is most susceptible to fracture in the midshaft region (Fig. 16–6). The ends of the clavicle are held firmly in place to the adjacent structures by multiple ligaments. **Clavicle fractures** may occur as a result of falling on an outstretched hand, direct trauma to the shoulder, or during childbirth (Eiff, 1997). In children, there is a high healing rate, but in adults, the healing rate is slower and sometimes compromised (Eiff, 1997). Operative treatment may be indicated for some clavicle fractures because of the potential of injury to other structures (e.g., the subclavian artery and brachial plexus). Satisfactory results have been reported (Edwards, 1992).

Distal third clavicle fractures are often categorized as type 1 to 3 fractures. These fractures are often overlooked, as they usually do not result in deformity. Type 1 fractures are most common, and the ligamentous connection is rarely disrupted. Type 2 fractures often result

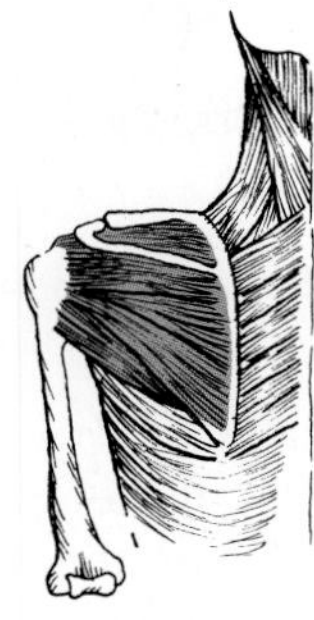

Figure 16–3 *Scapula fractures are rare owing to the large number of muscles that protect and surround the bone.*

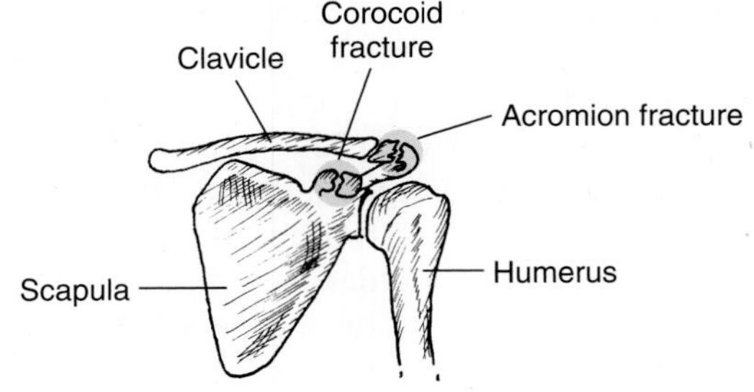

Figure 16–4 *Fractures of the acromion and coracoid process.*

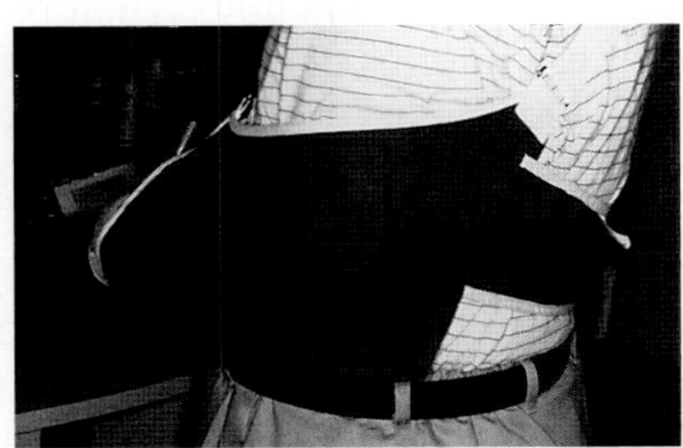

Figure 16–5 *A broad arm sling can be used for many diagnoses, including injuries to the scapula, clavicle, humerus, and elbow.*

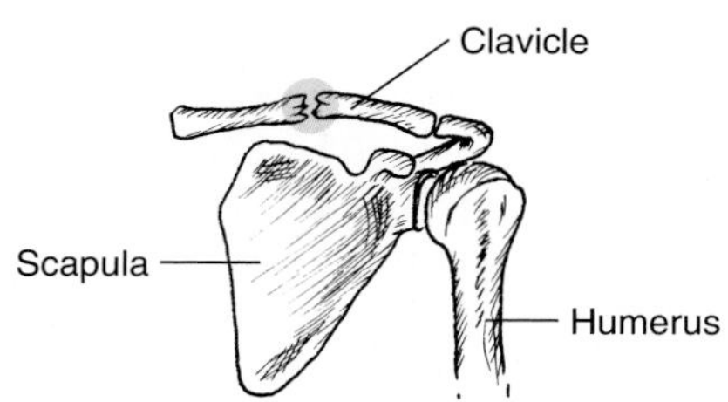

Figure 16–6 The middle third of the clavicle is the most common area of the clavicle to be injured.

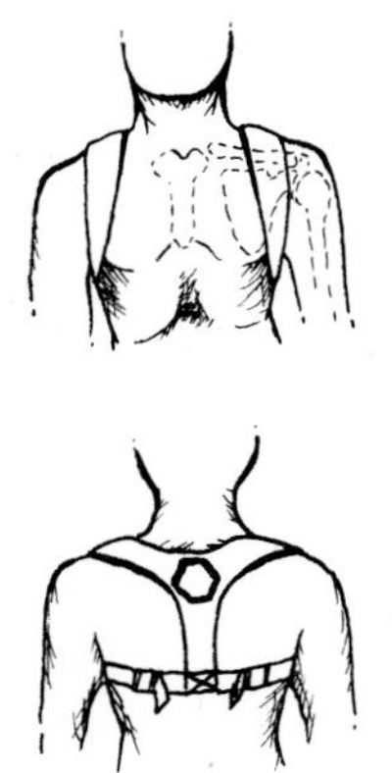

Figure 16–7 The Figure-8 strap places the shoulder in a retracted and upright position.

in proximal displacement of the upward fragment, while the attaching ligament holds the distal fragment down. Type 3 fractures are intra-articular.

Splinting Options

Splinting options for patients with a clavicle injury are the broad arm sling, Figure-8 strap, or taping. The broad arm sling is appropriate for all types of clavicle fractures, when used alone or in conjunction with a Figure-8 strap (Figs. 16.5 and 16–7). The Figure-8 strap is used for midshaft clavicle fractures and may be applied immediately or at 1 week postinjury, as edema subsides. This design places the shoulder region in the position of attention (Brown, 1983). The Figure-8 strap has also been shown to assist in reduction of a minimally displaced clavicle fracture (Brown, 1983). As the edema resolves, the splint loosens and the patient must be instructed to tighten the strap gently. When rehabilitating patients with these injuries, it is important not to allow the shoulder to abduct past 40 to 45°, because this puts a tremendous strain on the fracture site. Proximal third clavicle fractures are managed by immobilization in much the same way (Eiff, 1997).

Taping techniques have been used to manage midshaft fractures. One specific taping technique involves stabilizing the fracture site by taping in shoulder adduction, elbow at 90°, and forearm pronated (Fig. 16–8). Radial, ulnar, and anterior interosseous nerve (AIN) injuries have been reported as possible complications from taping this type of injury (Susso, 1994). Other supports have also been advocated for management of clavicle injuries (Craig, 1991). When treating proximal upper extremity injuries with external restraints (if appplicable), the therapist must instruct the patient in shoulder and distal extremity ROM to prevent stiffness. To avoid peripheral nerve compression from strap placement; the patient should be taught adaptive techniques for activities of daily living (ADLs) and work.

Humerus Fractures

The humerus is a long bone that articulates with the glenoid fossa of the scapula, connecting the shoulder girdle with the rest of the arm. **Humerus fractures** are caused by a variety of insults, including falls from a standing height or lower and from motor vehicle accidents (Biangini, 1991). Fractures commonly occur through the

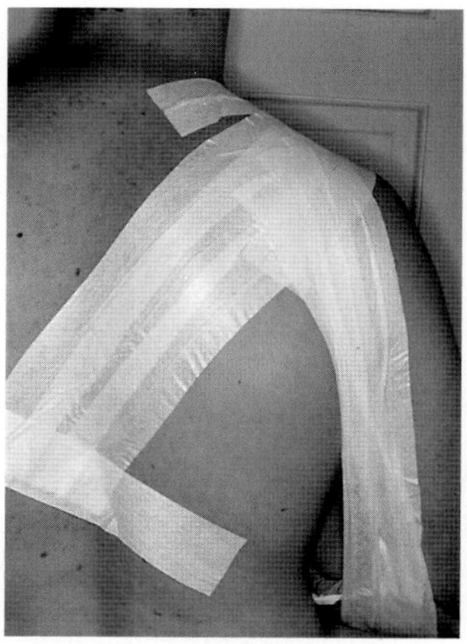

Figure 16–8 Taping techniques for midshaft clavicle fractures.

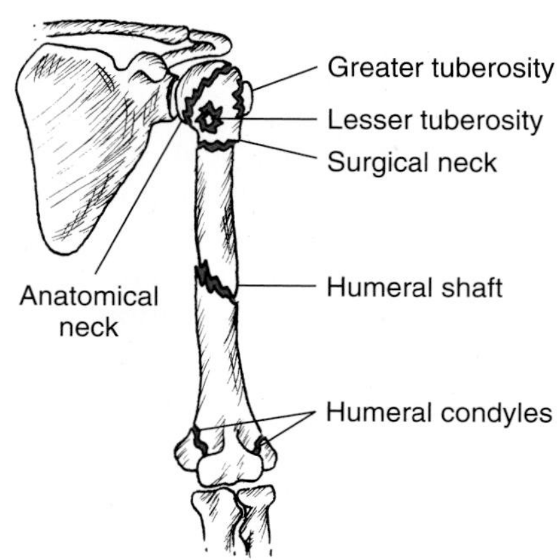

Figure 16–9 Areas of the humerus susceptible to fracture.

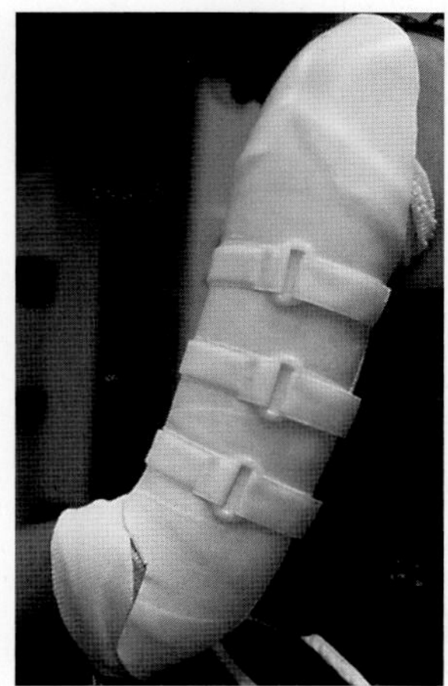

Figure 16–10 A custom-molded functional humeral brace (nonarticular humerus splint) that allows some shoulder and elbow ROM.

surgical neck, greater or lesser tuberosities, anatomic neck, humeral shaft, and distal humerus about the condyles (Fig. 16–9) (Brown, 1983). Patients with humeral shaft fractures can have an associated radial nerve injury; this nerve is susceptible to injury where it wraps around the humerus in the spiral groove at this level. Distal humerus fractures, commonly seen in children, usually present as comminuted fractures that are often difficult to manage (Sarmiento, 1990).

Splinting Options

Proximal fractures—involving the surgical neck, humeral head, or greater or lesser tuberosities—may be managed with a broad arm sling or its equivalent (Brown, 1983) (Fig. 16–5). Humerus shaft fractures may be successfully managed using a **functional fracture splint** or brace (Sarmiento, 1990). (The terms *fracture splint* and *fracture brace* are used interchangeably in this chapter.) Fracture braces are available commercially or can be fabricated by the therapist. The humeral shaft is a prime candidate for fracture bracing owing to its long length and because it is the only bone in this area (Fig. 16–10). The functional brace design is a circumferential splint that works by soft tissue compression of the fracture while restricting soft tissue movement, even when the muscles are actively contracting. The pressure from the splint stabilizes the fracture, and the assistance of gravity also helps correct angulation deformities (Camden & Nade, 1992; Sarmiento, 1990).

Many studies have documented that functional fracture bracing and splinting have proven to be the treatment of choice for fracture management at the midshaft level (Bleeker, 1991). Functional fracture bracing gained popularity in the 1970s. The primary benefit of this nonarticular splinting method is the freedom of motion afforded to the adjacent joints; articular splinting, such as slings or casts, usually immobilizes the joints proximal and distal to the fracture site (Sarmiento, Kinman, Galvin, Schmitt, & Phillips, 1977). Functional fracture bracing can be supplemented by the use of a sling or a U-shaped plaster of paris slab (U-slab or UPOP), which immobilizes the shoulder and elbow concurrently (Fig. 16–11) (Hunter, 1982). U-SLAB or UPOP casting has been shown to be a good immobilization technique, but poor ROM results have been reported (Hunter, 1982).

Functional fracture bracing for distal humerus fractures is helpful. Sarmiento (1990) demonstrated a 96% union rate in a study performed on 85 patients with extra-articular comminuted fractures. A restrictive elbow splint using a hinge device can also be fabricated to manage these fractures; they limit elbow mobility and minimize lateral forces about the elbow joint (Fig. 16–12) (Colditz, 1995). Table 16–2 summarizes splinting management of fractures in the shoulder region.

Elbow Fractures

"The elbow is the most inherently stable articulation" (Ring & Jupiter, 1998a). The elbow joint consists of articulations between the humerus (trochlea) and ulna (trochlear notch) as well as between the radius (radial head), ulna (ulnar notch), and humerus (capitulum). The radial head absorbs as much as 60% of the axial load transmitted throughout the elbow (Ring & Jupiter,

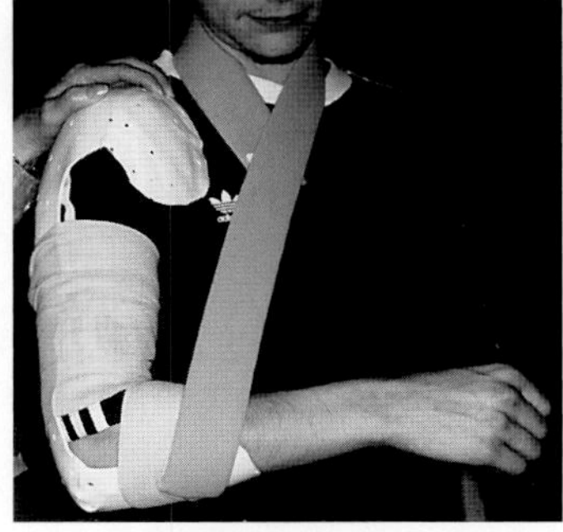

Figure 16–11 A variation of the U-slab casting, fabricated from thermoplastic, for a humerus fracture. Note that the joints adjacent to the fracture are immobilized.

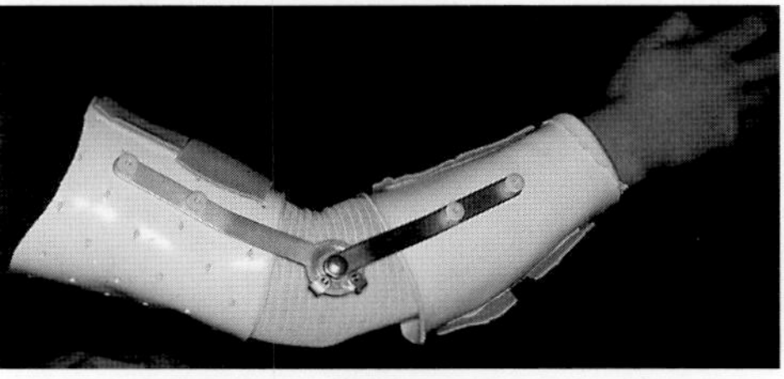

Figure 16–12 An elbow restriction splint using the Phoenix elbow hinge that permits protected elbow ROM. Note that the hinge is set to restrict elbow extension while allowing full flexion.

TABLE 16–2 Management of Shoulder Girdle, Clavicle, and Humerus Fractures[a]

Fracture	Splint Options	Time Frame	Figure
Shoulder girdle			
Scapula, acromion, coracoid	• Broad arm sling	2–3+ weeks	16-5
Distal third of clavicle			
Types 1 and 3	• Broad arm sling	3–6 weeks with gradual increase in activity	16-5
Type 2	• Broad arm sling (after surgical repair)	3–6 weeks with gradual increase in activity	16-5
Midshaft	• Figure-8 strap or taping	6–12 weeks or until no longer tender or without crepitation	16-7, 16-8
Humerus			
Surgical neck or greater tuberosity	• Sling (with or without surgical repair); humerus splint with proximal extension	Impacted: 7–10+ days; displaced: 3 weeks	16-5, 16-11
Shaft	• Humerus splint or functional fracture splint (with or without sling); U-slab; sling (after surgical repair)	6+ weeks	16-5, 16-10, 16-11
Distal	• Humerus splint with elbow hinge; broad arm sling; elbow and wrist immobilization splint or cast	Depends on severity	16-5, 16-12, 16-15, 16-18

[a]Note that the splinting options and time frames depend on the individual patient. Obtain clear orders from the referring physician before providing the patient with any therapy intervention.

1998a). Fractures usually occur as a result of a fall on an outstretched hand. **Radial head fractures** are divided into three types (Fig. 16–13). A type 1 fracture consists of a small fragment that does not interfere with ROM. A type 3 fracture is characterized by a fragment with greater than 2 mm of displacement, A type 3 fracture is comminuted (Ring & Jupiter, 1998a, 1998b). Type 1 fractures can be managed conservatively, including splinting, whereas type 2 and 3 fractures require surgical fixation. Postoperatively, protective splinting and casting may be used.

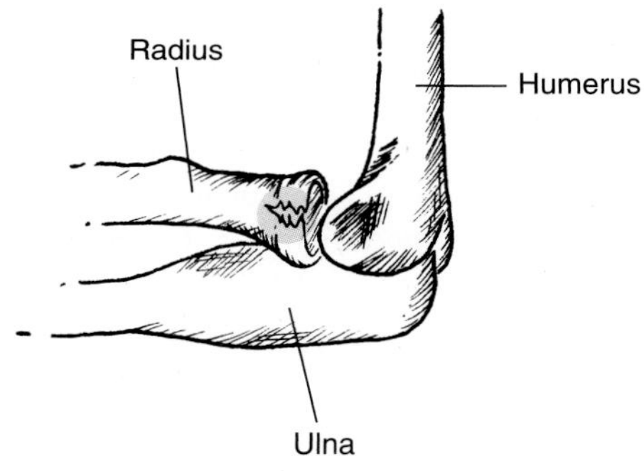

Figure 16–13 Type 3 radial head fracture.

An **olecranon fracture** often involves an avulsion of the triceps tendon (Fig. 16–14). When any avulsion injury occurs, the stability of the joint that it crosses often becomes jeopardized (Ring & Jupiter, 1998b). A **coronoid process fracture** may also occur. Little information is available on this type of fracture, but it is sometimes associated with a radial head fracture. Ligamentous structures may be involved, because the anular ligament connects the ulna and the radial head.

Splinting Options

The literature presents limited information on splinting fractures about the elbow. Most authors recommend slings or plaster elbow slabs that help protect the elbow, whether managed conservatively or postoperatively (total joint replacements excluded). Little research exists regarding the use of custom-molded elbow splints in the management of fractures about the elbow, probably because the focus of elbow management is on therapy (exercises after a short immobilization period). When applying either a cast or a custom-molded thermoplastic splint, a posterior elbow immobilization splint is usually indicated to provide rest or protection to the injured area. Inclusion of the wrist depends on the specific injury, the need to restrict forearm rotation, and the comfort level of the patient (Fig. 16–15). The exact position of the elbow and forearm depends on what structures are injured. For example, when splinting the elbow after an olecranon avulsion fracture, the therapist must appreciate the degree of elbow flexion in relation to the tension on the triceps. Splinting the elbow at 50° may place less tension on the healing structures versus positioning the elbow at 90°. Table 16–3 summarizes splinting management of fractures in the elbow region.

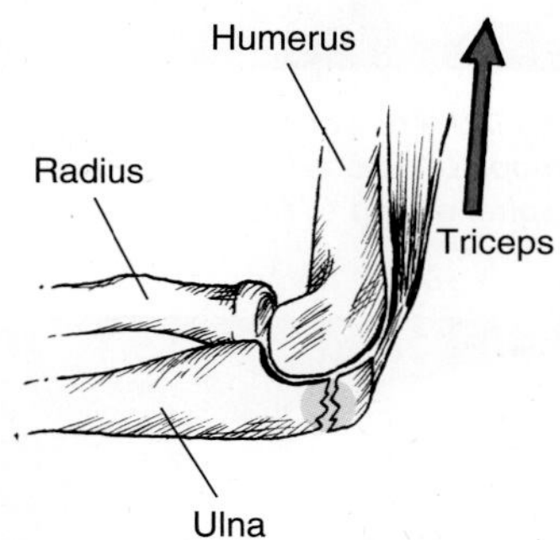

Figure 16–14 With an olecranon avulsion fracture, the triceps tendon pulls proximally with a fragment of bone.

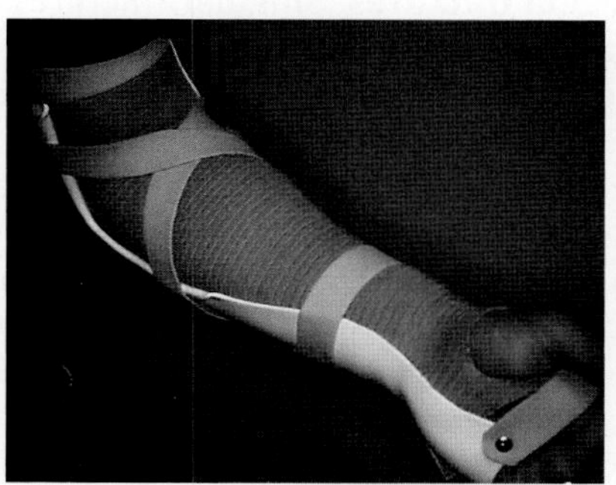

Figure 16–15 A posterior elbow/wrist immobilization splint is often used after radial head injuries and repairs. The wrist is included to restrict forearm rotation.

TABLE 16–3 Management of Radius and Ulna Fractures[a]

Fracture	Splint Options	Splint Position	Time Frame	Figure
Elbow				
Radial head	• Posterior elbow immobilization splint	Elbow: 90°; forearm: neutral	2 weeks (removed for exercise)	16-5, 16-15, 16-18
	• Sling	Elbow: 90°		
Olecranon (avulsion)	• Posterior or anterior elbow immobilization splint	Elbow: 40°; forearm: neutral	3+ weeks	16-15, 16-18
Coronoid	• Posterior or anterior elbow immobilization splint	Variable	2 to 3 weeks	16-15, 16-18
Forearm				
Ulna, midshaft	• Posterior elbow immobilization splint	Elbow: 90°; forearm: neutral	Variable	16-15, 16-18,
	• Nonarticular forearm splint	Forearm: neutral		16-19
Radius, midshaft	• Posterior elbow immobilization splint (after surgical repair)	Elbow: 90°; forearm: neutral	Variable	16-15, 16-18
Galeazzi	• Sugar-tong splint	Forearm: neutral	6 weeks	16-21,
	• Posterior elbow/wrist immobilization splint or cast	Elbow: 90°; forearm: neutral		16-15, 16-18
Monteggia types 1, 3, 4	• Long arm cast	Elbow: 110°; forearm: neutral	6 weeks	16-15, 16-18
Monteggia type 2	• Posterior elbow/wrist immobilization splint or cast	Elbow: 70°; forearm: maximum tolerated supination	6 weeks	16-15, 16-18
Distal radius				
Colles', Smith's, or Barton's	• Long then short arm cast	Variable, depends on radiograph	3 weeks; then 2–3 weeks	16-15, 16-18
	• Wrist immobilization splint (with or without clamshell)	Forearm: pronation; Wrist: (per physician)	4–6 weeks	16-23
	• Ulnar wrist immobilization splint (with external fixation)	Wrist: fixed (with hardware)	Variable 4–6 weeks	16-24 16-25

[a]Note that the splinting options and time frames depend on the individual patient. Obtain clear orders from the referring physician before providing the patient with any therapy intervention.

Forearm Fractures

This section focuses on the common fractures of the radius and ulna shafts. Fractures in the forearm include singular fractures of the radius and ulna, simultaneous fractures of the radius and ulna, **Galeazzi fractures,** and **Monteggia fractures.** Singular fractures usually result from a direct blow (e.g., getting struck by a bat); radius singular fractures are rare because of forearm muscle padding (Anderson & Meyer, 1991). Fractures of both bones can result from a motor vehicle accident, direct blow, or traumatic event (e.g., gunshot wound) (Anderson & Meyer, 1991). A Galeazzi fracture is a fracture of the lower third of the radial shaft, resulting in distal radioulnar disruption; it can be caused by a fall on an outstretched hand with simultaneous pronation (Fig. 16–16) (Anderson & Meyer, 1991; Brown, 1983). A Monteggia fracture involves the proximal third of the ulna with radial head dislocation; it can be caused by a direct blow to the arm (Fig. 16–17) (Anderson & Meyer, 1991). Monteggia fractures are classified into four types (Anderson & Meyer, 1991):

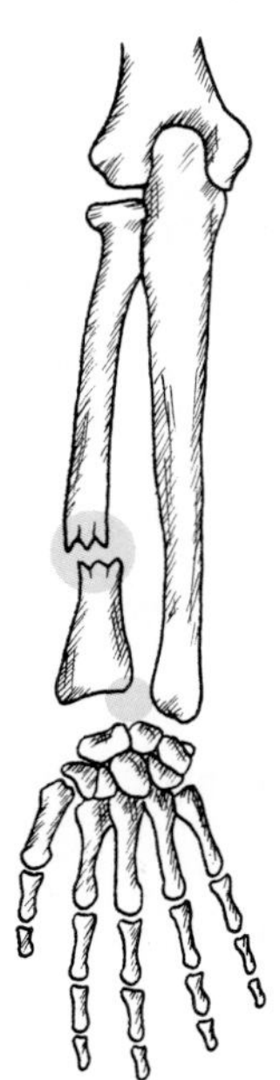

Figure 16–16 Galeazzi fractures affect the lower third of the radial shaft, resulting in distal radioulnar disruption.

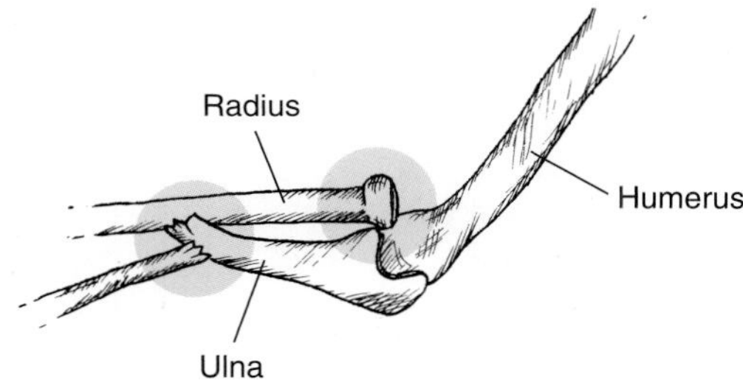

Figure 16–17 Monteggia fractures affect the proximal third of the ulna, resulting in radial head dislocation. These fractures often require open reduction and internal fixation.

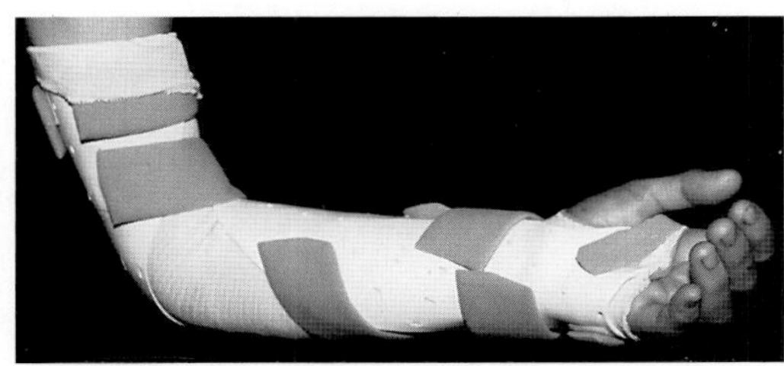

Figure 16–18 An elbow flexion/wrist immobilization splint can be made from thermoplastic material to maintain fracture reduction. Note the unique spiral design to facilitate supination positioning.

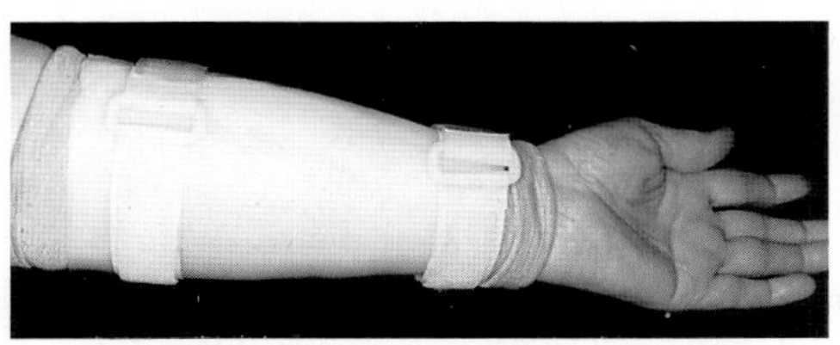

Figure 16–19 Be careful to apply pressure through the interosseous membrane region for proper positioning and fit of a functional fracture brace.

- *Type 1.* Dislocation of the radial head with fracture of the ulna diaphysis.
- *Type 2.* Posterior dislocation of the radial head with fracture of the ulna diaphysis.
- *Type 3.* Lateral dislocation of the radial head with fracture of the ulna metaphysis.
- *Type 4.* Anterior dislocation of the radial head with fracture of the proximal third radius and ulna.

These fractures usually require operative treatment, depending on the severity of the injury, but occasionally can be reduced by closed methods (Fig. 16–18) (Osterman, Ekkernkamp, Henry, & Muhr, 1994; Tang, Failla, & Contesti, 1999).

Splinting Options

Isolated stable fractures of the ulnar midshaft can sometimes be managed with functional fracture bracing (Fig. 16–19). This concept is similar to functional humeral fracture bracing: a circumferential custom or prefabricated splint is fit over the fracture site (Osterman, Ekkernkamp, Henry, & Muhr, 1994). This type of splint should place pressure along the interosseous membrane to provide soft tissue compression between the radius and ulna. Research has shown that the effectiveness of functional fracture bracing provides greater patient satisfaction, earlier return to work, and improved ROM than traditional forms of immobilization (Gebuhr, 1992).

Fractures that require open reduction and external fixation can be fit with a posterior elbow/wrist immobilization splint (Fig. 16–20). An optional thermoplastic cover may be fabricated for added protection and patient comfort. Galeazzi fractures may also be managed with a sugar-tong splint to stabilize the distal radioulnar joint but allow some elbow motion (Fig. 16–21). Table 16–3 summarizes splinting management of fractures in the forearm.

Distal Radius Fractures

Distal radius fractures can be challenging to manage. There are many confusing classification systems for these fractures, including Frykman, Melone, universal, and the Association for Study of Internal Fixation (AO) (Fernandez & Jupiter, 1995; Laseter & Carter, 1996). All of these systems define and group fractures at the distal radius as either extra-articular or intra-articular, and the AO classification system adds a third category (complex articular fractures). Within these categories are subsets of each fracture type. The specific systems are described in the literature.

Distal radius fractures have generally been referred to as **Colles' fractures.** But the term actually specifies fractures of the distal radius with dorsal displacement (Fig. 16–22) (Fernandez & Jupiter, 1995; Laseter & Carter, 1996). These fractures occur most frequently as a result of a fall on an outstretched hand. A **Smith's fracture,** also known as a reverse Colles' fracture, usually results from a fall on the dorsum of the hand. A **Barton's fracture** is an intra-articular fracture of the distal radius.

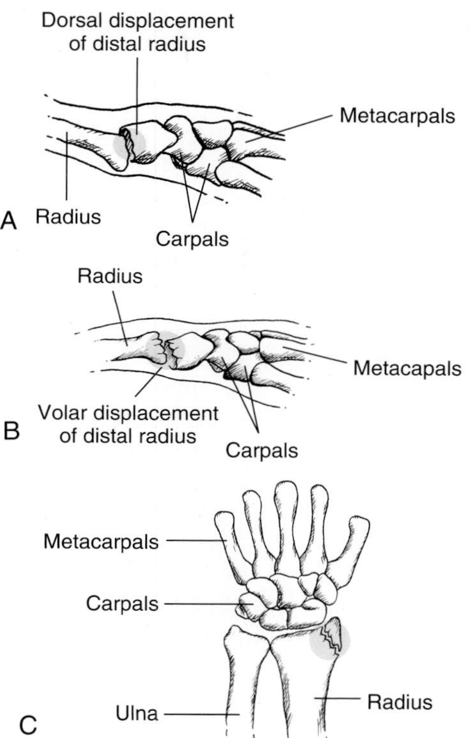

Figure 16–22 ***A,*** *Colles' fracture with dorsal displacement.* ***B,*** *Smith's fracture with volar displacement.* ***C,*** *A Barton's fracture is a displaced, unstable articular fracture.*

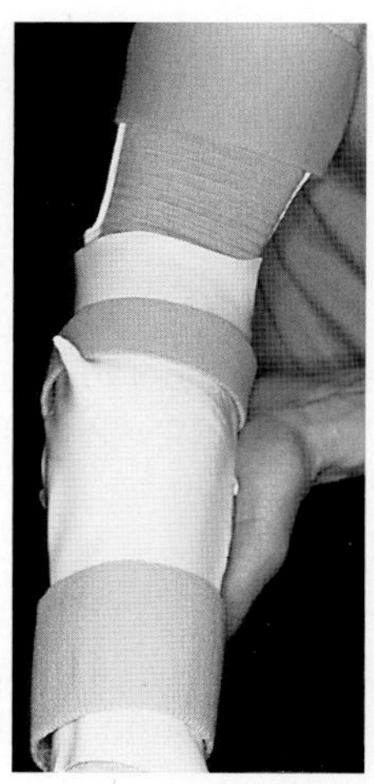

Figure 16–20 A dorsal elbow/wrist immobilization splint can include an optional pin cover for added protection.

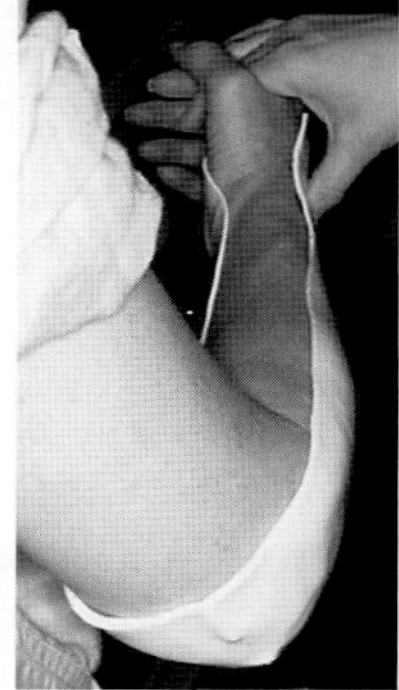

Figure 16–21 Sugar-tong splints allow limited elbow ROM but restrict forearm rotation.

The management of distal radius fractures is controversial (Fernandez & Jupiter, 1995; Laseter & Carter, 1996). Conservative treatment includes reduction and immobilization using casting materials. Long arm casts (above the elbow) are often applied for a 2- to 3-week period, followed by short arm casting (below the elbow) for 2 to 4 weeks. Fractures that require open reduction and internal fixation (ORIF) or percutaneous pinning are usually placed in a short arm cast.

For some displaced distal radius fractures, external fixation is used to produce ligamentotaxis (distracting tension on ligaments) of the joint to preserve fracture length. A bulky dressing is initially applied; this is followed by protective splinting or casting. A benefit of using an external fixation device is that angulation displacement can be corrected through distraction and any open wounds can be monitored.

Complications include index finger (IF) metacarpophalangeal (MP) joint stiffness, first web space contractures, radial sensory nerve irritation or injury, and pin tract infection. Functional casting and splinting for distal radius fractures has been discussed in the literature, but it is not widely accepted (Cohen & Frillman, 1997; Fernandez & Jupiter, 1995; Ledingham, Gorey, Mathieson, & Wardon, 1991; Moir, 1995).

Splinting Options

As noted, custom splinting for distal radius fractures is not often used in the acute stages (except for patients placed in an external fixator). After cast removal, the patient is often fitted with a custom or prefabricated wrist splint to provide protection and soft tissue support for an additional 2 to 4 weeks. The splint can be a forearm-based wrist immobilization splint (with or without a dorsal clamshell piece); the fingers and thumb should be free (Fig. 16–23). Patients with external fixation devices may be referred acutely for an ulnar wrist immobilization splint to support and protect the wrist. The splint may be forearm- or arm-based, depending on the patient's comfort level and the need to limit forearm rotation. A thermoplastic cover or hood can be fitted over the protruding pins to provide additional external protection (Fig. 16–24).

QuickCast can be used to maintain the reduction of distal radius fractures (Fig. 16–25). The wrist cast version was studied by Cohen and Frillman (1997) who concluded that QuickCast was just as effective as traditional casting in all cases in their study, except one. One benefit was the need for only one application versus the multiple cast changes with traditional plaster or fiberglass. This is because QuickCast can be easily reformed by heating with a hair dryer to adjust for changes in edema (see Chapter 12 for details) (Cohen & Frillman, 1997). Table 16-3 summarizes splinting management of distal radius fractures.

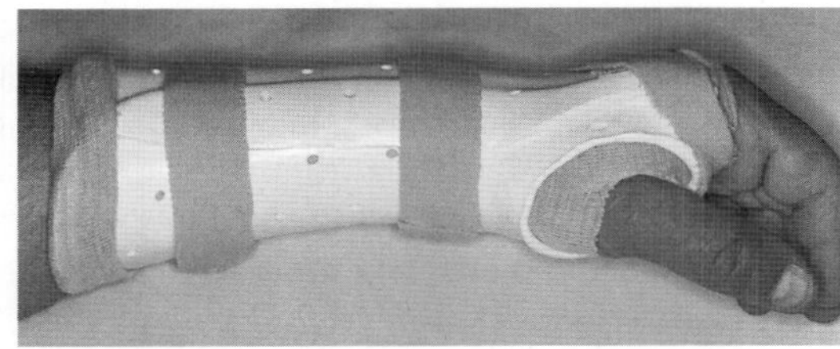

Figure 16–23 A dorsal clamshell piece added to a wrist immobilization splint provides stability at the fracture site. The dorsal section is simply an interlocking piece of thermoplastic material applied after the volar piece has been fabricated and is fully set. It overlaps the borders of the volar piece by approximately ½ in.

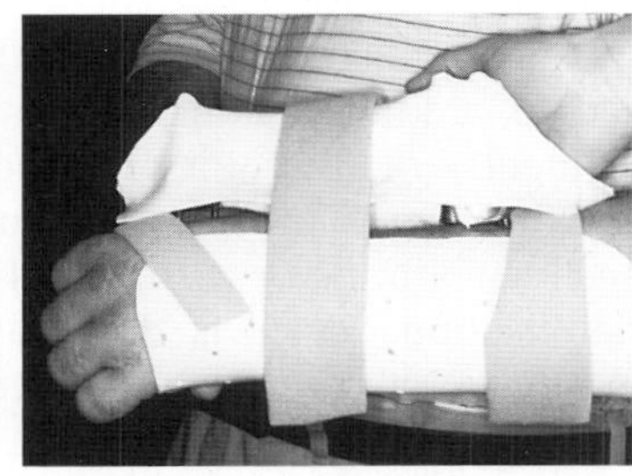

Figure 16–24 This ulnar wrist splint can be fabricated to incorporate the elbow as well as the wrist, depending on the patient's comfort level and whether forearm rotation needs to be limited. Note the pin cover fabricated to protect the pin sites.

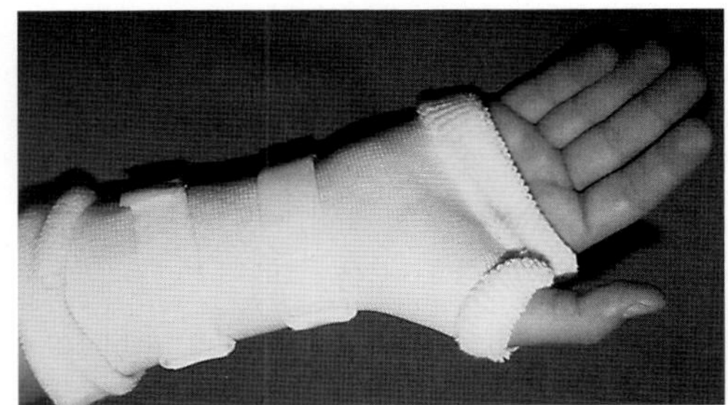

Figure 16–25 If not contraindicated, a QuickCast wrist splint can be univalved so it can be removed for bathing.

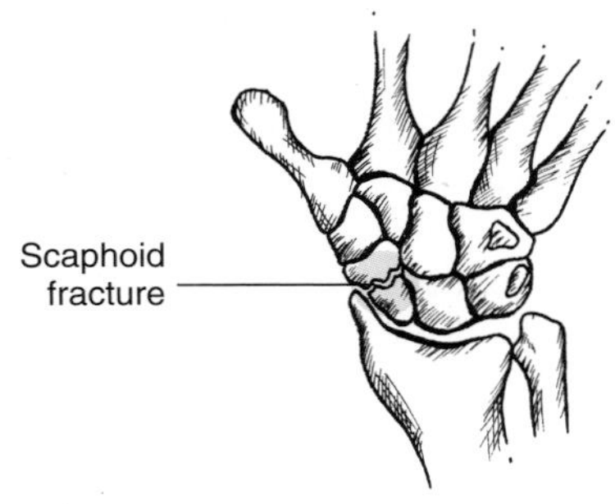

Figure 16–26 Scaphoid fractures commonly occur from a fall on an outstretched hand.

Carpal Fractures

The wrist is an intricately balanced structure, consisting of eight small bones bound by multiple ligaments that allow the motions of wrist flexion, extension, ulnar and radial deviation, and intercarpal rotation. Fracturing one of these bones will most likely disrupt the wrist kinematics and result in an alteration of hand function. The mechanism of fracture for each carpal bone is as follows (Hambridge, Desai, Schranz, Comson, Davis, & Barton, 1999; Prosser & Herbert, 1996):

- **Scaphoid fractures** are usually a result of a fall on an outstretched hand (fall off a ladder, playing football) (Fig. 16–26).
- **Trapezium fractures** usually occur from falling on a hyperextended and radially deviated wrist.
- **Triquetrum fractures** are most often associated with perilunate dislocations.
- **Lunate fractures** are commonly associated with a pathologic condition resulting from cystlike lesions in the lunate.

- **Pisiform fractures** are usually caused by direct trauma to the palm.
- **Hamate fractures** often occur as a result of a forceful swing of a golf club or baseball bat.
- **Trapezoid fractures** may occur from a direct high-velocity force to the IF.
- **Capitate fractures** are associated with wrist injuries, such as perilunate dislocations.

Splinting Options

Scaphoid

Options for the conservative treatment of scaphoid fractures are thoroughly presented in the literature. Most physicians advocate casting in either a long or a short arm cast with the whole thumb included, with the thumb included to the first metacarpal head, or with the thumb free (Hambridge, Desai, Schranz, Comson, Davis, & Barton, 1999). The therapist may be called on to splint the patient after the fracture has healed, or has nearly healed, when mobilization of the wrist is indicated (Fig. 16–27).

Surgery is often required to promote healing because of the poor blood supply in the proximal segment of this small bone. This may require a prolonged immobilization period to prevent disruption of healing. Postoperatively, splinting can be used as the means of immobilization. The immobilization splint choices include volar wrist/thumb immobilization with the thumb interphalangeal (IP) joint free, volar wrist/thumb immobilization splint with the MP joint free, or a simple volar wrist immobilization splint. Furthermore, a dorsal clamshell piece can be added to any of these splints to provide further protection and stabilization of the wrist within the splint (Fig. 16–23).

Other Carpals

The therapist does not often see fractures of the other carpal bones. Most of these fractures are easily managed with cast immobilization. Trapezium fracture management includes the use of a wrist/thumb splint or cast for 4 to 6 weeks (conservatively or with ORIF) (Fig. 16–27). Triquetrum fractures are usually managed with a wrist immobilization splint or cast for 3 weeks if stable, or treated with ORIF followed by splinting or casting until healed (Fig. 16–23 or 16–25).

Transverse and longitudinal lunate fractures are usually casted for 6 weeks if stable; ORIF is indicated if the fracture is unstable. If there is an avulsion fracture of the lunate, no formal treatment is indicated (Prosser & Herbert, 1996). Pisiform fractures can be either excised or casted for 3 weeks. Hamate fractures are generally casted or the hook of the hamate may be excised if problematic. If pisiform or hamate fractures are excised, a splint lined with silicone gel may offer protection and support to this vulnerable postoperative area. Trapezoid fractures are treated much the same as trapezium fractures, with 6 weeks of immobilization in a wrist/thumb immobilization splint or cast (Fig. 16–27). Capitate fractures are immobilized with a wrist immobilization splint or cast, with the thumb and digits free (Fig. 16–23 or 16–25). Table 16–4 summarizes splinting management for carpal fractures.

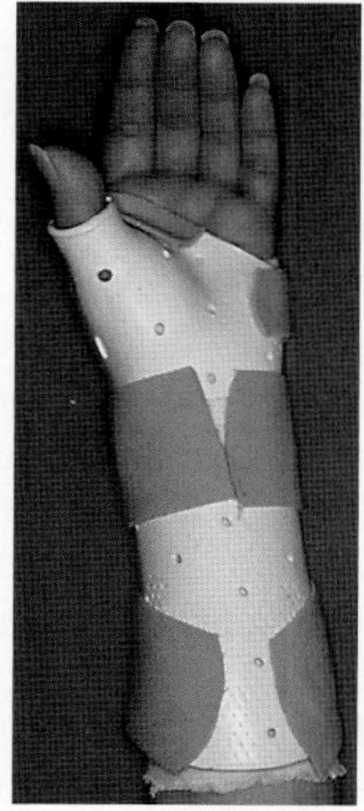

Figure 16–27 A wrist/thumb immobilization splint with a free thumb IP joint is a management option for a scaphoid or Bennett's fracture.

Metacarpal Fractures

Metacarpal (MC) fractures are frequently managed in the clinic for acute fracture bracing or splinting. MC fractures are classified according to their anatomic location: base, shaft, or neck. Base fractures tend to be stable and frequently require only splinting. Shaft fractures are either transverse, spiral, or oblique and often result in dorsal angulations; they are rarely functionally disabling (Jones, 1996). Neck fractures are the most common MC fracture and often present with apex dorsal angulation (Green & Rowland, 1991; Sorenson, Freund, & Keijla, 1993). Frequently, neck fractures require ORIF via plates and screws or pinning (Fig. 16–28).

Thumb MC fractures include **Bennett's, Rolando,** and **extra-articular fractures.** A Bennett's fracture occurs at the base of the first MC, usually as a result of an axial blow to the thumb (Fig. 16–29). Operative treatment may be considered to manage this fracture and includes closed reduction and percutaneous pinning. A Rolando fracture, which is a comminuted Bennett's fracture, usually requires operative treatment. Extra-articular fractures may be transverse or oblique. Transverse fractures are commonly managed with a wrist/thumb immobilization splint or cast for 4 weeks. Oblique fractures are usually fixed via percutaneous pinning for 4 weeks (Kaplan, 1940).

Splinting Options

MC fractures can be splinted using functional bracing methods or traditional immobilization methods (Fig.

TABLE 16–4 Carpal Fracture Management[a]

Fracture	Splint Options	Splint Position	Time Frame	Figure
Scaphoid	• Long to short arm cast	Wrist: extension	6+ weeks	
	• Wrist/thumb immobilization splint to IP or MP joint (with or without clamshell)		6 weeks	16-27
Trapezium	• Wrist/thumb immobilization splint or cast	Thumb: Midpalmar/ radial abduction	4–6 weeks	16-27
Trapezoid	• Wrist/thumb immobilization splint or cast	Wrist: extension	6 weeks	16-27
Capitate	• Wrist immobilization splint or cast	Wrist: extension	6+ weeks (depending on radiograph)	16-23, 16-25
Hamate				
Hook	• Soft splint (after excision - if needed)			
Body	• Wrist immobilization splint or cast	Wrist: extension	Variable	16-23, 16-25
Triquetrum	• Wrist immobilization splint or cast (after surgical repair)	Wrist: extension	3 weeks	16-23, 16-25
Pisiform	• Wrist immobilization splint or cast	Wrist: neutral	3 weeks	16-23, 16-25
Lunate	• Soft splint (after excision)			
Avulsion	• No treatment			
Longitudinal	• Wrist immobilization splint or cast (after surgical repair)		6 weeks	16-23, 16-25
Transverse	• Wrist immobilization splint or cast		6 weeks	16-23, 16-25

[a]Note that the splinting options and time frames depend on the individual patient. Obtain clear orders from the referring physician before providing the patient with any therapy intervention.

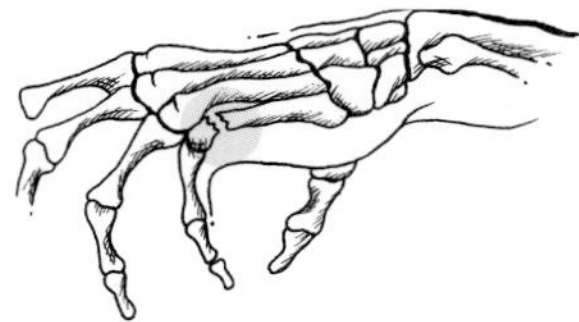

Figure 16–28 A boxer's or fighter's fracture involves the fifth metacarpal neck.

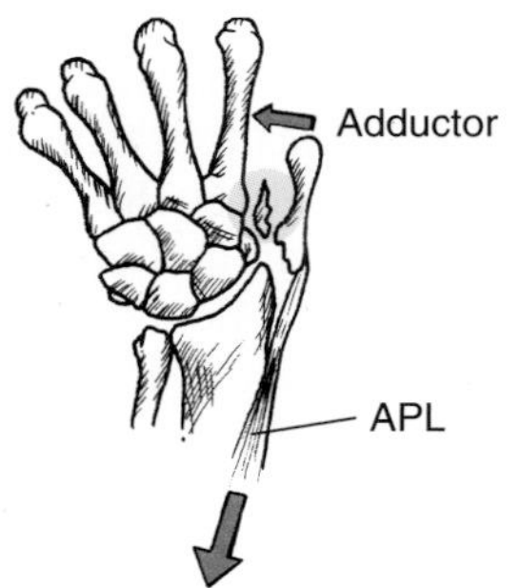

Figure 16–29 With a Bennett's fracture, the fractured fragment separates from the metacarpal shaft, which is further displaced by the pull of the abductor pollicis longus (APL) tendon dorsally and radially.

16–30). The following splinting recommendations may be used as a guideline for surgical and nonsurgical patients. Traditional management of the IF, middle finger (MF), ring finger (RF), and small finger (SF) MC fractures involves immobilization splinting using an ulnar or radial splint design with the MP joints at 60 to 70° of flexion and the IP joints at 0° extension—or with the proximal interphalangeal (PIP) joints at 0° and the distal interphalangeal (DIP) joints free or with the IP joints free (Fig. 16–31). It is important to hold these fractures in the described position to prevent MP joint extension contractures and maintain fracture stability.

Base and shaft fractures usually include the wrist for proper immobilization. First MC fractures require a wrist/thumb splint with the thumb IP joint free (Fig. 16–27). However, Colditz (1995) recommends that all metacarpal shaft fractures be immobilized in a hand-based splint (ulnar or radial design) with buddy taping of the injured and adjacent fingers (e.g., for a SF MC fracture, all MCs are included in the splint along with buddy taping of the SF to the RF). For neck fractures, the proximal phalanx needs to be included in the splint, with the IP joints free (if appropriate) (Colditz, 1995). This allows for functional ROM and can help prevent extensor tendon adherence to the fracture site.

Other splinting options for fractures of the second through the fifth MCs include the use of a prefabricated support, such as the Galveston brace. This splint consists of a plastic piece with padded disks that apply three-point pressure to the fracture. Caution should be employed when using this brace, because it has been found to produce excessive pressure and it holds the fracture reduction only marginally (Sorenson et al., 1993). Tables 16–5 and 16–6 summarize splinting management of metacarpal fractures.

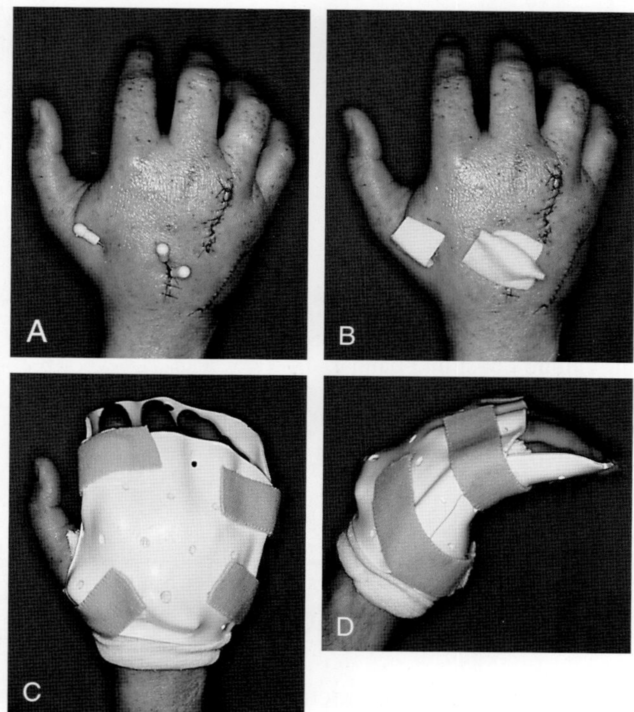

Figure 16–30 *A, Postoperative view of a patient with multiple MC fractures who underwent open reduction with percutaneous pinning. **B,** Padding is placed on the pins before molding the thermoplastic splint. **C,** A hand-based digit immobilization splint with a protective dorsal piece. **D,** Note the positioning of the MP joints in flexion and the IP joints in extension. The IP joint are left free to extend to promote tendon gliding.*

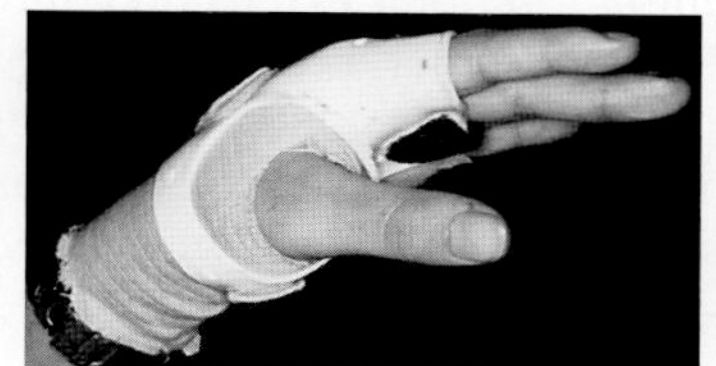

Figure 16–31 *A radial digit immobilization splint for an index MC neck fracture.*

Phalangeal Fractures

The therapist frequently splints finger fractures acutely. **Proximal** and **middle phalanx fractures** mainly involve the neck and the shaft. Shaft fractures may be transverse, spiral, oblique, or comminuted. Unstable proximal phalanx fractures often produce an apex volar angulation, owing to the pull of the interossei muscles onto the base of the proximal phalanx (Fig. 16–32). If unstable, operative techniques are used (Green & Rowland, 1991). Unstable middle phalanx fractures also present with volar angulation of the neck, caused by the strong pull of the flexor digitorum superficialis (FDS) tendon on the proximal side of the fracture. If the base of the middle phalanx is fractured, a dorsal angulation will likely occur (Fig. 16–33) (Green & Rowland, 1991). Management of these injuries can be extremely difficult because they are highly susceptible to tendon adherence. These patients may be candidates for a surgical tenolysis after the initial stages of healing are complete.

Distal phalangeal fractures commonly occur as a result of a crush injury and generally heal without complicated treatment (Kaplan, 1940) (Fig. 16–34). According to Kaplan (1940), distal phalanx fractures are classified as tuft, shaft, or base fractures. Tuft fractures do not necessarily require splinting, but splints may be used for patient comfort and protection. Shaft and base fractures require a brief period of splinting for protection and immobilization. Splinting may also be used after percutaneous pin fixation.

Phalangeal Fracture and Dislocations

PIP Joint

PIP fractures or dislocations are often problematic for the surgeon and therapist to treat. According to Kiefhaber (1966), there are three categories of these injuries. **Dorsal lip fractures** are hyperflexion injuries that cause avulsion-type fractures of the central tendon. If nondisplaced, they can be splinted in extension for 6 weeks; displaced fractures most often require

TABLE 16–5 Metacarpal Fracture Management[a]

Fracture	Splint Options	Splint Position	Time Frame	Figure
Head	• Radial/ulnar hand-based digit immobilization splint	MP: 60–70°, PIP/DIP: 0°; splint involved finger or with adjacent finger; include adjacent MC for stability	3–4 weeks	16-31, 16-35
Neck	• Radial/ulnar hand-based digit immobilization splint	MP: 60–70°, PIP/DIP: 0° or free	3–4 weeks	16-31
Shaft	• Radial/ulnar forearm-based wrist/digit immobilization splint	Wrist extension MP: 60-70°, PIP: 0°or free; with or without buddy taping	3–4 weeks	
Base	• Galveston brace • Wrist immobilization splint	Prefabricated splint Wrist: neutral, MPs: free	3–4 weeks	16-23

[a]Note that the splinting options and time frames depend on the individual patient. Obtain clear orders from the referring physician before providing the patient with any therapy intervention.

TABLE 16–6 Thumb Fracture Management[a]

Fracture	Splint Options	Splint Position	Time Frame	Figure
Bennett's	Wrist/thumb immobilization splint or cast	Wrist: neutral, Thumb CMC: mid-palmar and radial abduction	4–6+ weeks	16-27
Rolando	Wrist/thumb immobilization splint or cast	Wrist: neutral, Thumb CMC: mid-palmar and radial abduction	4–6+ weeks	16-27
Extra-articular				
Transverse	Wrist/thumb immobilization splint or cast	Wrist: neutral, Thumb CMC: mid-palmar and radial abduction MP: slight flexion	4 weeks	16-27
Oblique	Wrist/thumb immobilization splint or cast	Wrist: neutral, Thumb CMC: mid-palmar and radial abduction MP: slight flexion	4 weeks	16-27
Proximal phalanx	Thumb immobilization splint	MP: 10–20° flexion; IP: 0°; CMC: mid-palmar and radial abduction	4–6+ weeks	
Distal phalanx	Thumb immobilization splint	IP: 0°–5° hyperextension	3+ weeks	

CMC, carpometacarpal.
[a]Note that the splinting options and time frames depend on the individual patient. Obtain clear orders from the referring physician before providing the patient with any therapy intervention.

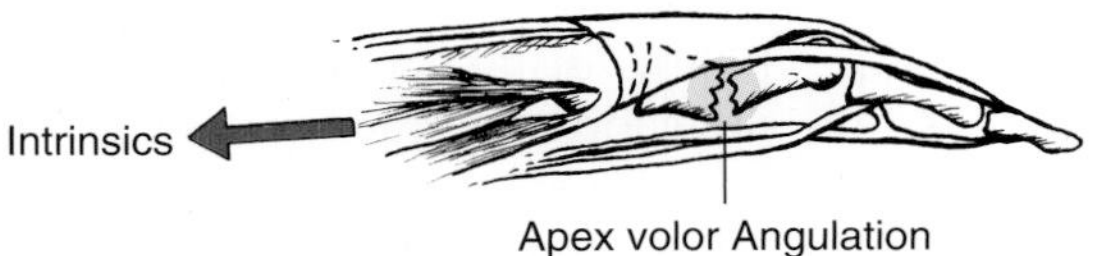

Figure 16–32 A proximal phalanx fracture with apex volar angulation. Note pull of intrinsic muscles.

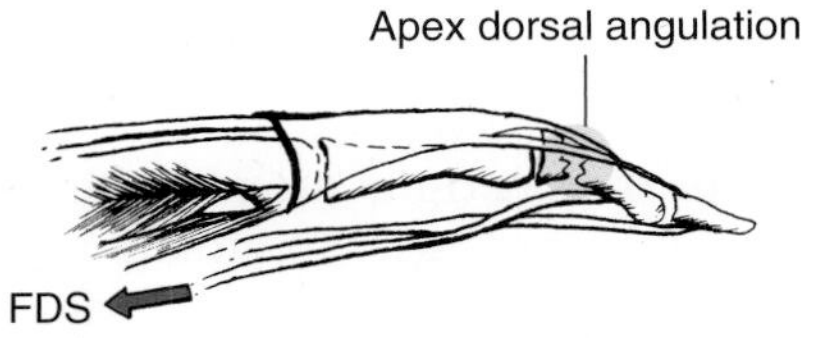

Figure 16–33 A middle phalanx fracture can produce apex dorsal angulation. Note the pull of the FDS tendon.

ORIF. **Palmar lip fractures** involve hyperextension injuries and cause palmar plate avulsions. They can be further divided into type 1 (stable), type 2 (tenuous), and type 3 (unstable) fractures. **Pilon fractures** are high-energy injuries causing severe comminution of the middle phalanx.

DIP Joint

Tension and compression forces often produce **DIP joint fracture and dislocations.** These injuries include extensor tendon avulsion, also known as mallet finger; volar margin fracture, consisting of a palmar plate avulsion fracture; and impaction shear fractures (Kiefhaber, 1996). Volar margin fractures may involve an FDP tendon injury, and palmar plate avulsion injuries result from a hyperextension force that causes dorsal DIP joint dislocation. A blow to the hand can cause impaction shear fractures when the fingertip is slightly flexed.

Splinting Options

Options for splinting phalangeal fractures (not fracture/dislocations) in this area vary greatly owing to differing physician preferences. In general, the optimal position for splinting the phalanx is to place the MP joints in flexion to keep the collateral ligaments at length, thereby preventing MP joint extension contractures, and to place the PIP/DIP joints in some degree of extension to prevent potential flexion contractures (Fig. 16–35).

For proximal phalanx fractures, hand-based digit immobilization splints are often used with the MP joints gen-

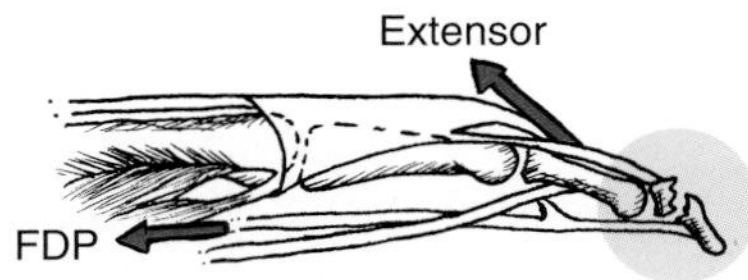

Figure 16–34 Distal phalanx avulsion fracture. Note the pull of the flexors and extensors and the resulting deformity.

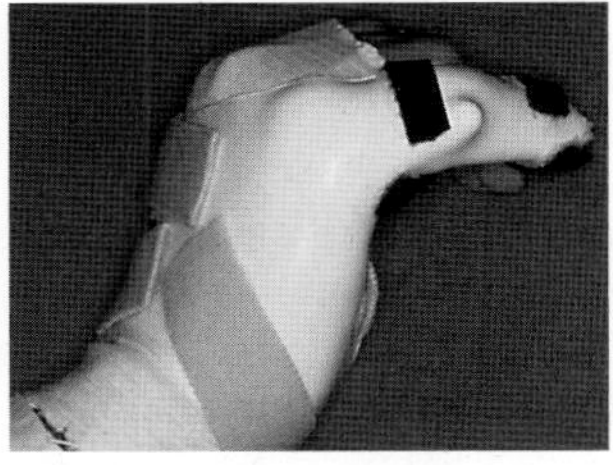

Figure 16–35 The adjacent metacarpals are often immobilized for added splint stability and patient comfort. Note how the splint was formed over a percutaneous pin.

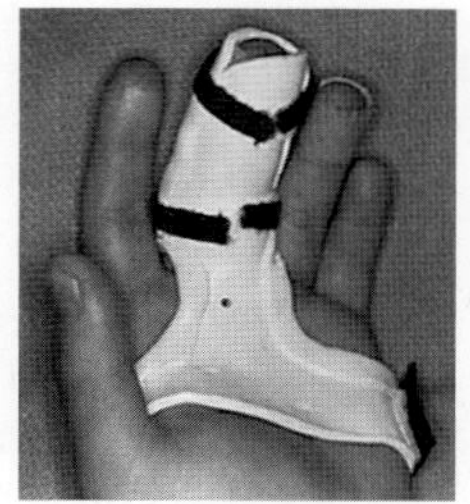

Figure 16–36 An interlocking dorsal piece, molded on top of a volar digit immobilization splint, may accommodate edema and provide circumferential support and protection for a proximal phalanx fracture.

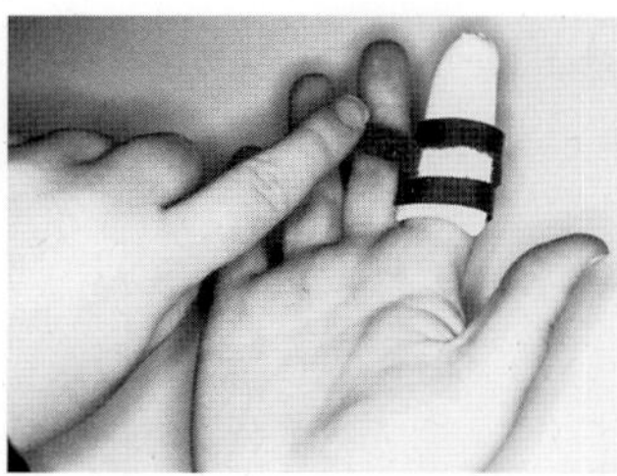

Figure 16–37 A digit immobilization splint for a middle phalanx fracture. Note the split strap design to prevent detachment.

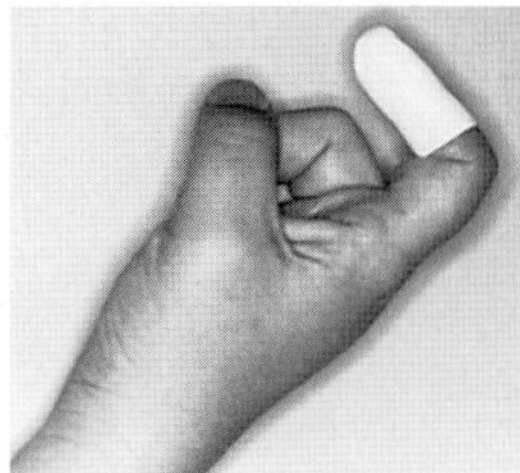

Figure 16–38 A DIP joint immobilization splint is commonly used to manage distal phalanx fractures.

erally positioned at 60 to 70° of flexion and the IP joints at 0° extension (Fig. 16–36). Other therapists advocate splinting the MP joints at 60 to 70° of flexion, the PIP joints at 15 to 20° of flexion, and the DIP joints at 5 to 10° of flexion, to assist in correcting or maintaining reduction of any angulation deformity (Green & Rowland, 1991). Some therapists include the wrist positioned in 30° of extension with the MP joints flexed and the IP joints at 0° (Green & Rowland, 1991). Nonarticular functional splinting may also be used as an option for stable proximal phalanx fractures, because it provides the immobilization necessary for the healing fracture yet allows tendon gliding and motion of uninvolved joints (Oxford & Hidreth, 1996).

Middle phalanx fractures can be successfully managed with a digit-based splint (Fig. 16–37). Sometimes, hand-based splints may be fabricated to provide additional support, protection, and rest. This may be necessary when treating the pediatric population or when splinting injuries that involve other structures and/or multiple digits.

Distal phalanx fractures may be splinted with a DIP immobilization splint (Fig. 16–38). Occasionally, the PIP joint is incorporated to improve splint stability and prevent the splint from sliding off the finger. This can be modified to free the PIP joint as healing progresses. A clamshell design can be used to provide further protection for a hypersensitive fingertip or to protect fracture reduction.

There are a variety of splinting options available for splinting both PIP and DIP joint fracture/dislocations (Fig. 16–39). A material that can withstand being repeatedly reheated is the material of choice for splinting these injuries. Frequently, the therapist is instructed by the physician to modify the splint as the fracture heals; therefore, an elastic or rubber material is preferable for convenience as well as cost-effectiveness. Table 16–7 summarizes splinting management of hand fractures.

Intra-Articular Fractures of the Hand

Intra-articular fractures of the hand are extremely difficult to manage because of the potential for poor outcomes. One method includes the use of dynamic traction splinting for postsurgical management (Fig. 16–40) (Schenck, 1994). This method provides passive motion to the injured area, while delivering ligamentotaxis (stress to maximize ligament length) to the joint. In some cases, the traction assists in stabilizing the fracture. If used for fracture reduction, passive motion is not used immediately (discussed in detail in the second case study).

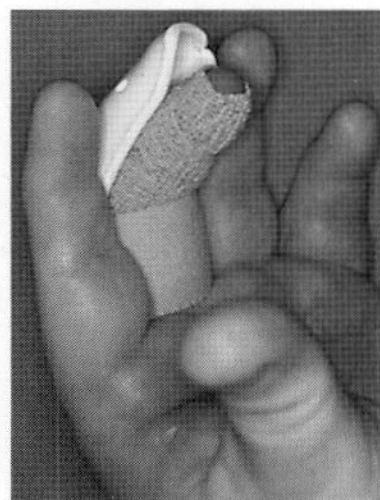

Figure 16–39 A dorsal PIP extension restriction splint is commonly used for a PIP joint dislocation to allow early protected motion.

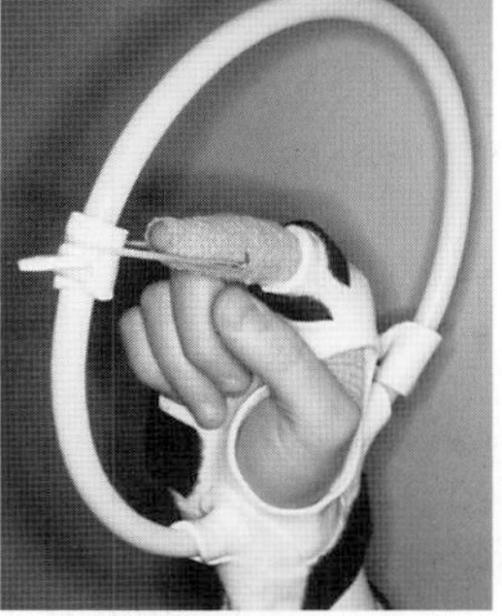

Figure 16–40 A dynamic traction splint maintains ligamentotaxis throughout a specific ROM.

TABLE 16–7 Phalangeal Fracture Management[a]

Fracture	Splint Options	Splint Position	Time Frame	Figure
Phalangeal				
Proximal	• Volar hand immobilization splint	MP: 60–70°; PIP: 0–15°; DIP: 5–10°	2–4 weeks	16-35, 16-36
Middle		MP: free, PIP: 0°; DIP: 0°	3+ weeks	
	• Digit immobilization splint	PIP/DIP 0°	3–4+ weeks	16-37
Distal	• Stax splint	Prefabricated	4–6 weeks	
	• DIP immobilization splint	DIP: 0°	4–6 weeks	16-38
Fracture or dislocation of PIP joint				
Dorsal lip				
Nondisplaced	• Digit immobilization splint	PIP/DIP: 0°	6 weeks	16-37
Displaced	• Digit immobilization splint after surgical repair	PIP: 30° for 3 weeks; 10° for 3 weeks	6 weeks	16-39
Palmar lip				
Type 1	• PIP extension restriction splint	Per physician (increase 10° each week until full extension achieved)	6 weeks	16-39
	• Buddy taping	To adjacent digit		
Type 2	• PIP extension restriction splint	PIP per physician; MP: 50–60°	6 weeks	16-39
Type 3	• Digit or hand-based immobilization splint	MP: 60°; PIP: 0° Per physician	Variable	16-35, 16-36, 16-37
	• Traction splint	Wrist extension MP: 60°; PIP per physician	6+ weeks	16-40, 16-42
Pilon	• Digit or hand-based immobilization splint	MP: 60°; PIP: 0°	Variable	16-35, 16-36, 16-37
Fracture or dislocation of the DIP joint				
Volar margin with FDP rupture	Wrist/hand extension restriction splint (Dorsal blocking splint)	Wrist: 30–45°flexion; MP: 45–60° flexion; PIP/DIP: 0°	4–6 weeks	
Palmar plate avulsion	Digit immobilization splint	PIP/DIP: 0°	4 weeks	16-37, 16-39
Impaction shear	Digit immobilization splint	Per physician (flexion initially; increase extension per physician until full extension achieved)	4 weeks	16-36, 16-37

FDP, flexor digitorum profundus.

[a]Note that the splinting options and time frames depend on the individual patient. Obtain clear orders from the referring physician before providing the patient with any therapy intervention.

CASE STUDY SECTION

The case studies presented here are meant as teaching guidelines only. Treatment and splinting protocols vary greatly from surgeon to surgeon and from therapist to therapist. Please check with the referring physician and colleagues to define the preferred treatment and splinting methods.

CASE STUDY 1: **Distal Radius Fracture with External Fixation**

DS is a 69-year-old semiretired male who sustained a distal radius fracture after falling on an outstretched hand. Closed reduction was attempted, but within 1 week, the fracture had collapsed, requiring surgery with external fixation and percutaneous pinning. DS was referred to therapy 3 days postsurgery, and the large bulky dressing was removed at that time. Digit ROM was extremely limited owing to severe pitting edema. Sensation was grossly intact. The patient reported his pain level as a 7 on a scale of 0 to 10.

A wrist immobilization splint was fabricated forearm in neutral rotation, and wrist in ulnar deviation with the fingers free (as per fixation) (Fig. 16-24). The splint was fabricated from a durable 1/8" rubber-like material. An external fixator protection cover was fabricated out of 1/16" material to fit over the pins. This cover provided protection for at-risk situations and for sleeping to prevent clothing and bedding from snagging on pins. To aid in managing the severe edema, an Isotoner glove was placed on the hand and an Ace bandage was used to circumferentially secure the splint.

The pins and fixator were removed at 6 weeks and a volar wrist immobilization splint was made with 3/32" elastic material (Aquaplast). Each week, as DS made gains in ROM, the material was reheated and refit to increase wrist extension optimally to 45°. Shortly thereafter, he regained full digital active and passive ROM as well as functional forearm rotation. He eventually required a wrist extension mobilization splint to aid in regaining wrist extension (Fig. 16–41). DS wore the mobilization splint three to five times a day for a minimum of 20 minutes per session. At 15 weeks postinjury, he had regained functional wrist extension and had begun an aggressive strengthening program.

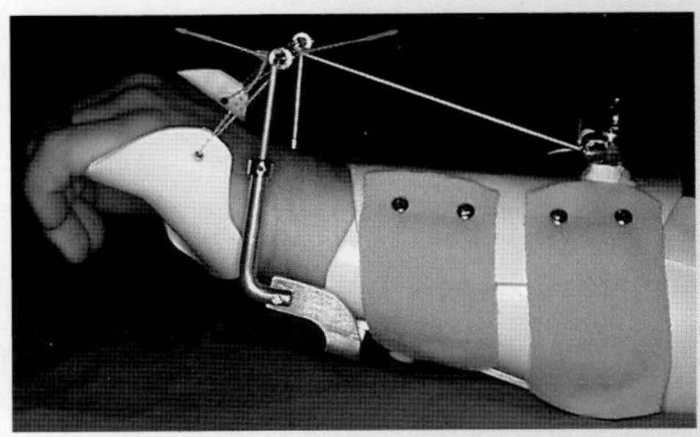

Figure 16–41 A static progressive wrist mobilization splint (here with a Phoenix wrist hinge and MERiT component) can be useful for gaining end range motion.

CASE STUDY 2: **Intra-Articular PIP Joint Fracture**

DG is a 49-year-old male who sustained a intra-articular fracture/dislocation of the IF PIP joint. He fell with his finger in a hyperextended position. He was initially seen at the emergency room of a community hospital where closed reduction was attempted. Upon returning home 2 days later, DG consulted his orthopedist, who scheduled surgery for fracture reduction/fixation. On the same day he saw the surgeon, DG was referred to therapy for preoperative fabrication of an intra-articular PIP (traction) mobilization splint (Fig. 16–40). The splint was to be applied in the operating room, and gentle therapy was to begin in the recovery room.

A radial wrist extension, MP flexion immobilization splint was fabricated with a hoop (outrigger) attachment for the application of dynamic tension. The hoop allows equal rubber band tension from the middle phalanx to the hoop, throughout PIP joint ROM. To achieve this tension, the surgeon placed a wire through the middle phalanx, leaving a small loop on each side of the protruding wire from which the rubber bands were attached and directed to the hoop. A variety of rubber bands were chosen to estimate the appropriate tension necessary to maintain fracture reduction. The rubber bands were given to the surgeon to attach to the splint in the operating room after reduction. An AlumaFoam duchess cap was fabricated for attachment of the rubber bands against the hoop (Fig. 16–42). The base was fabricated from a plastic material with moderate drapability. The hoop was made out of a 1/4" Aquatube for ease of fabrication.

DG wore the splint for 5½ weeks continuously, except for hygiene and skin inspection. The tension applied to the PIP joint was set at 300 g force as measured on a Haldux gauge to allow proper alignment of the joint, as well as to preserve the joint space (Oxford &

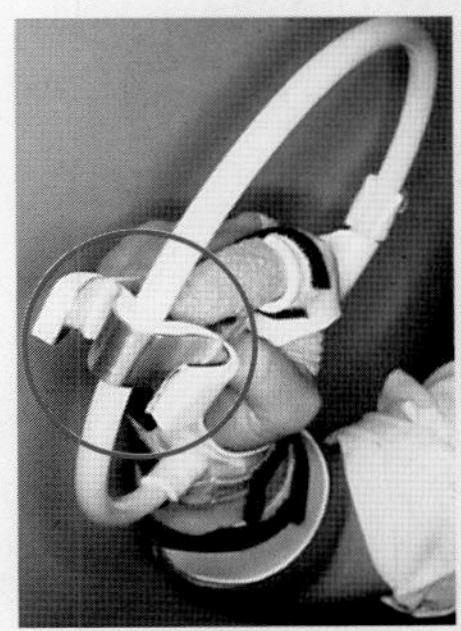

Figure 16–42 A duchess cap can be fabricated simply by bending AlumaFoam into the desired position and placing it directly onto the hoop.

Hidreth, 1996). Alignment was confirmed by x-ray postoperatively. After the splint was removed, a protective hand-based digit immobilization splint was fabricated with the IF MP flexed to 60° and the PIP/DIP joints gently flexed. DG was followed for an additional 2 months, as he regained ROM and strength, a mild PIP flexion contracture was managed with gentle serial static PIP extension casting (Fig. 16–43). The cast was changed weekly, and within 4 months of surgery the patient had obtained functional PIP joint ROM and strength.

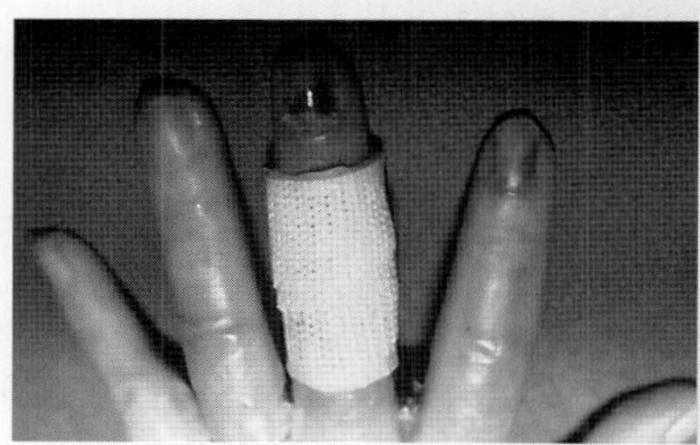

Figure 16–43 Casting to provide a serial static stretch is a useful way of improving extension of a PIP joint. (QuickCast used here.)

CONCLUSION

This chapter reviewed splinting interventions for common upper extremity fractures. The appropriate selection and judicious use of splints and strapping systems can aid in managing fractures early, while maximizing functional use of uninjured structures. In select cases, splints applied immediately postinjury can offer excellent conformability for secure fracture stabilization, while allowing joint mobility and gliding of surrounding soft tissue structures. Splints used during the rehabilitative phase are often to provide continued protection and guard against reinjury. Close communication with the physician regarding proper joint positioning within the splint is essential to prevent secondary problems such as joint or soft tissue contracture, tendon or nerve adherence, and chronic edema.

REFERENCES

Anderson, L., Meyer, F. N. (1991). Fractures of the shafts of the radius and ulna. In *Rockwood & Green's Fractures in adults*. Philadelphia: Lippincott.

Biangini, A. (1991). Part I: Fractures of the proximal humerus. In *Rockwood & Green's Fractures in adults*. Philadelphia: Lippincott.

Bleeker, W. A. (1991). Treatment of humeral shaft fractures related to associated injuries: A retrospective study of 237 Patients. *ACTA Orthopedics Scandinavian, 62,* 148–153.

Brown, P. S. H. (1983). *Basic facts of fractures.* Boston: Blackwell Scientific.

Butters, K. P. (1991). Fractures of the shoulder part III: Fractures and dislocations of the scapula. In *Rockwood & Green's Fractures in adults*. Philadelphia: Lippincott.

Camden, P., & Nade, S. (1992). Fracture bracing of the humerus. *Injury, 23,* 245–48.

Cohen, L. S., & Frillman, T. (1997). Distal radius fractures: A prospective randomized comparison of fiberglass tape with QuickCast. *Injury, 28,* 305–309.

Colditz, J. (1995). Functional fracture bracing. In J. M. Hunter, E. J. Mackin, & A. D. Callahan (Eds.). *Rehabilitation of the hand* (4th ed., pp. 395–406). St. Louis: Mosby Year Book.

Craig EV. (1991). Part II: Fractures of the clavicle. In *Rockwood & Green's Fractures in adults* (pp. 1041–1078). Philadelphia: Lippincott.

Edwards, D. E. (1992). Fractures of the distal clavicle: A case for fixation. *Injury, 23,* 44–46.

Eiff, M. P. (1997). Management of clavicle fractures. *American Family Physician, 55,* 121–128.

Fernandez, D., & Jupiter, J. (1995). *Fractures of the distal radius: A practical approach to management.* New York: Springer-Verlag.

Gebuhr, P. (1992). Isolated ulnar shaft fractures: Comparison of treatment by a functional brace and long arm cast. *Journal of Bone and Joint Surgery (British volume 5), 74,* 757–759.

Green, D. P., & Rowland, S, A. (1991). Fractures and dislocations in the hand. In *Rockwood & Green's Fractures in adults*. Philadelphia: Lippincott.

Hambridge, J., Desai, V. V., Schranz, P. J., Comson, J. P., Davis, T. R., & Barton, N. J. (1999). Acute fractures of the scaphoid. *Journal of Bone and Joint Surgery (British volume), 81,* 91–92.

Harkess, J. W., & Ramsey, W. C. (1991). Principles of fractures and dislocations. In *Rockwood & Green's Fractures in adults*. Philadelphia: Lippincott.

Hunter, S. G. (1982). The closed treatment of fractures of the humeral shaft. *Clinical Orthopaedics and Related Research, 164,* 192–198.

Jones, A. (1996). A custom brace for treatment of angulated fifth metacarpal fractures. *Journal of Hand Surgery, 21(2),* 319–320.

Kaplan, L. (1940). The treatment of fractures and dislocations of the hand and fingers. Technique of unpadded casts for carpal, metacarpal, phalangeal fractures. *Surgery Clinics of North America, 20,* 1695.

Kiefhaber, T. (1996). Phalangeal dislocation/periarticular trauma. In C. Peiner (Ed.). *Surgery of the hand and upper extremity* (pp. 939–972). New York: McGraw Hill.

Laseter, G., & Carter, P. R. (1996). Management of distal radius fractures. *Journal of Hand Therapy, 9,* 114–128.

Ledingham, W., Gorey, C. C., Mathieson, A. B., & Wardon, D. (1991). Immediate functional bracing of Colles fractures. *Injury, 22(3),* 197–201.

Moir, J. S. (1995). A new functional brace for treatment of Colles fractures. *Injury, 26(9),* 587–593.

Osterman, P. A., Ekkernkamp, A., Henry, S. L., & Muhr, G. (1994). Bracing of stable shaft fractures of the ulna. *Journal of Orthopaedic Trauma, 8,* 245–488.

Oxford, K., & Hidreth, D. (1996). Fracture bracing for proximal phalanx fractures. *Journal of Hand Therapy, 9,* 404–405.

Prosser, R., & Herbert, T. (1996). The management of carpal fractures and dislocations. *Journal of Hand Therapy, 9,* 139–148.

Ring, D., & Jupiter, J. (1998a). Restoring elbow stability after fracture dislocation Part I: Elbow anatomy and patterns of injury in fracture dislocation. *Medscape Orthopedics and Sports Medicine, 2.*

Ring, D., & Jupiter, J. (1998b). Restoring elbow stability after fracture-dislocation: Part II. *Medscape Orthopedics and Sports Medicine, 2.*

Sarmiento, A. (1990). Functional bracing for comminuted extra-articular fractures of the distal third of the humerus. *Journal of Bone and Joint Surgery (British volume), 72,* 283–287.

Sarmiento, A., Kinman, P. B., Galvin, E. G., Schmitt, R. H., & Phillipa, J. G. (1977). Functional bracing of fractures of the shaft of the humerus. *Journal of Bone and Joint Surgery, 59,* 596–601.

Schenck, R. (1994). The dynamic traction method: Combining movement and traction for intra-articular fractures of the phalanges. *Hand Clinics, 10,* 187–198.

Sorenson, J. S., Freund, K. G., & Keijla, G. (1993). Functional fracture bracing in metacarpal fractures. The Galveston brace versus plaster of paris in a prospective study. *Journal of Hand Therapy, 6,* 263–265.

Susso, S. (1994). Compression of the anterior interosseous nerve after use of a Robert-Jones type bandage for a distal end clavicle fracture: Case Report. *Journal of Trauma, 36,* 737–739.

Tang, P., Failla, J. M., & Contesti, L. A. (1999). The radio-ulnar joints and forearm axis: Surgeon's perspective. *Journal of Hand Therapy, 12,* 75–84.

SUGGESTED READINGS

Blackard, D., & Sampson, J. (1992). Management of an uncomplicated posterior elbow dislocation. *Journal of Athletic Training, 32,* 63–67.

Buckwalter, J. (1996). Effects of early motion on healing of musculoskeletal tissues. *Hand Clinics, 12,* 13–24.

Cabanela, M. E., & Morrey, B. F. (2000). Fractures of the olecranon. In B. F. Morrey (Ed). *The elbow and its disorders* (pp. 365–379). Philadelphia: Saunders.

Cohen, M. S., & Hastings, H. (1998). Acute elbow dislocations: Evaluation and management. Journal of the *American Academy of Orthopaedic Surgery, 6,* 15–23.

Cooney, W. P. (1998). Fractures of the distal radius. In W. P. Cooney, R. L. Linscheid, & J. H. Dobyns (Eds.). *The wrist* (pp. 310–355). St. Louis: Mosby.

Deitch, M. A., Keifhaber, T. R., Comisar, B. R., & Stern, P. J. (199?). Dorsal fracture dislocations of the proximal interphalangeal joint: Surgical complications and long-term results. *Journal of Hand Surgery, 24,* 914–923.

Faierman, E., & Jupiter, J. (1998). The management of acute fractures involving the distal radioulnar joint and distal ulna. *Hand Clinics, 14,* 213–229.

Freeland, A., & Benoit, L. (1994). Open reduction and internal fixation method for fractures of the proximal interphalangeal joint. *Hand Clinics, 10,* 239–250.

Gelinas, J. J., Faber, K. J., Patterson, S. D., King, G. J. W. (2000). The effectiveness of turnbuckle splinting for elbow contractures. *Journal of Bone and Joint Surgery (British volume), 82,* 74–78.

Jupiter, J. B., & Morrey, B. F. (2000). Fracture of the distal humerus in adults. In B. F. Morrey (Ed.). *The elbow and its disorders* (3rd ed.). Philadelphia: Saunders.

Kearney, L., & Brown, K. (1994). The therapist's management of intra-articular fractures. *Hand Clinics, 10,* 199–209.

Koval, K. J., Gallagher, M. A. (1997). Functional outcomes after minimally displaced fractures of the proximal part of the humerus. *Journal of Bone and Joint Surgery (American volume), 79,* 203–207.

Kozin, S. H., & Throder, J. J. (2000). Operative treatment of metacarpal and phalangeal shaft fractures. *Journal of the American Academy of Orthopaedic Surgery, 8,* 170–179.

Light, T., & Bednar, M. (1994). Management of intra-articular fractures of the metacarpophalangeal joint. *Hand Clinics, 10,* 303–314.

Meyer, F. N., & Wilson, R. L. (1995). Management of non-articular fractures of the hand. In J. M. Hunter, E. J. Mackin, & A. D. Callahan (Eds.). *Rehabilitation of the hand* (4th ed., pp. 353–375). St. Louis: Mosby Year Book.

Morrey, B. F. (2000). Splints and bracing at the elbow. In B. F. Morrey (Ed.). *The elbow and its disorders* (3rd ed., pp, 150–154). Philadelphia: Saunders.

Newport, M. L. (2000). Colles fracture: Managing a common upper extremity injury. *Journal of Musculoskeletal Medicine, 17,* 292–301.

Prosser, R., & Herbert, T. (1996). The management of carpal fractures and dislocations. *Journal of Hand Therapy, 9,* 139–147.

Rettig, A. C. (2000). Management of acute scaphoid fracture. *Hand Clinics,16,* 381–396.

Ring, D., Jupiter, J. B., Sanders, R. W., Mast, J., & Simpson, N. S. (1997). Transolecranon fracture-dislocation of the elbow. *Journal of Orthopaedic Trauma, 11,* 545–550.

Schenck, R. (1994). Classification of fractures and dislocations of the proximal interphalangeal joint. *Hand Clinics, 10,* 179–185.

Schneider, L. (1994). Fractures of the distal interphalangeal joint. *Hand Clinics, 10,* 277–285.

Wright, T. W., & Michlovitz, S. L. (1996). Management of carpal instabilities. *Journal of Hand Therapy, 9,* 48–156.

Arthritis

MaryLynn Jacobs, MS, OTR/L, CHT

INTRODUCTION

The word ***arthritis*** is derived from the Greek word *arthros* (joint) and *itis* (inflammation). Arthritis encompasses approximately 100 rheumatic diseases, all of which have joint disease as a prominent manifestation. In addition to the joints, the adjacent bones, tendons, and muscles are involved. The two most common rheumatic diseases are **osteoarthrosis (OA)** and **rheumatoid arthritis (RA).** For most kinds of arthritis there is as yet no cure; therefore, the main goals for treating these diseases are to minimize pain, control the inflammatory process, preserve joint structures, and maintain as much functional independence as possible.

The patient with arthritis of the upper extremity is best served by a supportive team approach, including primary care physician, rheumatologist, hand or orthopedic surgeon, physical therapist, occupational therapist, and family members. The therapist is uniquely qualified to educate the patient regarding joint protection, energy conservation, exercise programs, and splinting management (Estes, Bochenek, & Fasler, 2000; Kelley & Ramsey, 2000; Kozin, 1999; Kozin & Michlovitz, 2000; Poole & Pellegrini, 2000).

This chapter reviews joint disease, patient assessment, general characteristics of OA and RA, common surgical procedures, and the value of splints for these conditions. Specific rehabilitation techniques, therapeutic modalities, medical management, related inflammatory diseases, and detailed surgical procedures are not reviewed; see Suggested Readings for further study.

Splinting Goals

Initial conservative management of OA and RA may include splinting, often in combination with patient education, anti-inflammatory medication, and/or local steroid injection. Controversy in the literature exists regarding the efficacy of splinting interventions for the nonsurgical patient with arthritis, although there is agreement that splints can play a role in joint protection, pain relief, edema management, and functional performance (Barron, Glickel, & Eaton, 2000; Fess & Philips, 1987; Kozin & Michlovitz, 2000; Melvin, 1982; Philips, 1995; Seeger & Furst, 1987; Stern, Ytterbery, Krug, Larson, Portoghese, Kratz, & Mahowald, 1997; Swigart, Eaton, Glickel, & Johnson, 1999; Weiss, LaStayo, Mills, & Bramlet, 2000). Immobilization splints can be custom molded with thermoplastics or Neoprene material, or purchased prefabricated. The type of postsurgical splinting is determined by the procedure performed and the integrity of the patient's tissue. Some type of splint is usually introduced after the postoperative dressing is removed (Fess & Philips, 1987; Kozin & Michlovitz, 2000; Melvin, 1982; Philips, 1995; Seeger & Furst, 1987; Stern et al., 1997; Swigart et al., 1999; Weiss et al., 2000). General splinting interventions are discussed for each joint.

Goals for splinting patients with arthritis include the following (Fess & Philips, 1987; Melvin, 1982; Philips, 1995; Weiss et al., 2000):

- Reduce pain and inflammation of the involved joints.
- Rest and support the weakened structures.
- Position the involved joints as close to proper alignment as possible.
- Help prevent and/or minimize joint deformity.
- Provide external support (increase stability) to improve functional use of the hand.
- Position healing structures properly after postoperative procedures.

Joint Assessment

Components of a Normal Joint

Before discussing the diseased joint, normal joint anatomy must be understood. A joint is composed of many parts, each of which has a definite role and function (Fig. 17–1). All together, in a carefully orchestrated sequence, they provide smooth, fluid, pain-free joint motion. The main components of a joint are described below, along with their functions.

Bone is living tissue that provides the framework of the body. This hard porous material is composed of osteocytes that secrete a dense fibrous ground substance. This ground substance then calcifies into a strong and stiff material. Bone is considered the hardest structure in the body, except for parts of the teeth. Bones have a blood and nerve supply and are constantly being remodeled.

Articular cartilage is a tough connective tissue that covers the ends of the bones and functions as a cushion and shock absorber by lowering forces on adjacent bone. Cartilage goes through specific changes when the joint is loaded and possesses the ability to deform and reform many times. Cartilage has traditionally been thought to be incapable of regrowth, although some recent research may prove that cartilage has regenerative capacity.

The **fibrous joint capsule** is a thin layer of tissue that envelops the joint and maintains the integrity of the joint structure. The capsule consists of sheets of collagen, which supply stability and strength and the protein elastin, which gives the capsule its ability to stretch and return to its previous state. This elastic capability plays a significant role in joint mobility.

The **synovial membrane** lines the joint, just beneath the capsule, and produces **synovial fluid,** which nourishes and lubricates the joint. It also provides the mechanism by which fluid is removed from the joint.

Ligaments are strong fibrous bands that connect the bones together, reinforcing the joint and providing stability. Ligaments are composed of dense longitudinal connective tissue bundles with little ground substance.

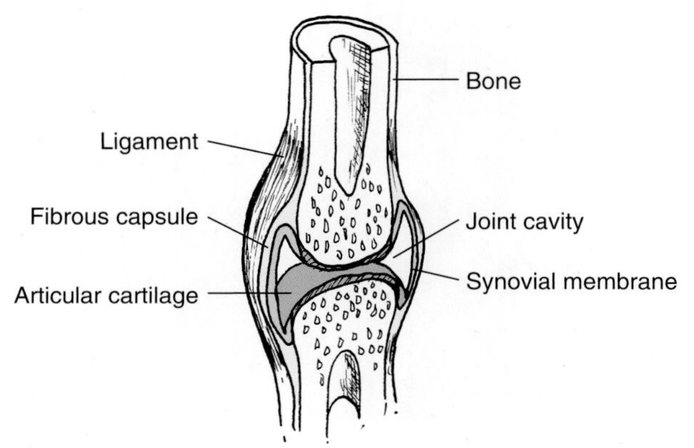

Figure 17–1 Normal joint anatomy and surrounding structures.

Muscles are the contractile tissue that provide joint motion. They attach to the bones on either side of the joint via cordlike **tendons.** Muscles provide dynamic stability to the joint.

Joint Disease and Inflammation

The disruption of any normal component of a joint, either through injury or a disease process, affects the quality of joint motion. This change in motion may significantly limit an individual's ability to perform even the simplest of daily tasks. OA is a noninflammatory joint disease that occurs specifically at the articular cartilage, which deteriorates over time. Simultaneously, bony osteophytes proliferate at the borders of the involved joint (Melvin, 1982; Poole & Pellegrini, 2000; Swanson, 1995a). RA is an inflammatory joint disease localized to the synovial lining. As the disease progresses, the synovial membrane stretches and fluid herniates from the fibrous capsule, causing damage to the capsule and supporting structures (Fig. 17–2) (Melvin, 1982; Swanson, 1995a).

Clinicians working with patients who have arthritis use their fundamental knowledge of normal joint anatomy and the consequences of joint disease to develop an effective therapeutic regime.

Osteoarthritis

Characteristics

Osteoarthritis is sometimes referred to as degenerative joint disease (DJD). It occurs as a chronic, noninflammatory disease that causes cartilage destruction and reactive changes about the periphery of joints and in subchondral bone. The most common sites are the weight-bearing joints (e.g., hips, knees, feet, and spine), and it may affect only one side of the body. The hand and wrist joints involved are the proximal interphalangeal (PIP) joints; the distal interphalangeal (DIP) joints; and the basal joint complex of the thumb, which includes the first carpometacarpal (CMC) joint, the trapeziometacarpal joint (TM), and the scaphotrapeziotrapezoid (STT) joint. (Fig. 17–3) (Melvin, 1982; Poole & Pellegrini, 2000; Swanson, 1995a). The cause of the disease may be genetic factors, trauma (via work or sports), mechanical problems, metabolic issues, and/or age. Onset usually occurs at 40 to 50 years of age, and there are generally no systemic features (Swanson, 1995a).

General Signs and Symptoms

Initially, patients may present with one or more of the clinical symptoms discussed below. Over time, radiographs may reveal actual joint damage; however, the degree of radiologic involvement may not always correspond with the patient's complaints.

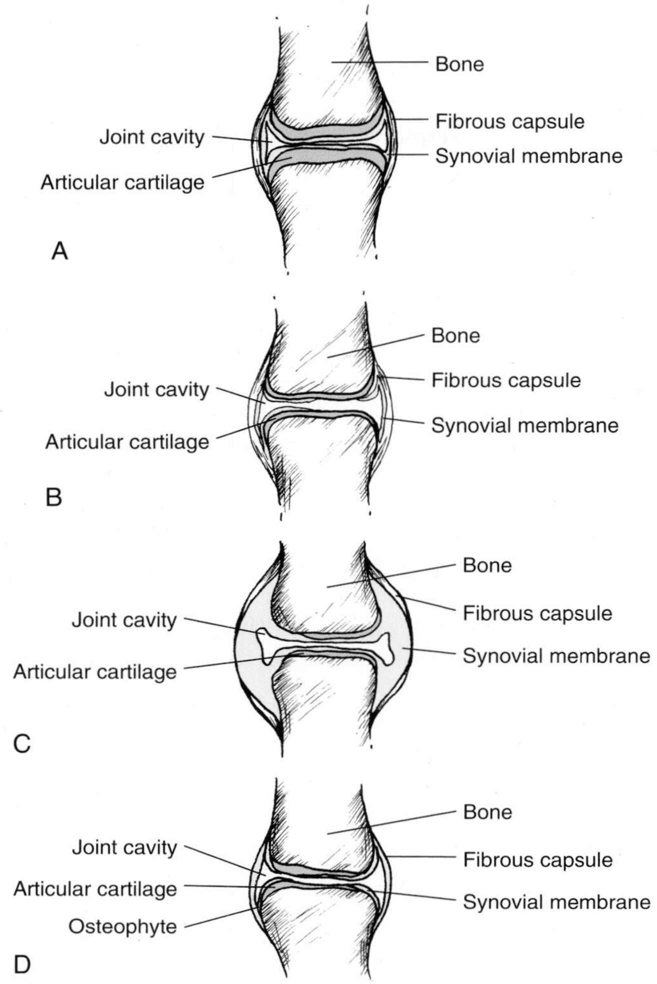

Figure 17–2 ***A,*** *Healthy joint surfaces. Changes owing to OA and RA: early inflammation (**B**), advanced inflammation with herniation of synovial fluid and bone and cartilage destruction (**C**), and noninflammatory disease with cartilage breakdown and osteophyte formation (**D**).*

Pain

Joint pain with motion, subsiding with rest, is one of the first symptoms. As the disease progresses, pain is noted during motion and rest, sometimes accompanied by muscle spasm.

Stiffness

Stiffness of the involved joints may occur, especially after an extended rest period. Active range of motion (AROM) and gross functional use of the involved joint may be limited and painful. As the disease progresses, strength may also diminish due to pain or disuse.

Crepitation

Crepitation may be noted in the joint or along the tendons as motion is performed. This is distinguished by a crunching sensation or sound produced as the joint or tendon moves.

Osteophytes

Bone spurs, or **osteophytes,** are common in the OA disease process, forming at the borders of the PIP and/or DIP joints of the fingers (Buckland-Wright, Macfarland, & Lynch 1991; Swanson, 1995a) (Fig. 17–2**D**). These bony enlargements can appear gradually over time or have a rapid onset. Discomfort resulting from bone spurs varies. Some patients describe a functional hindrance (e.g., putting on rings), while others describe episodes of pain (Buckland-Wright et al. 1991; Burkholder, 2000; Estes et al., 2000; Melvin, 1982). Osteophytes at the DIP joints are called **Heberden's nodes;** those at the PIP joints are referred to as **Bouchard's nodes** (Fig. 17–4) (Burkholder, 2000; Melvin, 1982).

Splinting Management

Early therapy is paramount. Conservative management for patients with OA may consist of supportive, protective, and preventive splinting; anti-inflammatory medications; exercise programs; and instruction in joint protection and activity modification. Patient education is imperative for

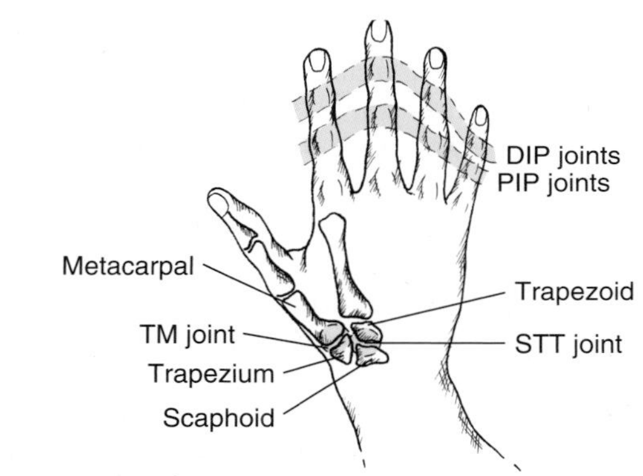

Figure 17–3 *Joints commonly affected by osteoarthritis.*

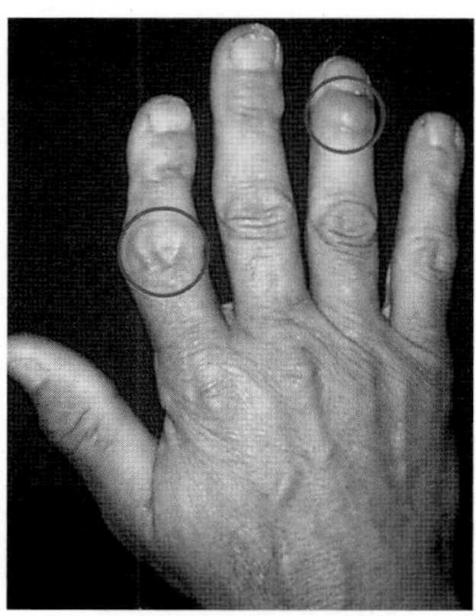

Figure 17–4 *Note the Heberden's and Bouchard's nodules at the PIP and DIP joints, respectively.*

providing information on compensatory techniques that decrease external forces on joints, which, if not addressed, may contribute to further deformity and/or pain (Estes et al., 2000; Kelley & Ramsey, 2000; Kozin, 1999; Poole & Pellegrini, 2000). Providing information on adaptive equipment and/or custom fabricating adaptations for activities of daily living (ADLs) may be extremely helpful in maintaining functional use of the hand (e.g., increasing the size of the grips on cooking or writing utensils, changing round door knobs to lever handles). Splinting with thermoplastic materials may not always be well tolerated by some individuals because of pressure at bony prominences, fragile skin, weight of the splint, or restrictive nature of the splint. Softer, more conforming splints may be substituted (see Chapter 11 for more information). Splinting, especially when applied early in the DJD process, can stabilize the involved joint during at-risk activities (situations that stress the involved joint), minimize further joint damage, and decrease pain during activity (Barron et al., 2000; Colditz, 2000; Weiss et al., 2000).

Material Selection

THERMOPLASTICS

Thermoplastic materials for the individual with OA should be carefully chosen. The selection ranges from heavyweight to lightweight materials, and the choice depends on the purpose of the splint and the individual's skin tolerance and joint integrity. A splint intended to provide gentle pressure for adequate joint stabilization might need to be of heavier weight than one used to position an inflamed joint (Colditz, 2000). Materials should easily contour about bony prominences, such as the ulnar styloid and the dorsal metacarpal heads. Because bony changes may occur over time in OA, consideration should be given to a material that can be reheated and reshaped repeatedly (Aquaplast).

Another consideration is material flexibility. Materials that are thin (1/16") and/or highly perforated tend to be more flexible than traditional (1/8") solid materials (see Chapter 5 for further details). However, a highly perforated material may irritate the fragile skin, owing to the friction of the perforations on the skin's surface. A cotton stockinette or padding about bony prominences can minimize this irritation. Materials may need to be popped apart to allow the splint to pass over an enlarged area. This can be done by using coated thermoplastic or by placing a wet paper towel or hand lotion between overlapping pieces of noncoated material. Not only does this provide a way for the patient to slip in and out of the splint, but it also provides a sense of security for the patient, who may be worried about being trapped in the splint. An excellent example involves splinting the MP joint of the thumb in some individuals; the interphalangeal (IP) joint can be significantly wider than the proximal phalanx, making removal of a thumb splint difficult unless it can be popped open (Fig. 17–5).

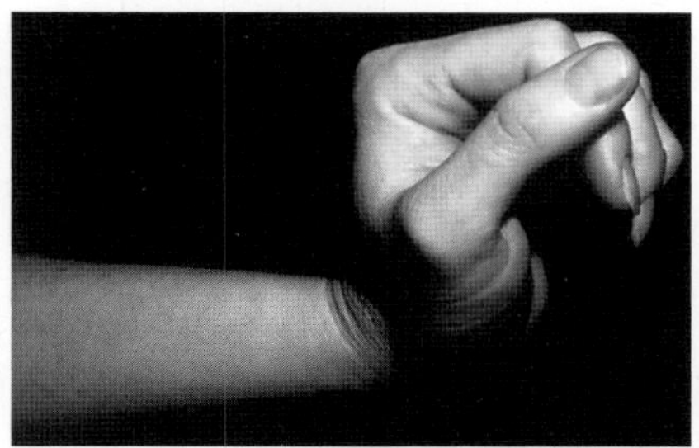

Figure 17–5 *Note the significant enlargement of the IP joint of the thumb of this patient with OA. Take care when splinting proximal to this joint to allow for easy splint don/doffing.*

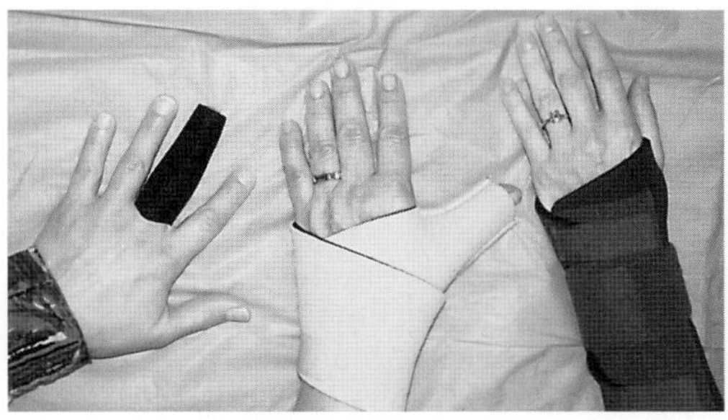

Figure 17–6 *Prefabricated splints used to manage the early intermittent symptoms of arthritis.*

STRAPPING

When securing straps onto the splint, consideration should be given to where the straps are going to traverse. Is the skin under the strap fragile? Are there bony prominences? Are Bouchard's or Heberden's nodes present? If so, are they tender and will straps irritate them? Strapping considerations for the extremity with arthritis should include soft, conforming, and flexible material. Straps can be lined with foam to soften the touch around bony areas. Consider soft 2" foam straps for night use, and less bulky elasticized straps for day use (such as thin Neoprene material). Both soft and elasticized strapping systems are comfortable, durable, and when applied correctly, contribute to minimizing shear and compression stress on tissue (see Chapter 4 for details).

PREFABRICATED SPLINTS

Prefabricated splints can be used for many patients with OA. Soft prefabricated wrist and thumb splints are a popular choice with physicians (Fig. 17–6) (Boozer, 1993; Murphy, 1996; Pagnotta, Baron, & Korner-Bitensky, 1998; Stern, Ytterberg, Krug, & Machowald, 1996). Most patients initially do well with these splints. However, if joint changes begin to alter the shape of the wrist and/or thumb, a more customized design may be necessary.

PIP and DIP Joints with OA

Osteoarthritis of the PIP and DIP joints can result in pain, edema, decreased digital AROM, and difficulty in tasks requiring gripping and pinching. The alterations in physical appearance that osteophytes can cause may be disturbing to some patients (Estes et al., 2000; Melvin, 1982). Such patients may see their fingers as becoming deformed, and they have great difficulty putting rings on because of the bony changes and swelling. Although osteophytes are not always painful, they can be episodically tender (Burkholder, 2000; Estes et al., 2000). Pain is reported as localized specifically to the involved joints during functional activities. The intensity of the pain does not necessarily indicate the amount of joint destruction or deformity as seen on a radiograph. Surprisingly, there are patients with minimal pain who have significant joint destruction on the radiograph (Estes et al., 2000).

Nonsurgical Splinting Guidelines

Splinting is usually reserved for the acutely painful PIP or DIP joint. Lightweight volar immobilization splints can be supportive (especially to prevent lateral movements of the PIP and DIP joints) (Fig. 17–7). The splints place the joints in comfortable extension and are worn mostly at night. Gel-lined products (such as the Silopad mesh digital cap or silicone-lined thermoplastic materials) may provide an absorbent cushion and layer of warmth to a painful joint (Fig. 17–8). A piece of silicone gel can be incorporated into a splint for added protection and cushioning.

Postsurgical Splinting Guidelines

There are few surgical options for the individual with DIP joint osteoarthritis, with the exception of **DIP joint arthrodesis** (fusion), because for this small, but important joint, stability takes priority over mobility (Estes et

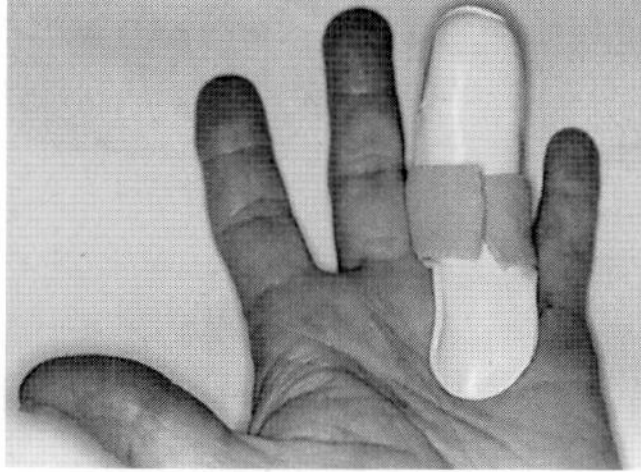

Figure 17–7 A volar RF digit immobilization splint that extends proximally to include the MP joint. This extension provides a longer lever arm for increased stability and comfort, especially for individuals with small hands or digits.

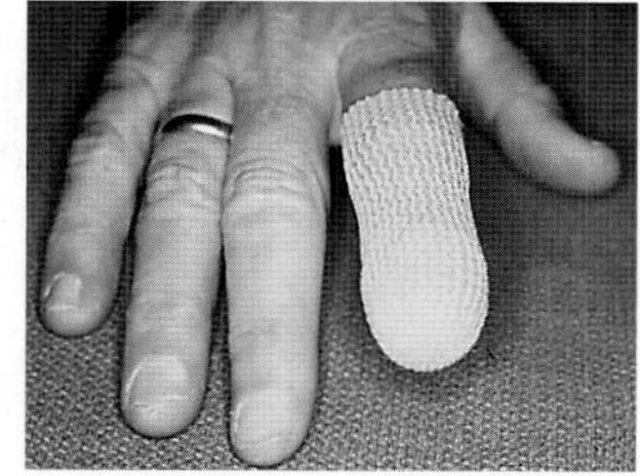

Figure 17–8 A Silopad mesh digital cap used to provide warmth and pain relief to a patient with OA of the IF DIP joint.

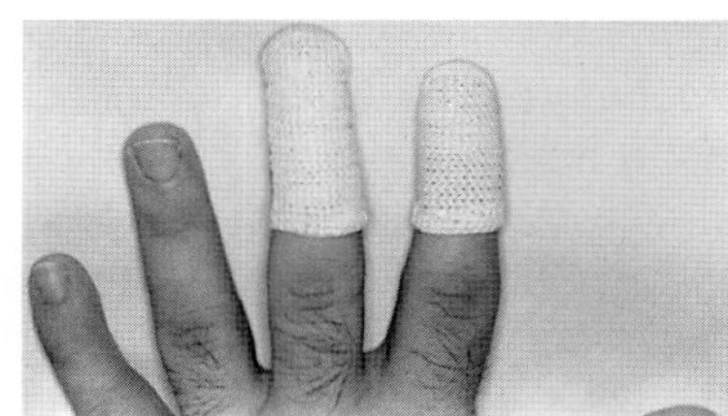

Figure 17–9 QuickCast used to fabricate DIP immobilization splints for protecting against DIP joint fusions.

al., 2000; Melvin, 1982; Pelligrini & Burton, 1990). An arthrodesis can provide this stability, along with decreasing intractable pain and enhancing cosmetic appearance (Pelligrini & Burton, 1990).

The DIP joint is protected after arthrodesis for 6 to 8 weeks until sufficient healing has occurred per radiograph (Pelligrini & Burton, 1990). Postsurgically, the patient can be placed in a DIP immobilization splint, which supports and protects the arthrodesis. For added length and support, the splint can include the PIP joint and then modified to include only the DIP joint once the patient is comfortably able to exercise and use the PIP joint (Fig. 17–9) (Rizio & Belsky, 1995).

PIP joint arthrodesis is considered for patients who use their hand for activities that require a forceful grip, such as in meat cutting or construction work. Surgical fusion has been recommended for several situations: to provide increased functional use of the hand when the soft tissues in the joint cannot support an implant, when stability is more important than mobility, and to provide for a pain-free joint. The postoperative splint should protect the PIP joint in the fused position for 6 to 8 weeks until the arthrodesis is solid per radiograph (in the latter weeks the DIP joint may be left free) (Estes et al., 2000; Rizio & Belsky, 1995). Lightweight thermoplastics or casting materials can be used (Fig. 17-7).

The position of fusion for the PIP or DIP joint is based on which digit is involved and the function of that particular joint as determined by preoperative discussion with the patient (Estes et al., 2000). In normal hand function, the index finger (IF) and middle finger (MF) are used mostly for prehension and do not require as much flexion as the RF and SF PIP joints. The ring finger (RF) and small finger (SF), on the other hand, require greater flexion, especially at the DIP joints, because they contribute greatly to grip strength (Estes et al., 2000; Rizio & Belsky, 1995).

PIP joint arthroplasty can be considered to gain PIP joint stability, increase functional ROM, and decrease overall pain. An arc of motion of 30 to 60° can be expected at the PIP joint (Kozin, 1999; Pelligrini & Burton, 1990; Rizio & Belsky, 1995; Swanson, Swanson, & Leonard, 1995). Exercise protocols vary and depend on postoperative joint stability. Therapeutic management should take into account other surgical procedures that may have been performed at the same time, such as tenolysis, extensor tendon reconstruction, or volar plate release. In general, AROM exercises are initiated between 2 and 7 days postoperatively. A recommended exercise schedule is 5- to 10-min sessions, four to six times a day.

A postoperative hand-based PIP extension immobilization splint is fabricated and worn at all times for 4 to 6 weeks; it is removed only for hygiene and exercise sessions (Fig. 17–10**A**). The MP joint is usually included, at least initially, for improved purchase and comfort. If the patient had a swan-neck deformity (PIP hyperextension, DIP flexion) before surgical implant, then consider positioning the involved joints in some degree of PIP flexion (approximately 10–30°) in the splint. This may help prevent the tendency for the PIP joint to rebound into hyperextension (Fig. 17–10**B**). Extension mobilization splints are an alternative postoperative management option (Fig. 17–10**C**). These splints are fabricated to position the PIP gently in extension yet allow gentle active flexion exercise against rubber band traction.

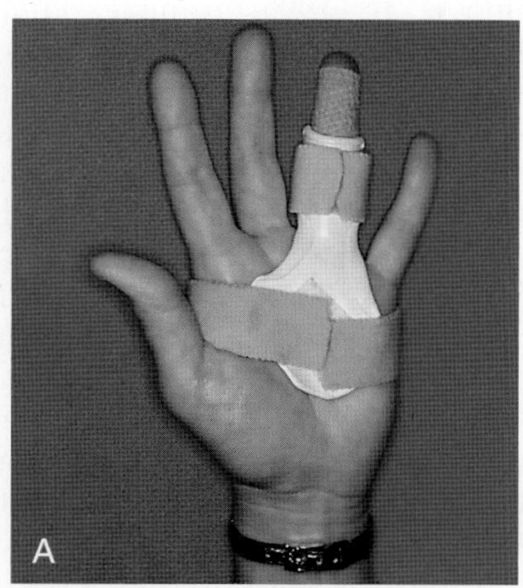

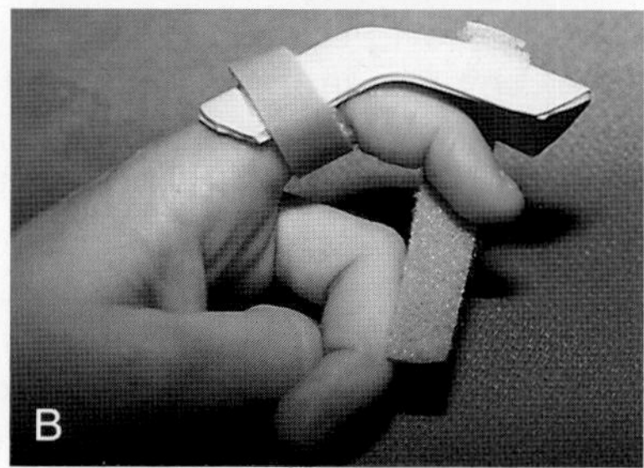

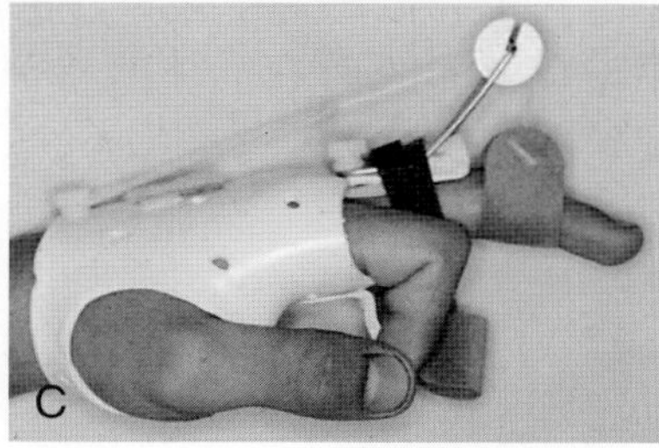

*Figure 17–10 PIP splints used after arthroplasty. **A,** This digit immobilization splint allows gentle DIP motion to facilitate tendon gliding. It can be removed for short periods of exercise per physician protocol. **B,** With this extension restriction splint, the patient is instructed to exercise into flexion from the dorsal block of the splint. **C,** A PIP extension mobilization splint may be indicated to allow frequent motion of PIP joint.*

Regardless of whether immobilization, mobilization, or restriction splints are used postoperatively, the splints should protect the joint from lateral stress and facilitate the encapsulation process (Estes et al., 2000). Immobilization and restriction splints should have sufficient depth for lateral protection. Mobilization splints should maintain the line of pull centrally over the middle phalanx and avoid any undesired rotation or lateral deviation stresses. It is important to recognize any tendon adherence, extension lag, and prolonged inflammation.

Thumb with OA

It is believed that ligamentous laxity and instability, either through the aging process or joint demands (wear and tear), are the initiators of OA at the base of the thumb (Barron et al., 2000; Boozer, 1993; Estes et al., 2000; Freedman, Eaton, & Glickel, 2000; Kelley & Ramsey, 2000; Pelligrini & Burton, 1990; Poole & Pellegrini, 2000). The thumb has a large arc of motion, allowing opposition to all the digits, which greatly influences overall hand function. A common site for OA in the thumb column is the TM joint; the STT joint is affected to a lesser degree (Poole & Pellegrini, 2000).

The TM joint is the key articulation responsible for imparting mobility to the thumb; although the trapezium also articulates with the scaphoid, trapezoid, and the index metacarpal (Poole & Pellegrini, 2000). This complex of articulations is also commonly referred to as the basal joint or the CMC joint (Poole & Pellegrini, 2000). Palpation may reveal tenderness over the TM joint, and in approximately half the population, concurrent pain is appreciated at the STT joint (Glickel et al., 1992; Kozin, 1999; Poole & Pellegrini, 2000). The patient may have a positive **grind test**—pain elicited when the examiner imparts gentle compression and rotation of the head of the first metacarpal into the trapezium (Estes et al., 2000). The typical patient notes pain during functional activities, such as opening jars, brushing teeth, and turning a doorknob. Pain is generalized to the thenar eminence but may also be noted proximal and distal to the involved joint.

Nonsurgical Splinting Guidelines

Splinting, along with anti-inflammatory medications, is often the initial treatment of choice for TM joint arthritis (Colditz, 1995, 2000; Swigart et al., 1999; Tomaino, Pelligrini, & Burton, 1995; Weiss et al., 2000). The purpose of splinting is to stabilize the base of the first metacarpal and inhibit joint motion during hand activity (Barron et al., 2000; Colditz, 1995, 2000; Poole & Pellegrini, 2000; Weiss et al., 2000). A variety of splint designs can be used. Common to most of

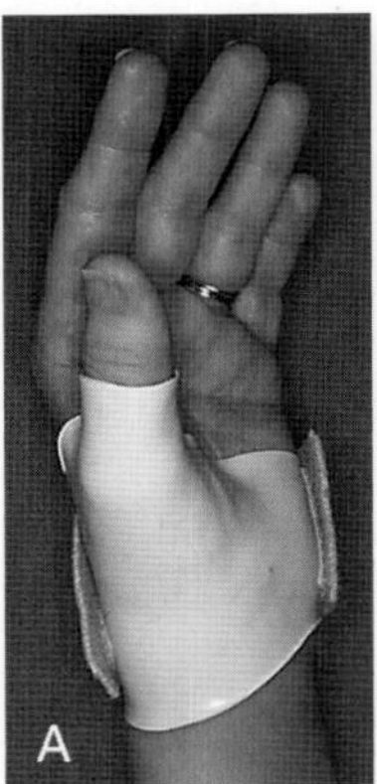

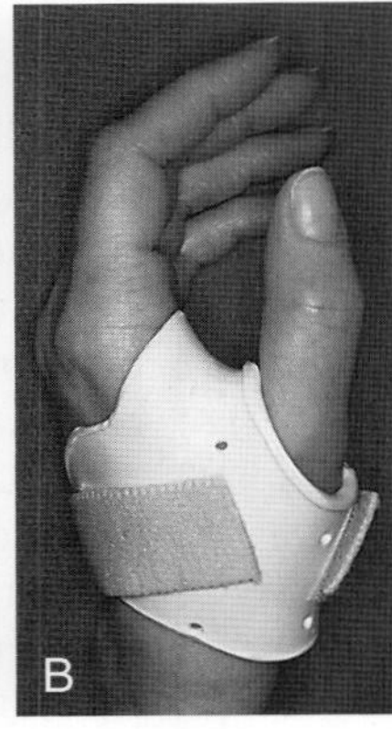

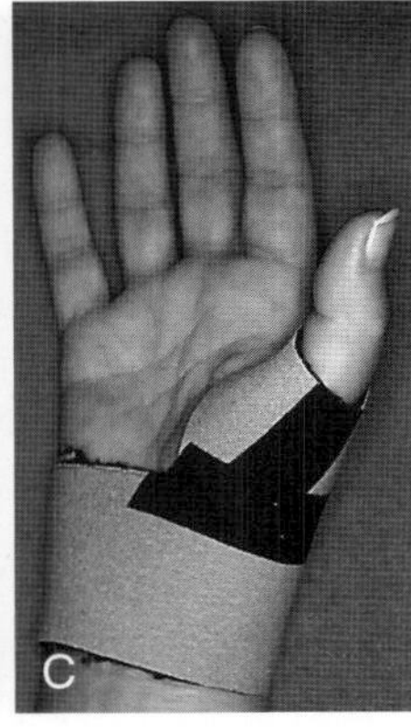

Figure 17–11 ***A,*** *Hand-based thumb TM immobilization splint to limit motion at the thumb first metacarpal and to place the thumb column in a position of function. Note the intimate contouring of the material about the proximal splint border.* ***B,*** *This splint (designed by Colditz) places an extension force to the volar/ulnar aspect of the distal metacarpal with counterpressure to the dorsal/radial portion of the metacarpal base.* ***C,*** *A custom splint fabricated from Neoprene may be appropriate when a nonrigid support is recommended.*

these splint designs is the maintenance of a wide first web space, because as the disease process advances, adduction and subluxation of the first metacarpal may occur, causing a contracture and/or narrowing of the first web space (Colditz, 2000; Diaz, 1994; Melvin, 1982; Melvin, 1995; Poole & Pellegrini, 2000; Swigart et al., 1999; Wajon, 2000; Weiss et al., 2000). Ideal splinting for TM joint arthritis involves positioning the thumb in palmar abduction and approximately 30° of MP flexion (Colditz, 1995; Poole & Pellegrini, 2000; Weiss et al., 2000). It may help to extend the splint border proximally on the radial aspect just beyond the STT joint to secure the thumb column. A conforming, lightweight material (e.g., 3/32" Aquaplast, Polyform light, Polyflex light, or TailorSplint) is an excellent choice for fabricating this splint (Melvin, 1995). Unfortunately, the material's thinness can make fabrication challenging to a novice splint maker and it may not offer the strength necessary to stabilize the first metacarpal (Fig. 17–11) (Colditz, 2000). These splints are used as functional day splints and are worn as needed to promote pain-free function.

Some physicians request that the day splint be complemented with a more inclusive resting splint for night use (Weiss et al., 2000). Forearm-based night splints can be fabricated to immobilize a wider or longer surface area, incorporating proximal and distal structures to achieve a greater degree of immobilization (Colditz, 2000; Fess & Philips, 1987; Leonard, 1995; Simmons, Nutting, & Berstein, 1996; Weiss et al., 2000). Therapists may find that patients become concerned about wearing splints too much, possibly leading to joint stiffness and/or weakness. In some cases, stiffness may be the desired outcome, because a decrease in joint motion may also produce a decrease in pain. If pain persists without relief from splinting and other interventions (use a trial period of 4 to 6 weeks), an injection or surgical consult should be considered (Barron et al., 2000; Estes et al., 2000; Kozin & Michlovitz, 2000).

Postsurgical Splinting Guidelines

Surgical intervention may be an option for patients with painful, progressive OA of the thumb. In these advanced cases, there usually has been a TM subluxation and/or dislocation; splinting is likely to be of little help (Fig. 17–12) (Colditz, 1995). Several surgical procedures (and variations of these procedures) for **ligament reconstruction of the TM joint** have been described (Estes et al., 2000; Freedman et al., 2000; Kozin, 1999; Poole & Pellegrini, 2000; Rozental & Bora, 2000; Tomaino & King, 2000; Tomaino et al., 1995; Trumble, Tafijah, Gilbert, Allan, North, & McCallister, 2000; Vartimidis, Fox, King, Taras, & Soreranes, 2000). All have the primary goals of pain relief, re-establishing the thumb/IF web space to provide a stable post for the digits to pinch against, and preventing further joint destruction. One such procedure uses a tendon interposition graft with a slip of the flexor carpi radialis (FCR) longus tendon with excision of the trapezium (Poole & Pellegrini, 2000; Tomaino et al., 1995). The successful outcome of ligament reconstruction of the thumb requires stabilization of the base of the thumb metacarpal and simultaneous adjustment of distal deformity (Colditz, 1995; Estes et al., 2000; Poole & Pellegrini, 2000; Tomaino et al., 1995).

Ligament reconstruction procedures of the TM joint normally require a short period of cast immobilization, which is followed by transition into a splint during the first 2 to 4 weeks postsurgery; however, protocols vary from surgeon to surgeon (Fig. 17–13) (Colditz, 1995; Kozin, 1999; Poole & Pellegrini, 2000; Tomaino et al., 1995; Weiss et al., 2000). From the cast, commonly a forearm-based wrist/thumb immobilization splint is fabricated that allows the IP joint to move freely. This splint is worn for 4 to 6 additional weeks after cast removal (Poole & Pellegrini, 2000). Some physicians prefer to shorten the splint after 6 to 8 weeks to allow wrist motion. After approximately 12 weeks, splinting

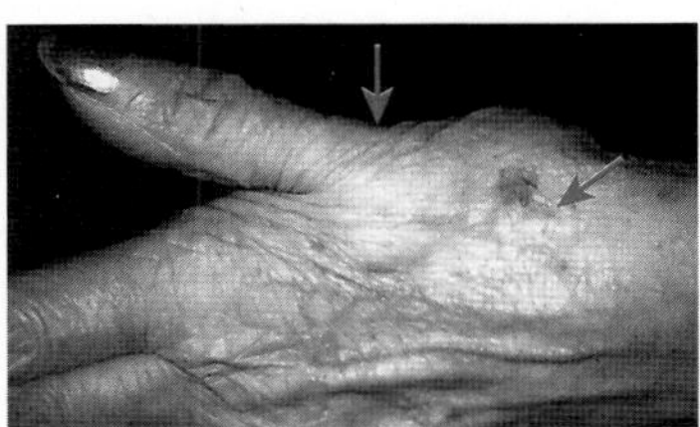

Figure 17–12 *The patient presented with exquisite joint pain with even light activity and was thus a strong candidate for TM joint arthroplasty.*

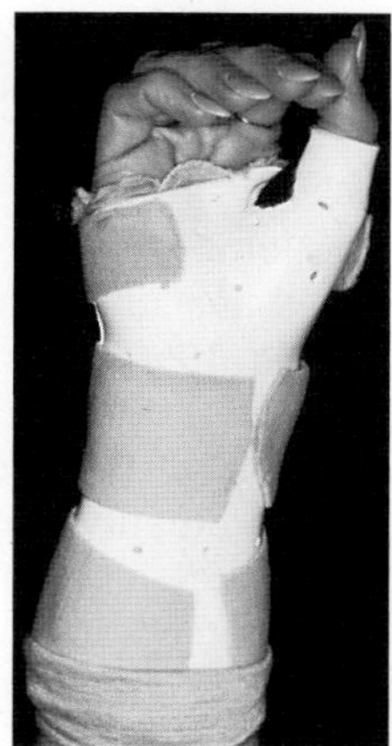

Figure 17–13 A wrist/thumb immobilization splint is often used after thumb TM joint arthroplasty.

can be discontinued or worn only at night, if necessary (Poole & Pellegrini, 2000).

Wrist with OA

Osteoarthritis of the wrist presents most often at the STT joint. Confusion can exist between STT arthritis and TM joint arthritis; the literature has clearly outlined clinical distinctions of each (Kozin & Michlovitz, 2000; Poole & Pellegrini, 2000). Patients with STT joint arthritis may exhibit pain with radial deviation (e.g., using scissors, pulling up socks), a decrease in active radial deviation, tenderness with palpation over the STT area, a positive grind test, joint space narrowing on radiograph, pain with the scaphoid shift test, and only occasional TM joint changes. Patients with TM joint arthritis (basal or CMC joint) may demonstrate difficulty with fine motor tasks (using clothespins, writing, doing needlepoint), a positive grind test, and subluxation of the TM joint with possible MP hyperextension; approximately half of patients with TM joint OA show STT space narrowing with possible osteophyte formation on radiographs (Kozin, 1999; Kozin & Michlovitz, 2000; Poole & Pellegrini, 2000; Weiss et al., 2000).

Nonsurgical Splinting Guidelines

Individuals with STT arthritis may find some temporary relief from such interventions as cortisone injection, pain modulating modalities, activity modification, and splint use (Kozin & Michlovitz, 2000). A recommended splint design is a wrist/thumb immobilization splint with the thumb IP free (Fig. 17–13). Wrist immobilization splints may also be successful in controlling pain and permitting hand use. Circumferential wrist splints (such as the Rolyan AquaForm zippered wrist splint) may be more appropriate for heavy labor workers, whereas a lightweight volar wrist immobilization splint will likely suffice for a person with less functional demands. There are several prefabricated splint designs that can work well for this population (Boozer, 1993; Stern et al., 1996, 1997; Trumble et al., 2000). See Chapter 11 for more options.

Postsurgical Splinting Guidelines

Several procedures have been described for managing OA of the wrist, including **scaphoid excision with four-corner fusion, proximal row carpectomy, wrist arthrodesis, arthrodesis of the distal radioulnar joint, arthrodesis of the STT joint, and distal ulna resection** (Beer & Turner, 1997; Feinberg, 1999; Kozin, 1999; Michlovitz, 1999; Shapiro, 1996; Swanson, 1995b; Tijhuis, Vliet Vlieland, Zwinderman, & Hazes, 1998; van-Vugt, van Jaarsveld, Hofman, Helders, & Bijlsma, 1999; Watson & Ballet, 1984; Watson, Weinzweig, Guidera, Zeppieri, & Ashmead, 1999; Wilson & Fredick, 1994). Common to these surgical procedures is the judicious postoperative splinting intervention. Splints are used after bulky dressing removal to further stabilize and protect the surgical site. Position of the wrist within the splint and the length of time the splint is worn depend on the exact procedure performed. A wrist/thumb immobilization splint with the IP joint free may be used 6 to 8 weeks after STT fusion, at which time gentle motion is most often begun (Fig. 17–13) (Kozin, 1999).

Rheumatoid Arthritis

Characteristics

Rheumatoid arthritis is an unpredictable, systemic, chronic, autoimmune, potentially debilitating disease of the synovial tissue of joints. It affects women more than men, in a 3:1 ratio (Melvin, 1982; Swanson, 1995a). The disease process is inflammatory and may be characterized by exacerbations and remissions that occur over the course of time. If the inflammation remains unchecked, the disease process may eventually cause severe joint destruction, attenuation or rupture of tendons, ligament laxity, joint deformity, and a generalized decrease in function (Kozin, 1999). Medical management includes a combination of anti-inflammatory medications and disease-modifying drugs, with the goal of reducing inflammation and joint damage (Fess & Philips, 1987; Massarotti, 1996; Melvin, 1982; Poole & Pellegrini, 2000; Swanson, 1995a, 1995b).

Early onset is often seen in the shoulders, wrists, and knees but may then involve other joints of the upper and lower extremities, including the MP and PIP joints of the hand (Fig. 17–14). RA is a systemic disease, and patients may also complain of intermittent fevers, weight loss, fatigue, muscle atrophy, and prolonged morning stiffness (Swanson, 1995a, 1995b).

In the early stages of the disease, splinting and medical management may be all that is required. As the disease progresses, surgical intervention, such as joint replacement and tendon transfer, may be considered, depending on the degree of functional impairment (Poole

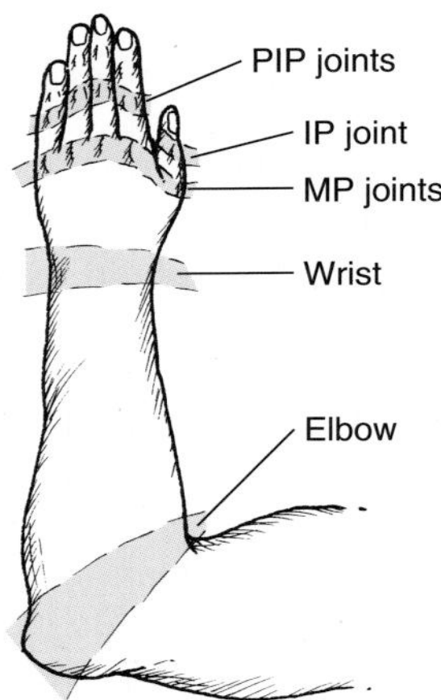

Figure 17–14 Upper extremity joints commonly affected by RA.

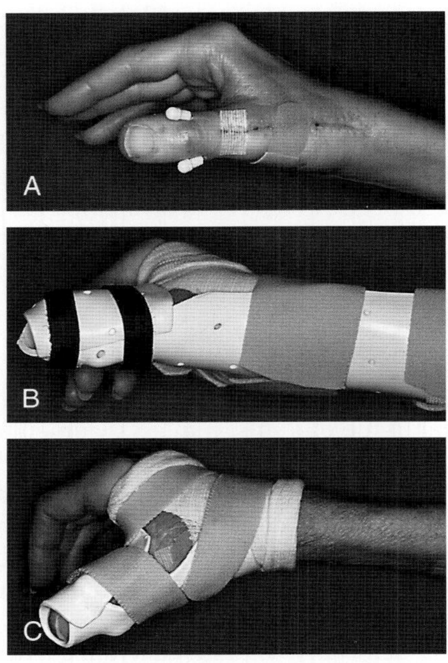

*Figure 17–15 TM joint arthroplasty with MP joint fusion. **A,** Note that pins secure the fusion during healing. **B,** At 6 days postsurgery, the patient was placed in a wrist/thumb immobilization splint with a protective cover for the pins. **C,** At 4–5 weeks postsurgery, the splint was modified to allow wrist motion per physician.*

& Pellegrini, 2000; Shapiro, 1996). A generally accepted operative sequence usually involves initially stabilizing the affected proximal structures (Wilson & Fredick, 1994). For example, procedures would commence at the wrist (arthrodesis), followed by the MP joints (arthroplasty). Some procedures can be performed simultaneously, such as a wrist and thumb MP fusion or a TM arthroplasty and thumb MP arthrodesis (Fig. 17–15) (Wilson & Fredick, 1994). When surgical intervention is planned, the ambulatory status of the patient must also be considered. If the patient is presently using a cane or crutches, he or she should be instructed in the use of platform crutches before surgery to allow ambulation with placing stress on surgical site.

General Signs and Symptoms

RA is characterized by joint redness, inflammation, and tenderness over involved areas on gentle palpation (Fess & Philips, 1987; Massarotti, 1996; Melvin, 1982; Swanson, 1995b). The involved joint(s) may be warm and swollen with a decrease in joint ROM. Unlike the normal healing process in which the inflammation subsides and the patient progresses through the stages of healing, patients with RA often remain in an extended inflammatory phase, which results in damage and deformity to the joints, pain, and impaired function (Swanson, 1995a).

Pain

Joint pain can occur during rest and may indicate acute inflammation (Melvin, 1982). Gentle pressure at the lateral aspects of an inflamed joint can cause some degree of pain, depending on the severity of the inflammation and joint damage. The joint(s) involved are generally described as sore with a notable decrease in AROM and functional use.

Stiffness and Decreased Function

Fluctuations in AROM can be related to joint pain and the extent of joint damage. Most individuals with RA describe an increase in joint stiffness in the morning, after prolonged inactivity, and during periods of exacerbation when pain limits functional use (Fess & Philips, 1987; Melvin, 1982).

Synovitis

Synovitis, inflammation of the joint lining (synovium), occurs slowly in the individual with RA. There are biochemical and autoimmune responses that cause changes in the synovium (Swanson, 1995). Inflammatory cells and enzymes attack the synovial lining of the joints, and the synovial tissues can eventually become fibrotic and form a scar tissue-like substance (pannus), which may invade tendons and ligaments (Fig. 17–2**B**). This process is progressive; continued swelling causes greater thickening of the synovium, capsular stretching, pain, and eventually destruction of the cartilage and bone (Fig. 17–2**C**) (Blank & Cassid, 1996).

The synovitis associated with RA may be divided into three phases: acute, subacute, and chronic active (Melvin, 1982). Each phase has the same symptoms of pain, tenderness, warmth, and limited ROM. The disease is most active in the acute phase, which leads to joint destruction. The symptoms begin to subside as the subacute phase is entered. The disease may be considered to be in the chronic active phase if the symptoms persist over a long period of time. The course of the disease varies and is unique to each patient; not all progress through these phases (Melvin, 1982; Swanson, 1995a).

Tenosynovitis

Tenosynovitis is an inflammation of the synovial lining of the tendon sheaths. In patients with RA, tenosynovitis usually occurs at the level of the flexor tendons, as they traverse the wrist (under the flexor retinaculum), and at the dorsum of the wrist, deep to the extensor retinaculum (Leslie, 1999; Wilson & Fredick, 1994). These tunnels are lined with the same synovial fluid that surrounds the joints. If left untreated, the lining becomes thickened and plaques and nodules may form, disrupting normal tendon excursion (Leslie, 1999). Some degrees of tendon impairment can result, leading to possible joint contracture. Tenosynovitis may develop at several sites.

Tenosynovitis in a *digit* usually appears as a sausage-type swelling, in which the entire digit may be enlarged and tender to palpation. Digital flexion can be significantly impaired by even a small amount of tenosynovitis (Leslie, 1999). Pain, mild triggering, and/or crepitation may be noted with attempted ROM (Ferlic, 1996; Melvin, 1982).

Tenosynovitis in the *volar wrist* can present with carpal tunnel syndrome. The group of thickened, enlarged flexor tendons within the small carpal canal secondarily places pressure on the median nerve as it passes through the shared carpal tunnel (Ferlic, 1996; Leslie, 1999).

Tenosynovitis in the *dorsal wrist* is quite evident by swelling, which can occur in one or all six dorsal compartments. Dorsal tenosynovitis can be distinguished from dorsal wrist synovitis by observing movement of the distended tenosynovium with active digital flexion and extension (Leslie, 1999; Wilson & Fredick, 1994).

DeQuervain's tenosynovitis is inflammation of the extensor pollicis brevis (EPB) and the abductor pollicis longus (APL) tendons within the first dorsal wrist compartment. Tenderness, thickening, and crepitation are often present over the radial styloid. Pain may radiate proximally and dorsally with active wrist radial/ulnar deviation (Kirkpatrick & Lisser, 1995).

Stenosing tenosynovitis, also known as *trigger finger,* commonly occurs at the RF and/or MF but can also occur in the thumb and other digits. Stenosing tenosynovitis is the result of swelling and thickening of the flexor tendon proximal to the A1 pulley (Ferlic, 1996; Kirkpatrick & Lisser, 1995). As the tendon attempts to traverse through the pulley, it catches, holding the digit in a flexed position that has to be manually released by the patient. Attempted movement and direct palpation over the A1 pulley can be painful.

Tendon Ruptures and Repairs

Tendon ruptures can occur when tendons are invaded by inflamed synovium or when tendons rub on a rough edge of a bone (Leslie, 1999). These rough edges or bony spurs are most likely the result of joint inflammation that has lead to joint damage (Fig. 17–16) (Ferlic, 1996; Shapiro, 1996; Swanson, 1995b; Wilson & Fredick, 1994). Tendon ruptures in the hand occur most commonly at prominent bony sites, such as the scaphoid waist, the distal ulna, and Lister's tubercle on the dorsal radius. As a result, most common ruptures are of the flexor pollicis longus (FPL), index flexor digitorum profundus (FDP), the extensor digiti quinti (EDQ), and the extensor pollicis longus (EPL) tendons (Ferlic, 1996; Katz & Moore, 2000; Leslie, 1999; Shapiro, 1996; Swanson, 1995b; Wilson & Fredick, 1994;).

Splinting Management

A combination of rest (splinting) and medical management can aid in reducing the symptoms of RA. Postsurgical patients should be instructed in digital motion to decrease the chance of adhesions and maximize movement. Gentle, early ROM and blocking exercises aid in optimizing tendon excursion. The therapist should teach the patient adaptations to ADLs and other techniques for joint protection and energy conservation; these tips help the patient cope with arthritis on a daily basis (Colditz, 2000; Fess & Philips, 1987; Massarotti, 1996; Poole & Pellegrini, 2000; Simmons et al., 1996; Terrono, Nalebuff, & Phillips, 1995).

Although splinting is a treatment component, it is rarely used alone. Other interventions should be integrated into the treatment plan. Thermal agents can be useful adjuncts in preparing the joints for exercise and reducing pain (e.g., paraffin, hot packs, ultrasound) (Katz & Moore, 2000). A well-instructed home exercise program can aid in maintaining joint flexibility and daily function. Physicians should be encouraged to refer patients early for therapy, patient education, joint protection, and splinting intervention. When used soon after diagnosis, splints can support weak structures around a joint, reduce stress to the joint capsule, decrease pain during use, and perhaps retard soft tissue damage (Blank & Cassid, 1996).

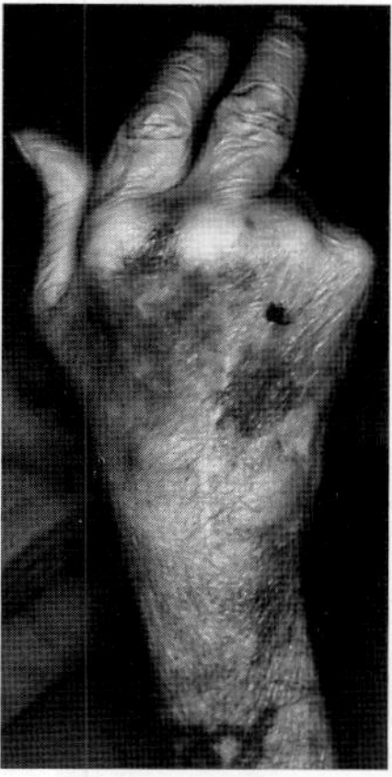

Figure 17–16 Rupture of the EDQ and EDC tendons of the RF and SF in a patient with RA.

Material Selection

THERMOPLASTICS

The need for and type of splint may change as the disease process evolves. The therapist must use his or her skill and experience to create the most appropriate splint and splinting regime. For example, a wrist/hand immobilization splint (resting hand splint) may be ordered for a patient, but lifestyle and daily demands may require at least some use of the hand. An option may be to fabricate a wrist immobilization splint for day use (digits free) and a wrist/hand immobilization splint for night use (Simmons et al., 1996). Before fabrication, consideration must be given to the acuteness of the disease, material choice, wearing schedules, patient's lifestyle, and ability to don and doff the splint(s) independently.

The choice of splint material should take into account conformability and weight. Splints should be lightweight and allow for fluctuating edema and synovitis whenever possible. Materials that are highly conforming (minimal resistance to stretch; plastic) may not be the best choice if joint swelling fluctuates or if frequent adjustments are anticipated to accommodate joint and soft tissue changes. Materials that are more rigid (high resistance to stretch; rubber) and do not fit as intimately into the contours of the body part being splinted may be a better choice. These materials provide joint support, are more forgiving than highly conforming materials, and accommodate fluctuations in edema. Splints that are fabricated for day and night use need to allow for possible nocturnal swelling (Melvin, 1982). This can be done during the fabrication process by having the patient wear several layers of cotton stockinette or an ace wrap over the intended area(s).

The therapist must also keep in mind that a splint worn for a specific problem may aggravate a proximal or distal condition. For example, a wrist immobilization splint may work well to stabilize the wrist; but during functional use, the forces may transfer proximally to the elbow, irritating existing elbow inflammation, or distally, increasing forces to the MP joints.

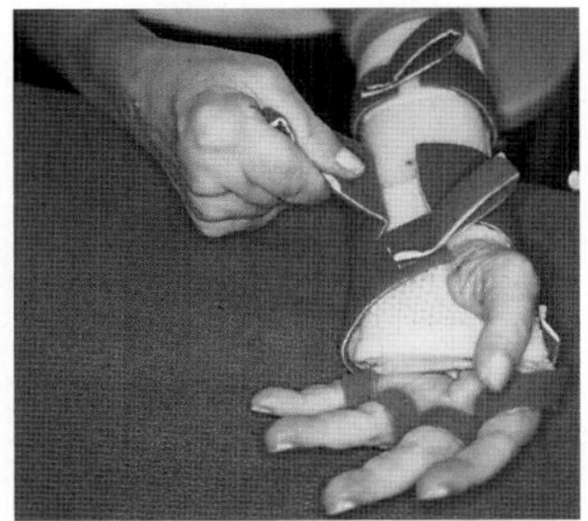

Figure 17–17 A patient with severe RA of the wrist and digits is able to don and doff a splint by using soft strap closures with loop attachments.

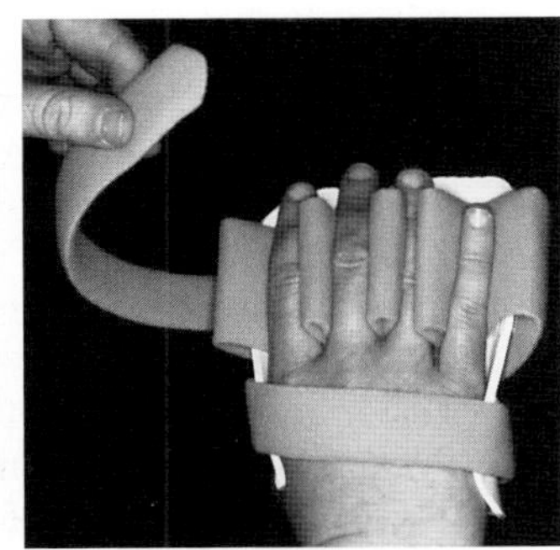

Figure 17–18 Soft 2-in. straps are used for a liner as well as to separate the digits in this splint to prevent maceration and provide comfort.

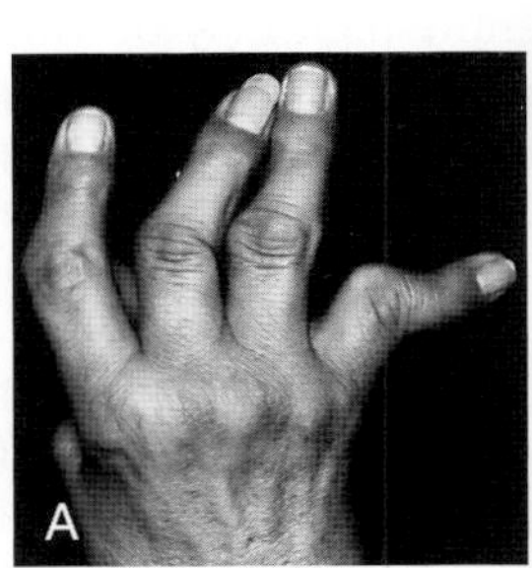

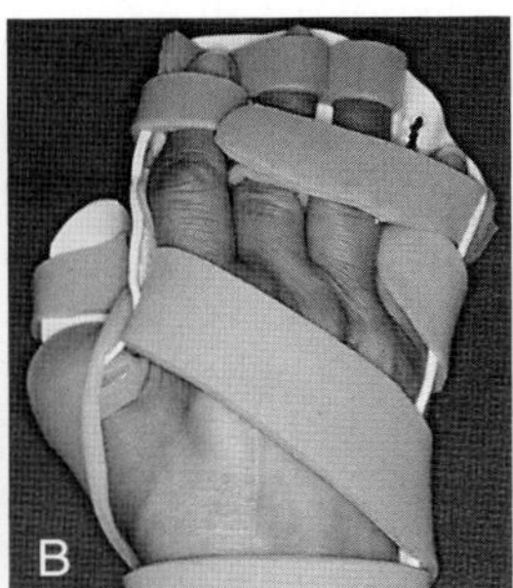

Figure 17–19 ***A,*** *A patient with psoriatic arthritis.* ***B,*** *A night resting splint with soft straps strategically placed to help improve joint alignment.*

STRAPPING

The strapping design of the splint should allow for easy independent donning and doffing. Straps should be wide, soft, and conforming, because patients with RA often have thin, fragile skin owing to their age, medications, or the disease process. Straps can be fabricated to allow extra length or loops on the end of the strap for easy application and removal (Fig. 17–17) (Philips, 1995).

Soft strapping material can also be used as digit dividers on wrist/hand immobilization splints. These dividers can aid in alignment and prevent maceration between the digits (Fig. 17–18). Care should be taken to place straps advantageously that can aid in gently directing joints into an antideformity position. Straps can successfully provide light joint positioning (Fig. 17–19).

PREFABRICATED SPLINTS

As discussed earlier, commercially purchased Neoprene splints can often work well to provide intermittent light support to joints during times of symptom exacerbation (Fig. 17–6). For some patients, these splints are easy to apply and care for.

Elbow with RA

Elbow involvement in the individual with RA can be noted as joint synovitis, and occasionally the presence of subcutaneous nodules at the posterior aspect of the elbow joint (Fig. 17–20). Chronic synovitis can lead to elbow flexion and extension contractures and to limitations in forearm rotation. These contractures tend to develop because of reduced motion secondary to joint pain. Ulnar nerve irritation may occur owing to tension on the nerve resulting from local trauma, static posturing, joint inflammation, osteophyte formation, or pressure from a subcutaneous nodule (McAuliffe & Miller, 2000).

Nonsurgical Splinting Guidelines

Conservative management for pain relief and edema control typically consists of anti-inflammatory medications and early referral for splint fabrication (McAuliffe & Miller, 2000; Nirschl & Moarrey, 1993). Splinting at the elbow joint is used cautiously and then only briefly because of the high risk of joint contracture (Morrey, 2000b). Soft devices can be used as an option in the early stages of the disease to provide protection and support to the painful elbow. A commercially available elbow protector, such as the Elbow/Heel Protector by Smith+Nephew (Germantown, WI), can limit flexion and extension and protect tender nodules. A custom-made donut design fabricated from T-Foam material or silicone gel sheets can absorb shock and cushion the ulnar nerve (Fig. 17–21). Neoprene splints produce gentle soft tissue compression and have the added benefit of neutral warmth and insulation (see Chapter 14) (McAuliffe & Miller, 2000).

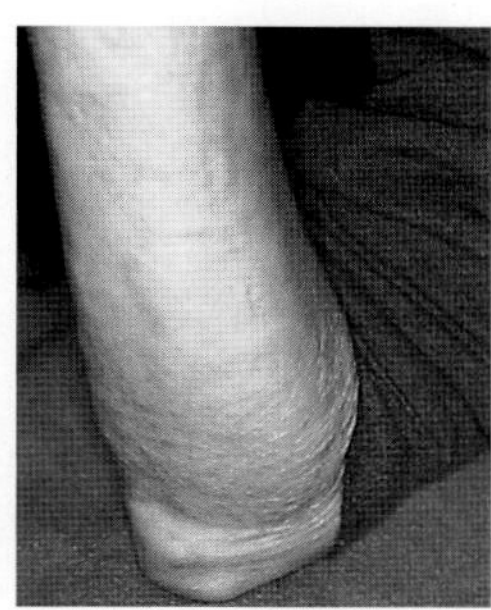

Figure 17–20 *Subcutaneous rheumatoid nodules are commonly seen at the posterior elbow.*

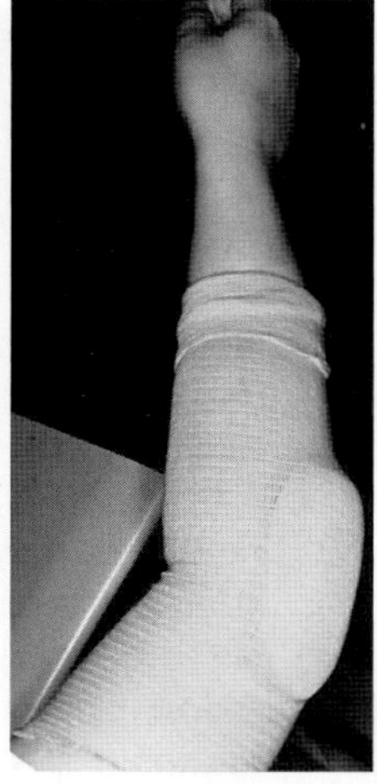

Figure 17–21 *Custom-made protection for a tender dorsal subcutaneous nodule is secured with an elasticized sleeve.*

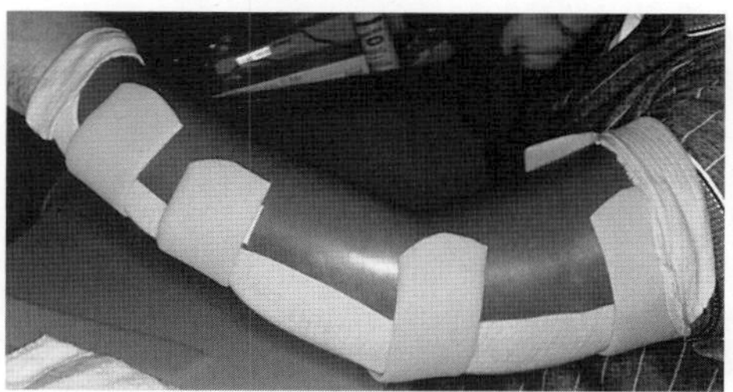

Figure 17–22 *An anterior elbow extension immobilization splint.*

When greater support is needed, anterior or posterior splints can be applied. An anterior elbow immobilization splint is recommended if nodules are present on the posterior elbow; it can be used during sleeping, since it allows the arm to relax on the bed rather than against hard material (Fig. 17–22) (McAuliffe & Miller, 2000). The anterior design may be less complicated to fit because there are fewer bony prominences and less potential for pressure areas.

When posterior splints are used, the wrist should be considered in the design. Patients with elbow arthritis may be more comfortable with the wrist included in the splint. Posterior splints should be cautiously molded and, if necessary, well padded about the condyles, ulnar styloid, and olecranon process. Contractures of the elbow can cause devastating limitations in ADLs and, if noted early, can be managed with gentle serial static splinting in the desired direction.

Postsurgical Splinting Guidelines

An **elbow joint synovectomy** can be performed to alleviate pain and increase functional joint ROM in the early stages of the disease, with or without a radial head resection (Varitimidis, Plakseychuk, & Sotereanos, 1999). Splinting after synovectomy is based on physician preference and is used with caution. The elbow joint commonly becomes stiff after surgical intervention; but if not treated early with ROM exercises, an irreversible loss of motion may result (Brach, 1999; Morrey, 2000b; Varitimidis, Plakseychuk, & Sotereanos, 1999). After surgery, the forearm is positioned in neutral rotation with the elbow comfortably positioned close to 90° of flexion (Melvin, 1982). The splint is worn for approximately 2 weeks.

Elbow joint arthroplasty is reserved for the severely involved joint. Pain, joint instability, ulnar nerve involvement, and the inability to perform simple ADLs may lead a patient to this decision. Several procedures have been described (Bryan & Morrey, 1982; Ferlic,

1999; Gill & Morrey, 1998; Morrey, 2000a; Wright, Froimson, & Stewart, 1993). Regardless of the procedure, early splinting and postoperative therapy can play significant roles in achieving maximal results (Ferlic, 1999; Gill & Morrey, 1998; Melvin, 1982; Morrey, 2000b; Nirschl & Morrey, 1993; Wolf, 2000). After arthroplasty, elbow immobilization or restriction splints are used cautiously and often in combination with a carefully guided exercise and edema-management program (Brach, 1999; Edmond, 1993; Wolf, 2000). The position of the elbow depends on the procedure(s) performed. For example, if the triceps tendon is detached and reattached as part of a joint replacement, the elbow may be splinted in some degree of extension (Bryan & Morrey, 1982; Edmond, 1993).

An anterior or posterior elbow splint should be removed three or four times a day for prophylactic ROM exercises. It should not be worn for extended periods of time (4 to 6+ weeks), unless there is a question of continued elbow joint instability or if reconstruction of ligaments was performed. Prolonged use of the splint carries the risk of joint contracture, as previously emphasized (Edmond, 1993; Wolf, 2000). The referring physician's input can help guide the specific parameters circumferentially wrapping the splint on the arm instead of using straps may aid in postoperative edema management and prevent migration of the splint as the edema subsides. Splinting over the midpoint of the olecranon, medial and lateral epicondyles, and the bony grooves of the cubital tunnel requires particular care, because these areas are prone to irritation from direct pressure.

Hinged splints (mobilization or restriction) allow a restricted amount of flexion and extension and can facilitate joint and tendon glide, increase blood flow and nutrition to the repair site, and aid in preventing joint

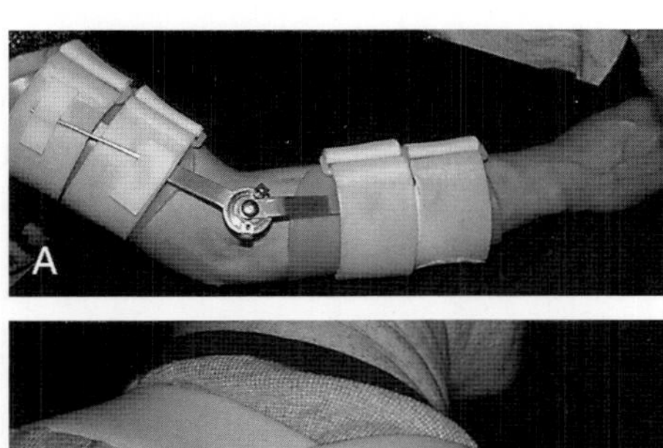

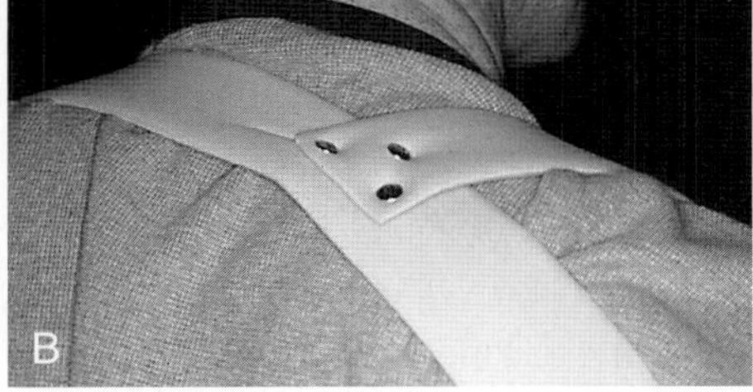

Figure 17–23 ***A,*** *This Phoenix elbow hinge splint, used after elbow reconstruction, restricts elbow AROM and prevents lateral stress.* ***B,*** *A shoulder harness can be secured to the proximal portion of an elbow hinge splint to prevent distal migration and maintain proper hinge alignment.*

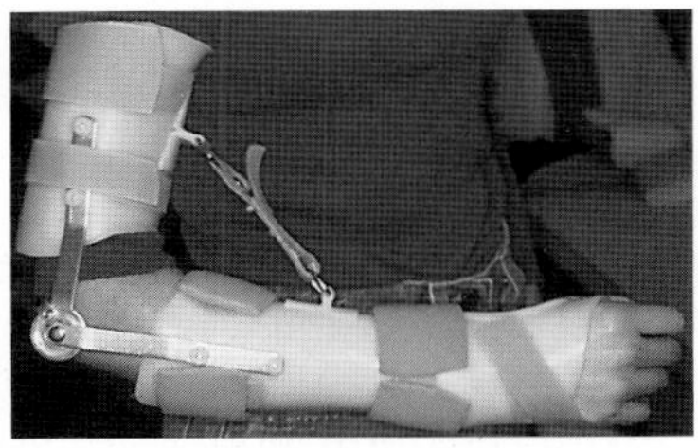

Figure 17–24 At 12 weeks after elbow arthroplasty, this patient was unable to gain functional elbow flexion. Thus a static progressive elbow flexion mobilization splint with a Phoenix elbow hinge was prescribed. Note the D-rings and loop strapping material that provide the mobilization force.

stiffness while healing (Fig. 17–23**A**). However, hinge splints at the elbow can be difficult to fit comfortably. There are few contours about the elbow that contribute to a congruent splint fit. Obtaining a secure mechanical hold of the splint in the proper position (axis of the elbow hinge lined up with the elbow's joint axis) may warrant fabrication of some type of shoulder harness to prevent migration as the forearm moves (Fig. 17–23**B**). Applying a mobilization force in the latter healing stages can elongate soft tissue in the event that a joint flexion or extension contracture has developed (Fig. 17–24). Both mobilization and immobilization splints should protect against lateral forces to the elbow joint (McAuliffe & Miller, 2000; Morrey, 2000a, 2000b).

Wrist with RA

Wrist and hand deformities caused by RA are often the first noticed, because these typically are the first joints affected in the upper extremity (Colville, Nicholson, & Belcher, 1999; Melvin, 1982; Swanson, 1995a, 1995b; Vamos, White, & Caughey, 1990; Wilson & Fredick, 1994). Deformity results from a combination of ligamentous laxity and the location of the synovitis. The individual with acute RA presents with diffusely swollen and red appearance of the involved joints (Fess & Philips, 1987). Any attempt to move the wrist or fingers may be exquisitely painful. On palpation, the wrist and hand may be warm, owing to a combination of joint and tendon inflammation. Rest (splinting) is one of the first treatment choices that may be prescribed (Blank & Cassid, 1996; Fess & Philips, 1987; Kozin, 1999; Melvin, 1982; Stirrat, 1996).

The wrist is a complex joint with multiple ligamentous connections on both the volar and dorsal surfaces. Many combinations of deformities may occur, depending on the location of the inflammation and the ligaments that have been injured. The three most common patterns of deformity are subluxation of the distal radioulnar joint, volar subluxation/supination of the carpus at the radiocarpal joint, and radial deviation of the wrist (Feinberg, 1999; Michlovitz, 1999; Rizio & Belsky, 1995;

Shapiro, 1996; Swanson, 1995b; Talesnick, 1989; van-Vugt et al., 1999; Wilson, 1986; Wilson & Fredick, 1994).

The triangular fibrocartilage complex (TFCC) stabilizes the distal radioulnar joint. If synovitis invades the TFCC, it can weaken and damage the supporting ligaments. As a result, the radius may sublux volarly and the ulna, dorsally (Shapiro, 1996; Swanson, 1995b). Wrist instability may eventually lead to tendon rupture. This deformity may be seen on radiographs or noted on simple palpation and visualization of a notably prominent distal ulna. The patient is likely to present with pain during active supination and wrist extension.

Synovitis in the radiocarpal joint also weakens the ligamentous structures surrounding it. There is often attenuation and laxity of the radioscapholunate and radiocapitate ligaments. This laxity, in combination with the natural volar inclination of the radius, may facilitate wrist volar subluxation. The direction of force of the extensor carpi ulnaris (ECU) tendon shifts from extension to flexion. Volar subluxation can contribute to carpal supination, ulnar translocation of the carpus, and radial shift of the metacarpals; all of these changes can decrease support to wrist extension and weaken the digital extensor tendons (Fig. 17–25) (Shapiro, 1996; Swanson, 1995b; Wilson & Fredick, 1994).

Radial deviation of the wrist is mainly caused by an ulnar translocation of the carpus with a radial shift of the metacarpals. The bones may displace in any number of directions. This shifting of the carpal bones can contribute secondarily to ulnar deviation of the digits, commonly referred to as **zigzag deformity.** In the normal resting hand, the wrist is positioned in about 10°of ulnar deviation, causing the radius to align with the index finger (Leslie, 1999; Swanson, 1995b). In the zigzag deformity, the body seems to attempt to re-create this balance (Fig. 17–26).

Nonsurgical Splinting Guidelines

Splinting options for RA of the wrist are similar even when the pathology is different. A wrist immobilization splint is often the treatment of choice for the individual with wrist inflammation (Blank & Cassid, 1996; Fess & Philips, 1987; Kozin, 1999; Melvin, 1982; Stirrat, 1996).

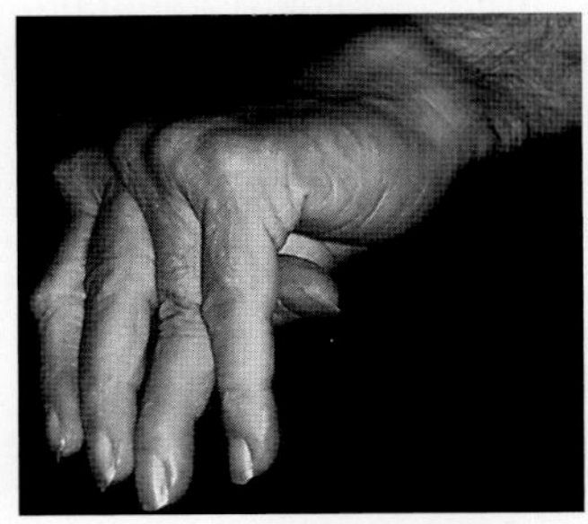

Figure 17–25 Synovitis in the radiocarpal joint weakens the surrounding ligamentous structures.

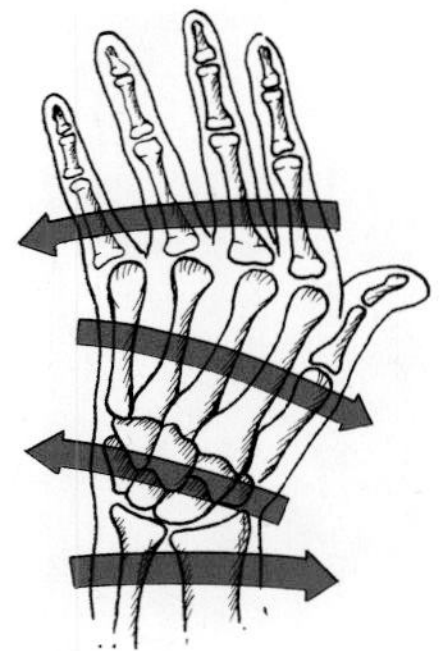

Figure 17–26 Typical deforming forces: The wrist deviates radially, the carpal bones deviate ulnarly, the metacarpals deviate radially, and the proximal phalanges deviate ulnarly.

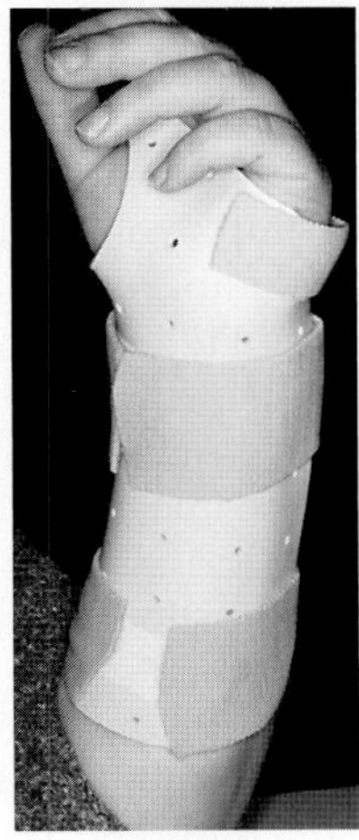

Figure 17–27 A wrist immobilization splint.

A lightweight, rubber material may be a good option for these immobilization splints (Orthoplast or Ezeform). To avoid increased pressure on the median nerve, the suggested wrist position is neutral to 10° of extension, if the deformity allows (Fig. 17–27) (Melvin, 1982).

Rigid splints that immobilize the wrist and hand may be initially recommended for night use because full-time wear can greatly limit any function of the hand(s) during the day (Leonard, 1995). It is important to incorporate volar support within the splint at the distal ulna and MP joints (Philips, 1995). This support helps protect against carpal and MP joint subluxation and MP joint ulnar deviation. A wrist/hand/thumb immobilization (resting hand) splint can provide this position for night use (Fig. 17–28). This design is selected because it positions the thumb comfortably between mid-palmar and radial abduction while supporting the wrist and digits. Suggested positions include the wrist at neutral to 10° extension, MP joints at 25 to 30° of flexion, and IP joints in a gentle, relaxed flexion (Fess & Philips, 1987; Melvin, 1982). The MP joints should be in no more than 30° of flexion because any greater flexion could force the joints

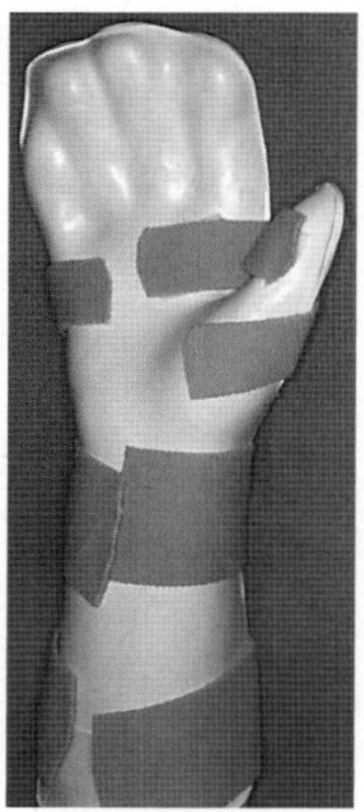

Figure 17–28 *A (mitten design) wrist/hand/thumb immobilization splint is generally worn at night to provide volar support to the wrist and MP joints and alignment to inflamed structures.*

into a position of deformity; volar subluxation of the MP joints and strained IP joint extension (Philips, 1995; Shapiro, 1996; Wilson & Fredick, 1994). Positioning the IP joints in full extension with the MP joints flexed may contribute to intrinsic muscle spasm and IP stiffness, which is difficult to overcome.

RA is often bilateral and symmetrical, requiring the patient to wear immobilization splints for both hands. Without assistance at home, it can be challenging to don or doff bilateral splints. Consider alternating the use of right and left splints each night. Wearing schedules depend on the presenting condition. If only wrist synovitis is present, the wrist splint may be worn as necessary. However, patients often present with coexisting MP joint synovitis, so immobilizing the wrist alone could place increased stress on the MP joints (Melvin, 1982; Philips, 1995). If MP pain and/or swelling become an issue, consideration should be given to alternating the splinting regime (wrist splint for functional day use, wrist/hand splint for night).

Prefabricated wrist splints with a removable metal stay can be an option for daytime activities that contribute to wrist pain (Leonard, 1995; Murphy, 1996; Pagnotta et al., 1998; Stern et al., 1996, 1997; Tijhuis et al., 1998). The metal stay can be removed, allowing a small amount of wrist motion when necessary, which may decrease the force placed on the MP joints. Neoprene wrist splints may also help provide a light support while allowing some degree of motion. Neoprene may provide some pain relief owing to its neutral warmth properties. Careful fitting of soft prefabricated splints is an important challenge. Not all of these splints fit well because of the often-encountered alteration in bony anatomy and size of the forearm in relationship to the wrist (Leonard, 1995). Neoprene splints can be custom fabricated to accommodate bony changes. Thermoplastic materials can be added to Neoprene to provide additional reinforcement and support (see Chapter 14).

Postsurgical Splinting Guidelines

There are many surgical procedures that have been described for managing pain, increasing stability, improving functional use, and minimizing deformity of the wrist with RA (Blank & Cassid, 1996; Colville et al., 1999; Linscheid, 2000; Nalebuff, 1990; Shapiro, 1996; Stirrat, 1996; Talesnick, 1989; vanVugt et al., 1999; Watson & Ballet, 1984; Watson et al., 1999; Wilson, 1986). Relevant surgical procedures include synovectomy, tenosynovectomy, tendon repair or transfer, arthroplasty, and arthrodesis (Shapiro, 1996).

SYNOVECTOMY OR TENOSYNOVECTOMY

Wrist synovectomy or tenosynovectomy is designed to decrease pain, increase function, prevent tendon rupture, and improve appearance. Synovectomy is not usually performed when there is advanced bony erosion, subluxation of the carpus, ruptured tendons, or flexion contractures (Wilson & Fredick, 1994). Splints are used to position the wrist joint after the postoperative dressing is removed (Fig. 17–27). If tenosynovectomy has been performed in combination with wrist synovectomy, the splinting protocol should protect the tendons as well (Fig. 17–28). Carefully instructed exercise sessions are essential for preventing tendon adherence postoperatively. The following are suggested positioning guidelines; however, the referring surgeon should recommend the positions of the involved joints (Leonard, 1995; Melvin, 1982; Philips, 1995).

- *Wrist synovectomy:* wrist splinted in neutral.
- *Dorsal wrist tenosynovectomy:* wrist splinted in gentle extension with the MP joints in 35 to 40° of flexion.
- *Volar wrist tenosynovectomy:* wrist splinted in neutral to 25° extension.
- *Digital flexor tenosynovectomy:* If wrist is included, wrist splinted in approximately 20° of extension, and MPs in 30° flexion. For a hand-based splint, MPs blocked at approximately 30°of flexion.

TENDON RUPTURES OR REPAIRS

The cause of **tendon rupture** in the individual with RA of the wrist results from rubbing of the tendons as they traverse over bony edges or from the destructive effects of chronic tenosynovitis (Ferlic, 1996; Leslie, 1999; Michlovitz, 1999; Shapiro, 1996; Wilson & Fredick, 1994). If tendon integrity permits, the ruptured tendon is usually repaired. Common sites for tendon rupture are the EDQ, extensor digitorum communis (EDC) to the SF at an eroded distal ulna, the FPL, and, less often, the flexor digitorum profundus (FDP) at the scaphoid level (Fig. 17-16) (Ferlic, 1996; Michlovitz, 1999; Shapiro, 1996; Wilson & Fredick, 1994). Splinting guidelines for tendon repairs and tendon transfers are similar to those described in detail in

Chapters 18 and 19. The therapist must keep in mind the extent of surgical intervention. If other procedures were done at the same time as the repair (e.g., tenosynovectomy or arthroplasty), postoperative splinting must consider these procedures (Fig. 17–29). Management of the tendon-repaired hand greatly depends on the extent of disease and surgical procedure; close communication with the referring surgeon is essential. Some physicians prefer complete cast immobilization for several weeks, whereas others prefer restrictive mobilization through a carefully guided splinting and therapy regime.

ARTHROPLASTY

There are several indications for **partial** or **total wrist arthroplasty:** Significant articular cartilage degeneration, pain, increasing difficulty with simple ADL tasks, and wrist deformity. The main goal is to preserve some painless wrist motion. After the postoperative dressing is removed, a wrist immobilization splint can be applied (Fig. 17–27). This splint can be removed for carefully guided exercises. AROM is generally initiated 2 to 6 weeks postoperatively, depending on soft tissue integrity and the prosthetic fit (Kozin, 1999; Michlovitz, 1999). The therapist's goal for flexion and extension arc should be approximately 60° (Feinberg, 1999; Michlovitz, 1999).

ARTHRODESIS

A **limited** or **total wrist arthrodesis** sacrifices motion for stability but provides maximal function of the distal and proximal joints for the severely arthritic wrist (Kozin & Michlovitz, 2000). This procedure is usually considered for patients with exquisite wrist pain, rupture of tendons, poor bone stock, and significant wrist deformity (Shapiro, 1996; Watson et al., 1999). It is often performed after other options have failed. A circumferential splint is sometimes used preoperatively to simulate the outcome of a wrist arthrodesis. Often, this same splint can be reheated and adjusted as a postoperative support (Fig. 17–30). Whether the arthrodesis is partial or total, postoperative splinting management is essentially the same. In general, the cast is removed 1 to 2 weeks after arthrodesis, and the patient is placed in a wrist immobilization splint. Digital tendon gliding exercises are performed to prevent tendon adherence over the fusion site.

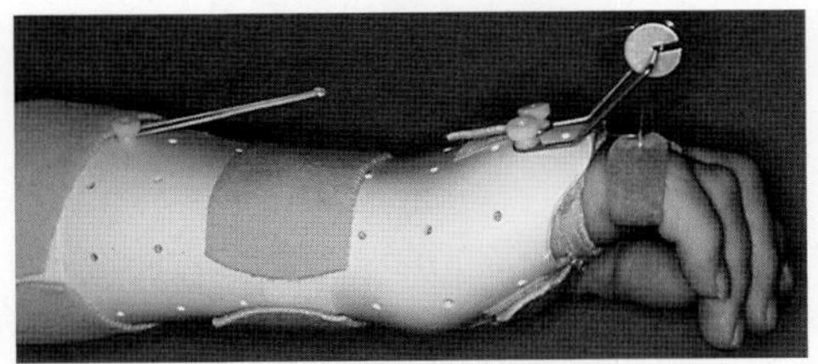

Figure 17–29 This patient underwent a SF MP joint implant arthroplasty and carpal tunnel release. The MP extension mobilization splint (with a Phoenix Outrigger) positions the wrist and supports the MP joint, allowing gentle ROM via rubber band traction.

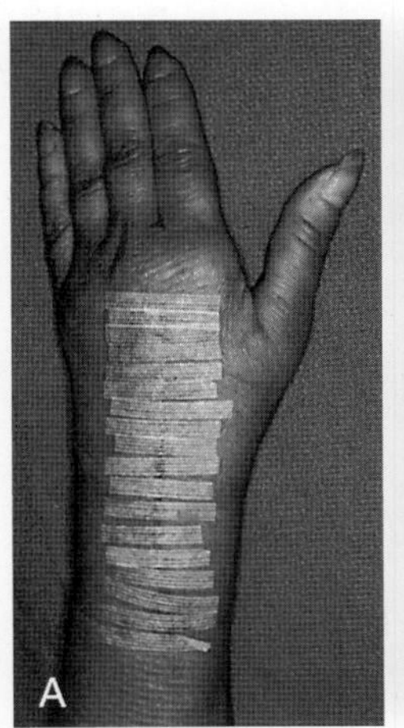

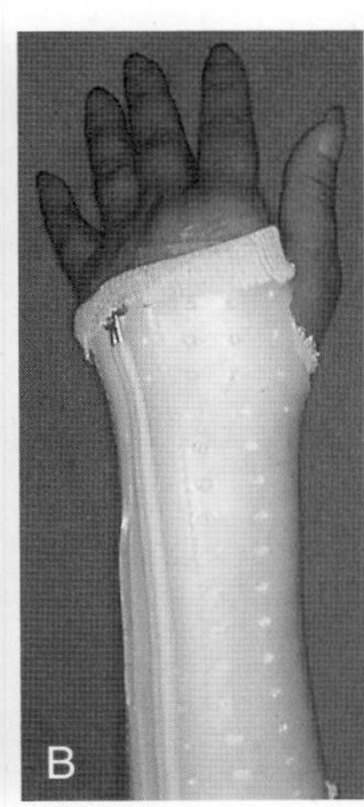

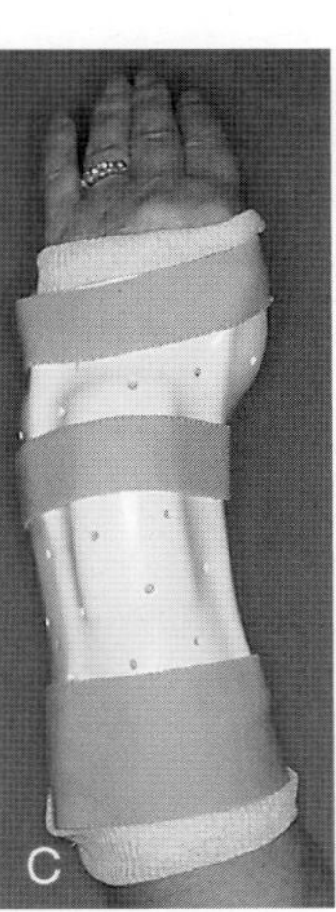

*Figure 17–30 **A,** A patient 2 weeks after undergoing a wrist arthrodesis. **B,** The same patient wearing a Rolyan zipper splint. The elastic material (Aquaplast) allows for easy remolding and refitting and the circumferential design ensures secure immobilization. **C,** A clamshell splint fabricated for a woman who underwent a wrist synovectomy and limited arthrodesis; she was exquisitely tender over the surgical site and slow to heal. The splint design allows the patient to remove the dorsal piece easily for wound care and dressing changes.*

The splint is generally worn until fusion is solid by radiograph (6 to 8 weeks) (Feinberg, 1999).

Thumb with RA

As with any chronic synovitis, the thumb may develop many different deformity patterns, well described in the literature (Nalebuff, 1968; Stein & Terrono, 1996). Any or all of the thumb joints may be involved to some degree. Management of the thumb with RA is based on the pattern of deformity and the functional needs of the patient. Splinting, used early on in the disease process, can enhance function and reduce pain of the thumb by stabilizing the joint(s) involved during hand use. Splinting is done as a conservative measure but can also be used to manage postoperative thumb procedures.

Boutonniere deformity of the thumb, characterized by MP flexion and IP extension, is commonly seen in RA (Gellman, Statson, Brumfield, Costigan, & Kuschner, 1997; Rizio & Belsky, 1995; Tomaino, Pelligrini, & Burton, 1995). Prolonged synovitis at the MP joint causes a stretching of the extensor mechanism, which results in decreased extension at the MP joint because the EPL tendon begins to migrate ulnarward and eventually displaces volarly, changing the vector of pull of the intrinsic muscles eventually leading to flexion at the MP joint (Stein & Terrono, 1996; Swanson, 1995; Terrono et al., 1995). This may gradually result in hyperextension of the IP joint (Nalebuff classification type 1) (Fig. 17–31) (Nalebuff, 1968; Rizio & Belsky, 1995; Stein & Terrono, 1996; Terrono et al., 1995). Simple pinching activities can further exacerbate the potential for collapse.

Swan-neck deformity of the thumb is also frequently seen in the RA population (Stein & Terrono, 1996). The

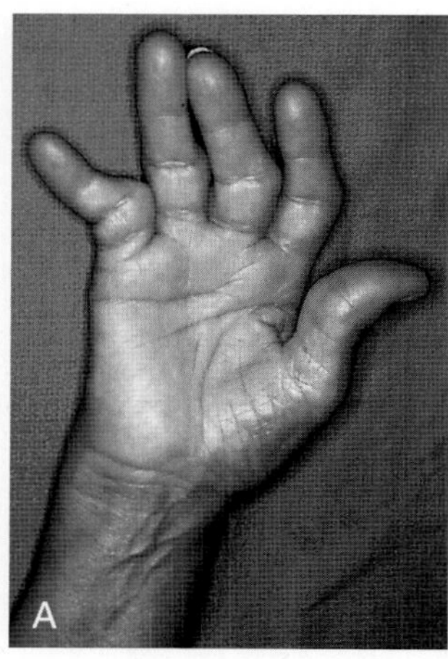

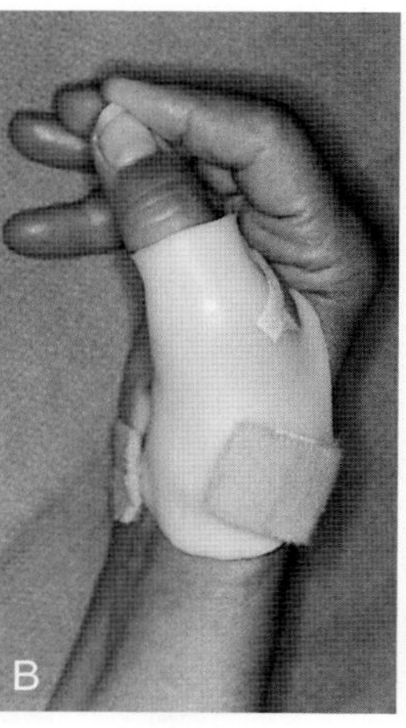

Figure 17–31 ***A,*** *Boutonniere deformity of the thumb can be exacerbated by tasks requiring pinch.* ***B,*** *A thumb immobilization splint supports the MP joint preventing further collapse during use.*

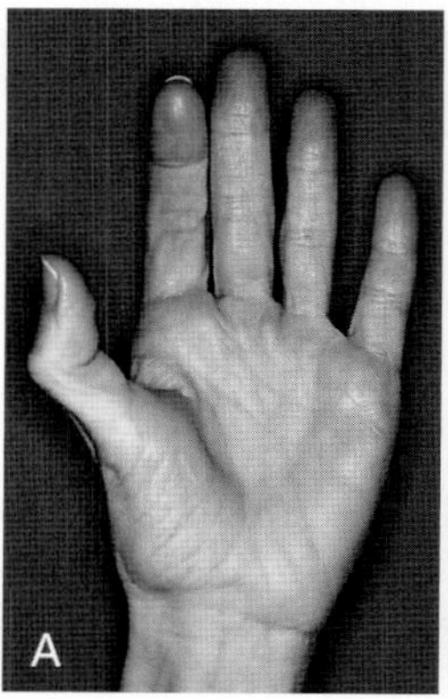

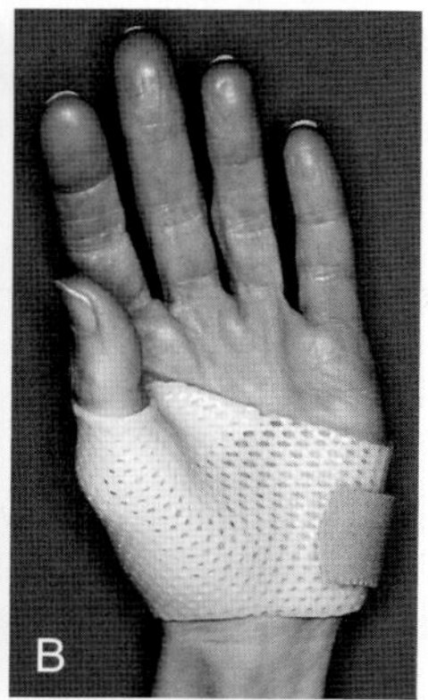

Figure 17–32 ***A,*** *Note the metacarpal adduction with MP joint hyperextension and IP flexion in this patient with a swan-neck deformity of the thumb. The initial stage of this deformity is CMC subluxation.* ***B,*** *This hand-based splint applies gentle three-point pressure to correct the CMC subluxation passively, which in turn aids in realignment of the MP and IP joints. The splint design allows the patient to perform light ADLs.*

deformity can be initiated by synovitis of the TM joint, followed by stretching of the joint capsule and radial subluxation of the base of the first metacarpal. This imbalance of forces may lead to adduction contracture of the first metacarpal joint. Eventually MP hyperextension develops as the patient makes an effort to abduct the contracted first metacarpal. The IP joint becomes flexed in an attempt to compensate for lack of movement at the base of the thumb (Nalebuff classification type 2) (Fig. 17–32) (Stein & Terrono, 1996; Swanson, 1995).

Deformity of the thumb MP joint can occur without TM involvement (Stein & Terrono, 1996). Synovitis can result in stretching of the ulnar collateral ligament (UCL) or the MP volar plate (Nalebuff classification type 3). The UCL injury causes the proximal phalanx to deviate radially. This in turn may cause the first dorsal interossei and the adductor muscles to become shortened and the web space contracted. With volar plate involvement, the MP joint hyperextends and the IP joint flexes. The pattern of thumb deformity is varied and may occur in different patterns and combinations. The goal of both conservative and operative treatment is restoration of pain-free balance and stability (Glickel et al., 1992; Stein & Terrono, 1996).

Nonsurgical Splinting Guidelines

Splinting can be used conservatively to protect the passively correctable joints from increased damage and to slow the progression of a fixed contracture (Stein & Terrono, 1996). In thumb boutonniere and swan-neck deformities, the goal is stabilization of the thumb in gentle abduction to prevent adduction contracture of the first web space, to provide pain relief, and to protect during rest and activity. A hand-based splint can allow for functional use, permitting full wrist mobility while performing ADLs (Fig. 17–31**B** and 17–32**B**). For advanced thumb boutonniere deformity—in which the IP joint significantly hyperextends—a splint that stabilizes the MP in slight flexion and provides a dorsal block to IP hyperextension may be of value for light use (Fig. 17–33). A forearm-based wrist/thumb immobilization splint is recommended for all other times to reduce pain and properly stabilize the CMC joint (Fig. 17–13) (Colditz, 1995; Terrono et al., 1995). Patients should be encouraged to wear this splint at night.

To address isolated thumb MP joint deformity, the joint should be splinted as close to extension as possible and the web space maintained, even if there is no pain (Colditz, 1995). The splint supplies the external stability to maintain the MP in extension and allows IP flexion; little motion is needed at the MP joint for good function. A variety of splint designs can be used, depending on the preference of the surgeon or therapist. Thinner materials ($^3/_{32}$") are recommended for fabrication if the deformity is easily passively correctable (Fig. 17–11**A**). If there are tight volar structures, a stronger material should be considered to provide adequate support ($^1/_8$").

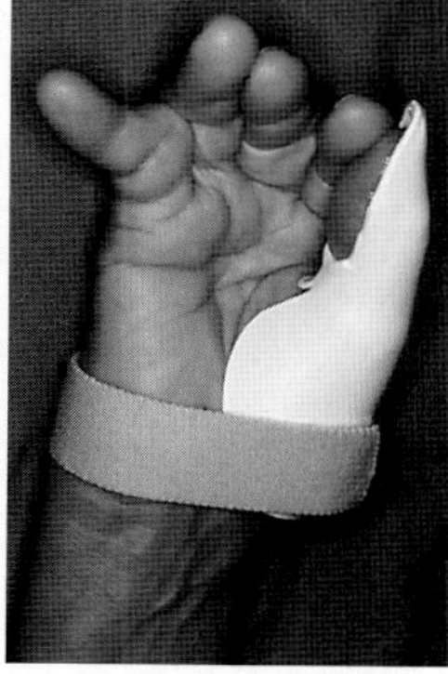

Figure 17–33 *A dorsal splint to hold the MP in slight flexion and prevent IP hyperextension.*

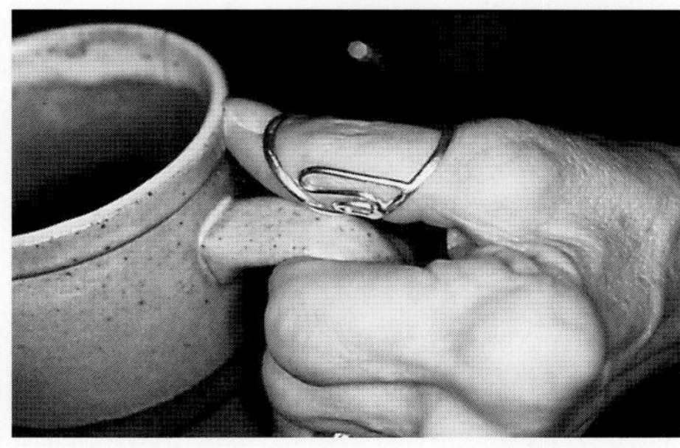

Figure 17–34 A thumb splint to prevent IP hyperextension and provide lateral joint stability. Ring splints can be custom fit and are durable, attractive, and low profile. Courtesy of Silver Ring Splint Company, Charlottesville, VA.

Protection can also be given to the thumb IP joint if instability occurs (Philips, 1995; Terrono et al., 1995). A small dorsal thermoplastic splint can be fabricated or commercially available splints (e.g., Silver Ring splints from Silver Ring Company, Charlottesville, VA) can be ordered to provide lateral support, prevent hyperextension, and provide stability for functional use or while awaiting surgical intervention (Fig. 17–34).

Postsurgical Splinting Guidelines

The goals of surgery for the individual with RA of the thumb depend on which joints are involved and how much the disease has progressed. The stability of each joint depends on the forces applied to it during use and the direction of the tendon forces that act on it (Stein & Terrono, 1996).

IP JOINT

Surgical intervention at the IP joint may consist of extrinsic **tendon reconstruction** if tendon integrity allows. Extensor tendon repairs should be splinted for at least 5 weeks in wrist extension, thumb radial abduction and extension, and MP/IP extension (Stein & Terrono, 1996). After flexor tendon repair, the patient is splinted in wrist flexion, thumb midpalmar/radial abduction, and slight MP/IP flexion (see Chapter 18 for details).

IP arthrodesis is reserved for the unstable, painful joint, providing there is minimal involvement of the TM, STT, and MP joints (Nalebuff, 1968). This procedure provides a stable joint for the digits to pinch against. A small thermoplastic splint can be applied to protect the IP joint during the healing phase.

MP JOINT

Surgical intervention for the thumb MP joint may include synovectomy, arthrodesis, relocation of EPL, capsulodesis, and arthroplasty (Chung et al., 2000; Rizio & Belsky, 1995; Terrono et al., 1995). **Synovectomy** is reserved for patients who have had chronic synovitis for 6 months or more (Chung et al., 2000). Splinting in extension is typically the postoperative position to prevent MP flexion contracture.

For severe instability and articular damage of the thumb MP, surgical options include **MP joint arthrodesis** or **arthroplasty.** The decision is influenced by vocational and avocational demands, the integrity of the MP joint, the condition of the bordering TM and IP joints, and the anticipated future activity level (Chung et al., 2000; Colditz, 1995; Rizio & Belsky, 1995). Some protocols limit the use of implant arthroplasty at the MP level to only those with flexion deformity (Chung et al., 2000; Terrono et al., 1995).

Thumb MP joint arthroplasty is done when the joint is painful, unstable, or shows articular destruction. If the thumb IP joint necessitates fusion, attempts may be made to preserve some motion of the MP joint through arthroplasty. The goal of the procedure is to gain stability with some motion, 10 to 35° of flexion (Chung et al., 2000; Swanson et al., 1995). Patients are splinted in close to full extension for 4 to 5 weeks, at which time AROM is begun (Chung et al., 2000).

The goal of thumb MP joint arthrodesis is to provide for thumb stability. The postoperative splinting program is based on the surgeon's protocol. In general, after the initial postoperative immobilization phase, the patient is placed in a hand-based protective splint that maintains the fused position and protects it from injury while allowing use of the proximal and distal joints (Fig. 17–35). Importance is placed on early IP joint motion to decrease the risk of extensor tendon adherence over the surgical site.

Digit MP Joints with RA

The other MP joints of the hand are frequently involved in patients with RA. Chronic inflammation with aggressive synovial proliferation may damage the surrounding structures (Flatt, 1996; Gellman et al., 1997; Nalebuff, 1968; Rothwell, Cragg, & O'Neil, 1997; Stirrat, 1996). Reasons for splinting the MP joints include: to rest the acutely inflamed hand, to minimize deformity, and to address for postoperative procedures such as MP joint arthroplasties (Boozer, 1993; Murphy, 1996; Rennie, 1996; Theisen, 1993).

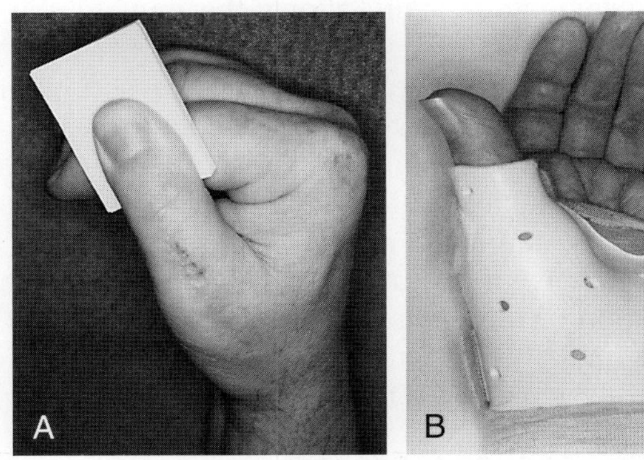

*Figure 17–35 **A,** Thumb MP joint fusion increases stability and improves the ability to pinch. **B,** Used after the postoperative immobilization period, this MP immobilization splint further protects the MP joint fusion during functional use.*

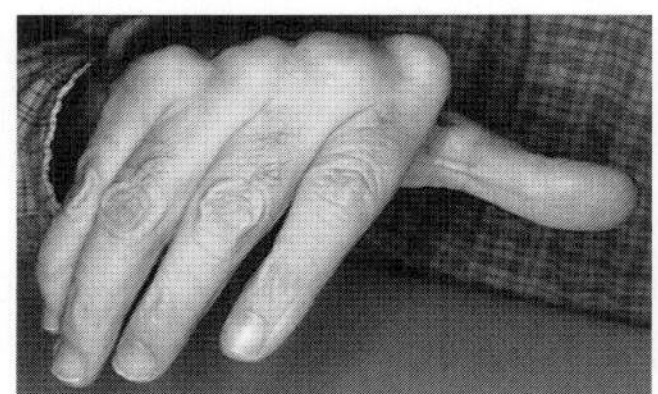

Figure 17–36 Volar MP subluxation and ulnar deviation of the proximal phalanxes.

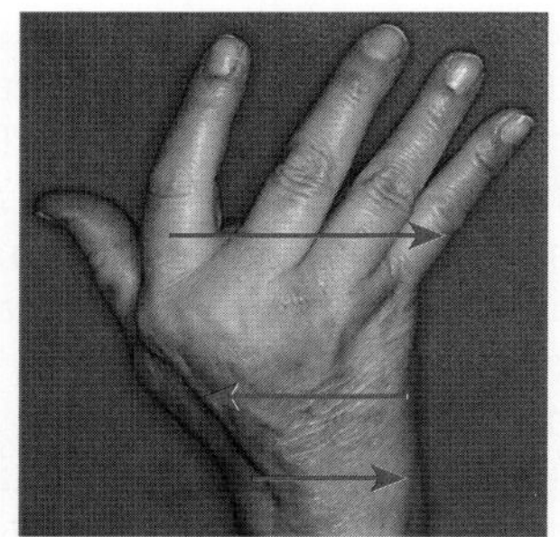

Figure 17–37 Zigzag deformity with radial deviation at the wrist and ulnar deviation at the MP joints. Note the tenosynovitis over the dorsal MP joints.

The two major deformities that occur at the digital MP joints are ulnar drift and MP volar subluxation/dislocation (Fig. 17–36). They may occur as a result of a number of factors (Rizio & Belsky, 1995; Shapiro, 1996; Stirrat, 1996; Swanson, 1995b; Swanson et al., 1995; Wilson & Fredick, 1994):

- The flexor tendons approach the MP joints from the ulnar side and, therefore, exert a stronger ulnar pull with muscular contraction.
- Most functional activities involving MP function (prehension) increase ulnar and palmar displacement of the flexor tendons across the MP joint.
- The shape of the metacarpal heads influences ulnar drift. The ulnar side of the metacarpal is shorter than the radial side, inducing the proximal phalanx to favor an ulnar-oriented position during flexion. Any ligamentous laxity allows the joint to slip to the ulnar side.
- Chronic synovitis weakens all of the soft tissues about the MP joint. Ulnarward tendon drift is a result of this weakening, distention of the capsular structures, laxity of the radial and ulnar collateral ligaments, and laxity of the radial sagittal bands.
- Wrist involvement can ultimately influence ulnar deviation of the digits. Often seen in early RA, the wrist radially deviates, and the digits position themselves ulnarly (Figs. 17-26 and 17–37).

Nonsurgical Splinting Guidelines

During periods of exacerbation the wrist should be included when splinting the MP joints to prevent or minimize any zigzag deformity (Stirrat, 1996). The optimal splint position includes wrist in 10 to 15° of extension and 10° of ulnar deviation, and MP joints in full extension (Stirrat, 1996). The MP joints should be positioned in extension to support weakened structures, prevent volar subluxation, minimize reflex intrinsic muscle contracture, and correct for ulnar drift (Boozer, 1993; Fess & Philips, 1987; Melvin, 1982; Murphy, 1996; Rennie, 1996). The splint is generally worn at night (Fig. 17–38). Carefully positioned straps can be the key to guiding the wrist and MPs gently into an antideformity position. A strap that attaches to the dorsum of the splint (just beneath the second metacarpal head) and traverses obliquely toward the fifth metacarpal can aid in gently directing the wrist and digits into antideformity position (Boozer, 1993; Flatt, 1996; Melvin, 1982; Philips, 1995).

Daytime functional splinting for ulnar drift can be difficult because the MP joints need to be supported in extension to maintain alignment, therefore making functional use a challenge. Various forms of prefabricated splints can be tried to aid in support and alignment (see Chapter 11) (Flatt, 1996; Rennie, 1996).

Postsurgical Splinting Guidelines

A surgical option for advanced MP joint arthritis is an **MP joint implant arthroplasty** (Fig. 17–39**A**). Indications for this procedure include ulnar drift not amenable to soft tissue repair alone, pain, subluxation or dislocation that severely limits function, and displeasing appearance (Fig. 17–36) (Flatt, 1996; Gellman et al., 1997; Melvin, 1982; Nalebuff, 1968; Rennie, 1996; Rizio & Belsky, 1995; Rothwell et al., 1997; Theisen, 1993; Wilson & Carlblom, 1989). MP arthroplasty involves resection of inflamed soft tissue, the metacarpal head, and the base of the proximal phalanx. A silastic implant is used as a spacer between these bones. During the healing process, a capsule typically forms about the new joint; this is referred to as encapsulation (Philips, 1995; Stirrat, 1996; Swanson, 1995; Tomaino et al., 1995).

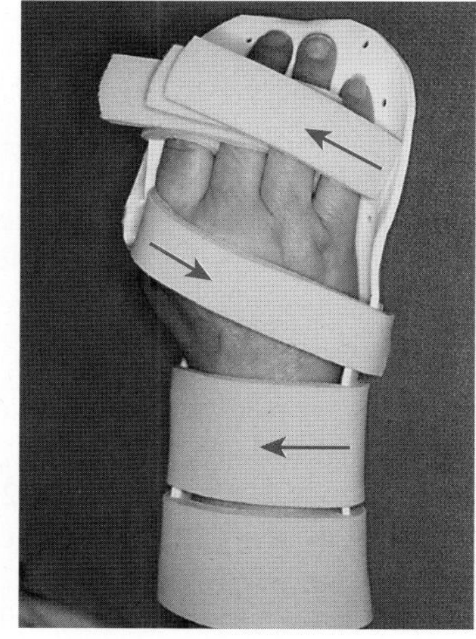

Figure 17–38 A night wrist/hand immobilization splint that uses straps to enhance the antideformity position of the wrist and digits.

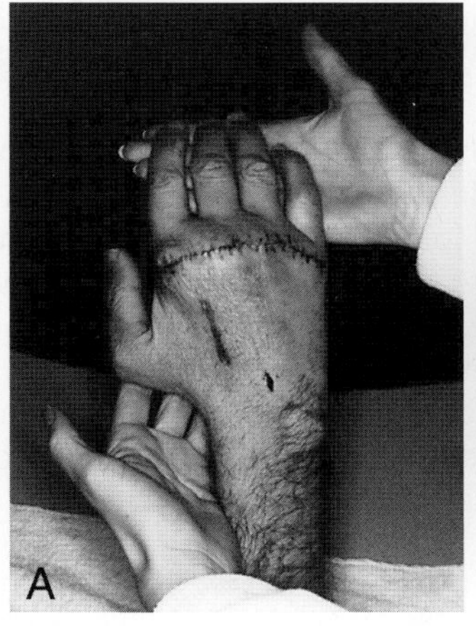

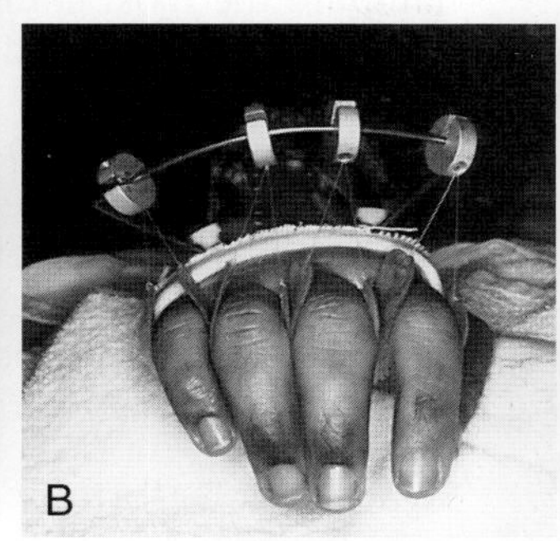

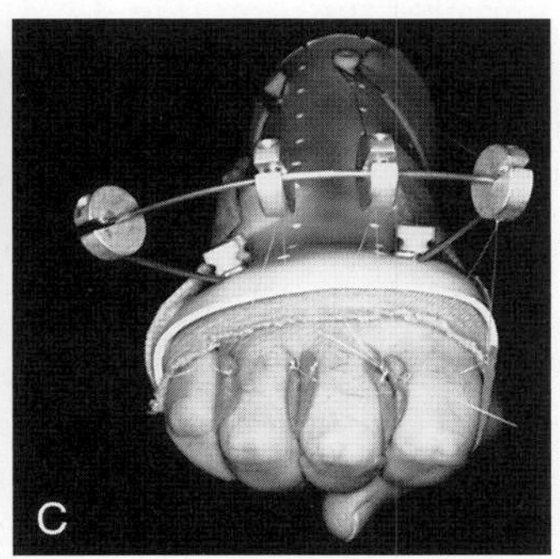

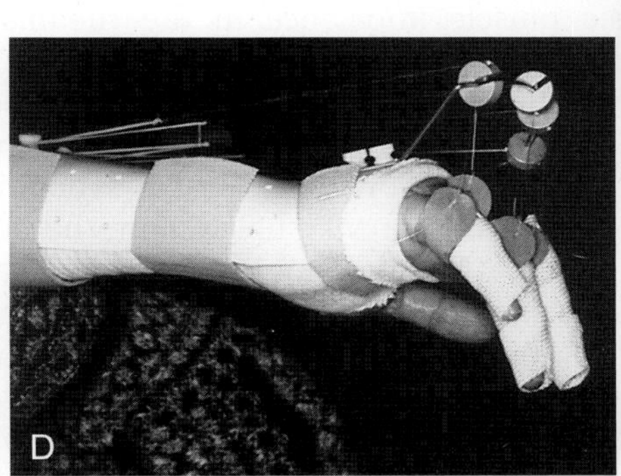

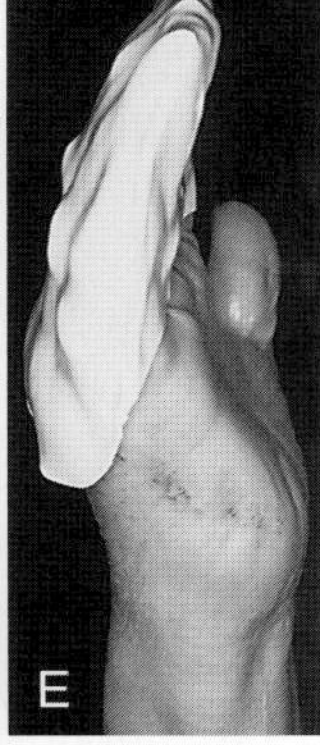

Figure 17–39 ***A,*** *Postoperative view of an IF-SF MP joint arthroplasty with reconstruction of all radial collateral ligaments of the MP joints.* ***B,*** *Dynamic MP extension mobilization splint applied 5 days postoperatively using Phoenix Outrigger kit. Note the slight radial pull at the proximal phalanges to protect the reconstructed MP joint radial collateral ligaments.* ***C,*** *Active MP flexion: caution not to place too much tension through the rubber bands; use just enough to hold the MPs in extension while allowing gentle gliding in flexion.* ***D,*** *PIP extension casts were added 2 weeks after surgery to gently direct greater flexion force to the MP joints during exercise.* ***E,*** *As healing allows, a composite PIP/DIP immobilization splint can be fabricated to concentrate the flexion forces uniformly to the MP joints during exercise.*

The therapist's role is critical in the postoperative management of these patients (Swanson et al., 1995). Usually a forearm-based MP extension mobilization splint is fabricated, allowing controlled and limited active MP flexion to facilitate the encapsulation process (Fig. 17–39**B–E**) (Melvin, 1982; Stirrat, 1996; Theisen, 1993; Wilson & Carlblom, 1989). If there has been reconstruction of the radial collateral ligament of the IF MP joint, a radial outrigger is used to prevent pronation and support the MP in slight radial deviation. The MP of the SF should be allowed unrestricted flexion, which may require removal from the extension component (sling) to that finger during exercise sessions (Stirrat, 1996). SF MP flexion can be inadequate because of the significant instability preoperatively or owing to weakness resulting from surgical release of the ulnar sided intrinsic muscles (Rizio & Belsky, 1995). If not carefully fitted, the sling may actually position the SF in MP hyperextension. The mobilization splint is normally worn during the day for a period of 4 to 6 weeks. The expected arc of flexion at the MP joints is approximately 40 to 60° (Kozin, 1999; Rizio & Belsky, 1995; Stirrat, 1996). This splint is often prescribed in combination with a less bulky night wrist/hand immobilization splint (Fig. 17–40) (Michlovitz, 1999; Stirrat, 1996; Theisen, 1993). The immobilization splint, maintains the wrist in slight extension while the MPs are slightly flexed to approximately 10° with the IPs gently extended. The immobilization splint is worn for months postoperatively to maintain good MP alignment (Terrono et al., 1995).

A hand-based splint can be fabricated from thermoplastic material 4 to 6 weeks postoperatively for intermittent light activity (Flatt, 1996; Kozin, 1999; Rennie, 1996; Rizio & Belsky, 1995; Stirrat, 1996). This small splint can provide external support for continued MP extension, pre-

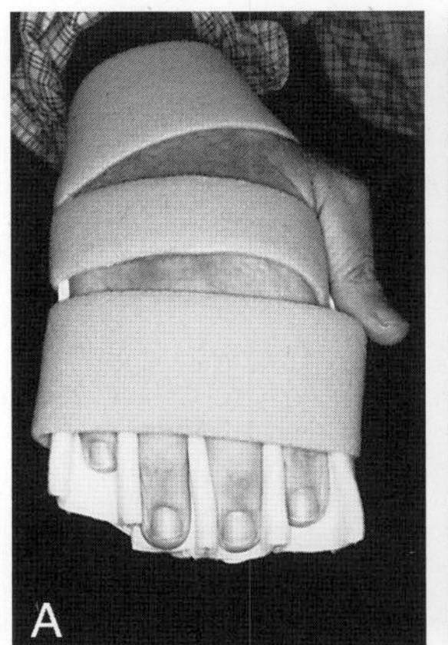

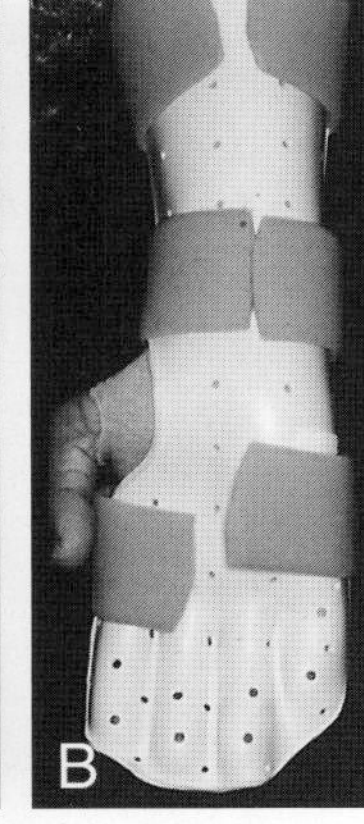

Figure 17–40 ***A,*** *Volar forearm-based design and dorsal view of hand-based design (**B**). Such splints are used to maintain MP extension alignment. Note the soft straps forming comfortable troughs for the digits to rest in.*

venting ulnar deviation, especially when the thumb attempts pinch against the IF. Care must be taken to decrease bulk and rough edges between the fingers, which can lead to discomfort and impaired function (Fig. 17–41). Soft Neoprene splints can also be used postoperatively to provide some volar MP support, guide against ulnar deviation, and increase ease of digital function (Fig. 17–42).

Digit PIP and DIP Joints with RA

Finger deformities as a result of RA impair function and appearance (Rizio & Belsky, 1995; Swanson et al., 1995). They can be difficult to treat because of the critical involvement of the extensor mechanism at this level. Synovitis of these small joints may cause pain, chronic edema, and stiffness (Wilson & Fredick, 1994). Swan-neck and boutonniere deformities of the rheumatoid hand are the most common finger pathologies. Implant arthroplasty or arthrodesis can be considered for the rheumatoid PIP or DIP joint and managed in the same way as discussed for OA, earlier in this chapter. Splinting intervention in the early stages of the disease process can be used as an external support to place joints in a mechanically advantageous position to enhance function. Splints can also be used as a postoperative tool to support and protect surgical procedures.

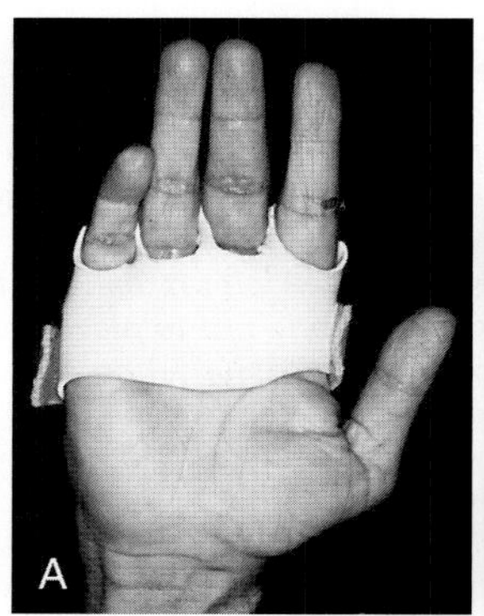

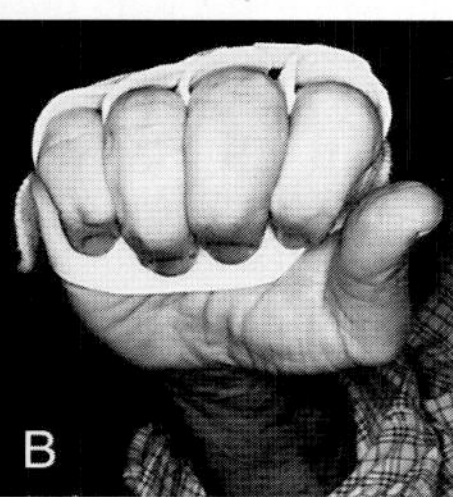

*Figure 17–41 At 4 to 6 weeks after MP joint arthroplasty, a small hand-based splint can be used for light functional tasks: digit extension (**A**) and flexion (**B**).*

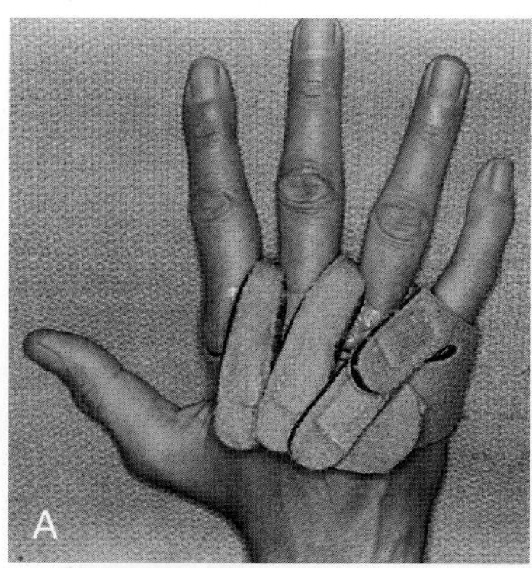

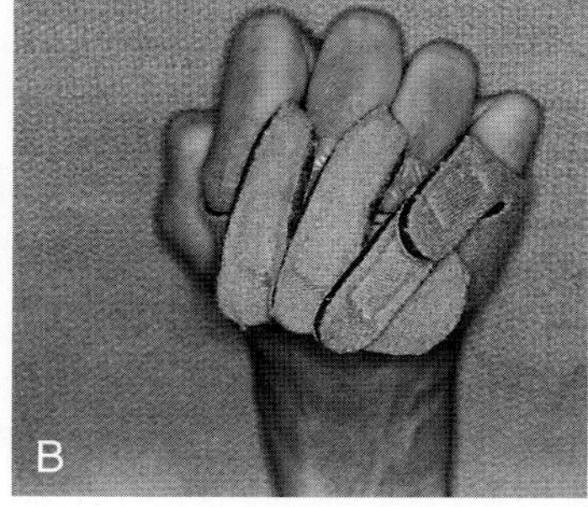

*Figure 17–42 Neoprene supports work well for some patients and allow an excellent ROM with continued light protection of the surgical procedure: digit extension (**A**) and flexion (**B**).*

Swan-Neck Deformity

Swan-neck deformity in the digit presents as PIP joint hyperextension and DIP flexion (Fig. 17–43**A**). This intrinsic/extrinsic muscle imbalance in the rheumatoid hand may occur from synovitis about the MP, PIP, or DIP joint or along the flexor tendon sheath as well (Eckhaus, 1993; Rizio & Belsky, 1995; Swanson, 1995b; Wilson & Fredick, 1994). The most common cause is synovitis at the MP joint; and with joint MP subluxation, the deformity is accentuated. Chronic synovitis appears to cause a reflex intrinsic muscle contracture. This contracture pulls on the PIP joint extensors, leading to volar plate laxity, PIP hyperextension, attenuation of the transverse fibers of the retinacular ligaments, dorsal subluxation of the lateral tendons, and attenuation of the oblique retinacular ligament distally (Swanson, 1995b). The DIP tends to flex secondarily to the proximal pathology (Melvin, 1982; Swanson, 1995b).

Swelling of the DIP joint may cause attenuation or a rupture in the terminal extensor tendon with resultant DIP flexion. The harmony of the entire extensor mechanism is disrupted, producing hyperextension at the PIP joint. Synovitis of the PIP joint itself may lead to stretching of the volar ligaments with a resultant dorsal migration of the lateral bands. Early management may consist of joint injections and swan-neck splints (Fig. 17–43**B**) (Rizio & Belsky, 1995).

NONSURGICAL SPLINTING GUIDELINES

The goal of splinting a passively correctable swan-neck deformity is to allow near to full flexion of the PIP joint while preventing PIP joint hyperextension (Eckhaus, 1993). A supple swan-neck deformity can be splinted with an extension restriction splint (Fig. 17–43**B**). These splints are good for short-term solutions. More permanent splints can be purchased (Silver Ring Company; 3-Point Products, Annapolis, MD) that are less bulky and work well for some patients. These tend to be more durable, fit well, and cosmetically pleasing.

POSTSURGICAL SPLINTING GUIDELINES

Surgical restoration of the hyperextended PIP joint may involve the use of a **tendon transfer,** such as a superficialis tendon. In some situations, DIP pin fixation in

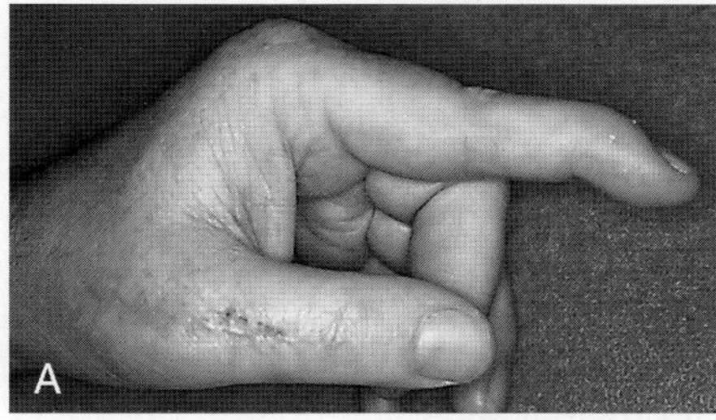

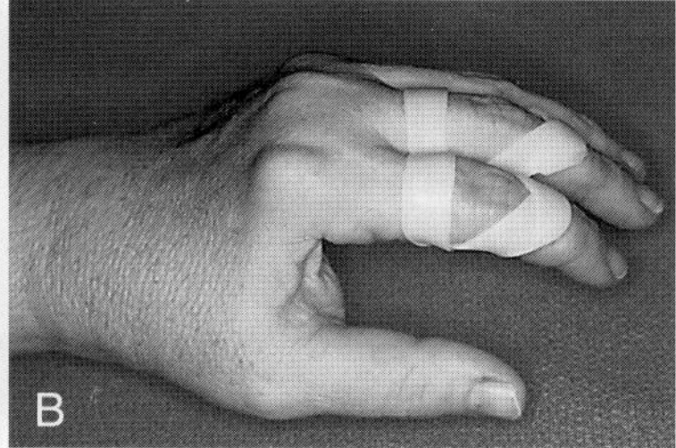

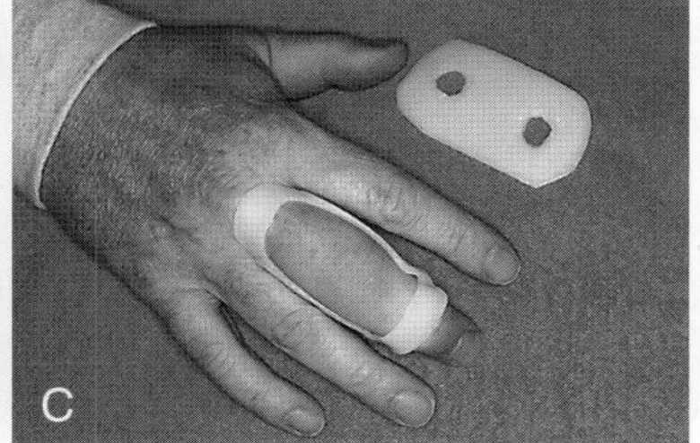

Figure 17–43 ***A,*** *Swan-neck deformity with hyperextension at PIP and flexion at DIP joint.* ***B,*** *This deformity be managed with an a extension restriction splint (Figure-8 design) that allows near full digital flexion, yet limits PIP joint hyperextension.* ***C,*** *Button-hole design.*

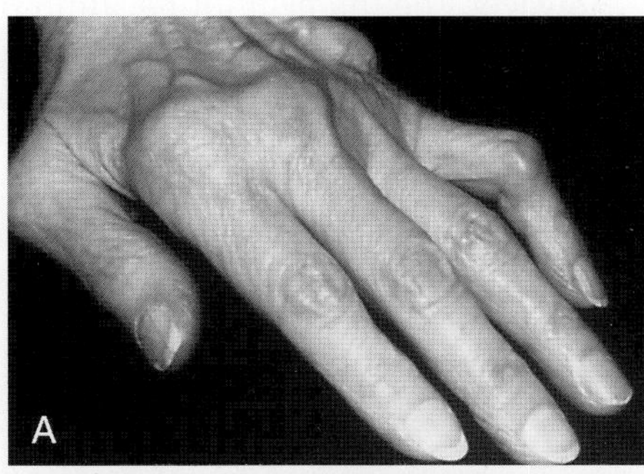

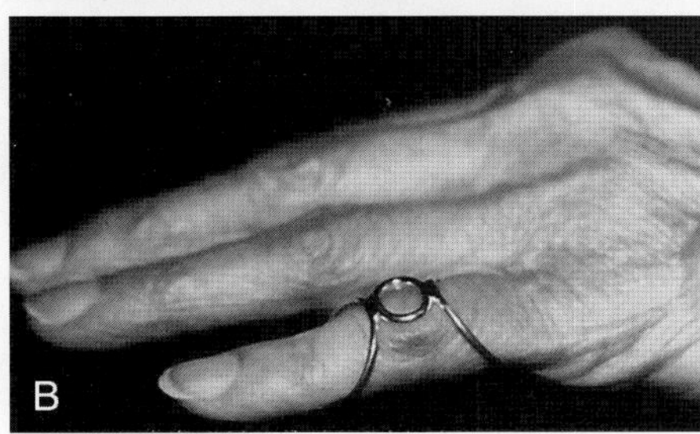

Figure 17–44 ***A,*** *Boutonniere deformity with flexion at the PIP joint. This deformity may be managed with a PIP extension splint on a long-term basis. Many patients find a ring splint* ***(B)*** *to be more cosmetically appealing than a thermoplastic PIP extension restriction splint, courtesy of Silver Ring Splint Company, Charlottesville, VA.*

0° is warranted. Postoperative splinting management depends on individual physician protocols; however, most include early fabrication of a splint that positions the wrist in neutral to slight extension, slight MP flexion, PIP flexion of 20 to 30°, and the DIP in neutral. If the PIP joint is pinned in flexion, the splint should support this position. This splint is worn for 2 to 3 weeks (Rizio & Belsky, 1995). The patient can then use a hand- or finger-based extension restriction splint. At approximately 6 weeks, the PIP joint can gently increase the amount of allowable extension. The splint should carefully accommodate these gradual changes per healing constraints.

Boutonniere Deformity

Boutonniere deformities of the digits are characterized by PIP flexion and DIP hyperextension (Fig. 17–44). The most common cause in the rheumatoid hand is chronic PIP joint synovitis (Eddington-Valdata, 1993; Nalebuff & Millender, 1975; Rizio & Belsky, 1995; Swanson, Maupin, Gajjar, Swanson, 1985; Wilson & Fredick, 1994). The synovitis migrates dorsally between the lateral bands, displacing them laterally and volarly (Swanson, 1995b). This, in turn, creates lengthening of the central tendon. The lateral bands eventually orient themselves below the axis of the PIP joint, becoming PIP joint flexors instead of extensors. This places a secondary pull on the DIP joint in extension. Left untreated, the oblique retinacular ligament shortens, causing the DIP joint to become tight in extension.

NONSURGICAL SPLINTING GUIDELINES

Splinting for a passively correctable boutonniere deformity is best achieved with a twofold process. The patient should have a digit immobilization splint for night use, which keeps the PIP joint in full extension (Fig. 17–45) (Glickel et al., 1992). An effective option for daytime splinting includes the use of a commercially purchased splint, or a custom-made PIP extension immobilization splint that allows full MP and DIP motion. If the deformity is the result of an attritional rupture of the central tendon, uninterrupted PIP extension must be maintained for approximately 6 weeks before motion is allowed

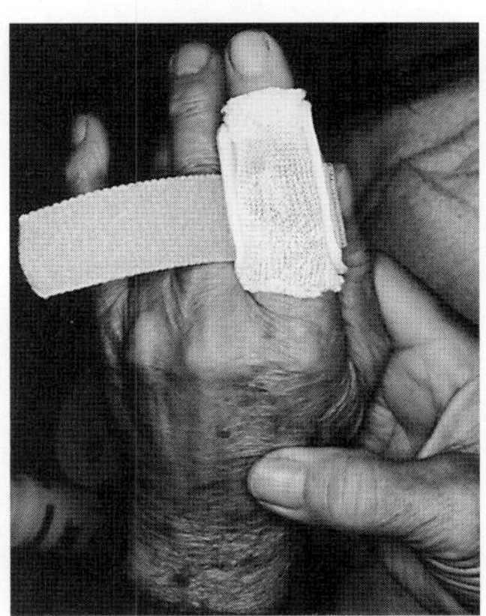

Figure 17–45 *Night extension splinting is important for reducing a PIP flexion contracture.*

(Eddington-Valdata, 1993). Gentle joint-blocking exercises at the DIP can help maintain the length of the extensor mechanism and oblique retinacular ligament, and mobility of the lateral bands (Poole & Pellegrini, 2000; Wilson & Fredick, 1994).

If the patient presents with a fixed flexion contracture of the PIP joint, a gentle serial static extension mobilization splinting approach may be implemented until full PIP extension is achieved (Eddington-Valdata, 1993). Full PIP extension is critical to achieve before the patient is considered for surgical intervention, such as a flexible implant arthroplasty (Nalebuff & Millender, 1975). Once fully extended, the PIP is held in extension for an additional 4 to 6 weeks (Eddington-Valdata, 1993). If, at that time, the patient cannot maintain extension, surgical intervention should be considered.

POSTSURGICAL SPLINTING GUIDELINES

Surgical intervention may be considered to re-establish PIP extension if conservative splinting has failed. Postoperative management varies, depending on the exact procedure, such as a **tenolysis** or **volar plate release** (Eddington-Valdata, 1993; Nalebuff & Millender, 1975; Rizio & Belsky, 1995). The PIP joint is positioned in extension for approximately 4 weeks, after which gentle active exercises are introduced (Fig. 17–45). Cautious active DIP joint flexion exercises should begin as soon as possible postoperatively to aid in advancing the extensor mechanism, allow for lateral band glide, and prevent tendon adherence (the PIP joint should be held in extension during this exercise) (Eddington-Valdata, 1993; Nalebuff & Millender, 1975; Wilson & Fredick, 1994).

CASE STUDY SECTION

The case studies presented here are meant as teaching guidelines only. Treatment and splinting protocols vary greatly from surgeon to surgeon and from therapist to therapist. The therapist should check with the referring physician and colleagues to define the preferred treatment and splinting methods.

CASE STUDY 1: **OA with TM Arthritis**

LS is a 45-year-old right-handed woman with a diagnosis of bilateral TM joint OA. She was referred to therapy for evaluation and treatment. She presented with bilateral thumb pain that was localized to the thenar eminences and reported pain with all functional activities involving grasp and pinch.

Clinical examination revealed tenderness with palpation and thickening at both TM joints. No acute swelling was noted. The patient had a positive grind test bilaterally. AROM was equal in both hands, with thumb opposition to the SF MP joint. Grip strength was bilaterally equal. Pinch strengths (lateral, tip, and 3-point) were decreased and associated with pain.

LS was referred to therapy with a prescription for bilateral hand-based, and forearm-based thumb immobilization splints. The hand-based splints were for daytime use and the forearm-based splints were to provide further support and protection at night. The day splints were fabricated from 1/16" Aquaplast (Fig. 17–11**A**). This elastic material provides the right amount of stretch and conformability to fit the first web space intimately and stabilize the TM joint. The night splints were made out of a plastic material with perforations (Fig. 17–13).

LS wore the splints with some pain relief at home and work. However, the intensity of her thumb pain climaxed to the point that even with splints she had consistent pain day and night. After 5 years of conservative management, LS opted for surgical intervention; her surgeon performed a ligament reconstruction with a tendon interposition graft.

The postsurgical wrist/thumb immobilization cast was worn for 4 weeks. At the time of cast removal, a wrist/thumb immobilization splint was applied and gentle wrist/thumb AROM was begun (Fig. 17–13). The splint was worn at all times except for hygiene and exercise. The same splint was cut down to a hand-based design at 6 weeks and a decrease in the wearing schedule was begun. At 8 weeks, therapy focused on grip and light pinch strengthening with splint use for only at-risk activities.

In addition to splinting, LS was instructed in joint protection principles and activity modifications to provide ways to decrease external stress on the thumb with ADLs. When last seen, 12 weeks after surgery, LS was able to do her normal activities with little discomfort.

CASE STUDY 2: **RA with MP Joint Arthroplasty**

PF is a 42-year-old right-dominant male who works days as a computer programmer and nights and weekends as a musician (drums and guitar). He had an 8-year history of RA and was referred for fabrication of day splints to address ulnar drift at the MP joints to enhance functional use. PF had limited digital ROM secondary to volar subluxation and ulnar drift of the proximal phalanxes. This deformity was passively correctable at that time (Fig. 17–36). Slight radial deviation was also noted at both wrist joints.

A hand-based MP extension and radial deviation immobilization splint was fitted for the patient (Fig. 17-41). The splint redirected the MPs in extension and neutral deviation (antideformity position). Although full MP flexion was not possible with this small splint design, the IP joints were free to fully flex and oppose the thumb for light functional use. Using this splint, PF was able to continue to use the computer keyboard. Thin thermoplastic material (3/32") was an excellent choice for this splint to avoid bulk between the digits. A forearm-based wrist/hand immobilization splint was fabricated for night use to complement the day splint (Fig. 17–38). A meticulous strapping technique aided in minimizing the zigzag deformity. This conservative treatment was satisfactory for 1 year until he began having difficulty with fine motor skills and was finding it nearly impossible to perform the simplest of work and ADL tasks. Because this decrease in function affected all aspects of his life, he sought surgical intervention.

An IF-SF MP joint arthroplasty was performed with reconstruction of all the radial collateral ligaments. The patient was seen 5 days postoperatively and was placed in a daytime MP extension mobilization splint and a night wrist/hand immobilization splint (Fig. 17–39**A**,**B**,**C** and 17–40**A**). At approximately 8 days, individual PIP/DIP extension casts were placed on the fingers so that the patient could gently direct flexion forces to the MP joints (Fig. 17–39**D**). These casts were used 3 times a day for short periods of exercise. At 2 weeks, SF MP joint was excluded from the day splint because of difficulty achieving MP flexion. At approximately 4 weeks postsurgery, PF was given a IF-SF IP extension splint to aid in achieving MP flexion (17.39**E**). This exercise splint is effective in blocking IP flexion, directing flexion force to the MP joint. At approximately 6 weeks the patient was placed into a Neoprene hand-based splint that supported the MPs in extension and prevented ulnar deviation (Fig. 17–42). He wore this for only light activity. PF continued to wear the forearm-based night immobilization splint. At 8 weeks postsurgery, he had functional MP motion. His night immobilization splint was cut back to a hand-based design, which was worn for several more months (Fig. 17–40**B**). The patient and his surgeon were delighted by the improvement in his hand function and appearance.

CONCLUSION

While medical options and surgical advances have combined to aid in the prevention and further progression of joint deformity in the patient with rheumatic disease, splinting remains both a valuable early modality and an important postoperative adjunct. Knowledge of the disease process, joint anatomy and function, and the patient's desired functional goals is crucial to providing effective and appropriate therapy interventions.

REFERENCES

Barron, O. A., Glickel, S. Z., & Eaton, R. G. (2000). Basal joint arthritis of the thumb. *Journal of American Academy of Orthopaedic Surgery, 8,* 314–323.

Beer, T. A., & Turner, R. H. (1997). Wrist arthrodesis for failed wrist implant arthroplasty. *Journal of Hand Surgery (American) 22,* 685–693.

Blank, J. E., & Cassidy, C. (1996). The distal radioulnar joint in rheumatoid arthritis. *Hand Clinics, 12,* 499–513.

Boozer, J. (1993). Splinting the Arthritic hand. *Journal of Hand Therapy, 6,* 46–49.

Brach, P. (1999). Reconstruction of the elbow: Therapist's commentary. *Journal of Hand Therapy, 12,* 73–74.

Bryan, R. S., & Morrey, B., F. (1982). Extensive posterior approach of the elbow—A triceps sparing approach. *Clinical Orthopaedics and Related Research, 166,* 188–192.

Buckland-Wright, J. C., Macfarland, D. G., & Lynch, J. A. (1991). Osteophytes in the osteoarthritis hand. Their incidence, size, distribution and progression. *Annals of Rheumatic Disease, 50,* 627–630.

Burkholder J. (2000). Osteoarthritis of the hand: A modifiable disease. *Journal of Hand Therapy, 13,* 79–90.

Chung, K. C., Kowalski, C. P., Myra, K. H., & Kazmers, I. S. (2000), Patient outcomes following Swanson silastic metacarpophalangeal joint arthroplasty in the rheumatoid arthritic hand: a systemic overview. *Journal of Rheumatology, 27,* 1395–1402.

Colditz, J. (1995), Anatomic considerations for splinting the thumb. In J. M. Hunter, E. J. Mackin, & A. D. Callahan (Eds.). *Rehabilitation of the hand* (4th ed., pp. 1161–1172). St. Louis: Mosby Year Book.

Colditz, J. C. (2000). The biomechanics of a thumb carpometacarpophalangeal immobilization splint: design and fitting. *Journal of Hand Therapy, 13,* 228–235.

Colville, R. J, Nicholson, K. S., & Belcher, H. J. (1999). Hand surgery and quality of life. *Journal of Hand Surgery (Edinburgh, Lotham), 24,* 263–266.

Diaz, J. A. (1994). Three point static splint for chronic volar subluxation of the thumb metacarpophalangeal joint. *Journal of Hand Therapy, 7,* 195–197.

Eckhaus, D. (1993). Swan-neck deformity. In G. Clark, W. Wilgis, B. Aiello, D. Eckhaus, & L. Eddington. Hand rehabilitation: A practical guide (pp. 137 –142). New York: Churchill Livingstone.

Eddington-Valdata, L. (1993). Boutonniere deformity. In G. Clark, W. Wilgis, B. Aiello, D. Eckhaus, & L. Eddington. Hand rehabilitation: A practical guide (pp. 143–152). New York: Churchill Livingstone.

Edmond, A. (1993). Total elbow arthroplasty. In G. Clark, W. Wilgis, B. Aiello, D. Eckhaus, & L. Eddington. Hand rehabilitation: A practical guide (pp. 235–240). New York: Churchill Livingstone.

Estes, J., Bochenek, C., & Fasler, P. (2000). Osteoarthritis of the fingers. *Journal of Hand Therapy, 13,* 108–123.

Feinberg, N. (1999). The carpus: Therapist's commentary. Arthroplasty of the hand and wrist. *Journal of Hand Therapy, 12,* 108–110.

Ferlic, D. C. (1996). Rheumatoid flexor tenosynovitis and rupture. *Hand Clinics, 12,* 561–572.

Ferlic, D. C. (1999). Total elbow arthroplasty for treatment of elbow arthritis. *Journal of Shoulder and Elbow Surgery, 8,* 367–378.

Fess, E. F., & Philips, C. A. (1987). *Hand splinting: Principles and methods* (2nd ed.). St. Louis: Mosby

Flatt, E. F. (1996). Ulnar Drift. *Journal of Hand Therapy, 9,* 282–292.

Freedman, D., Eaton, R., & Glickel, S. (2000). Long-term results of volar ligament reconstruction for symptomatic basal joint laxity. *Journal of Hand Surgery (America), 25,* 297–304.

Gellman, H., Statson, W., Brumfield, R. H., Costigan, W., & Kuschner, S. H. (1997). Silastic metacarpophalangeal joint arthroplasty in patients with rheumatoid arthritis. *Clinical Orthopaedics and Related Research, 342,* 16–21.

Gill, D. R., & Morrey, B. F. (1998). The Conrad-Morrey total elbow arthroplasty in patients who have rheumatoid arthritis. A ten to fifteen year follow-up study. *Journal of Bone and Joint Surgery, 80,* 1327–1335.

Glickel, S., Kornstein, A., & Eaton, R. (1992). Long-term follow-up of trapeziometacarpal arthroplasty with coexisting scaphotrapezial disease. *Journal of Hand Surgery (American), 17,* 612–620.

Katz, M. A., & Moore, R. S. (2000). Flexor tendon rupture and reconstruction of the rheumatoid hand. *Seminars Arthroplasty, 11,* 89–97.

Kelley, M., & Ramsey, M. (2000). Osteoarthritis and traumatic arthritis of the shoulder. *Journal of Hand Therapy, 13,* 148–162.

Kirkpatrick, W. H., & Lisser, S. (1995). Soft-tissue conditions: Trigger fingers and deQuervain's disease. In J. M. Hunter, E. J. Mackin, & A. D. Callahan (Eds.). *Rehabilitation of the hand* (4th ed., pp. 1007–1016). St. Louis: Mosby Year Book.

Kozin, S. (1999). Arthroplasty of the hand and wrist: Surgeon's perspective. *Journal of Hand Therapy, 12,* 123–132.

Kozin, S., & Michlovitz, S. (2000). Traumatic Arthritis and osteoarthritis of the wrist. *Journal of Hand Therapy, 13,* 124–136.

Leonard, J. B. (1995). Joint protection for inflammatory disorders. In E. J. Mackin & A. D. Callahan (Eds.). *Rehabilitation of the hand* (4th ed., pp. 1377–1384). St. Louis: Mosby.

Leslie, B. M. (1999). Rheumatoid tendinitis and tenosynovitis. *Atlas of Hand Clinics, 4,* 95–117.

Linscheid, R. (2000). Implant arthroplasty of the hand: retrospective and prospective considerations. *Journal of Hand Surgery (American), 25,* 796–816.

Massarotti, E. M. (1996). Medical aspects of rheumatoid arthritis: Diagnosis and treatment. *Hand Clinics, 12,* 463–475.

McAuliffe, F., & Miller, R. (2000). Osteoarthritis and traumatic arthritis of the elbow. *Journal of Hand Therapy, 13,* 136–147.

Melvin, J. (1982). Rheumatic disease: Occupational therapy and rehabilitation (2nd ed.). Philadelphia: Davis.

Melvin, J. (1995). Scleroderma: Treatment of the hand. In J. M. Hunter, E. J. Mackin, & A. D. Callahan (Eds.). *Rehabilitation of the hand* (4th ed., pp. 1385–1397). St. Louis: Mosby Year Book.

Michlovitz, S. (1999). Arthroplasty of the hand and wrist: Therapist's perspective. *Journal of Hand Therapy, 12,* 133–134.

Morrey, B. F. (2000a). Complications of elbow replacement surgery. In B. F. Morrey (Ed.). The elbow and its disorders (3rd ed., pp. 667–677). Philadelphia: Saunders.

Morrey, B. F. (2000b). Splints and bracing at the elbow. In B. F. Morrey (Ed.). The elbow and its disorders (3rd ed., pp. 150–154). Philadelphia: Saunders.

Murphy, D. (1996). Lycra working splint for the rheumatoid arthritis hand with MP ulnar deviation. *Australian Journal of Rural Health, 4,* 217–220.

Nalebuff, E. A. (1968). Diagnosis, classification and management of rheumatoid thumb deformities. *Bulletin of Hospital Joint Diseases, 24,* 119–137.

Nalebuff, E. (1990). Factors influencing the results of implant surgery in the rheumatoid hand. *Journal of Hand Surgery (British), 15,* 395–403.

Nalebuff, E., Millender, L. (1975). Surgical treatment of the boutonniere deformity in rheumatoid arthritis. *Orthopaedic Clinics of North American, 6,* 753–763.

Nirschl, R. P., & Morrey, B. F. (1993). Rehabilitation. In B. F. Morrey (Ed.). *The elbow and its disorders* (2nd ed., pp. 173–180). Philadelphia: Saunders.

Pagnotta, A., Baron, M., Korner-Bitensky, N. (1998). The effect of a static wrist orthosis on hand function in individuals with rheumatoid arthritis. *Journal of Rheumatology, 25,* 879–885.

Pelligrini, V., & Burton, R. (1990). Osteoarthritis of the proximal interphalangeal joint of the hand: arthroplasty or fusion? *Journal of Hand Surgery (American), 15,* 194–209.

Philips, C. (1995). Management of patients with rheumatoid arthritis. In J. M. Hunter, E. J. Mackin, & A. D. Callahan (Eds.). *Rehabilitation of the hand* (4th ed., pp. 1345–1350). St. Louis: Mosby Year Book.

Poole, J., & Pellegrini, V. (2000). Arthritis of the thumb basal joint complex. *Journal of Hand Therapy, 13,* 91–107.

Rennie, H. J. (1996). Evaluation of the effectiveness of a metacarpophalangeal ulnar deviation orthosis. *Journal of Hand Therapy, 9,* 371–377.

Rizio, L., & Belsky, M. (1995). Finger deformities in rheumatoid arthritis. In J. M. Hunter, E. J. Mackin, & A. D. Callahan (Eds.). *Rehabilitation of the hand* (4th ed., pp. 1385–1397). St. Louis: Mosby Year Book.

Rothwell, A. G., Cragg, K. J., & O'Neil, L. B. (1997). Hand function following silastic arthroplasty of the metacarpophalangeal joints in the rheumatoid arthritic hand. *Journal of Hand Surgery (Edinburgh, Lotham), 22,* 90–93.

Rozental, T. D., & Bora, F. W. (2000). Reconstruction of the rheumatoid thumb. *Seminars in Arthroplasty, 11,* 98–106.

Seeger, M. W., & Furst, D. E. (1987). Effects of splinting in the treatment of hand contractures in progressive systemic sclerosis. *American Journal of Occupational Therapy, 41,* 118–121.

Shapiro, J. (1996). The wrist in rheumatoid arthritis. *Hand Clinics, 12,* 477–498.

Simmons, B. P., Nutting, J. T., & Berstein, R. A. (1996). Juvenile rheumatoid arthritis. *Hand Clinics, 12,* 573–590.

Stein, A., & Terrono, A. (1996). The rheumatoid thumb. *Hand Clinics, 12,* 541–550.

Stern, E. B., Ytterbery, S. R., Krug, H. E., Larson, L. M., Portoghese, C. P., Kratz, W. N., & Mahowald, M. L. (1997). Commercial wrist extensor orthosis: A descriptive study of use and preference in patients with rheumatoid arthritis. *Arthritis Care Research, 10,* 27–35.

Stern, E. B., Ytterberg, S. R., Krug, H. E., & Machowald, M. L. (1996). Finger dexterity and hand function: effect of 3 commercial wrist extensor orthoses on patients with rheumatoid arthritis. *Arthritis Care Research, 9,* 197–202.

Stirrat, C. (1996). Metacarpophalangeal joints in rheumatoid arthritis of the hand. *Hand Clinics, 12,* 515–529.

Swanson, A. (1995a). Pathogenesis of arthritic lesion. In J. M. Hunter, E. J. Mackin, & A. D. Callahan (Eds.). *Rehabilitation of the hand* (4th ed., pp. 1307–1313). St. Louis: Mosby Year Book.

Swanson A. (1995b). Pathomechanics of deformities in hand and wrist. In J. M. Hunter, E. J. Mackin, & A. D. Callahan (Eds.). *Rehabilitation of the hand* (4th ed., pp. 1315–1328). St. Louis: Mosby Year Book.

Swanson, A., Maupin, B., Gajjar, N., & Swanson, G. P. (1985). Flexible implant arthroplasty in the proximal interphalangeal joint of the hand. *Journal of Hand Surgery (American),* 10, 796–804.

Swanson, A., Swanson, G., & Leonard, J. (1995). Postoperative rehabilitation programs in flexible implant arthroplasty of the digits. In J. M. Hunter, E. J. Mackin, & A. D. Callahan (Eds.). *Rehabilitation of the hand* (4th ed., pp. 1351–1376). St. Louis: Mosby Year Book.

Swigart, C., Eaton, R., Glickel, S., & Johnson, C. (1999). Splinting in the treatment of arthritis of the first CMC joint. *Journal of Hand Surgery (American),* 24, 86–91.

Talesnick, J. (1989). Rheumatoid arthritis of the wrist. *Hand Clinics, 5,* 257–278.

Terrono, A., Nalebuff, E., & Philips, C. (1995). The rheumatoid thumb. In J. M. Hunter, E. J. Mackin, & A. D. Callahan (Eds.). *Rehabilitation of the hand* (4th ed., pp. 1329–1344). St. Louis: Mosby Year Book.

Theisen, L. (1993). Metacarpophalangeal joint arthroplasty. In G. Clark, W. Shaw, B., Aiello, D. Eckhaus, & L. Eddington (Eds.). Hand rehabilitation: A practical guide (pp. 241–246). New York: Churchill Livingstone.

Tijhuis, G. J., Vliet Vlieland, T. P., Zwinderman, A. H., & Hazes, J. M. (1998). A comparison of the Futuro wrist orthosis with a synthetic ThermoLyn orthosis: utility and clinical effectiveness. *Arthritis Care Research, 11,* 217–222.

Tomaino, M. M., & King, J. (2000). Ligament reconstruction tendon interpositional arthroplasty for basal joint arthritis—simplifying FCR tendon passage through thumb metacarpal. *American Journal of Orthopaedics, 29,* 49–50.

Tomaino, M., Pelligrini, V., & Burton, R. (1995). Arthroplasty of the basal joint of the thumb. *Journal of Bone and Joint Surgery (American volume), 77,* 346–355.

Trumble, T., Tafijah, G., Gilbert, M., Allan, C., North, E., & McCallister, W. (2000). Thumb trapeziometacarpal joint arthritis: Partial trapeziectomy with ligament reconstruction and interposition costochondral allograft. *Journal of Hand Surgery (American), 25,* 61–76.

Vamos, M., White, G. L., & Caughey, D. E. (1990). Body image in rheumatoid arthritis: the relevance of hand appearance to desire for surgery. *British Journal of Medical Psychology, 63,* 267–77

vanVugt, R. M., van Jaarsveld, C. H., Hofman, D. M., Helders, P. J., & Bijlsma, J. W. (1999). Patterns of disease progression in the rheumatoid wrist: A long-term follow-up. *Journal of Rheumatology, 26,* 1467–73.

Vartimidis, S., Fox, R., King, J., Taras, J., & Soreranes, D. (2000). Trapeziometacarpal arthroplasty using the entire flexor carpi radialis tendon. *Clinical Orthopaedics and Related Research, 370,* 164–170.

Varitimidis, S., Plakseychuk, A., & Sotereanos, D. (1999). Reconstruction of the elbow: Surgeon's perspective. *Journal of Hand Therapy, 12,* 66–72.

Wajon, A. (2000). Clinical splinting successes: the "thumb strap" splint for dynamic instability of the trapeziometacarpal joint. *Journal of Hand Therapy, 13,* 236–237.

Watson, K., & Ballet, L. (1984). The SLAC wrist scapholunate advanced collapse pattern of degenerative arthritis. *Journal of Hand Surgery (American), 9,* 358–365.

Watson, K., Weinzweig, J., Guidera, M., Zeppieri, J., & Ashmead, D. (1999). One thousand intercarpal arthrodeses. *Journal of Hand Surgery (Edinburgh, Lotham), 24,* 307–315.

Weiss, S., LaStayo, P., Mills, A., & Bramlet, D. (2000). Prospective analysis of splinting the first carpometacarpophalangeal joint: An objective, subjective, and radiographic assessment. *Journal of Hand Therapy, 13,* 218–227.

Wilson, R. (1986). Rheumatoid arthritis of the hand. *Orthopaedic Clinics of North America, 17,* 313–343.

Wilson, R., & Carlblom, E. (1989). The rheumatoid metacarpophalangeal joint. *Hand Clinics, 5,* 223–237.

Wilson, R., & Fredick, H. (1994). Rheumatoid disease of the hand and wrist. In M. Cohen (Ed.). *Mastery of plastic and reconstructive surgery* (pp. 1710–1719). Boston: Little, Brown.

Wolf, A. (2000). Postoperative management after total elbow replacement. In *Techniques in hand and upper extremity surgery. (Quarterly Review Journal* by Lippincott Williams & Wilkins), *4,* 213–220.

Wright, P. E., Froimson, A. I., & Stewart, M. J. (1993). Interposition arthroplasty of the elbow. In B. F. Morrey (Ed.). *The elbow and its disorders* (2nd ed., pp. 611–622). Philadelphia: Saunders.

SUGGESTED READING

Bissell, J. H. (1999). Therapeutic modalities in hand surgery. *Journal of Hand Surgery (American), 24,* 435–448.

Brighton, S. W., & Louw, E. I. (1981). Social and rehabilitational aspects of rheumatoid arthritis. *South African Medical Journal, 60,* 103–104.

Goldenberg, D. (1992). Rheumatologic problems in the worker. In L. Millender, D. Louis, & B. Simmons (Eds.). *Occupational disorders of the upper extremity* (pp. 203–214). New York: Churchill Livingstone.

Kelley, M. J., & Ramsey, M. L. (2000). Osteoarthritis and traumatic arthritis of the shoulder. *Journal of Hand Therapy, 13,* 148–162.

Tucker, L. B., Allaire, S. H., DeNardo, B. A., Chernoff, M. C., Meenan, R. F., & Schaller, J. G. (1994). The role of subspecialty care for children with juvenile rheumatoid arthritis. Arthritis and Rheumatism, 37, 419.

Wolfe, T. (2000). Community resources and assistive devices for people with arthritis. *Journal of Hand Therapy, 13,* 184–192.

WORLD WIDE WEB RESOURCES

Arthritis foundation. www.arthritis.org. Accessed December 11, 2001.

ArthritisSupport. Arthritis Research and Treatment Resources. www.arthritissupport.com. Accessed December 11, 2001.

National Institute of Arthritis and Musculoskeletal and Skin Diseases www.nih.gov/niams. Accessed December 11, 2001.

CHAPTER 18

Splinting Tendon Injuries

Lisa M. Cyr, OTR/L, CHT

INTRODUCTION

An important component of a postoperative tendon repair regimen is the specific placement of joints within the postsurgical cast or splint. Customization of the proper splint can facilitate healing by enabling optimal approximation of the repaired tendon stumps. The splint helps prevent dehiscence of the wound by placing structures in a minimally stressed position, therefore permitting the process of tissue healing to begin. The splint can also function as protection from external forces, preventing a sudden movement away from the repair and causing possible tendon rupture.

This chapter addresses tendon anatomy, splinting techniques for flexor and extensor tendon injuries, and the specific needs relative to the particular zones of injury. The main emphasis of the postoperative splinting program is during the first 4 to 6 weeks after surgical repair. Suggestions for managing secondary problems, such as extrinsic tightness and joint contractures, will be briefly mentioned. However, these specific problems, along with the appropriate splinting intervention, are discussed in depth in Chapter 15. A brief overview of various protocols in relation to splinting concerns is presented. Further study is recommended for those who are not familiar with specific protocols, and the reader is referred to the Reference and Suggested Reading sections.

Postoperative management of repaired tendons requires the knowledge and skill of an experienced hand therapist and close communication with the referring hand surgeon. This exchange provides vital information regarding injuries to adjacent structures, such as bone, vessel, and/or nerve, as well as the condition of the tendon at the time of repair. This information and other factors—e.g., age, cognitive status, medical history (including smoking, caffeine, and alcohol intake), rate and quality of scar formation, motivation, and ability to participate in the rehabilitation process—help the therapist and surgeon select the most appropriate postoperative protocol.

Flexor Tendon Anatomy

Understanding the anatomy of the digit and wrist flexors is vital for accurate splint design and determination of proper postoperative care. There are two extrinsic digital flexor tendons—**flexor digitorum superficialis (FDS)** and **flexor digitorum profundus (FDP)**—one extrinsic thumb flexor—**flexor pollicis longus (FPL)**—and two extrinsic wrist flexors—**flexor carpi radialis (FCR)** and **flexor carpi ulnaris (FCU)** (the palmaris longus is not considered in this discussion because of its relative insignificance).

The FDP and FPL form the deep muscle layer in the flexor compartment of the forearm (Fig. 18–1). The FDP originates on the anterior surface of the shaft of the midulna, the interosseous membrane, and occasionally the proximal radius. Typically, the muscle belly of the FDP separates into a radial and ulnar bundle in the midforearm. The radial bundle becomes the tendon to the index finger (IF), and the ulnar bundle forms the tendons to the middle finger (MF), ring finger (RF), and small finger (SF). The muscle bellies transition to tendons in the

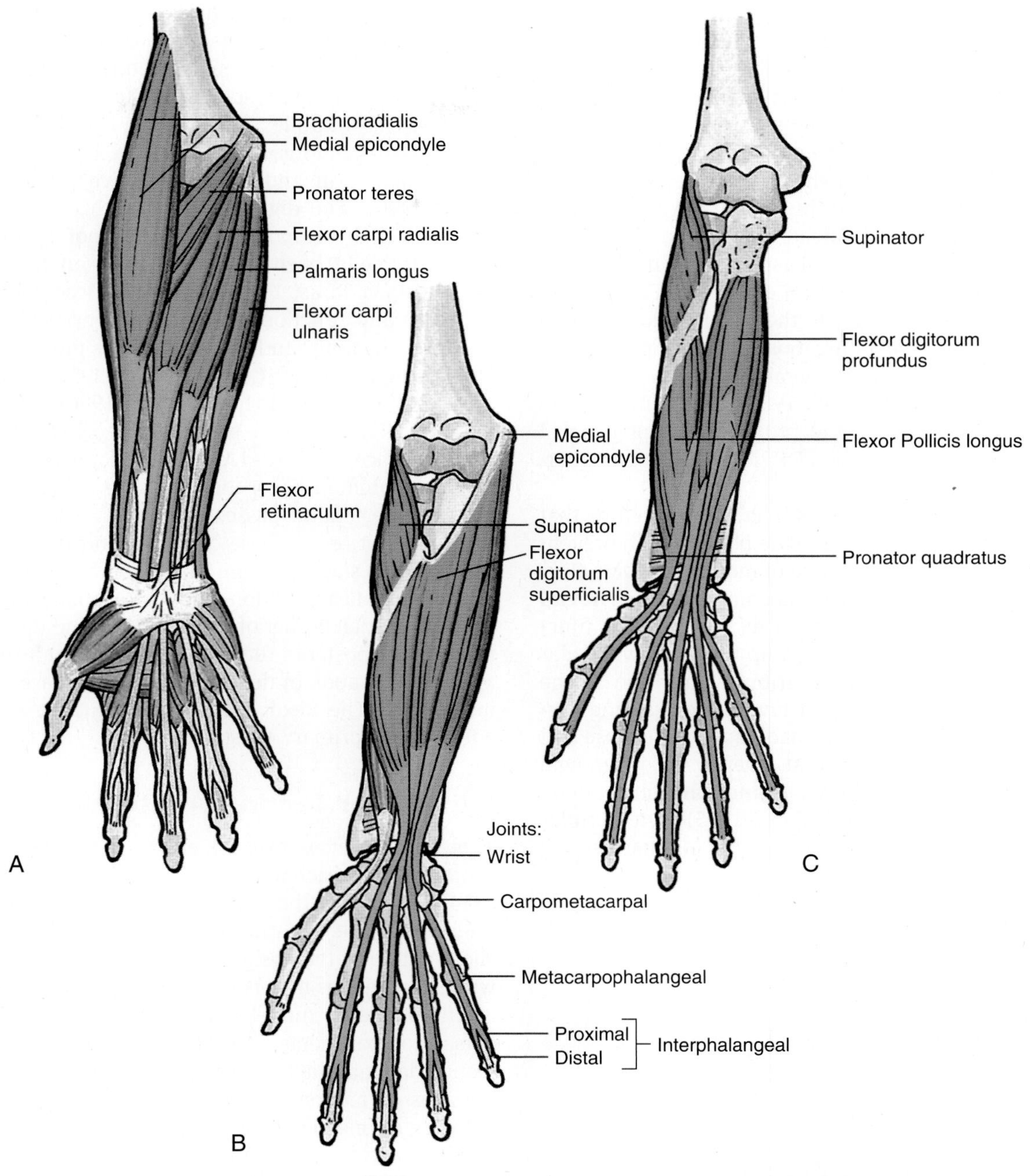

*Figure 18–1 Superficial (**A**), intermediate (**B**), and deep (**C**) layers of the flexor muscles of the forearm (volar view). Reprinted with permission from Moore, K. L. & Agur, A. M. (1995). Essential clinical anatomy. Baltimore: Williams & Wilkins.*

distal forearm. These four tendons traverse the carpal tunnel, occupying its floor, and then diverge to their respective digits in the palm. They enter the particular flexor sheaths at the level of the metacarpophalangeal (MP) joints and insert on the palmar base of the distal phalanx of each finger. Their primary function is to flex the distal joint of the fingers.

The FPL originates from the proximal radius and the interosseous membrane. The tendon also lies on the floor of the carpal tunnel and then enters the flexor sheath of the thumb and inserts on the proximal volar surface of the distal phalanx. Its primary function is to flex the IP joint of the thumb.

The FDS occupies the intermediate layer of the flexor compartment superficial to the FDP and FPL (Fig. 18-1**B**). Proximally, two separate heads originate from the elbow region. The humeroulnar head arises from the medial epicondyle of the humerus and the coronoid process of the ulna; the radial head originates from the proximal shaft of the radius. The FDS evolves into four distinct muscle bellies as it traverses distally in the midforearm and becomes four individual tendons in the distal forearm. The tendons travel through the carpal tunnel, with the tendons to the MF and RF, superficial and central to those of the IF and SF. The FDS enters the flexor sheath at the level of the MP joint with the FDP tendon. At the level of the midproximal phalanx, the FDS tendon bifurcates, and the radial and ulnar slips insert into the proximal aspect of the middle phalanx (Fig. 18–2). This bifurcation allows the FDP tendon to pass through on its course to the distal phalanx. When the digit is flexed, the bifurcation migrates proximally, making the FDP extremely vulnerable to injury in this position (Kleinert, Schepel, & Gill, 1981). The primary function of the FDS is to flex the proximal interphalangeal (PIP) joints of the fingers; the FDP flexes the dorsal interphalangeal (DIP) joints.

The **digital flexor sheath** is a critical structure that holds the flexor tendons close to the phalanges to prevent bowstringing during active range of motion (AROM) (Fig. 18–3). The digital flexor sheath is composed of **synovial** and **retinacular** tissue, each with its own distinct function. The synovial aspect is made up of a hollow tubular fibroosseous tunnel, which contributes nutrition to the tendons within and provides a low-friction gliding system. The retinacular portion is made up of transverse and crisscrossed fibrous bands that overlay this synovial sheath. These bands are known as **annular** and **cruciate pulleys,** respectively (Culp & Taras, 1995). The annular pulleys, notably A2 and A4, are critical for maintaining an efficient biomechanical relationship between the tendons and the phalanges. The flexor sheath in its entirety is important when considering postoperative treatment. The close contact between the tendons and the sheath makes this area highly susceptible to motion-limiting adhesions. Loss of pulley function can lead to bowstringing of the flexor tendons, resulting in an increased mechanical moment arm and impaired active motion (Culp & Taras, 1995). The digital flexor sheath occupies zone II and is partially responsible for the poor prognosis that has historically been associated with an injury to this area (Culp & Taras, 1995). Thorough descriptions of the structure and function of the sheath, as well as tendon nutrition, healing, and the role of the pulleys are available in the literature (Culp & Taras, 1995; Kleinert et al., 1981; Tubiana, Thomine, & Mackin, 1996).

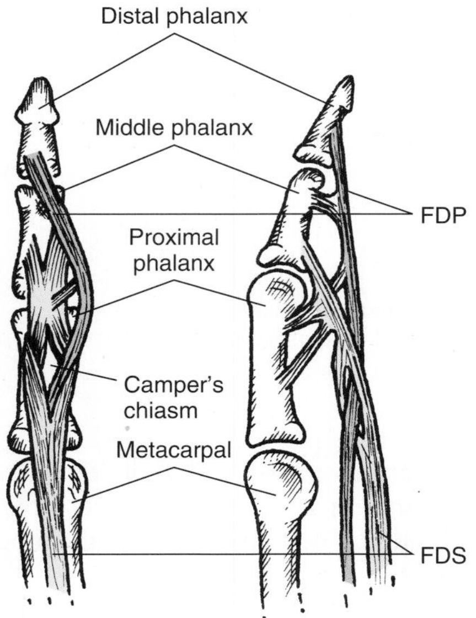

Figure 18–2 The bifurcation of the FDS tendon is also referred to as Camper's chiasm. The radial and ulnar slips insert into the proximal aspect of the middle phalanx and permit the FDP tendon to pass through.

The FCR and FCU are part of the superficial layer of the flexor surface (Fig. 18–1**A**). The FCR inserts proximally with the common flexor tendon at the medial epicondyle. Distally, the tendon passes through the **flexor retinaculum** to insert on the base of the second metacarpal. The FCU has two sites of origin: The humeral head arises from the common flexor tendon, and the second head originates from the medial border of the olecranon and the upper two thirds of the posterior ulna border. Distally, it inserts on the pisiform, the hook of the hamate, and the base of the fifth metacarpal. The flexor carpi radialis and flexor carpi ulnaris are the primary wrist flexors.

Extensor Tendon Anatomy

There are nine extrinsic extensors that are relevant for splinting: three each for the wrist, fingers, and thumb (Fig. 18–4). Similar to the extrinsic flexors, these muscles all originate in the forearm and insert distal to the wrist to elicit motion at the designated joint(s). At the level of the wrist, the tendons traverse the **extensor retinaculum.** This is a fibro-osseous tunnel system that is partitioned into six dorsal compartments (A-F) (Fig. 18–5). These compartments maintain the tendons in correct positions relative to the axes of motion and prevent the tendons from bowstringing during active digital extension (Doyle, 1999).

The longest wrist extensor, the **extensor carpi radialis longus (ECRL),** arises from the lower third of the supracondylar ridge of the humerus and inserts onto the dorsum of the base of the second metacarpal. The remainder of the extrinsic wrist and digit extensors, except for the **extensor indicis proprius (EIP),** originate from the common extensor origin on the lateral epicondyle (Fig. 18–4**A**). The **extensor carpi radialis brevis (ECRB)** inserts onto the dorsum of the base of the third metacarpal. The **extensor carpi ulnaris (ECU)** originates from the middle half of the posterior ulna as well as from the common extensor tendon. Distally, the tendon inserts onto the ulnar side of the base of the fifth metacarpal.

The **extensor digitorum communis (EDC)** arises from the common extensor origin and divides into four tendons

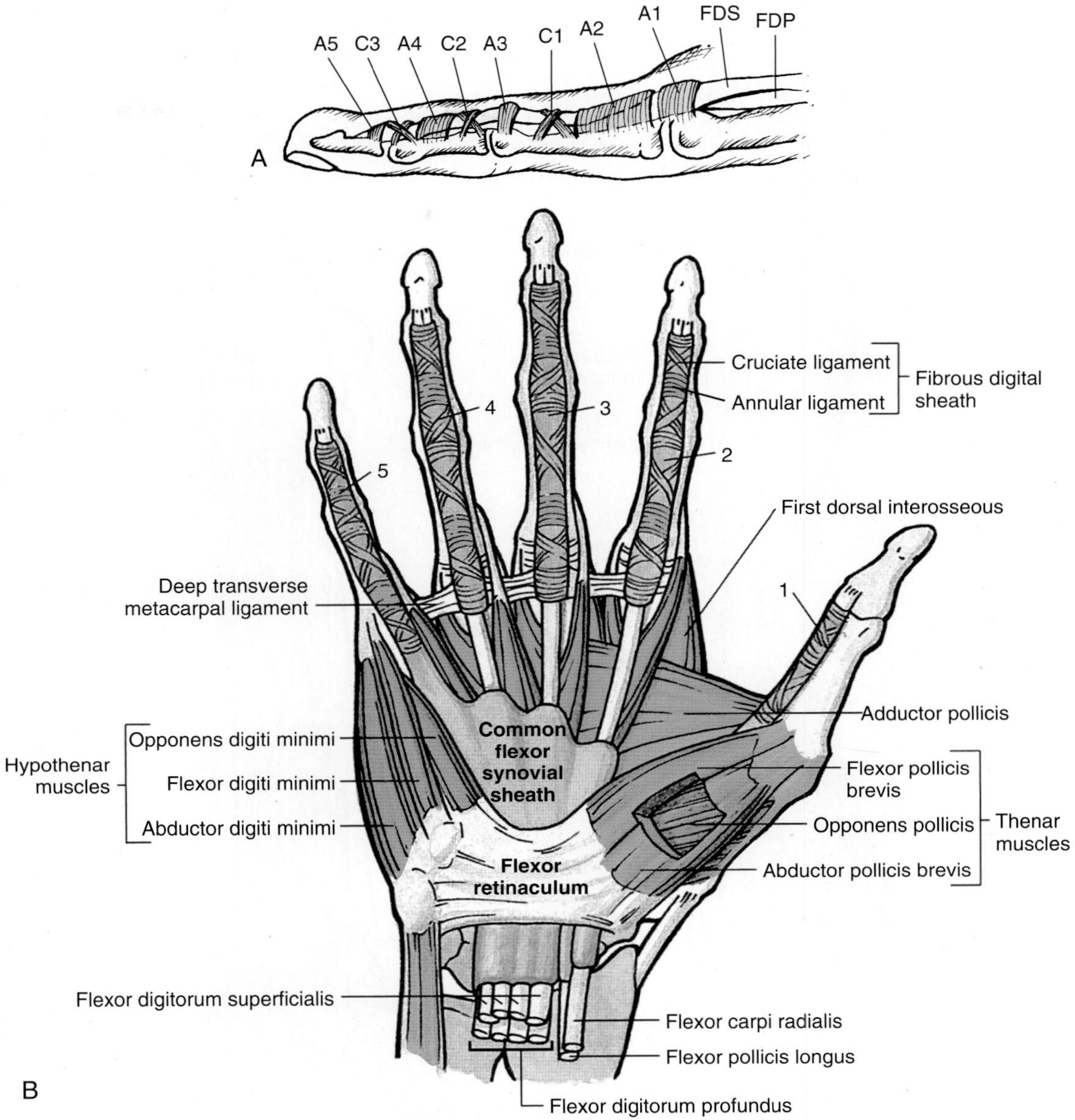

Figure 18–3 ***A,*** *The digital flexor synovial sheath has five annular (A1 to A5) and three cruciate (C1 to C3) pulleys surrounding it. Note the relative size of the A2 and A4 pulleys; biomechanically, they contribute greatly to maximizing tendon function.* ***B,*** *Dissection of hand showing the digital synovial sheath system. Reprinted with permission from Moore, K. L. & Agur, A. M. (1995). Essential clinical anatomy. Baltimore: Williams & Wilkins.*

in the distal third of the forearm. These tendons insert into the bases of the middle and distal phalanges of the IF through SF as part of the extensor apparatus. This muscle is unique in that there are intertendinous connections, the **juncturae tendinum,** on the dorsum of the hand that assist in extension of the adjacent digit by transferring forces and enabling the tendons to function as a unit (Fig. 18–5) (Netter, 1987; Rosenthal, 1995). This is significant when a laceration or rupture occurs, and may affect the design of the postoperative splint. For example, if the laceration is distal to the juncturae, the injured finger may be splinted with the MP at 0°, and the adjacent fingers positioned with the MP joints at 30° of flexion. This position reduces the tension on the EDC by advancing the proximal end of the severed tendon via the juncturae (Evans, 1991).

The **extensor digiti minimi (EDM)** is a slender muscle that is sometimes only partly separated from the EDC tendon to the SF. This tendon joins the ulnar side of the EDC to the SF, providing independent extension to this digit. The **extensor indicis proprius (EIP)** arises from the dorsal distal third of the ulna and the interosseous membrane. This tendon travels ulnar to the index finger

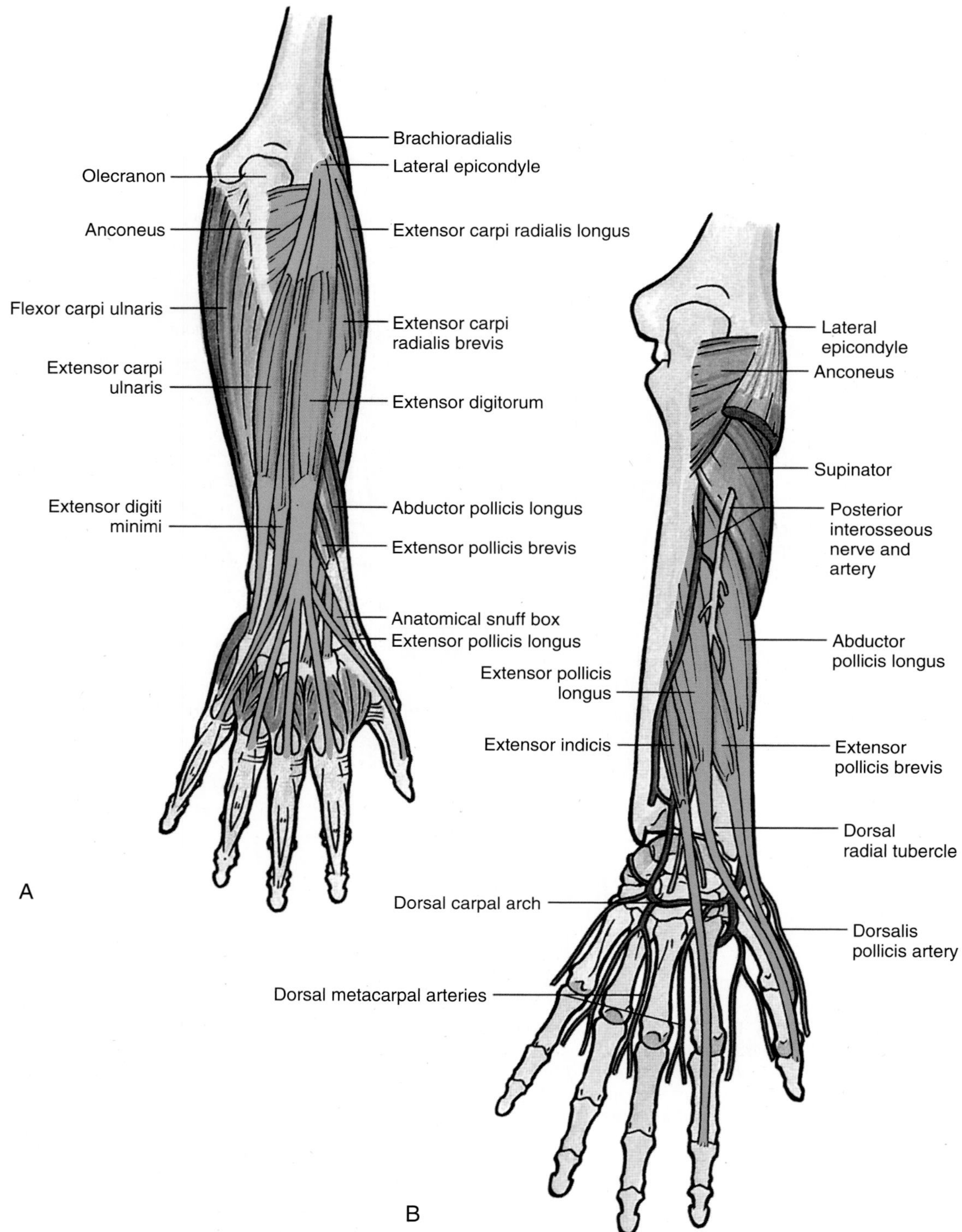

*Figure 18–4 Superficial (**A**) and deep (**B**) layers of the extensor compartment (dorsal view). Reprinted with permission from Moore, K. L. & Agur, A. M. (1995). Essential clinical anatomy. Baltimore: Williams & Wilkins.*

EDC and inserts into the extensor apparatus, allowing independent extension of the IF.

The digital extensor apparatus is a complex geometric arrangement of extrinsic, intrinsic, and retinacular fibers (Doyle, 1999; Rosenthal, 1995). At the MP level, the intrinsic tendons from the **lumbricals** and **interossei** muscles along with the **sagittal bands** maintain the central position of the extensor mechanism. The intrinsic tendons then converge with slips from the EDC at the level of the mid-portion of the proximal phalanx on both sides of the finger. These conjoined tendons continue distally as the **lateral bands** merge and connect with the **triangular (retinacular) ligament** and insert dorsally, as the **terminal tendon,** on the proximal aspect of the distal phalanx (Fig. 18–6).

The three extrinsic thumb muscles arise from the dorsal distal half of either the radius or ulna (Fig. 18–4). The **abductor pollicis longus (APL)** arises from the posterior surface of both bones and inserts on the radial side of the base of the first metacarpal. The **extensor pollicis brevis (EPB)** arises distal to the APL from the radius and interosseous membrane. Distally, the tendon inserts at the base of the proximal phalanx of the thumb. The **extensor pollicis longus (EPL)** originates from the ulna and the interosseous membrane also distal to the APL, terminating on the base of the distal phalanx of the thumb.

Zones of Injury

In June 1980, an international agreement on zones of anatomic nomenclature was established for both flexor and extensor tendon injuries to facilitate understanding

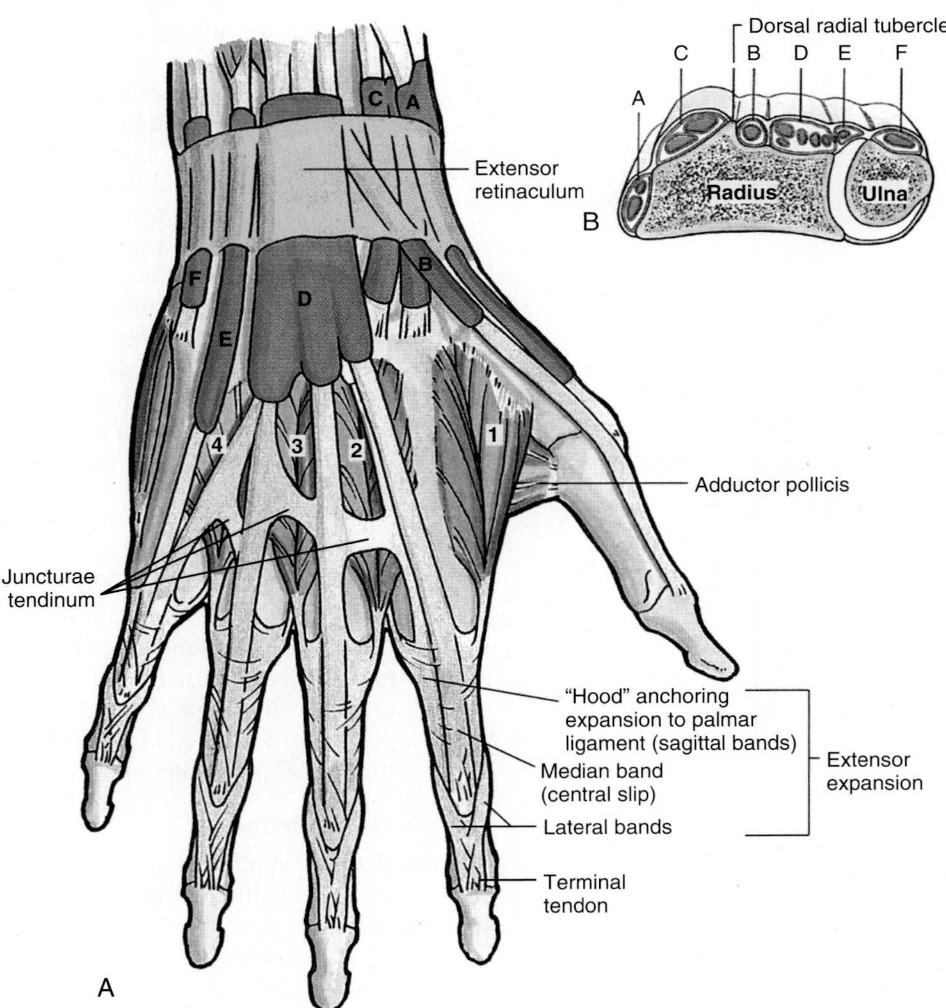

Figure 18–5 ***A,*** *Synovial sheaths of extensor tendons of the hand.* ***B,*** *The six dorsal compartments of the extensor tendons. A, abductor pollicis longus and extensor pollicis brevis; B, extensor pollicis longus; C, extensor carpi radialis longus and extensor carpi radialis brevis; D, extensor digitorum communis; E, extensor digiti minimi; F, extensor carpi ulnaris; 1–4, dorsal interossei. Reprinted with permission from Moore, K. L. & Agur, A. M. (1995). Essential clinical anatomy. Baltimore: Williams & Wilkins.*

and treatment of these problems (Kleinert & Verdan, 1983; Kleinert et al., 1981). An agreement was reached on distinguishing five zones for the flexor tendons of the digits and the thumb (Fig. 18–7), eight zones for the digital extensors, and six zones for the thumb extensors (Fig. 18–8). The particular zone of injury influences the complexity of the repair and the postoperative treatment protocol and splint selection.

General Splinting Considerations

The therapist should consider the following factors when splinting tendon injuries:

- Communicate closely with the surgeon. Operative findings may require special splint modifications (e.g., repair of neurovascular structures may necessitate a change in joint position).

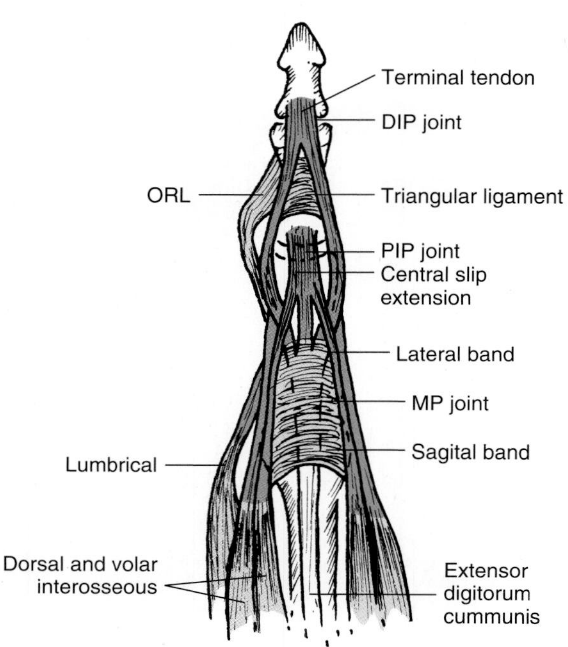

Figure 18–6 The intricate extensor apparatus. DIP, distal interphalangeal; ORL, oblique retinacular ligament.

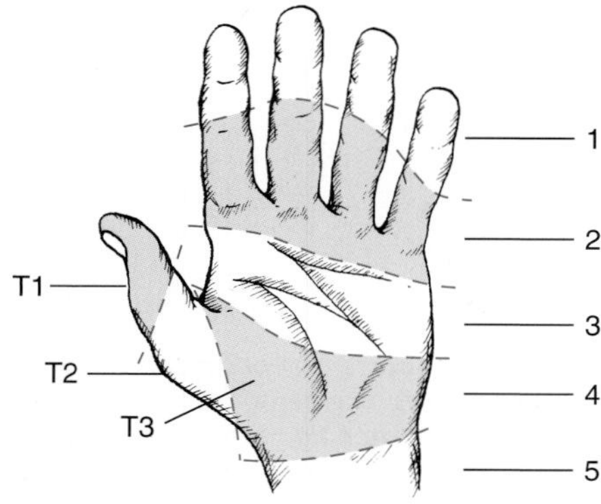

Figure 18–7 The flexor tendon zones.

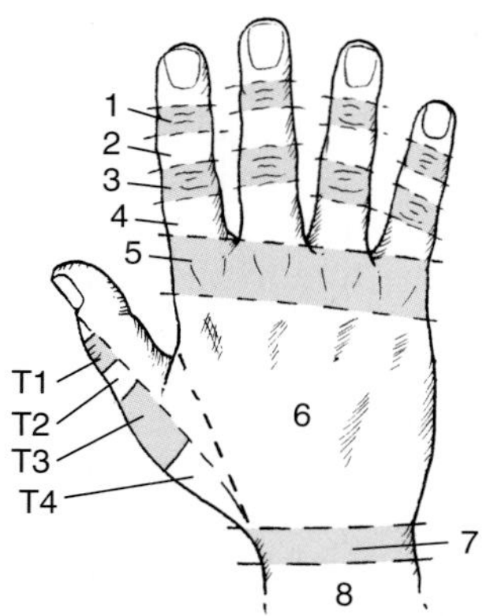

Figure 18–8 The extensor tendon zones.

- Protect the repaired tendon and associated injuries by carefully splinting the joints in a position that decreases tension on the repair site and other healing structures.
- Use a goniometer to preposition the wrist, digits, and thumb to aid in attaining proper joint alignment.
- For flexor tendons, consider fabricating a simple hand rest from rolled thermoplastic material to help properly maintain the exact position of the involved wrist, hand, or thumb. This allows the therapist to use both hands in the molding process.
- Consider using the unaffected hand to create the splint pattern when the injured hand is too painful to move or movement is contraindicated.
- Consider covering the body part with cotton stockinette, because splint material may adhere to postoperative dressings. When the splint is set, the stockinette can be simply cut off on the nonsplinted surface and gently pulled away from the splint.
- When appropriate, facilitate wound and tissue healing by utilizing protected early passive or early active motion within the confines of the splint.
- Patients who demonstrate exceptionally good AROM may not have formed sufficient intrinsic adhesions to safely discontinue splint use. Consider splinting protection for several more weeks to prevent tendon rupture. This concept applies to all protocols.

Material Selection

Consideration should be given to thermoplastic materials that can provide the required rigidity for maintaining appropriate joint positioning and air exchange to promote tissue healing. The forearm-based splints can be made from a variety of materials. Generally, 1⁄8" lightly perforated materials are good choices for supporting the forearm and the hand. There is occasion when a thinner material (3⁄32") can provide the required amount of rigidity. Plastic-like materials tend to have a high degree of conformability and drapability (thereby allowing less hands-on molding; Polyform), which can make the fabrication process less difficult when splinting postsurgical patients who present with a painful and edematous hand.

Elastic-like materials (Aquaplast) can provide another option. Although this material requires more aggressive handling during the molding process, the completed splint can be remolded and the splint angles adjusted more easily than their plastic counterparts. This can be extremely helpful, especially since many tendon splints require frequent splint angle adjustments. Because these splints need to be worn on a full-time basis, using perforated materials can help provide airflow to dressings and skin, reducing the problems associated with perspiration (e.g., tissue maceration, skin breakdown). Thinner materials—such as 1/16" thermoplastic or QuickCast—are excellent options for digit-based splints (zone I and II extensor tendon injuries) (Fig. 18–9). Chapter 5 provides a more in-depth discussion on material selection.

Strapping Selection

There are a variety of methods for securing the splint on the extremity. For the patient who presents with a postoperative edematous extremity, a distal to proximal circumferential wrap may be the most appropriate way to secure the splint until the edema subsides. Traditional hook-and-loop and soft straps are common methods for securing the splint to the extremity. For example, any wrist/hand immobilization splint, whether it is for a flexor or an extensor tendon injury, should have a minimum of three straps that traverse the splint: one strap at the distal portion of the splint, one at the wrist area (or middle of the splint), and one at the proximal margin of the splint. Additional straps can be added for further stabilization. For example, with flexor tendon splints, an additional strap can be riveted onto the palmar strap to secure the thumb in place, increase splint stability, and prevent splint migration (Fig. 18–10). The palmar strap should be contoured to prevent interference with the thumb motion (unless the FPL has also been repaired). Another strapping option, which increases conformity at the wrist level, is to make four tails at both ends of the wrist strap (Chow, Thomes, Dovelle, Monsivais, Milnor, & Jackson, 1988). This can be done by cutting approximately 2-in. longitudinal slits at the ends of the strap. This method tends to be more

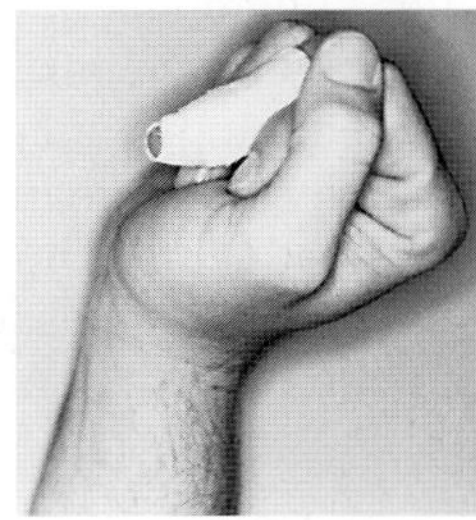

Figure 18–9 Zone I extensor tendon injury (Mallet finger) treated with QuickCast. Note the slight hyperextension at the DIP joint.

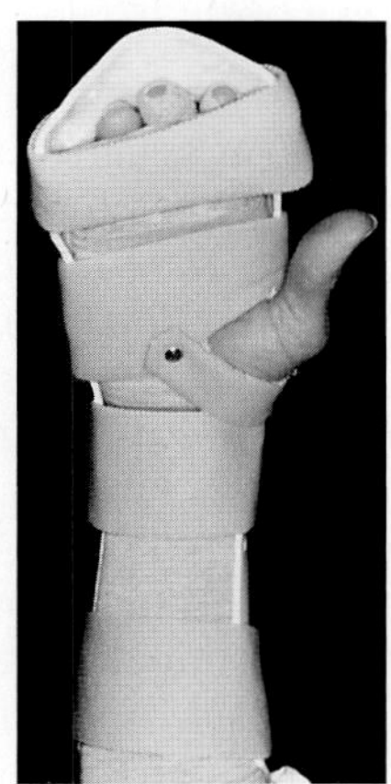

Figure 18–10 One method of strapping to prevent splint migration is to contour a palmar strap through the web space and rivet an additional attachment at the thenar crease. Secure it in place at the proximal dorsal border of the thumb.

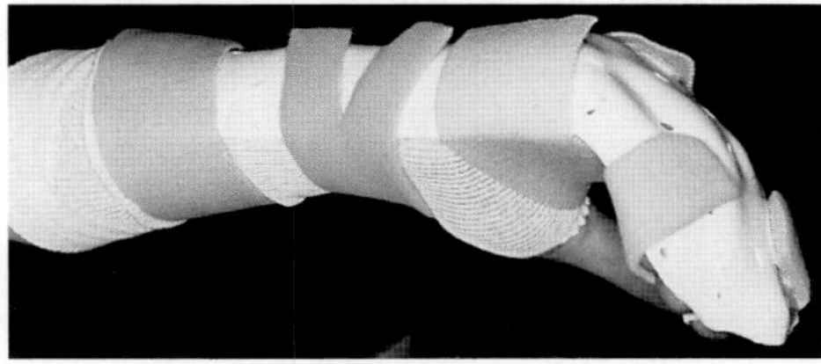

Figure 18–11 A split strap design may be a simple solution to securing the wrist position within the splint.

amenable with soft straps (Betapile and Velfoam) because there is little or no fraying, yet they are soft and conforming (Fig. 18–11). Additional techniques to prevent distal migration of the splint are to use 3/4" adhesive foam on the palmar and wrist straps (T-Foam) or to use 2" Neoprene straps. The Neoprene straps contour well about the base of the thumb and can provide additional warmth and gentle compression to sensitive scars.

Flexor Tendon Management

Although there are many protocols for guiding postoperative flexor tendon management, intervention should never follow only one particular approach. Frequently, the best approach combines techniques from several protocols. There are three protocols, or modes of intervention, for the initial 3 to 4 weeks of postoperative flexor tendon management; the intermediate (4 to 8 weeks) and late (8 to 12 weeks) phases of rehabilitation. The initial protective period encompasses the inflammatory and fibroblastic phases of wound healing and the beginning of scar maturation (Stewart & Van Stein, 1995). The rehabilitation techniques used during this phase are categorized into immobilization, early passive mobilization, and early active mobilization protocols.

- **Immobilization protocol.** Protects the surgical repair by preventing any movement of the fingers, thumb, or wrist until sufficient healing has occurred. This is accomplished by postoperative casting by the surgeon and is typically continued for 3 to 4 weeks.
- **Early passive mobilization protocol.** Begins 1 to 3 days after surgery and involves protected passive range of motion (PROM) of the interphalangeal (IP) joints to facilitate passive proximal gliding of the repaired tendon(s).
- **Early active mobilization protocol.** Begins 1 to 3 days after surgery and incorporates an active contraction from the muscle of the repaired tendon(s). This enables proximal glide of the repaired tendon with decreased risk of bunching, which may occur with passively mobilized tendons.

The decision to use a particular protocol is largely influenced by the referring surgeon. He or she makes this determination based on the nature of the tendon injury, the integrity of the tendon repair, any associated injuries, and the timing of the repair. Another important consideration when deciding on a postoperative protocol is the type of surgical repair performed. The suture technique greatly influences the ability of the tendon to withstand external forces (Bunnell, 1956; Evans & Thompson, 1993; Silfverskiold & May, 1994; Strickland, 2000; Strickland & Gettle, 1997; Taras, Raphael, Marczyk, Bauerle, & Culp, 1997; Taras, Skahen, Raphael, Marzyk, & Bauerle, 1996). This is a critical factor for early mobilization protocols, especially when opting for an early active regimen, because adequate suture strength is vital for decreasing the risk of rupture with an active contraction.

All of the protocols for postoperative flexor tendon injury or repair in zones I to V use a wrist/hand/thumb immobilization or restriction splint, commonly referred to as a dorsal blocking splint (DBS) (thumb included if FPL involved) (Fig. 18–12). This splint maintains the wrist and MP joints in moderate flexion and the IP joints in extension. This position protects the anastomosis of the repair by preventing simultaneous wrist, digit, and/or thumb extension. It also reduces the power of the flexor muscles in active contraction. When fabricating the dorsal MP portion of the splint, take care to position all MP joints in the desired amount of flexion, especially the RF and SF MP joints. These joints should be held in slightly more flexion than the other MP joints, if possible, because it mimics the natural position of the fisted hand. The position of the PIP and DIP joints depends on the injuries and specific protocol requested by the surgeon. This careful planning early on shortens the rehabilitation period by minimizing MP extension contractures and facilitating early active grasping.

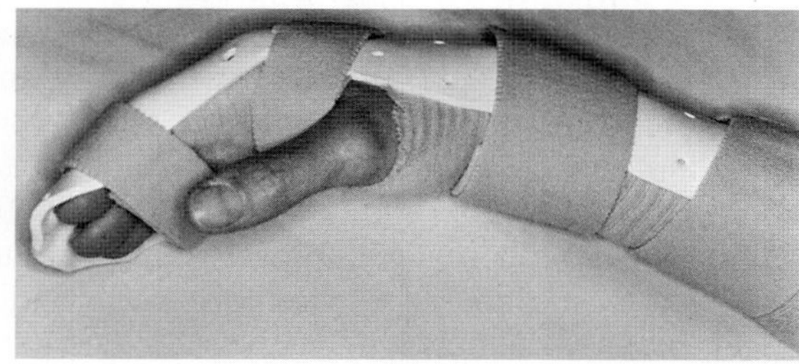

Figure 18–12 A wrist/hand extension restriction splint (dorsal blocking splint, DBS) is used after most flexor tendon repairs. The amount of wrist and MP flexion depend on the protocol used.

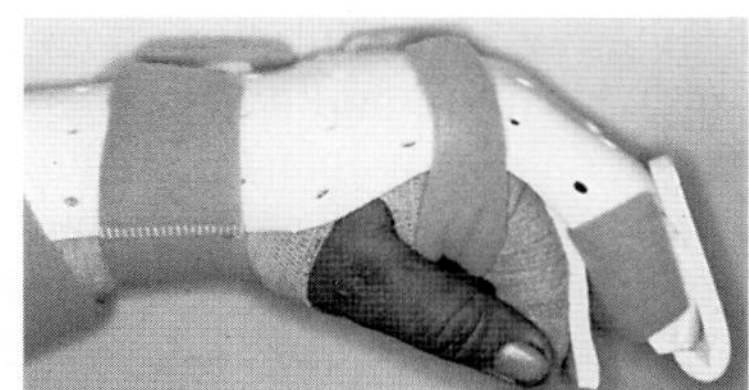

Figure 18–13 An AlumaFoam insert positions the MP joint in flexion, facilitating active PIP extension with exercise and allowing the PIP to be safely strapped into extension to prevent PIP flexion contracture.

Occasionally, the patient requires restriction of full PIP joint extension, owing to the nature and integrity of the surgical repair or to an associated digital nerve injury repaired under tension. In these cases, the splint must be modified to avoid stress to the repair site. This can be accomplished by adding adhesive foam to the inside of the splint or by fabricating an insert to provide dorsal support to the digit (Fig. 18–13).

Each protocol has specific guidelines and pertinent variations. The information presented below is based on a clean tendon repair without associated injuries. Detailed descriptions of each protocol are available in the literature. The therapist should review a protocol thoroughly with the referring physician before implementing it.

Immobilization Protocol

The immobilization protocol is used when circumstances preclude the use of early mobilization protocols. Such cases include young children, individuals with cognitive or behavioral problems, patients who are unwilling or unable to participate in a demanding rehabilitation program, and patients who have sustained associated injuries (e.g., fracture or replantation) (Stewart & Van Stein, 1995). Sometimes a patient who has been in a cast for several weeks after undergoing a tendon repair is referred to therapy. This may be the result of the surgeon's preference, difficulty obtaining a therapy appointment, insurance issues, or family/travel matters. Whatever the reason, the clinician treating the immobilized tendon should be aware of tendon healing issues and should use caution when guiding the rehabilitation program.

Zones I to V and TI to TV

Cast immobilization is most often the treatment of choice for immobilization. These patients are commonly casted with approximately 20° of wrist flexion, 50° of MP flexion, and 20° of IP flexion for 3 to 4 weeks (Cannon, 1991; Collins & Schwarze, 1991). If the FPL tendon is involved, the thumb is positioned in a comfortable degree of palmar abduction with gentle MP and IP flexion. Isolated lacerations to the FCR and/or FCU are usually immobilized for 4 to 6 weeks in a cast or wrist flexion immobilization splint, which needs to include only the wrist, positioned at approximately 30° of flexion (Cannon & Strickland, 1991).

When the patient arrives to therapy (3 to 4 weeks postsurgery), sufficient healing may have occurred to begin PROM and AROM within a protected range. However, tissue healing depends on the individual and related factors (see Chapter 3), and initiation of exercise must be approved by the physician. The cast is removed and a protective splint is fabricated; the wrist is positioned in 0 to 30° flexion, MP joints at approximately 50° of flexion, and the IP joints as close to 0° as comfortably allowable (Fig. 18–12) (Cannon, 1991; Collins & Schwarze, 1991).

If **extrinsic flexor tightness** has developed during the immobilization phase, then the patient may require a gentle volar wrist/hand extension mobilization splint (serial static approach), initiated at approximately 6 weeks postsurgery (check with physician first) (Fig. 18–14) (Collins & Schwarze, 1991). This splint is remolded into more composite wrist, digit, and/or thumb extension as the healing time frame allows. PIP flexion contractures are not uncommon after a period of immobilization. These can be addressed with PIP extension mobilization splinting or casting after 6 weeks (check with physician first) (Fig. 18–15). Depending on the density of the contractures, these splints or casts may be worn throughout the day and night, taken off only for exercise and hygiene. The position of the PIP joint is changed during therapy visits until the desired amount of extension (preferably 0°) is achieved. Graded resistive exercises are introduced as healing continues, and the protective splint is discontinued at approximately 6 weeks after the repair. Mobilization splints may continue until residual extrinsic tightness and joint contractures have resolved.

The **distal biceps brachii** can be traumatically lacerated or ruptured through attrition. When repaired, some surgeons prefer to immobilize the elbow in 90° of flexion and almost full supination (Sleeboom & Regoort, 1991). The wrist is often included for comfort. This can be achieved with either cast immobilization or a thermoplastic splint. The elbow is generally immobilized for 3 to 4 weeks; then, depending on the surgeon's preference, guarded motion is begun. The protective splint is continued for an additional 3 to 4 weeks.

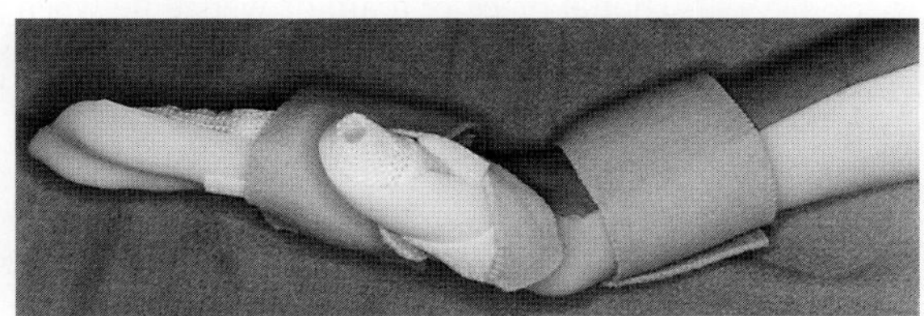

Figure 18–14 A serial static wrist/hand/thumb extension mobilization splint for extrinsic flexor tightness is remolded as the tissues gently elongate. Note the use of QuickCast serial static digit extension splints to direct corrective force to the extrinsic flexors.

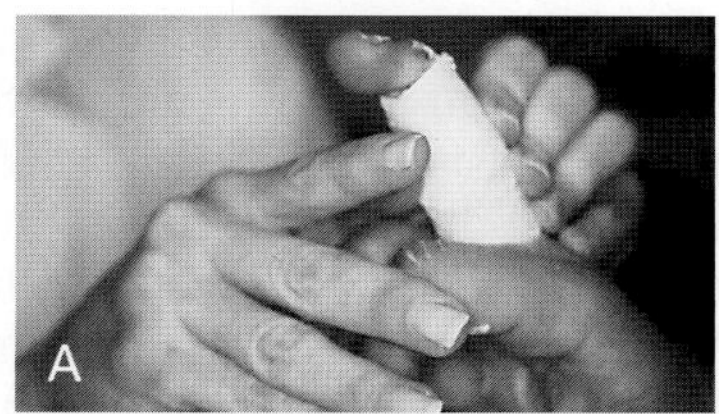

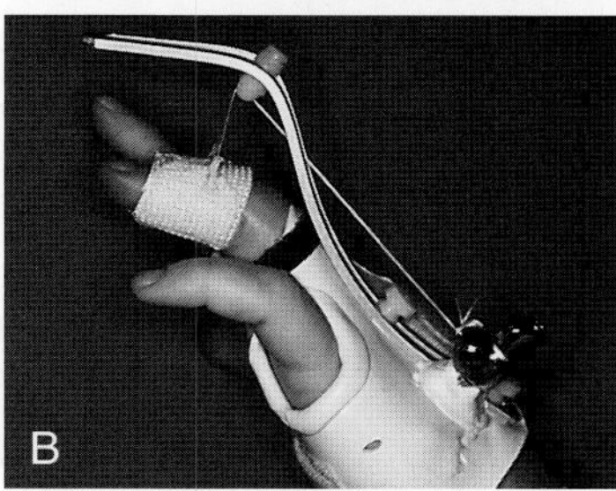

*Figure 18–15 **A,** Serial static PIP extension mobilization splint using plaster. Note the DIP is left free to allow for FDP gliding exercises. **B,** Static progressive PIP extension mobilization splint using a Splint Tuner component and Base2 outrigger.*

Early Passive Mobilization Protocol

The trend toward using an immediate controlled passive mobilization protocol evolved during the late 1970s from the work of Gelberman and others (Gelberman, Manske, Akeson, & Woo, 1986; Hitchcock, Light, Bunch, Knight, Sartori, Patwardhan, & Hollyfield, 1987; Woo, Gelberman, Cobb, Amiel, Lothringer, Akeson, 1981). Their classic studies demonstrated that immobilization is deleterious to repaired tendons and that early mobilization has many significant benefits. These include better excursion properties, increased vascularity, increased tensile strength, and decreased adhesion formation, all contributing to a better functional outcome. Duran, Houser, Coleman, and Stover (1978) determined that only 3 to 5 mm of motion away from the repair site is necessary to elicit desirable responses in a repaired digit.

There are a few basic early passive mobilization (EPM) protocols that are familiar to most therapists who work in a hand setting. Kleinert and co-workers advocated dynamic flexion traction as a way to protect the repair while eliciting synergistic relaxation of the flexors with active digit extension to the dorsal block of the splint (Kleinert et al., 1981; Lister, Kleinert, Kutz, & Atasoy, 1977). Duran and co-workers (1978) used dynamic traction to maintain the digit(s) in relaxed flexion to prevent stress at the repair site. These protocols use dynamic flexion traction by attaching a rubber band, monofilament, or elastic thread to a suture placed through the fingernail during surgery. As an alternative, a dressing hook, adhesive hook, or the rubber band itself can be glued onto the nail. The proximal aspect of the traction line is secured to a strap at the wrist level with a safety pin or line guide (Fig. 18–16) .

A prefabricated brace is another option. Kleinert developed the postoperative flexor tendon traction brace (DeRoyal; Powell, TN). The advantages of this brace are that the digit(s) can extend easily against minimal resistance; and with passive flexion, near full tendon excursion is achieved through increasing DIP flexion (Dovelle & Heeter, 1989; Evans, 1990; Peck, Bucher, Watson, & Roe, 1998; Schenck & Dennis, 1996).

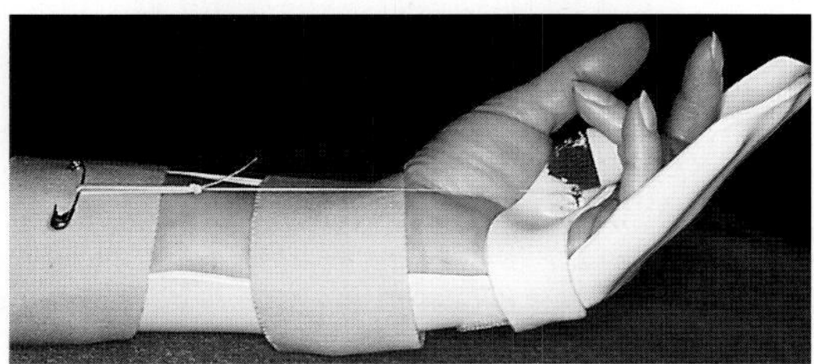

Figure 18–16 Rubber band traction is used for gentle digital flexion in an early passive flexion/active extension program (shown is a modified splint with palmar pulley).

In 1981, the Washington regimen, a protocol incorporating features from both the Duran and Kleinert protocols was developed (Chow et al., 1988; Dovelle & Heeter, 1989; Schenck & Dennis, 1996). The splint includes a palmar pulley and soft strapping with a split tail design to secure it to the forearm. Dynamic traction is composed of two rubber bands. A #18 rubber band is used during rest in flexion, and a single-strand #18 rubber band (a rubber band cut in half) is used during active extension exercises. The palmar pulley increases passive flexion of the IP joints in the involved digit(s). Through this technique, DIP joint motion is maximized and PIP joint contractures are minimized.

Although these classic protocols are widely recognized, many therapists now combine and/or modify elements of each to manage their patients. Table 18–1 summarizes the differences between the common flexor tendon protocols used with early passive motion.

TABLE 18–1 Tendon Protocols

Protocol	Positions[a]	Theory	Possible Modifications
Kleinert	Wrist: 45° flexion; MP: 40° flexion; IP: dynamic flexion traction	Protect the repair from stress; facilitate active extension against the rubber band to relax the flexor tendon synergistically	• Decrease wrist flexion • Increase MP flexion • Consider a distal palmar guide to increase composite digit flexion vs a rubber band going directly to the wrist crease • Help minimize PIP flexion contractures placed into a modified Duran splint for night use (or use the same splint and strap digits gently into extension)
Duran–Houser	Wrist: 20° flexion; MP: relaxed flexion; IP: dynamic flexion traction	Maintain the digit in relaxed flexion via dynamic traction; prevent stress to the repair	• Strap IP joints into extension for night use to minimize PIP flexion contractures • Consider increasing MP joint flexion and IP joint extension at night by adding an additional piece of foam or wedge between the splint and the dorsal proximal phalanges
Modified Duran	Wrist: 20° flexion; MP: relaxed flexion (~45°); IP: strapped into extension	Prevent and/or minimize PIP flexion contractures	• Consider increasing MP joint flexion and IP joint extension at night by adding an additional piece of foam or wedge between the splint and the dorsal proximal phalanges
Washington	Wrist: 45° flexion; MP: 40° flexion; IP: dynamic flexion traction	Prevent and/or minimize IP flexion contractures via active digital extension against minimal resistance; relax tension on the repair via passive composite flexion; increase passive excursion of the involved tendon	• May use any of the above

[a]All use a wrist/hand/thumb extension restriction splint.

Zones I and II and TI to TIV

Therapeutic intervention for EPM protocols begins 1 to 3 days postsurgery, with removal of the bulky surgical dressing and fabrication of a protective wrist/hand/thumb flexion extension restriction splint. The exact position of the splinted joints depends on the operative factors and associated injuries. For example, associated digital nerve repairs may initially require the involved PIP joint(s) to be positioned in 10 to 30°of PIP flexion. The joint(s) can be gently and serially extended over the following 6 weeks, depending on the surgeon's preference (Cannon & Strickland, 1991). In general, the postoperative splint positions the wrist between 20 and 45° of flexion, the MP joints between 30 and 60° of flexion, and the IP joints in near full extension (Fig. 18-12) (Cannon, 1991; Duran et al., 1978; Stewart & Van Stein, 1995). If the FPL tendon is involved, the thumb should be held in some degree of palmar abduction, with all joints flexed.

For protocols that use rubber band traction, the splint base is the same as described above; however, the digits and/or thumb are dynamically held in gentle composite flexion (Fig. 18-16) (Cannon, 1991; Chow et al., 1988; Dovelle & Heeter, 1989; Evans, 1990 Kleinert & Verdan, 1983; Kleinert et al., 1981; Lister et al., 1977; Peck et al., 1998). Evans designed a protocol for zone I injuries that includes an additional DIP extension restriction splint to further decrease tension on the repaired FDP tendon (Fig. 18–17) (Schenck & Dennis, 1996).

Passive mobilization protocols rely on the patient to perform regular, controlled passive flexion and active extension of the injured and adjacent fingers within the confines of the splint (Cannon, 1991; Duran et al., 1978; Stewart & Van Stein, 1995). At 4 to 6 weeks, the protective splint is discontinued. Many therapists use a protective wrist cuff (or wristlet), recommended by Duran, in place of the splint after this time (Fig. 18–18) (Duran et al. 1978). Worn for an additional few weeks, the wristlet allows full digit extension with the wrist in neutral but prevents simultaneous wrist and digit extension.

Isolated FPL repairs are splinted with the wrist in 20 to 30° flexion, the thumb in palmar abduction, and both MP and IP joints in approximately 15° of flexion (Fig. 18–19) (Cannon, 1991; Cannon & Strickland, 1991). It is important to ensure that the IP joint is flexed, or it may be difficult to regain active flexion later. In cases in which excursion is limited by adhesions, a volar wrist/thumb extension mobilization splint can be fabricated after 4 to 6 weeks (Fig. 18–20).

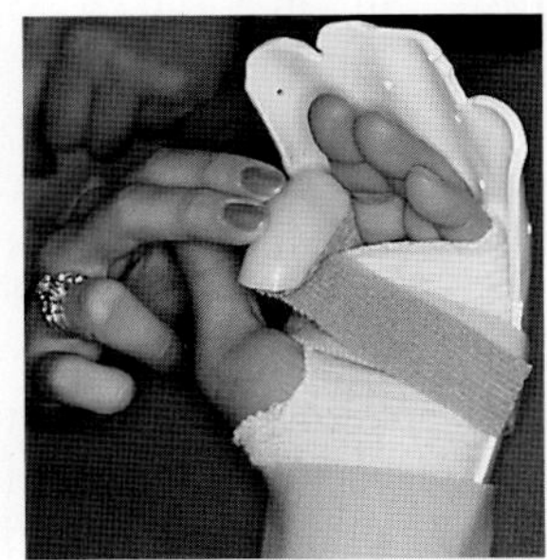

Figure 18–17 A DIP extension restriction splint to position the repaired tendon proximal to the site of the injury, decreasing adhesion formation.

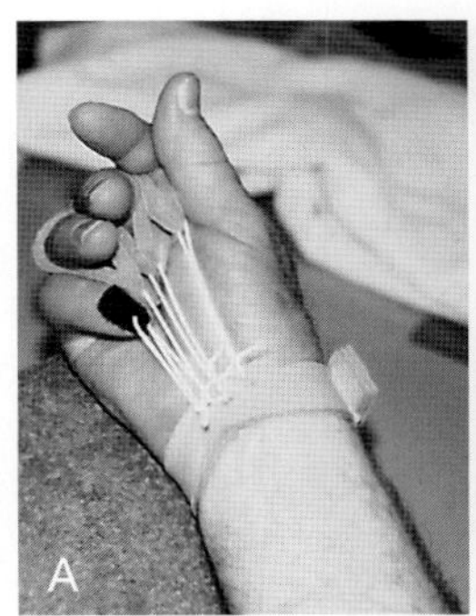

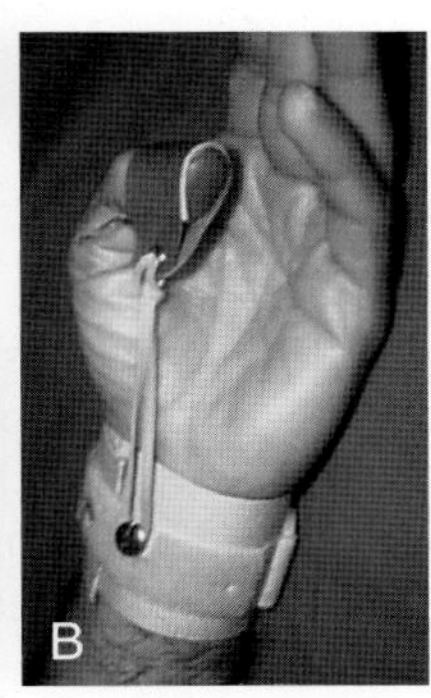

*Figure 18–18 A wristlet is worn during the intermediate phase of treatment with the modified Duran protocol. **A,** The force can be secured distal to the proximal phalanx directly to the nail (SF) or applied via a sling on the proximal phalanges (IF, MF and RF). **B,** FPL repairs can be managed in a similar fashion with a passive thumb IP flexion cuff.*

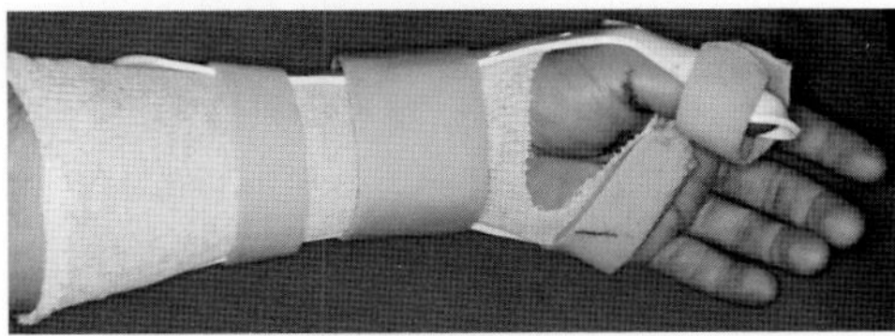

Figure 18–19 Thumb extension restriction splint for a repaired FPL tendon.

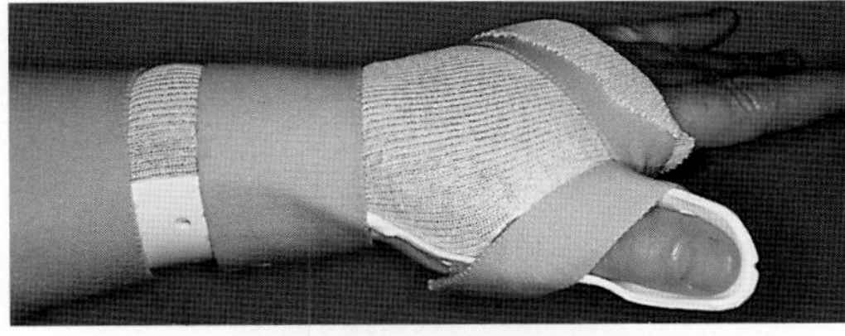

Figure 18–20 A thumb extension mobilization splint gently elongates thumb joint contractures and FPL tightness (serial static approach).

Most EPM protocols advocate initiation of AROM exercises between 3½ to 5 weeks. During this time, joint contractures and extrinsic tightness are also initially addressed. An MP immobilization splint used during exercise sessions after 4 to 5 weeks can sometimes be beneficial to block motion at the MP joints and facilitate stronger FDS and FDP excursion (Fig. 18–21) (Cannon & Strickland, 1991).

Similar to the immobilization protocols, the presence and extent of intrinsic and extrinsic adhesions guide the rehabilitation process during the intermediate and late stages and help determine the appropriate time to discontinue protective and initiate mobilization splinting.

Zones III to V and TV

Tendon injuries occurring in zones III to V tend to have more successful outcomes than those in zones I and II. This may be attributed to absence of the fibroosseous canals in these zones, which create less potential for tendon adherence. Postoperative complications arise when multiple tendons and/or any of the neurovascular structures within these zones are also injured. The decision to incorporate early passive mobilization after injury in these zones is determined by the referring surgeon and follows the same postoperative course as for zone II injuries.

If the ulnar or median nerve has been repaired, splinting may continue for additional weeks to protect the healing nerve. Isolated lacerations to the FCR and/or FCU are usually immobilized for 4 to 6 weeks in a wrist flexion immobilization splint. This splint needs to include only the wrist, which is positioned at approximately 30° of flexion (Cannon & Strickland, 1991). If the median nerve is involved, thumb positioning is critical to prevent possible thumb adduction contractures. A dorsal splint can be used with the thumb positioned in comfortable palmar abduction and opposition (Fig. 18–22). When healing allows, flexible opposition splints made from Neoprene or similar materials can be fabricated to facilitate thumb abduction and opposition. These small splints can optimize position of the hand to improve overall functional performance (see Chapter 19 for details).

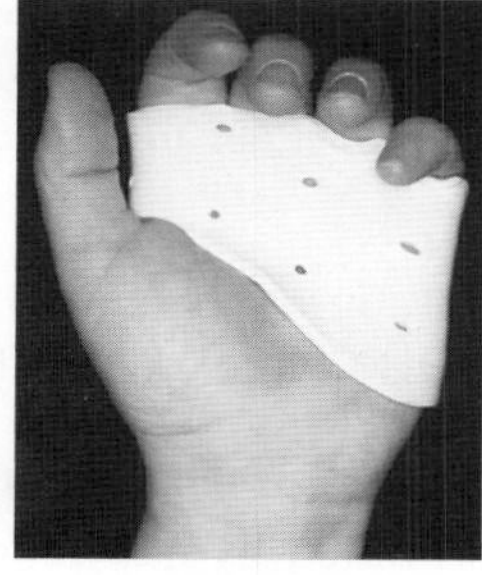

Figure 18–21 An exercise splint can be fabricated to block MP flexion and improve IP flexion. The one shown isolates the FDS and FDP to enhance tendon excursion.

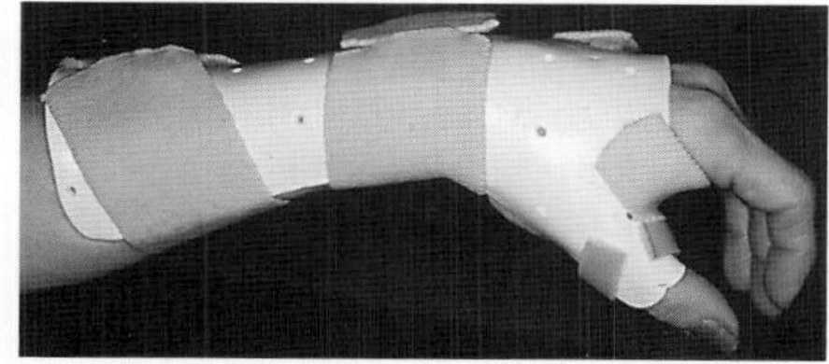

Figure 18–22 A dorsal splint is used to protect a combined repair of the FCR tendon and the median nerve. Note the thumb position in palmar abduction and opposition to maintain first webspace.

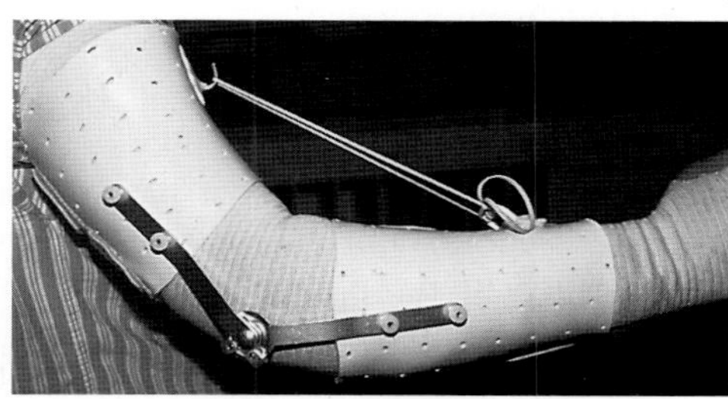

Figure 18–23 An elbow flexion mobilization/extension restriction splint is used to manage a repair of the distal biceps tendon. Note that extension is blocked by the hinge mechanism.

Morrey (1993) advocates an EPM program for distal biceps tendon repairs. These patients are casted for a short period of immobilization (2 to 4 weeks) and then are referred to therapy for a dynamic elbow flexion mobilization/extension restriction splint (Fig. 18–23). The splint positions the elbow in approximately 90° of flexion and the forearm in near full supination. Pain and edema may limit the ability of the patient to achieve full supination; if this is an issue, try to splint in no less than forearm neutral. Incorporating the wrist in the splint is optional, although initial inclusion may help prevent distal splint migration and edema pooling. This splint allows passive flexion through rubber band traction and active extension (permitting limited passive excursion of the biceps tendon) against the rubber band to the splint limits.

Active extension is usually limited to 45° during weeks 3 and 4. As tolerated and per the surgeon's recommendation, small increments of extension are permitted until full extension is achieved. During rest (elbow flexion) two thick rubber bands can be used to position the elbow at 90°. During exercise sessions, only one rubber band is necessary. This lessens resistance to the traction and minimizes distal migration of the proximal segment of the splint. A Figure-8-type shoulder harness can be used to prevent further distal migration of the splint.

Early Active Motion Protocol

The use of early active motion (EAM) protocols was resurrected in the late 1980s (Cullen, Tolhurst, Lang, & Page, 1989; Elliot, Moiemen, Flemming, Harris, & Foster, 1994; Gratton, 1993; Silfverskiold & May, 1994; Sirotakova & Elliot, 1999; Small, Brennen, Colville, 1989; Strickland & Gettle, 1997). These protocols require a suture technique that can withstand the force of controlled active motion without increasing the risk of tendon rupture (Evans, 1997; Strickland & Gettle, 1997). It has been determined that a four-strand core suture combined with certain types of peripheral epitendinous sutures can withstand the force associated with a light composite grip for the entire healing period (Strickland, 2000). Controlled EAM is effective in producing proximal translation of the repair site via active contraction and stimulates intrinsic healing (Kubota, Manske, Mitsuhiro,

Pruitt, & Larson, 1996; Tanaka, Manske, Pruitt, & Larson, 1995). Conversely, with EPM, the tendons are pushed proximally, and there is the potential for folding or bunching up rather than smooth gliding (Kleinert & Verdan, 1983). A study by Elliot and co-workers (1994) found similar results in terms of outcomes and rupture rates as described for EPM protocols. Other studies have determined that the higher rupture rates associated with EAM are largely the result of inappropriate use of the injured hand (Evans, 1990; Harris & Harris, 1999). Early active mobilization is appropriate only if both the surgeon and the therapist have expertise in tendon management and communicate closely with each other. The patient should be motivated, compliant, and knowledgeable about the principles of the rehabilitation program.

Zones I to II, TI to TII

Patients are generally seen in therapy 1 to 3 days post-surgery for fabrication of a wrist/hand/thumb extension restriction splint and initiation of a passive and controlled active exercise program. Wrist position in the splint varies from 0 to 40° flexion, the MP joints are in 45 to 90° of flexion and the IP joints are held in near full extension (Fig. 18-12) (Evans, 1997; Strickland & Gettle, 1997). Some surgeons prefer to apply a plaster cast at the time of surgery; the cast is used during the rehabilitation phase instead of a thermoplastic splint; a removable window is cut out at the volar distal cast to allow for digit exercise. It is wise to be aware of these protocols since many surgeons follow them (Cullen et al., 1989; Gratton, 1993; Silfverskiold & May, 1994; Small et al., 1989).

Evans (1997) uses the zone I protocol described previously, with an active hold component for zone I repairs. For zone II repairs, Evans (1997) recommends a palmar pulley to protect the repair and decrease the risk of PIP flexion contracture with active extension exercises.

Strickland and Cannon developed an EAM protocol based on research that theorizes how combined wrist extension and MP flexion produces the least tension on a repaired tendon during active digital flexion (Savage, 1988). They recommend a resting splint with the wrist in 20° of flexion, the MP joints in 50° of flexion, and the IP joints at 0° between exercises and for the PROM portion of the protocol (Fig. 18–12). The patient is to remove the splint and apply a hinged wrist splint during the place and hold portion of the exercise program (Fig. 18–24) (Strickland, 2000; Strickland & Gettle, 1997). Although this can be an effective approach, the patient must be highly motivated and must thoroughly understand the exercise program. The use of two splints can be cumbersome to some; therefore, patient selection is critical for a good outcome.

Siritakova and Elliot (1999) compared several combinations of suture techniques and splint mobilization protocols before discovering a splint that provides optimal results with EAM of a repaired FPL. The splint holds the wrist in 10° extension and 10° of ulnar deviation, the

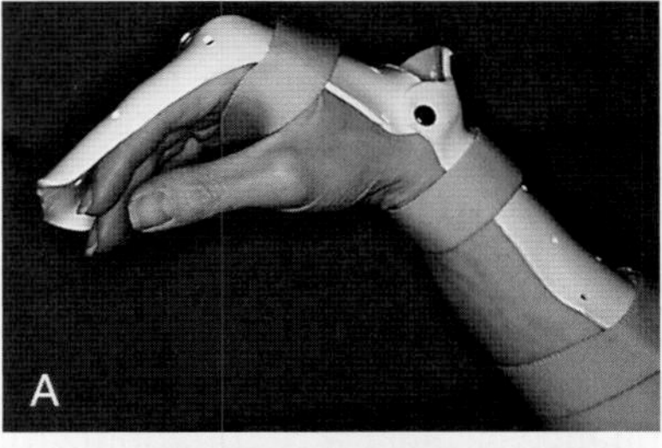

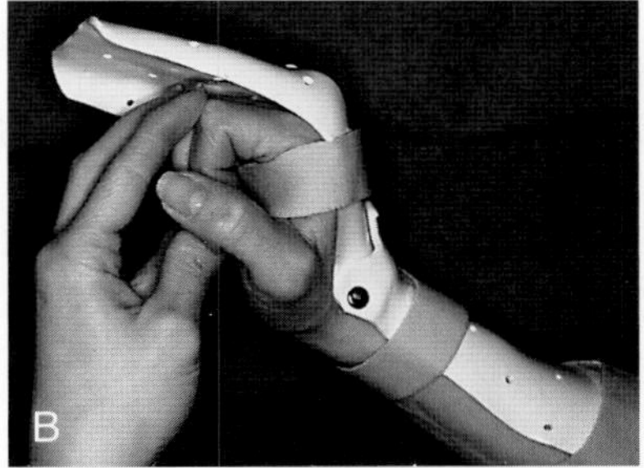

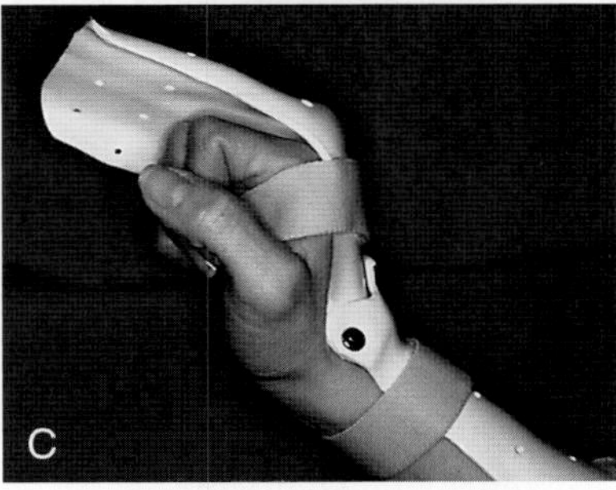

*Figure 18–24 This tenodesis splint allows full flexion of the wrist, but blocks extension at 30°. **A,** Wrist flexion with digit extension. **B,** Passive digit flexion with wrist extension. **C,** Active digit flexion hold.*

thumb in 30 to 35° of radial abduction, the carpometacarpal (CMC) in 10° of flexion, and the MP and IP joints at 0°.

All of these protocols recommend that the splint be discontinued between 4 and 8 weeks and that the patient continue with a guarded graded exercise program. Extrinsic tightness and joint contractures, although uncommon, are addressed as previously described.

Extensor Tendon Management

A postoperative extensor tendon program follows the same guidelines as a postoperative flexor tendon management program. Intervention is divided into three phases—initial (first 3 to 4 weeks), intermediate (4 to 8 weeks), and late (8 to 12 weeks)—and may involve immobilization, EPM, or EAM treatment programs. The referring physician ultimately decides which protocol to follow based on factors such as the nature of the tendon injury, timing of repair, integrity of the repaired structures, and repair technique used as well as other pertinent psychosocial, cognitive, and behavioral factors.

Splint design is critical to minimize stress to the repair site, prevent gap formation, and/or prevent or minimize extensor lag of the involved tendons (Evans, 1991).

Immobilization Protocol

An immobilization protocol for extensor tendon laceration is often the preferred choice of treatment for complex injuries when caring for young children or patients whose compliance is suspect. Immobilization remains the treatment of choice for extensor tendon injuries in zones I, II, TI, and TII and is frequently used for conservative management of closed injuries in zones III and IV. Positioning the DIP (or PIP with zone III and IV injuries) in extension is normally sufficient to restore continuity to the injured tendon.

Zones I to IV and TI to TII

Laceration at the level of zones I and II is often referred to as a mallet or baseball finger. This is a traumatic injury to the terminal extensor tendon; if left untreated, it will result in a DIP flexion deformity and the inability to extend the DIP joint. Uninterrupted splinting or casting of the DIP joint in extension or in slight hyperextension for 6 weeks or longer is a common treatment method (Fig. 18–9) (Cannon, 1991; Doyle, 1999; Evans, 1991). The PIP joint is left free unless a posture of hyperextension develops. In this case, consider inclusion of the PIP in approximately 30° of flexion within the splint to help rebalance the extensor mechanism.

Skin maceration may become problematic under a thermoplastic splint or cylindrical cast. The patient should be instructed to return to therapy for re-evaluation and cast change at least weekly. If thermoplastic material is used to immobilize the DIP joint, the patient should be taught careful splint removable for hygiene purposes. There are several ways to complete uninterrupted splint removal. One method is to have the patient rest the tip on a counter's edge while removing the splint. While maintaining the DIP joint hyperextension position, the skin is inspected and cleansed, after which the splint is carefully reapplied. Once the tendon has healed, gentle guarded AROM into flexion can begin (normally 6 weeks). The patient is often instructed to continue splint use at night and for at-risk activities for an additional 2 weeks.

As with zone I and II extensor tendon injuries, closed zone III and IV (acute boutonniere) injuries generally use a similar immobilization protocol of uninterrupted splinting or casting for 6 weeks. A circumferential, dorsal, or volar immobilization splint or cast can be used to position the PIP at 0° (Fig. 18–25) (Cannon, 1991; Doyle, 1999; Evans, 1991). The DIP can be included if injury to the lateral bands has occurred or is suspected. The DIP is left free when the lateral bands are intact, which helps keep the DIP supple, avoids loss of extensibility of the oblique retinacular ligament, and prevents adherence of the lateral bands (Evans, 1991). Open injuries may require earlier active mobilization to prevent tendon adherence (discussed below).

Immobilization for TI and TII repair of the EPL requires a volar or dorsal immobilization splint maintaining the CMC joint in radial abduction with the thumb MP and IP joints at 0° (IP can be slightly hyperextended) (Fig. 18–26) (Evans, 1991). These splints are worn continuously for 4 to 6 weeks. After that time, protected ROM is initiated, and the patient is gradually weaned from the splint over the next few weeks.

Flexion mobilization splinting may be indicated at 6 to 8 weeks after a zone III or IV injury to address possible PIP and IP/MP thumb extension contractures (Fig. 18–27) (Evans, 1991). At this same time, the therapist should also monitor closely for any developing PIP ex-

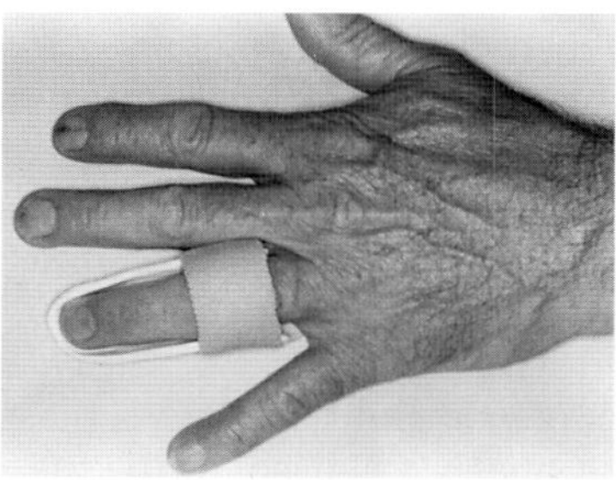

Figure 18–25 A volar digit immobilization splint used for a boutonniere injury (zones III and IV).

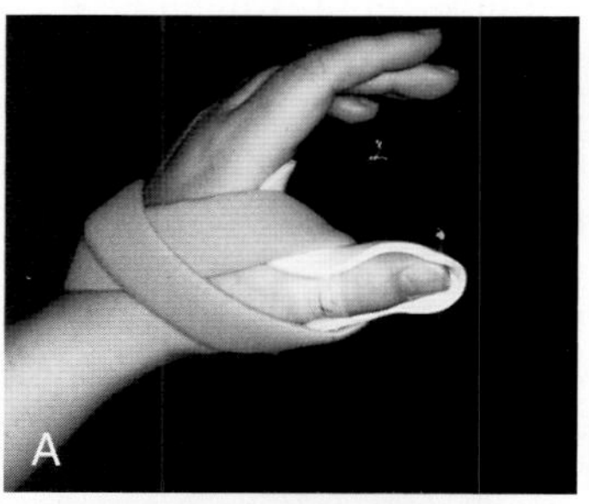

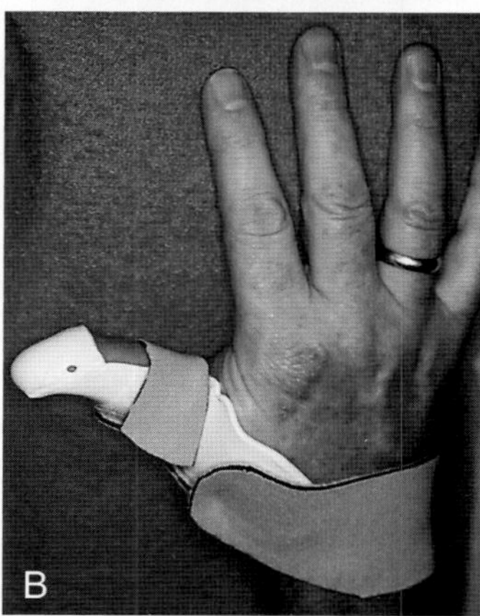

*Figure 18–26 Volar (**A**) and dorsal (**B**) thumb extension immobilization splints used with zones TI and TII EPL injuries during the initial stages of healing.*

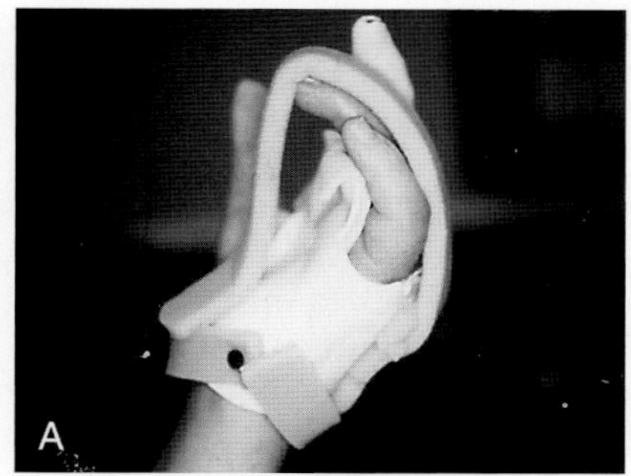

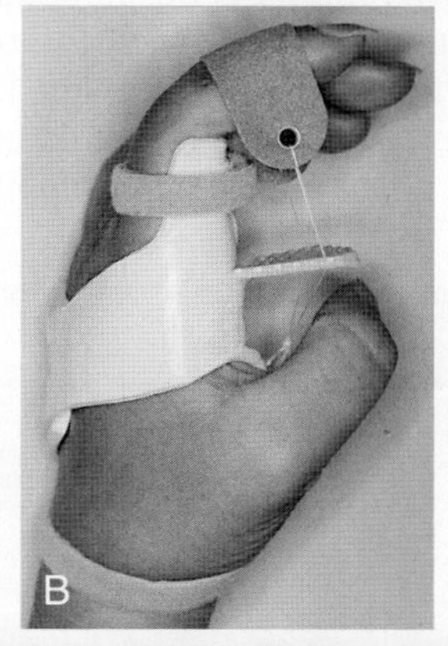

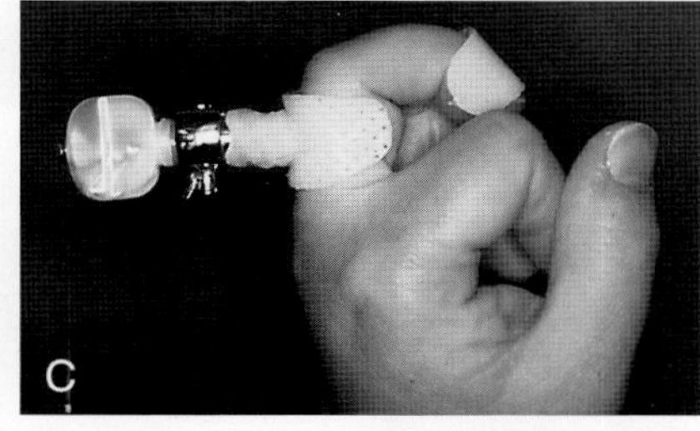

*Figure 18–27 PIP flexion mobilization splints used for PIP extension contractures. Static progressive using soft foam strapping (**A**), dynamic approach with rubber band (**B**), and static progressive (**C**). The patient must have at least 60% of total flexion at each joint, or the splint will slide off the finger.*

tension lag(s) to address overstretching, and/or permanent attenuation of the involved extensor tendon(s).

Zones V to VIII and TIII to TV

Closed sagittal band injuries (zone V) are often treated with about 6 weeks of immobilization splinting in a splint that positions the MP joint at approximately 20° of flexion and in slight deviation in the direction of the injured sagittal band to decrease tension. The IP joint(s) are usually left free (Fig. 18–28) (Doyle, 1999).

Immobilization protocols for extrinsic extensors in zones V to VII recommend that the patient be seen in therapy 3 to 7 days postsurgery for splint fabrication. The splint should position the wrist in 20 to 45° of extension, the MP joints at 0 to 20° of flexion, and the IP joints are free or held at 0° with a removable volar component that can be applied between exercise sessions (Fig. 18–29) (Evans, 1991; Slater & Bynum, 1997). The volar component helps avoid the development of an extensor lag at the level of the PIP joint and helps prevent PIP flexion contractures commonly caused by edema and posturing. Many authors advocate splinting the MP joints in 20° of flexion to prevent contracture of the collateral ligaments. Although this is an important consideration, the therapist must carefully monitor the patient for adverse development of an extensor lag at the MP joint level. If the laceration of the tendon is distal to the juncturae tendinum, the injured finger can be splinted with the MP joint at 0° with the adjacent MP joints splinted in approximately 30° of flexion. This position reduces the tension on the EDC by advancing the proximal end of the severed tendon via the juncturae (Fig. 18–30) (Evans, 1991).

Isolated EPL repairs can be managed postoperatively by splinting or casting the wrist in 30° of extension, the CMC joint in midradial abduction, and the MP and IP joints of the thumb as close to 0° as possible for 4 to 6 weeks (Fig. 18–31) (Evans, 1991; Slater & Bynum, 1997). Care should be taken to avoid excessive pressure on the radial sensory nerve when molding the splint about the radial aspect of the wrist.

Gentle flexion mobilization splinting for MP joint stiffness can be initiated as early as 4 to 6 weeks with the wrist in extension (check with physician prior to initia-

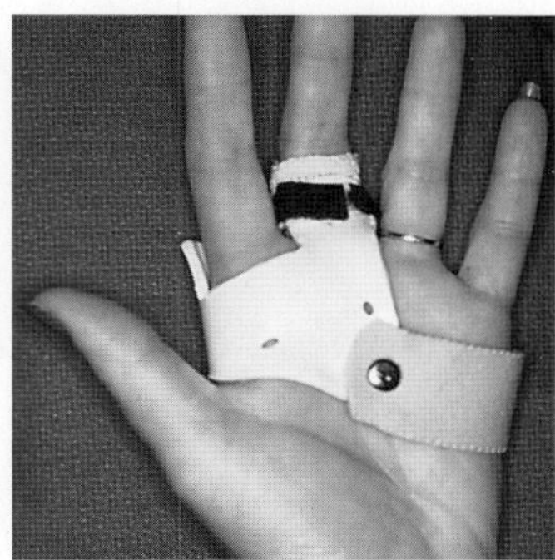

Figure 18–28 MP immobilization splint used with closed sagittal band injuries. This can often be effective if the patient is seen acutely after injury. If surgery is required, the patient wears the splint for 3 to 4 weeks postsurgery; then the patient wears buddy straps for an additional 4 weeks to protect against abduction forces.

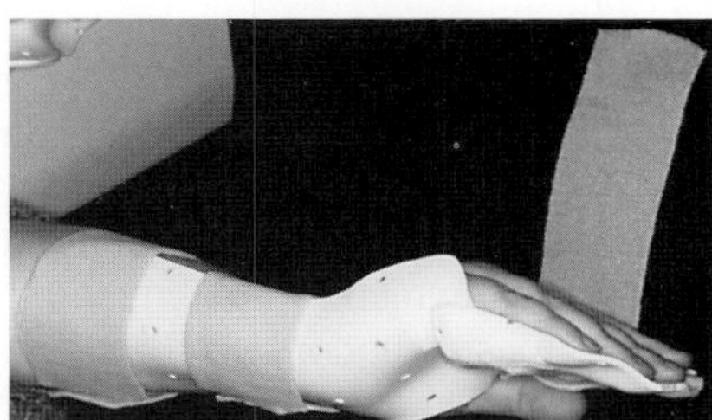

Figure 18–29 A volar wrist/MP extension immobilization splint used for zone V to VII extensor tendon lacerations. An IP joint extension component can be applied at night to minimize IP joint flexion contractures.

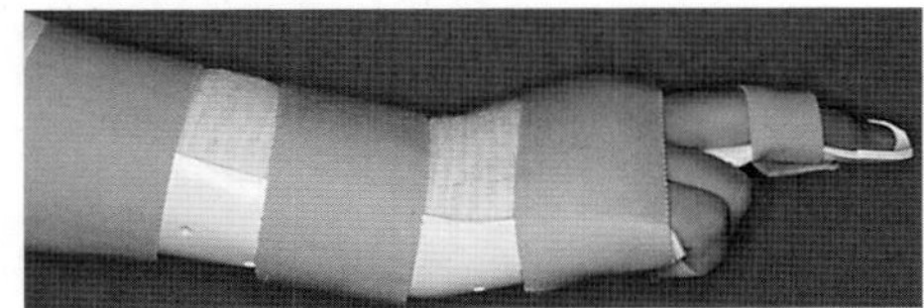

Figure 18–30 *This extended position of the middle finger relieves stress at the anastomosis while allowing gentle flexion of the adjacent digits to prevent collateral ligament shortening.*

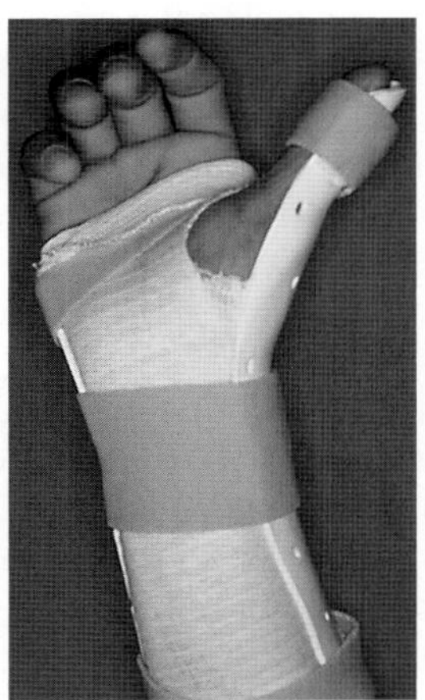

Figure 18–31 *A dorsal extension immobilization splint used for an EPL repair in zones TIV and TV.*

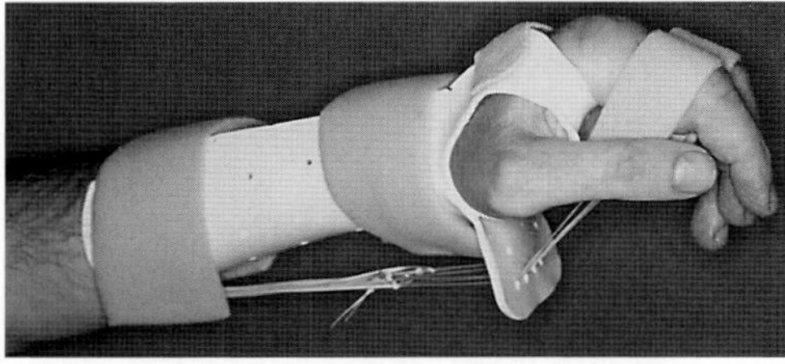

Figure 18–32 *An MP flexion mobilization splint to mobilize adherent extensor tendons and shortened collateral ligaments.*

tion of mobilization splinting) (Fig. 18–32). This splint is worn only as a daytime intermittent exercise splint and its effectiveness is monitored closely and adjusted as necessary. The original protective splint is discontinued at approximately 6 weeks.

Extra care must be taken when immobilizing the repaired thumb and digital extensors in zones VII and TV. This is the location of the extensor retinaculum, and prolonged immobilization may create dense adhesions between the tendons and the fibroosseous canals. Therapists should also be aware of potential disruption of the retinaculum with a laceration, which can potentially lead to bowstringing of the extensor tendons at the wrist level, presenting as an extensor lag at the MP level (Evans, 1991).

Though complete immobilization is not the treatment of choice for zones V to VII and TV, it may be necessary with young or noncompliant patients. Injuries to the ECRL, ECRB, and ECU in zone VII are typically immobilized in a cast with the wrist extended to 40 to 45° for 4 to 5 weeks (Doyle, 1999). Gentle range of motion is initiated at that time, and the splint is continued at night for approximately 2 more weeks.

For injuries to zone VIII and the proximal muscle bellies, the sutures are not strong enough to permit early mobilization (Doyle, 1999). Repairs to this area should be splinted or casted for 4 weeks with the wrist at 30 to 45° of extension, the MP joints at 10 to 20° of flexion, and the IP joints free (Fig. 18–33C) (Cannon, 1991; Doyle, 1999). If the EPL is also involved, the thumb is positioned in extension and midradial abduction. The elbow is immobilized at 90° if the injured muscles arise at or above the lateral epicondyle (Doyle, 1999). Protected ROM is started at 4 weeks, and a protective night wrist extension immobilization splint is

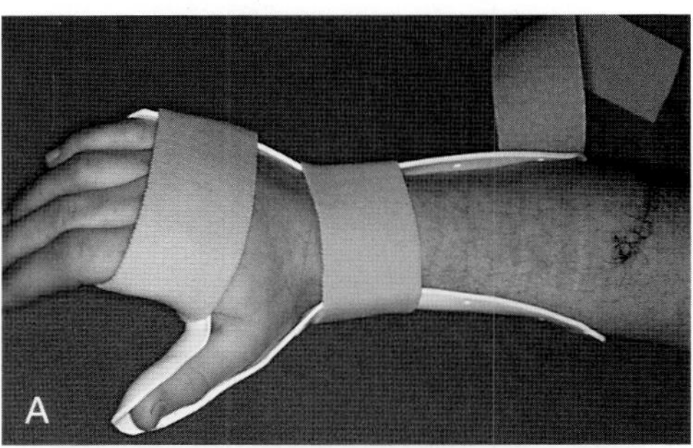

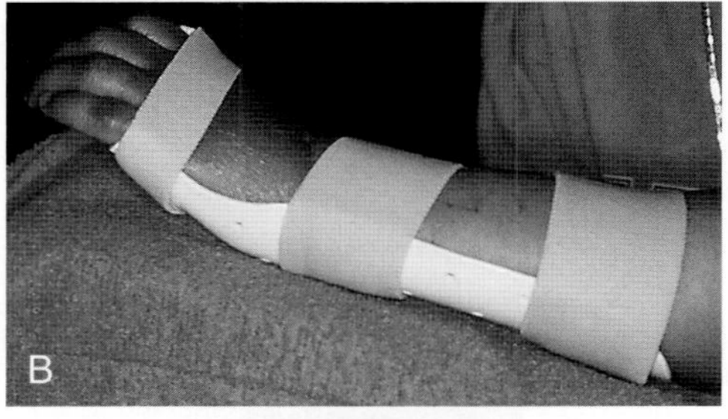

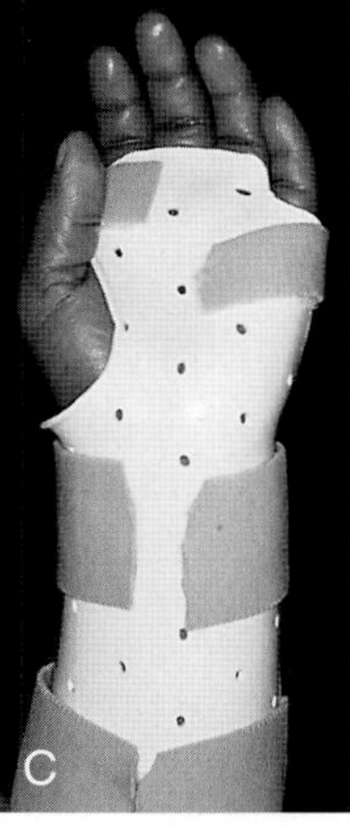

Figure 18–33 *Management of a proximal forearm (zone VIII) tendon laceration.* ***A,*** *A wrist/thumb extension immobilization splint is used to hold the MP joints from 0 to 20° of flexion.* ***B,*** *A wrist/MP extension immobilization splint. Note the extended position of wrist.* ***C,*** *Note the clearance for unrestricted IP range of motion accommodates differing heights of the digit flexion creases.*

typically used for 2 more weeks. Mobilization splinting for the wrist and/or MP joints can begin after 6 weeks if extrinsic extensor tightness is present (Fig. 18–32).

Early Passive Motion

Optimally, early mobilization protocols are used with most patients. Protected motion elicits gliding of the repaired tendon(s) to maximize tendon excursion, increase tensile strength, minimize formation of adhesions, and improve vascularity (Evans, 1991; Gelberman et al., 1986; Hitchcock et al., 1987; Woo et al., 1981). Early passive motion is desirable with extensor tendons for the same reasons it is advocated for flexor tendons. These factors are all important to maximize the functional outcome. EPM for extensor tendons can be accomplished via restrictive splinting, as done with the modified Duran protocol for flexor tendons, or by using mobilization splinting.

Zones III to VII and TIV to TV

EPM protocols for zones III and IV most often use a hand-based, dorsal splint that supports the MP joint at 0° and some type of dynamic traction to position the PIP at 0° (Fig. 18–34). A line stop or bead can be applied to limit the excursion of PIP flexion (Thomes & Thomes, 1995; Walsh, Rinehimer, Muntzer, Patel, & Sitler, 1994). The stop bead can be adjusted weekly to allow more flexion progressively, until the splint is discontinued after 4 to 5 weeks. A basic hand-based digit extension immobilization splint is fabricated for night use to maintain full extension. Exercises are progressed, and PIP flexion mobilization splinting is initiated after 6 weeks, if indicated (Walsh et al., 1994).

Repaired extensor tendons in zones V and VII are usually seen in therapy 0 to 5 days after surgery for fabrication of a dorsal digit extension mobilization splint. This splint positions the wrist at 30 to 45° of extension, and the MP and IP joints in 0° of extension via dynamic traction. Take care to avoid placing the ulnar MP joints in hyperextension through the dynamic tension. This posturing can jeopardize the mechanics of the arch system of the hand and may contribute to MP collateral ligament shortening (Evans, 1991).

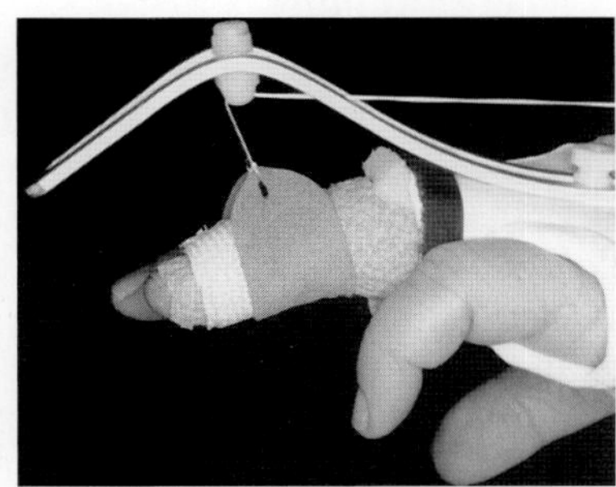

Figure 18–34 *A PIP extension mobilization splint is used for zones III and IV extensor tendon injuries. The position of the MP joint should be near full extension.*

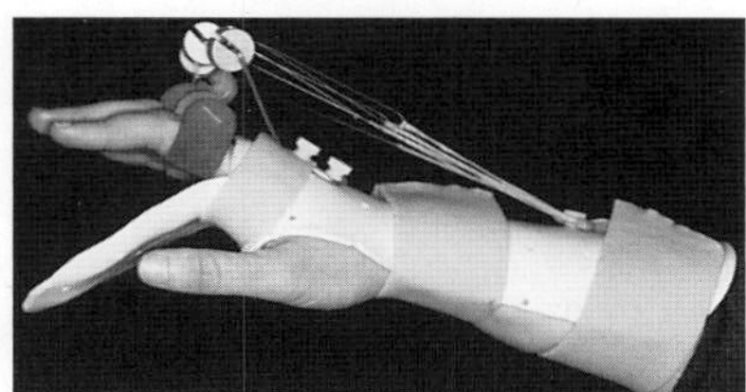

Figure 18–35 *A dynamic MP extension mobilization/flexion restriction splint used for an EPM program for zone V to VII extensor tendon repair.*

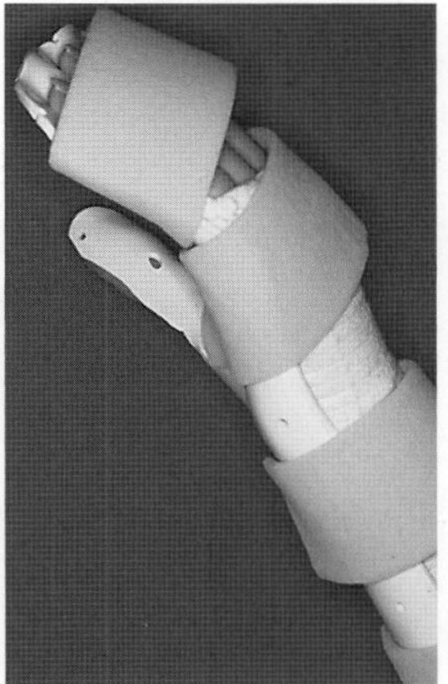

Figure 18–36 *A wrist/hand extension immobilization splint is worn during rest to complement an EPM program for zone V to VII extensor tendon repair.*

A volar MP flexion block splint can be fabricated and then attached onto the dorsal splint to limit MP flexion during exercise (Fig. 18–35) (Cannon, 1991; Evans & Thompson, 1997; Taras, Skahen, Raphael, Marzyk, & Bauerle, 1996). The addition of a volar block splint allows the safe passive mobilization of the extensor tendons through the action of the contracting flexors tendons. Restricting MP flexion can also be accomplished by applying a line stop or bead to the static line, limiting flexion as the line stop abuts the pulley. The suggested general initial limits of allowable MP flexion are IF and MF 30° and RF and SF 35° (Cannon, 1991). Evans and Thompson (Evans, 1991; Evans & Thompson, 1997) prefer a moving outrigger (made from spring steel) rather than a static outrigger (made from rolled thermoplastic or commercially purchased), because it offers less resistance to active flexion with AROM.

During rest periods and sleep, patients use a wrist/hand immobilization splint with the wrist at 30 to 40° of extension, the MP joints at 0 to 10° flexion. and the IP joints in neutral (Fig. 18–36) (Cannon, 1991). Gentle flexion mobilization splinting of the MP and wrist joints may be initiated at 6 to 8 weeks to address extrinsic extensor tightness that may be limiting composite flexion.

EPL repairs in zone IV or V are splinted with the wrist in approximately 40° of extension, the CMC joint in midradial abduction, the MP joint at 0°, and the IP joint held at 0° or slight hyperextension. A volar block splint or line stop can also be applied for the same reasons as noted earlier, restricting flexion of the thumb MP and IP joints. Evans and Thompson (Evans, 1991; Evans & Thompson, 1997) recommend a maximum of 60° of IP flexion (Fig. 18–37). The volar component is discontinued at 3 to 3½ weeks, and exercises are progressed. Protective splinting should continue for another 2 to 3 weeks. Mobilization splinting can begin at 6 to 8 weeks for extrinsic tendon and capsular tightness, if necessary.

Early Active Motion

The trend toward EAM of tendons has progressed as tendon suture techniques have improved. Active contraction of the muscle/tendon unit is the only way to ensure true proximal migration of a repaired tendon. Many studies conducted by Evans and co-workers revealed that extensor tendons treated with EAM demonstrated modest to significant improvement compared to those treated with EPM or immobilization, respectively (Evans, 1991; Evans & Thompson, 1993). Similar to flexor tendon early active motion programs, patient selection is crucial. Patients participating in EAM protocols must be motivated and compliant to prevent tendon rupture and maximize functional gains.

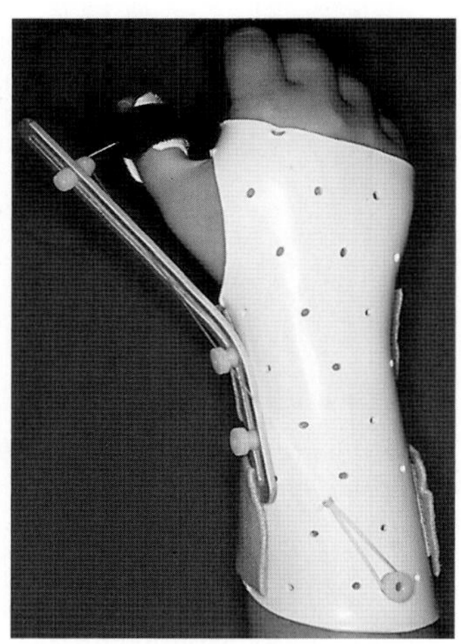

Figure 18–37 A dorsal thumb extension mobilization splint is used for an early passive mobilization program for an EPL repair.

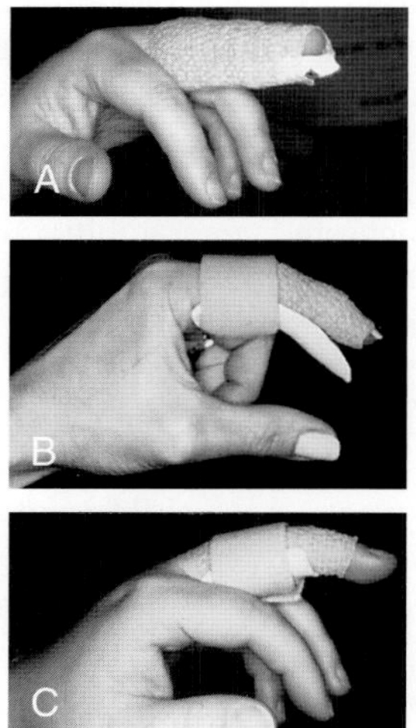

*Figure 18–38 Three splints used for the SAM protocol. **A,** A volar PIP/DIP immobilization splint is used between exercise sessions. **B,** The first exercise splint allows 30° of flexion at the PIP joint and 20 to 25° of flexion at the DIP joint. **C,** The second exercise splint blocks the PIP joint so that the lateral bands can glide distal to the repair site.*

Zones III to VII and TIV to TV

EAM for zone III and IV extensor tendon injury is known as the short arc motion (SAM) protocol (Evans, 1991; Evans & Thompson, 1997). This protocol is initiated between 24 and 48 hours postsurgery and uses three splints. The immobilization splint, worn between exercises, positions the PIP and DIP at 0° of extension. Patients are instructed to remove this hourly for controlled active motion, which is delineated specifically in the protocol (Fig. 18–38) (Evans, 1991; Evans & Thompson, 1997). There are two exercise splints. The first is modified biweekly to allow progressive PIP flexion. The second positions the PIP at 0° with DIP free to elicit AROM at the DIP level and to encourage gliding of the lateral bands. The splints are discontinued at 6 weeks unless an extensor lag is present.

The EAM splinting regimens for zones V to VII and TIV to TV are exactly the same as described for EPM protocols. The only difference is the active component occurs out of the splint and under the supervision of a therapist (Evans, 1991; Evans & Thompson, 1997).

CASE STUDY SECTION

The case studies presented here are meant as teaching guidelines only. Treatment and splinting protocols vary greatly from surgeon to surgeon and from therapist to therapist. The therapist must check with the referring physicians and colleagues to define the preferred treatment and splinting methods.

CASE STUDY 1: **FDP Rupture**

ML is a 12-year-old right-handed boy who sustained a closed rupture of the right RF FDP tendon at its insertion site (zone I) while playing football; this injury is referred to as the classic jersey finger. He underwent surgical exploration and repair. The tendon was reattached to the distal stump and secured with a pull-through wire and button on the dorsal nail. The C4 and A4 pulleys were repaired as was the flexor sheath. ML was referred to therapy 2 days after surgery.

A dorsal wrist/hand extension restriction splint was fabricated (the wrist and MP joints in approximately 30° of flexion; the IP joints extended) (Fig.

18–12). ML and his mother were instructed in a passive flexion/active extension program within the confines of the splint for home exercise. Because of patient's age and the severity of the repair, he was seen in therapy three times a week for PROM by the therapist, including wrist tenodesis, PROM of the digit with the splint off, and gentle protected PIP active extension. Wound care, scar management, and edema control were also addressed, as was PROM of the uninvolved digits.

AROM was initiated at 4 weeks. At that time, the splint was remolded to place the wrist in a neutral position. The splint was discontinued except for night use at 6 weeks postoperatively. Blocking exercises, strengthening, and use of the right hand in ADL activities were gradually progressed.

At 8 weeks, ML was fit with a circumferential PIP immobilization splint (Fig. 18–15**A**) to encourage FDP pull through via blocking exercises and to decrease the small residual PIP flexion contracture. The patient was discharged from therapy with full AROM of the RF PIP, and a 25° DIP active flexion deficit (compared to the contralateral RF). He had full hand function, including confident participation in all sports activities.

CASE STUDY 2: **Central Slip Laceration**

TG is a 42-year-old right-handed female who cut her left MF PIP with a knife while camping. Emergency room evaluation the following day revealed a lacerated extensor tendon in zone IV. The patient underwent surgical repair of the MF extensor mechanism and was referred to hand therapy the next day to begin an EAM program. She was shown the use of Coban to aid in controlling edema.

Three splints were fabricated per the SAM protocol, and TG was instructed in a detailed hourly exercise program (Evans, 1991; Walsh et al., 1994). She was first splinted with the PIP and DIP joints in extension in a volar immobilization splint (Fig. 18–38**A**). Both joints were able to rest comfortably at 0°. This was the patient's primary splint and was worn continuously when not using the exercise splints.

Two exercise splints were also fabricated. The goals of these splints were to allow gentle gliding of the repaired central tendon and to apply controlled stress the repair site. The first exercise splint allowed PIP flexion to a maximum of 30°. The second exercise splint allowed DIP flexion (with the PIP extended) to tolerance (Fig. 18–38**A,B**).

TG was monitored in therapy 2 times a week and encouraged to use her left hand in light ADLs while avoiding heavy lifting or grasping. At 2 weeks postinjury, the first exercise splint was remolded to allow increased PIP flexion; however, the therapist monitored for an extensor lag. PIP blocking exercises and light strengthening exercises were initiated after 5 weeks.

Upon discharge from therapy 8 weeks postsurgery, TG had −5° PIP extension and 100° flexion. She was able to resume full work and home responsibilities without difficulty.

CONCLUSION

Treatment of tendon injuries is challenging and provides many opportunities to use clinical reasoning skills. It is critical for the therapist to communicate closely with the referring surgeon, assimilate all the factors associated with a particular injury, and then use clinical judgment to design the optimal rehabilitation protocol.

REFERENCES

Bunnell, S. (1956). *Surgery of the hand.* Philadelphia: Lippincott.

Cannon, N. M. (Ed.). (1991). *Diagnosis and treatment manual for physicians and therapists* (3rd ed.) Indianapolis: Hand Rehabilitation Center of Indiana.

Cannon, N. M., & Strickland, J. W. (1985). Therapy following flexor tendon surgery. *Hand Clinics, 1,* 147–164.

Chow, J. A., Thomes, L. J., Dovelle, S., Monsivais, J., Milnor, W. H., & Jackson, J. P. (1988). Controlled motion rehabilitation after flexor tendon repair and grafting. *Journal of Bone and Joint Surgery (British), 70,* 591–595.

Collins, D. C., & Schwarze, L. (1991). Early progressive resistance following immobilization of flexor tendon repairs. *Journal of Hand Therapy,* 111–116.

Cullen, K. W., Tolhurst, P., Lang, D., & Page, R. E. (1989). Flexor tendon repair in zone 2 followed by controlled active mobilisation. *Journal of Hand Surgery (Edinburgh, Lotham), 14,* 392–395.

Culp, R. W., & Taras, J. S. (1995). Primary care of flexor tendon Injuries. In J. M. Hunter, E. J. Mackin, & A. D. Callahan (Eds.). *Rehabilitation of the hand* (4th ed., pp. 417–431). St. Louis: Mosby Year Book.

Dovelle, S., & Heeter, P. K. (1989). The Washington regimen: Rehabilitation of the hand following flexor tendon injuries. *Physical Therapy, 69,* 1034–1040.

Doyle, J. R. (1998). Extensor tendons, acute injuries. In D. P. Green, R. N. Hotchkiss, & W. C. Pederson (Eds.). *Operative hand surgery* (4th ed., Chapter 51). New York: Churchill.

Duran, R. J., Houser, R. G., Coleman, C. R., & Stover, M. G. (1978). Management of flexor tendon lacerations in zone 2 using controlled passive motion postoperatively. In J. M. Hunter, L. H. Schneider, E. J. Mackin (Eds.). *Tendon surgery in the hand* (pp. 178–182). St. Louis: Mosby.

Elliot, D., Moiemen, N. S., Flemming, A. F. S. , Harris, S. B., & Foster, A. J. (1994).The rupture rate of acute flexor tendon repairs mobilized by the controlled active motion regimen. *Journal of Hand Surgery (Edinburgh, Latham), 19,* 607–612.

Evans, R. B. (1997). Rehabilitation techniques for applying immediate active tension to zone I and II flexor tendon repairs. *Techniques in Hand and Upper Extremity Surgery, 1,* 286–296.

Evans, R. B. (1990). A study of zone I flexor tendon injury and implications for treatment. *Journal of Hand Therapy, 3,* 133–148.

Evans, R. B. (1995). An update on extensor tendon management. In J. M. Hunter, E. J. Mackin, & A. D. Callahan (Eds.). *Rehabilitation of the hand* (4th ed., pp. 565–606). St. Louis: Mosby Year Book.

Evans, R. B., & Thompson, D. E. (1993). The application of force to the healing tendon. *Journal of Hand Therapy, 6,* 266–284.

Evans, R. B., & Thompson, D. E. (1997). Immediate active short arc motion following tendon and nerve repair. In J. M. Hunter, L. H. Schneider, E. J. Mackin (Eds.). *Tendon surgery in the hand* (Chapter 43). St. Louis: Mosby.

Gelberman, R. H., Manske, P. R., Akeson, W. H., Woo, S. L.-Y., Lundborg, G., & Amiel, D. (1986). Flexor tendon repair. *Journal of Orthopaedic Research, 4,* 119–128.

Gratton, P. (1993). Early active mobilization after flexor tendon repairs. *Journal of Hand Therapy, 6,* 285–289.

Harris, S. B., & Harrism D. (1999). The etiology of acute rupture of flexor tendon repairs in zones 1 and 2 of the fingers during early mobilization. *Journal of Hand Surgery (Edinburgh, Latham), 24,* 275–280.

Hitchcock, T. F., Light, T. R., Bunch, W. H., Knight, G. W., Sartori, M. J., Patwardhan, A. G., & Hollyfield, R. L. (1987). The effect of immediate constrained digital motion on the strength of flexor tendon repairs in chickens. *Journal of Hand Surgery (American), 12(4)* 590–595.

Kleinert, H. E., Schepel, S., & Gill. T. (1981). Flexor tendon injuries. *Surgery Clinics of North America, 61,* 267–286.

Kleinert, H. E., & Verdan, C. (1983). Report of the committee on tendon injuries. *Journal of Hand Surgery (American), 8(5 pt 2)* 794–798.

Kubota, H., Manske, P. R., Mitsuhiro, A., Pruitt, D. L., & Larson, B. J. (1996). Effect of motion and tension on injured flexor tendons in chickens. *Journal of Hand Surgery (American), 21,* 456–463.

Lister, G. D., Kleinert, H. E., Kutz, J. E., & Atasoy, E. (1977). Primary flexor tendon repair followed by immediate controlled motion. *Journal of Hand Surgery (American), 2,* 441–451.

Morrey, B. F. (1993). Tendon injuries about the elbow. In B. F. Morrey (Ed.). The elbow and its disorders (2nd ed.). Philadelphia: Saunders.

Netter, F. H. (1987). *The CIBA collection of medical illustrations* (vol. 8). New Jersey: CIBA-GEIGY.

Peck, F. H., Bucher, C. A., Watson, J. S., & Roe, A. (1998). A comparative study of two methods of controlled mobilization of flexor tendon repairs in zone 2. *Journal of Hand Surgery (Edinburgh, Latham), 23,* 41–45.

Rosenthal, E. (1995). The extensor tendons; anatomy and management. In J. M. Hunter, E. J. Mackin, & A. D. Callahan (Eds.). *Rehabilitation of the hand* (4th ed., pp. 519–564). St. Louis: Mosby Year Book.

Savage, R. (1988). The influence of wrist position on the minimum force required for active movement of the interphalangeal joints. *Journal of Hand Surgery (Edinburgh, Latham), 13,* 262–268.

Schenck, R. R., & Dennis, E. L. (1996). Results of zone II flexor tendon lacerations in civilians treated by the Washington regimen. *Journal of Hand Surgery (American), 21,* 984–987.

Silfverskiold, K. L., & May, E. J. (1994). Flexor tendon repair in zone II with a new suture technique and an early mobilization program combining passive and active flexion. *Journal of Hand Surgery (American), 19,* 53–60.

Sirotakova, M., & Elliot, D. (1999). Early active mobilization of primary repairs of the flexor pollicis longus tendon. *Journal of Hand Surgery (Edinburgh, Latham), 24,* 647–653.

Slater, R. R., & Bynum, D. K. (1997). Simplified functional splinting after extensor tenorrhaphy. *Journal of Hand Surgery (American), 22,* 445–45.

Sleeboom, C., & Regoort, M. (1991). Rupture of the distal biceps tendon of the biceps brachii muscle. *Netherlands Journal of Surgery, 43,* 195–197.

Small, J. O., Brennen, M. D., & Colville, J. (1989). Early active mobilization following flexor tendon repair in zone 2. *Journal of Hand Surgery (Edinburgh, Latham), 14,* 383–391.

Stewart, K. M., & Van Strein, G. (1995). Postoperative management of flexor tendon injuries. In J. M. Hunter, E. J. Mackin, & A. D. Callahan (Eds.). *Rehabilitation of the hand* (4th ed., pp. 433–462). St. Louis: Mosby Year Book.

Strickland, J. W. (2000). Development of flexor tendon surgery: twenty five years of progress. *Journal of Hand Surgery (American), 25,* 214–235.

Strickland, J. W., & Gettle, K. H. (1997). Flexor tendon repair the Indianapolis method. In J. M. Hunter, L. H. Schneider, E. J. Mackin (Eds.). *Tendon and nerve surgery in the hand* (Chapter 42). St. Louis: Mosby.

Tanaka, H., Manske, P. R., Pruitt, D. L., (1995). Larson, B. J. Effect of cyclic tension on lacerated flexor tendons in vitro. *Journal of Hand Surgery (American), 20,* 467–473.

Taras, J. S., Raphael, J. S., Marczyk, S. D., Bauerle, W., & Culp, R. W. (1997). Evaluation of suture caliber in flexor tendon repair. In J. M. Hunter, L. H. Schneider, E. J. Mackin (Eds.). *Tendon and nerve surgery in the hand* (Chapter 37). St. Louis: Mosby.

Taras, J. S., Skahen, J. R. III, Raphael, J. S., Marzyk, S., & Bauerle, W. (1996). The double-grasping and cross-stitch for acute flexor tendon repair. Applications with active motion. *Atlas of the Hand Clinics,* 1, 13–28.

Thomes, L. J., & Thomes, B. J. (1995). Early mobilization method for surgically repaired zone III extensor tendons. *Journal of Hand Therapy, 8,* 195–198.

Tubiana, R., Thomine, J. M., & Mackin, E. (1996). *Examination of the hand and wrist.* St. Louis; Mosby.

Walsh, M. T., Rinehimer, W., Muntzer, E., Patel, J., & Sitler, M. R. (1994). Early controlled motion with dynamic splinting versus static splinting for zones III and IV extensor tendon lacerations. *Journal of Hand Therapy, 7,* 232–236.

Woo, S. L.-Y., Gelberman, R. H., Cobb, N. G., Amiel, D., Lothringer, K., & Akeson, W. (1981). The importance of controlled passive mobilization on flexor tendon healing. A biomechanical study. *Acta Orthopaedics Scandinavia, 52,* 615–622.

SUGGESTED READING

Alba, C. D., & LaStayo, P. (2001). Postoperative management of functionally restrictive muscular adherence, a corollary to surgical tenolysis: A case report. *Journal of Hand Therapy, 14,* 43–50.

Durr, H. R., Stabler, A., Pfahler, M., Matzko, M., & Reifior, H. J. (2000). Partial rupture of the distal biceps tendon. *Clinical Orthopaedics and Related Research, 374,* 195–200.

Khandawaka, A. R., Webb, J., Harris, S. B., Foster, A. J., & Elliot, D. (2000). A comparison of dynamic extension splinting and controlled active mobilization of complete divisions of extensor tendons in zones 5 and 6. *Journal of Hand Surgery (Edinburgh, Latham, 25,* 140–146.

Lester, B., Jeong, G. K. (2000). A simple splinting technique for the mallet finger. *American Journal of Orthopedics, 29,* 202–206.

Moiemen, N. S., & Elliot, D. (2000). Primary flexor tendon repair in zone 1. *Journal of Hand Surgery (Edinburgh, Latham), 25,* 78–84.

Purcell, T., Eadie, P. A., Murugan, S., O'Donnell, M., & Lawless, M. (2000). Static splinting of extensor tendon repairs. *Journal of Hand Surgery (Edinburgh, Latham), 25,* 180–182.

Scott, S. C. (2000). Closed injuries to the extension mechanism of the digits. *Hand Clinics, 16,* 367–374.

Strickland, J. W. (2000). Development of flexor tendon surgery. *Journal of Hand Surgery (American), 25,* 214–235.

CHAPTER 19

The need for corrective splintage in peripheral nerve injuries has been recognized for a long time, but only recently has it been appreciated that a good splint should do more than merely prevent deformity, it should also encourage function.

WYNN PARRY

Peripheral Nerves Injuries

MaryLynn Jacobs, MS, OTR/L, CHT

INTRODUCTION

Splinting for **peripheral nerve injury (PNI)** is challenging, thought provoking, and always specific to the individual. This chapter describes splinting management for deficiencies of the three main peripheral nerves: median, ulnar, and radial. Nerve lacerations, common mixed lesions, compression neuropathies, lesions associated with other injuries, and tendon transfers are addressed. A table is provided to aid the therapist in nerve injury identification and appropriate splint selection.

Assessment of the nerve-injured hand requires sound knowledge of functional anatomy, physiology, and kinesiology as well as a thorough understanding of motor, sensory, and vasomotor pathways. With this information, the therapist can recognize abnormalities and determine the appropriate therapeutic and splinting intervention. The therapist must appreciate motor and sensory loss, protection of the healing nerve, prevention of deformity, adaptive techniques, exercise, and continual reassessment of nerve return to achieve the best functional results for the patient (Fig. 19–1).

Definition

Peripheral nerve injuries commonly seen by a therapist are either **traumatic** in nature or as a result of an **entrapment** or **compression neuropathies.** Most traumatic injuries occur in association with other injuries, such as fractures or tendon lacerations. Compression neuropathies usually occur in specific anatomic areas where the nerve is vulnerable as it passes through a soft tissue restraint, such as the median nerve as it traverses beneath the transverse carpal ligament in carpal tunnel syndrome (American Society for Surgery of the Hand [ASSH], 1995; Eaton, 1992; Mackinnon, 1992; Thomas, Yakin, Parry, Lubahn, 2000). A nerve can also be entrapped at more than one site along the nerve's pathway resulting in a **double-crush** or **multiple-crush syndrome** or **phenomenon** (Mackinnon, 1992). Nerves are vulnerable to injury as they pass and/or rub over or between bony prominences and grooves (e.g., ulnar nerve at the cubital tunnel and Guyon's canal). Neuropathies can occur secondary to endocrine disorders (e.g., diabetes or hypothyroidism), hormonal changes (e.g., pregnancy or menopause), electrical injury, traction, ischemia, rheumatoid arthritis, or tumors (Dellon, 1992; Smith, 1995).

A nerve injury produces changes within the nerve itself and in the tissues that it innervates. Symptoms of nerve in-

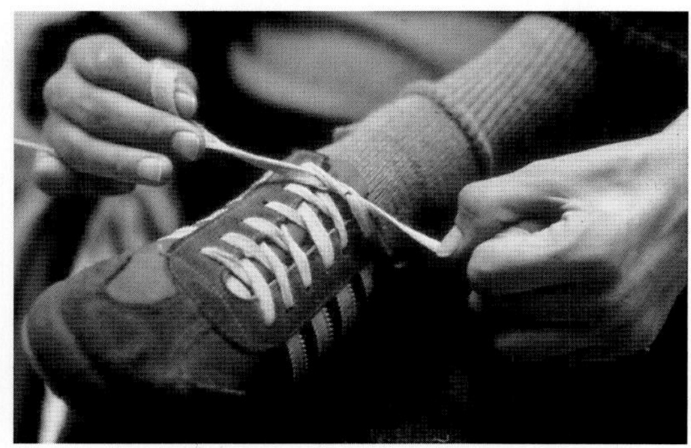

Figure 19–1 Although nerve injuries are devastating, many patients can learn adaptive methods for functioning independently. Note the ulnar nerve atrophy on the patient's left side.

jury include weakness or paralysis of the muscles innervated by the motor branches of that particular nerve and sensory loss to areas innervated by the sensory branches of the injured nerve. Early symptoms of compression neuropathy may be more vague but usually include some combination of pain, tingling, numbness, and weakness. Pain may be sharp and burning with accompanying paresthesias over the corresponding **dermatome** or sensory distribution. These signs may occur proximal and/or distal to the site(s) of compression (Mackinnon, 1992; Smith, 1995). Applying a splint that positions the limb in such a way that tension or compression stress is decreased on the nerve may relieve some, or all, of the nerve symptoms.

Nerve Anatomy

The nervous system is made up of two parts: the **peripheral nervous system (PNS)** and the **central nervous system (CNS).** The PNS consists of the spinal and cranial nerves, and the CNS incorporates the brain, and spinal cord (Carpenter, 1978). The PNS serves as the mediator (or transporter) of neural impulses traveling between the sensory receptors, muscles, and CNS. A bundle of **axons** (nerve fibers) in the PNS is called a nerve, and a network of nerves is referred to as a **nerve plexus.** A collection of nerves outside the cell bodies is a **ganglion.** Peripheral nerve fibers are made of an axon, **myelin sheath,** and **neurolemma** or sheath of **Schwann cells.** After a nerve has been injured, the changes that happen to the nerve are collectively termed **Wallerian degeneration** (Boscheinen-Morrin, Davey, & Conolly, 1985; Carpenter, 1978; Mackinnon, 1994; Parry, 1981; Smith, 1995).

Figure 19–2 shows the anatomy of a nerve cell and its pathway to the target organ. A peripheral nerve is protected by the three layers of connective tissue that surround it (Boscheinen-Morrin et al., 1985). The layers are the **epineurium,** a sheath that encompasses the entire nerve; the **perineurium,** which encloses a small bundle (fasciculus) of nerve fibers and forms a more fragile connective tissue sheath than the epineurium; and the **endoneurium,** a thin connective tissue sheath that surrounds the individual nerve fibers.

Figure 19–3 illustrates nerve injury and regeneration (Boscheinen-Morrin et al., 1985). After any significant neural insult, degeneration of the axon and myelin sheath occurs distal to the injury site. Degeneration also occurs proximal to the injury and to the previous node of Ranvier (constrictions of the myelin sheath). During this process of Wallerian degeneration, the axon atrophies but the connective tissue sheath remains open to accept regenerating axonal fibers.

Different types of nerve lesions result in different prognoses; therefore, it is important to appreciate the effect and extent that each type of nerve injury may have on its respective nerve cell, axon, and target organ. This information is also important for assessing nerve regeneration, applying appropriate splinting intervention, and timely splint modifications. The more proximal the injury, the worse the prognosis is, possibly because there is a greater distance from the site of insult to the target organ (Lundborg, 1988; Moore & Agur, 1995). By the time the regenerated axon reaches the end organ, significant muscular atrophy may have occurred. Regenerated axons may not always find their end organs. For example, a sensory axon may reach a motor plate or visa versa. Age can be a significant factor in potential

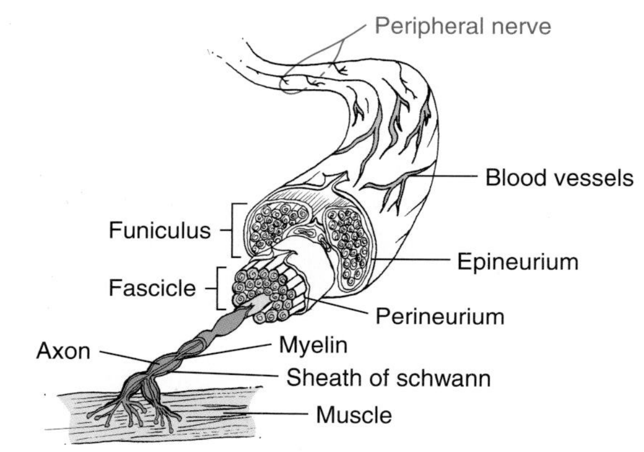

Figure 19–2 Anatomy of a nerve cell and its pathway to the target organ.

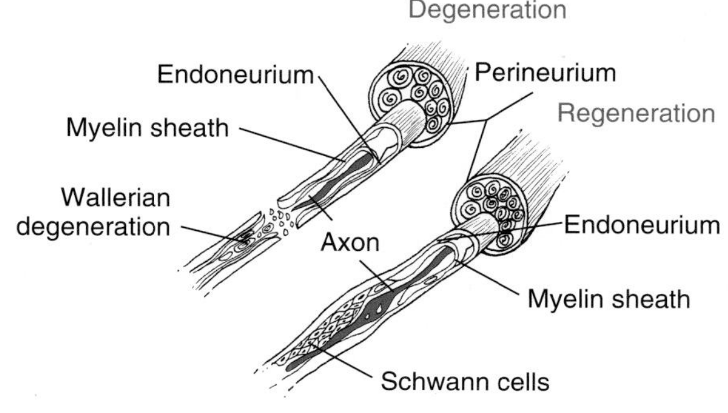

Figure 19–3 Nerve degeneration and regeneration.

nerve recovery. In general, young children have a better functional result than adults. This may be due to the shorter distances axons have to grow to reach their target organ and for the great capacity young brains have to integrate centrally and reorganize incoming information (Parry, 1981). Proximal injury in adults may require that functional or antideformity splints be worn for extended periods of time.

A crush or compression injury may cause damage to the axon but can leave the connective tissue layers of the nerve intact, maintaining a conduit to guide the growing axons to their ultimate destinations. However, when a nerve is severed, the part distal to the injury degenerates, and only careful surgical anastomosis will provide a chance of functional recovery (Lundborg, 1988; Mackinnon, 1994; Moore & Agur, 1995).

Nerve Injury Classification

Seddon (1943) was the first to classify nerve injuries (Smith, 1995), using the terms **neuropraxia, axonotmesis,** and **neurotmesis.** In 1951, Sunderland (1952) expanded this classification to five degrees of injury (Fig. 19–4) (Horn & Crumley, 1984; Smith, 1995). Mackinnon (1994) identified a sixth lesion, a mixed injury that includes normal fascicles with some or all of Sunderland's five degrees.

First-Degree Injury (Neurapraxia)

First-degree injury involves a localized area of conduction block, which is reversible. Recovery is quick, usually complete within 12 weeks. Wallerian degeneration does not occur in neurapractic lesions, because the perineurium is left intact.

Second-Degree Injury (Axonotmesis)

In the **second-degree injury,** damage to the axon occurs and regeneration of the nerve proceeds at the standard rate of approximately 1 mm per day, or 1" per month. An advancing **Tinel's sign** is present. The Tinel's sign is a common technique used to assess nerve regeneration; a gentle tapping is performed along the nerve's pathway, distal to proximal (although many therapists perform this proximal to distal), which, when performed carefully, should elicit poresthesias into innervated tissue (Lundborg, 1988; Mackinnon, 1994; Parry, 1981). The recovery rate for second-degree injuries is slow; yet complete return of function can be expected. If the injury occurs so proximal to the distal target, the time required to reach the end organ makes the recovery pattern slower than normal (Lundborg, 1988).

Third-Degree Injury (Axonotmesis or Neurotmesis)

Third-degree injuries have the most unpredictable degree of recovery, which ranges from almost normal to no

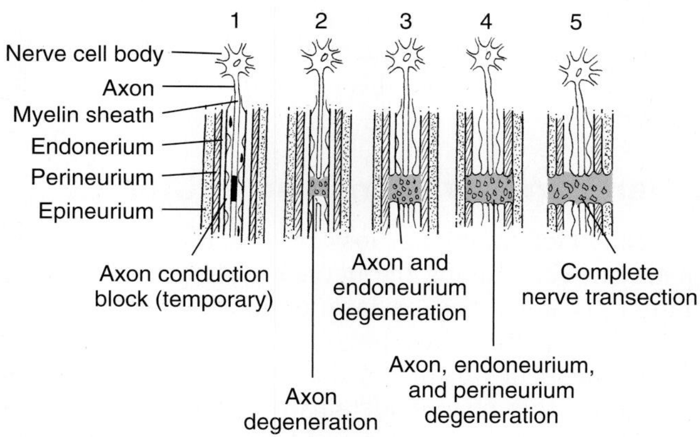

Figure 19–4 Sunderland's five degrees of nerve injury: 1, conduction block; 2, axonal degeneration; 3, axonal and endoneurial degeneration; 4, axonal, endoneurial, and perineurial degeneration; 5, complete nerve transection.

recovery at all. With this type of injury, there is some scarring within the endoneurium, making it difficult for the axon to reach the appropriate receptor. The lesion may be iatrogenic in nature, occurring when a patient sustains a nerve injury during a surgical procedure. These injuries recover slowly, and patients eventually achieve some, but usually not all, function.

Fourth-Degree Injury (Neurotmesis)

In a **fourth-degree injury,** a segment of the nerve is completely blocked by scar. The nerve is in continuity, but only because of the fibrous bond. The internal structure of the nerve is severely damaged. There is no function or nerve conduction through the fibrous block of scar. Surgical repair or grafting is most often recommended.

Fifth-Degree Injury (Neurotmesis)

In **fifth-degree injuries,** the nerve is completely severed. The patient must undergo surgical intervention, which may include direct repair or a nerve graft, depending on the size of the deficit. Functional recovery depends on factors such as the time since injury and/or repair, wound status, patient's age, surgeon's skill, and the degree of tension on the repair.

Sixth-Degree Injury (Mixed Injury or Neuroma in Continuity)

The **sixth-degree injury** is a mixed lesion that includes some normal fascicles in combination with all or any of Sunderland's five degrees of injury (Mackinnon, 1994). This lesion includes several patterns of injury from fascicle to fascicle. The variation in injury can also be seen along the length of the nerve. Complicated upper extremity lesions are often the result of devastating injuries such as gunshot wounds, traumatic crushing and traction injuries, or they can occur from a combination of the above mechanisms. Surgical intervention may include a combination of procedures such as neurolysis, nerve graft, and/or direct repair. Mixed lesions are challenging injuries for the surgeon to treat and the therapist to rehabilitate, owing to the variability of injury, repair, and recovery.

Nerve Innervations and Pathology

The extent of functional loss from a nerve injury depends on where along the nerve's pathway it has been injured. Lesions and/or lacerations are generally referred to as high (injury proximal to the elbow) or low (injury near or distal to the elbow joint). Figures throughout this chapter detail the specific muscles an individual nerve innervates and at what level the innervation generally occurs. There can be variations in nerve innervations that can be functionally significant. Clinicians should be aware of these possible connections and how they may complicate the clinical presentation (Bas & Klienert, 1999). One such example is the link between the median and ulnar nerves in the proximal forearm. The motor portion of the median nerve can communicate with the ulnar nerve; this association is termed the **Martin–Gruber anastomosis.** When this anastomosis is present, a complete lesion of the median nerve may not cause paralysis in all the median-nerve-innervated muscles because some of the muscles may be receiving innervation from the ulnar nerve. This puzzling presentation may make the therapist question whether the nerve has been completely severed (Matloub & Yousif, 1992; Moore & Agur, 1995).

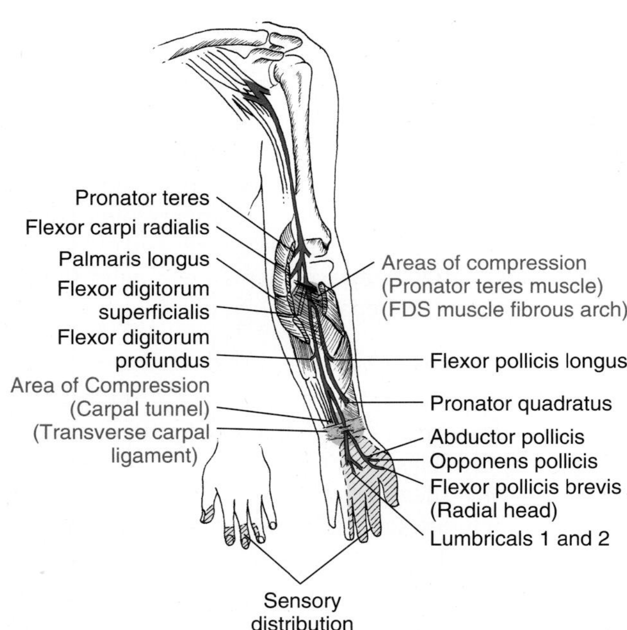

Figure 19–5 The motor portion of the median nerve innervates the majority of the wrist and digital flexors. The sensory distribution of the median nerve plays an integral role in providing sensation to the volar radial aspect of the hand.

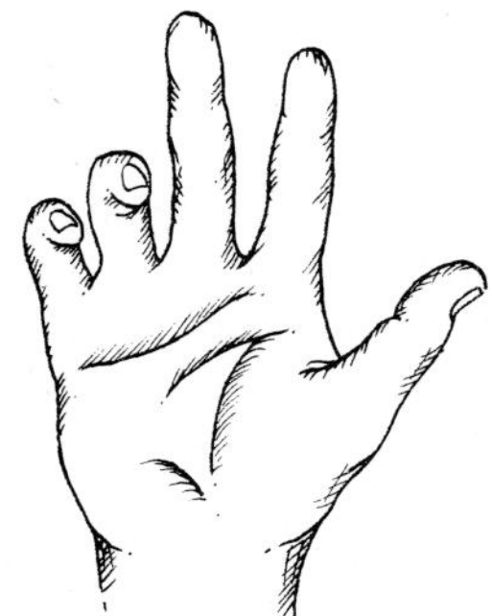

Figure 19–6 A high median nerve laceration causes a peace sign posturing of the hand, owing to the loss of the flexor digitorum profundus (FDP), flexor digitorum superficialis (FDS), and intrinsics of the IF and MF.

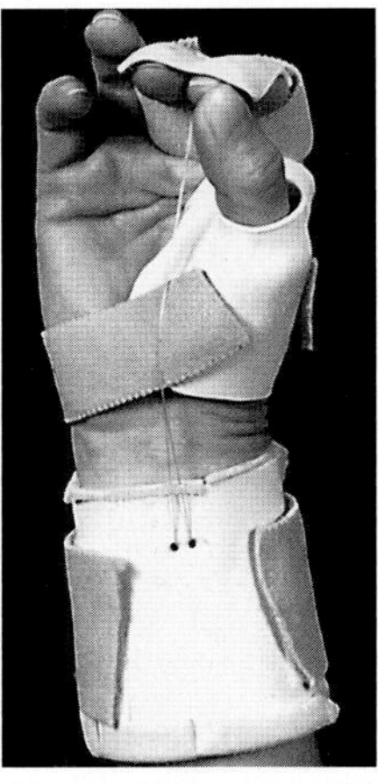

Figure 19–7 A wrist and IF/MF finger extension restriction splint. This tenodisis splint employs power from the radial nerve to allow light functional pinch of the IF and MF to the thumb.

Median Nerve Injuries

High Laceration

High median nerve injury is often associated with traumatic injury of the upper extremity, which may include several neurovascular structures (Fig. 19–5). Clinical signs of isolated high median nerve injury are a loss of:

- Forearm pronation.
- Wrist radial flexion.
- Independent proximal interphalangeal (PIP) joint flexion from the index finger (IF) through the small finger (SF).
- IF and middle finger (MF) distal interphalangeal (DIP) and metacarpophalangeal (MP) joint flexion.
- Thumb interphalangeal (IP) flexion, opposition, and palmar abduction.
- Thumb MP flexion weakness caused by the partial innervation of the flexor pollicis brevis (FPB) radial head.
- Sensation to the volar radial aspect of the hand.

The hand will posture in a **peace sign**-like posture (Fig. 19–6). This devastating injury robs the hand of normal function. Rehabilitation should involve preservation of joint range of motion (ROM), education on sensory precautions, and careful splinting intervention to maximize function and prevent deformity (Fig. 19–7).

Low Laceration

Low median nerve injury, at the level of the wrist, may be associated with flexor tendon injury. Motor, sensory, and sometimes vascular innervation to all structures distal to the injury site may be affected. In this laceration, there may loss of:

- IF and MF MP flexion (lumbricals IF and MF).
- Thumb opposition and palmar abduction.
- Thumb MP flexion (weakness caused by partial innervation of the FPB radial head).
- Sensation to the volar radial aspect of the hand.

The sensory loss is extremely disabling because there is no sensory input to the majority of the volar surface of the hand. The clinical presentation of this injury is often referred to as **ape hand** because of the loss of stabilizing thenar musculature to the volar radial aspect of the hand (Fig. 19–8).

If wrist, thumb, or digital flexor tendons are involved, treatment includes a wrist/hand flexion immobilization or restriction splint (dorsal blocking splint) to decrease tension on the nerve repair and associated soft tissue structures (Fig. 19–9). If the median nerve was repaired in isolation, a splint that positions the radial aspect of the wrist and MPs in flexion (allowing IP motion) with the thumb in opposition and palmar abduction is often acceptable (Fig. 19–10). When healing allows (at 4 to 6 weeks), a small opposition strap can be used to enhance and facilitate opposition (Fig. 19–11). Splinting is used in combination with the referring physician's postoperative protocol, which may include such techniques as wound care, edema reduction, and guarded active or passive ROM.

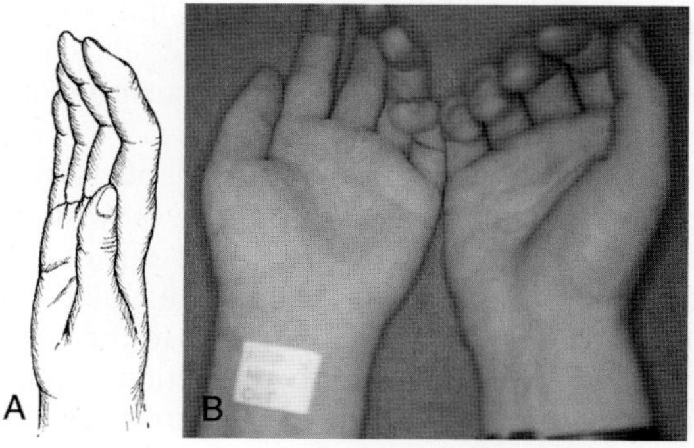

Figure 19–8 *A low median nerve laceration leaves an ape-like hand.*

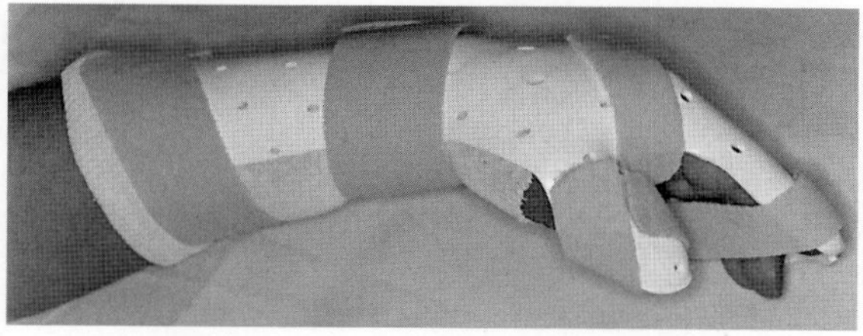

Figure 19–9 *A wrist/hand flexion immobilization or restriction splint (dorsal blocking splint).*

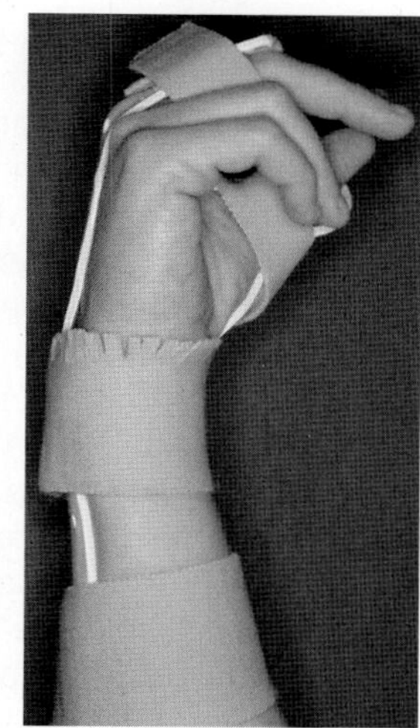

Figure 19–10 *A wrist/MP flexion, thumb opposition/abduction immobilization splint to protect an isolated median nerve repair.*

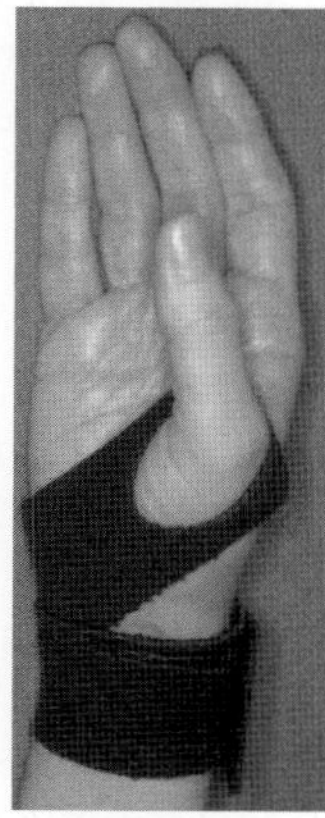

Figure 19–11 *A simple strap can be used to allow functional opposition. This Neoprene strap allowed an OB/GYN surgeon to resume limited work activities.*

Compression Neuropathies

PRONATOR SYNDROME

In the volar, proximal forearm region, the median nerve can be compressed by the ligament of Struthers, lacertus fibrosis, proximal arch of the flexor digitorum superficialis (FDS), or pronator teres muscle (Eversmann, 1992; Hartz, Linscheild, Gramse, & Daube, 1981). Compression in this region is referred to as **pronator syndrome.** Symptoms may include intermittent or consistent pain and parerethises in the volar forearm and hand, which increases with active use or provocative positioning. The thenar muscles may feel weak and fatigued with only an occasional loss of sensation in the median nerve distribution of the hand. There is often a positive Tinel's sign in the volar forearm, negative **Phalen's and reverse Phalen's tests** (positioning in extreme wrist flexion/extension creating parerethises in the median nerve distribution), pain with resistive pronation, and pain in the forearm with resistance to the flexor digitorum superficialis (FDS) of the MF and ring finger (RF).

Pronator syndrome is often seen in patients who do heavy manual labor; those whose jobs require resistive, repetitive forearm rotation; and in musicians who maintain awkward postures or bear the weight of their instruments on their hands for long periods of time (Charness, 1992; Eversmann, 1992; Mackinnon & Novak, 1997). Care must be taken to examine and rule out carpal tunnel syndrome and cervical radiculopathy. Splinting management is usually in combination with rest, activity modification, appropriate therapeutic modalities, gentle nerve gliding exercises, and anti-inflammatory medication. Suggested splint positioning includes elbow flexion, forearm pronation, and wrist neutral.

ANTERIOR INTEROSSEOUS NERVE SYNDROME

The anterior interosseous nerve (AIN) is a motor branch of the median nerve, originating 5 to 8 cm distal to the level of the lateral epicondyle (Lundborg, 1988). **Anterior interosseous nerve syndrome** is purely a motor lesion and may occur secondary to trauma (fracture, puncture, compression), vascular insult, or compression under tendinous bands. Symptoms can include weakness or paralysis of the flexor pollicis longus (FPL), FDP of the IF and MF, and pronator quadratus muscle. Injury to the AIN results in the inability to perform tip and three-point pinch properly (Eversmann, 1992). If the patient is unable to make the okay sign, it is likely he or she has AIN loss (Fig. 19–12).

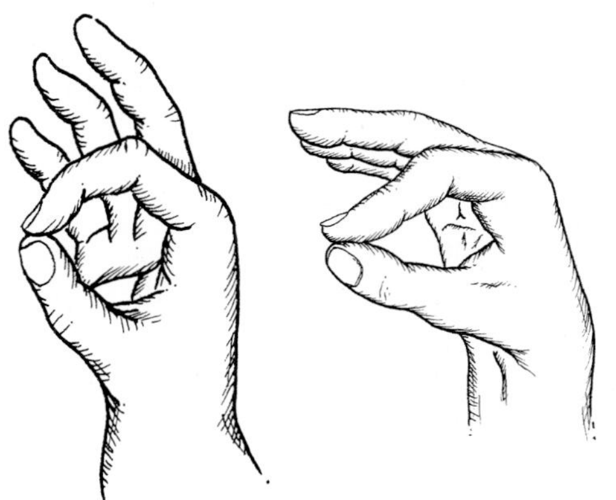

Figure 19–12 With an AIN injury, loss of thumb IP and IF DIP flexion results in the inability to perform the okay sign.

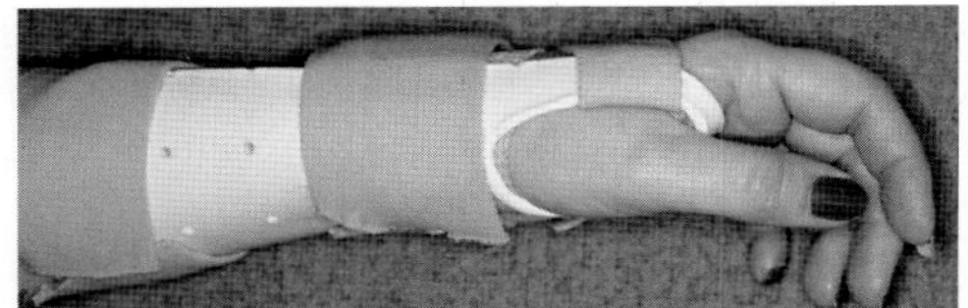

Figure 19–13 When the median nerve is compressed at the level of the wrist, a splint that positions the wrist in neutral can decrease symptoms.

Splinting intervention is not common but may be considered to prevent thumb IP, IF, and sometimes MF DIP extension contractures if applicable. If nerve regeneration is not noted after a reasonable amount of time, other treatment options for complete loss of this branch may be considered, including surgical decompression or tendon transfer.

CARPAL TUNNEL SYNDROME

Carpal tunnel syndrome (CTS) may be recognized as one of the most common compression neuropathies of the upper extremity. The carpal tunnel is a narrow space in which the median nerve and nine digital flexor tendons traverse. The tunnel is bordered on three sides by carpal bones and on the volar aspect by the thick, dense **transverse carpal ligament** (Lundborg, 1988). This narrow space is just wide enough for the structures within it to pass. Any additional pressure, inflammation, or obstacle—such as an osteophyte or scar tissue—within this space, may cause compression of the nerve. Compression of the median nerve at this level may occur owing to a multitude of factors, including inflammatory conditions, metabolic disorders, status post fracture or dislocation of the distal radioulnar joint, and tenosynovitis of the digits and wrist flexors caused by arthritis or repetitive stress motions (Lundborg, 1988).

Initially, the patient may experience nocturnal burning pain and paresthesias, clumsiness with routine tasks (e.g., drying hair, taking dishes out of the dishwasher), or radiating pain along the volar forearm. Continued compression and irritation to the nerve may result in weakness of thumb abduction, opposition, and the median nerve innervated intrinsics. The patient may have difficulty with fine motor manipulation because of the described weak musculature and the sensory disturbance to the volar thumb, IF, MF, and radial half of the RF (Boscheinen-Morrin et al., 1985). The patient may have a positive Tinel's sign with tapping over the carpal tunnel and a positive Phalen's test. Conservative treatment consists of rest, activity modification, a volar wrist immobilization splint with the wrist in neutral for night use, nerve gliding exercises, and anti-inflammatory medication (Fig. 19–13) (Sailor, 1996). Surgical intervention is an option if symptoms persist.

Ulnar Nerve Injuries

High Laceration

Lacerations of the ulnar nerve at or above the elbow result in loss of (Fig. 19–14):

- Ulnar wrist flexion.
- DIP and MP flexion of RF and SF.
- Abduction and adduction of all digits.
- Adduction of thumb.
- Thumb MP flexion (weakness owing to partial innervation of the FPB ulnar head).
- Sensory loss of the dorsoulnar aspect of the hand, radiating along the ulnar side of the forearm.
- Significant loss of grip and pinch strength.

Clinical signs of chronic **high-level ulnar nerve injury** may include a mild **clawing deformity** of the hand (hyperextension of the RF and SF MP joints secondary to loss of the stabilizing intrinsics, weakened or stretched MP joint volar plates, and overpull of the intact extensor tendons) with a loss of the hypothenar and interosseous muscles (Fig. 19–15). The patient may be unable to adduct the SF secondary to paralysis of the third volar interossei (**Wartenberg's sign**) and abduct the IF owing to paralysis of the first dorsal interossei (Lundborg, 1988). The patient may also exhibit the inability to contract the adductor pollicis; and when combined with the loss of the first dorsal interossei, attempted lateral pinch is significantly impaired. Lateral pinch is compensated for by the median-nerve-innervated FPL, causing extreme flexion of the thumb IP joint during attempted pinch (**Froment's sign**); and with chronic loss of innervation, this clinical picture may eventually include hyperextension of the thumb MP joint (**Jeanne's sign)** (Lundborg, 1988; Parry, 1981).

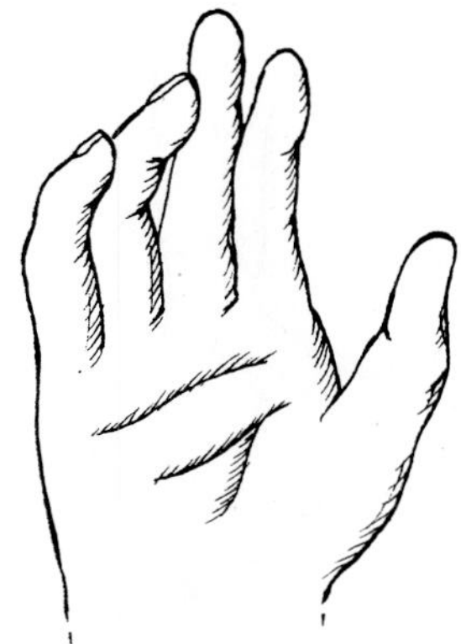

Figure 19–15 A high ulnar nerve laceration does not cause the pronounced RF and SF PIP/DIP flexion posturing that is seen with a lower ulnar nerve lesion secondary to the paralysis of the associated FDP tendons.

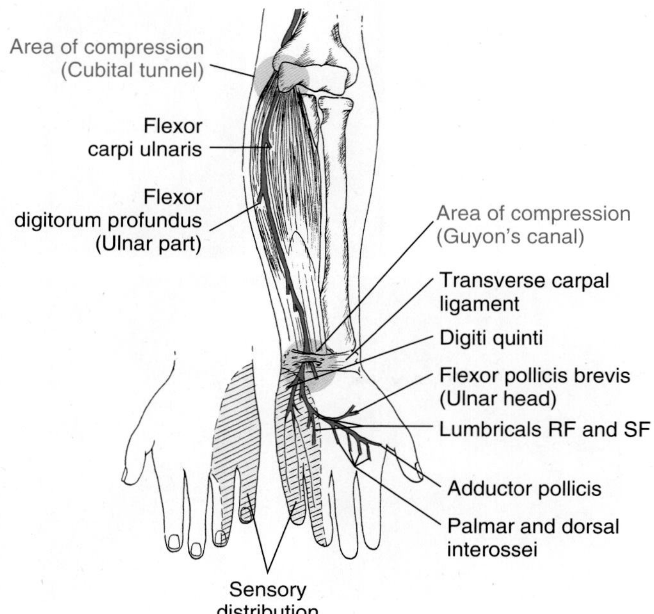

Figure 19–14 The ulnar nerve provides innervation to the ulnar aspect of the wrist and hand. The sensory branches innervate the dorsal ulnar and the volar aspect of the SF and the ulnar half of the RF.

Treatment may consist of education regarding sensory precautions, preservation of ROM, and splinting of the distal extremity to maximize functional use and prevent joint contractures while waiting for nerve regeneration.

Low Laceration

Low ulnar nerve injury, at the wrist, is often seen in combination with flexor tendons, median nerve, and vascular injury. Injury of the ulnar nerve at this level results in loss of:

- MP flexion of RF and SF.
- Abduction and adduction of all digits.
- Adduction of thumb.
- Sensory loss of the ulnar aspect of the hand.
- Thumb MP flexion (weakness caused by partial innervation of the FPB ulnar head).
- Significant loss of grip and pinch strength.

A clawing deformity of the RF and SF is more prominent than with a high lesion, secondary to the intact profundus tendon to these digits (Fig. 19–16**A,B**). In chronic conditions, the patient may progress to the point that the Wartenberg's, Froment's, and Jeanne's signs are present. Splinting the MPs in flexion, can prevent overstretching of the volar soft tissue supports and facilitate functional use while waiting for nerve return (Fig. 19–16**C,D**).

Combined Ulnar and Median Nerve Injury

A **combined median and ulnar nerve injury** can result in a claw hand deformity. In a low lesion, clawing of all the digits occurs secondary to complete loss of intrinsic control and a functioning profundus tendons

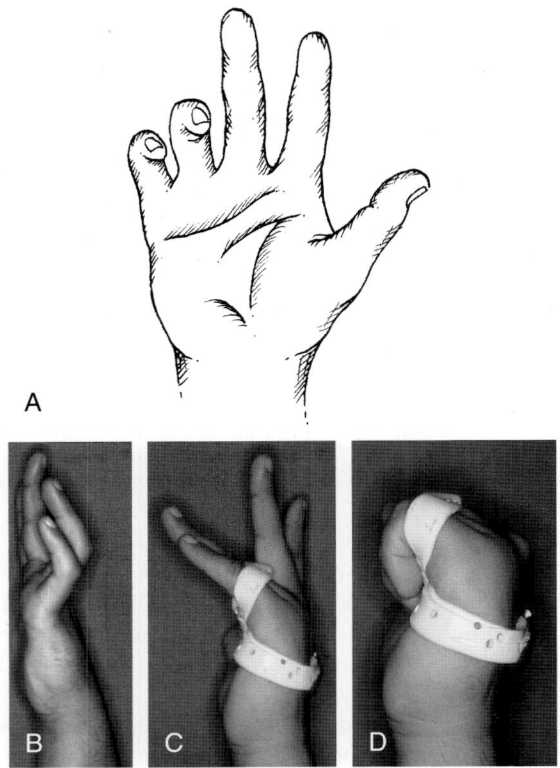

Figure 19–16 ***A and B,*** *A low ulnar nerve laceration leads to partial claw deformity. An RF/SF MP extension restriction splint allows RF and SF digit extension* ***(C)*** *and flexion* ***(D).***

(Fig. 19–17**A,B**). If the injury is high, clawing still occurs but is significantly less pronounced.

Intervention (for high and low combined lesions) includes patient education regarding sensory precautions as well as daytime functional splinting that includes all the MPs in flexion (and thumb abduction/opposition if necessary) to prevent MP joint extension/PIP flexion contractures while providing a position for functional use. Furthermore a nighttime wrist/hand immobilization splint is used to place the structures in an antideformity position while waiting for nerve return (Fig. 19–17**C–E**).

Compression Neuropathies

CUBITAL TUNNEL SYNDROME

The cubital tunnel is formed by a tendinous arch joining the ulnar and humeral attachments of the flexor carpi ulnaris (FCU) tendon. The boundaries of the cubital tunnel are the medial epicondyle, the ulnohumeral ligament, and the fibrous arch formed by the two heads of the FCU tendon (Rayan, 1992). Many factors can cause or contribute to **cubital tunnel syndrome,** a common compression neuropathy, including direct trauma; fracture or fracture and dislocation of the medial or lateral epicondyles; arthritis; a subluxating ulnar nerve; or postural stress caused by sleeping positions, vocational demands, or recreational activities.

The clinical symptoms of cubital tunnel syndrome are paresthesias and numbness in the ulnar portion of the hand and forearm, vague ulnar-sided arm pain that is sometimes described as a sharp radiating pain that may worsen with an increase in activity level, and reported weakness of grip and pinch strength. Novak, Lee, Mackinnon, and Lay (1994) found that the cubital tunnel can be quickly screened by performing an **elbow flexion test** (prolonged elbow flexion positioning resulting in paresthesias along the ulnar nerve distribution) combined with pressure on the ulnar nerve. A positive Tinel's sign over the ulnar nerve at the elbow, sensory changes in the ulnar nerve distribution, decreased grip and pinch strength, and atrophy of the intrinsic muscles of the hand are also common indicators (Novak et al., 1994). In some cases, chronic compression may lead to positive Wartenberg's, Froment's, and Jeanne's signs. The differential diagnosis should rule out thoracic outlet syndrome, C8/T1 nerve root compression, and compression of the ulnar nerve distally at the Guyon's canal.

Conservative management usually involves rest, and avoidance of provocative activities (e.g., prolonged elbow flexion, repetitive elbow flexion/extension, and weight bearing on the medial elbow), gentle nerve gliding exercises, anti-inflammatory medication if appropriate, and some type of night elbow immobilization splint

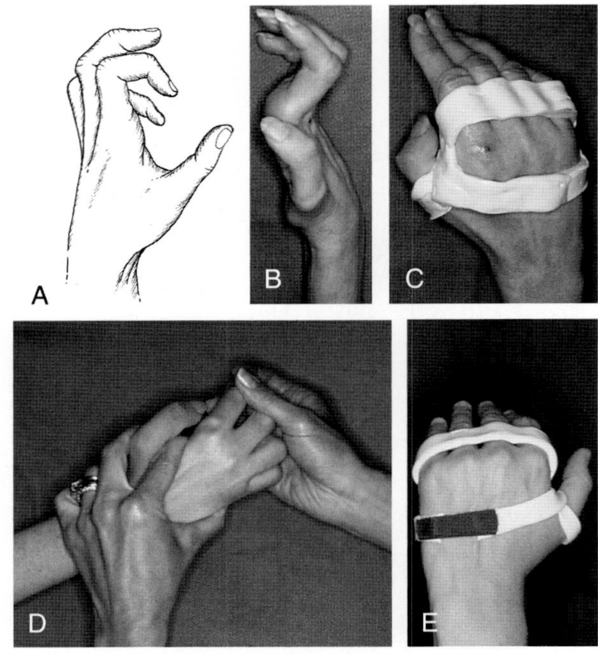

Figure 19–17 ***A and B,*** *A combined median and ulnar nerve injury leads to a claw hand deformity.* ***C,*** *An IF/SF MP extension restriction splint.* ***D,*** *Atrophy of the hypothenar and the first dorsal interossei muscles may cause an indenting along the lateral borders of the hand, making application and removal quite difficult.* ***E,*** *A trap door helps with splint application.*

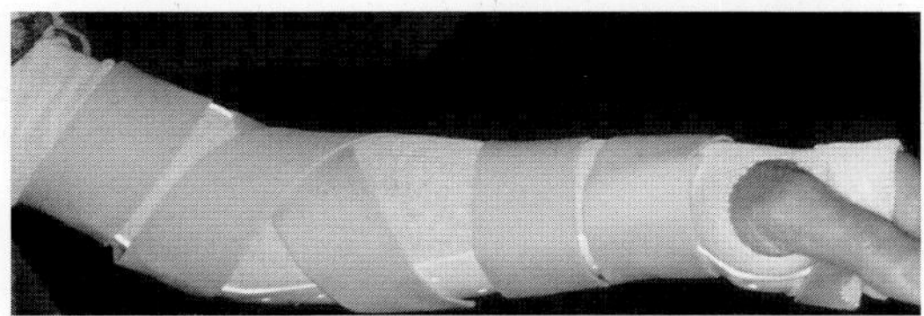

Figure 19–18 A night resting elbow immobilization splint minimizes compression on the nerve as it passes through the cubital tunnel. Restriction of elbow flexion during sleep may decrease irritation in this area.

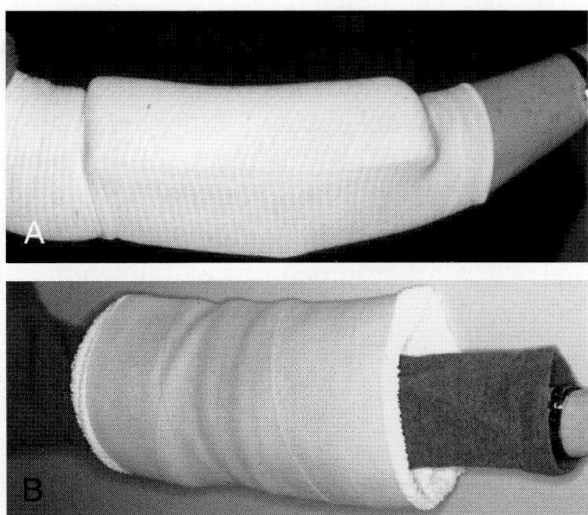

*Figure 19–19 **A,** A foam pad applied to the anterior aspect of the elbow can provide some light resistance to full elbow flexion. **B,** A towel wrapped about the elbow can also prevent full elbow flexion while sleeping, allowing a less restraining option to rigid immobilization.*

(slight elbow flexion, neutral forearm to slight pronation, and wrist neutral with slightly ulnar deviation) (Fig. 19–18) (Harper, 1990; Sailor, 1996; Tetro & Pichora, 1996; Warwick & Seradge, 1995).

If the patient cannot tolerate thermoplastic splinting for nighttime use (or insurance will not cover it), other options can be considered. A piece of foam can be placed on the anterior aspect of the elbow crease to prevent elbow flexion. The foam should extend proximally to the middle upper arm and distally to the midforearm; it can be held in place with a stockinette or light circumferential wrap. Another option is to wind a towel around the elbow, securing it with a circumferential wrap (Fig. 19–19). Both these methods restrict full elbow flexion and may be tolerated better than a rigid splint. During the day, soft padding (foam or silicone) about the posterior and medial elbow (cubital tunnel region) may protect the nerve from further trauma and provide a sense of security for the patient (Fig. 19–20). If symptoms continue, surgical decompression or transposition of the nerve may be warranted.

ULNAR TUNNEL (GUYON'S CANAL) SYNDROME

The **ulnar tunnel,** also referred to as **Guyon's canal,** is formed by the volar carpal ligament, hook of the hamate, and the pisiform bones. This space is small and somewhat superficial, making the nerve vulnerable to injury. Just proximal to the wrist, the nerve divides into a dorsal superficial sensory branch and a volar deep motor branch. Compression of the sensory branch, motor branch, or both branches may occur, depending on the level of the impingement. If only the motor branch is involved, the intrinsic muscles are affected but sensation is left intact. An isolated lesion to the deep motor branch may be seen in individuals who use tools intensively, such as a screwdriver or pruning sheers. They do not usually complain of pain, just weakness and atrophy (Boscheinen-Morrin et al., 1985; Matloub & Yousif, 1992).

The compression of the ulnar nerve at this level can be caused by repetitive trauma (cycling, hammering, use of vibrating tools), fracture of the hook of the hamate or pisiform bones, arthritis in the pisohamate joint, ganglion, anomalous muscle or ligament, or possibly an ulnar artery aneurysm or thrombosis (Lundborg, 1988; Moore & Dalley, 1999). Symptoms include vague pain, paresthesias or numbness of the SF and ulnar half of the RF, and weakness of the intrinsic muscles. In some cases, the patient may demonstrate positive Wartenberg's, Froment's, and Jeanne's signs owing to the weakness of the ulnar innervated muscles. When the sensory branch is involved, examination may reveal a positive Phalen's test and Tinel's sign over the ulnar tunnel.

Treatment of these low lesions focuses on rest, immobilization, avoidance of symptomatic activities, and anti-inflammatory medication. If symptoms persist, surgical intervention may be necessary. Splints may be used initially to immobilize the wrist and ulnar aspect of the hand for symptom relief. Once symptoms subside, splints can be fabricated to protect the ulnar tunnel during vocational or recreational activities. Padding the ulnar wrist over the ulnar tunnel area with gel or high dense foam may aid in absorbing vibration and compression stress to this vulnerable area. A splint can then be formed directly over this padded area (Fig. 19–21).

Radial Nerve Injuries

The radial nerve innervates the triceps muscle, which provides elbow extension, and innervates all of the

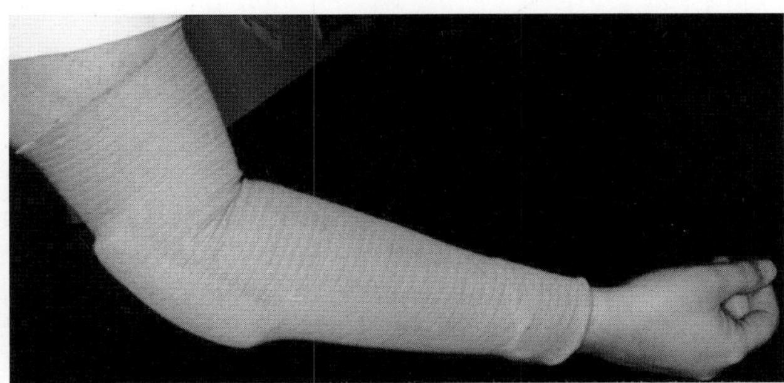

Figure 19–20 Soft padding or use of silicone gel sheets over the cubital tunnel area may help protect and absorb forces to a hypersensitive ulnar nerve.

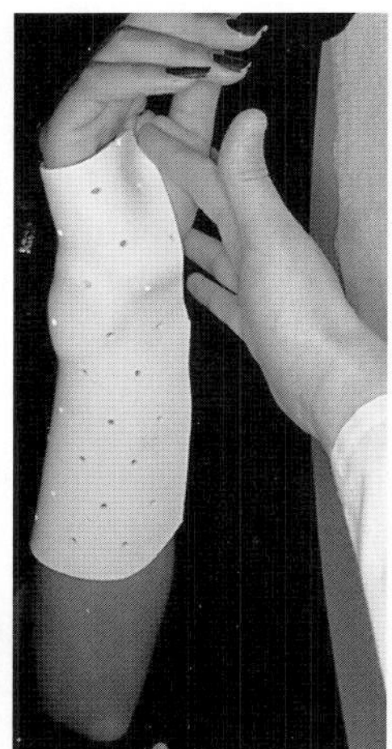

Figure 19–21 An ulnar wrist immobilization splint can be fabricated by incorporating silicone gel or high dense foam over the volar ulnar aspect of the wrist to protect the ulnar nerve in this region.

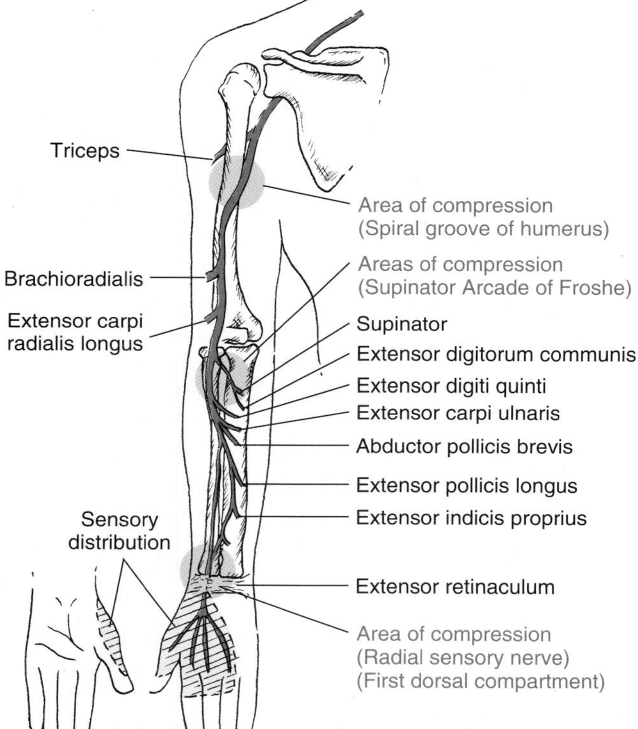

Figure 19–22 Injury to the motor potion of the radial nerve is functionally disabling.

wrist, digit, and thumb extensors as well as the supinator muscle (Fig. 19–22). Sensory loss of the radial nerve is much less functionally significant than that of the ulnar or median nerve.

High Laceration

Laceration to the radial nerve in the upper arm is often associated with a midshaft humerus fracture or traumatic injury to the nerve from a gunshot or stabbing injury. The radial nerve travels in close proximity to the humerus and is extremely vulnerable to injury if the humerus is involved. If lacerated at this level, the patient experiences loss of:

- wrist extension.
- forearm supinator (weak).
- thumb and digital extension.
- independent IF and SF digital extension.
- sensation over the dorsal radial aspect of the forearm and hand.

This clinical presentation is often referred to as **wrist drop** (Fig.19–23). The radial nerve cannot innervate its distal musculature, making wrist and digital extension impossible. Splinting intervention can be used to place the wrist and digits in a functional position to prevent overstretching of the involved extensor muscle tendon units, prevent joint contractures, and provide a mechanical advantage for the flexor tendons while waiting return of radial nerve function (Fig. 19–24). A wrist extension immobilization splint can

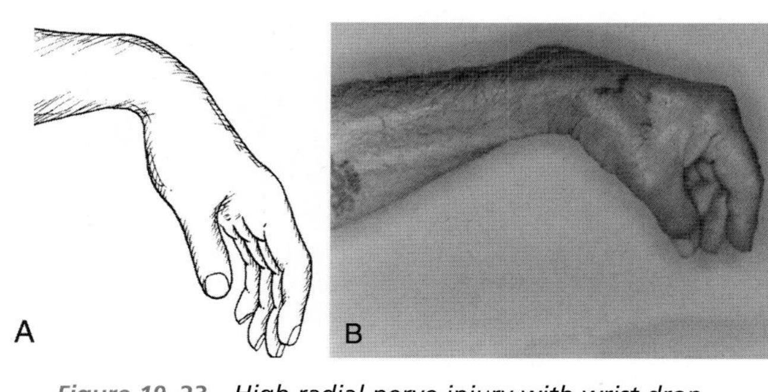

Figure 19–23 High radial nerve injury with wrist drop.

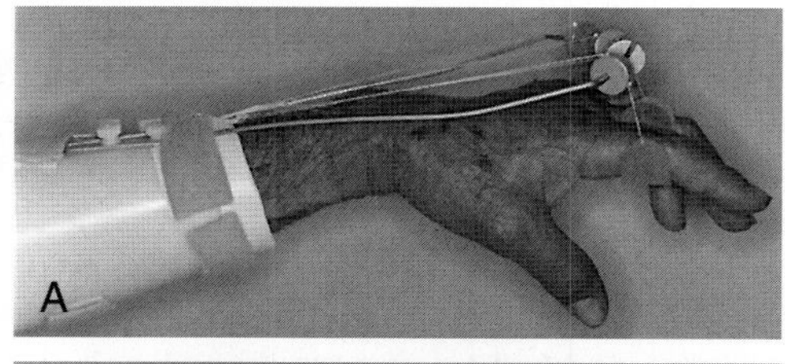

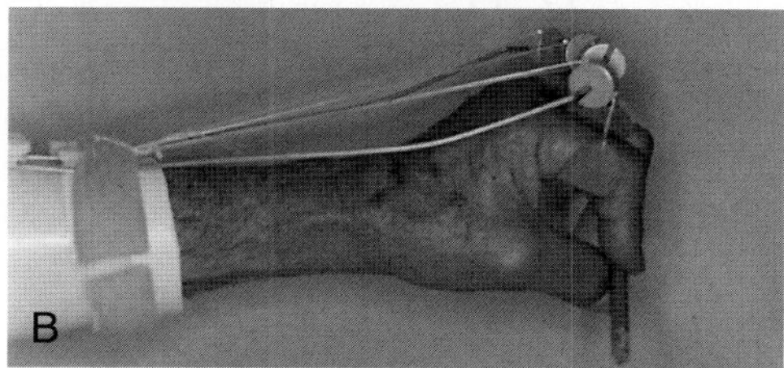

*Figure 19–24 A wrist/MP/thumb extension mobilization splint (for radial nerve palsy) is used to enhance hand function for a patient waiting for radial nerve reinnervation. When the wrist is passively extended, the digits flex **(A)**; and when the wrist actively flexes, the digits passively extend **(B)**. The proximal dorsal splint was fabricated out of 3⁄32" material; the mobilization component is a Phoenix Extended Outrigger Kit. Colditz, J. C. (1995). Splinting the hand with a peripheral nerve injury. In J. M. Hunter, E. J. Mackin, & A. D. Callahan (Eds.).* Rehabilitation of the hand *(4th ed., pp. 679–692). St. Louis: Mosby Year Book.*

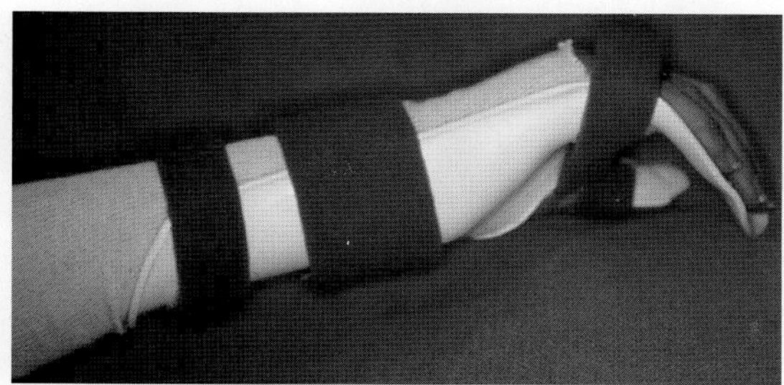

Figure 19–25 A wrist/hand immobilization splint can be used at night to position the wrist in extension, the MPs in flexion, and the IPs extended. This position may help prevent the MP collateral ligaments from shortening and PIP flexion contractures, which can occur as a consequence of this injury.

also be used for day functional use; however, the therapist should caution the patient on potential MP and PIP flexion contractures due to loss of active extension. Nighttime splinting may consist of a simple wrist/hand/thumb immobilization splint (Fig.19–25). When surgical tendon transfer or repair is warranted, similar splinting intervention is appropriate after the initial postoperative phase. Postoperative splints can be used to facilitate muscle re-education and functional use, maintain balance of muscle tendon unit length(s), and prevent joint contractures.

Low Laceration

Distal and anterior to the lateral epicondyle (at 8 to 10 cm), the radial nerve divides into a sensory and a motor branches. The sensory branch provides innervation to the dorsoradial forearm while the motor branch (PIN) continues distally to innervate the digit and thumb extensors. The radial wrist extensors—the extensor carpi radialis longus (ECRL) and extensor carpi radialis brevis (ECRB)—are innervated proximal to this bifurcation. Therefore, with low injury to the posterior interroseous nerve (PIN) wrist extension is normal with only the loss of digit and thumb extension. The intrinsics attempt to extend the PIP and DIP joints, but the MPs cannot be extended by the inactive extrinsic extensor tendons. Splinting management is essentially the same as for a low lesion. The inclusion of the wrist is optional and not recommended if there is adequate wrist extension strength (Fig. 19–26).

Compression Neuropathies

HIGH COMPRESSION

The radial nerve courses about the humerus at the level of the spiral groove. Injury may occur owing to local compression of the radial nerve against the humerus for an extended period of time, also known as **Saturday night palsy** (i.e., falling asleep with arm against a hard object; a forceful squeeze). There may be tenderness directly over the compression site with little other pain noted. This area of compression block may cause a neuropraxia, resulting in impairment of the muscles innervated below this level. With time this weakness or paralysis may resolve with little or no functional deficit (Eaton & Lister, 1992; Lundborg, 1988; Moore & Dalley, 1999; Parry, 1981). The goals of splinting intervention consist of prevention of joint contractures, protection against overstretching of the involved extensor muscle-tendon units, and maximizing functional use of the hand and wrist while waiting for nerve return.

RADIAL TUNNEL SYNDROME

The PIN passes deep to the origin of the ECRB and the arcade of Frohse (proximal margin of the supinator) and then passes between the two heads of the supinator to supply the supinator (Lundborg, 1988; Moore & Dalley, 1999). Compression can occur at any one of the sites through which the nerve passes; however the arcade of Frohse is by far the most likely anatomic structure to compress the PIN (Lundborg, 1988; Moore & Dalley, 1999). **Radial tunnel syndrome,** also known as **resistant tennis elbow,** is often characterized by pain with repetitive rotational movement of the forearm (Roles & Manudsley, 1972; Simmons & Wyman, 1992). Pain is described as aching and radiating toward the dorsal part of the wrist. There is profound tenderness on palpation directly over the extensor muscle group and supinator, 3 to 4 cm distal (over the arcade of Frohse) to the lateral epicondyle (Lundborg, 1988; Rayan, 1992). Resistance to supination, wrist extension, and MF extension usually reproduces the pain. Pain can occur during the day with forearm rotation activities; however, it is usually most evident at night. Radial tunnel can be misdiagnosed as lateral epicondylitis (tennis elbow). A careful differential diagnosis should be done. In lateral epicondylitis, pain is directly over the lateral epicondyle, wrist extension may be weak and painful, and pain is most often during and/or after work or recreational activity (Eaton & Lister, 1992; Lundborg, 1988). Note that controversy exists

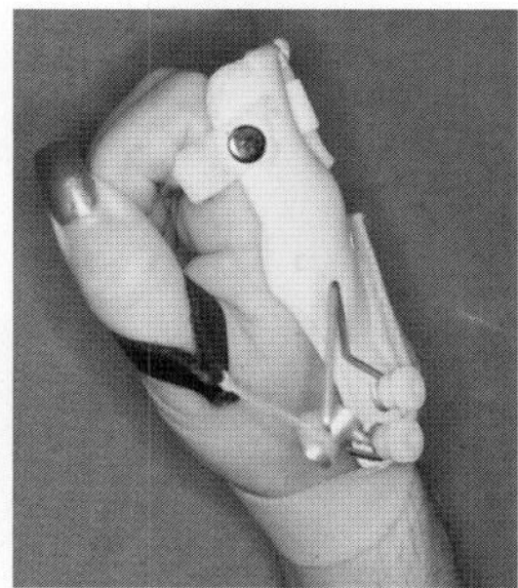

Figure 19–26 PIN injury can be managed with a hand-based MP/thumb extension mobilization splint. This splint maintains passive MP/thumb extension while allowing active digital and thumb flexion until the nerve recovers. A lightweight material is used to contour to the dorsum of the hand. A thumb extension outrigger is not always necessary and may be cumbersome to some patients; however, here it helped the patient carry out work responsibilities. Prepadding the dorsal MPs may assist in decreasing migration and increasing comfort.

in the literature regarding whether compression of the radial nerve at this level actually exists.

Management should include rest, avoidance of provocative positions, activity modification, anti-inflammatory medication or modalities, nerve gliding exercises, and splinting with the elbow gently flexed (optional) and forearm supinated with wrist extension.

POSTERIOR INTEROSSEOUS NERVE SYNDROME

The same pathology and therapeutic intervention as described for the low radial nerve laceration applies to **posterior interosseous nerve syndrome.** Although not common, the PIN can be damaged, compressed, or lacerated at this level (Thomas et al., 2000). Injury may occur from a mass pressing on the nerve (e.g., ganglion, lipoma, or fibroma), from a traumatic incident (e.g., an injection, plate or pin fixation while repairing a proximal radius or ulna fracture), rheumatoid arthritis of the elbow, or a forearm compression injury (Dell & Guzewicz, 1992). Symptoms usually include some degree of pain and weakness. Physical examination reveals no sensory deficit and a temporary partial or complete paralysis of the extrinsic digit and thumb extensors.

SUPERFICIAL RADIAL SENSORY NERVE SYNDROME (WARTENBERG'S SYNDROME)

The sensory branch of the radial nerve is vulnerable to injury as it approaches the radial styloid of the wrist. Therapists and surgeons often see injury and/or irritation at this level. In **superficial radial sensory nerve syndrome** or **Wartenberg's syndrome,** the nerve can become entrapped in scar from a laceration or from a surgical incision, as occasionally seen with a deQuervain's release. Irritation to this branch can also be caused by friction from by pin placement, jagged splint edges, sharp or compressive splint straps, or excessive edema (Colditz, 1995). Sensory alterations (paresthesias and numbness) occur in the dorsoradial aspect of the hand (Lundborg, 1988). Intervention focuses on splinting, with a silicone gel cushion or pad placed directly over the radial styloid (Fig. 19–27). For an acute, painful injury, a doughnut may be used over this area

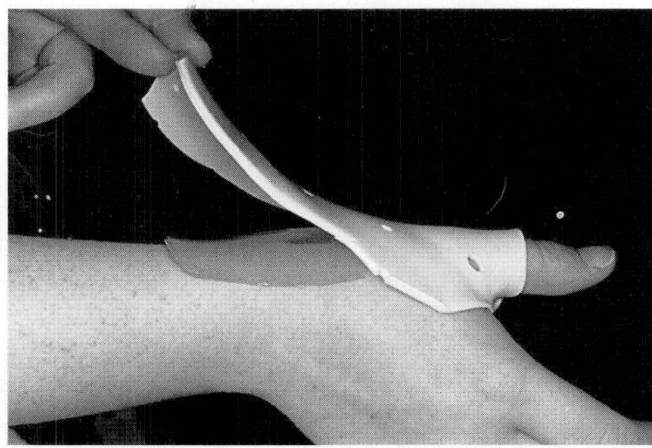

Figure 19–27 Place a silicone gel cushion or pad directly over the radial styloid process and under the splint.

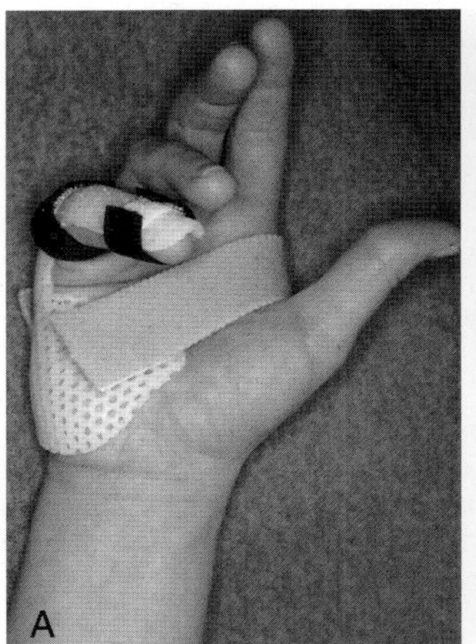

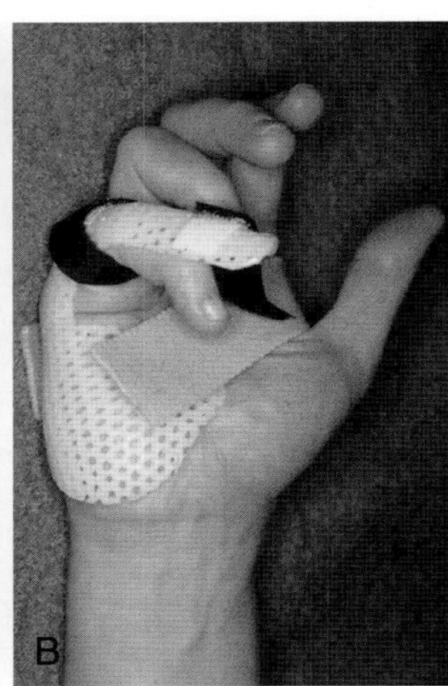

*Figure 19–28 This splint positions the repaired digital nerve in a shortened position (**A**) while allowing periodic gentle ROM within the splint confines (**B**).*

to avoid direct contact. A splint can offer protection and decreased tension on the nerve. Other therapeutic modalities may be used as warranted. Surgical decompression is considered when all conservative management fails.

Digital Nerve Laceration

Digital nerves can be lacerated in isolation but most often are seen in combination with tendon injury in zones II to IV. If seen in isolation, they are carefully placed into a hand-based immobilization or restrictive splint (depending on the physician's protocol), in a gently flexed position, to minimize stress on the surgical anastomosis. Protective splinting is used for 4 to 6 weeks; the patient is put into progressively greater extension per physician's orders (Fig. 19–28).

During the initial weeks, a guarded ROM program is begun, which usually involves unrestricted flexion and some degree of restricted extension. If tendons are involved, the wrist and/or thumb must be incorporated into the splint following the physician's preferred tendon protocol. Patient education regarding sensory precautions, wound care, edema control, and ROM protocols must be reviewed.

Brachial Plexus Injury

Injuries to the **brachial plexus** are extremely varied, ranging from simple compression and irritation injuries to complex traumatic lacerations. Although a review of this nerve complex is beyond the scope of this chapter, it is relevant to mention that splinting intervention is based on the anticipated distal pathology and potential deformity (Hunter & Whitenack, 1995; Lowe & O'Toole, 1995). Pain is often a consequence of these injuries and can play a major role in the therapist's ability to manage the patient. The therapist should appreciate that the peripheral nerves, nerve plexuses, spinal nerves, and nerve roots may all become a source of pain and thus may limit the therapeutic intervention plan (Barbis & Wallace, 1995; Elvey, 1997).

The same general splinting principles, considerations, and precautions discussed in this chapter apply to brachial plexus injuries as well. The level at which the brachial plexus is injured determines the most appropriate splinting intervention for preventing deformity and maximizing function (Hunter & Whitenack, 1995; Lowe & O'Toole, 1995). For example, a patient with an injured medial cord of the brachial plexus has involvement of the ulnar nerve as well contributions to the median nerve. This type of injury results in remarkable loss of the ulnarly innervated intrinsic hand muscles and causes some median nerve deficits as well. The patient essentially presents with a claw hand deformity (Fig. 19–17**B**). Applying an IF through SF MP flexion restriction splint may preserve function while the patient waits for nerve return (Fig. 19–17**C** and **E**).

Injury to the posterior cord of the brachial plexus results in damage to all of the extensors of the forearm, wrist, thumb, and fingers and to the deltoid, which abducts the shoulder at the glenohumeral joint. The patient presents with a wrist drop deformity that can be managed with a wrist/MP (optional thumb) extension mobilization splint (radial nerve palsy) (Figs. 19–23 and 19–24). Such a splint allows for a light functional grasp using the natural tenodesis of the hand. The therapist should teach the patient sensory precautions, passive ROM exercises for the involved joints, carefully guided nerve-gliding exercises, adaptive techniques and postural awareness (Barbis & Wallace, 1995; Lowe & O'Toole, 1995).

General Splinting Principles for Peripheral Nerve Injuries

Table 19–1 summarizes peripheral nerve injury management, including splinting considerations. The therapist should have the following goals in mind:

- Provide a balance among the innervated and denervated muscle/tendon structures while waiting for motor return.
- Keep denervated muscles from remaining in a lengthened position.
- Prevent joint stiffness and contractures.
- Prevent development of abnormal substitution patterns.
- Position the hand and wrist to maximize functional use and substitute for loss of motor function.
- Decrease pain and paresthesias associated with nerve compression injuries.
- Protect the surgically repaired or injured nerve and associated injuries.
- Protect insensate areas.

TABLE 19–1 PNI: Splinting Management and Considerations[a]

Diagnosis	Therapy Goals	Splinting Guidelines	Considerations
Median Nerve			
High and low lacerations	• Prevent adduction contractures of the thumb • Prevent overstretching of the thenar muscles • Prevent IF MP joint contractures • Prevent tension on the surgical repair	• Week 1 (postsurgery): elbow flexed (high lesion only), wrist flexed, thumb midpalmar/radial abduction immobilization splint • Week 3: increase wrist extension of splint to tolerance • Weeks 4–5: discontinue elbow for high lesions • Week 5–6: discontinue wrist, continue protective splinting for night and at-risk situations only; children and tenuous repairs 1 week longer; thumb abduction/opposition mobilization strap for day; maintain thumb abduction at night • Week 8: begin gentle mobilization splinting, if necessary	• Maintain IF PROM: extend distal borders of thumb abduction portion of the splint (for comfort) • Apply soft material under web portion of splint to provide intimate fit (Elastomer or silicone gel) • Weeks 5–6: attempt thumb opposition to MF with day splint to allow functional pinch through the common origin of the FDP

[a]This table is meant as only a guideline for injury management. Keep in mind that other nerve innervations may be present, and the pattern of nerve return is never predictable. This table does not include all possible mixed lesions. Remember that splint modifications occur frequently to accommodate motor return. Evaluate for sensory loss, and teach patients careful skin inspection.

[b]Data from Colditz, J. C. (1995). Splinting the hand with a peripheral nerve injury. In J. M. Hunter, E. J. Mackin, & A. D. Callahan (Eds.). *Rehabilitation of the hand* (4th ed., pp. 679–692). St. Louis: Mosby Year Book.

[c]Data from Matloub, H. S., Yousif, N. J. (1992). Peripheral nerve anatomy and innervation patterns. *Hand Clinics, 8,* 203–214.

Continued

TABLE 19–1 Continued			
Diagnosis	**Therapy Goals**	**Splinting Guidelines**	**Considerations**
Pronator syndrome	• Relieve pain and paresthesias • Rest inflamed structures • Prevent provocative motions of the wrist and forearm	• Day: forearm pronation, wrist neutral to slight flexion, immobilization splint • Night: for severe symptoms, include elbow in slight flexion	• Fabricate with patient in supine for gravity assist • Careful placement of straps to prevent direct pressure over tender area • The splint should be worn until symptoms have subsided and should be only part of a comprehensive rehabilitation program
Anterior interosseous syndrome	• Simulate pinch while waiting for nerve return • Prevent thumb IP and IF DIP extension contracture	• IF DIP/thumb IP flexion immobilization splints (or casts); optional	• Consider splinting in this position if thumb IP and IF DIP function is required for vocational functional tasks • Thin thermoplastic materials or QuickCast can be used, leaving volar pads free for sensory input
Carpal tunnel syndrome	• Decrease pain and paresthesias • Avoid repetitive and/or provocative motions • Rest inflamed structures	• Mild symptoms: day use is optional or depends on physician preference; wrist immobilized in neutral • Severe symptoms: consider night wrist/hand splint to immobilize entire muscle-tendon length.	• Allow unimpeded MP flexion and thumb mobility • The splint should be worn until symptoms have subsided and should be only part of a comprehensive rehabilitation program
Ulnar Nerve			
High and low lacerations	• Prevent RF/SF MP extension, PIP flexion contractures • Prevent overstretching of intrinsic muscles • Prevent RF/SF MP collateral ligament shortening • Protect and decrease the tension on surgical repair	• Week 1 (postsurgery): elbow flexed (high lesion only), wrist flexed, immobilization splint • Week 3: increase wrist extension in splint to tolerance • Weeks 4–5: discontinue elbow for high lesions • Weeks 5–6: discontinue wrist; continue MP flexion protective splinting for night and at-risk situations only; children and tenuous repairs 1 week longer; use RF/SF MP extension restriction splint for day • Week 8: begin gentle mobilization splinting, if necessary	• Allow for full RF/SF MP flexion • The dorsal component should be well molded to distribute pressure • Prevent RF/SF collateral ligament shortening • Atrophy of the hypothenar muscles may make the day splint difficult to don and doff; incorporate an opening (on dorsal aspect) to ease application
Cubital tunnel syndrome	• Prevent repetitive and prolonged elbow flexion • Decrease shearing stress on the nerve as it travels through the cubital tunnel • Position the nerve in a resting state	• Day: posterior medial elbow pad; buddy tape SF to RF (if needed) • Night: elbow at 30 to 40°; wrist neutral with slight ulnar deviation immobilization splint • Alternative: elbow flexion restriction splint to allow a protected, limited ROM, avoiding full elbow flexion • Alternative: foam on anterior elbow or towel wrap around elbow to prevent elbow flexion at night	• Severe symptoms may require splint use during day • Avoid pressure over epicondyles • Posterior splint designs should be well padded over cubital tunnel • Restriction splint may be used for intermittent symptoms and does not allow elbow flexion beyond 90°[b] • Avoid straps directly over tender or inflamed areas. • The splint should be worn until symptoms have subsided and should be only part of a comprehensive rehabilitation program

[a]This table is meant as only a guideline for injury management. Keep in mind that other nerve innervations may be present, and the pattern of nerve return is never predictable. This table does not include all possible mixed lesions. Remember that splint modifications occur frequently to accommodate motor return. Evaluate for sensory loss, and teach patients careful skin inspection.

[b]Data from Colditz, J. C. (1995). Splinting the hand with a peripheral nerve injury. In J. M. Hunter, E. J. Mackin, & A. D. Callahan (Eds.). *Rehabilitation of the hand* (4th ed., pp. 679–692). St. Louis: Mosby Year Book.

[c]Data from Matloub, H. S., Yousif, N. J. (1992). Peripheral nerve anatomy and innervation patterns. *Hand Clinics, 8,* 203–214.

TABLE 19–1 Continued

Diagnosis	Therapy Goals	Splinting Guidelines	Considerations
Ulnar tunnel/ Guyon's canal syndrome	• Decrease stress on the ulnar nerve as it passes through the ulnar tunnel • Protect from direct forces over the pisiform • Avoid provocative activities	• Day and night: immobilization splint with wrist 0° to slight flexion; consider padding ulnar/volar wrist area • Alternative: soft Neoprene splint for work and leisure activities	• Consider applying a silicone gel patch directly over the sensitive area before splint fabrication, or use a foam doughnut • The splint should be worn until symptoms have subsided and should be only part of a comprehensive rehabilitation program
Combined Median and Ulnar Nerves			
High and low lacerations	• Same goals as listed for each nerve • Maintain three-point pinch	• Week 1 (post surgery): elbow flexed (high lesion only), wrist flexed, thumb midpalmar and radial abduction immobilization splint • Week 3: increase wrist extension in splint to tolerance • Weeks 4–5: discontinue elbow for high lesions • Weeks 5–6: discontinue wrist, continue with IF-SF MP flexion/thumb abduction splint for night and at-risk situations only; children and tenuous repairs 1 week longer; use IF-SF MP extension restriction splint for day, with or without thumb • Week 8: begin gentle mobilization splinting, if necessary	• Splinting may be difficult; some patients may benefit from a splint that recruits power from the radial nerve[c] • These injuries most often occur in combination with tendon and vascular injury; check with physician for specific protocol • Paramount to maintain PROM of all involved joints
Radial nerve			
High laceration or compression injury	• Re-create tenodesis action while waiting for nerve return • Prevent overstretching of the wrist, thumb, and digital extensors • Prevent joint contractures (wrist, MP, and PIP flexion)	• Week 1 (postsurgery): if repair is proximal to the elbow, consider splinting or casting as follows—elbow flexion/wrist extension/digit and thumb extension immobilization • Week 2–3 or nonsurgical or compressive injury; use wrist/MP/thumb extension immobilization splint (IPs are free) for day; use wrist extension/MP flexion/IPs and thumb extension immobilization for night • Alternative: tenodesis splint (wrist flex/MP extension; MP flex/wrist extension) • Alternative: consider fabricating a wrist immobilization splint for work if the tenodesis splint is too cumbersome or not appropriate. • Alternative: InRigger radial nerve glove with wrist (AliMed)	• Avoid pressure over ulnar styloid, consider prepadding • Take care when fitting all the proximal phalanx slings • Check for appropriate tension when fabricating tenodesis splint • The splint should be worn until symptoms have subsided and should be only part of a comprehensive rehabilitation program • Prolonged splint use may contribute to weakened extensors

[a]This table is meant as only a guideline for injury management. Keep in mind that other nerve innervations may be present, and the pattern of nerve return is never predictable. This table does not include all possible mixed lesions. Remember that splint modifications occur frequently to accommodate motor return. Evaluate for sensory loss, and teach patients careful skin inspection.

[b]Data from Colditz, J. C. (1995). Splinting the hand with a peripheral nerve injury. In J. M. Hunter, E. J. Mackin, & A. D. Callahan (Eds.). *Rehabilitation of the hand* (4th ed., pp. 679–692). St. Louis: Mosby Year Book.

[c]Data from Matloub, H. S., Yousif, N. J. (1992). Peripheral nerve anatomy and innervation patterns. *Hand Clinics, 8,* 203–214.

Continued

TABLE 19–1 Continued

Diagnosis	Therapy Goals	Splinting Guidelines	Considerations
Low laceration and posterior interosseous nerve injury	• Re-create tenodesis action while waiting for nerve return • Prevent overstretching of the wrist, thumb, and digital extensors • Prevent joint contractures	• Day: wrist flexion/MP extension; MP flexion/wrist extension mobilization splint (tenodesis splint) • Night: wrist/thumb/digit extension immobilization splint • Alternative: hand-based MP extension mobilization splint, with or without thumb extension outrigger • Alternative: InRigger radial nerve glove (AliMed)	• Take care when fitting all the slings • Avoid pressure over the ulnar styloid, consider prepadding • Check for appropriate tension when fabricating tenodesis splint • For hand-based splint, avoid MP irritation • Correct thumb position
Radial tunnel syndrome	• Prevent repetitive resisted supination • Avoid provocative positions • Position the nerve in a resting state	• Day and night: wrist extension (30 to 40°), forearm neutral rotation immobilization splint	• When in combination with lateral epicondylitis, splint the elbow in 60–90° flexion, and the forearm in supination • Avoid strap compression over tender area • The splint should be worn until symptoms have subsided and should be only part of a comprehensive rehabilitation program
Superficial radial nerve syndrome, Wartenberg's syndrome	• Eliminate irritation of the cutaneous branch of the radial nerve about the radial styloid • Protect the area from direct trauma while healing	• Day and night: radial wrist immobilization splint that positions the wrist and thumb column to minimize tension on the radial sensory nerve	• Take care when molding; avoid direct pressure over the radial styloid • For severe irritation, consider lifting the material up by making a doughnut to relieve pressure on the entrapped nerve • Alternative: apply silicone gel or padding over this area before splinting
Digital nerves			
Lacerations	• Protect and decrease tension on the surgical repair • Prevent joint MP, PIP, or DIP contractures • Sensory precautions	• Day and night: hand-based MP/PIP/DIP extension restriction splint (MP: 45°, PIP: 30°; DIP slight flexion)	• Splint position depends greatly on level of digital nerve injury and involvement of other structures (e.g., neurovascular, tendon, ligament) • When splinting, pay extra attention to the splint's borders, making sure they do not dig into insensate areas

[a]This table is meant as only a guideline for injury management. Keep in mind that other nerve innervations may be present, and the pattern of nerve return is never predictable. This table does not include all possible mixed lesions. Remember that splint modifications occur frequently to accommodate motor return. Evaluate for sensory loss, and teach patients careful skin inspection.

[b]Data from Colditz, J. C. (1995). Splinting the hand with a peripheral nerve injury. In J. M. Hunter, E. J. Mackin, & A. D. Callahan (Eds.). *Rehabilitation of the hand* (4th ed., pp. 679–692). St. Louis: Mosby Year Book.

[c]Data from Matloub, H. S., Yousif, N. J. (1992). Peripheral nerve anatomy and innervation patterns. *Hand Clinics, 8,* 203–214.

Splinting Considerations and Precautions

The therapist should keep the following considerations and precautions in mind when splinting this patient population:

- Sensory and motor return should be monitored and splints modified accordingly.
- Watch for deformities that may not initially be clinically or functionally evident. As reinnervation occurs, the deformity may become apparent and corrective splinting mandatory (e.g., in a returning high ulnar nerve lesion, the FDP eventually becomes innervated and the distal claw deformity becomes more prominent) (Dell & Guzewicz, 1992).
- If patients with nerve injuries must wear splints for function, keep the design simple and low profile. A splint that is cumbersome and bulky may interfere with the function of uninvolved joints. Patients are less likely to comply with splint schedules when the splint is big and cumbersome.

- Educate patients regarding any sensory deficits, teaching careful skin inspection to prevent excess pressure and potential breakdown from extended splint wear (Blackmore & Hotchkiss, 1995).

Material Selection

Lightweight, contouring, and highly drapable materials may be the most appropriate choice for splinting the nerve-injured hand. Many of these injuries have accompanying sensory loss, which limits the patient's ability to detect sheer or compressive stress. Great care should be taken to ensure proper length, width, and weight distribution. Corners and borders should be rounded and flared to maximize splint strength, comfort, and cosmesis. Patient education regarding skin inspection is paramount.

Materials that tend to retain heat may be uncomfortable and even painful for some patients with nerve involvement. Select a material that has a lower heating temperature, but can still provide an intimate fit with minimal handling.

Component Selection

The use of components, such as outriggers, slings, and line guides, should be minimized. Every additional component makes the splint more complicated to apply and wear. Finger and hand slings should be cautiously applied to the insensate hand. Close attention should be given to avoid creation of sheer and/or compression stress under these slings. If components are necessary to maintain active function, the therapist ought to review with the patient the correct application and wearing schedule, as well as stress the precautions of the splint. The selection of the components should be as low profile as possible. Many companies carry their own designs of splinting components. Carefully read instructions for applications and precautions. Commonly, mobilization splints are worn for functional day use, complemented by a night immobilization splint to prevent joint contractures.

Strapping Selection

Straps should be conforming and soft. They should be strategically placed to minimize migration and increase comfort. Neoprene and soft straps conform nicely around joints and through web spaces with little skin irritation.

Other Management Options:

Other options to manage peripheral nerve injuries include simple prefabricated splints such as a wrist support following radial nerve injury. The Robinson InRigger soft leather glove is another option for management of such nerve injuries (AliMed, Inc., Dedham, MA). A low-profile spring outrigger fits within a leather glove to provide digit extension after active flexion. This glove was initially created to manage posterior interosseous nerve injuries but has since been developed to include designs for other nerve injuries (see Chapter 11 for details).

Various types and applications of tape can be used to help position and increase the function of the hand. For example, the thumb can be taped in abduction and opposition after a median nerve injury. A Figure-8 design around the proximal phalanx can enhance tip pinch during wrist extension (Fig. 19–29) (see Chapter 13 for additional information).

Tendon Transfers

Tendon transfers are surgical procedures that re-establish balance and active motion to a nerve-injured hand or one that has experienced a tendon avulsion or rupture. A tendon transfer procedure uses the tendon of a functioning muscle; it is detached, mobilized, rerouted, and resutured to the tendon of a muscle that has lost innervation or into a bony insertion (Brand, 1995; Jones, 1994). Here, only common tendon transfers related to median, ulnar, and radial nerve injuries will be discussed. The reader is referred to the suggested reading list for a more in-depth anatomic review and detailed discussion of splinting intervention.

Patients may undergo tendon transfers to substitute for motion of a paralyzed muscle in which peripheral nerve function has not been restored within a reasonable period of time (Jones, 1994). The best functional results seem to occur when ulnar and median nerve sensation is at least partially present, though some patients seem to do quite well despite a sensory loss. In most cases, the patient cannot maximize use of the hand without adequate sensory feedback; therefore, the results of the surgical reconstruction will be marginal at best.

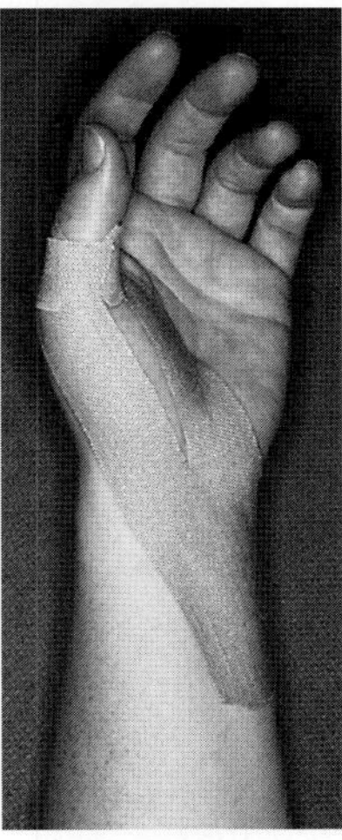

Figure 19–29 For a returning median nerve, Kinesio tape is used to position the thumb gently in palmar abduction and opposition. As the wrist is extended, the thumb is carried farther into opposition and abduction, providing the capacity for light tip pinch. This taping technique can be used in conjunction with other splinting interventions.

Tendons are transferred and repaired with a distinct degree of tension, and the postoperative splinting program should adequately protect the surgical reconstruction during the healing period (Barbis & Wallace, 1995; Blackmore & Hotchkiss, 1995; Brand, 1995; Chan, Jaglowski, & Kaplan, 1994; Colditz, 1995; Elvey, 1997; Hunter & Whitenack, 1995; Jones, 1994; Lowe & O'Toole, 1995; Smith, 1987). The postoperative splint should relax tension on the surgically transferred muscle(s) by placing the joint that the transferred muscle/tendon unit crosses in a shortened position to allow rest. It is also important that the splint positions the joint(s) in a manner that protects the proper direction of the transferred tendon's pull. For example, when an opponensplasty has been performed using a slip of the RF FDS tendon guided through a FCU pulley, then the splint should hold the thumb in a palmar abduction/opposition with the wrist in neutral to slight flexion and ulnar deviation.

The therapist should review with the surgeon the exact reconstruction that was performed before seeing the patient. With good surgeon–therapist communication, a clear picture can be established regarding which muscle/tendon unit was used, what function has been restored, and what the appropriate splint design should be (e.g., dorsal versus volar design). This information can guide the therapist in thorough patient education, proper splint fabrication, and optimal therapeutic intervention.

This section reviews functional deficits relative to specific levels of nerve injury. A general discussion is presented; the reader must fully research the specific tendon transfer preformed for each patient. The splint recommendations given here are meant as only guidelines. Each patient must be evaluated and immobilized or mobilized according to his or her needs and in accordance with the surgeon's protocol. Table 19–2 summarizes splinting management for common tendon transfers.

Selection of Tendon Transfers

In an ideal situation, the therapist, patient, and surgeon decide on what function is to be restored and what is available to use as a possible donor. The selection process includes the analysis of the anticipated strength of a donor muscle after the transfer, its potential excursion, how many joints it must cross, the direction it must pull in to be effective, and the overall effect the transfer has on the balance of other muscle/tendon units in the extremity (Brand, 1995; Colditz, 1995; Jones, 1994; Mackinnon, 1994; Smith, 1987). Before surgical intervention the following therapy considerations should have been met:

- Prevent or correct substitution patterns from developing or progressing while awaiting transfer by providing preoperative therapy and splinting to encourage the natural use of the hand.
- Achieve and maintain full passive ROM of all involved joints.
- Elongate the involved skin and soft tissue adhesions and joint contractures (Brand, 1995; Colditz, 1995; Jones, 1994).
- Strive to achieve maximal strength (4+) of the donor muscle(s) considered for transfer (Brand, 1995).
- Patient education regarding postoperative course of the therapy and the importance of splinting compliance.

Postoperative Therapy Considerations

If a tendon transfer is performed on a young child, splinting the hand postoperatively may not be appropriate. Children do quite well with the use of a cast for the required healing time (4 to 8 weeks) and then progress directly into the rehabilitation phase. Applying splints that are potentially removable on a young person may tempt him or her to take it off, possibly jeopardizing the surgical reconstruction. The stiffness encountered while wearing the cast is a small price to pay for the security the cast provides to the parents and physician. Joint and musculotendinous tightness can be addressed readily in the young patient.

Splinting should protect and position the joints properly to avoid too much or too little tension at the transfer site. Too much tension can cause attenuation, rupture, or gap at the anastomosis site. Too little tension can cause excessive tightness and tissue contracture.

All fabricated splints should be carefully inspected for possible areas of compression. Depending on the nerve deficit, sensation can be greatly impaired. It is the therapist's responsibility to teach the patient vigilant skin inspection under the confines of the splint and its straps.

Splints can be used to initiate limited, guarded active exercise under supervision of a therapist. For example, exercising within a protective splint after an opponensplasty can retrain the transferred muscle tendon unit, minimize adhesion formation, and increase nutrition to the repair site while protectively positioning the thumb. (Fig. 19–30).

Splints are generally worn for 3 to 4 weeks; then active motion is begun. Protective splinting continues for an additional 3 to 6 weeks during at-risk activities and while sleeping.

Extensor tendons used as transfers are generally weaker than flexor tendons. The therapist must consider this when fabricating a splint design. Extensors are often immobilized a few weeks longer (about 2 weeks) and held in a shorter resting state than flexor tendons (Smith, 1987; Stanley-Goodwyn, 1995).

Mobilization splinting can be initiated after the initial phase of immobilization (8 to 12 weeks) to gently stretch tight structures, such as tight intrinsic muscles

TABLE 19–2 Tendon Transfers[a,b]

Nerve Involved	Functional Loss	Common Tendon Transfer Options	Splint
Median Nerve			
High	• Flexion of the thumb IP joint • Flexion of the IF and possibly MF PIP and DIP joints • Thumb opposition and palmar abduction • Wrist radial flexion (FCR)	• BR to FPL to restore IP joint flexion of the thumb • IF and MF FDP side-to-side suture to RF and SF FDP to restore FDP flexion • See also low median nerve tendon transfers	• The wrist, digits, and thumb are immobilized in some degree of flexion (wrist: 20–30°; MP: 40–60°; PIP/DIP: neutral to slight flexion; thumb MP and IP: 30°; CMC: midabduction) • Maintain for approximately 4 weeks, with an additional 1–2 weeks for protection only • Consideration should be given to providing a comfortable balance between wrist, digit, and thumb position when this procedure is done in combination with an opponensplasty • Transfers restore opposition and palmar abduction
Low	• Thumb opposition and palmar abduction • Thumb MP joint flexion may or may not be noticed secondary to the dual innervation from the ulnar nerve	• EIP to APB or proximal phalanx • FDS RF to FCU pulley, to base of thumb proximal phalanx or into APB • PL to APB	• The wrist from neutral to approximately 30°of flexion; exact position depends on whether a flexor or extensor tendon was used as the donor • EIP: wrist approximately 30° flexion, thumb full abduction, slight palmar flexion, and opposition to approximately MF tip, for 4–5 weeks; use as additional protection for 2 weeks. • FDS: wrist neutral, thumb full abduction, slight palmar flexion, and opposition to approximately MF tip, for 3–4 weeks; use as additional protection 1–2 weeks.
Ulnar nerve			
High	• Ulnar wrist flexion (FCU) • DIP joint flexion of RF and SF • See also low lesion	• High ulnar nerve injury can be functionally devastating, grip strength is severely affected; transfers restore grip capabilities and balanced wrist function • FDS MF or IF to FDP RF and SF to restore digit flexion • FCR to FCU to restore ulnar deviation and wrist flexion	• The wrist is immobilized in neutral to slight extension, the MPs are flexed, and the PIP/DIPs are extended. Immobilization is mandatory for 3 weeks with an additional 3 weeks for protection

[a]This table is meant as only a guideline for injury management. It provides the basic background information needed for challenging cases. Remember that the exact design and position of joints within the splint must be determined by close communication with the surgeon. This table does not include all possible tendon transfers and does not list all available splinting interventions.

[b]Data from American Society for Surgery of the Hand. (1995). *Regional review courses in hand surgery* (vols. 4 & 21). Englewood, CO: Author; Jones, N. F. (1994). Tendon transfers. In M. Cohen (Ed.). *Mastery of plastic and reconstructive surgery* (pp. 1579–1597). Boston: Little, Brown; and Smith, R. J. (1987). *Tendon transfers of the hand and forearm.* Boston: Little, Brown.

[c]Data from Jones, N. F. (1994). Tendon transfers. In M. Cohen (Ed.). *Mastery of plastic and reconstructive surgery* (pp. 1579–1597). Boston: Little, Brown; Brand. P. W. (1995). Mechanics of tendon transfers. In J. M. Hunter, E. J. Mackin, & A. D. Callahan (Eds.). *Rehabilitation of the hand* (4th ed., pp. 715–727). St. Louis: Mosby Year Book.

[d]Data from Blackmore, S. M., & Hotchkiss, R. N. (1995). Therapist's management of ulnar neuropathy at the elbow. In J. M. Hunter, E. J. Mackin, & A. D. Callahan (Eds.). *Rehabilitation of the hand* (4th ed., 665–677). St. Louis: Mosby Year Book.

APB, abductor pollicis brevis; *APL,* abductor pollicis longus; *BR,* brachioradialis; *CMC,* carpometacarpal; *EIP,* extensor indices proprius; *EPL,* extensor pollicis longus; *FCR,* flexor carpi radialis; *PL,* palmaris longus; *PT,* pronator teres.

Continued

TABLE 19–2 Continued

Nerve Involved	Functional Loss	Common Tendon Transfer Options	Splint
Low	• Digital abduction or adduction • MP joint flexion of RF and SF • PIP and DIP joint extension of RF and SF • Thumb adduction	• Transfers provide MP flexion and PIP extension (prevent clawing) • FDS MF to radial lateral bands of RF and SF • FDS MF or IF to pulleys of RF and SF (Zancolli lasso operation) • ECRL or ERCB (with tendon graft) to lateral bands of RF and SF (Brand transfer)[c] • ECRB to AP with APL accessory to first dorsal interosseous to restore thumb adduction	• See high lesion
Combined median and ulnar nerves			
Low and high	• Thumb abduction and adduction (lateral pinch and opposition) • Thumb IP and IF/MF DIP flexion (tip and three-point pinch) • SF adduction • MP IF through SF flexion and PIP and DIP extension (claw hand) • Wrist flexion • Volar hand sensory loss	• Transfers provide balance and at least partial function • Low: (1) ECRB to APB for lateral pinch; (2) EIP to APB/EPL for thumb opposition; (3) APL to first dorsal interossei (possible arthrodesis of MP joint) to restore tip pinch; (4) ECRL or BR to IF through SF A2 pulley area for MP flexion • High: (1) see low injury; (2) BR to FPL for thumb IP joint flexion; (3) ECU to FCU for wrist flexion	• The wrist is positioned in neutral; the MPs are flexed; the PIP/DIPs are extended; and the thumb is held in slight flexion, abduction, and opposition. • Check with surgeon for specific positioning measurements
Radial nerve			
High	• Wrist extension • Digit extension and thumb extension • Radial thumb abduction.	• The inability to actively control or position the wrist makes grasp and release activities nearly impossible • Common transfers restore wrist, digit, and thumb extension[d] • PT to ECRB, FCU to EDC, PL to EPL • PT to ECRB, FCR to EDC, PL to EPL • PT to ECRL plus ECRB, FDS MF to EDC MF/SF, FDS RF to EIP and EPL, FCR to APL and EPB	• Postoperative cast position includes elbow flexion to 90°, maximum pronation, wrist extension to 30–40°, MPs at 0°, CMC in extension and abduction, and PIP/DIP joints free • Maintain in a cast for 3–4 weeks, unless the protocol differs • After 4 weeks, splint for 3–4 weeks, in the same position with gradual weaning for supervised exercise and hygiene
Low	• Digit extension • Thumb extension	• Transfers restore digit and thumb extension • FCU to EDC, PL to EPL • FDS MF to EDC MF/SF, FDS RF to EIP and EPL, FCR to APL and EPB • FCR to EDC, PL to EPL	• Same position and time frame as for high lesion with exclusion of the elbow

[a]This table is meant as only a guideline for injury management. It provides the basic background information needed for challenging cases. Remember that the exact design and position of joints within the splint must be determined by close communication with the surgeon. This table does not include all possible mixed tendon transfers and does not list all available splinting interventions.

[b]Data from American Society for Surgery of the Hand. (1995). *Regional review courses in hand surgery* (vols. 4 & 21). Englewood, CO: Author; Jones, N. F. (1994). Tendon transfers. In M. Cohen (Ed.). *Mastery of plastic and reconstructive surgery* (pp. 1579–1597). Boston: Little, Brown; and Smith, R. J. (1987). *Tendon transfers of the hand and forearm.* Boston: Little, Brown.

[c]Data from Jones, N. F. (1994). Tendon transfers. In M. Cohen (Ed.). *Mastery of plastic and reconstructive surgery* (pp. 1579–1597). Boston: Little, Brown; Brand. P. W. (1995). Mechanics of tendon transfers. In J. M. Hunter, E. J. Mackin, & A. D. Callahan (Eds.). *Rehabilitation of the hand* (4th ed., pp. 715–727). St. Louis: Mosby Year Book.

[d]Data from Blackmore, S. M., & Hotchkiss, R. N. (1995). Therapist's management of ulnar neuropathy at the elbow. In J. M. Hunter, E. J. Mackin, & A. D. Callahan (Eds.). *Rehabilitation of the hand* (4th ed., 665–677). St. Louis: Mosby Year Book.

APB, abductor pollicis brevis; *APL,* abductor pollicis longus; *BR,* brachioradialis; *CMC,* carpometacarpal; *EIP,* extensor indices proprius; *EPL,* extensor pollicis longus; *FCR,* flexor carpi radialis; *PL,* palmaris longus; *PT,* pronator teres.

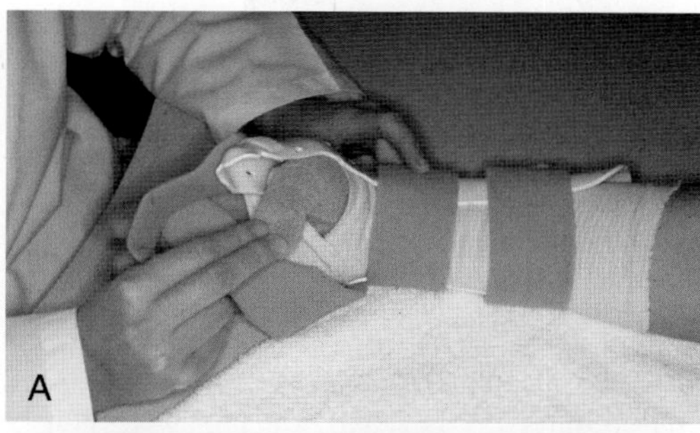

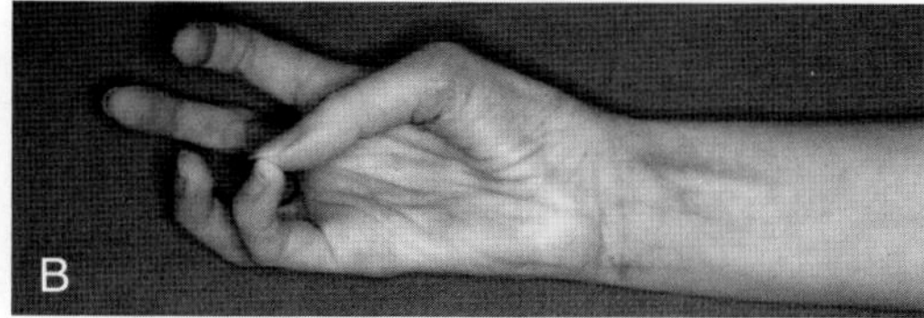

Figure 19–30 ***A,*** *With protective splinting after opponensplasty, gentle motion can be begun under supervision.* ***B,*** *At 6 weeks postsurgery, functional pinch has returned.*

after an extensor tendon transfer. Splints used to encourage motion can be fabricated out of lightweight material and used for a home program. For example, immobilizing the IP joint of the thumb can prevent the FPL from overpowering a weak opponensplasty. A variety of taping and strapping techniques can also be used to facilitate appropriate movement, such as thumb abduction and opposition (Fig. 19–11).

CASE STUDY SECTION

The case studies presented here are meant to be used as teaching guidelines only. Treatment and splinting protocols vary greatly from surgeon to surgeon and from therapist to therapist. The therapist must check with the referring physicians and colleagues to define the preferred treatment and splinting methods.

CASE STUDY 1: **High-Level Nerve Injury**

GH is a 39-year-old, right-dominant female who sustained a right midhumeral fracture, right distal radius fracture, and radial nerve injury during a hit-and-run accident. In the emergency room, she was placed in a long arm cast with her elbow at 90°, forearm pronated, wrist in slight flexion, and digits left free. Because of the edema in her hand and digits, and her inability to extend her digits, she was referred to hand therapy with a question of radial nerve injury.

Upon clinical examination, it was noted that she did indeed have symptoms consistent with radial nerve compression or injury. GH was unable to extend her digits or thumb actively within the cast. Therefore, an MP extension mobilization splint was fabricated to fit directly over the cast. This allowed the patient to use her digits purposefully and prevent overstretching of the digit and thumb extensors (Fig. 19–31).

The cast was removed 6 weeks later. Upon examination, GH demonstrated weak triceps function and no active wrist, digit, or thumb extension. She had impaired sensibility over the dorsoradial aspect of her forearm. She required continued splinting to substitute for loss of muscle function. A wrist flexion/MP extension, wrist extension/MP flexion splint was chosen (radial nerve splint). This design allowed the patient to take advantage of the natural tenodesis effect of the digits with wrist movement. When the wrist extends, the digits flex; when the wrist flexes, the digits extend (Fig. 19–24). This splint design allows full use of the palmar surface of the hand and is light in weight. GH continued with the splint for approximately 6 weeks. At night, she wore a simple wrist/hand/thumb immobilization splint (Fig. 19–25), which she found did not disrupt her sleep. In therapy, the patient worked on regaining wrist motion and strength.

When her wrist extensors were strong enough to support themselves against gravity, she was placed in a hand-based MP/thumb extension mobilization splint (Fig. 19–26), while waiting for the return of the distal motor branch of the PIN. GH wore the splint for ADLs and work-related tasks. Compliance with wearing the splint was not an issue because of its low profile design. She was able to take it off with increased frequency while waiting return of nerve function, which took an additional 5 weeks. Eventually, she discarded all splinting and worked on a general strengthening program.

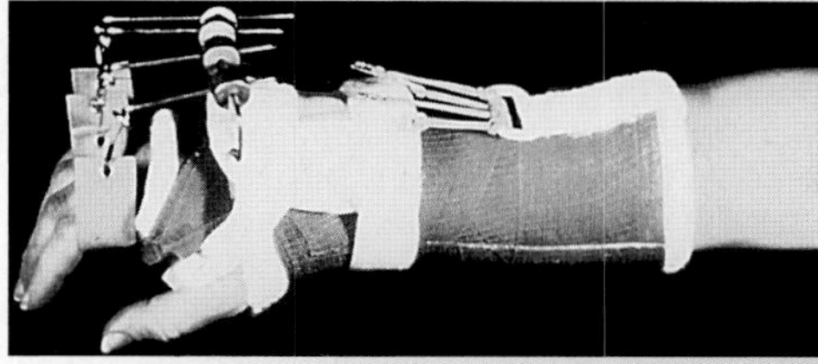

Figure 19–31 Extension mobilization splinting can be fabricated over a cast to maximize functional hand use while waiting for nerve return. For this splint, a drapable, 1/8" plastic material was used to contour to the ridges of the fiberglass. Roylan adjustable outrigger kit shown here.

CASE STUDY 2: **Median Nerve Compression (Carpal Tunnel Syndrome)**

In her fifth month of pregnancy NA began having numbness and tingling in the median nerve distribution of her hands bilaterally. She was experiencing nighttime symptoms that were so severe she woke up several times during the night. She was experiencing pain and paresthesias during the day while driving, holding a book to read, pushing a grocery cart, and even putting on jewelry. She was referred by her primary care physician to therapy with a diagnosis of carpal tunnel syndrome.

Upon evaluation, NA had an acutely positive Phalen's test and thenar weakness bilaterally. She was placed into bilateral wrist immobilization splints that held the wrists in neutral. In this position, compression of the median nerve is significantly decreased (Fig.19–13). The splints also kept her from placing her wrists in provocative positions. She was instructed to wear the splints at all times initially, taking them off for hygiene purposes only. As her symptoms subsided, splint use was decreased to nighttime only.

The therapist taught NA about carpal tunnel syndrome and how to avoid activities and static postures that could irritate the nerve. The patient had great relief of symptoms with the use of the splints, nerve gliding exercises and continued the nighttime regime through out the remainder of her pregnancy.

REFERENCES

American Society for Surgery of the Hand. (1995). *Regional review courses in hand surgery* (vols. 4 & 21). Englewood, CO: Author.

Barbis, J. M., & Wallace, K. A. (1995). Therapist's management of brachioplexopathy. In J. M. Hunter, E. J. Mackin, & A. D. Callahan (Eds.). *Rehabilitation of the hand* (4th ed., pp. 923–950). St. Louis: Mosby Year Book.

Bas, H., & Klienert, J. M. (1999). Anatomic variations in sensory innervation of the hand and digits. *Journal of Hand Surgery (24)6, 24,* 1171–1184.

Blackmore, S. M., & Hotchkis, R.N. (1995). Therapist's management of ulnar neuropathy at the elbow. In J. M. Hunter, E. J. Mackin, & A. D. Callahan (Eds.). *Rehabilitation of the hand* (4th ed., pp. 665–677). St. Louis: Mosby Year Book.

Boscheinen-Morrin, J., Davey, V., & Conolly, W. B. (1985). Peripheral nerve injuries. In The hand: Fundamentals of therapy (pp. 53–90). Boston: Butterworth.

Brand, P. W. (1995). Mechanics of tendon transfers. In J. M. Hunter, E. J. Mackin, & A. D. Callahan (Eds.). *Rehabilitation of the hand* (4th ed., pp. 715–727). St. Louis: Mosby Year Book.

Carpenter, M. B. (1978). Gross anatomy of the brain In Core text of neuroanatomy (2nd ed., pp. 15–40). Baltimore: Williams & Wilkins.

Chan, S. W., Jaglowski, J. M., & Kaplan, R. (1994). Rehabilitation of hand injuries. In M. Cohen (Ed.). *Mastery of plastic and reconstructive surgery* (pp. 1755–1757). Boston: Little, Brown.

Charness, M. E. (1992). Unique upper extremity disorders of musicians. In L. H. Millender, D. S. Louis, & B. P. Simmons (Eds.). *Occupational disorders of the upper extremity* (227–252). New York: Churchill Livingston.

Colditz, J. C. (1995). Splinting the hand with a peripheral nerve injury. In J. M. Hunter, E. J. Mackin, & A. D. Callahan (Eds.). *Rehabilitation of the hand* (4th ed., pp. 679–692). St. Louis: Mosby Year Book.

Dell, P. C., & Guzewicz, R. M. (1992). Atypical peripheral neuropathies. Nerve compression syndromes. *Hand Clinics, 8,* 275–282.

Dellon, L. A. (1992). Patient evaluation and management considerations in nerve compression. *Hand Clinics, 8,* 229–238.

Eaton, R. G. (1992). Entrapment syndromes in musicians. *Journal of Hand Therapy, 5,* 91–99.

Eaton, C. J., & Lister, G. D. (1992). Radial nerve compression. Nerve compression syndromes. *Hand Clinics, 8,* 345–352.

Elvey, R. L. (1997). Physical evaluation of the peripheral nervous system in disorders of pain and dysfunction. *Journal of Hand Therapy, 10,* 122–129.

Eversmann, W. (1992). Proximal median nerve compression. *Hand Clinics, 8,* 307–315

Harper, B. (1990). The drop out splint: an alternative to the conservative management of ulnar nerve entrapment at the elbow. *Journal of Hand Therapy, 3,* 199–201.

Hartz, C., Linscheild, R., Gramse, R., & Daube, J. (1981). The pronator teres syndrome: Compressive neuropathy of the median nerve. *Journal of Bone and Joint Surgery (American volume), 63,* 885–890.

Horn, K. L., & Crumley, R. L. (1984). The physiology of nerve repair. *Otolaryngologic Clinics of North America, 17,* 319–332.

Hunter, J. M., & Whitenack, S. H. (1995). Traction neuropathies of the brachial plexus and its terminal nerves. In J. M. Hunter, E. J. Mackin, & A. D. Callahan (Eds.). *Rehabilitation of the hand* (4th ed., pp. 885–904). St. Louis: Mosby Year Book.

Jones, N. F. (1994). Tendon transfers. In M. Cohen (Ed.). *Mastery of plastic and reconstructive surgery* (pp. 1579–1597). Boston: Little, Brown.

Lowe, C, & O'Toole, J. (1995). Therapist's management of brachial plexus injury. In J. M. Hunter, E. J. Mackin, & A. D. Callahan (Eds.). *Rehabilitation of the hand* (4th ed., pp. 647–664). St. Louis: Mosby Year Book.

Lundborg, G. (1988). Nerve entrapment. In Nerve injury and repair (pp. 111–148). New York: Churchill Livingston.

Mackinnon, S. E. (1992). Double and multiple crush syndromes. *Hand Clinics, 8,* 369–380.

Mackinnon, S. E. (1994). Nerve injuries: Primary repair and reconstruction. In M. Cohen (Ed.). *Mastery of plastic and reconstructive surgery* (pp. 1598–1624). Boston: Little, Brown.

Mackinnon, S. E., & Novak, C. B. (1997). Repetitive strain in the workplace. *Journal of Hand Surgery (American), 22,* 2–18

Matloub, H. S., & Yousif, N. J. (1992). Peripheral nerve anatomy and innervation patterns. *Hand Clinics, 8,* 203–214.

Moore, K. L., & Agur, A. M. (1995). Introduction to clinical anatomy. In *Essential clinical anatomy.* Baltimore: Williams & Wilkins.

Moore, K. L., & Dalley, A. F. (1999). *Clinically oriented anatomy* (4th ed.). Philadelphia: Lippincott, Williams & Wilkins.

Novak, C. D., Lee, G. W., Mackinnon, S. E., & Lay, L. (1994). Provacative testing for cubital tunnel syndrome. *Journal of Hand Surgery (American) 19,* 817–820.

Parry, W. (1981). Peripheral nerve injuries. In Rehabilitation of the Hand (4th ed., pp. 78–204). London: Butterworth.

Rayan, G. M. (1992). Proximal ulnar nerve compression, cubital tunnel syndrome. Nerve compression syndromes. *Hand Clinics, 8,* 325–331.

Roles, N. C., & Manudsley, R. H. (1972). Radial tunnel syndrome: Resistant tennis elbow as a nerve entrapment. *Journal of Bone and Joint Surgery (British volume), 54,* 400–508.

Sailor, S. M. (1996). The role of splinting and rehabilitation in the treatment of carpal and cubital tunnel syndrome. *Hand Clinics, 12,* 223–241.

Seddon, H. J. (1943).Three types of nerve injury. *Brain, 66,* 237.

Simmons, B. P., & Wyman, E. T. (1992). Occupational injuries of the elbow. In L. H. Millender, D. S. Louis, & B. P. Simmons (Eds.). *Occupational disorders of the upper extremity* (pp. 155–175). New York: Churchill Livingston.

Smith, K. L. (1995). Nerve response to injury and repair. In J. M. Hunter, E. J. Mackin, & A. D. Callahan (Eds.). *Rehabilitation of the hand* (4th ed., pp. 609–626). St. Louis: Mosby Year Book.

Smith, R. J. (1987). Tendon transfers of the hand and forearm. Boston: Little, Brown.

Stanley-Goodwyn, B. (1995).Preoperative and postoperative management of tendon transfers after median nerve injury. In J. M. Hunter, E. J. Mackin, & A. D. Callahan (Eds.). *Rehabilitation of the hand* (4th ed., pp. 765–778). St. Louis: Mosby Year Book.

Sunderland, S. (1952). Factors influencing the course of regeneration and the quality of recovery after nerve suture. *Brain,* 75, 19.

Tetro, A. M., & Pichora, D. R. (1996). Cubital tunnel and the painful upper extremity. *Hand Clinics, 12,* 665–678.

Thomas, S. J., Yakin, D. E., Parry, B. R., & Lubahn, J. D. (2000).The anatomical relationship between the posterior interosseous nerve and the supinator muscle. *Journal of Hand Surgery (American), 25,* 936–941

Warwick, L., & Seradge, H. (1995). Early versus late range of motion following cubital tunnel surgery. *Journal of Hand Therapy, 8,* 245–248.

SUGGESTED READING

Bell-Krotoski, J. A. (1995). Preoperative and postoperative management of tendon transfers after ulnar nerve injury. In J. M. Hunter, E. J. Mackin, & A. D. Callahan (Eds.). *Rehabilitation of the hand* (4th ed., pp. 753–763). St. Louis: Mosby Year Book.

Brand, P. W. (1993).Biomechanics of balance in the hand. *Journal of Hand Therapy, 6,* 247–251.

Brand, P. W., & Hollister, A. (1993). Operations to restore muscle balance in the hand. In Clinical mechanics of the hand (pp. 179–222). St. Louis: Mosby.

Burke, D. T., Burke, M. M., Stewart, G. W. (1994). Splinting for carpal tunnel syndrome: in search of the optimal angle. *Archives of Physical Medicine and Rehabilitation, 75,* 1241–1244.

Chusid, J. G. (1982). Peripheral nerves and autonomic system. Correlative neuroanatomy and functional neurology (pp. 85–139). Los Altos: Lange Medical.

Kasch, M. C. (1995).Therapists evaluation and treatment of upper extremity cumulative trauma disorders. In J. M. Hunter, E. J. Mackin, & A. D. Callahan (Eds.). *Rehabilitation of the hand* (4th ed., pp. 1731–1732). St. Louis: Mosby Year Book.

Klienart, J. M., & Mehta, S. (1996). Radial nerve entrapment. *Orthopedic Clinics of North America, 27,* 305–315.

Mackinnon, S. E., Dellon, A. L. (1988). *Surgery of the peripheral nerve.* New York: Thieme.

Millender, L. H., & Louis, D. S., Simmons BP. (1992). *Occupational disorders of the upper extremity.* New York: Churchill Livingston.

Omer, G. E., Jr, Spinner, M., Van Beek, A. L. (1997). *Management of peripheral nerve problems* (2nd ed.). Philadelphia: Saunders.

Omer, G. E., Jr. (1980). Tendon transfers for reconstruction of the forearm and hand following peripheral nerve injuries. In G. E. Omer, Jr & M. Spinner (Eds.). *Management of peripheral nerve problems* (pp. 817–846). Philadelphia: Saunders.

Reynolds, C. C. (1995). Preoperative and postoperative management of tendon transfers after radial nerve injury. In J. M. Hunter, E. J. Mackin, & A. D. Callahan (Eds.). *Rehabilitation of the hand* (4th ed., pp. 729–744). St. Louis: Mosby Year Book.

Ristic, S., Strauch, R., & Rosenwasser, M. (2000). The assessment and treatment of nerve dysfunction after trauma around the elbow. *Clinical Orthopaedics and Related Research, 370,* 138–153.

Serror, P. (1993).Treatment of ulnar nerve palsy at the elbow with a night splint. *Journal of Bone and Joint Surgery (British volume), 75,* 322–327.

Tardif, G. Nerve injuries. Testing and treatment tactics. *Physician and Sportsmedicine, 23,* 61–72.

Zancolli, E. A. (1957). Claw hand caused by paralysis of the intrinsic muscles a simple surgical procedure for it's correction. *Journal of Bone and Joint Surgery (American volume), 39,* 1076.

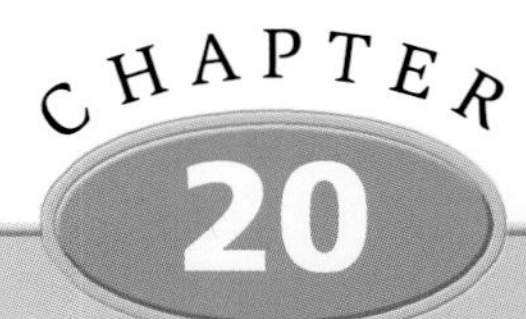

The Athlete

Lisa Schulz Slowman, MS, OTR/L, CHT

INTRODUCTION

Splinting upper extremity injuries in athletes poses unique challenges for the therapist. These splinting challenges do not arise primarily from the injuries seen but are often related to the unique demands of the athlete. Approximately one in four injuries sustained in sports involves the hand and wrist (Barton, 1997). The injured athlete, whether high school, collegiate, professional, or recreational, is generally eager to return to activity and competition as soon as possible. Often the therapist is asked to provide splinting that offers adequate protection to facilitate the early return to sports but that does not interfere with the athlete's performance.

The purpose of this chapter is to highlight common sport-specific injuries and review options in splinting management. Common upper extremity injuries seen in athletes are listed in Table 20–1 and include bony and ligamentous injuries to the elbow, forearm, wrist, hand, thumb, and digits in addition to a variety of other soft tissue injuries.

Splinting Implications

As with any condition, the splinting requirements for upper extremity injuries in athletes change as the athlete progresses through the phases of rehabilitation, from acute injury to return to sport (Schulz, Busconi, & Pappas, 1995). Special considerations include a history of similar injuries, the athlete's age and level of competition, the sport-specific demands of the athlete, and the rules established by the governing bodies relating to the use of protective devices during competition.

General Splinting Considerations

After injury, an athlete progresses through the phases of rehabilitation, which are acute injury, initial rehabilitation, progressive rehabilitation, integrated functions, and return to sport (Skerker & Schulz, 1995). In the early phases of rehabilitation, splinting goals are generally to provide rest and protection to the injured structure(s) while allowing easy removal of the splint for initiation of a range of motion (ROM) program. Other rehabilitation goals during this period are to decrease edema and pain.

As the athlete progresses, splinting goals begin to focus on providing protection to the injured structure(s) while minimally interfering with the upper extremity function of the athlete. For example, a hockey player who sustains a metacarpal fracture initially requires a wrist extension/metacarpophalangeal (MP) flexion immobilization splint to protect the fracture; the player removes the splint to do protected ROM exercises. As the athlete progresses to return to competition, he or she is fitted with a similarly positioned hand-based splint that fits into the hockey glove; this facilitates early return to competition.

Any splint or protective device provided to an athlete should protect the injured structure and prevent reinjury, allow safe and effective participation, not pose an injury threat to an opposing athlete, and meet the demands of the governing bodies for the sport and the local game officials (DeCarlo, Malone, Darmelio, & Rettig, 1994). The specific rules regarding the use of splints, casts, and other types of protective equipment depend on the sport and the level of competition. Information regarding the rules and guidelines is readily available; some sources are listed in Table 20–2.

Communication with the treating physicians, team athletic trainers, and/or coaches is important. These team members provide valuable information regarding the injury and help the therapist gain an understanding of the sport-specific demands to help maximize the splinting intervention. Specific demands include the level of competition, type of sport, and position played.

TABLE 20–1 Common Upper Extremity Sports Injuries

Sport	Injuries	
Baseball	Elbow • Medial tension overload syndrome (medial epicondylitis, ulnar neuropathy, ulnar collateral ligament instability)	Hand • Mallet finger • Phalangeal fractures • Hamate hook fractures
Basketball	Hand • Proximal or middle phalanx fracture • PIP joint sprain, fracture, or dislocation • Mallet finger • Acute Boutonniere injury	
Biking	Wrist • Ulnar neuropathy at Guyon's canal • Distal radius and/or ulna fracture • Scaphoid fracture • Hamate hook fracture • Hypothenar hammer syndrome	
Football	Wrist • Distal radius and/or ulna fracture • Scaphoid fracture • Triangular fibrocartilage (TFCC) complex injury	Hand • Metacarpal fracture • PIP sprain, fracture or dislocation • Flexor digitorum profundus (FDP) avulsion injury (jersey finger) • Mallet finger • Acute Boutonniere injury
Golf	Elbow • Medial epicondylitis (golfer's elbow) • Lateral epicondylitis Wrist • Intersection syndrome	Hand • Hypothenar hammer syndrome • Hamate hook fracture
Gymnastics	Elbow • Fracture and/or dislocation	Wrist • Dorsal impaction syndrome (gymnast's wrist) • TFCC injury
Hockey	Hand • Metacarpal fracture	
Lacrosse	Forearm • Radius and/or ulna midshaft fracture	Hand • Phalangeal fracture
In-line skating, roller skating, or skate boarding	Elbow • Radial head fracture • Radius and/or ulna shaft fracture	Wrist • Distal radius and/or ulna fracture • Scaphoid fracture • TFCC injury
Skiing	Hand • Thumb MP ulnar collateral ligament injury or avulsion fracture (skier's thumb)	
Snowboarding	Elbow • Radial head fracture	Wrist • Distal radius and/or ulna fracture • TFCC injury

Continued

TABLE 20–1 Continued

Sport	Injuries	
Tennis and racquet sports	Elbow • Lateral epicondylitis (tennis elbow) • Medial epicondylitis • Radial tunnel syndrome • Pronator syndrome	Wrist • Tendonitis • Intersection syndrome
Volleyball	Hand • Proximal or middle phalanx fracture • PIP sprain, fracture or dislocation • Mallet finger • Acute Boutonniere injury	

TABLE 20–2 Sports Rules and Regulations

National Collegiate Athletic Association (NCAA)
6201 College Blvd.
Overland Park, KS 66211-2422
913-339-1906
www.NCAA.org
College sports

National Federation of State High School Associations (NFHS)
P.O. Box 20626 [64195-0626]
11724 Northwest Plaza Circle
Kansas City, MO 64153
816-464-5400
www.NFHS.org
High school sports

American Alliance for Health, Physical Education, Recreation and Dance (AAHPERD)
1900 Association Dr.
Reston, VA 20191
703-476-3400
www.AAHPERD.org
High school sports

It is also important to know the athlete's goals for continued participation in the sport. For example, a high school field hockey player with the prospect of a collegiate sports scholarship may have a stronger desire to return to competition compared to a high school freshman trying field hockey for the first time.

If the athlete uses gloves or other equipment (e.g., sticks, clubs, bats, braces, handlebars), it is important that the athlete has them with him or her when any splint is fabricated. This allows the therapist to make any necessary modifications to permit continued effective use of the equipment without creating pressure areas or impingement from the splint (Fig. 20–1).

Finally, educating the athlete about the splint's purpose is imperative. The athlete should understand why the splint is necessary, when and how it should be used and cared for, and the plan for duration of use and weaning from the splint. The better the athlete understands the purpose of the splint, the greater the chance for compliance and the lower the patient's risk for reinjury. It is also important that the athlete's coach, athletic trainer, team members, and family understand the purpose and importance of the splint to help reinforce its use.

Materials Selection

A variety of splinting materials may be appropriate when splinting upper extremity injuries in athletes. The choice of material depends on the objective for the splint. For example, in the initial phases of rehabilitation, the goal for the splint may be to provide protection during daily activities and to allow removal for hygiene and ROM exercises. A ⅛" material typically used for a protective splint is appropriate. As the athlete returns to practice and competition, a **playing splint** (or cast) may be suitable. This type of splint can be made with a silicone rubber material, such as **room-temperature vulcanizing (RTV) material** (Canelon,

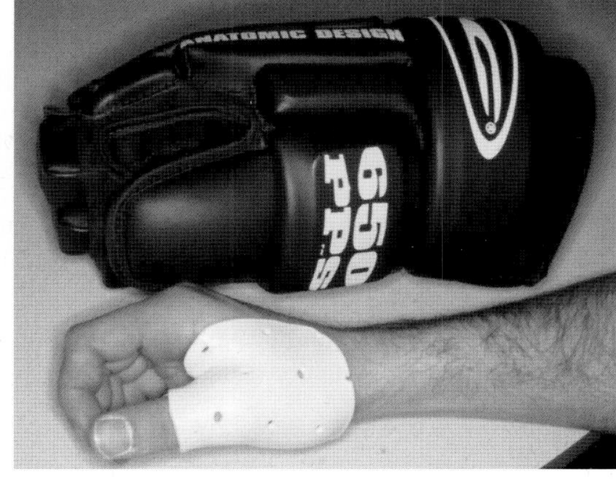

Figure 20–1 The therapist must consider the injured athlete's sports equipment when fabricating or fitting a splint. This thumb immobilization splint is protecting a healing UCL injury in this professional hockey player.

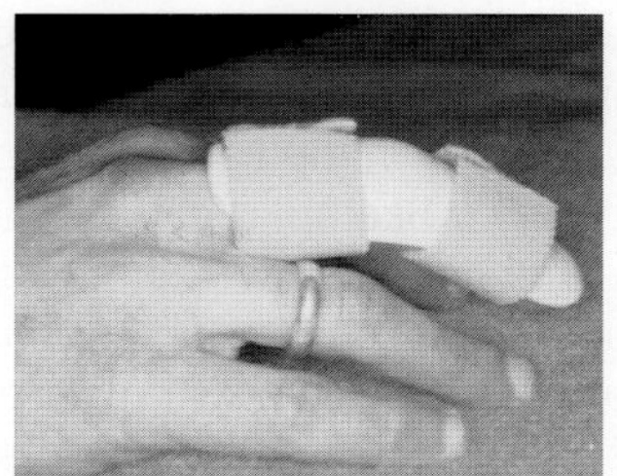

Figure 20–2 A PIP extension restriction splint for a volar plate avulsion fracture fabricated from 1/16" material.

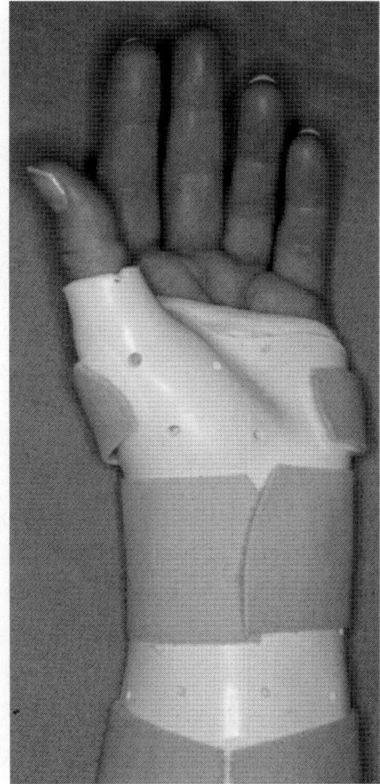

Figure 20–3 Wrist/thumb immobilization splint fabricated from 1/8" perforated material for a schaphoid fracture.

1995). This material works well as a transition splint providing impact absorption while continuing to protect healing structures. If only soft support is necessary, a **Neoprene splint** may be appropriate. Neoprene material is a synthetic, latex-free rubber that is available in a variety of thickness, densities, elasticity, and perforations. It is able to provide flexible support and compression via prefabricated or custom-fabricated splints (see Chapter 14 for details).

The body part being splinted also influences the material selection. A thinner material with memory, such as 1/16" or 1/32" Aquaplast, is a good option for digit-based immobilization splints used after a fracture (Fig. 20–2), but it may not be appropriate for a wrist/thumb immobilization splint following a scaphoid fracture, which requires greater durability, stability, and protection (Fig. 20–3).

When determining the best material to use for a protective splint for an athlete returning to competition, the therapist should consider the hardness of the material (must be strong enough to protect and stabilize the injured structures), the ability of the material to absorb an impact, and the rules of the sport's governing body and local officials regarding playing with splints and/or casts (DeCarlo et al., 1994). For example, professional and collegiate athletes can usually return to competition with a hard cast or splint provided that it is covered with soft padding, but this is generally not allowed in high school contact sports. The sport's governing body may dictate the thickness and type of padding material, but generally closed-cell foam at least 3/4" thick is appropriate. If the athlete requires padding only in competition, consider securing the padding in place with an elastic wrap so that it can be removed when the patient is not competing.

Material options include low-temperature thermoplastics, RTV silicone rubber, tape, fiberglass-based materials (Scotchrap and Plastazote), and Neoprene materials (Bouvette, Malanga, Cooney, Stuart, & Miller, 1994; Canelon, 1995; Colditz, 1999). QuickCast, a combination of rubber and fiberglass, has simplified many splint applications. Circumferential splints fabricated from this material provide immobilization and protection of the involved structure(s), eliminating the need for straps. If the splint is made without a liner, the athlete does not have to remove the cast for hygiene because of the material's mesh-like quality. In addition to the benefit of allowing air exchange, the material is extremely durable, allowing the athlete to bathe or swim with it on. This works especially well for acute boutonniere and mallet injuries, because the ability to get the hand wet is appreciated along with the slim custom fit (Fig. 20–4).

Additional considerations for splinting materials include the use of perforated materials to decrease perspiration and minimize skin irritation and the use of colored materials and strapping to coordinate with uniforms, which may improve splint compliance.

Strapping Selection

The strapping systems used for athletic splints are unique, especially for splints used in conjunction with other protective equipment. For example, a thumb immobilization splint fabricated for a ski racer returning to competition may not require a strap; rather the splint is held in place by the ski glove (Fig. 20–5). A strap in this case is unnecessary and could interfere with the skier's feel of the ski pole in the palm. But if strapping is to run

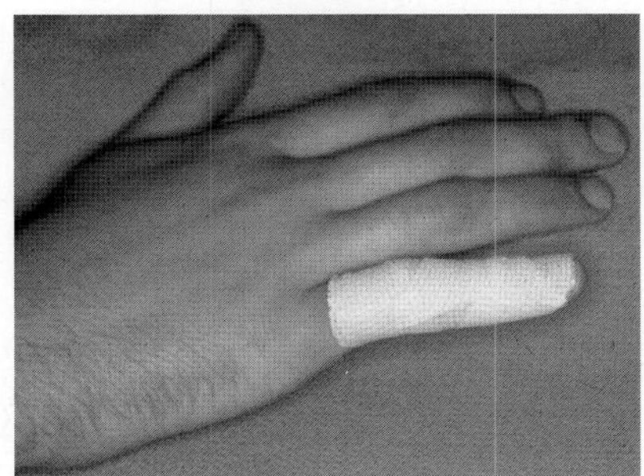

Figure 20–4 A QuickCast circumferential digit immobilization splint allows the patient to bathe with the splint on.

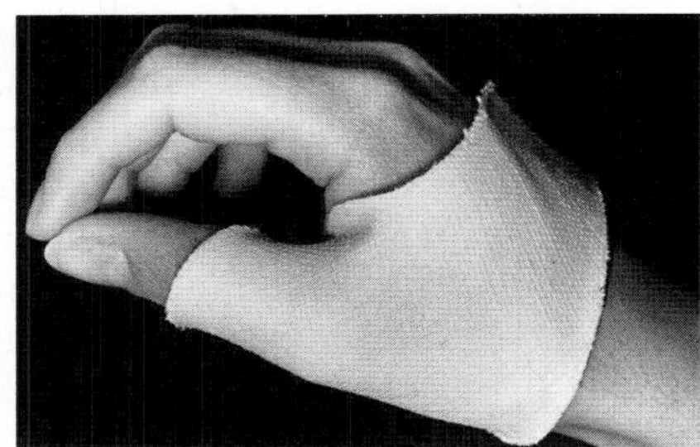

Figure 20–5 A hand-based thumb immobilization splint using Fabriplast that can be secured inside a ski glove without additional strapping.

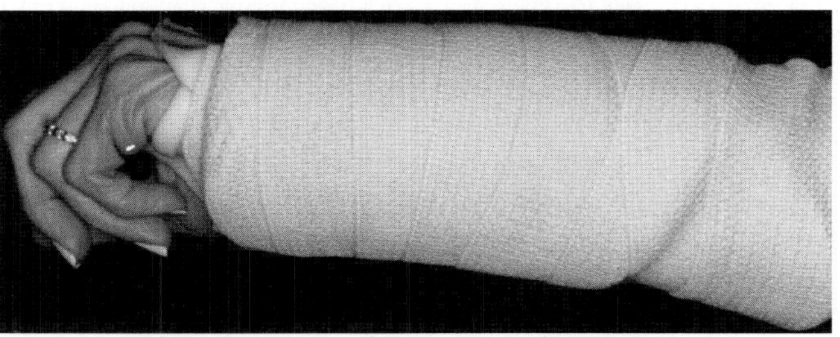

Figure 20–6 A padded wrist immobilization splint secured with a circumferential elastic wrap.

under equipment, consider soft strapping material to minimize the risk of skin irritation.

Sometimes, it is appropriate to use a circumferential elasticized wrap, such as an Ace wrap or Coban, to hold a splint in place. This secures the splint while distributing the pressure evenly on the body part. For example, when splinting the hand of a football blocker, a padded wrist splint used during practice or competition may best be secured with an elasticized bandage (Fig. 20–6).

It is important that the strapping best suits the athlete's needs. Whenever possible, the athlete should bring to the clinic the sports equipment he or she will use while wearing the splint. The athlete should practice using the splint with the equipment. The therapist must work with the athlete to customize the strapping system and allow maximal upper extremity use while maintaining the function of the splint. It may be necessary to secure the splint with tape or an elasticized wrap to decrease bulk. Two sets of straps are useful for athletes involved in aquatic activities such as rowing, kayaking, swimming, water polo, and diving so that dry straps are always available for securing the splint. This is necessary for maintaining good skin integrity under the straps.

Splinting Options

Common splints fabricated for athletes with upper extremity injuries include articular and nonarticular immobilization and restriction splints for the elbow, forearm, wrist, hand, thumb, and digits. Example of articular splints are a thumb MP immobilization splint used to protect the healing ulna collateral ligament (UCL) of a skier and a proximal interphalangeal (PIP) joint extension restriction splint used to prevent reinjury of the volar plate in a soccer player (Figs. 20–2 and 20–5). Examples of nonarticular splints are a proximal phalanx splint (pulley ring) for a rock climber to protect against flexor tendon sheath injury and a proximal forearm splint (epicondylitis strap) used to absorb and disperse forces of the forearm muscles as they approach the medial and/or lateral epicondyle(s) (Fig. 20–7) (Warme & Brooks, 2000; Wichmann & Martin, 1996).

Sport-Specific Injuries

Management of specific common upper extremity injuries such as fractures, fracture/dislocations, ligamentous injury, and muscle/tendon ruptures are discussed in detail elsewhere in this book (see Chapter 16 and Chapter 18). A brief description of common sport-related injuries are reviewed below. Table 20–3 summarizes splinting for sport-related injuries.

Fractures

When treating an athlete with an acute fracture, the therapist must consider the stability of the injury as well as the patient's age, level of competition, position played, and desire to return to sport. Most fractures sustained by athletes during competition are stable injuries owing to the relatively low impact forces involved, and they can be treated with immobilization followed by a transition into a playing splint with early return to competition (Rettig, 1991). Unstable fractures may require surgical intervention, resulting in a more variable course of treatment (see Chapter 16).

Distal Radius

Distal radius fractures are common in sporting activities; the usual mechanism of injury is a fall on an outstretched hand (FOOSH). These injuries tend to be high-energy fractures and involve the articular surfaces causing disruption of the distal radioulnar and distal radiocarpal joints (Rettig & Raskin, 2000). After cast removal, a wrist immobilization splint with a circumferential design may offer the most protection for the athlete while he or she begins to progress through the later stages of rehabilitation (Fig. 20–8). Returning to full sport participation depends on

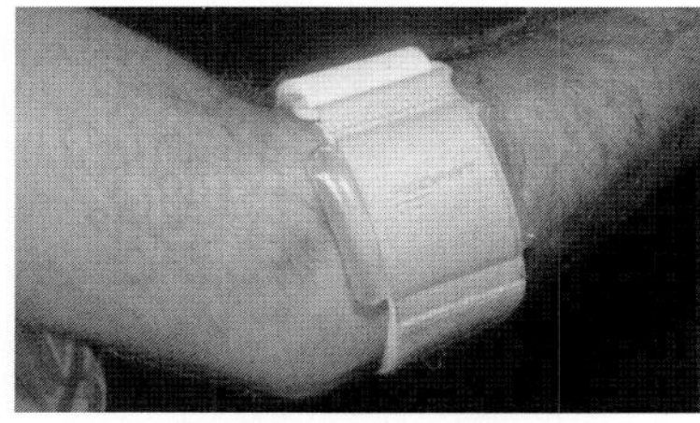

Figure 20–7 A proximal forearm splint (also known as an epicondylitis strap or counterforce brace) used to reduce stress at the epicondyle. (An Aircast Pneumatic Airband is shown; North Coast Medical, Morgan Hill, CA.)

TABLE 20–3 Splinting for Sports Injuries

Diagnosis	Splint Options	Considerations	Time Frame
Distal radius and/or ulna fracture	After ORIF or cast removal: • Wrist immobilization splint Return to sport: • Circumferential wrist splint (primarily with contact sports)	• Adapt playing splint to athlete's upper extremity demands • Well padded on outside for contact sports	• With confirmed healing, protective splint worn for 2–4 weeks per physician recommendation and sports-specific position requirements
Scaphoid fracture	After ORIF or cast removal: • Wrist/thumb MP immobilization splint Return to sport: • Circumferentially padded wrist/thumb immobilization splint or an RTV playing cast • Neoprene wrist/thumb wrap • Taping to restrict thumb motion	• Adapt playing splint to athlete's upper extremity demands • Trim thumb portion of Neoprene wrap to allow necessary motion • Tape to limit full thumb motion, protecting against hyperextension and radial deviation forces	• Per physician recommendation and sports-specific position requirements • Use of playing splint depends on status of scaphoid healing
Metacarpal fracture	After ORIF or cast removal: • wrist extension/MP flexion or MP flexion immobilization splint Return to sport: depending on fracture stability and sport-specific demands • Buddy taping • Wrist/hand or hand immobilization splint	• Make sure splint is adapted to equipment used by athlete (hockey stick and glove, bicycle handle bars, ski glove and pole)	• Per physician recommendation and sports-specific position requirements
Phalangeal fracture	After ORIF or cast removal: • Hand-based digit immobilization splint • Buddy taping Return to sport: depends on fracture stability and sport-specific demands • Digit or hand immobilization splint for injured digit(s) only • Digit or hand immobilization splint for injured and adjacent digits • Buddy taping to adjacent digits	• Splint should provide enough stability to protect fracture and adapted to allow athlete to meet upper extremity demands • Adapt splint to equipment as necessary	• Per physician recommendation and sports-specific position requirements
PIP fracture and/or dislocation (volar plate injury)	Acute (nonoperative management): • Hand-based PIP extension restriction splint (extension allowed is increased weekly until full extension is attained) Return to sport: • Buddy taping to adjacent digit	• Splint should position PIP in appropriate degree of flexion determined by fracture reduction • Early motion program and edema management important	• PIP extension restriction splint used for initial 2–4 weeks • Buddy taping continues for 4–6 months during competition

AROM, active range of motion; *DIP,* distal interphalangeal; *FDP,* flexor digitorum profundus; *IP,* interphalangeal; *ORIF,* open reduction and internal fixation; *PROM,* passive range of motion.

Continued

TABLE 20–3 Continued			
Diagnosis	**Splint Options**	**Considerations**	**Time Frame**
Acute Boutonniere injury	Acute (nonoperative management): • PIP or IP extension immobilization splint	• Watch for problems with skin maceration or breakdown at dorsal PIP joint • Changes in edema require splint adjustments • Splint must maintain PIP in full extension when DIP is actively flexed with exercise	• Used 4–6 weeks (day and night) • Used 4–8 weeks between ROM exercises and at night • Used 8+ weeks at night and as required during the day
Mallet finger	Acute (nonoperative management): • DIP extension immobilization splint	• Watch for problems with skin maceration or breakdown at dorsal DIP joint • Changes in edema require splint adjustments • Watch for inadvertant removal of splint if used under glove	• Use 6 weeks (day and night) • Use 6–8 weeks ROM exercise and at night • Use 8+ weeks at night and as needed during the day
FDP avulsion (jersey finger)	After surgical repair: wrist flexion/MP flexion/IP extension immobilization splint	• With repaired tendon, follow protocol precautions • Generally, athlete will not return to competition for at least 12 weeks	• Use 4–6 weeks (day and night) • Use 6–8 weeks: for additional protection only
Thumb UCL injury (skier's or gamekeeper's thumb)	After surgical repair (Stenar lesion): • Wrist/thumb MP immobilization splint After cast immobilization: • Thumb immobilization splint Return to sport: • Hand-based splint during sport for 1–2 months Partial tear: hand-based thumb MP immobilization splint • Taping (Chapter 13)	• Adapt splint to equipment used by athlete	• After surgery: use ~8 weeks • After casting: use 6–8 weeks • Partial tear: use 4–6 weeks
Medial epicondylitis (golfer's elbow)	• Proximal forearm splints (counterforce brace: Epitrain, Nirschl brace) or custom made • Taping (Chapter 13)	• In addition to bracing, patient education, anti-inflammatory treatment, massage, ice, activity modification, and equipment modification (wider handle) may help	• Depends on symptoms
Lateral epicondylitis (tennis elbow)	• Proximal forearm splints (counterforce brace: Epitrain, Nirschl brace) or custom made • Taping (Chapter 13)	• In addition to bracing, patient education, anti-inflammatory treatment, massage, ice, and activity modification, and equipment modification (wider handle, string tension) may help	• Depends on symptoms

AROM, active range of motion; *DIP,* distal interphalangeal; *FDP,* flexor digitorum profundus; *IP,* interphalangeal; *ORIF,* open reduction and internal fixation; *PROM,* passive range of motion.

TABLE 20–3 Continued

Diagnosis	Splint Options	Considerations	Time Frame
Guyon's canal syndrome (handlebar palsy)	Acute symptoms: • Wrist immobilization splint in neutral to slight flexion and ulnar deviation Return to sport: • Padded biking gloves	• Padding may require modification (doughnut) to relieve pressure on the nerve	• Depends on symptoms
Dorsal impaction syndrome (gymnast's wrist)	Return to sport: • Wrist immobilization splint to decrease wrist hyperextension • Neoprene splint • Taping (Chapter 13)	• Minimize palmar contact area in the hand with splint material and strapping • Patient education regarding changing hand position and periodic stretching • Consider prefabricated or Neoprene splint to limit hyperextension	• Continuous use for practice and competition • Not used for daily activities

AROM, active range of motion; *DIP*, distal interphalangeal; *FDP*, flexor digitorum profundus; *IP*, interphalangeal; *ORIF*, open reduction and internal fixation; *PROM*, passive range of motion.

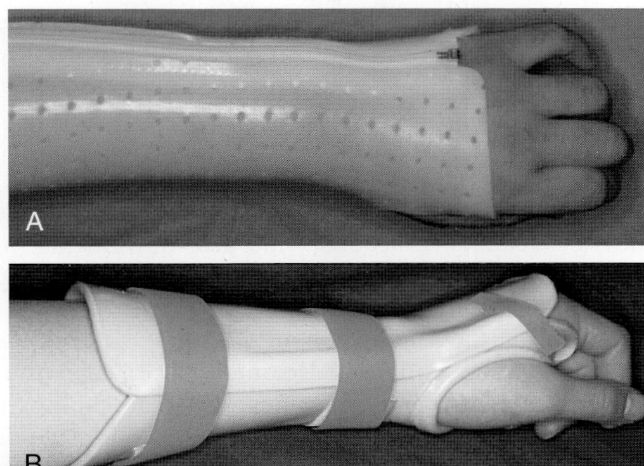

*Figure 20–8 Circumferential wrist immobilization splints. **A,** Roylan AquaForm Zippered Wrist Splint (Smith+Nephew, Germantown, WI). **B,** Clamshell design with interlocking volar and dorsal pieces.*

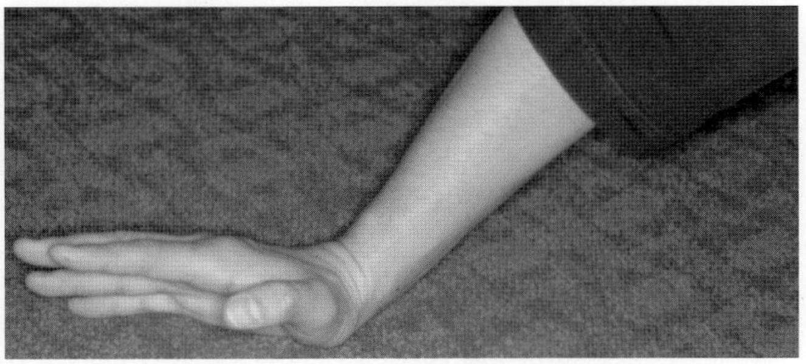

Figure 20–9 Scaphoid and distal radius fractures are commonly caused by a fall on an outstretched hand.

the sport-specific activities and the demands placed on the healing extremity. For example, a soccer player (except the goalie) may be able to return to play before a football player, because of the individual natures of the sports.

Scaphoid

A **scaphoid fracture** in sports can occur with a fall on an outstretched arm with maximum wrist dorsiflexion (football, soccer, biking) (Fig. 20–9). Stable nondisplaced fractures are often immobilized in either a long arm or a short arm thumb spica cast, followed by splint application during the initial return to play (Fig. 20–3) (Rettig, 1991). If bone healing is slow and both the physician and the athlete agree that return to a guarded level of performance may be of benefit, then a protective playing cast—made from silicone rubber—may be appropriate (Canelon, 1995; Rettig, 1991). In the collegiate or professional athlete, percutaneous fixation of nondisplaced scaphoid fractures may be done to facilitate early return to competition in a playing cast.

Bennett's

Fracture of the base of the first metacarpal, a **Bennett's fracture,** is often associated with a fall on a hyperextended thumb, as in a baseball player diving for a ball. The fracture is accentuated by the strong pull of the abductor pollicis longus (APL) tendon as it inserts on the base of the first metacarpal. The athlete generally undergoes a period of cast immobilization; after this, he or she is fitted with a return-to-sport splint (Fig. 20–3). For unstable first metacarpal fractures in athletes, especially for the professional athlete, surgical fixation may be the primary treatment of choice, because surgical fixation may facilitate an earlier return to play.

Metacarpal

Fracture of the neck, shaft, or base of the metacarpal bone(s) can be sustained from blunt trauma (hit with a lacrosse stick, goalie block in soccer) and, more commonly, from punching-type sports (boxing, karate). **Metacarpal shaft fractures** may be adequately treated with a simple nonarticular metacarpal immobilization splint that traverses the involved metacarpal and adjacent structures. When treating a young athlete, the therapist should consider adding the proximal phalanx within the splint and buddy taping the injured finger to the adjacent finger (Fig. 20–10). Including the MP joint in the splint provides greater protection and stability against external forces (Colditz, 1995).

A **metacarpal neck fracture** of the ring (RF) or small (SF) fingers can be managed with a splint that immobilizes the metacarpals along with the middle metacarpal and positions the MP joints in flexion. Anchoring the RF and SF to the MF decreases the natural mobility of the ulnar side of the hand. **Metacarpal base fractures** are treated in the same manner; however, the wrist is included in the splint to provide optimal fracture alignment.

Phalangeal

Fracture of the proximal or middle phalanges are common in the athlete. **Phalangeal fractures** can occur in a variety of sports, including tumbling events in gymnastics, wrestling maneuvers, football, and lacrosse. Fracture management using splints depends on the location (articular versus nonarticular), type of fracture, presence of dislocation or subluxation, and need for surgical intervention. Of the many options for splinting these fractures, fracture bracing, circumferential casting, restrictive splinting, and buddy taping are examples (Fig. 20–2 and 20–4).

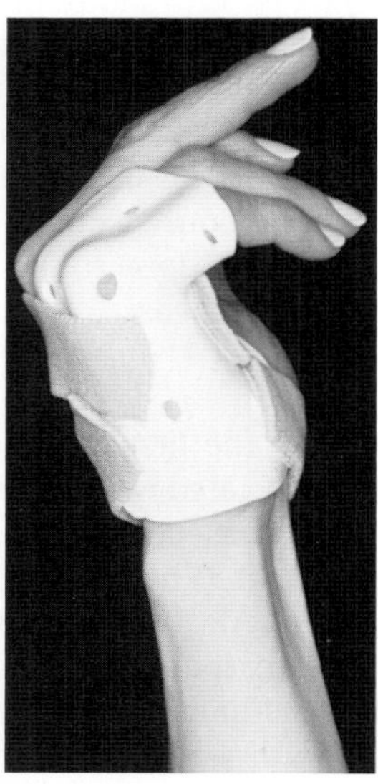

Figure 20–10 A hand-based splint, designed to fit into a hockey glove, made from perforated ⅛" material to allow for air exchange. Notice how the PIP joints are free to move.

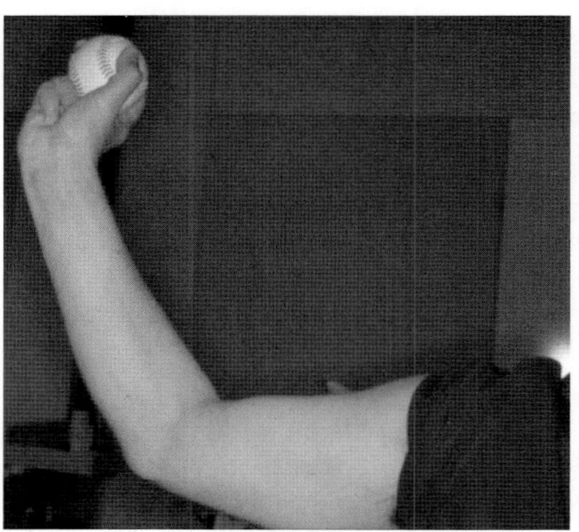

Figure 20–11 Pitching places tremendous stress on the medial structures about the elbow.

Sprains, Ligamentous Injuries, Dislocations

Injury to ligamentous structures are common in athletes. The degree of injury depends on the amount of force applied to the body part and directly effects the recommended medical intervention.

Elbow Ulnar Collateral Ligament Injuries

Medial-side elbow injuries are common in any sport requiring forceful overhead or side arm movements, for example with baseball pitching (Fig. 20–11). Owing to the combination of forces on the elbow during the final stages of cocking and initiation of the acceleration phase, the **ulnar collateral ligament (UCL)** and **ulnar nerve** can undergo significant microtrauma, resulting in both acute and chronic injuries, such as progressive degeneration of the UCL. Rest (immobilization in a splint to limit lateral stress to the elbow), followed by strengthening of the flexor pronator mass, is the initial treatment. In chronic cases, reconstruction of the UCL may be indicated. Symptoms of ulnar neuropathy often occur simultaneously; therefore, an ulnar nerve transposition may be performed at the same time (Alley & Pappas, 1995). Postoperative management involves protection in a long arm splint immediately after surgery and initiation of gentle elbow flexion and extension 1 week later. Protection against lateral stresses is accomplished with an articulating (hinged) brace once the athlete begins full ROM and activity (Fig. 20–12).

Triangular Fibrocartilage Complex Tears

Injury to the **triangular fibrocartilage complex (TFCC),** a stabilizer and cushion for the ulnar carpus, is often caused by a fall on an outstretched hand resulting in compression of the TFCC between the head of the ulna and the carpus. This injury is seen in athletes who break a fall with the hand (gymnasts) or who undergo excessive rotational force (e.g., racket and throwing sports) (Howse, 1994). A nonsurgical or surgical approach may be taken with this population, depending on the severity of the disruption. Splinting can be an important component of the rehabilitation plan. Initial injury may require a rigid cast for complete immobilization. As rehabilitation progresses, a less rigid support, such as taping or Neoprene, may be appropriate to allow initiation of guarded activity with continued protection (Fig. 20–13).

Thumb MP Joint Injury

Thumb MP joint sprain most often occurs from forceful thumb MP hyperextension, resulting in a MP volar dislocation. Lateral forces at the MP joint can disrupt the collateral ligaments, resulting in joint instability. A UCL sprain—also known as gamekeeper's or skier's thumb—occurs commonly in sports after a fall onto the hand with the thumb in abduction, such as when gripping a ski pole or racquet (Fig. 20–14) (Melone, Beldner, & Basuk, 2000). Splints can be used to place the ligament in a tension-free position while healing occurs (Fig. 20–5). As with other ligamentous injuries, a range of damage can occur, from a midsubstance tear of the ligament to a fracture avulsion of the ligament as it inserts on the thumb proximal phalanx. In a pure ligamentous injury, a Stenar lesion can occur (the adductor is interposed between the UCL and its insertion). A rotated fracture or a Stenar lesion is generally an indication for surgery (Melone et al., 2000). Patients who require surgery should undergo a period of postoperative immobilization in a splint that can be used for protection during sport and to prevent reinjury. Radial collateral ligament disruptions can also occur, but those injuries are much less common.

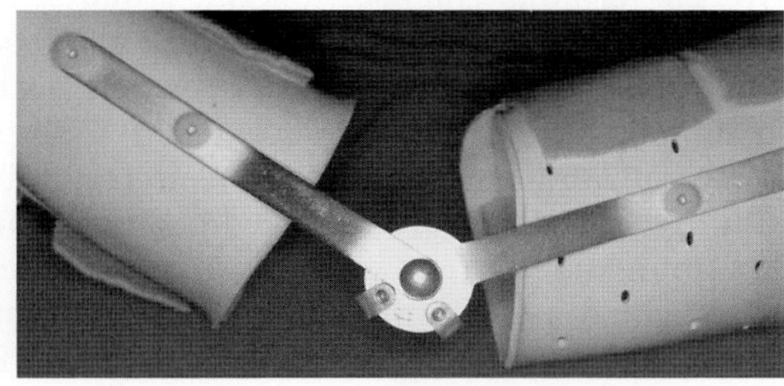

Figure 20–12 A Phoenix Elbow Hinge prevents lateral forces about the elbow and allows the therapist to restrict specific degrees of motion.

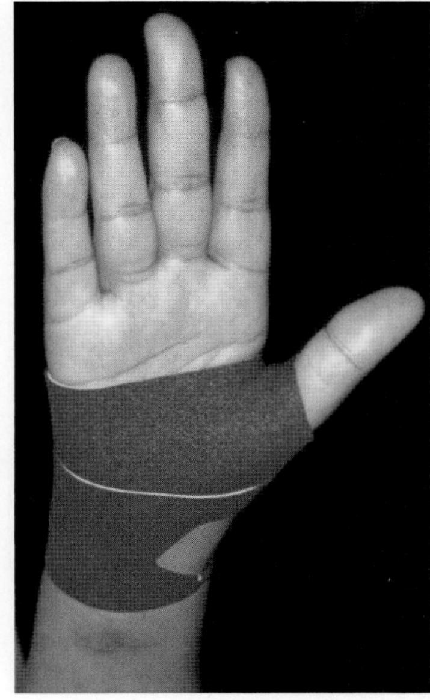

Figure 20–13 A Neoprene wrist wrap provides warmth and light support to the wrist.

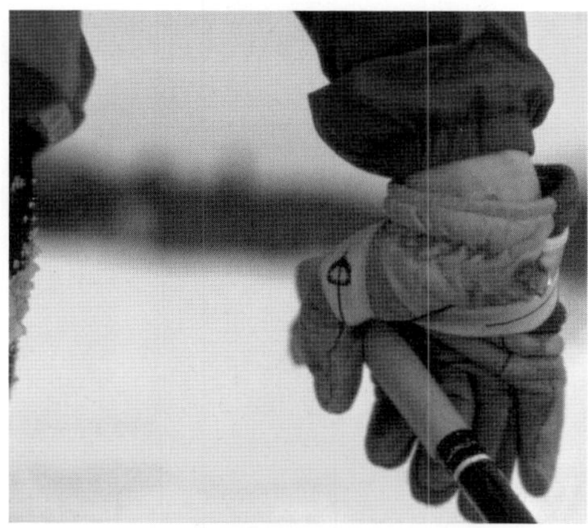

Figure 20–14 Note that holding a ski pole places the thumb MP joint at risk for injury.

PIP Joint Dislocations

PIP joint dislocation can result from an axial load or hyperextension force applied to the PIP joint in sports such as volleyball, basketball, soccer (primarily goalie), rock climbing, and gymnastics (Fig. 20–15). The severity of this injury depends on the amount of force applied and the direction of the force (Glickel & Barron, 2000). Injury can occur to a single collateral ligament, to both collateral ligaments, and/or to the volar plate. If the volar plate is disrupted, then at least one of the collateral ligaments is usually involved. This injury can include a fracture of the middle phalanx associated with the volar plate (fracture dislocation of the PIP joint).

Splint needs are affected by the degree of injury and stability of the joint. Collateral ligament injuries may be managed with buddy taping or Figure-8 splinting (Fig. 20–16), whereas volar plate involvement usually requires dorsal PIP extension restriction splinting (Fig. 20–2). Splinting after surgical intervention may also be necessary.

Distal Interphalangeal Joint Dislocations

A forceful blow to the distal finger is most often the cause of **distal interphalangeal (DIP) joint disloca-**

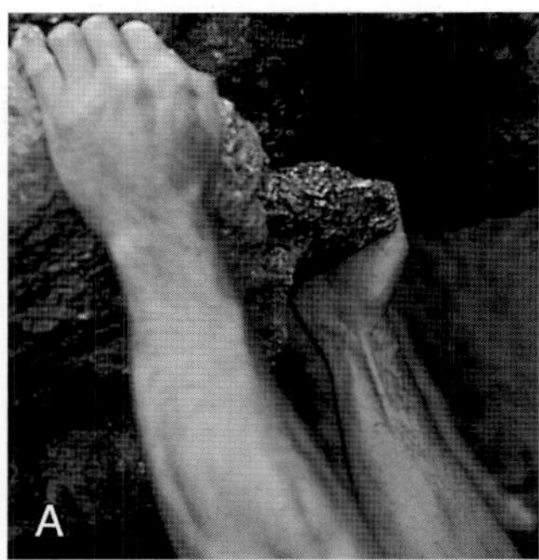

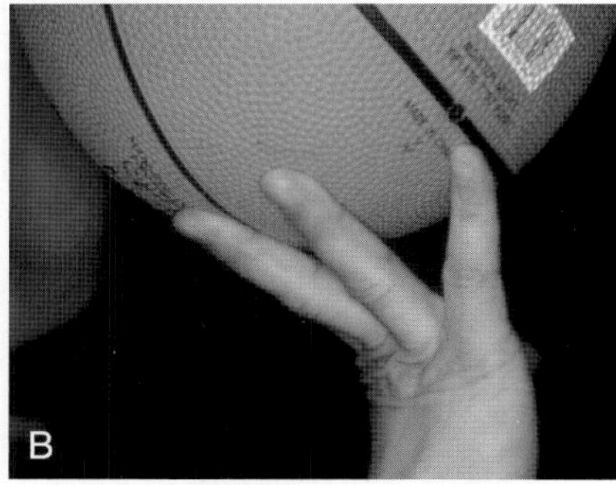

Figure 20–15 ***A,*** *The IP joints are stressed during rock climbing, placing them at risk for injury.* ***B,*** *PIP hyperextension injuries are common in basketball players.*

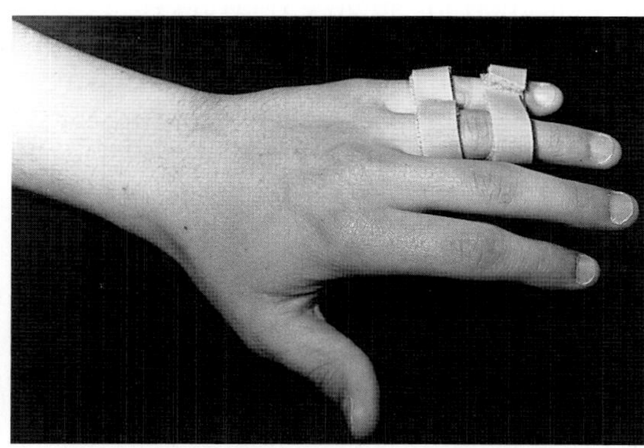

Figure 20–16 *Buddy taping the ring and small fingers, while allowing unrestricted digit motion, can be challenging because of the difference in the lengths of the fingers. Custom straps to accommodate this difference is necessary to allow full joint motion.*

tion. Sprain and/or dislocation of the DIP joint can occur in many sports, but these injuries are most often associated with ball-handling sports such as volleyball, basketball and football. Thermoplastic materials, taping techniques, and silicone-lined products are a few options available for protecting an injured distal phalanx.

Tendon Injuries

Tendon injuries can occur in any sport in which the tendon is placed in a vulnerable position (e.g., excessive force loading, forceful hyperextension or flexion).

Distal Biceps Tendon Rupture

Distal **biceps tendon rupture** can occur after a fall on a hyperextended elbow or a sudden eccentric load to the biceps brachii muscle during a sport such as snowboarding, rock climbing, and bodybuilding (Williams, Hang, & Bach, 1996). Athletes usually note that a pop occurred during the activity and present with a deformity of the upper arm with pain and difficulty supinating forearm. Management of these patients can be surgical or nonsurgical. Surgical repair to preserve elbow flexion and supinating strength is one option for the highly competitive athlete. Rehabilitation protocols after surgical repair of the ruptured biceps tendon depends on the method and stability of the repair. Newer protocols advocate early restricted ROM, whereas older protocols favor an extended period of immobilization (Fig. 20–12). Return to the preinjury level of competition is dictated by the surgeon and may warrant several months of rehabilitation for regaining full strength for sports participation (Morrey, 1993).

Terminal Extensor Tendon Rupture (Mallet Finger)

Injury to the terminal extensor tendon, a **mallet finger,** can occur from hitting the fingertip against an oncoming ball (volleyball, baseball) or on an opponent's athletic equipment helmet (Fig. 20–17) (Scott, 2000). The athlete should wear a DIP extension immobilization splint, with the DIP in a neutral to hyperextended position, continuously for approximately 6–8 weeks to allow for adequate healing (Wichmann & Martin, 1996). Splints can be custom fabricated from thin thermoplastic material or QuickCast, or a prefabricated splint such as a Stax or AlumaFoam splint can be fit to the digit (Fig. 20–18). The splint can be secured with cloth tape, Coban, or hook-and-loop straps.

Profundus Avulsion (Jersey Finger)

Flexor digitorum profundus (FDP) avulsion usually occurs when a player grabs the jersey of another player and gets the fingertip caught in the shirt while the opposing player continues to run (Fig. 20–19). This is most commonly seen in the RF FDP tendon (Stamos &

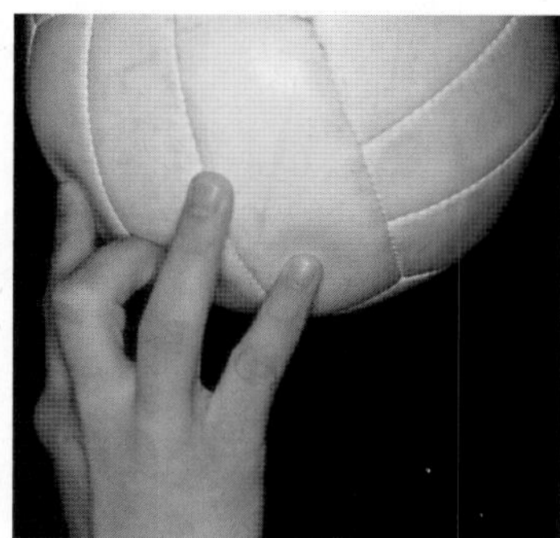

Figure 20–17 *Force directed at the DIP joint into flexion can result in a mallet finger deformity.*

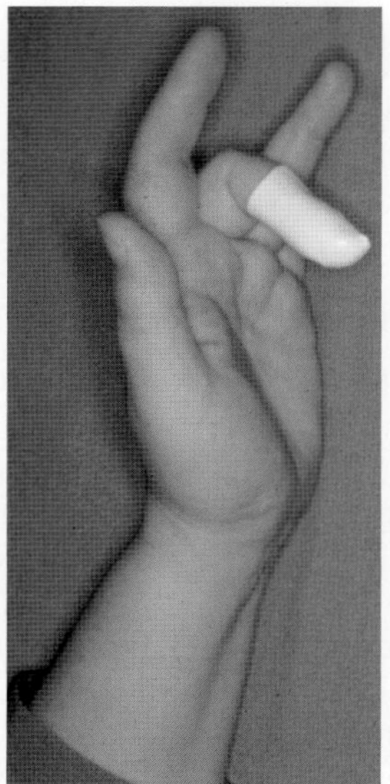

Figure 20–18 *A DIP immobilization splint fabricated from 1/16" material. Note clearance of PIP joint.*

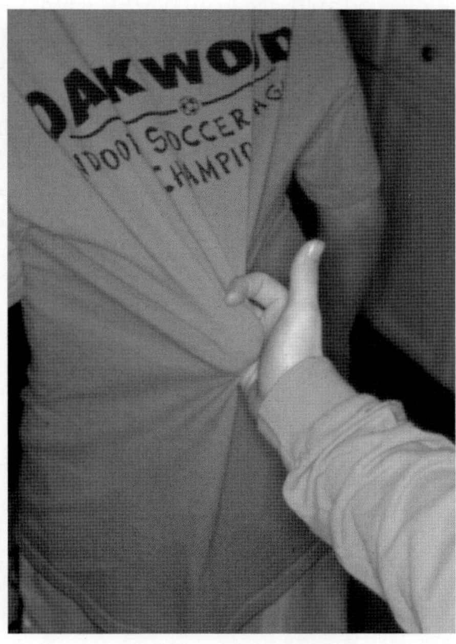

Figure 20–19 *If a player has a finger stuck in an opponent's jersey, the DIP joint will be forced to flex strongly if the opponent continues to run. This may result in a rupture of the FDP tendon.*

Leddy, 2000). This is a severe injury and should be managed according to the treating physician's flexor tendon protocol (see Chapter 18). For professional athletes and promising collegiate athletes, the option to not repair the ruptured tendon may be exercised. The athlete may require taping of the digits upon return to sport. Postseason or at the end of the athlete's career, secondary tendon repair options or a DIP fusion may be considered.

Acute Boutonniere Injury

Rupture of the extensor mechanism at the PIP joint can result in flexion posturing of the PIP, a **boutonniere deformity,** owing to rupture of the insertion of the central tendon and volar migration of the lateral bands (Fig. 20–20) (Scott, 2000). These injuries can occur from a fall or from striking the hand against another player or ball. Immobilization of the PIP joint in extension for 6 to 8 weeks is necessary for the management of these injuries. A variety of splint designs can be fabricated to achieve this goal. In most cases, the DIP joint is left free for ROM to encourage and facilitate gliding of the lateral bands dorsally. Splinting may be continued throughout the rest of the sport season as a precautionary measure (Wright & Rettig, 1995).

Other Soft Tissue Injuries

Overuse injuries in athletes can result from repetitive microtrauma that leads to inflammation of the involved muscle/tendon units and local tissue irritation and/or damage. These injuries are most likely to occur when an athlete changes the mode, intensity, or duration of training. Soft tissue injuries can occur from a single traumatic event or from repetitive stress.

Olecranon Bursitis

The olecranon bursa is a fluid-filled sac at the posterior elbow that may become inflamed from pressure or a direct blow to the olecranon process, with resultant **olecranon bursitis.** This is sometimes seen in golfers with repeated grounding of the club or during athletic competition from direct blows sustained to this region from a piece of playing equipment (hockey stick, baseball bat, tennis racket). Treatment options include aspiration, cortisone injection, edema control techniques, and the use of a soft elbow protective pad. Return to sport is recommended when the athlete can use the piece of sporting equipment with adequate force and no pain. Weight bearing should be performed painlessly before returning to any sport requiring such maneuvers (e.g., gymnastics).

Epicondylitis

Injury to the muscles and tendon origins at both the medial and lateral elbow are seen in a variety of athletes (Fig. 20–21). Repetitive microtrama to either the wrist extensors (**lateral epicondylitis**) or the flexor pronator mass (**medial epicondylitis**) can result in injury, ranging from acute inflammation to chronic degeneration and fibroblastic

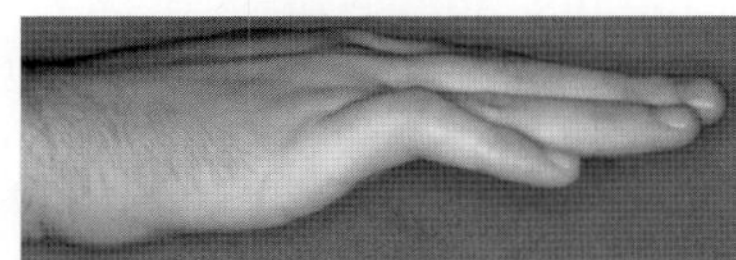

Figure 20–20 *Acute boutonniere injury results in PIP flexion and occasionally DIP extension.*

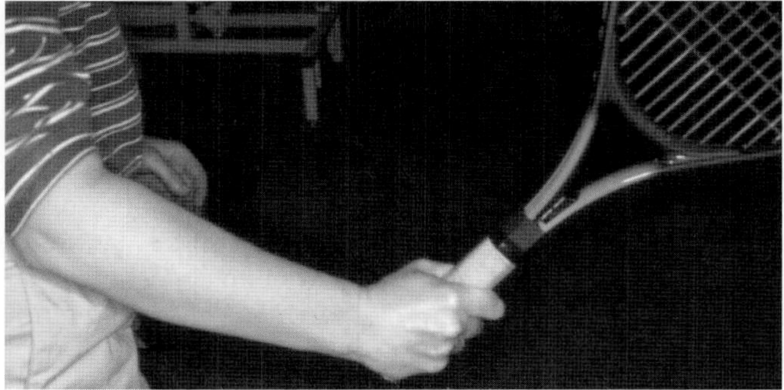

Figure 20–21 When treating a tennis player with lateral epicondylitis, the therapist should critique his or her technique and equipment offering suggestions for modification.

changes (Anderson, Hall, & Martin, 2000). Management of these injuries focuses on rest (refraining from the sport), nonsteroidal anti-inflammatory drugs (NSAIDs), and/or corticosteroid injection. Splinting or taping of the wrist to decrease activity of the involved muscle/tendon units and the use of a nonarticular proximal forearm splint (counterforce brace) may help (Fig. 20–7). It is important for the athlete and therapist to determine the factors that may be contributing to the development of the epicondylitis—e.g., grip size, racquet stringing, and technique (Alley & Pappas, 1995). Appropriate changes should be made.

DeQuervain's Tenosynovitis

DeQuervain's tenosynovitis involves the tendon and synovial sheath of two thumb muscles: the extensor pollicis brevis (EPB) and the abductor pollicis longus (APL). These tendons share a common tendon sheath (first dorsal compartment), which can become irritated and inflamed when there is too much friction within the sheath as a result of activities such as improperly using a golf club or racquetball racket. A direct blow to this area can result in an acute onset of DeQuervain's tenosynovitis. Pain usually occurs with ulnar deviation of the wrist and thumb flexion (a positive Finkelstein test) and most often radiates proximally along the thumb column into the forearm. Management is similar to other tendonopathies, including rest (splinting and activity modification), NSAIDs, corticosteroid injection, and equipment modification. The appropriate splint for this condition is one that immobilizes the wrist and thumb (Fig. 20–3). Taping can also be considered.

Intersection Syndrome

Intersection syndrome is inflammation or tenosynovitis at the junction of the first and second dorsal compartments of the wrist (Servi, 1997). Intersection syndrome most often occurs from overuse of the radial wrist extensors, for example in skiing when the pole is pulled from deep snow. It may also be seen in weightlifters, rowers, and indoor racket sport players (Servi, 1997). Signs and symptoms include tenderness, crepitus, and swelling over the dorsal radial aspect of the forearm. Crepitation, or squeaking, may be noted with active wrist extension or passive motion. Treatment is similar to that for DeQuervain's tenosynovitis: splinting, NSAIDs, and activity/equipment modification. Splinting should incorporate the wrist positioned in extension (Fig. 20–22).

Extensor Carpi Ulnaris Tenosynovitis

The extensor carpi ulnaris (ECU) tendon is a prime mover for wrist extension and ulnar deviation. **ECU tenosynovitis** can occur in athletes who participate in racket and rowing sports, because of the repetitive ulnar deviation involved in these activities. Management consists of rest, evaluation of equipment, and technique modification. The wrist should be splinted in extension and slight ulnar deviation (Fig. 20–22). Transition athlete to a strengthening program once the inflammation and pain have been controlled.

Distal Ulna Instability

Distal ulna instability can be acute or chronic in nature. Acute instability is often associated with a fracture of the ulna styloid and disruption of the TFCC. Treatment of this type of injury may be surgical or may require 6 weeks of cast immobilization (Morgan, 1995). Chronic instability often results from a late diagnosis after a "wrist sprain"—e.g., in gymnasts or snowboarders. Treatment of these injuries is generally surgical and involves a period of immobilization after surgery. A Neoprene or leather extension restriction splint may be recommended when the athlete returns to practice and competition.

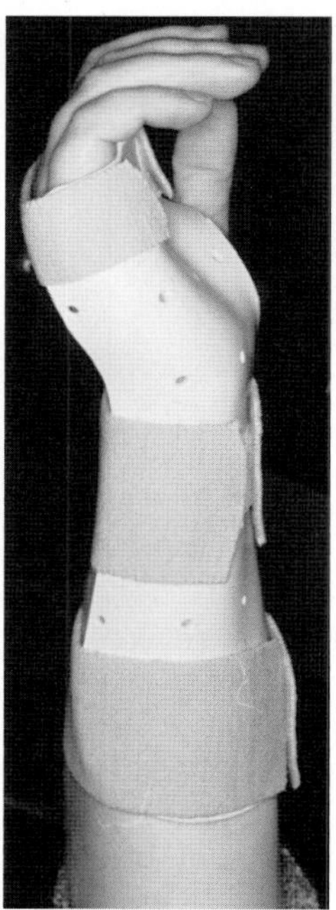

Figure 20–22 A wrist immobilization splint is commonly used to treat tendonitis about the wrist, forearm, and elbow region.

Pisotriquetral Joint Synovitis

Pisotriquetral joint synovitis, or degeneration between the pisiform and triquetrum, can cause pain with activities that require gripping or pressure along the volar ulnar aspect of the palm. Arthritic changes in this joint are often an indication for pisiform excision. A gel-lined or cushioned splint may be helpful to protect this area from direct trauma during competition.

Hypothenar Hammer Syndrome

Athletes exposed to blunt trauma to the hands, for example catchers in baseball, are at risk for injury to the ulnar artery, called **hypothenar hammer syndrome.** This can result in ischemia to one or more digits, depending on the athlete's palmar arch configuration. Use of custom padding (i.e., donut) in the glove to minimize trauma may be necessary to alleviate symptoms (Mueller, Mueller, Degreif, & Rommens, 2000).

Nerve Injuries

Sports related nerve injuries are not as common as the bony and soft tissue injuries described previously. Many sports activities lead to compression and direct trauma to the nerves of the upper extremity (see Chapter 19).

Ulnar Nerve

Injury to the **ulnar nerve** in athletes most commonly occurs either at the elbow (**cubital tunnel syndrome**) or in the hand at Guyon's canal (**handlebar syndrome**) (Wright & Rettig, 1995). Ulnar neuropathy at the elbow is often seen in throwing athletes secondary to the significant valgus stretch placed on the elbow and its surrounding soft tissue structures during the late cocking and acceleration phases of the pitch. In professional and collegiate athletes, ulnar nerve transposition surgery is often the treatment of choice. Splinting after surgery depends on the type of transposition and involvement of other structures (UCL reconstruction). Often an elbow immobilization splint with the wrist included is fabricated for use during the early phases of rehabilitation.

Compression of the ulnar nerve at Guyon's canal is seen most commonly in cycling. Positioning and pressure of the hands on the handlebars is usually the biomechanical cause of injury. Management consists of making adjustments to the type and position of the handlebars as well as use of padded cycling gloves or custom splints (Fig. 20–23).

Median Nerve

Neuropathy of the **median nerve** at the wrist (**carpal tunnel syndrome**) can have a significant effect on the athlete's performance. Nighttime volar wrist immobilization splinting, with the wrist in a neutral position, is the initial treatment for carpal tunnel syndrome (Lawrence, Mobbs, Fortems, & Stanley, 1995).

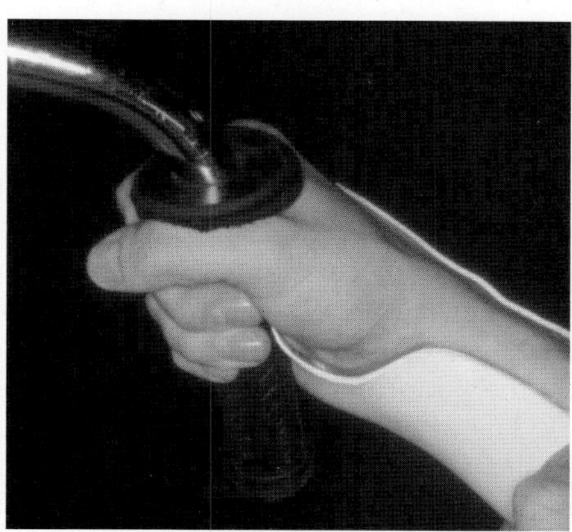

Figure 20–23 Gel-lined thermoplastic material is molded on the wrist of a biker to reduce stress on the ulnar palm region.

Pronator syndrome, or entrapment of the median nerve in the vicinity of the elbow, can occur at a number of sites including pronator teres, lacertus fibrosis, and proximal portion of the flexor digitorum superficialis (Lawrence et al., 1995). (Refer to Chapter 19 for more details.) An arm- or forearm-based splint may be helpful to place the structures at rest.

Radial Nerve

Acute trauma can occur to the **radial nerve** at multiple locations along its course, but acute injury usually occurs at the spiral groove of the humerus and in the proximal forearm. Compression of the radial nerve, **radial tunnel syndrome,** can occur where the nerve enters the intermuscular septum or at the radial tunnel. These injuries are uncommon in sports but may be seen in athletes who perform repetitive pronation and supination (Jebsib & Engber, 1997; Long, 1995). An arm- or forearm-based splint may be helpful to place the structures at rest.

Digital Nerves

One of the most common sites of neuropathy in the **digital nerves** is the thumb of bowlers (**bowler's thumb**) (Wright & Rettig, 1995). A painful neuroma can develop in these athletes. Widening the size of the thumbhole in the bowling ball may be necessary to decrease pressure on the nerve. The use of padding or a silicone gel sleeve at the base of the thumb may be useful for management of this condition.

Treatment and Return to Sport

Exercises are critical to the successful return to sport; they include eccentric and concentric loading and sport-specific drills. The clinician or athletic trainer should review proper technique, provide information for equipment modification, teach adequate warmup and cooldown exercises specific to the injury, and if appropriate, provide splinting or taping for use during and/or after exercise. The athlete should initially monitor the intensity and duration of exercise and report any signs and symptoms of reoccurring pain.

Other Management Options

Communication with the physician, athlete, coaching staff, and trainers ensures that the most appropriate splinting options are being considered. Appropriate prefabricated splints or sport-specific equipment that is not commonly used (skiing gloves with thumb MP support) may be available to meet the performance demands of the athlete (see Chapter 11). The athlete, coaches, or trainers may be familiar with such equipment, and it is important for the therapist to investigate these options. If other management options are explored, the therapist must make sure that the equipment meets the medical needs of the athlete.

In some cases, taping may be an option for protection of the injured structures. For example, after acute management of volar plate injuries, buddy taping adjacent fingers helps prevent undue stress to healing structures (Fig. 20-16). Some of the goals that can be met with taping are restriction of ROM, managing edema, providing anatomic support, and protecting against reinjury (Birrer & Poole, 1994). Taping of the wrist, thumb, and digits is common after injuries to these parts (see Chapter 13) (Birrer & Poole, 1996; Dievert, 1994).

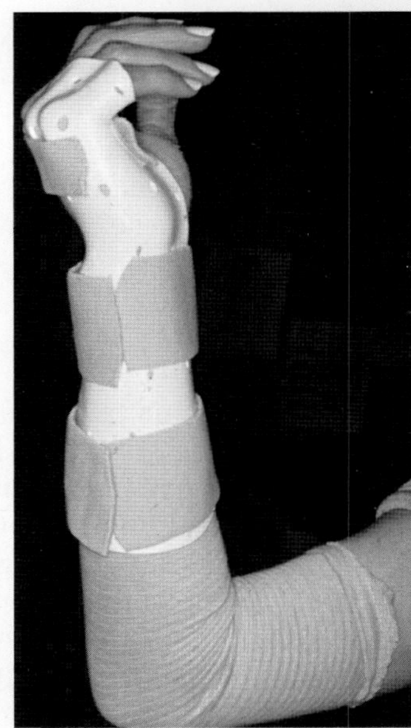

Figure 20–24 A forearm-based ulnar wrist and RF/SF immobilization splint with the IP joints free.

CASE STUDY SECTION

The case studies presented here are meant as teaching guidelines only. Treatment and splinting protocols vary greatly from surgeon to surgeon and from therapist to therapist. The therapist must check with the referring physicians and colleagues to define the preferred treatment and splinting methods.

CASE STUDY 1: **Fifth Metacarpal Fracture**

RP is a 25-year-old right-handed professional hockey player. He sustained a fifth-metacarpal base fracture to his right SF during a fight. The fracture was managed by cast immobilization. The patient was referred to hand therapy at 3 weeks postinjury. RP presented with evidence of early fracture healing.

RP was placed in an ulnar wrist extension/RF-SF MP flexion immobilization splint (wrist: 20° extension; MP: 60° flexion; PIP/DIP: free) (Fig. 20–24). He was instructed in splint removal for AROM exercises of the wrist and digits. At 4 weeks after injury, his splint was modified to include only the hand (fifth MP joint). The splint was small enough to fit into the hockey glove (Fig. 20–10) and was used for protection during practice and, eventually, for safe return to competition.

CASE STUDY 2: **Mallet Finger**

ML is a 28-year-old right-hand-dominant professional baseball player. He sustained a mallet injury (rupture of the terminal extensor tendon) to his left MF while sliding into base during a game. He was immobilized for 8 weeks in a prefabricated Stax splint. After that time, he was referred to hand therapy for ROM and splint fabrication. He presented with limited DIP motion, but was nontender over the dorsum of the DIP. A DIP immobilization splint that easily slid into ML's baseball glove was fabricated (Fig. 20–18). This small splint allowed the patient to continue playing ball and provided him with the additional protection he needed to prevent reinjury of the newly healed dorsal structures.

CASE STUDY 3: **Thumb UCL Injury**

RS is a 24-year-old highly competitive ski racer who sustained a right thumb MP joint UCL avulsion injury in a skiing accident. Surgery was performed to repair the ligament using a suture anchor. Postoperatively, she was placed in a wrist/thumb cast.

After cast removal (5 days postsurgery), RS was placed in a wrist/thumb immobilization splint (wrist: extension; carpometacarpal [CMC]: midpalmar and radial abduction; MP: slight flexion and ulnar deviation; IP: free) and was instructed in daily wrist and gentle thumb CMC, MP, and IP ROM exercises (avoiding MP radial deviation) (Fig. 20–3). The splint was fabricated from a 1/8" material.

At approximately 4 weeks, the splint was modified to allow unrestricted wrist motion. To return RS safely to competition with minimal risk of reinjury, a thumb MP splint was fabricated out of Fabriplast (a thin fabric-based material) material to be worn in the ski glove (Fig. 20–5). Both the glove and the ski pole were brought to therapy for splint fabrication. This allowed the therapist to fabricate the splint to conform comfortably inside the patient's ski glove and to permit correct ski pole grip. The glove held the splint firmly in place so straps were not required. Caution was used to make sure there were no jagged edges on the splint that would irritate the patient's skin while skiing. RS returned to ski racing with no complications.

CASE STUDY 4: **Scaphoid Fracture**

TB is a 30-year-old professional football player who sustained a right scaphoid fracture from a fall during practice. The patient underwent open reduction and internal fixation (ORIF) of the fracture; an interosseous screw was used. He was placed in a wrist/thumb cast after suture removal.

At 4 weeks postsurgery, TB was referred to therapy for a circumferential wrist/thumb immobilization splint along with a ROM program. The splint was made in two sections, a volar and a dorsal piece, and was fabricated out of a perforated ⅛" material. The dorsal component was added to the splint after the volar piece was molded and set. The therapist was careful to pad the ulnar styloid before applying the dorsal piece. This circumferential design further protected the wrist from moving dorsally out of the splint.

At 6 weeks, TB regained full wrist and thumb ROM. At that time, a silicone playing cast was fabricated, which allowed the patient to return to practice and competition (Fig. 20–25). He continued to use the thermoplastic splint for protection when not participating in football for an additional 3 weeks. The silicone cast was used for the rest of the football season.

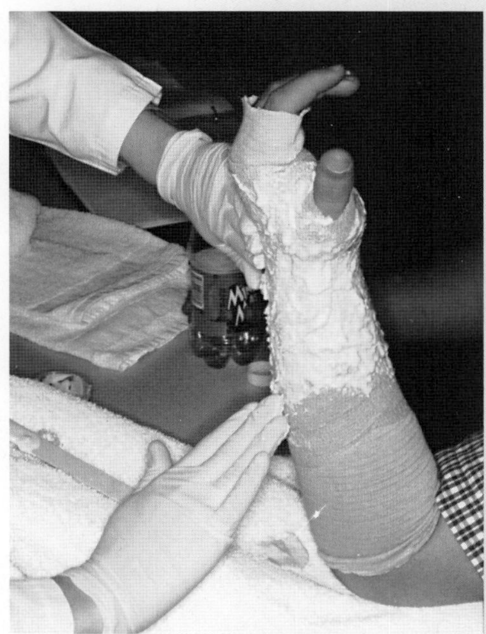

Figure 20–25 Fabrication of a forearm-based wrist/thumb silicone cast.

CONCLUSION

Upper extremity injuries in athletes confront therapists with a variety of splinting situations. Knowledge of the demands of the sport and a thorough understanding of the athlete's injury guide the therapist to appropriate splint selection. This chapter reviewed some of the common injuries therapists see in clinical practice and provided general guidelines for splinting intervention. For information about other injuries, see other chapters in the book and the suggested reading list.

REFERENCES

Alley, R. M., & Pappas, A. M. (1995). Acute and chronic performance-related injuries of the elbow. In A. M. Papas & J. Walzer (Eds.). *Upper extremity injuries in the athlete* (pp. 339–364). New York: Churchill Livingstone.

Anderson, M. K., Hall, H. J., Martin, M. (2000). *Sports injury management* (2nd ed.). Philadelphia: Lippincott Williams & Wilkins.

Barton, N. J. (1997). Sports injuries of the hand and wrist. *British Journal of Sports Medicine, 31,* 191–196.

Birrer, R. B., & Poole, B. (1996). Athletic taping. Part 5: The wrist, thumb and fingers. *Journal of Musculoskeletal Medicine, 13,* 48–50.

Birrer, R. B., & Poole. B. (1994). Taping of sports injuries: Review of a basic skill. *Journal of Musculoskeletal Medicine, 11,* 56–68.

Bouvette, C. M., Malanga, G. A., Cooney, W. P., Stuart, M. J., & Miller, R. W. (1994). A new protective soft splint for contact sports. *Journal of Sports Rehabilitaion, 3,* 282–291.

Canelon, M. F. (1995). Silicone rubber splinting for athletic hand and wrist injuries. *Journal of Hand Therapy, 8,* 252–257.

Colditz, J. C. (1995). Functional fracture bracing. In J. M. Hunter, E. J. Mackin, & A. D. Callahan (Eds.). *Rehabilitation of the hand* (4th ed., pp. 395–406). St. Louis: Mosby Year Book.

Colditz, J. C. (1999). *Splinting with neoprene.* Morgan Hill, CA: North Coast Medical.

DeCarlo, M., Malone, K., Darmelio, J., & Rettig, A. (1994). Casting in sport. *Journal of Athletic Training, 29,* 37–43.

Dievert, R. G. (1994). Functional thumb taping procedure. *Journal of Athletic Training, 29,* 357–359.

Glickel, S. Z., & Barron, A. (2000). Proximal interphalangeal joint fracture dislocations. *Hand Clinics, 16,* 333–344.

Howse, C. (1994). Wrist injuries in sport. *Sports Medicine, 17,* 163–175.

Jebsib, P., & Engber, W. (1997). Radial tunnel syndrome: long term results of surgical decompression. *Journal of Hand Surgery (American), 22,* 889–896.

Lawrence, T., Mobbs, P., Fortems, Y., & Stanley, J. (1995). Radial tunnel syndrome. *Journal of Hand Surgery (British), 4,* 454–459.

Long, R. R. (1995). Nerve Injuries. In A. M. Papas & J. Walzer (Eds.). *Upper extremity injuries in the athlete* (pp. 61–76). New York: Churchill Livingstone.

Melone, C. P., Beldner, S., & Basuk, R. S. (2000). Thumb collateral ligament injuries. *Hand Clinics, 16,* 345–357.

Morgan, W. J. (1995). Injuries of the distal radius and distal radioulnar joint. In A. M. Papas & J. Walzer (Eds.). *Upper extremity injuries in the athlete* (pp. 393–412). New York: Churchill Livingstone.

Morrey, B. F. (1993). Tendon injuries about the elbow. In B. F. Morrey (Ed.). The elbow and its disorders (2nd ed.). Philadelphia: Saunders.

Mueller, P., Mueller, L., Degreif, J., & Rommens, P. (2000). Hypothenar hammer syndrome in a golf player. *American Journal of Sports Medicine, 28,* 741–745.

Rettig, A. C. (1991). Current concepts in management of football injuries of the hand and wrist. The Hand in Sports. *Journal of Hand Therapy* [Special Issue: *The Hand in Sports*], *4,* 42–50.

Rettig, M. E., & Raskin, K. B. (2000). Acute fractures of the distal radius. *Hand Clinics, 16,* 405–415.

Schulz, L. A., Busconi, B., & Pappas, A. M. (1995). Protective equipment. In A. M. Papas & J. Walzer (Eds.). *Upper extremity injuries in the athlete* (pp. 90–100). New York: Churchill Livingstone.

Scott, S. C. (2000). Closed injuries to the extension mechanism of the digits. *Hand Clinics, 16,* 367–373.

Servi, J. T. (1997). Wrist pain from overuse: detecting and relieving intersection syndrome. *The Physician and Sports Medicine, 25,* 41.

Skerker, R. S., & Schulz, L. A. (1995). Principles of rehabilitation of the injured athlete. In A. M. Papas & J. Walzer (Eds.). *Upper extremity injuries in the athlete* (pp. 30–33). New York: Churchill Livingstone.

Stamos, B. D., & Leddy, J. P. (2000). Closed flexor tendon disruption in athletes. *Hand Clinics, 16,* 359–365.

Warme, W., & Brooks, D. (2000). The effect of circumferential taping on flexor tendon pulley failure in rock climbers. *American Journal of Sports Medicine, 28,* 674–678.

Wichmann, S., & Martin, D. R. (1996). Bracing for activity. *Physician and Sports Medicine, 24,* 9.

Williams, J. S., Hang, D. W., & Bach, B. R. (1996). Distal biceps rupture in a snowboarder. *Physician and Sports Medicine, 24,* 12.

Wright, H. H., & Rettig, A. C. (1995). Management of common sports injuries. In J. M. Hunter, E. J. Mackin, & A. D. Callahan (Eds.). *Rehabilitation of the hand* (4th ed., pp. 1809–1838). St. Louis: Mosby Year Book.

SUGGESTED READING

Alexy, C., & DeCarlo, M. (1998). Rehabilitation and use of protective devices in hand and wrist injuries. *Clinic in Sports Medicine, 17,* 635–655.

Altchek, D. W., & Andrews, J. R. (2001). *The athlete's elbow.* Philadelphia: Lippincott, Williams & Wilkins.

Altchek, D. W., Hyman, J., Williams, R., Levinson, M., Allen, A. A. (2000). Management of MCL injuries of the elbow in throwers. In R.F. Warren (Ed.). Techniques in shoulder and elbow surgery. Philadelphia: Lippincott, Williams & Wilkins.

American College of Sports Medicine. (1996). *ACSM's handbook for the team physician.* Baltimore: Williams & Wilkins.

Canelon, M. F., & Karus, A. J. (1995). A room temperature vulcanizing silicone rubber sport splint. *American Journal of Occupational Therapy, 49,* 244–249.

Cassidy, C., & Chung, A. N. (1999). Diagnosis and management of medial epicondylitis. In D. S. Zelouf (Ed.). *Atlas of the hand clinics: Tendinitis and tenosynovitis* (vol. 4, pp. 61–67). Philadelphia: Saunders.

Dobyns, J. (1991). Cumulative trauma disorder of the upper limb. *Hand Clinics, 7(3).*

Ellenbecker, T. S., & Mattalino, A. J. (1997). *The elbow in sport: injury, treatment and rehabilitation.* Champaign, IL: Human Kinetics.

Fu, F. H., & Stone, D. A. (1994). *Sports injuries.* Baltimore: Williams & Wilkins.

Groppel, J. L., & Nirschl, R. P. (1986). A mechanical and electromyographic analysis of the effects of various counterforce braces on the tennis player. *American Journal of Sports Medicine, 14,* 195–200.

Honing, E. W. (1998). Wrist injuries. Part 2: Spotting and treating troublemakers: The recreational athlete. *Physician and Sports Medicine, 16,* 10.

Journal of Hand Therapy. (1991). *The Hand in Sports* [Special Issue].

Kahn, K. M., & Cook, J. L. (2000). Overuse tendinosis, not tendonitis. *Physician and Sports Medicine, 28,* 38–48.

Kirkpatrick, W. H. (1999). Intersection syndrome. In D. S. Zelouf (Ed.). *Atlas of the hand clinics: Tendinitis and tenosynovitis* (vol. 4, pp. 55–60). Philadelphia: Saunders.

McKoy, B. E., Benson, C. V., & Hartsock, L. A. (2000). Fractures about the shoulder: Conservative management. *Orthopedic Clinics of North America, 31,* 205–216.

Melone, C. P. (2000). Update on management of sports injuries. *Hand Clinics, 16(3).*

Meredith, R. M., & Butcher, J. D. (1997). Field splinting of suspected fractures: preparation, assessment, and application. *Physician and Sports Medicine, 25,* 10.

Morrey, B. F. (2000). *The elbow and its disorders.* Philadelphia: Saunders.

O'Connor, F., Howard, T., Fieseler, C., & Nirschl, R. (1997). Managing injuries: A systematic approach. *Physician and Sports Medicine, 25,* 5.

Rettig, A. C., & Kollias, S. C. (1996). Internal fixation of acute stable scaphoid fractures in the athlete. *American Journal of Sports Medicine, 24,* 182–186.

Rettig, A., Stube, K., & Shelbourne, K. (1997). Effects of finger and wrist taping on grip strength. *American Journal of Sports Medicine, 25,* 96–98.

Sailer, S. M., & Lewis, S. B. (1998). Rehabilitation and splinting of common upper extremity injuries in athletes. *Clinics in Sports Medicine, 14,* 411–445.

Stamos, B. D., & Leddy, J. P. (2000). Closed flexor tendon disruption in athletes. *Hand Clinics, 16,* 359–356.

Whiteside, J. A., Andrews, J. R., & Fleisig, G. S. (1999). Elbow injuries in young baseball players. *Physician and Sports Medicine, 27,* 6.

Wilk, K. E., & Levinson, M. (2001). Rehabilitation of the athlete's elbow. In D. W. Altchek & J. R. Andrews (Eds.). The athlete's elbow. Philadelphia: Lippincott, Williams & Wilkins.

Wright, H. H. (1991). Hand therapist set the pace in sports medicine. *Journal of Hand Therapy* [Special Issue: *The Hand in Sports*], *4,* 37–41.

CHAPTER 21

Adult Neurologic Dysfunction

Sue Ann Ordinetz, MS, CAS, OTR/L

INTRODUCTION

This chapter addresses splinting interventions for adults with **central nervous system (CNS) disorders** (see Chapter 22 for the pediatric population). This chapter discusses the common manifestations of neurologic dysfunction, focusing primarily on the clinical-reasoning and problem-solving aspects of splinting this unique population. A wide variety of splints have been developed for use with these clients. Support for the use of many of the available interventions is primarily anecdotal.

It is beyond the scope of this chapter to extensively evaluate the literature; thus the reader is encouraged to explore current research. Milazzo and Gillen (1999) provide an extensive review of the literature related to splinting and abnormal muscle tone. Wilton (1997) provides a thorough description of abnormal upper extremity positioning related to neurologic disorders and offers specific recommendations for several presentations. Hill and Presperin (1986) provide recommendations for deformity management in **spinal cord injury (SCI),** and Hill (1988) specifically addresses splinting and casting issues for **traumatic brain injury (TBI).** Given the complexity and variety of presentation seen with CNS disorders, the therapist is encouraged to seek out and make use of all the available resources to assist in the clinical-reasoning process.

Central nervous system disorders can lead to problems such as spasticity, flaccidity, weakness, incoordination, tremors, contractures, pain, sensory dysfunction, and cognitive loss; all involve decreased functional abilities. Splinting patients with neurologic disorders, particularly spasticity, is highly controversial (Fess & Philips, 1987; Hill, 1988; Milazzo & Gillen, 1999; Lohman, 1996; McKee & Morgan, 1998; Wilton, 1997). Developing splinting interventions for these individuals requires a thorough understanding of the diagnosis, prognosis, goals, and functional abilities. Because of the variety of presentations for most neurologic disorders, the therapist's use of problem-solving and clinical-reasoning skills is critical.

Specific Conditions Related to Neurologic Disorders

The three primary problems resulting from neurologic dysfunction for which splinting is commonly used are flaccidity, spasticity, and contractures..

Flaccidity

Recovery from a neurologic insult such as SCI, TBI, brain surgery, or **cerebral vascular accident (CVA)** typically progresses in stages. The acute stage is often characterized by **flaccidity,** or loss of muscle tone. Minimal activity is seen in the skeletal muscles, and joint malalignment occurs through loss of soft tissue support as a result of muscle weakness and the effects of gravity. Secondary complications related to lack of muscle activity include edema, pain, and contracture.

The shoulder, wrist, and thumb are apt to be unstable during the flaccid stage. The flaccid shoulder is susceptible to subluxation owing to the downward rotation of the

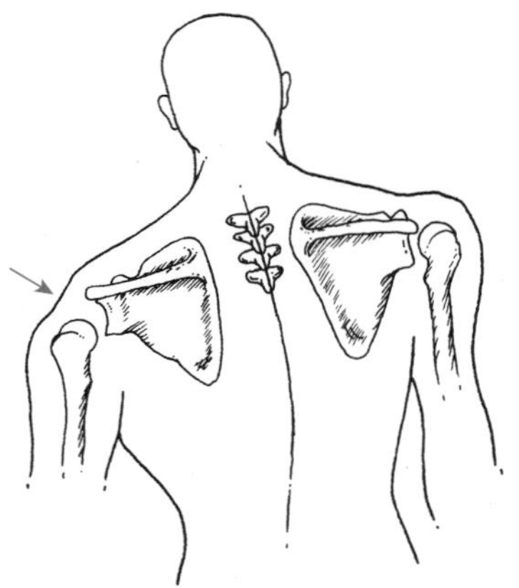

Figure 21–1 Note the flaccid left shoulder and the indentation just proximal to the humeral head.

scapula and weight of the arm putting a prolonged stretch on the soft tissue surrounding the shoulder (Fig. 21–1). The individual is at risk for injury to an unstable, malaligned joint through either traction (e.g., a caregiver pulling on a flaccid extremity) or misuse (e.g, weight bearing on a malaligned flexed wrist) (Gillen, 1998a). It is critical to maintain joint alignment and soft tissue length during the flaccid period to promote full use of the upper extremity during and after recovery. Caregiver education on proper positioning and how to assist the patient during activities is crucial during this stage of recovery.

Splinting Considerations

Primary goals for splinting the flaccid upper extremity are protection of unstable joint structures, prevention of injury to vulnerable structures, maintenance of proper joint alignment, prevention of soft tissue contractures, and improving function. Splints and/or **slings** should be considered only when appropriate to achieve these goals. Prolonged static immobility can actually contribute to soft tissue stiffening and, therefore, should be avoided. Splints or slings should be used as one component of a total 24-hr active positioning plan that incorporates passive range of motion (PROM) and proper positioning in a variety of resting postures throughout the day. Splinting should not take the place of an appropriate positioning program.

Splinting Options

SHOULDER SUPPORTS

Use of a sling to support the flaccid shoulder is a controversial treatment intervention. The intent of the sling is to support the glenohumeral joint in proper alignment and prevent subluxation. However, to accomplish this, the following criteria must be met: the humerus must be elevated, the head of the humerus must be properly aligned in the glenoid fossa, the scapula must be aligned on the thorax, and the lost support of the rotator cuff must be replaced (Cailliet, 1980; Gillen, 1998b,1999). At best, a sling can provide vertical support, but no sling can realign the scapula on the trunk. Cailliet (1980) and Gillen (1998b, 1999) reviewed the literature and note there is no hard evidence that slings can prevent or reduce long-term shoulder subluxation and that improper sling use can cause or exacerbate subluxation. Ridgeway and Byrne (1999) evaluated and compared two different types of slings and treatment options for hemiplegia. Their results are summarized in Table 21–1.

Typical positioning recommendations for the affected upper extremity are elbow/wrist extension and shoulder abduction and external rotation. Slings typically position the patient in elbow flexion and shoulder adduction and internal rotation. Worn for long periods, the sling acts as an immobilizer and can contribute to contractures of the shoulder and elbow (Fig. 21–2). Shoulder supports that bear the weight of the upper extremity, via a humeral or distal cuff attached to a shoulder saddle, allow for more normal movement patterns and do not hold the extremity in a flexion pattern (Fig. 21–3). Shoulder taping may also be used to provide support while allowing for functional use and range of motion (ROM) of the extremity (Fig. 21–4). These supports can often be worn under loose-fitting clothing, which may increase wearer compliance.

TABLE 21–1 Comparison of Shoulder Slings

Characteristic	Unilateral Cuff	Hemi Sling
Pros		
Permits ROM of all joints	X	
Reduces inferior subluxation	X	
Reduces anterior subluxation		X
Decreases bicipital tendonitis		X
Permits functional use of upper extremity	X	
Aesthetic, low profile	X	
Allows arm swing in gait	X	
Cons		
Promotes unilateral neglect		X
Limits sensory input		X
Can exacerbate impingement		X
Promotes contractures		X
Requires firm contact for support	X	
Difficult to don	X	
Can promote flexion synergy		X
Can facilitate anterior subluxation		X
Pressure on contralateral neck		X
Pressure on contralateral axilla	X	

ROM, range of motion.

Modified with permission from Ridgeway, E. M., & Byrne, D. P. (1999). To sling or not to sling? *Occupational Therapy Practice, 1*, 38–42.

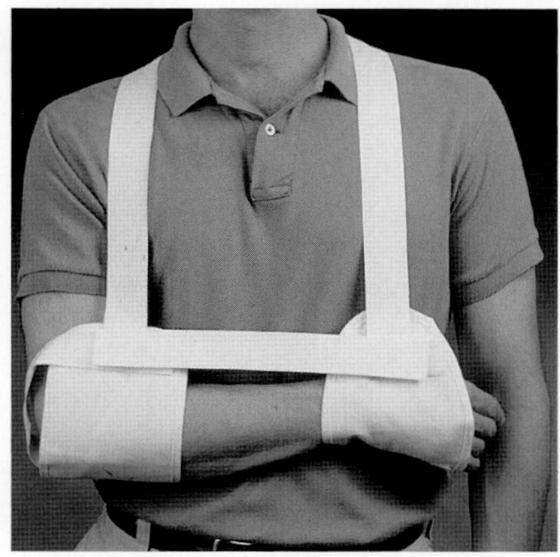

Figure 21–2 A Standard Hemi Arm Sling promotes a pattern of shoulder adduction and internal rotation as well as elbow flexion. Courtesy of North Coast Medical (Morgan Hill, CA).

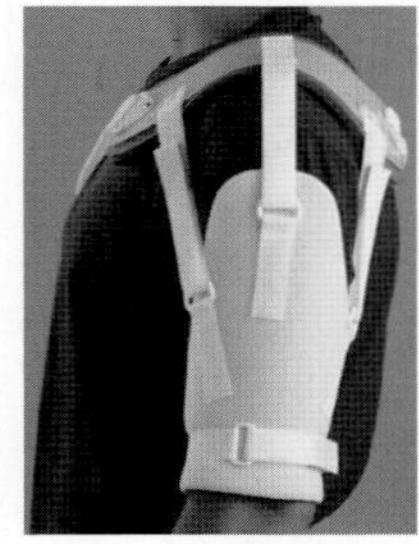

Figure 21–3 A Hemi Shoulder Sling with a humeral cuff to support the weight of the affected extremity in a functional position. Courtesy of Sammons Preston (Bolingbrook, IL).

Slings or shoulder supports can be beneficial when used correctly and to meet specific goals. They must be applied properly to be effective; so the therapist must teach the patient and caregiver about correct donning and adjustment of the sling. Ease of donning and doffing needs to be considered to ensure compliance. Slings that support the extremity in a flexed position should be used initially only during upright activities, such as ambulation, transfer, and gait training and then removed after the activity ends. Alternate positioning options should be used throughout the day to prevent contractures and promote proper alignment; tables, lap trays, and arm troughs can be adjusted to the proper position or the patient can use bed positioning (Eggers, 1983; Gillen, 1999; Ridgeway & Byrne, 1999). There is no one sling that is appropriate for every patient. The need for a sling must be evaluated carefully and selected to meet the specific goals for the individual. Sling use must be evaluated frequently and discontinued as soon as it is no longer meeting the goals.

WRIST/HAND SUPPORTS

Immobilization splints are typically used to position the flaccid wrist and hand. The standard resting pan splint, or **wrist/hand immobilization splint,** may be used as a nighttime splint to protect unstable joint structures and prevent contracture. The wrist should be positioned in 20 to 30° of extension, metacarpophalangeal (MP) joints in 40 to 45° of flexion, interphalangeal (IP) joints in 10 to 20° of flexion, and the thumb in palmar abduction to maintain the first web space. However, wrist and hand immobilization splints are not appropriate for daytime wear, because they block sensory input and prevent any attempt at movement or function (Milazzo & Gillen, 1999).

Prefabricated hard resting splints are often issued as a cost-saving measure; unfortunately, these splints often do not fit properly. Preformed splints with memory characteristics are preferable, as the fit can be adjusted by heating and molding to the patient. Prefabricated soft resting splints are generally comfortable with a more forgiving fit (Fig. 21–5). Some have removable pieces or wire foam inserts that allow adjustment of fit. Others contain air bladders that can be inflated to provide gentle stretch to the wrist and/or fingers. Soft splints may be

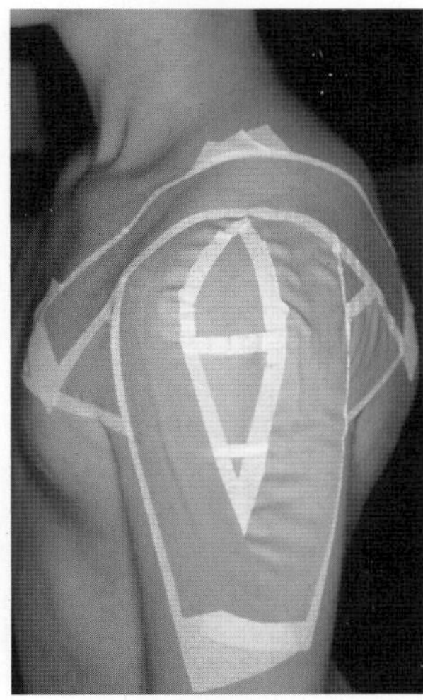

Figure 21–4 With this McConnell taping technique, the tape should be applied distal to proximal to provide proper support when correcting an anterior inferior shoulder subluxation.

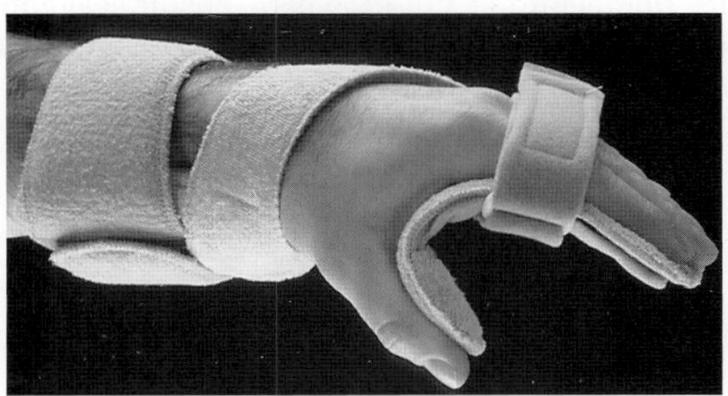

Figure 21–5 A soft resting splint can be more comfortable than a thermoplastic splint. The Freedom Omni Progressive Wrist/hand/thumb Orthosis (shown here) allows the therapist to adjust the digit, thumb, and wrist positions. Courtesy of AliMed (Dedham, MA).

appropriate for individuals with sensitive or fragile skin, such as the geriatric population. Soft splints may be unable to provide adequate support for a large or heavy individual. Resting splints must be carefully evaluated for fit to prevent slippage during wear. A dorsal strap may be placed just proximal to the carpometacarpal (CMC) joint to prevent splint migration (Fig. 21–6).

Wrist immobilization splints may be used to provide protection to the flaccid wrist during functional activities. A dorsal design should be considered when edema is present to allow for better pressure distribution, sensory input and edema control. Wide straps or circumferential wrapping may be used to help control edema. A volar splint can provide better conformity and support to the arch system in the hand. Many patients with flaccidity develop a flattened hand. Care must be taken to provide adequate support and definition to the palmar arches when fabricating any splint incorporating the hand. In either design, the wrist should be supported in neutral to 20° extension, neutral forearm rotation, and neutral ulnar/radial deviation. It is often not necessary to provide finger support during the flaccid stage of recovery (Gillen, 1998b, 1999).

Because of the increased risk of injury to joint structures and soft tissue during the flaccid stage, it is crucial for the therapist to train the patient and caregiver in proper techniques for ROM, positioning, and splint wearing. When the patient's cognitive status is intact, the patient should be taught to direct others in splint application, to self-position the extremity, and to follow the wearing schedule.

Spasticity

As recovery progresses, flaccidity can give way to **spasticity.** Spasticity is commonly described as a pathologic increase in muscle tone to passive stretch. In the upper extremity, spasticity typically presents as a pattern of scapular protraction and depression, internal rotation and adduction of the shoulder, elbow flexion, forearm pronation or supination, wrist flexion with ulnar deviation, finger flexion, and thumb flexion with adduction (Fig. 21–7). Multiple factors influence the abnormal posturing of the spastic upper extremity, including the site and severity of the neurologic damage, environmental factors (temperature, noise levels), postural alignment, movement of other body parts, and psychological factors

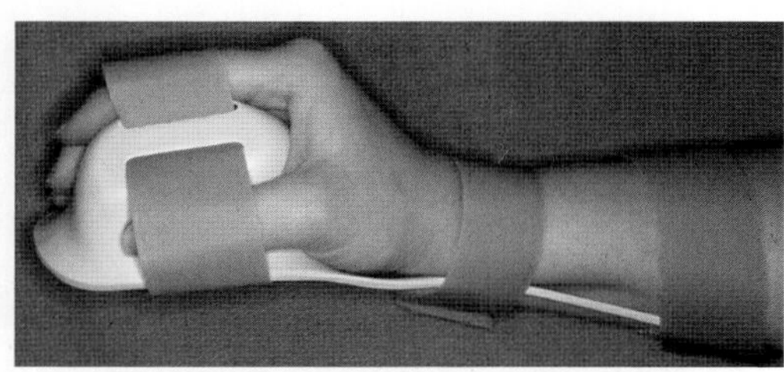

Figure 21–6 A dorsal wrist strap placed just proximal to the thumb CMC joint can help prevent splint migration. Shown here is a Preformed Neutral Position Hand Splint (by DeRoyal; Powell, TN.)

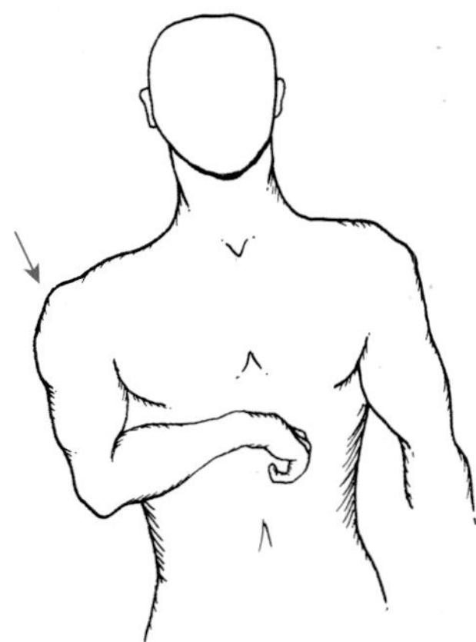

Figure 21–7 Typical flexion synergy posturing of the spastic upper extremity. Note the depression of the right shoulder.

(arousal level, anxiety, excitement). Spasticity is often seen to some degree with SCI, TBI, CVA, brain tumors, multiple sclerosis (MS), and other degenerative central nervous system disorders.

Splinting Considerations

Goals for splinting the spastic upper extremity are reduction of muscle tone; lengthening of soft tissue; maintenance of joint alignment, prevention of pain, contractures, and skin breakdown; and increasing function. There is a lack of consensus on the methods for achieving these goals and even whether the spastic extremity should be splinted. McKee and Morgan (1998) provide a nice summary of the areas of controversy, including volar versus dorsal application, maximal versus submaximal stretch to spastic muscles, and static versus dynamic splinting. Milazzo and Gillen (1999) provide a thorough review of the literature and common splint designs used to treat spasticity. Their analyses support the controversial nature of splinting the spastic upper extremity.

Splints must be designed for the environment in which they will be worn. A splint may fit well when fabricated and issued to the patient, who may be in a relaxed state; however, if the patient must wear the splint during functional activities, the muscle tone may be affected, which in turn may affect the fit and usefulness of the splint. The client and/or caregivers must be taught to employ tone-reduction techniques, if necessary, before donning the splint.

The therapist must be prepared to define the goals of the splint clearly and to be willing to use a trial-and-error approach. Often, a variety of splints may be needed over time; a splint may eventually lose its effectiveness, and other options will need to be explored.

Splinting Options

Splints are used to achieve proper joint alignment (immobilization splints) and provide a gentle stretch to tight soft tissues (mobilization splints via a serial static approach). **Low-load, prolonged stretch (LLPS)** at end range has been shown to reduce both spastic hypertonicity and contractures (Milazzo & Gillen, 1999). Splinting should begin early, before the severity of the spasticity increases, to prevent the deforming influences of prolonged hypertonicity. Controversy regarding splinting to reduce mild to moderate spasticity centers around the need to provide maximal or submaximal stretch to the muscles. Some therapists advocate prolonged stretch at end range, and others believe that maximal stretch actually increases muscle tone (Gillen, 1998b; McKee & Morgan, 1998). Advocates of a submaximal stretch recommend splinting each joint at 5 to 10° less than the available range, or at the position of stretch reflex activation (Hill, 1988; McKee & Morgan, 1998; Milazzo & Gillen, 1999; Wilton, 1997). Splinting is not recommended for severe spasticity. Medical management, such as antispasticity medication and nerve blocks, are recommended to control severe spasticity. Splinting after medical management may be indicated to increase or maintain ROM or to promote function.

Splints for spasticity typically consist of either a dorsal or volar application, although some designs provide circumferential support. Supporters of the dorsal-based splint believe that sensory input from the contact of the splint over the dorsal forearm and hand may stimulate weak extensors and may leave the palm of the hand open for sensory input. Advocates for the volar-based splint contend that the splint material blocks sensory input to the flexor surface, thus preventing stimulation of already spastic flexors. There are no conclusive data at this time to support one method over the other (Fess & Philips, 1987; Hill, 1988; Lohman, 1996; Milazzo & Gillen, 1999; Wilton, 1997). Wilton (1997) advocates use of a dorsal/volar immobilization splint (dorsal forearm trough with volar finger support) that supports the fingers in extension but leaves the volar forearm uncovered (Fig. 21–8) (Wilton, 1997).

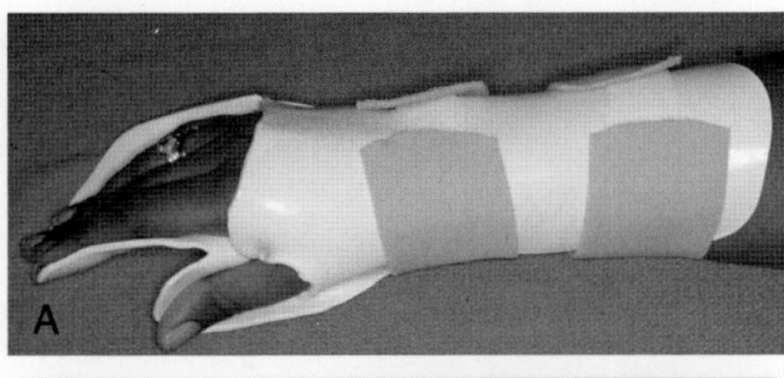

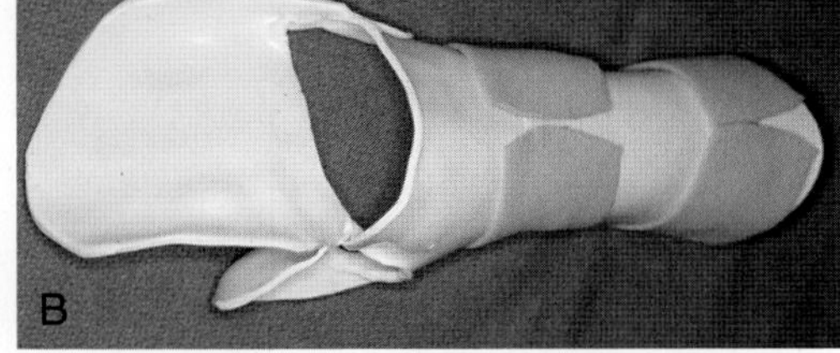

Figure 21–8 ***A,*** *The rubber-like material used to fabricate this splint provides maximal durability and strength.* ***B,*** *Note that the dorsum of the hand was left uncovered.*

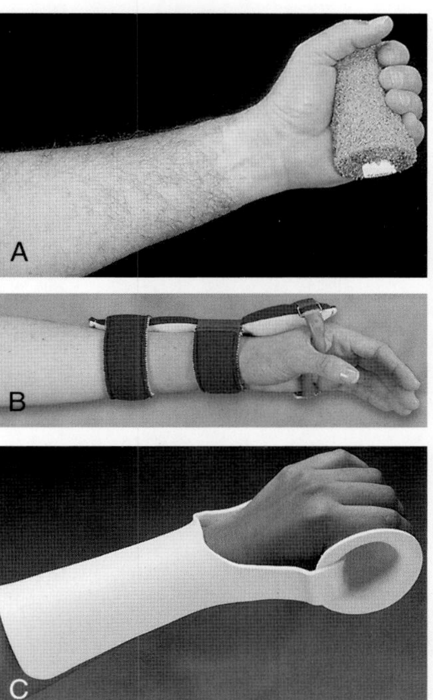

Figure 21–9 Hand cone-based splinting interventions to inhibit spasticity. ***A,*** *The Economy Terry Cloth Cone is a typical design. Courtesy of AliMed (Dedham, MA).* ***B,*** *A variation of the Mackinnon splint (the LMB Air-Soft Dorsal Wrist Support) uses a hard dowel. Courtesy of DeRoyal (Powell, TN).* ***C,*** *This splint, made of Omega Plus splinting material, includes a dorsal forearm trough. Courtesy of North Coast Medical (Morgan Hill, CA).*

HAND-BASED SPLINTS

Hand-based volar splints usually consist of a **hard cone** or **thumb and finger spreader.** The rationale behind the hard cone is that when the spastic hand grips the cone, deep pressure to the flexor tendons in the hand will inhibit the flexor tone (Fig. 21–9**A**). Drawbacks of the hard cone are that it interferes with function and does not directly act on the wrist. A variation of the hard cone concept was created by Mackinnon, Sanderson, and Buchanan (1975) and modified by Exner and Bonder (1982). This splint consists of a dorsal forearm trough and a hard dowel positioned to place pressure on the palmar surface of the metacarpal heads (Fig. 21–9**B**). This configuration is thought to activate the intrinsics and inhibit the long finger flexors (Lohman, 1996). Lohman (1996) incorporated the hard cone into a forearm-based immobilization splint with a dorsal forearm trough (Fig. 21–9**C**).

Positioning the thumb and/or fingers in abduction is thought to inhibit flexor tone in the hand through the use of **reflex-inhibiting postures** (Lohman, 1996). Although the concept of static positioning for reflex inhibition is debatable, some therapists now believe that the prolonged

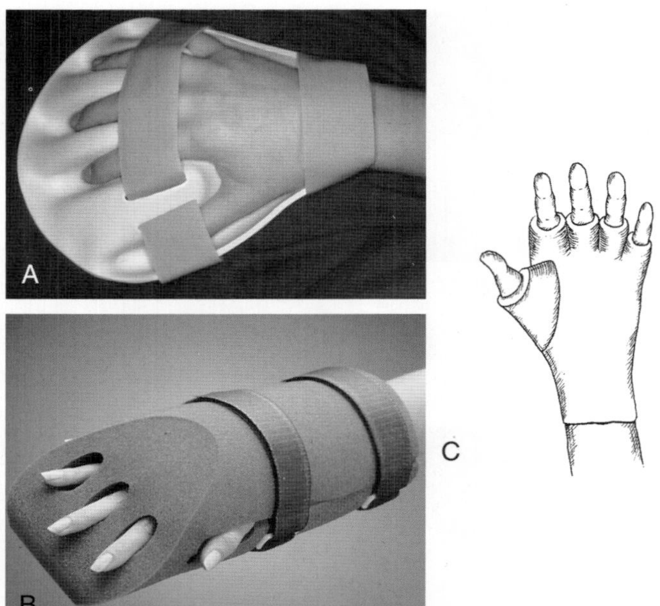

Figure 21–10 *Hand-based digit abduction interventions to inhibit spasticity.* ***A,*** *An Antispasticity Ball Splint (by DeRoyal; Powell, TN).* ***B,*** *A foam wrist/hand orthosis (Finger Spreader). Courtesy of Sammons Preston (Bolingbrook, IL).* ***C,*** *A padded stretch glove.*

stretch provided by this splint may explain its effectiveness in temporarily decreasing muscle tone (Milazzo & Gillen, 1999). Variations of this concept include the antispasticity ball splint, foam finger spreaders, thumb abduction splints, and designs using a padded stretch glove (Fig. 21–10) (O'Connell, 1998). Splint selection must take into consideration the severity of the spasticity and the specific muscles involved. Functional use of the extremity should always be a goal, and splinting interventions must support, and not block, function.

Maintaining soft tissue length is a goal of treating spasticity, and LLPS has been shown to reduce spasticity initially (Gillen, 1998b). However, the reduction in tone has not been shown to be maintained once the splint is removed (Fess & Philips, 1987; Lohman, 1996; Milazzo & Gillen, 1999; Wilton, 1997). Splinting must be considered an adjunct to other tone-reduction techniques and may be appropriate in conjunction with functional training of the upper extremity.

SEMIDYNAMIC SPLINTS

Another mobilization approach for treating spasticity is a group of splints referred to as **semidynamic splints** (Milazzo & Gillen, 1999). Examples of this type of splint are air splints, orthokinetic splints, and tone and positioning splints. Their designs are based on neurophysiologic principles of facilitation and inhibition and reflex-inhibiting postures. According to Wilton (1997), the use of a dynamic or elastic material provides significant sensory input that "has an impact on muscle physiology associated with abnormal tone such that changes are seen in the posture of the limb, the presence of tone, and the agonist-antagonist balance in muscle action."

Inflatable air splints are often used to reduce flexor tone and facilitate elbow extension. Although original beliefs that the air splint reduced spasticity and increased function have not been supported by research, the splint may be used as a dynamic assist to elbow extension during upper extremity weight-bearing activities (Fig. 21–11) (Milazzo & Gillen, 1999). Air pressure in the splint should not exceed 40 mm Hg (Milazzo & Gillen, 1999).

Orthokinetic splints attempt to re-establish a balance between muscle groups by providing facilitation to the weaker target muscles and neutral to inhibitory stimulation to their antagonists. Orthokinetic cuffs consist of an elastic component over the muscle belly to be facilitated (active field) and a nonstretch material covering the antagonist (inactive field). Orthokinetic splints have been shown to be effective in restoring muscle balance and allowing increased function (Fig. 21–12) (Milazzo & Gillen, 1999).

Tone and positioning (TAP) splints are constructed of a heavy-duty stretch material, typically Neoprene or

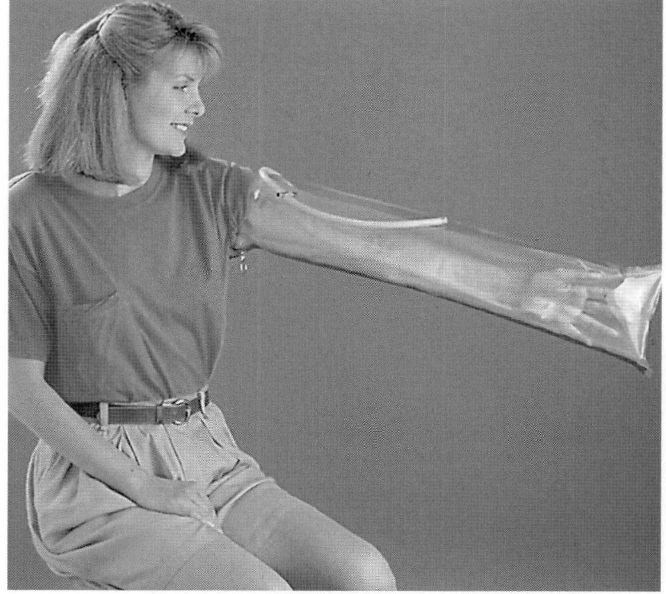

Figure 21–11 *The Urias Pressure Splint for promoting elbow extension can be used during weight-bearing activities. Courtesy of AliMed (Dedham, MA).*

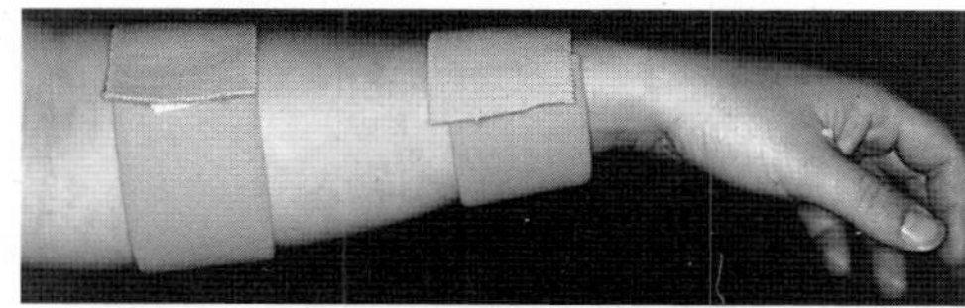

Figure 21–12 *An orthokinetic splint is used to re-establish balance between opposing muscle groups. Notice elastic material over dorsal extensors and nonelastic foam strap on flexor surface.*

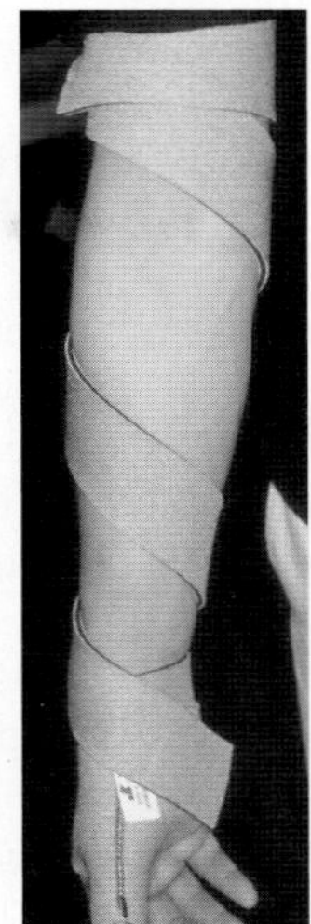

Figure 21–13 Neoprene's flexibility allows voluntary movement while its elastic properties facilitate movement away from a spastic pattern. Shown is the Roylan tone and positioning (TAP) splint (by Smith+Nephew; Germantown, WI).

Lycra. They can be hand-based, supporting the thumb in abduction and extension, or forearm-based, including a spiral wrap that provides a dynamic assist into thumb abduction and extension, and forearm supination or pronation (Fig. 21–13). Although these splints can be fabricated by the therapist, they are commercially available through rehabilitation vendors. Care must be taken to apply these splints properly, wrapping in the direction of thumb abduction/extension and placing the limb in the desired wrist and forearm positions. Wilton (1997) also describes the use of Lycra splints to achieve more normalized active movement patterns of the upper extremity, including a sleeve-length (axilla to wrist) dynamic assist (elbow extension forearm supination or elbow flexion forearm pronation) model, a gauntlet style with a thumb abduction sleeve, and a full glove style (Fig. 21–14).

Semidynamic splints are indicated when there is some functional movement of the limb (Milazzo & Gillen, 1999; Wilton, 1997). Wilton (1997) reports a high patient acceptance rate with the Lycra splints owing to minimal problems with pressure and increased comfort and cosmesis. A drawback of these splints is that they can be difficult to apply properly, so thorough patient and caregiver education in donning the splints is critical (Milazzo & Gillen, 1999; Wilton, 1997).

Reducing muscle tone and subsequently improving function are often goals of splinting for spasticity. Current research on motor control is questioning the relationship between spasticity and function (Gillen, 1998b). Therapists must be aware of the complex nature of these issues and current research, and they must select splinting interventions according to clearly established goals and an understanding of current theory.

Contractures

Contracture, commonly defined as a stiffening of tissues, can result from any type of immobility, including spasticity; flaccidity; poor positioning; and prolonged immobilization from splints, braces, or slings. Contractures can affect both soft tissue and joint structures, and the formation of contractures in neurologic diagnoses indicates a poor prognosis for return of limb function (Gillen, 1998b). Contracture formation can also be a secondary complication of advanced stages of degenerative neurologic conditions (e.g., MS and dementia, owing to increased muscle tone) or from immobility (owing to loss of the volition to move, resulting from the global deterioration of the cerebral cortex). While the relationship between spasticity and function is currently in question, the relationship between spasticity and contracture is well established (Gillen, 1998b; Hill, 1988; Hill & Presperin, 1986; Milazzo & Gillen, 1999; Wilton, 1997).

Splinting Considerations

Preventing and ameliorating contractures are important aspects of splinting for the patient with neurologic dysfunction. Soft tissue contracture interferes with attempts at normal movement. Often seen contracture sites are the shoulder, elbow, wrist, thumb, and fingers. Flexion contractures are the most common; however, extension contractures can also occur.

Contracture management involves two components: moving a joint through its full ROM and maintaining the full length of soft tissues. Active or passive ROM exercises are necessary to maintain joint fluid and lubrication. Mobilization splinting can help accomplish the second component through the application of LLPS.

The major difference between contracture management for patients with neurologic impairment and patients with an intact nervous system is that the underlying reason for the contracture risk often remains active in the former (e.g., spasticity or abnormal posturing). Contracture management is an ongoing consideration.

Goals for splinting contractures are maintenance of joint integrity, prevention of pain, maintenance of maximum length in soft tissue structures, prevention of skin

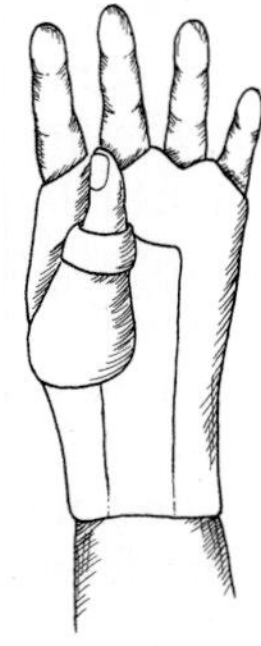

Figure 21–14 A hand-based Lycra tone-reduction splint.

maceration and breakdown, allowance for air circulation and hygiene, and promotion of function.

Splinting Options

Prolonged immobilization causes changes in the properties of muscle tissue. Prolonged immobilization from static splints, casts, slings, or infrequent position changes may result in spasticity and contractures. Research has shown that the pathologic changes are more likely when the tissue is shortened rather than lengthened and the changes are reversible (Gillen, 1998b; McKee & Morgan, 1998; Wilton, 1997).

Mobilization splinting using a serial static approach can provide the LLPS necessary to effect the muscle tissue. A prolonged stretch of 30 minutes has been shown to be effective for mild contractures; more severe contractures require more time (Milazzo & Gillen, 1999). Milazzo and Gillen (1999) recommend that the optimal duration for a LLPS is 5 to 7 hours, which must be built up slowly from an initial 1 to 2 hours. Other therapists recommend that the orthotic should be in place for up to 12 hours (McKee & Morgan, 1998). Pressure from the splint should be felt as a gentle stretch, but never painful. Caution must be taken when using this intervention with neurologically impaired patients. Sensory deficits in this population are common, so frequent monitoring for pressure areas and skin breakdown is critical. Splints must be readjusted frequently as the contracture lessens.

The best treatment for contractures is prevention. Joint mobility is best maintained through active and passive ROM. It is important to maintain shoulder mobility, particularly scapular mobility, abduction, and external rotation through ROM activities, proper bed and wheelchair positioning, and mobilization techniques (Cailliet, 1980; Gillen, 1998b, 1999). Treating a contracted (frozen) shoulder is often difficult and painful for the patient.

Preventing or alleviating contractures in the neurologic patient is often compounded by abnormal muscle tone, causing contractures in positions of abnormal posturing. Correcting abnormal posturing often involves splinting more than one joint. If abnormal tone is present, attempting to correct more than one joint at a time can lead to added deformity. It may be preferable to correct the more proximal joint first, then address the more distal malalignment (Milazzo & Gillen, 1999).

Methods for reducing contractures include serial static splinting and serial casting. If abnormal tone and posturing is present, it is usually impossible for the individual to hold his or her extremity in the correct position. In this case, it is necessary for two people to be involved in the fabrication: one to hold the extremity in the correct position and one to apply the splint or casting material. If possible, the patient should be observed during sleep to note if spasticity is evident. If spasticity is not present, the contracture can be most effectively addressed during sleep (Wilton, 1997).

ELBOW SPLINTS

Elbow flexion contractures can be a common result of both increased tone in the elbow flexors and prolonged positioning in elbow flexion (through use of a sling or positioning on the armrests or lap tray of a wheelchair). Severe elbow flexion contractures not only interfere with function but can put the individual at risk for skin breakdown and hygiene problems at the elbow crease. Traditional elbow extension splints may be used, although severe contractures may need to be treated with serial casting. An anterior elbow splint should be fabricated with the humerus in external rotation and forearm in as much supination as possible. The splint should provide a gentle stretch at the elbow. If necessary, extend the splint just proximal to the distal palmar crease to support the wrist and encourage the elbow extension/forearm supination position to counteract the spastic elbow flexion/forearm pronation pattern (Fig. 21–15) (Milazzo & Gillen, 1999). Perforated thermoplastic is recommended to provide air circulation, and the skin should be monitored closely for maceration or breakdown. Wide straps or circumferential wrapping can be used to distribute the pressure over a wide area or to control edema if present.

Progressive elbow orthotics are another option. These orthotics are typically made of metal supports and locking elbow hinges with humeral and forearm cuffs. These either can be fabricated by an orthotist or therapist or can be purchased prefabricated from a rehabilitation supplier. A variety of prefabricated elbow orthotics exist with removable metal or thermoplastic struts that can be adjusted by the therapist as ROM increases. Circumferential padded cuffs provide neutral warmth, which may also assist in tissue relaxation (Fig. 21–16) (Wilton, 1997). As in other prefabricated splints, fit can be a problem. Commercial splints also tend to be heavier and more cumbersome than custom-made splints, increasing the risk of discomfort or noncompliance.

WRIST AND HAND SPLINTS

There are a variety of splint designs to treat contractures of the wrist and hand. Most common are variations of traditional immobilization splints. It is important to determine whether the contracture exists in the wrist, fingers, and/or thumb to prescribe the appropriate splint.

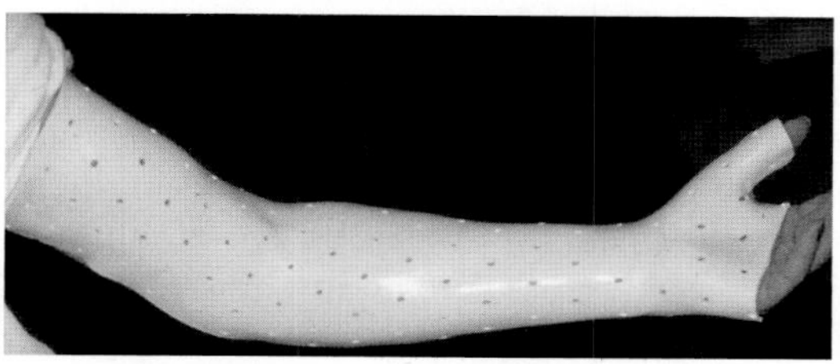

Figure 21–15 An anterior elbow mobilization splint used to stretch a contracture of the elbow flexors and forearm pronators. Note the inclusion of the thumb to maintain the first web space.

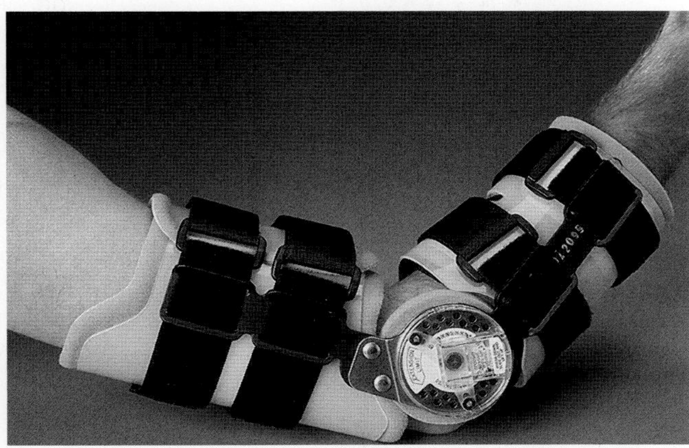

Figure 21–16 When applying a commercially available elbow orthotic, the therapist should consider the splint's weight, ease of adjustment, and fit. A proper fit is essential to prevent migration. The IROM Elbow Brace shown here locks to restrict flexion and extension to specific limits. Courtesy of the Rehabilitation Division of Smith+Nephew (Germantown, WI).

Many of the immobilization splints discussed for spasticity are also appropriate for treating contractures. The joint angles must be determined based on careful attention to the amount of stretch needed (maximal versus submaximal) and the purpose of the splint (spasticity reduction or contracture management). Because of the controversy and lack of hard evidence regarding the most effective stretch for the spastic muscle, clinical observation is needed to determine the specific effects of a given splint on a particular individual, and adjustments should be made as indicated by achieving the desired results.

Wrist and hand immobilization splints may need to be adapted to accommodate for both contracture and spasticity. Overstretching spastic finger flexors can cause distal interphalangeal (DIP) hyperextension against the splint as the proximal interphalangeal (PIP) joints pull into flexion. Rolling the finger platform of a resting splint to form a cylinder or cone may provide a gently stretch to the finger flexors without overstretching them (Fig. 21–17) (Hill, 1988). The dorsal/volar hand immobilization splint design is recommended for addressing both contracture and spasticity in the wrist and hand, because it creates an effective lever system to provide extension forces to the fingers and wrist (Fig. 21–8). It also widely distributes the pressure across the dorsal forearm and volar hand, is easily adjustable, and can be independently donned with one hand by the wearer (Wilton, 1997).

Severe multiple finger flexion contractures may be seen in individuals with long-standing TBI or CVA and with progressive neurologic disorders, such as end-stage MS and dementia. Often this type of deformity is seen in long-term care settings that have minimal access to therapy services. This type of contracture puts the individual at high risk for skin maceration and breakdown in the palm and makes nail care and hygiene difficult. Often the fingernails may dig into the palm, causing pain and compromising skin integrity. A small hard cone may be used, but often the commercially available cones are too large. Smaller cones may need to be constructed out of thermoplastic or a high-density foam.

Commercially available inflatable resting splints provide a LLPS to the fingers. The stretch can be adjusted by the progressive inflation of an air bladder placed in a palmar roll. These splints come with washable covers and a padded forearm platform. Some styles also allow wrist position adjustments through a removable strut. The Therapy Carrot Finger Orthosis is a tapered, carrot-shaped device that allows progressive stretching of contracted hands (Fig. 21–18). It comes

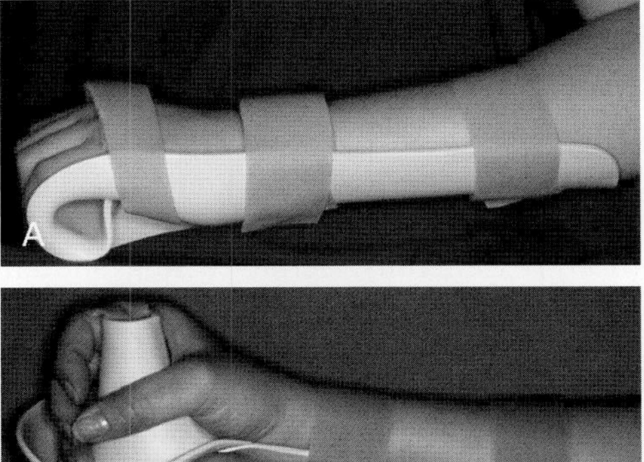

*Figure 21–17 Rolling the finger platform on a wrist/hand immobilization splint (**A**) or forming a cone (**B**) in the hand portion of a wrist/hand immobilization splint may provide LLPS to spastic finger flexors without overstretching them. Shown in **B** is a Preformed Spasticity Splint (by DeRoyal; Powell, TN).*

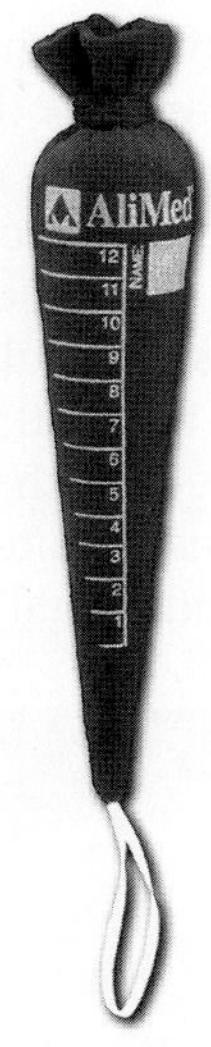

Figure 21–18 A Freedom Finger Contracture Orthosis is recommended for patients who cannot be splinted with more conventional orthoses. Courtesy of AliMed (Dedham, MA).

with a wand to assist in placement of the hand without causing discomfort.

SERIAL AND INHIBITORY CASTING

Serial casting, based on biomechanical principles of tissue elongation to effect change in length, is considered to be an effective means of treating contractures. **Inhibitory casting,** which is based on neurophysiologic principles of sensory input, neutral warmth, and effects on muscle and tendon stretch receptors, is used to treat spasticity. Serial and inhibitory principles are often used simultaneously when treating individuals with CNS disorders (Hill, 1988; Hill & Presperin, 1986; Joachim-Grizzaffi, 1998; Wilton, 1997). Progressive casting over a period of days to weeks provides the best opportunity to take full advantage of the LLPS.

Although an effective treatment, the pros and cons need to be considered before selecting this intervention. The drawbacks to casting include the effects of immobilization, limited use of the extremity, possible problems with pressure and skin integrity, limited means of monitoring, and poor tolerance (Joachim-Grizzaffi, 1998; Wilton, 1997). Generally, serial casting should not be used when there is edema, subluxation, fracture, heterotrophic ossificans, significant agitation, or open wounds. Joachim-Grizzaffi (1998) provides an extensive list of precautions and contraindications of casting patients who have suffered a CVA (Hill, 1988). Casting should be used as a last resort, if splinting and other interventions to increase ROM are not effective (Hill, 1988; Joachim-Grizzaffi, 1998; Wilton, 1997).

Usually, casts are applied at submaximal range for contractures and/or at or just below the point where the stretch reflex is activated for spasticity. Casts may be left on anywhere from 5 to 10 days, depending on the patient, the diagnosis, the reasons for casting, and the patient's response to treatment (Fig. 21–19). In between casts, ROM and activation of the stretch reflex are remeasured. The limb is cleaned, the skin is checked, and PROM is completed to alleviate joint stiffness; then the next cast is applied. Progressive casts are applied weekly for 3 to 5 weeks (Hill, 1988; Joachim-Grizzaffi, 1998; Wilton, 1997). A successful result per cast, according to Hill (1988), is a gain of 10 to 20° or a gain of 10 to 20° in the angle at which the stretch reflex is elicited.

Serial casting is terminated after full ROM is achieved, functional ROM for the individual's goals are achieved, or no improvement is seen after two casts (Hill & Presperin, 1986). A holding cast is applied for a final 1 to 2 weeks to maintain gains, after which the holding cast can be bivalved and used at night to maintain ROM gains (Joachim-Grizzaffi, 1998). Immobilization splints can also be used to maintain gains from casting. Some individuals may need to wear immobilization splints long term to maintain gains made through casting (Wilton, 1997). See Chapter 12 for detailed information on fabrication of casts.

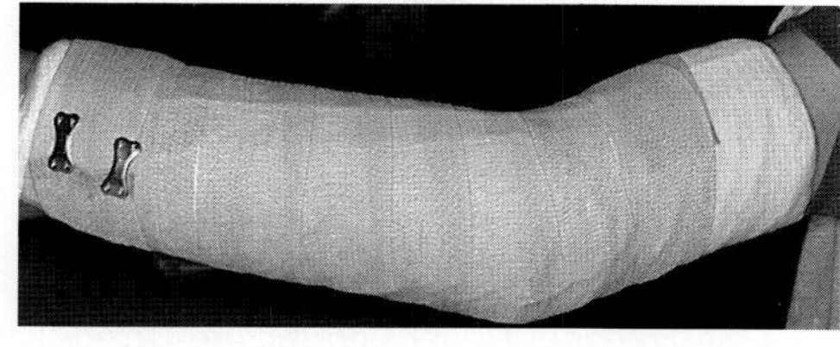

Figure 21–19 Elbow serial casting used for contracture management. Note use of circumferential elasticized wrap for securing splint.

CASE STUDY SECTION

The case studies presented here are meant as teaching guidelines only. Treatment and splinting protocols vary greatly from surgeon to surgeon and from therapist to therapist. The therapist should check with the referring physician and colleagues to define the preferred treatment and splinting methods.

CASE STUDY 1: **CVA with Spastic Hemiplegia**

MG is a 72-year-old right-dominant male. He was admitted to a rehabilitation facility 10 days after a left middle cerebral artery CVA and 14 days after a coronary artery bypass graft.

On evaluation, the therapist noted that MG had dysarthric speech and receptive language appeared functional. He presented with a right spastic hemiplegia with spasticity evident in the scapular rotators, elbow, wrist, and finger flexors. All joints of the upper extremity had full PROM. Attempts at voluntary movement elicited a flexor synergy in the upper extremity. Sensation was impaired in both upper and lower extremities. He was dependent for all activities of daily living (ADLs).

Therapy interventions included neuromotor retraining—focusing on re-establishing trunk control, symmetry, and weight bearing on the right upper extremity to reduce spasticity and promote normal motor patterns—and ADL retraining. A positioning program was developed, and MG and his caregivers were trained to change his position regularly to prevent contractures.

At 2 weeks after admission, a volar wrist/hand immobilization splint was fabricated to wear during rest to prevent contractures while providing gentle stretch to spastic muscles. As spasticity increased, MG's fingers and wrist began pulling away from the splint. A dorsal/volar wrist mobilization splint (Fig. 21–8) was fabricated to better inhibit the spasticity by providing LLPS to the wrist and digital flexors. The splint was tolerated well, and the patient was able to wear it throughout the night and for 2-hr intervals throughout the day when not involved in therapy.

At 4 weeks after admission, MG was able to control actively shoulder and elbow movements in a gravity-eliminated plane. He was taught self ROM and weight-bearing exercises for inhibiting tone, which he performed several times a day. He continued to wear the dorsal/volar wrist mobilization splint at night, but was no longer wearing it during the day.

At 6 weeks after admission, MG was able to ambulate with a quadcane, and was able to complete all basic ADLs while sitting and with supervision for showering. The right upper extremity continued to exhibit mild flexor spasticity, especially during ambulation and functional activities. At rest, the wrist and digits postured in flexion with the thumb tightly adducted and flexed. MG expressed concern about this posturing, but did not want to wear his night splint during the day.

A trial with a Neoprene TAP splint was well tolerated. The soft splint consisted of a half glove, which positioned the thumb and index MP joint in extension and abduction. A wrist-based Neoprene strap was directed from the wrist, across the palm, through the first web space, and wrapped around the distal ulna. The strap was then guided up the forearm into a supinated direction (Fig. 21–13). Wearing the TAP splint, MG was able to use his right hand voluntarily in a gross grasp pattern, which was previously impossible.

MG was discharged after 6 weeks with a home exercise program and continued use of both splints. At 6 months after discharge, he remained active in his avocational activities and had adapted household tools to accommodate his limited grasp.

CASE STUDY 2: **End-Stage MS with Contractures**

VC is a 68-year-old female long-term resident of a nursing home, who was referred to therapy for contracture management. The primary diagnosis was end-stage MS. She was dependent in all ADL activities, and her caregivers found it increasingly difficult to bath and dry her upper body adequately, resulting in poor hygiene and skin breakdown in the palm. VC spent her days supine in bed or propped up with pillows in a recliner chair. Active and passive ROM was significantly limited secondary to spasticity and joint contractures of the shoulder internal rotators and adductors and the elbow wrist and digital flexors. At rest, the hands were fisted with the thumb adducted and flexed into the palm. Skin inspection revealed maceration in both palms and elbow creases, with fingernail marks evident bilaterally.

Therapy interventions for VC included a positioning program, PROM, and splinting to provide LLPS to reduce contractures primarily at the elbows and hands. Owing to the patient's discomfort and resistance to passive movement, the therapist focused on one elbow at a time, giving priority to the left elbow, which had less PROM and was at immediate risk for further skin breakdown. An orthotist was consulted, and VC was fitted for a custom elbow brace. The therapist was responsible for adjusting, monitoring, and developing a maintenance program for the caregivers to follow. Since VC was a small woman, it was determined that a custom orthotic would provide a better fit than a prefabricated one (Fig. 21–16). Additional padding was placed on all of the hardware that was in contact with VC's body. The area over the elbow crease remained open to air to allow healing of the skin breakdown.

By the end of 1 week, VC was tolerating the orthotic for 2 hours, and PROM had increased by 5°. She wore the orthotic for 2 hours each in the morning and afternoon. Each week, PROM was measured and the orthotic was adjusted to accommodate for changes.

Simultaneously, VC's caregivers were trained in techniques to open her hands gently, wash and dry thoroughly, and to provide nail care. Bilateral palm protectors were placed in each hand secured with hook and loop strapping (Fig. 21–20). VC tolerated the palm protectors and wore them throughout the day. The staff carried out skin inspection every 2 hours to prevent skin breakdown in her palms and maintain adequate PROM for hygiene and ADLs.

PROM of the left elbow increased a total of 20° over the course of 6 weeks. At that point it was determined that a bony contracture existed and maximum benefit had been achieved. The skin remained free of breakdown and PROM was maintained through positioning and passive exercises during daily care, so the orthotic was discontinued.

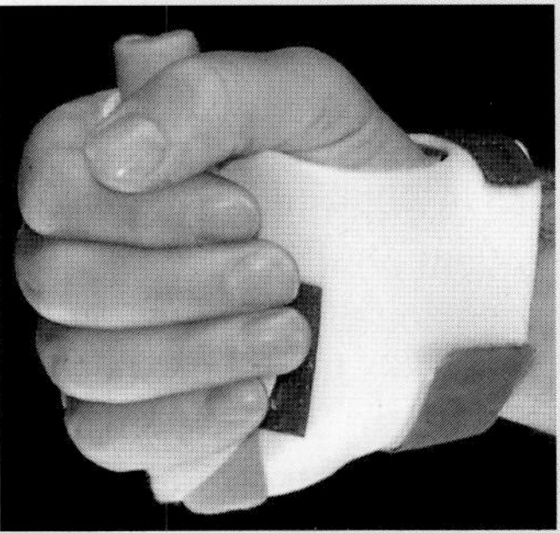

Figure 21–20 A Freedom Progressive Palm Guard Kit allows gradual alterations in position. A roll or cone can be fabricated from hard foam, shaped as needed, and secured to the splint with glue or hook and loop straps. Courtesy of AliMed (Dedham, MA).

CASE STUDY 3: **CVA with Flaccid Hemiplegia**

PP is a 36-year-old female who had suffered a massive right CVA secondary to an occluded right carotid artery 4 months earlier. She was an avid cyclist and employed full time in an office. Immediately after the infarct, she was hospitalized and nonresponsive for approximately 1 week; after 2 weeks of acute hospitalization, she was discharged to a rehabilitation facility where she participated in therapy for 6 weeks, at which time functional progress had reached a plateau. She was discharged to a skilled nursing facility for an additional 6 weeks and was subsequently discharged home with a referral for home care services.

On evaluation by the home care therapist, PP was ambulating independently with a hemiwalker, was independent in transfers, and able to complete basic ADLs with some clothing adaptations and compensatory techniques. PPs family members completed all home management activities. The patient was unable to return to work and was despondent about her disabled status and appearance.

PP demonstrated a left unilateral neglect and left field cut in the lateral half of her left visual field. Cognitively, she was able to articulate an understanding of her deficits; however, she was observed bumping into things on the left and was noncompliant with wearing several splints that had been issued to her.

Upper extremity evaluation revealed a flaccid left upper extremity with tight finger flexors but no contractures. Moderate edema was noted in the left wrist and hand. The left shoulder was observed to have a three-finger's-width subluxation with downward rotation of the scapula. The patient complained of generalized excruciating pain throughout her entire left side; however, she was also seen moving her flaccid arm with her nonaffected arm without any indication of pain. When ambulating, PP's flaccid arm hung dependently at her left side.

When questioned about previous splinting, PP reported that she had received several slings and a splint, but that she didn't use them. Upon investigation, it was found that the patient had a standard hemiplegic sling, a humeral cuff sling (Fig. 21–2 and 21–3), and a wrist/hand immobilization splint for night wear to prevent contractures of the left hand. PP noted that she occasionally wore the splint, but that it was uncomfortable. She stated she did not use the hemiplegic sling because her arm "fell out of it," and she did not use the humeral cuff sling because she and her family members found it "impossible" to don.

Therapy interventions consisted of teaching safety awareness and compensatory techniques to accommodate for the visual neglect, client and family education about edema management and protection of the flaccid extremity, and splinting and positioning interventions. A new wrist/hand immobilization splint was tried (Fig. 21–21). This splint design was comfortable and provided her the appropriate wrist support and digital positioning. A program of decongestive massage and elevation was taught to the client and her family as part of the edema management program.

The previously issued humeral cuff sling was not acceptable to the client because it had complex strapping and was difficult to don. The humeral head could be passively elevated to approximate the glenoid fossa, and since PP was an active ambulator it was beneficial to try another sling. Even though it was impossible for PP to localize her pain, the therapist reasoned that the traction on the soft tissues of the shoulder could be contributing to the general upper extremity pain. A shoulder support with a distal cuff (Fig. 21–22) was worn on a trail basis during upright activities, including ambulation. Although unable to identify a localized reduction in her pain, the patient stated that the sling "felt good" and was much easier to manage.

PP received home therapy three times a week for approximately 1 month. On discharge, she was correctly donning the sling with minimal assistance from family members, and donning the splint independently. Compliance with the nighttime splint was excellent. Visual scanning techniques were being used spontaneously when ambulating; thus PP was able to avoid bumping into things. Edema remained an intermittent problem that continued to be managed with massage and positioning, although compliance was a problem.

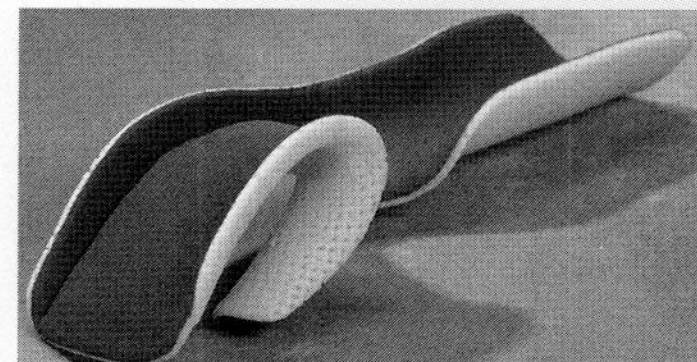

Figure 21–21 The Roylan AirThru Functional Position Splint is a preformed splint that can be easily modified to alter the wrist, digits, and/or thumb position. The splint shown is prepadded for improved patient comfort. Courtesy of the Rehabilitation Division of Smith+Nephew (Germantown, WI).

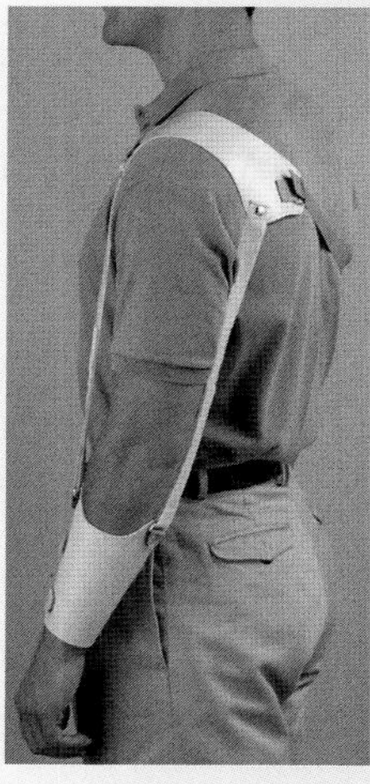

Figure 21–22 A Shoulder Saddle Sling with distal cuff permits some elbow flexion and extension while maintaining shoulder support. It can be worn under loose clothing for improved acceptance. Courtesy of Sammons Preston (Bolingbrook, IL).

CONCLUSION

In summary, the decision to use splinting interventions for the neurologically impaired adult is complex and needs to be made on an individual basis, taking into account the particular diagnosis, prognosis for recovery, functional abilities, patient goals and motivation, the purpose of the splint, patient and caregiver ability to manage the intervention, and the environment in which the splint is to be used. The lack of research supporting many splint interventions for this population points to the need for clinicians to document interventions and changes objectively and to conduct or participate in the necessary research. Good clinical reasoning, observation, and documentation skills are essential. Until more objective evidence is available to justify one intervention over another, therapists must keep up with current research in neuroscience and motor control science and be able clearly to articulate the rationale and objectives for using a particular intervention.

REFERENCES

Cailliet, R. (1980). *The shoulder in hemiplegia.* Philadelphia: Davis.

Eggers, O. (1983). *Occupational therapy in the treatment of adult hemiplegia.* Oxford, UK: Butterworth-Heinemann.

Exner, C., & Bonder, B. (1982). Comparative effects of three hand splints on bilateral hand use, grasp, and arm-hand posture in hemiplegic children: A pilot study. *Occupational Therapy Journal Research, 3,* 75–92.

Fess, E. E., & Philips, C. A. (1987). *Hand splinting: Principles and methods.* St. Louis: Mosby-Yearbook.

Gillen, G. (1999). *The hemiplegic shoulder: current concepts and management.* Paper presented at the annual conference of the American Occupational Therapy Association, Indianapolis.

Gillen, G. (1998a). Managing abnormal tone after brain injury. Occupational *Therapy Practice, 8,* 18–24.

Gillen, G. (1998b). Upper extremity function and management. In G. Gillen, & A. Burkhardt (Eds.). *Stroke rehabilitation: A function-based approach* (pp. 109–151). St. Louis: Mosby-Yearbook.

Hill, J. (1988). Management of abnormal tone through casting and orthotics. In K. M. Kovich & D. E. Bermann (Eds.). *Head injury: A guide to functional outcomes in occupational therapy* (pp. 107–124). Gaithersburg, MD: Aspen.

Hill, J. & Presperin, J. (1986). Deformity control. In J. P. Hill (Ed.). *Spinal cord injury: A guide to functional outcomes in occupational therapy* (pp. 49–85). Gaithersburg, MD: Aspen.

Joachim-Grizzaffi, L. (1998). Casting applications. In G. Gillen, & A. Burkhardt (Eds.). *Stroke rehabilitation: A function-based approach* (pp. 185–204). St. Louis: Mosby-Yearbook.

Lohman, M. (1996). Antispasticity splinting. In B. M. Coppard & H. Lohman (Eds.). Introduction to splinting: A critical-thinking & problem-solving approach (pp. 194–251). St. Louis: Mosby-Yearbook.

Mackinnon, J., Sanderson, E., & Buchanan, D. (1975). The Mackinnon splint: a functional hand splint. *Canadian Journal of Occupational Therapy, 42,* 157–158.

McKee, P., & Morgan, L. (1998). *Orthotics in rehabilitation: Splinting the hand and body.* Philadelphia: Davis.

Milazzo, S., & Gillen, G. (1999). Splinting applications. In G. Gillen, & A. Burkhardt (Eds.). *Stroke rehabilitation: A function-based approach* (pp. 161–184). St. Louis: Mosby-Yearbook.

O'Connell, B. (1998, January–February). Tru-grasp: a new form of hand splinting. *NDTA Network,* 1–5.

Ridgeway, E. M., & Byrne, D. P. (1999). To sling or not to sling? *Occupational Therapy Practice, 1,* 38–42.

Wilton, J. C. (1997). Splinting and casting in the presence of neurological dysfunction. In J. C. Wilton (Ed.). Hand splinting: Principles of design and fabrication (pp. 168–197). Philadelphia: Saunders.

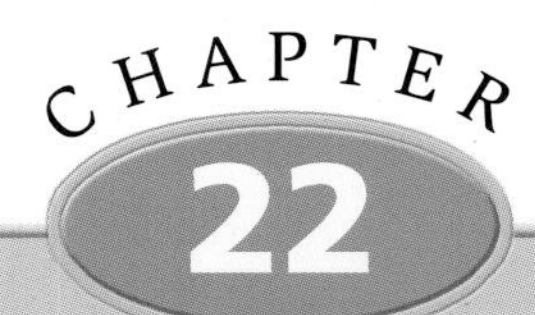

The Pediatric Patient

Elaine Charest, MA, MBA, OTR/L

INTRODUCTION

"To splint a child I just have to make a tiny splint, right?" Actually, it is not that simple. Splinting a child can be difficult, the therapist must rely on two foundations: splinting fundamentals (see Section I) and normal child development, particularly hand development.

Many researchers have written about the normal development of **grasp patterns** and hand use as well as the role **gross motor development** plays in skill acquisition. Table 22–1 is a summary of normal fine and gross motor skills seen in a child's first 15 months of life. Although all of the children who may require splinting are not younger than 1 year, some of them may be developmentally delayed and have delayed integration of the primitive reflexes, which affects splint selection and fabrication. Table 22–2 briefly defines commonly encountered pediatric diagnoses and recommendations for splinting intervention.

This chapter reviews the purpose of splinting the pediatric population, special considerations when working with children (including strapping suggestions and appropriate material selection), and tricks of the trade (including tried-and-true methods of getting a child to wear a splint). When choosing a splint for a child, the splinting objective(s) must first be identified. The objectives are related to issues of position, function, hygiene, and protection.

Splinting for Position

A positional splint can prevent or decrease contractures, provide stability, improve joint alignment, rest affected structures, and allow wound healing.

Contractures

"A **contracture** is a chronic or permanent tightening of soft tissues, causing decreased range of motion (ROM) at a particular joint" (Ratliffe, 1998). Immobilization splinting can prevent contracture formation by maximizing ROM, thereby preventing soft tissue shortening. A mobilization splint can also help elongate soft tissues over an extended period of time, decreasing an existing contracture (Fig. 22–1).

Stability

Injury to the ligaments, tendons, joints, or neurovascular structures can affect **joint stability.** An unstable joint significantly alters the biomechanics of the hand and thus affects function. A splint may provide external support to a joint, or series of joints, improving the overall biomechanical function of the hand (Fig. 22–2).

Alignment

A splint can aid in properly aligning joints and preventing the progression of **deformity.** The maintenance of normal anatomic relationships is important after injury, illness, or surgery to prevent permanent contracture, pseudoarthrosis, and subsequent loss of function (Fig. 22–3).

Rest

Rest is an integral part of healing, whether needed because of a traumatic event, disease process, or a surgical intervention. A splint can hold the hand in proper anatomic alignment while soft tissues are allowed to heal and inflammation and edema diminish. For example, a teenager who has undergone a procedure to increase active elbow flexion, which was nonexistent as a result of polio, must be maintained in approximately 110° of flexion for an extended period of time to allow the transferred pronator mass to heal (Fig. 22–4).

TABLE 22–1 Pediatric Upper Extremity Gross and Fine Motor Skills

Age Skill Appears, Months	Upper Extremity Gross and Fine Motor Skill
0–2	Physiologic flexion
2	Grasp reflex
3	Hands together on chest in supine position
4	Grasp reflex diminishing; objects held in both hands at midline; in supine position bears weight on forearm, more weight on the ulnar side than the radial side; pats sides of bottle with hands
5	Two-handed approach to objects, but grasp is unilateral; bilateral transfer extended-arm weight bearing in prone position; places two hands on bottle with some forearm supination
6	Weight shifts on extended arms in prone position; sits with a straight back; elbows fully extend when reaching
7	First purposeful release; pulls self to stand
8	Crawls on hands and knees
9	Active forearm supination when reaching
10	Pokes with index finger
12	Uses hands in a coordinated manner in which one hand stabilizes and the other manipulates; begins to scribble
15	Releases a pellet with wrist extension and precision

Modified from Hogan, L., & Uditsky, T. (1990). *Pediatric splinting: Selection, fabrication and clinical application of upper extremity splints.* San Antonio, TX: Therapy Skill Builders.

TABLE 22–2 Splinting Intervention for Common Pediatric Diagnoses

Diagnosis	Description	Suggested Splints
Cerebral palsy	Group of nonprogressive conditions occurring in young children; characterized by poor motor control owing to damage to motor centers of brain[a]	Functional splints if necessary
Hemiplegia	Involvement of upper and lower extremity on same side; typically includes wrist flexion and ulnar deviation with fisted posture or thumb in palm deformity[a]	Wrist/hand immobilization splint; wrist immobilization splint; Neoprene splint; hand-based thumb abduction immobilization splint; serpentine splint; Joe Cool splint (Joe Cool Company, South Jordan, UT)
Quadriplegia	Involvement of all four limbs, head trunk and neck;[a] posture same as for hemiplegia	Wrist/hand immobilization splint; wrist immobilization splint; antispasticity ball splint; Neoprene splint; Comfy splint (AliMed, Dedham, MA); Pucci splint (DeRoyal, Powell, TN); carrot splint (AliMed, Dedham, MA); cone splint
Duchenne muscular dystrophy	"General muscle weakness and wasting, affecting pelvis, upper arms and upper legs first. Duchenne progresses slowly, yet eventually involves all voluntary muscles. Survival is rare beyond the 20's"[b]	Wrist/hand immobilization splint; wrist immobilization splint; ring splint (Three Point Products, Annapolis, MD) (Silver Ring Splint Company, Charlottesville, VA)
Rett syndrome	Progressive encephalopathy characterized by autistic features, loss of purposeful hand movements with characteristic hand ringing, ataxia, and spastic paraparesis[c]	Elbow sleeve
Polio	Viral infection of spinal cord, resulting in asymmetrical ascending paralysis[c]	Not usually needed (except postoperatively)

[a]Bleck, E. E. (1987). *Orthopedic management in cerebral palsy.* Philadelphia: Lippincott.
[b]Muscular Dystrophy Australia. (2001). *Disorder description.* www.mda.org.au/general/descript.html. Accessed December 12, 2001.
[c]Batshaw, M. L. (1998). *Children with disabilities* (4th ed.). Baltimore: Brookes.
[d]Flatt, A. E. (1994). *The care of congenital hand anomalies* (2nd ed.). St. Louis: Quality Medical.
[e]Thomas, C. L. (Ed.). *Taber's cyclopedic medical dictionary.* Philadelphia: Davis.
[f]Charcot-Marie-Tooth Association. (2001). *What is CMT?* www.charcot-marie-tooth.org/site/content/what_is_cmt.asp. Accessed December 12, 2001.
[g]Avenues. (1992). *What is arthrogryposis?* www.sonnet.com/avenues/pamphlet.html. Accessed December 12, 2001.
[h]Melvin, J. L. (1982). *Rheumatic disease in the adult and child: Occupational therapy and rehabilitation* (3rd ed.). Philadelphia: Davis.

Continued

TABLE 22–2 Continued

Diagnosis	Description	Suggested Splints
Thumb hypoplasia	Underdevelopment of thumb, ranging from slight shortening to floating or absent thumb[d]	Thumb immobilization/mobilization splint (before surgery to preserve and increase first web space); hand-or forearm-based thumb immobilization splint (after pollicization or opponensplasty)
Radial deficiency	Congenital malformation characterized by shortening or absence of radius, radial-sided carpal bones, and possibly thumb; clinical deformity includes wrist flexion and radial deviation[d]	Forearm-based wrist immobilization splint to correct radial wrist deviation and flexion
Ulnar deficiency	Congenital malformation characterized by shortening/absence of the ulna, ulnar-sided carpal bones, and possibly the small finger; clinically deformity includes ulnar deviation[d]	Forearm-based wrist immobilization splint to correct ulnar deviation
Osteogenesis imperfecta	Hereditary connective tissue disorder characterized by defect in bone matrix calcification, resulting in some degree of bone fragility and deformity[c,e]	Nonarticular humerus splint for fracture management; wrist/hand immobilization splint for infants
Charcot-Marie-tooth disease	Hereditary neural muscular atrophy characterized by slow loss of normal use of feet/legs and hands/arms as nerves to extremities degenerate[f]	Wrist/hand immobilization splint; wrist immobilization splint; ring splint (Three Point Products, Silver Ring Splint Company); Figure-8 splint
Arthrogryposis	Group of congenital anomalies characterized by joint contractures at birth; severity varies by number of joints involved—from few to nearly all; joint contractures are frequently accompanied by muscle weakness, which further limits movement;[g] characteristically includes wrist flexion, elbow extension, and thumb in palm deformity with or without finger flexion contractures	Wrist/hand immobilization splint; wrist immobilization splint; Neoprene splint; elbow extension mobilization splint to maintain or improve elbow extension (after triceps plasty/lengthening); elbow flexion mobilization splint to maintain or improve elbow flexion (after Steinler flexorplasty); forearm-based thumb abduction immobilization splint with elastomer insert (after first web space z-plasty)
Brachial plexus palsy	Upper extremity paralysis, resulting from damage to nerves of brachial plexus[h]	Wrist/hand immobilization splint; wrist immobilization splint; elbow extension immobilization splint; Neoprene wrist splint; shoulder abduction immobilization splint (after L'Episcopo procedure)
Radial ulnar synostosis	Union of radius and ulna by osseous tissue[e]	Arm-based elbow/wrist immobilization splint (after rotational osteotomy of forearm)
Juvenile rheumatoid arthritis	Onset before age 16; may range from polyarticular onset to involving only one joint[h]	Wrist/hand immobilization splint; wrist immobilization splint; ring splint; Neoprene wrist splint; elbow extension immobilization splint; MP joint extension mobilization splint (after MP arthroplasty); Dynasplint (Dynasplint, Severna Park, MD)
Thumb duplication	Doubling of thumb, ranging in severity from "varying degrees of longitudinal splitting to abnormal delta phalanges and triphalangeal thumbs"[d]	Hand-based thumb immobilization splint; forearm-based thumb immobilization splint (after excision of rudimentary digit or closing wedge osteotomy); thumb immobilization splint (after ulna collateral ligament repair or tightening)

[a]Bleck, E. E. (1987). *Orthopedic management in cerebral palsy.* Philadelphia: Lippincott.
[b]Muscular Dystrophy Australia. (2001). *Disorder description.* www.mda.org.au/general/descript.html. Accessed December 12, 2001.
[c]Batshaw, M. L. (1998). *Children with disabilities* (4th ed.). Baltimore: Brookes.
[d]Flatt, A. E. (1994). *The care of congenital hand anomalies* (2nd ed.). St. Louis: Quality Medical.
[e]Thomas, C. L. (Ed.). *Taber's cyclopedic medical dictionary.* Philadelphia: Davis.
[f]Charcot-Marie-Tooth Association. (2001). *What is CMT?* www.charcot-marie-tooth.org/site/content/what_is_cmt.asp. Accessed December 12, 2001.
[g]Avenues. (1992). *What is arthrogryposis?* www.sonnet.com/avenues/pamphlet.html. Accessed December 12, 2001.
[h]Melvin, J. L. (1982). *Rheumatic disease in the adult and child: Occupational therapy and rehabilitation* (3rd ed.). Philadelphia: Davis.

TABLE 22–2 Continued

Diagnosis	Description	Suggested Splints
Brachydactyly	Congenital shortening of phalanges[d]	Opposition post of fingers so short that there is no functional grasp; hand-based digit immobilization splint (clamshell design) (while applying external fixator for distraction and after removal of device for protection)
Camptodactyly	Congenital PIP contracture, usually of small finger[d]	Ring splint if slight (Three Point Products, Silver Ring Splint Company); hand-based finger extension mobilization splint; may use ulnar design if splint is difficult to maintain on hand
Clinodactyly	Congenital curvature of finger, usually small finger, with deviation of tip toward ring finger[d]	Finger extension immobilization splint (after osteotomy)
Myelodysplasia	Defect in formation of spinal cord, resulting in some degree of paralysis, sensory loss, and urinary/bowel dysfunction; may include hydrocephalus, cognitive impairments, seizure disorders, visual impairments, and other musculoskeletal deformities[c]	Wrist/hand immobilization splint; Neoprene splint

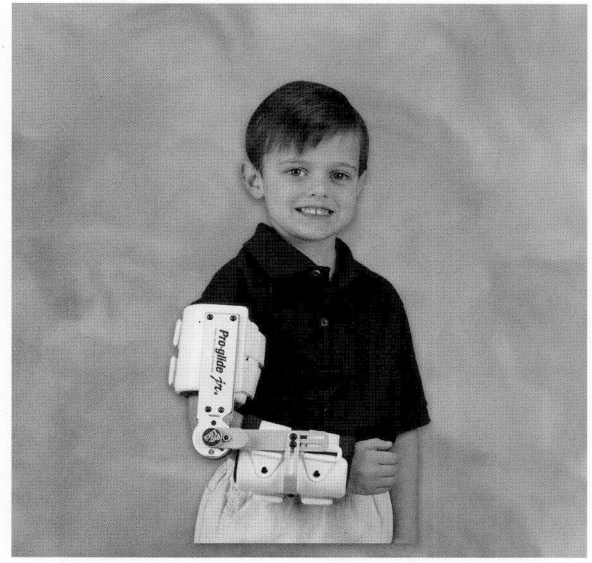

Figure 22–1 A Pro-glide Junior Dynamic Elbow ROM Orthosis can help reduce an existing joint contracture by providing a low load prolonged stretch. Courtesy of DeRoyal (Powell, TN).

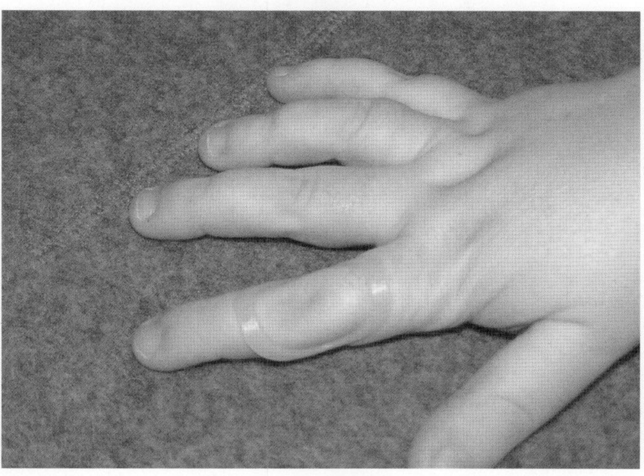

Figure 22–2 Oval 8 ring splints can provide external support to maximize function. This restriction splint is used to prevent PIP hyperextension in this child with a Swan neck deformity. Courtesy 3-Point Products (Annapolis, MD).

Splinting for Function

A **functional splint** can augment existing function by substituting for weak or absent muscles caused by peripheral nerve dysfunction, neuromuscular disorders, or spinal cord injuries. The therapist can design a splint to hold a pencil or eating utensil (Fig. 22–5). Splints can be fabricated for other specific purposes, such as supporting the index finger (IF) in extension for computer or communication system access.

Splinting for Hygiene

A splint may improve or prevent a potential hygiene problem. Hands that remain fisted during most, if not all, of the day owing to posturing secondary to severe spasticity or obligatory reflexes are at high risk for skin breakdown. The inability to extend the fingers also makes nail clipping difficult. Long and/or jagged fingernails can cut into the palm of the hand, leading to infection. Splints can be fabricated to protect the

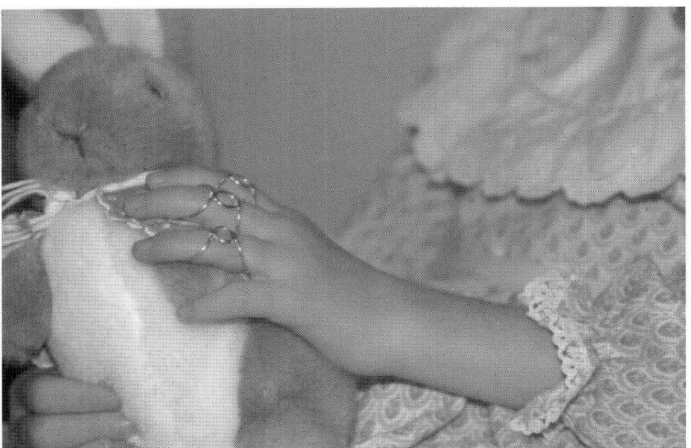

Figure 22–3 *These Silver Ring splints provide stabilization to prevent progression of boutonniere deformities. Courtesy of Silver Ring Splint Company (Charlottesville, VA).*

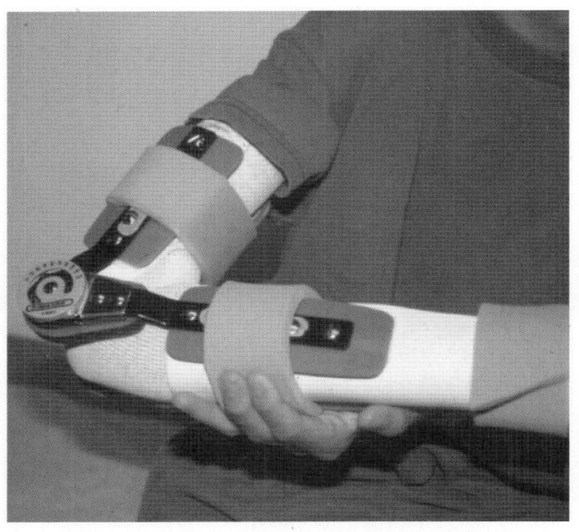

Figure 22–4 *A splint with a lockable component allows for rest immediately after surgery yet provides freedom of movement later in the rehabilitation process.*

palm and minimize the risk of skin breakdown (Fig. 22–6).

Splinting for Protection

A splint may be used for protection, either after a surgical procedure or to prevent a child from self-abusive or interfering behaviors. A **bivalve splint** can be used to protect a postoperative area after the cast has been removed but before complete healing has occurred (Fig. 22–7). Children will be children, and once the discomfort from a surgical procedure subsides, they will not always understand why they cannot resume their typical play activities.

Some children with developmental disabilities demonstrate self-abusive behaviors. These behaviors can affect the child socially as well as academically and medically. Splinting can be used to minimize or diminish these behaviors. For example, a child who tends to bite his or her thumb metacarpophalangeal (MP) joint when upset may have open wounds that are prone to infection; a simple hand-based thumb immobilization splint allows use of the thumb while protecting the open area, allowing healing, and assisting in the prevention of infection (Fig. 22–8).

The therapist must be careful not to cross the line between splints and restraints. The purpose and wearing schedule for such splints needs to be carefully documented. The therapist should refer to his or her specific facility's policies and procedures for clarification.

Other Considerations

Once the therapist has identified the goal of the splint and has an idea of the splint's style, he or she must focus on several other factors, discussed below.

Anatomic Structures

The therapist must assess the child to determine if all anatomic structures are present. Children with **congenital**

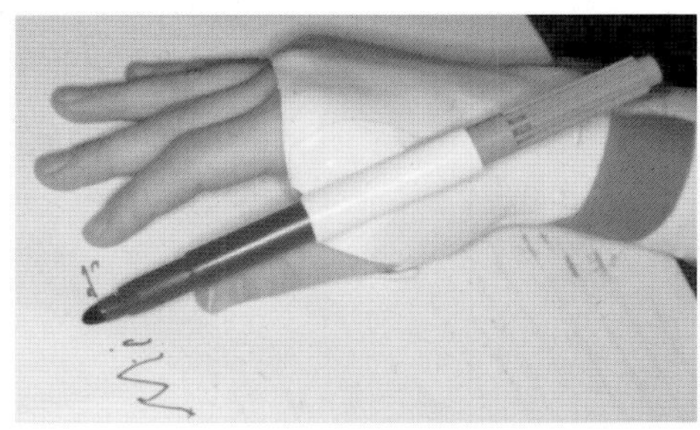

Figure 22–5 *This splint was adapted to hold a pen.*

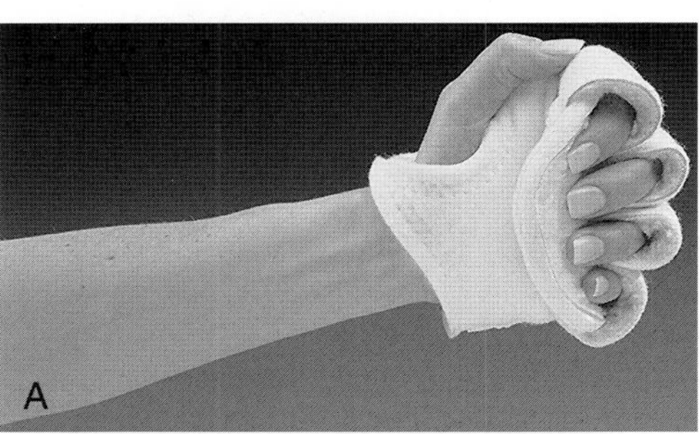

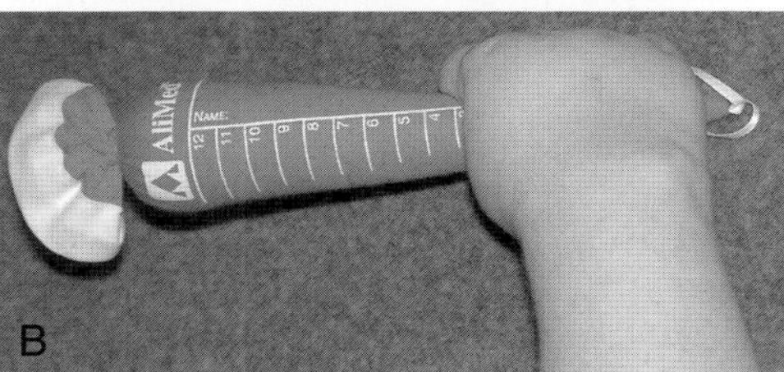

Figure 22–6 *Splints to protect the palm.* ***A,*** *The Roylan Palm Protector can prevent fingernails from cutting into the palm, thus helping prevent skin breakdown. Courtesy of the Rehabilitation Division of Smith+Nephew (Germantown, WI).* ***B,*** *The Freedom Finger Contracture Orthosis, which is also known as the carrot splint can be used to progressively increase space in palm (by AliMed; Dedham, MA).*

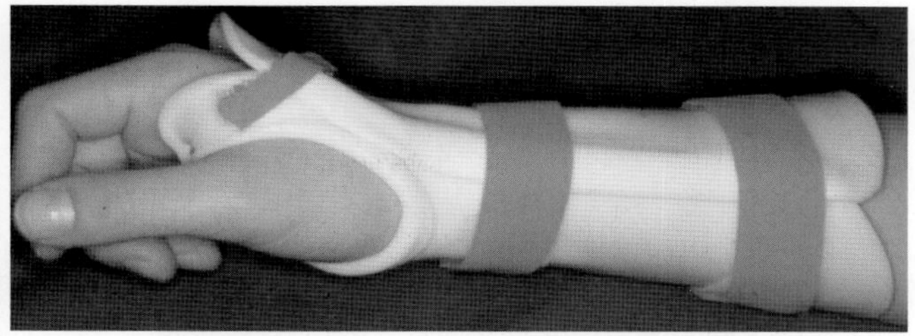

Figure 22–7 A bivalved or clamshell splint with interlocking segments can provide additional protection when a cast is removed from an active child.

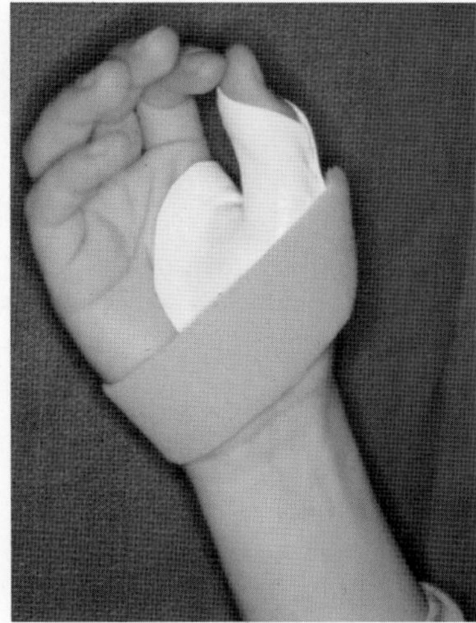

Figure 22–8 A hand-based opponens splint may diminish hand biting behavior while allowing current wounds to heal.

hand anomalies have unusual anatomy that will most likely alter the splint plan. Depending on the type of splint, absent digits or bony structures can make the purchase or fit of a splint more difficult to achieve and maintain. The unique contours of the patient's limb may make splint stabilization a challenge. For example, the goal of splinting a child with a radial deficiency who does not have a thumb may be to stretch out the severe radial deviation seen at the wrist; but adequate purchase is difficult because of the limited digits and baby fat. Sometimes, the immobilization of an additional joint—such as the elbow, in this example—may be needed to gain leverage and optimize the effectiveness of the splint. Consider a simple solution, such as using Dycem as a splint liner to prevent slippage.

Healing Time Frames

Healing rates in a child are different from those in adults. Children's healthy bones, ligaments, tendons, nerves, and blood vessels tend to heal quickly, allowing shorter immobilization times (Putnam & Fischer, 1996). On the other hand, children tend to remain in plaster casts longer than adults because it is often difficult for children to follow through on the precautions associated with their injuries and surgeries. Adults may be placed in a splint before the soft tissues are completely healed; this allows an early start to therapy and decreased possibility of contractures and stiffness. Children generally do not respond the same as adults to prolonged immobilization; most children can be casted for as long as 6 to 8 weeks without adverse consequences.

It is commonly known that children's soft tissues are more elastic than those of an adult. For example, an adult who undergoes a tendon transfer may be placed in a splint as early as 1 week after surgery (Bishop, Topper, & Bettinger, 1996). A child who undergoes the same procedure is generally casted for 3 to 6 weeks until the tendon has time to heal; then splinting is initiated (Idler, 1996). In these cases, children do not usually suffer any loss of ROM as result of the longer immobilization period.

Nerve regeneration is another area in which children fare far better than adults. It has been estimated that children recover three times faster than adults, based on comparisons of sensory action potential amplitudes. In addition, it is known that cellular activity depends on age, which again puts children at an advantage (Watchmaker & Mackinnon, 1996).

Abnormal Tone

The presence of **spasticity** may require a rigid splinting material to prevent the child from bending or cracking the splint during normal wear. A moderately to severely spastic hand may put enough stress on the distal portion of a resting splint to crack it. Reinforcing the splint with additional splinting material may help. Splints that reduce tone by placing the hand in a **reflex inhibiting position,** such as an antispasticity ball splint, may be the wisest choice (see Chapter 21 for details). (Fig. 22–9).

Swelling

Edema management in a child is similar to that in an adult: ice, elevation, and compression (elasticized

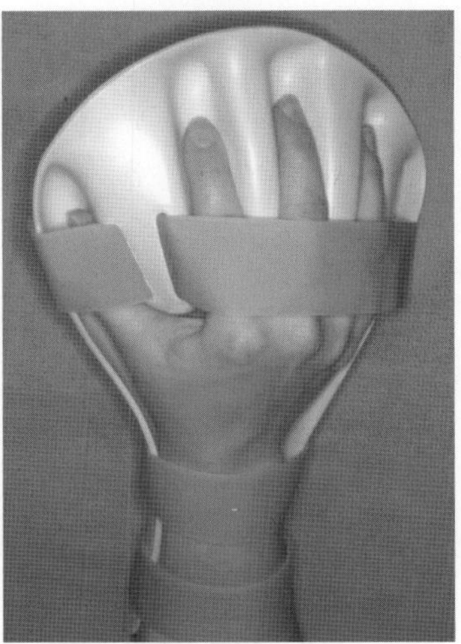

Figure 22–9 An antispasticity ball splint helps reduce tone by placing the hand in a reflex-inhibiting position.

wraps) being the key treatment interventions. However, it is important to supervise a child to make sure he or she is maintaining an elevated position. In some cases, a sling can be made from stockinette: Insert the postoperative hand and arm into the stockinette, and affix it to the opposite shoulder, placing the elbow in 120° of flexion. This prevents the child from holding the extremity in a dependent position (Fig. 22–10). Family involvement is essential; careful instruction and explanation are the keys to success.

Compliance

The therapist must take a multifaceted approach when encouraging compliance for a pediatric patient. First and foremost, it is important that the child accept the splint. If a child is not willing to wear a splint, he or she will find ways not to. If the child is able to take the splint off independently, the splint may come off as soon as they are out of the therapist's or caregiver's sight. Children have even been known to flush splints down the toilet. When possible, the therapist and parents must explain why the splint is necessary in terms that the child understands.

Understanding the rationale is not always enough for a child. Many young patients have been exposed to medical professionals all of their lives. Someone has always been telling them what to do, what not to do, how to stretch, what to wear, etc. Giving these children some degree of control can sometimes improve compliance. For example, the therapist can offer choice of colors for the thermoplastic, strapping, and Neoprene materials; this may give young patients enough ownership to get them to buy into the therapy program.

For older children, the therapist should focus on fabricating the splint to be as low profile and cosmetically appealing as possible. The fashion police are alive and well among children today. Children understand that not

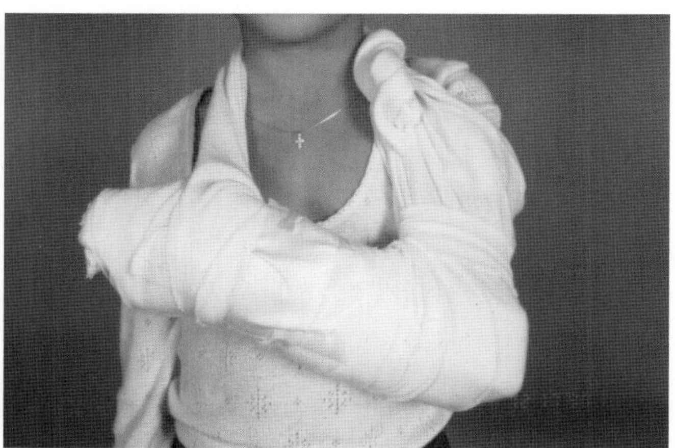

Figure 22–10 A sling can be made from stockinette to hold a child's elbow in 120° of flexion and position the hand out of a dependent position (above heart level).

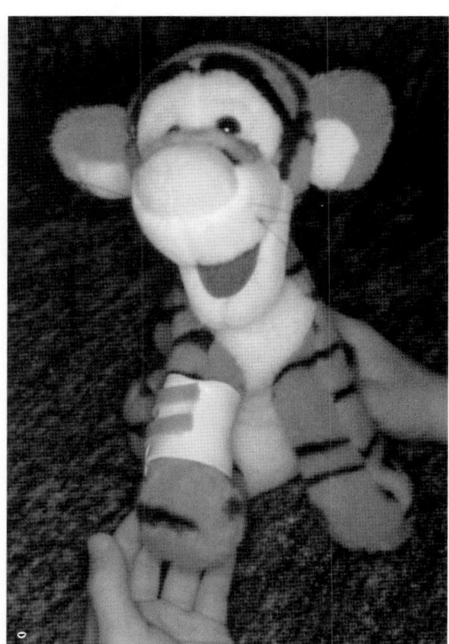

Figure 22–11 Putting a splint on the child's stuffed animal or doll may assist in compliance.

everyone has to wear a splint and many do not want to be different from their peers.

Here are some other creative ways to gain compliance in the pediatric population:

- Issue bilateral hand-based Neoprene splints so the child can tell his or her friends that they are sports, biking, or in-line skating gloves.
- Splint a teddy bear or doll with scrap materials so the child can apply a splint to his or her toy while a parent or caregiver applies a splint to the child (Fig. 22–11),
- Encourage the child to decorate the splint with stickers or markers.
- Apply colorful cut out designs made of scrap thermoplastic material to the splint base.

Compliance goes beyond the child. The patient's family and school (teacher, aide, school therapist) must understand and comply with the splinting program. Without carryover, the program will not be successful. The therapist can facilitate compliance by constructing the splint as simply as possible. Most families and school professionals do not have clinical degrees and are often too busy to wrestle with a difficult splint. Splints should be easy and quick to don and doff.

Written and verbal instructions should be provided. Sometimes the child, parent, and/or caregiver is able to apply the splint in the presence of the therapist but then encounters difficulty when at home or at school. Pictures may help facilitate the process. Other ideas that may help get the splints on properly are marking the splints for right and left, indicating which end of an elbow splint is for the forearm or upper arm, and numbering or lettering loop strapping and corresponding hook to ensure the straps are applied appropriately.

The therapist should remember, that adults—not just children—have different levels of literacy. The instructions should be simple and include diagrams whenever possible. Note that for some adults English is a second language. The therapist should be aware that the most important members of the child's treatment team are the family.

Sensory Factors

Some children present with a **hypersensitivity** to touch. Having a splint on their hand may be irritating. To maximize the success of the intervention, sensory processing issues should be identified and addressed before initiating the splinting program. For example, a child who does not tolerate wearing a hand splint before surgery will, in all likelihood, not tolerate a splint after surgery. If wear issues can be identified and treated before the procedure, postoperative compliance may not affect outcome.

Some children are nonverbal and are unable to articulate if they are experiencing pain or discomfort. Careful padding of bony prominences, during and after fabrication, can help prevent skin breakdown. Even some children without sensory issues are afraid of being burned by the splinting material. Although the therapist knows the material will not hurt the child, the child may become afraid when he or she sees the steaming water bath. Allow the patient to touch and play with heated scraps of splinting material so he or she can be assured that the material is not too hot. A piece of stockinette placed over that patient's body part before splinting may alleviate some of their fears.

The therapist should take some time to develop a rapport with the child, playing with the patient for a couple of minutes before starting the fabrication process. While playing with the child, explain the process. Then remind the child at the start of each step of what's to come.

Cognition and Developmental Age

The **developmental level** of the child to be splinted is important. If the child is still mouthing objects, avoid any small parts that may be sucked or bitten off the splint. At this stage, the therapist must also avoid glues and adhesives that may be toxic. Children who have reached a developmental age of 8+ years, depending on the expected compliance, can be taught self-donning and care of the splint, which may increase the child's sense of independence.

The presence of primitive reflexes may also influence splint design and fabrication. For example, an infant with a strong grasp reflex may require a dorsal-based splint to prevent stimulation of the palm. The obligatory positioning of the upper extremities in the presence of an **asymmetrical tonic neck reflex (ATNR)** may require positioning of the head or asking the child to look at the affected hand to facilitate molding. This position elicits the extension patterns, rather than the flexion patterns, imposed by the ATNR (Fig. 22–12). A child who is old enough to follow commands but is still bound by primitive reflexes owing to neurologic impairments, may participate in the positioning when asked to look at the involved hand.

Many children have difficulty sitting still during splinting. Having small toys or bubbles available may help keep the child distracted. If the child is particularly squirmy, the therapist should concentrate on molding one part of the splint at a time, which may avoid the need for remolding the entire splint several times. This allows the child to take small breaks during the fabrication process.

A cold spray can speed material setting time, which reduces the amount of time the child needs to stay still. Cold spray should be used cautiously around children with asthma or other medical conditions that cause a sensitivity to inhalants. Alternatives are to run the splint under cold water or to submerge the child's hand and splint into a cool water bath.

Latex Allergies and Precautions

In 1979, Nutter described an allergic reaction to **latex.** Since that time, many other reports have been substantiated. The reaction varies from a rash, hives, edema, watery eyes, and respiratory symptoms to anaphylaxis. High-risk groups for the allergy include children or adults

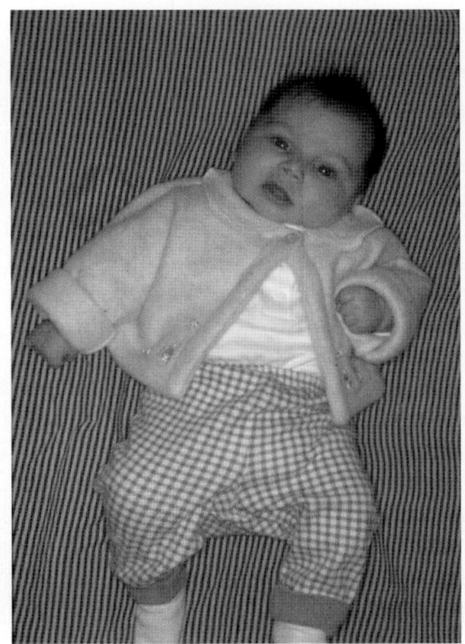

Figure 22–12 When splinting, the ATNR can be used to help with positioning. Notice the extension pattern on the baby's right side.

with myelodysplasia or spina bifida, cerebral palsy, and bladder extrophy. Frequent exposure to latex products (via bladder catheterization, ventriculoperitoneal shunt, or surgical procedures) is a predisposing factor (Delfico, Dormans, Craythorne, Templeton, 1995; Meeropol, 1996; Meeropol, Frost, Pugh, Roberts, & Ogden, 1993).

When splinting a child with any of these conditions, the therapist must take care to avoid the use of latex products. Many pediatric hospitals have become latex-safe environments, limiting the products available for use. Most major supply companies are now aware of latex sensitivity and provide information about latex content on request. Many companies such as TheraBand have reformulated their products to be latex-free. The National Spina Bifida Association (2001) posts a list of latex-safe medical and therapy supplies on their Web site. When in doubt, the therapist should ask the manufacturer or distributor for additional information.

Home Environment

Geographic location may influence the types of splints and materials the therapist chooses for a child. Patients who live in warmer climates may benefit from perforated thermoplastic material, rather than solid material, to allow air flow and help prevent skin maceration. If a patient has a tendency toward excessive perspiration, a dorsal-based splint may help, since the tendency to perspire is less on the dorsal surface than on the volar surface of the hand. This benefit must be weighed against the fact that there are more bony prominences to accommodate dorsally.

Material Selection

The type of material selected for a splint depends on the child's age, muscle tone, level of cooperation, and level of pain. Children tend to be less forgiving in regard to any discomfort associated with the splinting process, such as for positioning strategies or heat from the splint material. If a child is in pain and is cooperative, a drapable plastic-like material allows minimal contact from the therapist during the molding process. A child who is squirming around during fabrication, but who is not in pain, may require a more forgiving material, such as those in the rubber category, which allow the therapist to hold on to the splint and the limb with more force while molding.

The weight of the splint can be significant for very young children and patients with weak muscles. The thinner materials (1/16" and 3/32") often provide adequate positioning while minimizing weight. Thinner materials also allow better conformability for smaller hands (e.g., molding into a web space).

Neoprene splints tend to be more comfortable for children who have minimal, if any, fixed deformity, such as a child with spastic hemiplegia who tends to posture

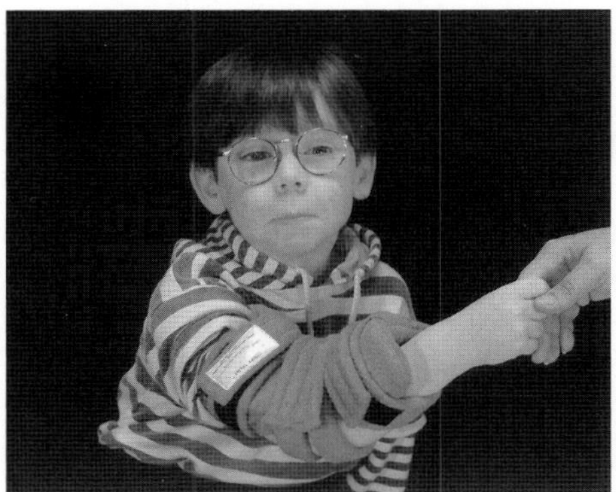

Figure 22–13 A Pedi-Comfy Elbow Splint with a machine-washable terry cloth cover. Courtesy of AliMed (Dedham, MA).

in a wrist flexion/thumb in palm position when actively using the involved hand. Because of the soft nature of the material, severe spasticity and rigid deformity cannot be controlled adequately with Neoprene (see Chapter 14 for information).

At times, perforated materials are the most appropriate choice to improve the dissipation of heat because this is a problem for children with congenital or traumatic amputations and osteogenesis imperfecta. The autonomic nervous systems of these patients perceive that all limbs are present even when they are not; thus these children tend to perspire excessively to reduce body temperature. This is of significant importance when fabricating functional splints for a child who has a quadrimembral limb deficiency.

There are many prefabricated splints on the market; however, most of them do not come in pediatric sizes. Prefabricated Neoprene splints may be purchased for hand-based thumb abduction, wrist support, and thumb/wrist support. Carrot splints to protect the palm of a patient with extreme fisting can be used for school-aged and older children, owing to the size of the smaller end of the carrot. Comfy makes prefabricated resting hand and wrist supports, with a machine-washable terry cloth cover in pediatric sizes (Fig. 22–13). Sometimes items originally fabricated for another purpose can be used for splinting. For example, infant-size knee immobilizers can be used for elbow extension splints on a small child.

Component Selection

With few exceptions, outriggers and splint attachments are not recommended for the young pediatric population. These attachments tend to have small pieces that can become detached, presenting a choking hazard. Outriggers can cause injury to the eyes, ears and other areas if the child is running and falls on the splint. If mobilization splinting is recommended by the physician, serial static splinting may be the safest choice for this population. For the older child, outriggers made from thermoplastic tubing serve the same purpose as their metal counterparts, minimizing the risk of injury.

Strapping Selection

As mentioned, a child can get out of almost any splint if he or she really wants to. The trick is to get the child to *want* to wear the splint. Traditional straps come in a variety of colors; allowing the child to pick his or her favorite and thus to participate in the creation of the splint may increase the patient's willingness to wear the splint. Circumferential splint designs offer an alternative option that may be more difficult for a child to remove.

At times, a child's functional limitation can be used to ensure splint compliance. Children who have a weak pinch or grasp may not be able to remove the strap from a Dual-Lock or Poly-Lock strapping system, which results in a stronger attachment than standard hook and loop. Note that "the closure strength of standard Velcro hook to loop for lengthwise peel is 1 pound per square inch (psi) while Poly-Lock requires 25 psi" (Hogan & Uditsky, 1998).

There are however, a few drawbacks to a lock system. First, it can also be difficult for caretakers to remove the loop; this can be countered by leaving a small tab at the end of the loop for easier grasping. But remember, if it is easier for the parent, it is also easier for the child. Second, the loop material wears out quickly with lock systems, so additional straps must be issued. Finally, the Dual-Lock straps do not conform about the forearm as well as other types of straps; this can be overcome by placing a thinner strip of Dual-Lock along this region. Sometimes, heating the adhesive surface of the Dual-Lock assists with obtaining strong adhesion.

Another Houdini-proof method of applying splints is resorting to riveted straps and buckles. Developmentally, children learn to unfasten traditional loop-and-hook systems long before they learn to unbuckle. Be sure these are securely fastened to the splint to prevent any choking hazard. One word of caution: When splinting for a hereditary condition such as Charcot-Marie-Tooth syndrome, make sure the parents have the hand function needed to manipulate the straps and splint since they are likely to be affected by the condition as well.

Foam strapping tends to be tolerated better than traditional loop by the sensitive skin of an infant or young child. These straps need to be changed frequently because they are made of an open-cell foam, which absorbs salvia and other liquids quite readily.

Another possible way to make sure the splint is not taken off is to place a sock over the child's hand. Sometimes, when it comes to straps, out of sight is out of mind. The therapist may encourage the child to wear a watch over a strap to convince him or her to leave the splint on. Fastening splints with zippers or laces may prevent some children from removing the device.

CASE STUDY SECTION

The case studies presented here are meant to be used as teaching guidelines only. Treatment and splinting protocols vary greatly from surgeon to surgeon and from therapist to therapist. The therapist must check with the referring physicians and colleagues to define the preferred treatment and splinting methods.

CASE STUDY 1: **Spastic Quadriplegic Cerebral Palsy**

TW is a 7-year-old male with a history of neonatal sepsis, resulting in spastic quadriplegic cerebral palsy. He attends a special needs program at the local elementary school where his cognitive abilities are reported to be at a 1-year-old level. On physical examination, TW had significantly increased bilateral tone in his upper extremities, including the elbow, wrist, and digital flexors. He maintained a thumb in palm posture while in a wheelchair and when lying supported on an examining table. He had full passive ROM of both upper extremities with diminished selective active motor control.

Given the increased tone, TW was at high risk for developing fixed contractures in his upper extremities. Through parental interview, it was determined that TW also fisted his hands when sleeping, although his elbows could easily be ranged at that time. Bilateral resting splints were issued for night wear to provide a prolonged gentle stretch to the spastic muscles and prevent the fisted posture (Fig. 22–14). The therapist suggested that the splints be donned after the patient fell asleep. Soft Neoprene thumb abduction splints were prescribed for day wear to keep TW's thumb out of the palms and encourage grasping activities.

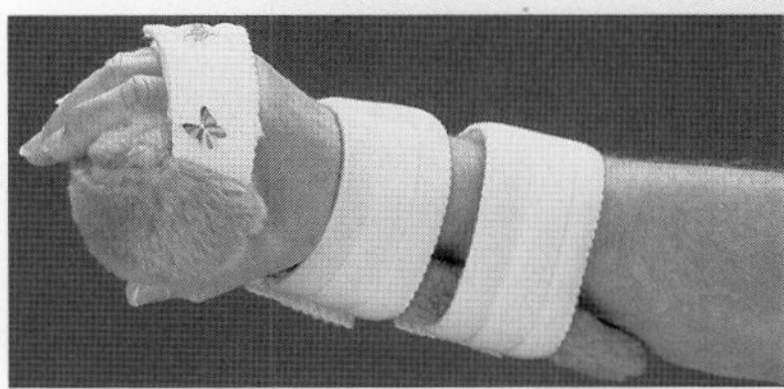

Figure 22–14 A Pucci Air-T WHO Splint may be worn at night to provide a low load prolonged stretch of spastic muscles. Courtesy of AliMed (Dedham, MA).

CASE STUDY 2: **Duchenne Muscular Dystrophy**

LR is a 12-year-old male with Duchenne muscular dystrophy. His progressive muscular weakness was beginning to involve the hands, as demonstrated by the mild swan-neck posturing of the middle and ring fingers during active digit extension. The patient was fitted with Silver Ring splints for wear during waking hours to restrict hyperextension at the proximal interphalangeal (PIP) joints of the involved fingers (Fig. 22–15).

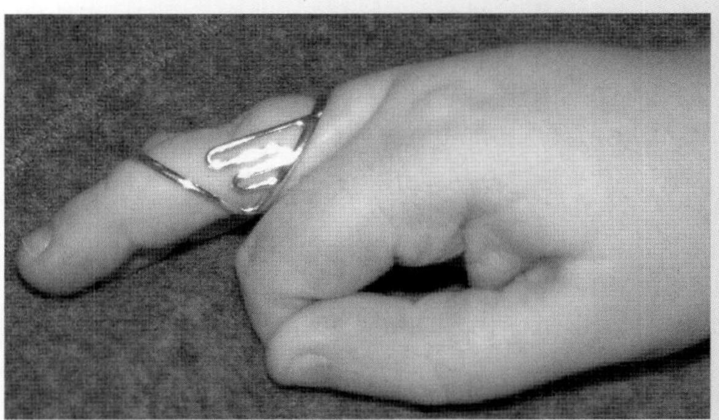

Figure 22–15 This particular Silver Ring splint blocks hyperextension of the PIP joints while allowing full active flexion for a teen with muscular dystrophy. Courtesy Silver Ring Splint Company (Charlottesville, VA).

Full active flexion was still attainable, which allowed LR to continue feeding himself, participate in school activities, and steer his power wheelchair. The goal of the splints was to provide better digital tendon balance and mechanical advantage, while positioning the joints for function, therefore preventing undue joint stress and possible long-term deformity.

CASE STUDY 3: **Left Hemiplegia**

SS is a 14-year-old male with left hemiplegia. He had a normal developmental history until age 3, when he fell out of a shopping cart onto his head, sustaining a large epidural hematoma that required surgical evacuation. SS's primary complaint was the lack of functional use of the left hand. When trying to stabilize an object to be manipulated by his right hand, SS had to trap the object either between his left forearm and body or against an external surface.

On physical examination, SS was able to preposition the hand in space but tended to go into a wrist flexion, thumb in palm, fisted posture when he attempted to use the hand. He had full passive ROM, although increased tone was noted in the wrist and finger flexors. Stereognosis was intact, increasing the likelihood that SS could use the hand if he had better selective motor control.

The patient was fitted with a Neoprene wrist/thumb splint (Fig. 22–16). The splint contained an aluminum stay to hold his wrist in a neutral position. The thumb was prepositioned in abduction and opposition. While using the Neoprene support, SS was able to oppose his thumb to his fingers actively. There was enough support to the wrist and thumb that the abnormal pattern was minimized.

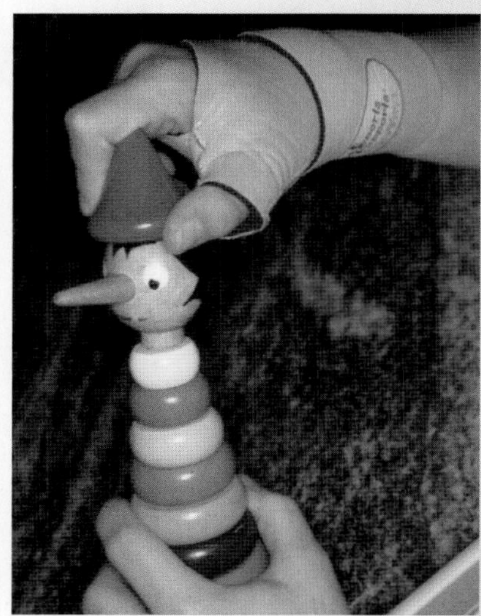

Figure 22–16 A Neoprene wrist support with a thumb abduction component improves hand function in a child with hemiplegia.

CASE STUDY 4: **Hyperlaxity Syndrome**

EH is an 11-year-old girl with a hyperlaxity syndrome involving most joints, a right transverse deficiency of the metacarpals, and a right elbow flexion contracture. Her bilateral upper extremity shoulder active ROM was limited to 115° of flexion; she had no abduction and minimal internal and external rotation. On her left side, she demonstrated full elbow active ROM with no active supination. EH had a hypoplastic hand, involving a small palm, no fingers, and a hypoplastic thumb without joints. On her right side, a 75° elbow flexion contracture was present with active flexion to 110°, which progressed during the past year, and no active supination. The patient did demonstrate active wrist extension to neutral after undergoing a flexor carpi radialis (FCR) to extensor carpi radialis brevis (ECRB) transfer several years earlier. EH presented with significant hyperlaxity of her lower extremities and required knee/ankle/foot orthoses to ambulate short distances; she used a wheelchair for long distances.

EH was a remarkably bright girl who was highly motivated to be independent. She used a wrist immobilization splint on the right when she began to fatigue and assume a wrist drop position. During the day, she wore an elbow Dynasplint on the right to diminish the elbow

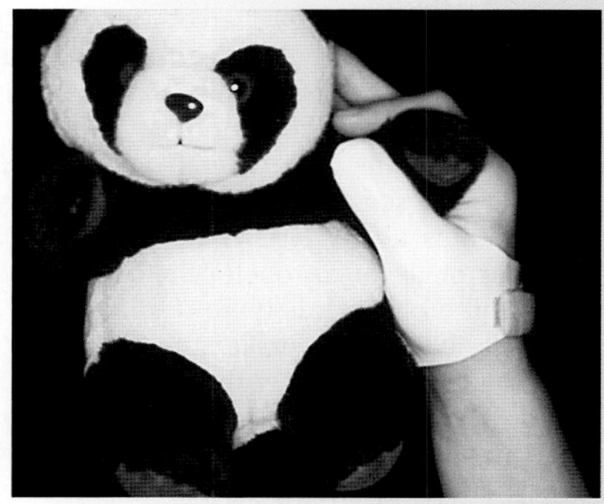

Figure 22–17 An opposition post can aid in manipulating objects.

flexion contracture (Fig. 22–1). At night, she used an elbow mobilization splint (serial static) to maintain tissue length and prevent further loss of elbow ROM.

The primary complaint for EH and her family was difficulty performing bilateral tasks. The question of a prosthesis had been raised in the past, but owing to arm length on the right side and the decreased strength and stability of the upper body, a prosthesis was not a feasible option. An opposition post was fabricated for EH, which was attached to her forearm. This allowed her to use the active wrist flexors and hypoplastic thumb to grasp objects (Fig. 22–17). The patient was able to wear the post as needed to become independent in most activities of daily living.

CASE STUDY 5: **Radial Club Hand**

JS is a 6-year-old boy who was born with a left unilateral cleft lip and palate and bilateral radial club hands. He presented after bilateral pollicizations and opponensplasties to increase hand function. JS's resting posture was 15° of radial deviation. Night wrist/thumb immobilization splints were prescribed to position his wrists in neutral while maintaining the opposition gained through the surgery (Fig. 22–18).

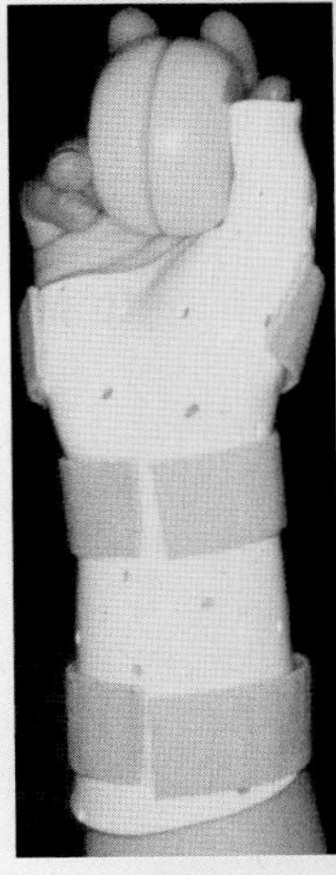

Figure 22–18 A wrist/thumb splint maintains positioning after pollicization and opponensplasty.

CONCLUSION

To splint children is a challenge. The therapist must use clinical judgement, creative problem solving, and have knowledge of all the resources available to splint these small extremities. It is of paramount importance that the therapist has a solid appreciation of child development as well as advanced skills in splint fabrication. Family and/or caregivers play a significant role in compliance and positive outcomes for this very special population.

REFERENCES

Avenues. (1992). *What is arthrogryposis?* www.sonnet.com/avenues/pamphlet.html. Accessed December 12, 2001.

Batshaw, M. L. (1998). *Children with disabilities* (4th ed.). Baltimore: Brookes.

Bishop, A. T., Topper, S. M., Bettinger, P. C. (1996). Flexor mechanism reconstruction & rehabilitation. In C. A. Permer (Ed.). *Surgery of the hand and upper extremity* (pp. 1133–1188). New York: McGraw-Hill.

Bleck, E. E. (1987). *Orthopedic management in cerebral palsy.* Philadelphia: Lippincott.

Charcot-Marie-Tooth Association. (2001). *What is CMT?* www.charcot-marie-tooth.org/site/content/what_is_cmt.asp. Accessed December 12, 2001.

Delfico, A. J., Dormans, J. P., Craythorne, C. B., & Templeton, J. J. (1995). Intraoperative anaphylaxis due to allergy to latex in children who have cerebral palsy: a report of six cases. *Developmental Medicine and Child Neurology, 39(3)* 194–197.

Flatt, A. E. (1994). *The care of congenital hand anomalies* (2nd ed.). St. Louis: Quality Medical.

Hogan, L., & Uditsky, T. (1998). *Pediatric splinting: Selection, fabrication and clinical application of upper extremity splints.* San Antonio: Therapy Skill Builders.

Idler, R. S. Pediatric tendon injuries. (1996). In C. A. Permer (Ed.). *Surgery of the hand and upper extremity* (pp. 2165–2178). New York: McGraw-Hill.

Meeropol, E. (1996). Latex allergy update: Clinical practice and unresolved issues. *Journal of Wound Ostomy and Continence Nursing, 23(4),* 193–196.

Meeropol, E., Frost, J., Pugh, L., Roberts, J., & Ogden, J. A. (1993). Latex allergy in children with myelodysplasia: A survey of Shriners hospitals. *Journal of Pediatric Orthopaedics, 13(1)* 1–4.

Melvin, J. L. (1982). *Rheumatic disease in the adult and child: Occupational therapy and rehabilitation* (3rd ed.). Philadelphia: Davis.

Muscular Dystrophy Australia. (2001). *Disorder description.* www.mda.org.au/general/descript.html. Accessed December 12, 2001.

Nutter. (1979). Contact urticoria to rubber. *British Journal of Dermatology, 101,* 597–598.

Putnam, M. D., & Fischer, M. (1996). Forearm fractures. In C. A. Permer (Ed.). *Surgery of the hand and upper extremity* (pp. 599–635). New York: McGraw-Hill.

Ratliffe, K. T. (1998). *Clinical pediatric physical therapy: A guide for the physical therapy team.* St. Louis: Mosby Year Book.

Spina Bifida Association of American. (2001, spring). *The latex issue.* www.sbaa.org/html/sbaa_latex.html. Accessed December 12, 2001.

Thomas, C. L. (Ed.). *Taber's cyclopedic medical dictionary.* Philadelphia: Davis.

Watchmaker, G. P., & Mackinnon, S. E. (1996). Nerve injury and repair. In C. A. Permer (Ed.). *Surgery of the hand and upper extremity* (pp. 1251–1276). New York: McGraw-Hill.

SUGGESTED READING

Buck-Gramcko, D. (Ed.). (1998). *Congenital malformations of the hand and forearm.* London: Churchill Livingstone.

Byron, P. M. (1995). Splinting the hand of a child. In J. M. Hunter, E. J. Mackin, & A. D. Callahan (Eds.). *Rehabilitation of the hand* (4th ed., pp. 1443–1450). St. Louis: Mosby Year Book.

Henderson, A., & Pehoski, C. (1995). *Hand function in the child: Foundations for remediation.* St. Louis: Mosby- Year Book.

Manske, P. R., & Strecker, W. B. (1996). Cerebral palsy, brain injury, stroke: Spastic disorders of the upper extremity. In C. A. Permer (Ed.). *Surgery of the hand and upper extremity.* New York: McGraw-Hill.

Osterhout, B. M. (1990). Postoperative splinting of the pediatric upper extremity. *Hand Clinics, 6,* 693–695.

CHAPTER 23

Burns

Reg Richard, MS, PT

INTRODUCTION

The use of splints to treat patients with **burn injuries** is one approach in a cornucopia of treatment interventions that may be used in the rehabilitation of these patients. Construction of burn splints employs the basic splinting principles described in Section I. Because the focus of this text is on how to splint patients, and not on the treatment of patients overall, this chapter addresses the nuances of splinting that are unique to patients with burns and highlights particular principles that can contribute to successful patient outcome. The most significant characteristic of splints fabricated for patients with burns is that the splint is individualized to the specific needs of each patient. However, before focusing on aspects of splinting that apply to burns, some fundamental information about when and why patients need a splint is presented.

Burn Injury Considerations

Objectives when splinting a patient with burns are to prevent burn scar contracture deformity; preserve range of motion (ROM) achieved in exercise sessions or through surgical release of a contracture; correct a scar contracture; and protect tenuous joints and other delicate structures such as tendons, vessels, nerves, skin grafts, and flaps. The decision to splint a patient with a burn injury is based on the patient's age, level of cooperation, and three aspects particular to the burn injury itself. Those aspects are the severity of the patient's injury, the patient's point of recovery in regard to the phases of wound healing, and the different biomechanical principles that are associated with the rehabilitation strategy of splint application.

Burn Wound Severity

The severity of a patient's injury is judged by the extent, depth, and location of the burn wounds. Extent of injury involves the surface area of the body burned. A direct relationship exists between how much surface area of the body was burned and the number of scar tissue contractures a patient may develop (Kraemer, Jones, & Deitch, 1988). The depth of the burn injury is classified into one of four categories relative to the level of skin damage (Richard, in press). From a rehabilitation perspective, the location of the burn injury is of concern when it involves skin creases overlying or adjacent to joint areas.

Depth of burn is classified as **superficial, partial-thickness, full-thickness,** and **subdermal** (Fig. 23–1). Partial-thickness burns can be subdivided into **superficial** and **deep. Depth of injury** is important from a wound-healing perspective, because it relates to the formation of scar tissue and the potential for subsequent contracture development. Superficial and superficial partial-thickness burns are of little consequence from a splinting perspective, because minimal scar tissue is formed during the healing of these types of injuries. Deep partial-thickness burns that heal by secondary intention do so by production of dense scar tissue. Full-thickness burns, which typically require a skin graft to heal, have a far greater predilection for contracture formation than partial-thickness injuries (Dobbs & Curreri, 1972; Kraemer et al., 1988). Finally, subdermal burns, commonly caused by electrical injury and followed by extensive tissue damage underlying the skin, likewise can cause functional deficits that require splints.

A consideration over the early application of splints centers around a decrease in blood perfusion to areas of deep partial-thickness burns. These burns have been noted to possess questionable blood flow (Rutan, 1998).

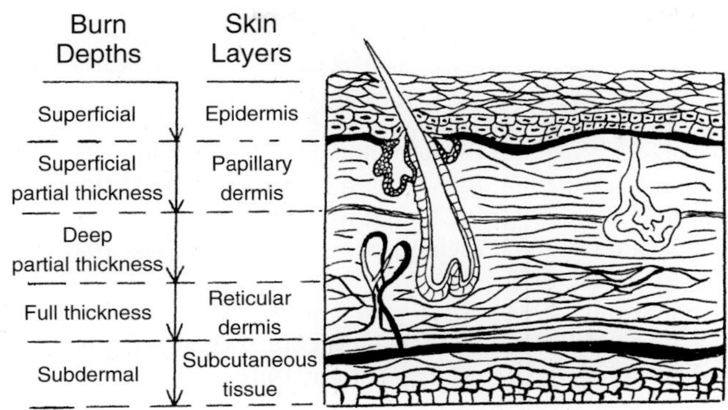

Figure 23–1 Layers of the skin and depth of tissue damage from different burn injuries.

In this event, splints applied with too much pressure can obliterate an already compromised blood flow and cause the initial burn area to convert to a full-thickness injury. Conversion of a partial-thickness burn to a full-thickness burn can be caused by termination of blood flow with subsequent tissue necrosis. Therefore, until a burn wound has fully demarcated itself within the first few days after injury, splints should be judiciously applied.

The depth of injury is directly related to the potential for involvement of other structures in addition to the skin layers. Splinting approaches must take into account any involvement of tendon, joint capsule and ligaments, and neurovascular structures. In general, the structures should be positioned to prevent any excess stress that may disrupt their integrity or maintain a functional position if the structures have been disrupted. For example, when deciding on the optimal joint positions when splinting a dorsal hand burn with questionable extensor tendon integrity, there are many issues to consider. Ideally, the wrist and metacarpophalangeal (MP) joints should be positioned to place the tendons in a slack position (wrist and MP extension); however, this position encourages the development of wrist and MP joint extension contractures. Therapists must use their clinical judgment and constantly re-evaluate their patient's needs, which change as tissue healing evolves.

Another aspect to be aware of with splint use on patients with burns is the development of **neuropathies.** A frequent site for an upper extremity neuropathy to develop as a result of a splint is at the brachial plexus with the use of a shoulder abduction immobilization, or airplane, splint. Brachial plexus injury may result from the patient being positioned in pure shoulder abduction over an extended period of time. The usual recommended position of the shoulder is 90°, but pressure on the brachial plexus can be relieved by horizontally adducting the upper extremity 10 to 15°. However, children have been positioned higher than this angle without any reported detrimental effects (Fig. 23–2).

A final factor that applies to the use of splints for patients with burn injuries is the variability of **wound location.** Burn splints can have a wide dispersion of designs and configurations, depending on the burn wound site. Table 23–1 lists splint designs that have been suggested for use with upper extremity burns. In general, splints are applied on the surface of a burn to oppose the direction of the anticipated deformity. For example, a burn to the elbow antecubital surface, requires an elbow extension immobilization splint placed on the anterior surface of the extremity to prevent an elbow flexion **contracture** from occurring. Circumferential burns involving joints may require alternating flexion/extension immobilization splints to oppose the direction of the anticipated deformity.

The most common contractures associated with upper extremity burns are the following:

- Shoulder adduction/extension.
- Shoulder internal rotation.
- Elbow flexion.
- Forearm pronation.
- Wrist flexion.
- MP joint extension.
- Digit interphalangeal (IP) joint flexion.
- Thumb adduction.

Basic Burn Splints

An extensive review of designs for basic burn splints is available (Richard, Staley, Daugherty, Miller, & Warden, 1994c). Although hand splints are considered standard therapy practice, no consensus was found for a specific design. Splints in this category are referred to by a variety of names, but they essentially sort out into two groups: **position of function splints** and **antideformity splints.**

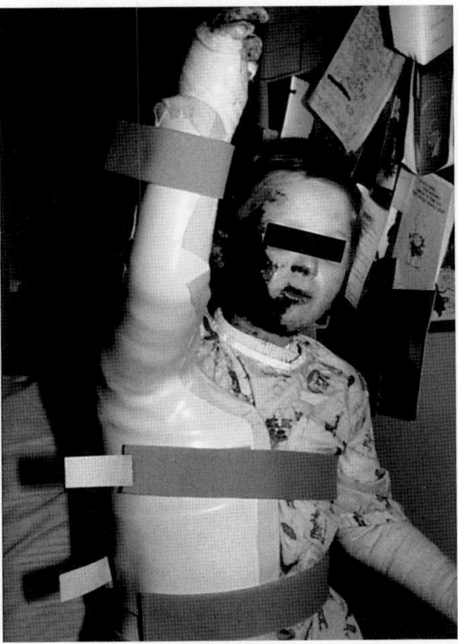

Figure 23–2 Example of a pediatric axillary, or airplane, splint (shoulder abduction/elbow extension immobilization splint) fabricated for more than 90° of shoulder flexion and abduction.

TABLE 23–1 Common Upper Extremity Burn Splints

Burn Wound Location	Common Splint Name	Reference
Axilla or shoulder	• Airplane	• Malick & Carr, 1982; Richard et al., 1994b; Walters, 1987
	• Conformer	• Malick & Carr, 1982; Richard et al., 1994b; Walters, 1987
	• Abduction	• Malick & Carr, 1982; Richard et al., 1994b
	• Clavicular strap	• Malick & Carr, 1982; Richard et al., 1994b; Walters, 1987
Elbow	• Dynamic	• Richard et al., 1995
	• Gutter or trough	• Richard et al., 1994b
	• Conformer	• Richard et al., 1994b, Malick & Carr, 1982, Walters, 1987
	• Three point	• Richard et al., 1994b, Malick & Carr, 1982
	• Spiral	• Richard et al., 1994b
Wrist and hand	• Palmar pan	• Richard et al., 1994b, Malick & Carr, 1982, Walters, 1987
	• Position of function	• Richard et al., 1994b, 1994c
	• Antideformity	• Richard et al., 1994b, 1994c
	• Thumb spica	• Daugherty & Carr-Collins, 1994; Richard et al., 1994b
	• C-bar thumb web spacer	• Richard et al., 1994b; Walters, 1987
	• Palmar or dorsal extension	• Malick & Carr, 1982; Richard et al., 1994b; Schwanholt et al., 1992; Yotsuyanagi, Yokoi, Omizo, 1994
	• Traction or banjo	• Malick & Carr, 1982; Richard et al., 1994b
	• Halo	• Richard et al., 1994b; Walters, 1987
	• Flexion glove	• Richard et al., 1994b
	• Sandwich	• Gilliam et al., 1993; Richard et al., 1994b; Walters, 1987
	• Bivalve	• Richard et al., 1994b
	• Gutter	• Rivers, Collin, Fisher, Solem, & Ahrenholz, 1984

Several suggested positions for the thumb were noted, which probably coincided with burn location based on clinical experience. Both types of splints position the wrist in some degree of extension. In general, position of function splints allow for some degree of flexion at the proximal interphalangeal (PIP) and distal interphalangeal (DIP) joints, whereas antideformity splints hold those joints in extension. The discriminating factor between the splints is the amount of flexion allowed at the MP joints.

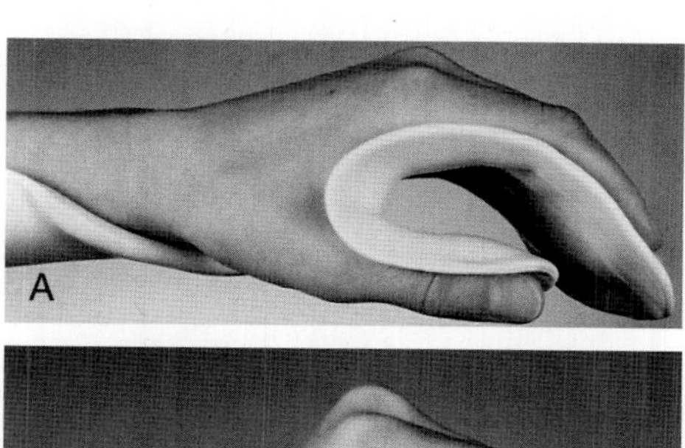

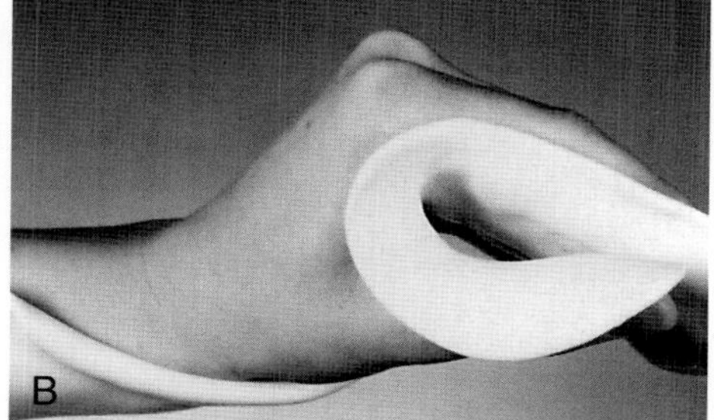

Figure 23–3 ***A,*** *A position of function splint.* ***B,*** *An antideformity splint. Note the differences in degree of MP and IP joint flexion.*

Position of function splints hold the joints at 60° or less of flexion, whereas antideformity splints position the MP joints in greater than 60° of flexion (Fig. 23–3).

A further consideration related to burn location is when the injury involves skin creases over multiple, consecutive joints. Previous work has shown that the position of an adjacent joint has an influence on skin excursion at the next joint in the series (Richard, Ford, Miller, & Staley, 1994a). Therapists need to consider splint designs that incorporate all areas of involvement to ensure maximal benefit of a splint program by placement of an elongation stress over multiple, consecutive joint surface areas (discussed below) (Coonwy, 1984).

Wound Healing Phases

Wound healing can be divided into three phases that have some amount of overlap (see Chapter 3 for details) (Greenhalgh & Staley, 1994). During the **inflammatory stage,** edema develops, which can be quite severe, especially in the hand (Fig. 23–4). During the initial stage of wound repair, which lasts 3 to 5 days under normal circumstances, splints should be avoided primarily for two reasons, unless needed to stabilize a joint. First, a splint fabricated and applied too early can cause vascular compromise when edema increases, making the splint too small. For the same reason, straps used to hold the splint in place can become constrictive, potentially impeding circulation. Second, a splint applied to the hand during the early stage of healing can limit active ROM, which in turn inhibits the muscle pump activity necessary to rid the area of edema. If splints are used during the acute phase of injury, they should be nonconforming to accommodate for fluctuations in edema.

The use of splints for patients who have moved beyond the emergent phase of treatment and into the **proliferative** and **wound maturation phases** depends on several factors (Richard, Staley, Miller, & Warden, 1996, 1997a, 1997b). In the past, splints were applied routinely at the time of patient admission and after skin graft surgery, especially when the hand was involved. Currently, therapists tend to delay the application of splints until the patient demonstrates a decrease in ROM (Richard et al., 1996). Recently, a splint algorithm was proposed to help the therapist in the decision-making process for treatment of acute burn injuries (Heidenrich & Hansbrough, 1999). In general, immobilization splints are commonly used to prevent scar contractures, whereas mobilization splints are used to correct an existing scar contracture (Richard, Shanesy, & Miller, 1995). Part of the reason for this difference is based on the biomechanical principles that underlie each type of splint.

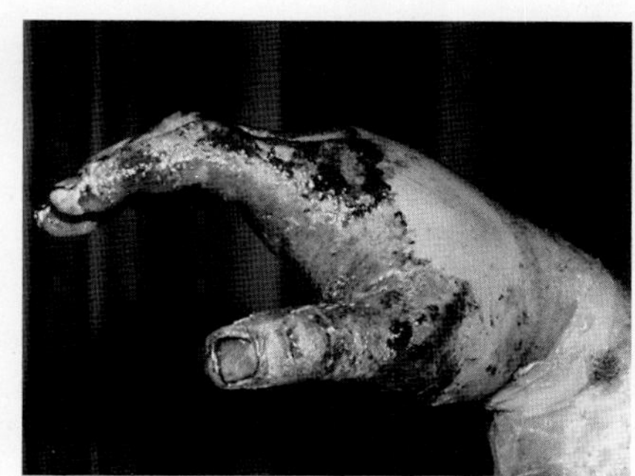

Figure 23–4 Massive edema as a result of a burn injury places the hand in a position that predisposes the development of claw hand deformity (MP extension, IP flexion).

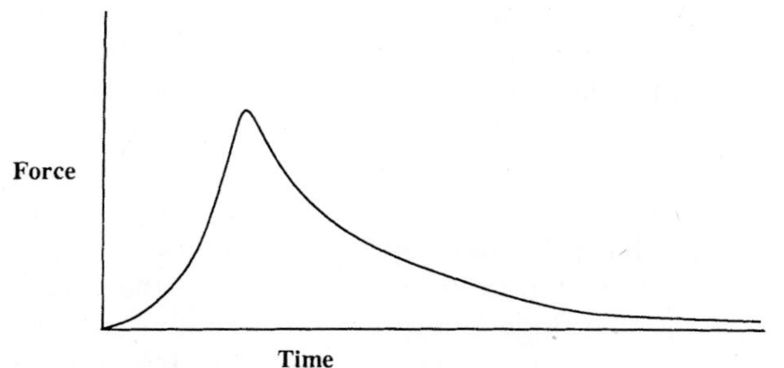

Figure 23–5 Soft tissue stress relaxation. After the peak stress is reached from the application of an immobilization splint, the amount of stress experienced by the tissue decreases. Reprinted with permission from Richard, R.L., Staley, M.J. (1994). Biophysical aspects of normal skin and burn scar. In Richard, R. L., & Staley, M. J. (Eds.). Burn care and rehabilitation—Principles and practice (p. 65). Philadelphia: Davis.

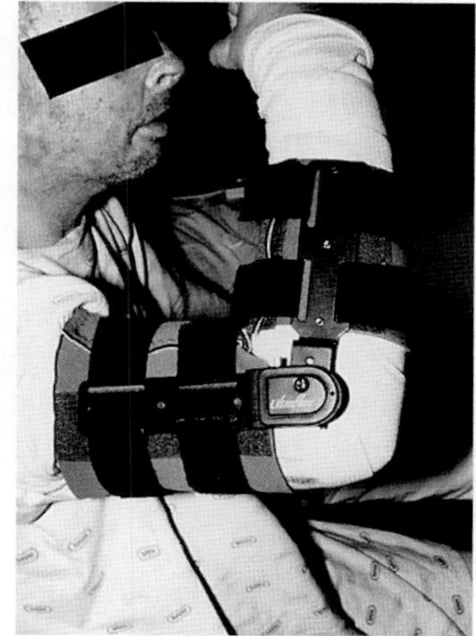

Figure 23–6 A commercial elbow mobilization splint.

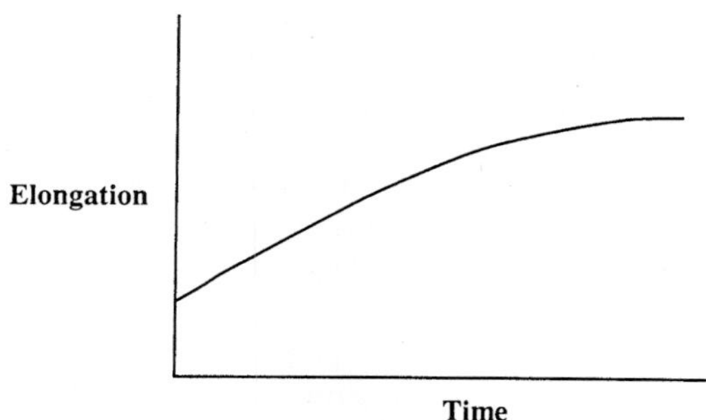

Figure 23–7 Continual tissue elongation, or creep, in response to a constant force applied to tissue over a prolonged period of time. Reprinted with permission from Richard, R.L., Staley, M.J. (1994). Biophysical aspects of normal skin and burn scar. In Richard, R. L., & Staley, M. J. (Eds.). Burn care and rehabilitation—Principles and practice (p. 64). Philadelphia: Davis.

Biomechanical Principles

Immobilization splints, which statically place a joint in a specific position, use the principle of stress relaxation on scar tissue (Richard & Staley, 1994b). Based on this principle, the amount of force required to maintain a given position of angularity decreases over time (Fig. 23–5). Essentially, tissues adapt to the stress placed on them. Burn wounds that remain open during the healing process are painful. Forceful stress on the tender tissues may increase the amount of pain experienced by the patient. When an immobilization splint is initially applied to a patient, there should be only slight discomfort, which lessens in a short period of time, owing to accommodation of the tissues. To avoid generating too much stress on delicate tissue, there is a tendency to use immobilization splints more than mobilization splints during this time.

After burn wound closure, as scar tissue continues to mature and contract, the ongoing biologic force needs to be counteracted by an equal or greater force. Once a burn wound is covered with new tissue, the primary source of pain is essentially removed and a greater demand can be placed on the tissue with less discomfort. If the patient has developed a scar tissue contracture during this phase of scar maturation, mobilization splints that operate under the principle of tissue creep are suggested (Fig. 23–6). Tissue creep is the process whereby the length of biologic tissue continues to elongate if tension is kept constant and maintained over a prolonged period of time (Fig. 23–7) (Richard & Staley, 1994b). The key to this principle is the constant application of force, which provides a stimulus for the tissue to lengthen by production and growth of additional tissue.

Splinting Implications

General Splinting Considerations

Burn care literature commonly refers to splints as either **nonconforming** or **conforming.** Nonconforming splints are usually fabricated off the patient; conforming splints are molded directly to an area and result in a more intimate fit. Conforming splints have better pressure distribution than nonconforming splints and less tendency to migrate on a limb. Caution should be used when applying nonconformed splints, because their more generalized fit may lead to excessive pressure along the splint borders. Furthermore, there is a tendency for the splint to migrate along the extremity. Special attention also should be afforded when splinting over bony prominences to prevent skin breakdown. A positive side to prefabricated nonconforming splints is they can be made readily available to clinicians during emergencies. They may be useful at other times when therapists are not available, such as nights, weekends, and holidays. These splints can be applied relatively safely over bulky dressings by nursing personnel. Staff should, of course, be instructed in proper application, fit, and precautions with use.

A common concern regarding splinting is whether splints can be used over fresh **skin grafts.** Generally, the area that has received a skin graft is heavily padded with dressings to absorb wound drainage and provide protection. Splints can be applied safely over skin grafts, particularly if the splint's intent is to immobilize the area of injury until adherence of the graft to the wound bed is evident (Engrav, 1983; Friang, 1986). Caution should be

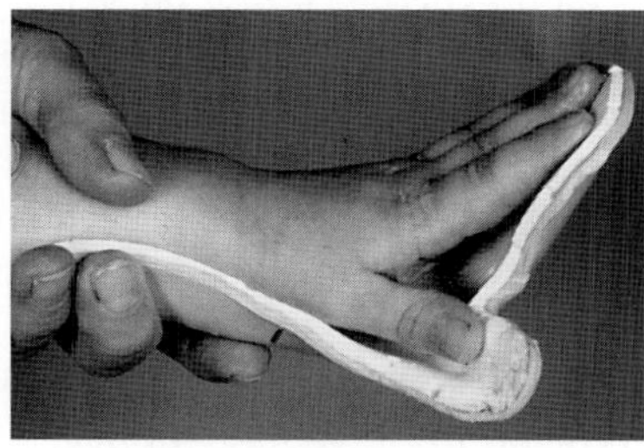

Figure 23–8 A pediatric volar splint for combined palmar expansion and finger/thumb hyperextension.

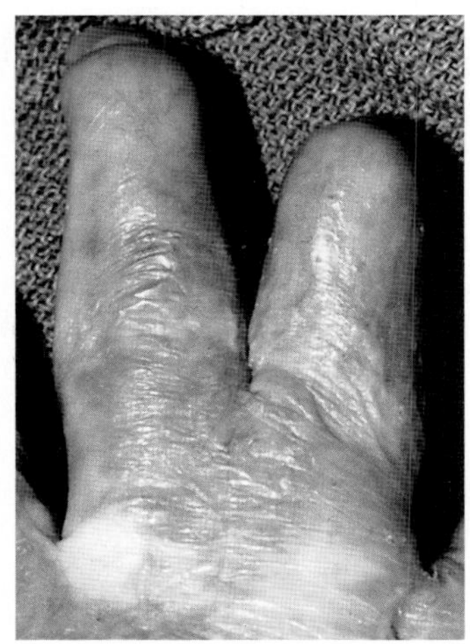

Figure 23–9 Dorsal hand scar tissue overgrowth of the web space between the middle and ring fingers.

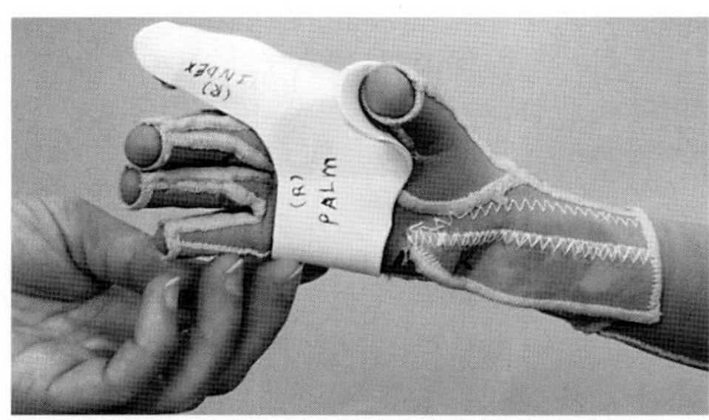

Figure 23–10 A pediatric CMC abduction immobilization splint (C-bar splint) for treating burns to the first web space.

used to avoid sheer and/or compressive stress on any grafted site. Often, a splint may not be used because the bulkiness of the postoperative dressings alone can act as a block to prevent excessive joint motion.

A major consideration when splinting the burned hand is the patient's age. With older patients who may have preexisting problems (e.g., arthritis), the degree to which fingers and other joints can be stressed and held immobile is less than for younger patients. Conversely, young children typically possess flexible joints. In these cases, positions of hyperextension of the MP joints can be made for palmar burns with minimal potential for causing MP extension contractures (Fig. 23–8) (Schwanholt, Daugherty, Gaboury, & Warden, 1992).

A scar contracture problem that is unique to patients with hand burns is a **web space syndactyly** (Fig. 23–9). This condition can occur on the dorsum of the hand between any two fingers, but it is functionally most problematic at the first web space. A burn in this area may cause the thumb to contract into adduction or hyperextension. When splinting the thumb, caution is needed to avoid damage to the collateral ligaments and subsequent instability of the thumb (Fig. 23–10).

The optimal amount of time that a splint should be worn has yet to be determined. Each patient presents differently and should be approached individually. Initially, adults and children should wear splints at night and, for children, during naps. Depending on the area of the body involved and the depth of injury, uncooperative patients may need to be splinted continuously until they are able to actively participate in the therapy regime.

Unconscious patients may or may not need splinting. If the patient can be positioned properly, avoid splint use, because the patient cannot communicate any problems with the device. This situation is especially important for skin grafts, which need close monitoring. These patients are at high risk for developing contractures and demand a therapist's attention in regard to proper positioning, splinting, and exercise.

Splints should be checked frequently for proper fit and adjustments made accordingly. During the day, mobility of alert patients should be encouraged until a decrease in ROM becomes apparent. (However, splint wear should be continuous except for dressing changes when exposed joints are present.) Clinically, a patient's ROM guides the wearing schedule of a splint. If ROM is decreasing, then the time in splints should be increased with all other treatment interventions and activity programs considered. Frequently, a 2-hour-on and 2-hour-off schedule is advocated, but no research exists to support this regimen. A review of the literature to find the origin of this approach reveals only a recommendation that splints made of thermoplastic material should be removed every 2 hours for cleaning (Willis, 1969). In regard to the latter, disinfectant cleaning of splints was found more beneficial than air drying for burn splints (Richard & Staley, 1994a; Staley, Richard, Daugherty, Warden, 1991).

If the patient is wearing pressure garments for scar control, pieces of loop strapping material can be sewn to the garment material. The hook portion of the strap is then attached to the splint material in a mirrored position. This technique is especially useful to ensure that the splint is placed correctly each time it is worn.

Oftentimes when burns affect several areas, it is helpful to incorporate multiple splints into one design pattern. The more splints there are, the greater the chance of losing one.

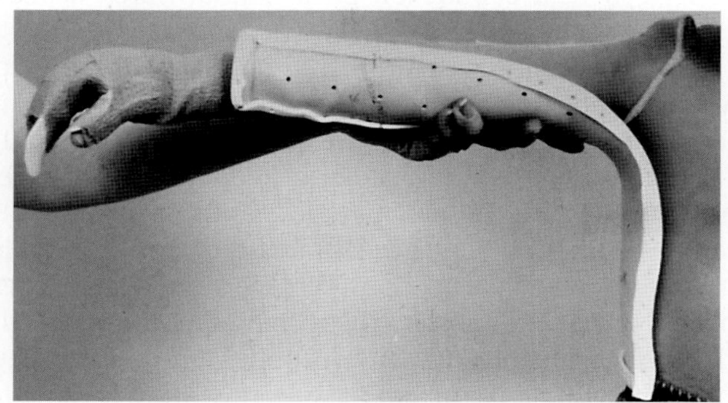

Figure 23–11 A combination of axillary and elbow extension splints.

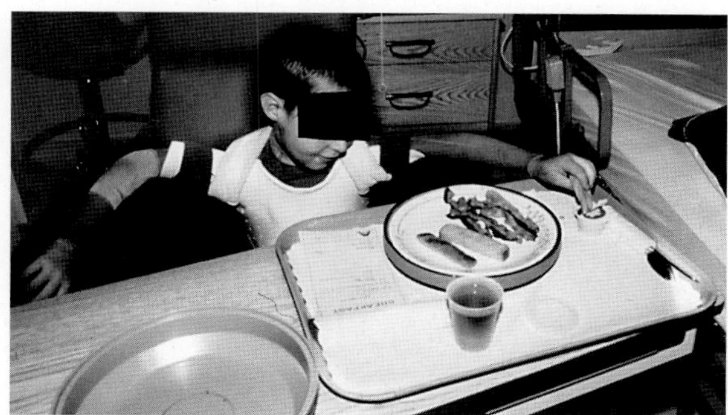

Figure 23–12 A T-shirt splint (bilateral shoulder abduction immobilization splint) used to position both extremities after a burn injury.

TABLE 23–2 Thickness of Burn Dressings

Burn Dressing or Splint Material	Thickness, [a]mm
Self-adherent wrap	0.25
Elastic wrap	0.40
Surgical net	0.50
6-ply gauze	0.40
12-ply gauze	0.80
1/8" splint material	3.20

[a]Used to calculate the placement of MP joint flexion in the splint. Each additional layer of material must be taken into account.

Reprinted with permission from Richard, R., Schall, S., Staley, M., & Miller, S. (1994). Hand burn splint fabrication: Correction for bandage thickness. *Journal of Burn Care and Rehabilitation, 15,* 370.

Furthermore, an all-inclusive splint design makes donning the splint easier for caregivers. For example, with small children particularly, a shoulder abduction and an elbow immobilization extension splint can be combined (Fig. 23–11) (Richard, Schall, Staley, Miller, 1994b). As another example, the hand, wrist, and elbow can be incorporated into one splint (Richard et al., 1994b). A novel splint for treating bilateral axillary burns simultaneously is the T-shirt splint (Fig. 23–12) (Daugherty & Carr-Collins, 1994). The splint is worn on the anterior torso and secured with straps that crisscross over the back.

Materials Selection

Commercially available splints can be used to treat patients with burns, if fit properly. Acutely, prefabricated splints are often difficult to fit on the extremity owing to the bulkiness of wound dressings and the frequent change in the amount of dressings that patients require. Dressing thickness must be accounted for, because of the influence it can have on achieving an acceptable splint fit, especially when the hand is involved (Tables 23–2 and 23–3) (Howell, 1994; Richard et al., 1994b).

Owing to the small anatomic structures of patients younger than 1 year of age, fabrication of splints is diffi-

TABLE 23–3 Proximal Displacement of Hand Splint from Palmar Crease[a]

Total Bandage Thickness[b]	Degree of Desired MP Flexion												
	30	35	40	45	50	55	60	65	70	75	80	85	90
3.2	0.9	1.0	1.2	1.3	1.5	1.7	1.8	2.0	2.2	2.5	2.7	2.9	3.2
3.4	0.9	1.1	1.2	1.4	1.6	1.8	2.0	2.2	2.4	2.6	2.9	3.1	3.4
3.6	1.0	1.1	1.3	1.5	1.7	1.9	2.1	2.3	2.5	2.8	3.0	3.3	3.6
3.8	1.0	1.2	1.4	1.6	1.8	2.0	2.2	2.4	2.7	2.9	3.2	3.5	3.8
4.0	1.1	1.3	1.5	1.7	1.9	2.1	2.3	2.5	2.8	3.1	3.4	3.7	4.0
4.2	1.1	1.3	1.5	1.7	2.0	2.2	2.4	2.7	2.9	3.2	3.5	3.8	4.2
4.4	1.2	1.4	1.6	1.8	2.1	2.3	2.5	2.8	3.1	3.4	3.7	4.0	4.4
4.6	1.2	1.5	1.7	1.9	2.1	2.4	2.7	2.9	3.2	3.5	3.9	4.2	4.6
4.8	1.3	1.5	1.7	2.0	2.2	2.5	2.8	3.1	3.4	3.7	4.0	4.4	4.8
5.0	1.3	1.6	1.8	2.1	2.3	2.6	2.9	3.2	3.5	3.8	4.2	4.6	5.0
5.2	1.4	1.6	1.9	2.2	2.4	2.7	3.0	3.3	3.6	4.0	4.4	4.8	5.2
5.4	1.4	1.7	2.0	2.2	2.5	2.8	3.1	3.4	3.8	4.1	4.5	4.9	5.4
5.6	1.5	1.8	2.0	2.3	2.6	2.9	3.2	3.6	3.9	4.3	4.7	5.1	5.6
5.8	1.6	1.8	2.1	2.4	2.7	3.0	3.3	3.7	4.1	4.5	4.9	5.3	5.8
6.0	1.6	1.9	2.2	2.5	2.8	3.1	3.5	3.8	4.2	4.6	5.0	5.5	6.0
6.2	1.7	2.0	2.3	2.6	32.9	3.2	3.6	3.9	4.3	4.8	5.2	5.7	6.2
6.4	1.7	2.0	2.3	2.7	3.0	3.3	3.7	4.1	4.5	4.9	5.4	5.9	6.4
6.6	1.8	2.1	2.4	2.7	3.1	3.4	3.8	4.2	4.6	5.1	5.5	6.0	6.6
6.8	1.8	2.1	2.5	2.8	3.2	3.5	3.9	4.3	4.8	5.2	5.7	6.2	6.8
7.0	1.9	2.2	2.5	2.9	3.3	3.6	4.0	4.5	4.9	5.4	5.9	6.4	7.0

[a]To determine the proper placement of MP flexion in the splint, find the intersection of the bandage thickness and desired degree of splint flexion.
[b]Derived from Table 23-2.
Reprinted with permission from Richard, R., Schall, S., Staley, M., & Miller, S. (1994). Hand burn splint fabrication: Correction for bandage thickness. *Journal of Burn Care and Rehabilitation, 15,* 370.

cult and requires some splinting experience to achieve a successful outcome. Therefore, it may be easier to position the extremity with the use of bulky dressings or insert material, such as Elastomer or foam, in lieu of a splint. Splints that do not fit correctly can place body segments in positions that encourage development of scar tissue contractures. Therefore, the adage "no splint is better than a poorly fitted splint" is one to heed in burn care.

If therapists fabricate custom splints early during a patient's hospitalization, then a material that can be frequently remolded is recommended, because of the number of modifications that may be needed to accommodate fluctuations in edema and bandage thickness. In 1969, the first use of a thermoplastic material to customize a burn splint was described (Costa, Nakamura, & Engrav, 1999). Since that time, a host of splinting materials have been advocated and used (Cox, Taddonio, & Thompson; Willis, 1970). Generally, 1⁄16" material can be used with the pediatric population and in areas that do not bear much weight, such as the fingers. Thicker materials—3⁄32" or 1⁄8"—should be used for adult splints to ensure a rigid splint with adequate positioning. The inception of colored splint material and strapping has allowed patients to participate in creating the device, which may assist in compliance, especially for children.

Perforated or open weave splint material is best used for patients who have a large amount of wound exudate or transudate and when topical antibiotic solutions are in use; the perforations allow the former to escape and the latter to penetrate through the dressings. Perforated material also allows for some air to reach the dressings, drying them and preventing wounds from becoming macerated.

A major consideration with the use of thermoplastic material and its immediate fabrication at a patient's bedside is the anxiety evoked in patients with burns by the thought of having hot material placed on their wounds. This situation is especially heightened in children. To circumvent this issue, educate the patient and apply ample padding between the patient and splint material when fabricating the splint. A successful approach is to demonstrate the lack of heat conduction on a nonburn area using a piece of scrap splint material.

Traditional plaster cast material provides a cost-effective alternative to thermoplastics in some cases. The technique may not be the best choice during the acute phase of wound healing, because frequent cast changes would be required. Cast material tends to absorb the wound exudate, which necessitates removal and application of a new cast. Consider thermoplastics when splint hygiene is an issue. These materials can be easily wiped clean, disinfected, and reapplied to the extremity. Casting may help in the later stages of wound healing to position joint(s) for mobilization splinting using serial static stress to improve ROM (Daugherty & Carr-Collins,

1994). See Chapter 11 and Staley and Serghiou (1998) for more information.

Component Selection

Occasionally, dress hooks are glued to the fingernails so a traction force can be applied. The hooks act as terminal attachments for rubber bands that originate at the end of the pan portion of a hand or banjo splint (Fig. 23–13). This technique is useful when the finger joints are placed in extension. As an alternative, hook material can be glued to the fingernails. A primary consideration before using any of these approaches is to ensure that the fingernails are viable and intact, otherwise the traction force may disrupt the nail from its bed (Richard et al., 1994b; Wright, Taddonio, Prasad, & Thompson, 1989). This technique also should be avoided in very young children because of the instability of their fingernails.

For scar management, inserts made of putty (Elastomer or Otoform) can be incorporated into a splint nicely if perforated material is used (Richard et al., 1994b). Before the insert material hardens, it can be pushed through the interstices of the splint material. The excess material that extrudes through the perforations is then flattened to form a rivet that secures the insert material in place (Ward, Schnebly, Kravitz, Warden, & Saffle, 1989).

For children under the age of 3, therapists should avoid the use of small parts when making a splint (Richard et al., 1994b). If one of these pieces came loose, it would be a potential choking hazard.

Strapping Selection

The strapping methods used in adult and pediatric populations may differ. For compliant adults, a rolled gauze bandage, elastic wrap (e.g., Ace or Coban), or foam straps (e.g., Velfoam) offer an effective means to secure a splint. Caution must be taken not to compress any superficial nerves or vascular structures; frequent monitoring is necessary.

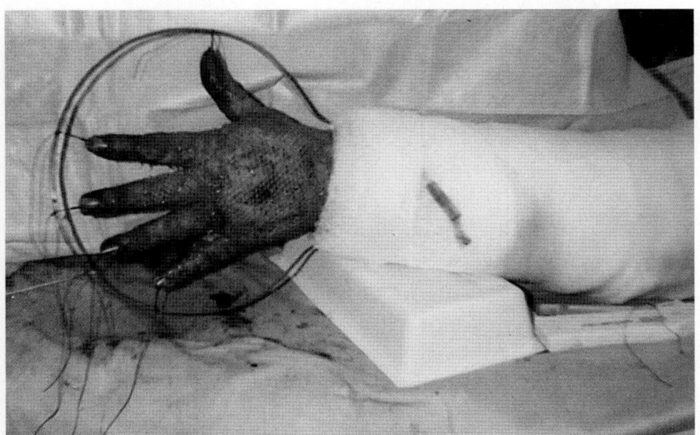

Figure 23–13 Dress hooks are applied to the fingernails to position the digits in extension for this digit extension/abduction immobilization splint.

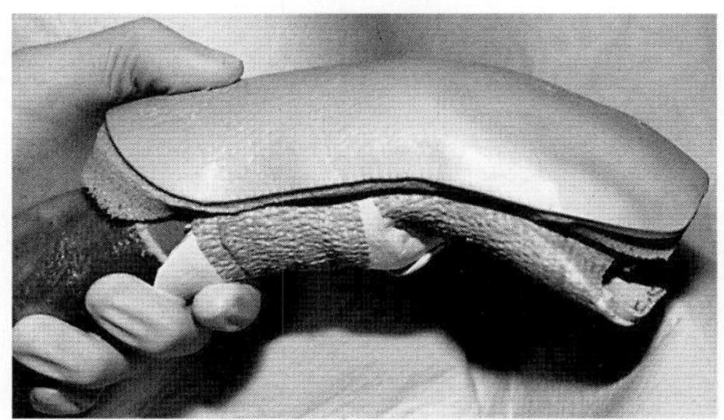

Figure 23–14 A sandwich splint (hand immobilization splint), also called a clamshell splint, includes two interlocking segments.

A splinting difficulty that often arises with children is getting the child to keep a splint on for extended periods of time. In burn care, splints are needed daily and for an extended period of time. The longer the child wears the splint, the greater the likelihood that he or she will find a way to remove it. Several methods can make the process of splint removal more difficult for the pediatric patient.

One method is to use a self-adherent elastic wrap, such as Coban, to hold the splint in place, instead of applying ordinary elastic wraps that fasten with clips or tape, as commonly used for adults (Richard et al., 1994b; Schwanholt et al., 1992). A second method is to use a sandwich splint (Fig. 23–14) (Gilliam, Hatler, Adams, & Helm, 1993). With this type of splint, recommended for use with the hand, a dorsal and volar piece is made that encases the hand. The use of self-adherent elasticized wrap is suggested for holding this splint together and in place. As an alternative, a bivalve hand cast can act as a type of sandwich splint.

Another technique for holding a splint in place and preventing distal slippage is to line the splint with Dycem or a similar nonskid material. This tacky material acts as a good interface between the splint and material in which it comes into contact, especially slick pressure garments commonly employed for burn management. Finally, simply increasing the angle of wrist extension in a hand splint, if appropriate, can prevent distal migration of the hand beyond the end of the splint.

CASE STUDY SECTION

The case study presented here is meant to be used as a teaching guideline only. Treatment and splinting protocols vary greatly from surgeon to surgeon and from therapist to therapist. The therapist must check with the referring physicians and colleagues to define the preferred treatment and splinting methods.

CASE STUDY 1: **Upper Extremity Burn Injury with Skin Grafting**

MJS, a 41-year-old, left-dominant female, was preparing supper and used an accelerant on smoldering bri-

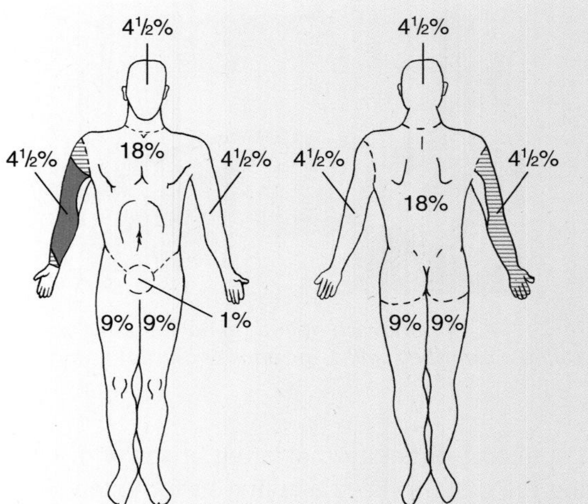

Figure 23–15 Distribution and depth of burns. The hatched areas represent partial-thickness burns, and the solid areas represent full-thickness burns.

quettes in her outdoor barbecue grill when the charcoal suddenly erupted into flames.

The previously healthy patient was estimated to have experienced a 7% surface area burn of her dominant upper extremity. The palm of her hand was spared along with an area of skin on the medial aspect of her upper arm. She was diagnosed as having mixed deep-partial and full-thickness burns throughout (Fig. 23–15). When the therapist first evaluated the patient the morning after the injury, the patient's hand and remaining upper extremity were markedly edematous and the hand and fingers were in a slightly flexed position. Joint motion was moderately restricted throughout, secondary to edema and pain. Surgery to apply skin grafts to the areas of full-thickness injury was scheduled for 2 days after injury. Owing to the swelling and impending surgery, the therapist placed the upper extremity in an elevated position with external compression bandages, and instructed MJS to perform limited active ROM to aid in edema reduction, and maintenance of ROM.

By the time of surgery, the edema had subsided remarkably, and the areas of full-thickness burn had demarked themselves and were confined to the volar aspect of the arm and forearm, which involved the antecubital space. These areas were excised and covered with split-thickness sheet skin grafts harvested from a suprapubic donor site. The surgeon requested the therapist's attendance in the operating room, where a position of function hand splint was fabricated to immobilize the deep-partial thickness burns (Fig. 23–3**A**), and an elbow extension immobilization splint was formed and applied over the bulky dressings. MJS's elbow area was kept immobile for 3 days to allow for adherence of the skin graft.

After surgery and throughout the remainder of MJS's hospitalization, the hand splint was modified into more of an antideformity position (Fig. 23–3**B**). The patient's finger ROM increased through a program of progressive exercise. At 2 weeks after surgery, the patient wore the splint at night; the schedule progressed to an as-needed basis after the patient was discharged from the hospital.

When the elbow area was undressed for the first time after surgery and ROM was reinitiated, the patient lacked 25° of elbow extension with noticeable blanching of the skin graft when stress was applied. Apparently, her elbow had been slightly flexed when the bulky outer bandages were applied in the operating room, which was not apparent by visual inspection. MJS's existing postoperative elbow splint was remolded to form an elbow extension mobilization splint (Fig. 23–16).

The patient received twice-daily therapy treatments. She showed minimal improvements in ROM, and the splint was modified as necessary. The nurses began having difficulty applying the splint at night owing to increasing elbow flexion tightness. A decision was made to change the intervention to a commercial elbow extension mobilization splint (Fig. 23–6). The rationale was that MJS could receive gentle stress applied intermittently throughout the day to the tight skin grafted area while retaining functional use of the extremity. She continued to wear the serial static elbow mobilization splint at night.

The patient was compliant with the commercial splint program, and within 3 weeks had regained full extension of her elbow. At that time, the splint was formally discontinued with instructions to continue the night splint regime for an additional month to maintain tissue length.

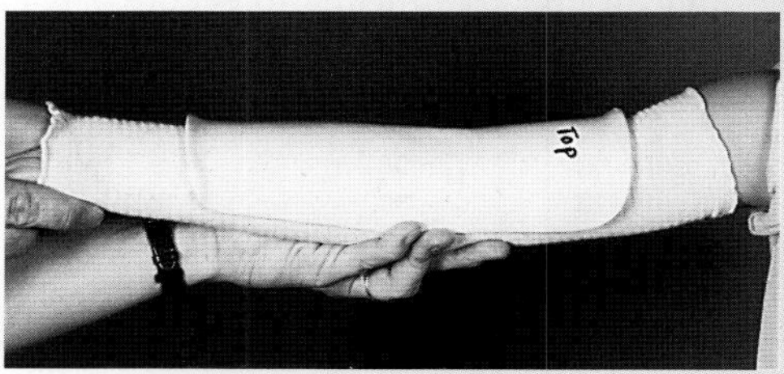

Figure 23–16 An elbow extension immobilization splint applied directly over healing skin grafts.

CONCLUSION

The use of splints in the rehabilitation of patients with burn injuries is an integral part of a comprehensive treatment program. Specific considerations for splint use includes burn wound extent, depth, and location as well as anatomic sites and phase of healing. Biomechanical principles should be taken into account based on the treatment objectives. Special con-

siderations should be extended to pediatric and geriatric patients and the age-specific characteristics these populations possess.

Successful strategies demand a decision on whether to custom fabricate a splint or to use a prefabricated or commercially available splint. If a splint is custom made, attention should be paid to design and the type of material selected. The use of inserts, splint wear in conjunction with skin grafts, pressure garments, and the method used to secure splints can challenge a therapist's creativity. Treatment parameters, such as optimal duration of splint wear and ideal design, need further investigation and research.

REFERENCES

Cooney MA. (1984). Splinting the pediatric patient with multiple joint involvement. *Journal of Burn Care and Rehabilitation, 5,* 215–217.

Costa, B. A., Nakamura, D. Y., & Engrav, L. H. (1999). Self "riveting" silicone to make palm burn splints. *Journal of Burn Care and Rehabilitation, 20,* S250.

Cox, N. Y., Taddonio, T. E., & Thompson, P. D. (1991). Decontamination procedures of six thermoplastic splint materials used in burn care. *Proceedings of the American Burn Association, 23,* 179.

Daugherty, M. B., & Carr-Collins, J. A. (1994). Splinting techniques for the burn patient. In Richard, R. L., & Staley, M. J. (Eds.). *Burn care and rehabilitation—Principles and practice* (pp. 242–323). Philadelphia: Davis.

Dobbs, E. R., & Curreri, P. W. (1972). Burns: analysis of results of physical therapy in 681 patients. *Journal of Trauma, 12,* 242–248.

Engrav, L. H. (1983). Do splinting and pressure devices damage new grafts? *Journal of Burn Care and Rehabilitation, 4,* 107–108.

Friang, J. (1986). The effects of splinting on graft take. *Proceedings of the American Burn Association, 18,* 22.

Gilliam, K. S., Hatler, B., Adams, S., & Helm, P. (1993). T-shirt splint for prevention of burn scar contracture of the neck, chest and axillas. *Proceedings of the American Burn Association, 15,* 213.

Greenhalgh, D. G., & Staley, M. J. (1994). Burn wound healing. In Richard, R. L., & Staley, M. J. (Eds.). *Burn care and rehabilitation—Principles and practice* (pp. 70–102). Philadelphia: Davis.

Heidenrich, L., & Hansbrough, J. (1999). Guidelines for splint assessment: An algorithm. *Journal of Burn Care and Rehabilitation, 20,* S252.

Howell, J. W. (1994). Management of the burned hand. In Richard, R. L., & Staley, M. J. (Eds.). *Burn care and rehabilitation—Principles and practice* (pp. 531–575). Philadelphia: Davis.

Kraemer, M. D., Jones, T., & Deitch, E. A. (1988). Burn contractures: Incidence, predisposing factors, and results of surgical therapy. *Journal of Burn Care and Rehabilitation, 9,* 261–265.

Malick, M. H., & Carr, J. A. (1982). *Manual on management of the burn patient, including splinting, mold and pressure techniques.* Pittsburgh: Harmarville Rehabilitation Center .

Richard, R. (2000). Burn characteristics by type. *Advances in Wound Care. 13,* 87.

Richard, R. L., Staley, M. J. (1994a). Appendix H: Splinting materials. In Richard, R. L., & Staley, M. J. (Eds.). *Burn care and rehabilitation—Principles and practice* (pp. 658–666). Philadelphia: Davis.

Richard, R. L., Staley, M. J. (1994b). Biophysical aspects of normal skin and burn scar. In Richard, R. L., & Staley, M. J. (Eds.). *Burn care and rehabilitation—Principles and practice* (pp. 49–69). Philadelphia: Davis.

Richard, R., Ford, J., Miller, S. F., & Staley, M. (1994a). Photographic measurement of volar forearm skin movement with wrist extension: The influence of elbow position. *Journal of Burn Care and Rehabilitation, 15,* 58–61.

Richard, R., Schall, S., Staley, M., Miller, S. (1994b). Hand burn splint fabrication: Correction for bandage thickness. *Journal of Burn Care and Rehabilitation, 15,* 369–371.

Richard, R., Shanesy, C. P. III, & Miller, S. F. (1995). Dynamic versus static splints: A prospective case for sustained stress. *Journal of Burn Care and Rehabilitation, 16,* 284–287.

Richard, R., Staley, M., Daugherty, M. B., Miller, S. F., & Warden, G. D. (1994c). The wide variety of designs for dorsal hand burn splints. *Journal of Burn Care and Rehabilitation, 15,* 275–280.

Richard, R., Staley, M., Miller, S., & Warden, G. (1996). To splint or not to splint—Past philosophy and present practice: Part I. *Journal of Burn Care and Rehabilitation, 17,* 444–453.

Richard, R., Staley, M., Miller, S., & Warden, G. (1997a). To splint or not to splint—Past philosophy and present practice: Part II. *Journal of Burn Care and Rehabilitation, 18,* 64–71.

Richard, R., Staley, M., Miller, S., & Warden, G. (1997b). To splint or not to splint—Past philosophy and present practice: Part III. *Journal of Burn Care and Rehabilitation, 18,* 251–255.

Rivers, E., Collin, T., Fisher, S., Solem, L. D., & Ahrenholz, D. H. (1984). The use of individual gutter splints to preserve exposed PIP joints: A case presentation. *Proceedings of the American Burn Association, 16,* 88.

Rutan, R. L. (1998). Physiologic response to cutaneous burn injury. In G. J. Carrougher (Ed.). *Burn care and therapy* (pp. 1–33). St. Louis: Mosby.

Schwanholt, C., Daugherty, M. B., Gaboury, T., & Warden, G D. (1992). Splinting the pediatric palmar burn. *Journal of Burn Care and Rehabilitation, 13,* 460–464.

Staley, M., Richard, R., Daugherty, M. B., & Warden, G. (1991). A comprehensive evaluation of available splinting materials. *Proceedings of the American Burn Association, 23,* 178.

Staley, M. J., & Serghiou, M. (1998). Casting guidelines, tips, and techniques from the 1997 American Burn Association PT/OT casting workshop. *Journal of Burn Care and Rehabilitation, 19,* 254–260.

Walters, C. J. (1987). *Splinting the burn patient.* Laurel, MD: RAMSCO.

Ward, R. S., Schnebly, W. A., Kravitz, M., Warden, G. D., & Saffle, J. R. (1989). Have you tried the sandwich splint? *Journal of Burn Care and Rehabilitation, 10,* 83–85.

Willis, B. (1970). Follow-up: The use of orthoplast isoprene splints in the treatment of the acutely burned child. *American Journal of Occupational Therapy, 23,* 187–191.

Willis, B. (1969). The use of orthoplast isoprene splints in the treatment of the acutely burned child: Preliminary report. *American Journal of Occupational Therapy, 23,* 57–61.

Wright, M. P., Taddonio, T. E., Prasad, J. K., & Thompson, P, D. (1989). The microbiology and cleaning of thermoplastic splints in burn care. *Journal of Burn Care and Rehabilitation, 10,* 79–83.

Yotsuyanagi, T., Yokoi, K., & Omizo, M. (1994). A simple and compressive splint for palmar skin grafting in young children with burns. *Burns, 20,* 55–57.

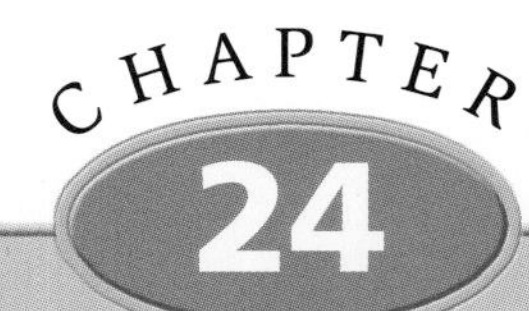

The Musician

Caryl Johnson, OTR/L, CHT

INTRODUCTION

Injured musicians are a patient population with unique needs and expectations. Instrumental musicians place remarkable repeated stresses on their upper extremities. If they suffer an injury to any part of their upper extremities, it can be a devastating problem (Johnson, 1992b; Quarrier, 1993). To care for their injuries effectively, the therapist must know how specific instruments are played and what demands are placed on the patient's body.

Musical instruments require specialized and repetitive use of shoulders, elbows, wrists, and hands. Some instruments stand alone and must be reached, touched, or otherwise caused to sound (piano, harp, drums); others are held for playing (violin, clarinet, guitar). Some instruments require a combination of facial motor control and upper extremity action (French horn, trumpet, trombone); others require elaborate fine motor control of the hand (flute, cello, organ). Therefore, an ergonomic approach to body and upper extremity use adds specificity to understanding and treating a musician's injuries.

General Considerations

When treating musicians' injuries, knowledge of correct playing technique is combined with clinical problem solving and treatment modalities. Pain, muscle spasms, numbness, paresthesias, and tenderness are often treated with anti-inflammatory medication, immobilization, modalities, and soft tissue techniques, followed by gentle remobilization. After the acute stage of treatment, the therapist assists in establishing more efficient body mechanics and playing habits along with initiating a practical long-term conditioning program to prevent further injury.

Certain helpful parallels may be drawn between treating musicians and treating athletes. The fine motor control and elaborate coordination used to play an instrument require regular physical conditioning—training such as that required to achieve skill in a sport. Musicians and athletes spend many hours each day training to improve their specific physical skills and enhance their innate talent. For both of these patient groups, external or internal demands for performance success may drive the patient beyond his or her conditioning and/or abilities. Information about the patient's level of skill and the role music plays in his or her life help the therapist determine a realistic plan of treatment. Along with upper extremity exercise to recover full use of the involved tissues, a generalized conditioning program should be implemented to improve overall strength and endurance. A plan for a whole body warm up before playing and a home program of whole body strengthening help the patient avoid reinjury.

A graded plan for return to the instrument, in addition to a conditioning program, is important to a successful recovery. It is not enough simply to tell the patient to return to playing. The amount of playing he or she can do should be progressive, based on the injury, preinjury practicing habits, length of time played on a reduced schedule, and general physical status. This author recommends practicing in units of not less than 15 minutes, preceded by whole body and upper extremity warm-up exercises. Units of practice time should not be lengthened more often than once a week. In this author's experience, most patients are able to tolerate two 5- to 15-minute units of practicing with 1 hour rest between units.

From the student, to the amateur, to the professional performer, musicians as patients usually have strong emotional drives to play their instruments. This drive adds intensity and anxiety to their responses to injury, including fears about losing the ability to play. Frequent reassurance and sympathetic understanding during the course of rehabilitation are important to the recovery of these patients.

Indications for Playing Splints

Musicians of all levels, like the general population, are subject to traumatic upper extremity injuries. The most frequently seen are fractures, sprains, lacerations, crush injuries, and contusions. Although the initial phases of treatment are the same as those for a similar injury in any patient, a musician's urge to return to playing may put pressure on the therapist to speed up the steps of recovery. Progress of healing as determined by the treating physician and the therapist should still be the deciding factor in treatment planning and return to the instrument.

In addition to traumatic injuries, musicians frequently present with conditions directly related to playing their instruments, such as inflammation of muscle and tendon (usually the result of insufficient conditioning or increased use), compression neuropathies (related to repeated motion in extreme joint angles), and soft tissue injuries (due to repeated impact to palm or finger). The most common repetitive use injuries, tendonitis and synovitis, are usually the result of misuse of the upper extremity or of insufficient conditioning for the physical demands placed on the player (e.g., increased playing time and intensity before an audition or performance). The complicated coordination and specialized repetitive use of the musician's body and upper extremity require sound technical training and a conditioning program to prevent injury. If the player's instrument must be lifted or supported while it is played, this prolonged positioning can also cause reactive inflammation.

Whether it is a traumatic or repetitive use injury, the resulting limits on playing time can represent a significant emotional and financial loss (Wilson, 1998). Splints that can be worn by the instrumentalist during recovery have been used successfully. This chapter describes the possibilities and practical considerations of creating **playing splints** for musicians, which are splints made to be worn and used while playing an instrument. Playing splints maximize extremity function by providing some degree of immobilization while protecting areas of healing, reducing inflammation, stabilizing joints, reducing tendencies toward deformity, improving joint alignment, and/or assisting and training muscle action.

Playing splints are immobilization or restrictive devices that serve a dynamic function. They can be constructed for the wrist, hand, fingers, or thumb. The upper extremity motions for playing, together with the clinical purpose for a splint, determine its design (Johnson, 1992a). The playing splint should

- Limit joint motion only as much as needed.
- Be as lightweight as possible.
- Utilize minimal or no strapping.
- Conform closely to the splinted area.
- Not touch the instrument or interfere with its moving parts.
- Not chafe the skin or rub against bony prominences.
- Minimally interfere with the body motions of playing (Van Lede & Veldhoven, 1998).

Splinting Traumatic Injuries

Patients who have suffered **traumatic injuries,** including nondisplaced and/or stable upper extremity fractures, can be fitted with playing splints that brace the fracture against stressful motions. This can allow safe use of a healing bone on the instrument. Gutter playing splints (three-sided U-shaped splints) can be used on long bones (distal radius or distal ulna) and on the phalanges.

For example, a recorder player with a fractured proximal phalanx may be immobilized in a volar hand-based splint that is removed only for exercise (Fig. 24–1**A**). In the later stages of healing, the patient may be able to safely return to the instrument by being fitted with a dorsal nonarticular proximal phalanx splint to support the fractured area (Fig. 24–1**B**). Theoretically, longitudinal stress can hasten the formation of callus if alignment is not disturbed (Schenk, 1992). Such a nonarticular splint allows playing and provides additional longitudinal stress to the fracture. An immobilization splint is worn when the patient is not playing to provide support and protection.

Many traumatic ligament injuries are amenable to splinting in a way that allows the performer to continue

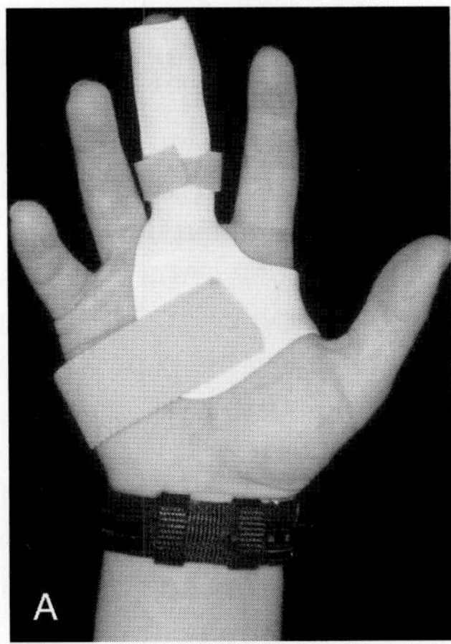

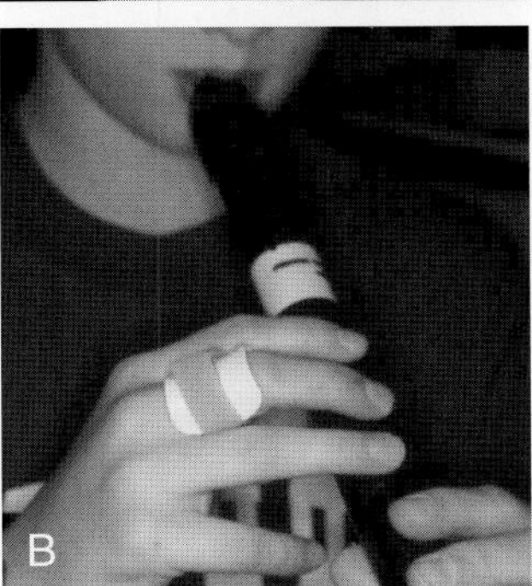

*Figure 24–1 In this musician with a proximal phalanx fracture, a volar digit immobilization splint (**A**) and playing splint (**B**) were used to protect the healing fracture.*

playing. The necessary alignment, degree or nature of instability, and amount of swelling determine the choice of splint design (Mayer & McCue, 1990; Sadler & Koepfer, 1992). A double ring playing splint (proximal interphalangeal [PIP] extension restriction splint or Figure-8 splint) for PIP joint volar plate injuries is a good example (Fig. 24–2). Splints used for acute injuries must be adjusted as swelling and contours change to ensure an appropriate fit. Although musicians who are able to make an earlier return to music will be more able to cope with the psychological feelings of loss caused by the injury, the use of playing splints should create no disruption to alignment, bony reduction, or healing. Lacerations or other skin lesions may be splinted to provide wound protection or to avoid overstretching of healing tissues.

Splinting Repetitive Use Injuries

Repetitive use injuries, including tendonitis, synovitis, myositis, and compression neuropathies, are frequent presenting diagnoses for musicians (Johnson, 1992a, 1992b). A broad spectrum of therapy modalities can be used to treat these conditions, including heat/ice, soft tissue and joint mobilization, therapeutic exercise, and splints. Complete immobilization is used as an early intervention to rest inflamed tissues and block provocative motions. After the acute phase, when pain has receded, a playing splint can be used to block extreme or symptom-producing motions and allow the patient to return to his or her instrument. For example, a patient with extensor carpi ulnaris (ECU) tendonitis may be fitted with a wrist playing splint (wrist immobilization splint) (Fig. 24–3). The wrist should be positioned in 30° of extension and the splint molded generously around the hypothenar eminence to restrict ulnar deviation. This splint supports the wrist in extension and prevents repetitive ulnar deviation, thus training the musician to avoid ulnar deviation when playing.

Progressive ligament injuries that result from playing can be considered an overuse injury. Woodwind players who bear the instrument on their right thumb are often found to have injured the ulnar collateral ligament

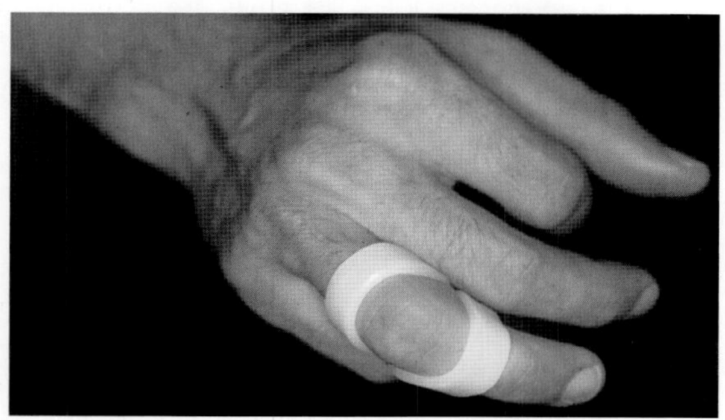

Figure 24–2 A PIP extension restriction splint for the middle finger PIP joint fabricated from 1/16" Aquaplast, cut 1/4" wide.

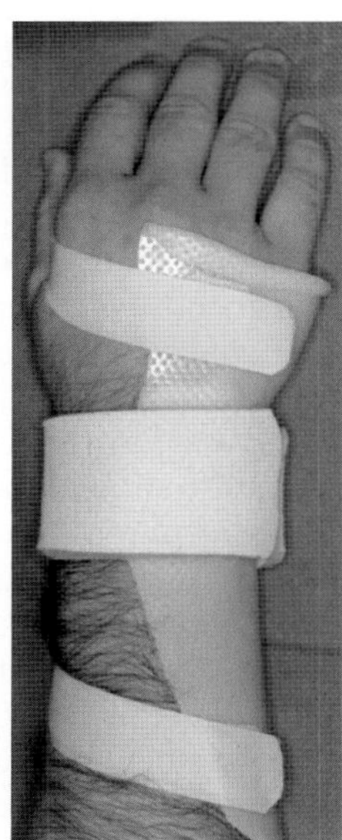

Figure 24–3 Because it is lightweight and has some flexibility, 1/16" perforated Orfit was used to support the wrist in slight ulnar deviation in this wrist immobilization splint.

(UCL) by repetitive stretching of the thumb at the metacarpophalangeal (MP) joint. A hand-based thumb immobilization playing splint can provide static alignment to the thumb MP (and IP if needed) joint (Fig. 24–4). This splint can be used to decrease inflammation and retard progressive deformities at the thumb MP joint in the same way that a wrist/thumb immobilization splint may be used to decrease inflammation and retard deformity at the thumb carpometacarpal (CMC) joint (Swigart, Eaton, Glickel, & Johnson, 1999). Many variations of a thumb MP immobilization playing splint can be used to treat musicians with overuse or cumulative trauma injuries. Playing splints can be constructed to stabilize any of the thumb joints laterally or longitudinally. The CMC can be blocked from excess adduction and/or dorsal subluxation, and the MP and IP joints can be stabilized laterally to prevent stress on the collateral ligaments (Bean, Tencer, & Trumble, 1999; Brandsma, Oudenaarde, Oostendorp, 1996; Glickel, Malerich Pearce, & Littler, 1993; Haelterman, 1996; Heyman, Gelberman, Duncan, & Hip, 1993).

Soft tissue impact injuries are also seen in musicians. The palmar skin, fingertips, and sides of the fingers are areas that receive repetitive mechanical stresses from some instruments. They are subject to reactive injury, painful and inflamed soft tissues, or development of small masses. Reactive soft tissue problems on the finger or fingertips of players may be successfully protected with soft materials, such as Leuko tape or Steri-strips. String players are subject to painful fingertip subcallus blisters, neuromas, or small glomus tumors on the finger pads of the left hand from the repeated blows struck against sharp metal strings. Callus injuries tend to resolve over a period of months if they are not irritated further (R. G. Eaton, personal communication, 1997). Many patients try taping the fingertip, but sharp strings quickly cut through the tape. Although the use of any material on the fingertip can be unacceptable to some players, in a concert such musicians can often tolerate the use of a silicone-lined finger cap (Fig. 24–5) (Manske, 1999).

Splinting Injuries Related to Handling Instruments

Many instruments must be held to the mouth or lifted in some way for playing, resulting in **injuries related to lifting and positioning the instrument.** Woodwind instruments are good examples; all must be supported and held near the body and mouth for playing. Lifting the weight of these instruments places stress on the whole upper extremity, especially the joints of the thumb. Playing splints can assist instrument support by transferring part of the instrument weight to a more proximal joint

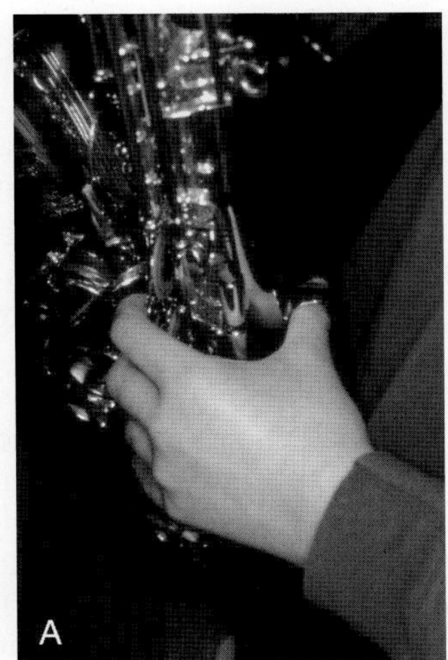

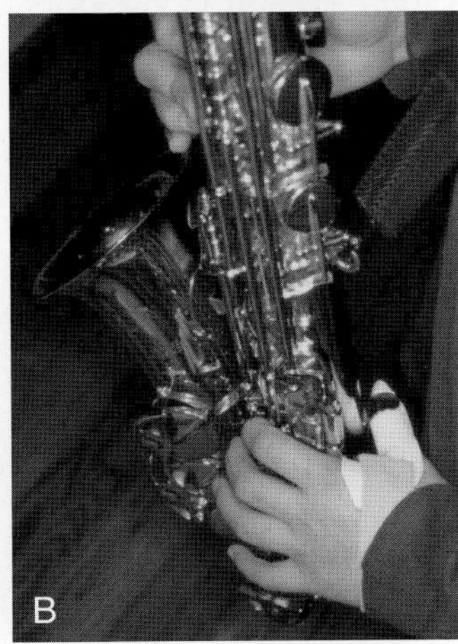

Figure 24–4 ***A,*** *Note the lateral stress on thumb from holding a saxophone.* ***B,*** *A hand-based thumb immobilization splint that includes the IP joint helps support the weight of instrument thereby decreasing stress on the MP joint UCL.*

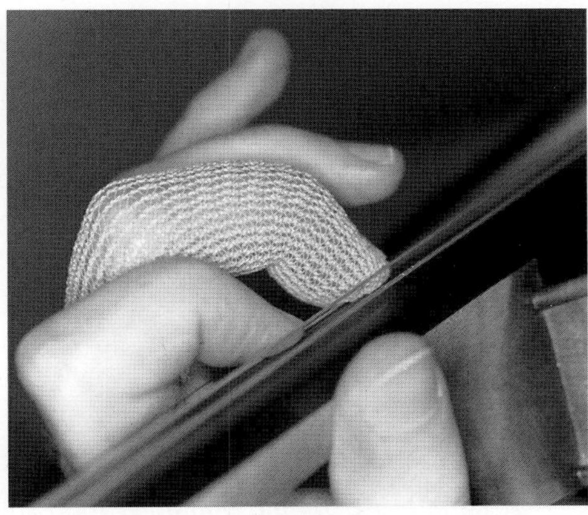

Figure 24–5 A Silipos Digital Cap used to protect a violinist who has a middle finger neuroma. The sleeve can be trimmed to the DIP or PIP crease to allow greater freedom of movement.

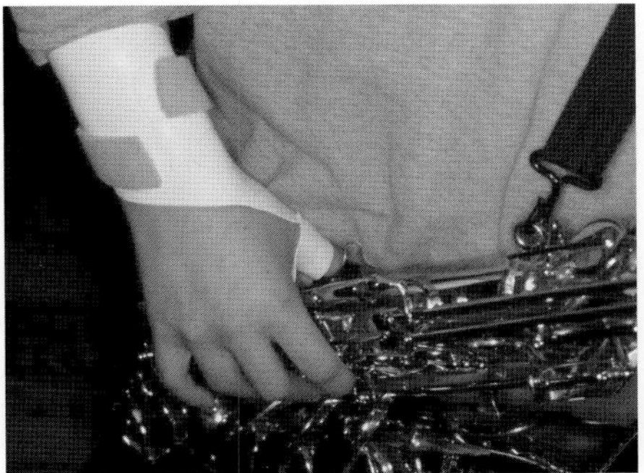

Figure 24–6 This spiral design of a wrist/thumb immobilization splint decreases the lateral stress on the thumb.

and muscle group (Johnson, 1992a). Two types of custom-molded playing splints can be used to assist instrument support for the thumbs of woodwind players. The more supportive splint is a variant of a wrist/thumb immobilization splint and transfers part of the instrument's weight from the thumb to the dorsal ulnar wrist (Fig. 24–6). The other splint is a hand-based thumb MP immobilization splint; wrapped from ulnar to radial and around the thumb (Fig. 24–7).

There are no prefabricated splints that provide as much assistance to instrument support as a well-molded custom fabricated thumb immobilization splint. However, in the absence of a custom option, a nonbulky prefabricated thumb splint may give partial support to the MP and IP joints (Fig. 24–8). When choosing a prefabricated splint, it is helpful to consider the same factors as when designing a custom splint: avoid any obstruction to the instrument or its moving parts and respect the player's customary hand and wrist position (see Chapter 11 for additional information).

Other commercially available adaptive devices used for instrument support include neck straps, the FHRED oboe or English horn support (rests on the chair and

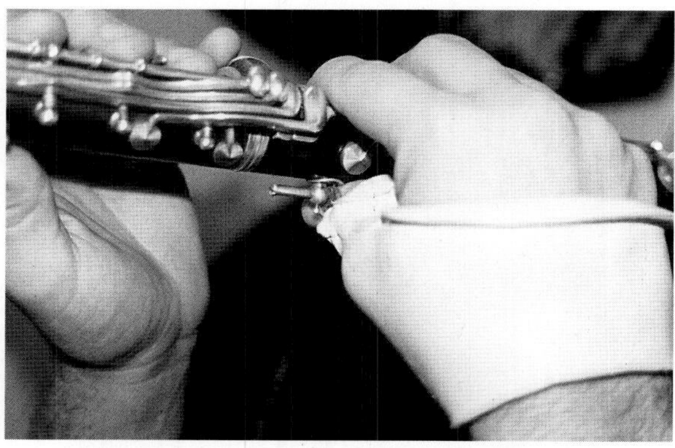

Figure 24–7 A hand-based thumb immobilization splint fabricated for the right hand of a clarinet player. By wrapping distal and radialward around the thumb and crossing the thenar crease, this splint stabilizes the CMC and MP joints. In addition, part of the weight of the instrument is transferred to the ulnar border of the hand.

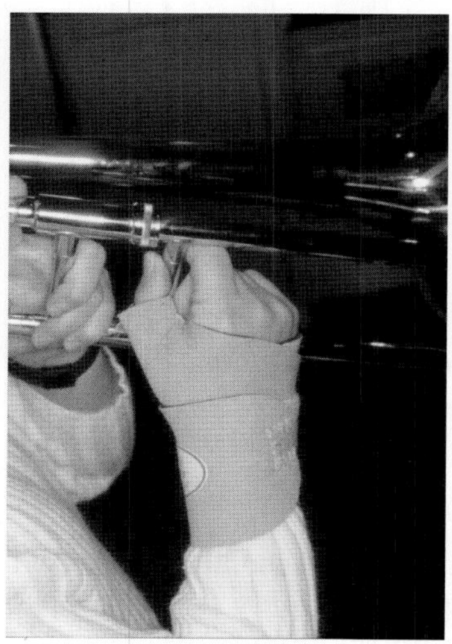

Figure 24–8 If the prefabricated splint has a wrist component, as shown, it will assist CMC stability and may decrease wrist symptoms.

supports the instrument on a rigid stem), and the post (holds the instrument out from the body braced against the player's abdomen). Instrument catalogs offer many solutions to this common problem.

Splint Fabrication

Material Selection

Drapable materials with a prolonged setup time are usually preferred for playing splints. A high degree of conformability is necessary to ensure comfort and optimal fit (Fig. 24–9). A longer setup time allows for adjustments before the position of the splint is finalized. Thick 1/8" materials, with some degree of conformability, such as Tailor Splint or NCM Clinic, are best used for instrument-weight-bearing splints or splints that cross the wrist. Thicker materials are more suited to larger hands. Thinner materials, such as 1/16" and 3/32" Aquaplast or Orfit are best used for alignment splints on the fingers or thumb, Figure-8 splints for IP joints, and light thumb supports. Sometimes a thin material, such as 1/16" perforated Orfit or Fabriplast, is best used for a training splint—not to provide rigidity but to serve as a gentle reminder of proper joint position.

The choice of perforated or nonperforated materials depends on the splint's function and the amount of splint adjustment time needed for construction. Perforated materials tend set up more quickly and may not allow for the multiple adjustments needed when making a playing splint comfortable. Whether to use coated or uncoated material depends on splint structure and the need for bonding (Breger-Lee & Buford, 1992; Moberg, 1984). Often musicians who perform in public prefer a splint material that is close to their skin color to minimize visibility.

Strapping Selection

Straps are best made of traditional hook and loop when firm stabilization is required. When soft tissues have to move beneath the straps, softer materials, such as elastic or foam, are a more appropriate choice. Finger splints that require stabilization can be applied with an elasticized wrap such as Coban or elastic tape. Wrap these materials without applying too much tension to avoid any impairment of neurovascular structures.

Certain types of taping techniques are suitable as playing splints. Taping can often substitute for splint use. This gives the patient a chance to try playing with some degree of restriction. Taping may also be appropriate as a form of emergency immobilization if a player must perform with an injury and there is no time to fabricate a protective splint. Useful taping patterns for musicians include X taping to allow a joint to move while being supported laterally (Fig. 24–10**A**). The X pattern can be combined with lateral or longitudinal taping for firmer support (Fig. 24–10**B**). On the thumb, basket-weave taping can be used for partial stability and can be combined or reinforced with longitudinal strips to support areas of stress (Fig. 24–10**C**). Taping is not a long-

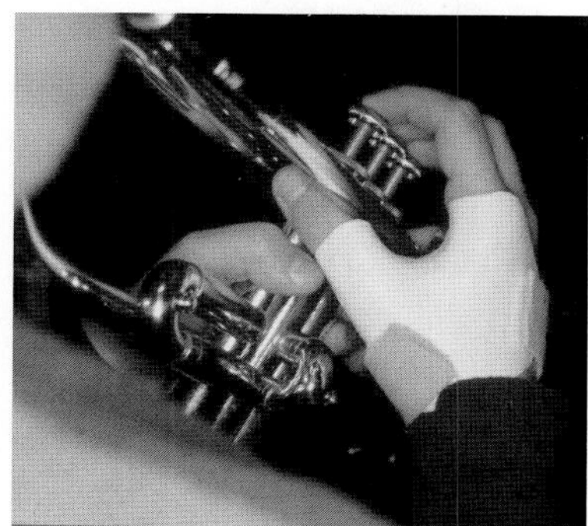

Figure 24–9 Note the precise fit achieved with the use of plastic material on this hand-based thumb immobilization splint.

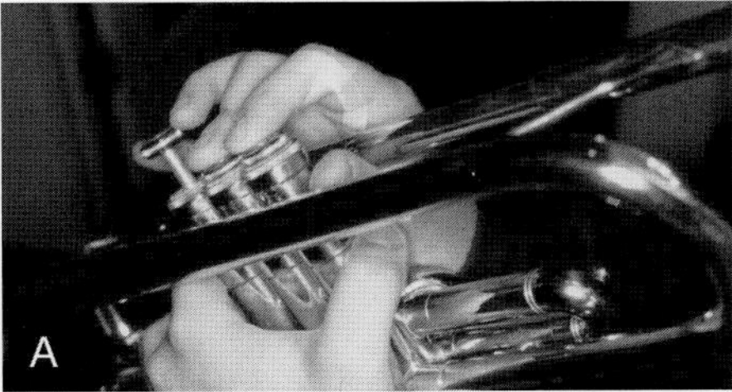

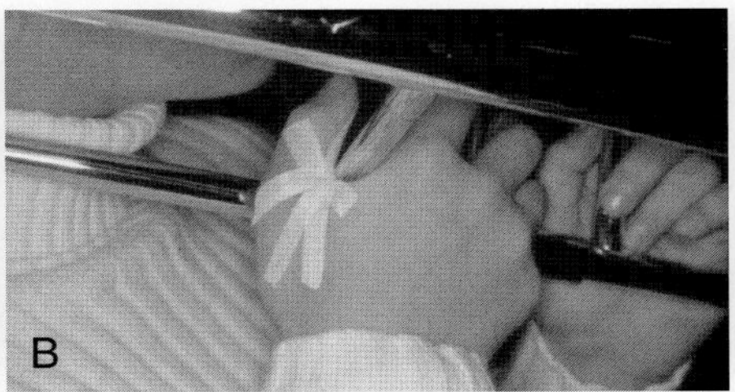

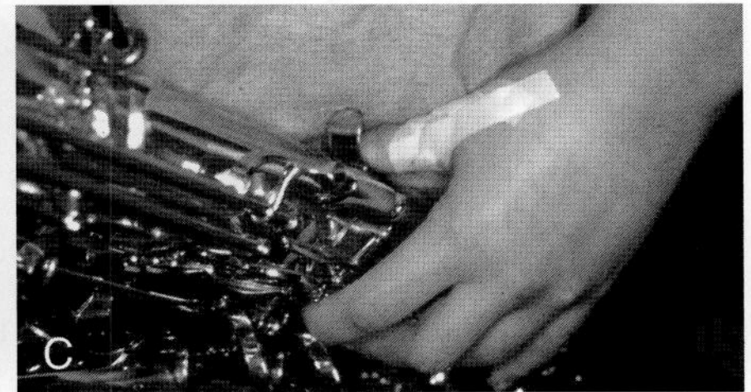

Figure 24–10 ***A,*** *X taping to improve lateral stability of the right index finger PIP joint in a trumpet player.* ***B,*** *X taping with additional lateral strips to improve thumb MP joint stability in a trombone player.* ***C,*** *Basket-weave taping to support the thumb of a saxophone player.*

term solution for musicians because it must be applied and removed frequently; this medium can also be irritating to the skin (Reese, Burruss, & Patten, 1990).

Constructing a Playing Splint

Taking a thorough history and completing a physical examination precede construction of a playing splint. If the patient has an acute or traumatic injury he or she needs two splints: a resting or protective splint and, when the injury allows, a playing splint to hasten return to the instrument. If the patient has an inflammatory or chronic problem, an audition and observation of the playing should be included in the initial evaluation. Useful information is collected about the patient's body mechanics, posture, head position, balance, joint positions during playing; excessive tension in muscle groups; increases in body or facial tension; endurance; and correctness of technique.

The therapist must determine the treatment plan and consider the use of playing splints as soon as clinically possible. A playing splint should also be approved by the referring physician (Stephens & Leilich, 1998; Stotko, 1998). The patient should bring the instrument to the splint fabrication appointment. The therapist should schedule a generous amount of time if possible. The following is a step-by-step procedure for evaluating for and constructing a playing splint:

1. Observe the patient as he or she plays the instrument. Note the required motion of the bones, joints, and soft tissues in relation to the instrument.
2. Determine an appropriate splint pattern by taking into account the goals of the playing splint, based on the diagnosis and treatment plan.
3. Choose a suitable material based on the function and fit needed.
4. Measure to fabricate a splint pattern from a paper towel.
5. Again, observe the patient playing the instrument and review the rationale for the design. Try on the pattern and test for interference with instrument parts.
6. Cut and prepare the splint material. The patient should be ready to play the instrument for the fitting.
7. Mold the splint material on the patient's extremity while he or she maintains a playing position with the instrument; take great care when conforming to avoid the moving parts of the hand and instrument.
8. Apply straps or tape if needed, making sure they do not interfere with the hand or instrument; the material used should be the patient's choice.
9. Test the splint. Ask the patient to try playing with the splint firmly in place. Encourage him or her to identify any parts that are uncomfortable or hinder playing. Take time with this step; if the patient does not use the splint, it was a waste of time and money.
10. Test the splint while the patient plays in several musical contexts: a slow passage, a fast passage, and a technically demanding section. Note: Some players have to change instruments or costumes in the course of a performance; test the patient's ability to doff and don the splint.
11. Plan a follow-up visit for the patient and instrument to make any necessary alterations. Be sure the patient is really able to play in the splint.

CASE STUDY SECTION

The case studies present here are meant to be used as teaching guidelines only. Treatment and splinting protocols vary greatly from surgeon to surgeon and from therapist to therapist. The therapist should check with the referring physicians and colleagues to define the preferred treatment and splinting methods.

CASE STUDY 1: **Violinist with Distal Radius Fracture**

JP is a 42-year-old violinist who fell and sustained a nondisplaced fracture of the left distal radius. He was placed in a short arm plaster cast with the fingers and thumb free. The patient was started on a program of exercise to maintain range of motion (ROM), strength, and muscle balance of all uninvolved joints. At 1 month postinjury, x-rays demonstrated no loss of fracture reduction; the cast was removed, and a wrist immobilization splint was ordered to provide continued protection of the fracture site.

Eager to return to work, JP was fitted with an additional playing splint that allowed him to start practicing (Fig. 24–11). Based on left-hand use for violin playing, a radial wrist immobilization playing splint was constructed to protect and maintain fracture alignment and to prevent disruption of the newly formed callus. With the splint in place, JP could start to regain finger strength and facility. After 2 weeks of using the transitional playing splint, he was able to return unencumbered to his instrument and to work.

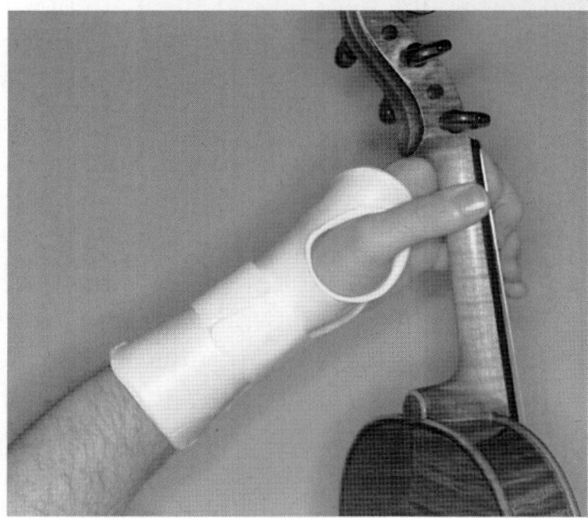

Figure 24–11 A wrist immobilization splint (radial design) for a violinist with a left distal radius fracture. The splint was cut away on the ulnar side, allowing motion into moderate ulnar deviation and full finger use in the first four positions.

CASE STUDY 2: **Bass Player with Distal Phalanx Fracture**

BRT is a 40-year-old double bass player who fractured the distal phalanx of his left middle finger (MF) when he was thrown off a horse. Radiographs revealed a bony mallet injury that did not require surgical intervention. Because the DIP joint of the MF moves very little during string depression on the bass, it was safe to fabricate a playing splint without risking disruption of the healing tendon/bone interface.

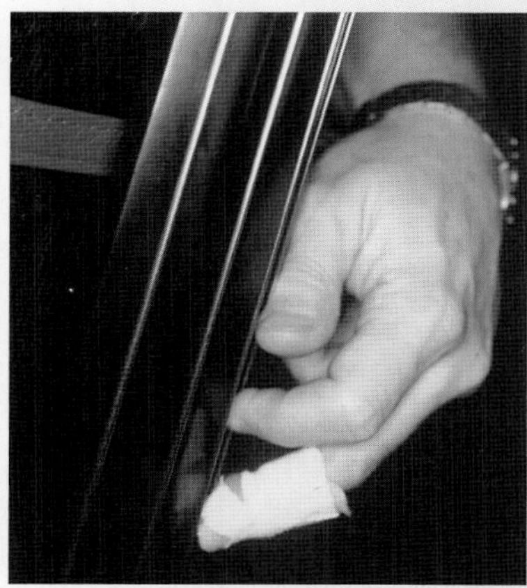

Figure 24–12 A dorsal DIP immobilization splint fabricated from 1/16" Aquaplast for the MF of a double bass player. Special considerations included acceptable protection of the fracture during impact on the string and soft but stable strapping that would not interfere with sensory input from the string.

A simple dorsal DIP immobilization splint allowed an early return to work (Fig. 24–12). The splint was conformed to the dorsum and lateral borders of the DIP joint. Elastic tape was directed diagonally to ensure maximum conformity with the finger pulp; DIP joint hyperextension was maintained and the fracture was protected during instrument use. BRT was able to return to work 3 days after the injury, the fracture remained aligned and healed without incident.

CASE STUDY 3: **Percussion Player with PIP Joint Sprain**

FW is a 23-year-old percussion player who was injured in a basketball game when he jammed his right ring finger (RF) against another player, spraining the radial collateral ligament (RCL) of the PIP joint. After x-rays determined there was no fracture, he was referred for a PIP joint immobilization splint. A splint was molded dorsally over the proximal and middle phalanges with the PIP in maximum achievable extension to provide lateral support and complete immobilization. This splint was worn full time for 10 days.

FW expressed great concern over an upcoming audition that was scheduled for 3 weeks later; if the patient was to audition, he must return to practicing. A PIP extension restriction splint was constructed to maintain lateral support while allowing a limited flexion/extension arc of motion (Fig. 24–13). He was able to control the stick while wearing the splint and returned to practicing for the audition on a modified schedule. Before FW's treatment was complete, he had several playing splints constructed because the joint edema fluctuated with increased use. The injured joint, held in alignment, progressed satisfactorily to well-aligned healing, and the patient was able to play at his audition.

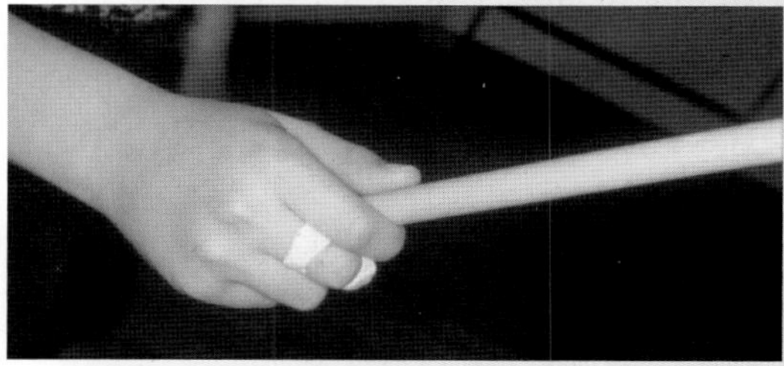

Figure 24–13 A PIP extension restriction splint for the MF PIP joint of a percussion player. After the material was molded to the PIP joint, but before the material had hardened, the patient gripped a drumstick so the splint conformed to the stick.

CASE STUDY 4: Guitarist with Wrist Tendonitis

PCG is a 32-year-old guitar player who presented with complaints of burning and pain at the right medial epicondyle that extended distally along the ulnar border of the forearm. These problems had developed over the previous 3½ months, during which time his job schedule had increased from two to six nights a week. He was started on anti-inflammatory medication and fitted with a dorsal wrist immobilization splint that kept the wrist in 5 to 10° of flexion. Pain kept PCG from returning to his instrument for 2 weeks, at which time he believed it was imperative to start to play again.

At his instrument evaluation, PCG was observed to use extreme ulnar deviation in forceful repeated swipes for strumming. When questioned about this style of playing, he reported that his band had been working on a new strident style of playing and had asked him to slap the strings more and more forcefully. When he began to repeat this motion, he realized it was directly related to his pain. At 2 weeks into his treatment, PCG was fitted with a playing splint designed to provide a partial restriction of ulnar deviation (Fig. 24–14). He was able to play in the splint and the restriction of extreme ulnar deviation helped him revise his right-hand technique. He used the splint for practicing and part of his performing hours until he accomplished the modification of technique. After 4 weeks of tapered use, the splint was discontinued.

CASE STUDY 5: Bassoonist with Thumb Instability

SD is a 40-year-old bassoonist who was referred to therapy with a 4-month history of progressive pain in the left thumb. This problem had finally led her to take a leave of absence from her full-time orchestra job. Physical findings included pain along the thenar eminence, dorsally over the first metacarpal, and proximally into the CMC and radiocarpal joint with tenderness over the ulnar collateral ligaments of the MP and IP joints. Passively, both the MP and IP joints could be moved 20° and 15°, respectively, into radial deviation, demonstrating a significant laxity at both joints compared to the other side. Bassoonists use the left thumb to depress many different keys (Fig. 24–15**A**).

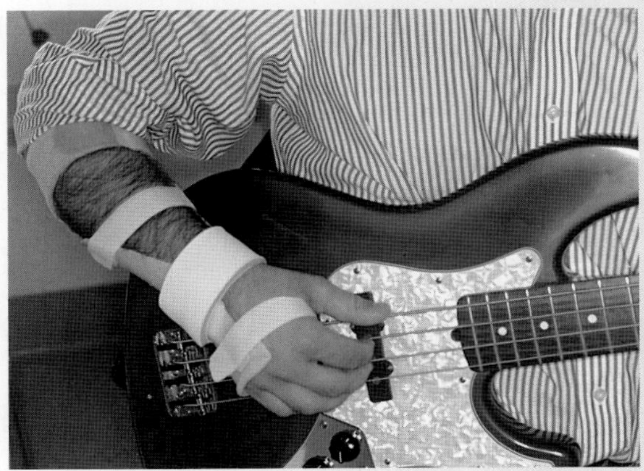

Figure 24–14 A wrist immobilization splint (ulnar design) for the right wrist of guitar player with flexor carpi ulnaris (FCU) tendonitis.

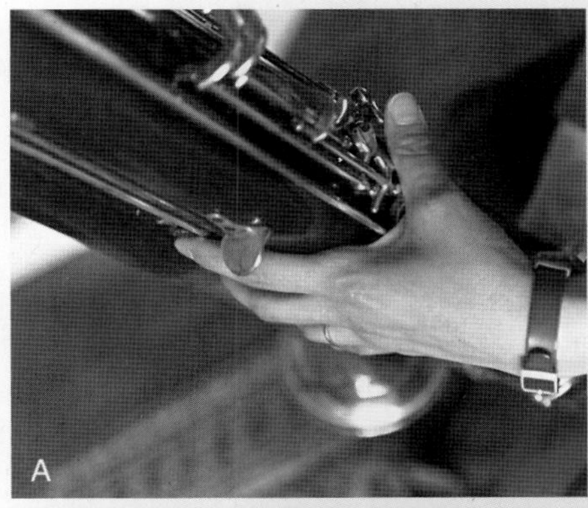

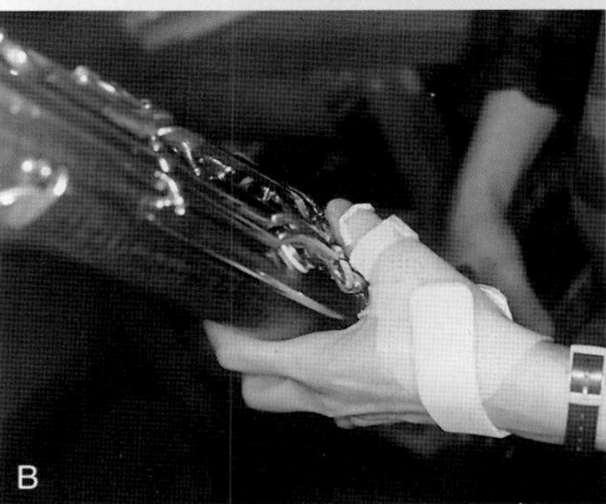

*Figure 24–15 **A,** Note the stress to the left thumb of this bassoonist. **B,** A variant of a hand-based thumb-immobilization splint constructed from 1/16" perforated Orfit with lateral support to the MP and IP joints. The splint includes a slim volar opening to allow variable IP joint flexion and a protective palmar lip to block the first metacarpal from maximum adduction. Soft material was used for strapping, and the contact edges were bound with adhesive-backed 1/16" liner.*

SD's painful thumb was treated for 8 weeks, progressing from immobilization, to partial immobilization, and then to gradual strengthening. A playing splint was then designed to assist her thumb joint stability at the instrument (Fig. 24–15**B**). Owing to the progressive nature of this problem, SD continued to wear her playing splint and thus avoided further acute episodes.

CASE STUDY 6: Woodwind Player with Thumb Pain and Lateral Epicondylitis

LT is a 45-year-old professional musician who plays clarinet and saxophone. He was referred with two diagnoses: thumb pain and lateral epicondylitis in his right upper extremity. Symptoms included diffuse pain along the thumb and radialward after 30 min of playing, pain on palpation at the CMC and MP joints of the right thumb, and pain on resisted thumb extension and adduction. Provocative testing of resisted extensor carpi radialis longus (ECRL) and extensor carpi radialis brevis (ECRB) was also positive, with increased pain at the lateral epicondyle. LT was not tender over the first dorsal compartment, and the Finkelstein's test was negative, suggesting that he did not have DeQuervain's tenosynovitis. The patient also tested positive to resisted isometric thumb extension and adduction.

Both the clarinet and saxophone are constructed with a thumb support on the back of the instrument that rests on the ulnar border of the player's right thumb. Much of the instrument's weight transfers to the thumb, stressing the MP and CMC thumb joints. Although playing his instrument caused pain, LT was unwilling to take more than an occasional night off from his job playing on stage in a Broadway show. Taping (thumb basket-weave taping with vertical supports to the radial and ulnar collateral ligaments) was used as a trial immobilization and was found to be somewhat helpful, providing partial support to the MP and IP joints (Fig. 24–10**C**). Therefore, a hand-based thumb immobilization splint was constructed to assist the thumb in supporting the instrument (Fig. 24–7). This splint requires exact molding to the instrument for the thumb support to be successful. No good skin match was available in splinting material of the required consistency, so the splint and straps were painted with acrylic paint, making it invisible to the audience.

LT was also placed on a program to reduce the inflammation, including anti-inflammatory medication, isometric strengthening exercises, and the use of a wrist/thumb immobilization splint when not playing. He progressively returned to the show while wearing the splint, starting with four shows a week, making weekly increases. The splint was worn onstage for 3 months; then wear was tapered over a period of 4 weeks. LT stores the splint in his dressing room so he can use it if he becomes symptomatic.

CASE STUDY 7: **Drummer with Ulnar Neuritis**

TF is a 58-year-old drummer who presented with a painful palm 2 months after the excision of a reactive inflammatory mass over the digital ulnar nerve in the right palm. The drumstick hit the excision area with each stroke, repeating the original cause of injury. Unwilling to give up any more playing time, TF requested a mechanism for softening the stick's impact without interfering with touch and control. A light leather golf glove was chosen as the base for the playing splint (Fig. 24–16). A patch of thicker leather was used to cover a piece of 1/8" Styrofoam padding cut to align with the stick-striking area. TF was able to play while wearing the glove, because it did not interfere with motion or sensation in the fingers or thumb.

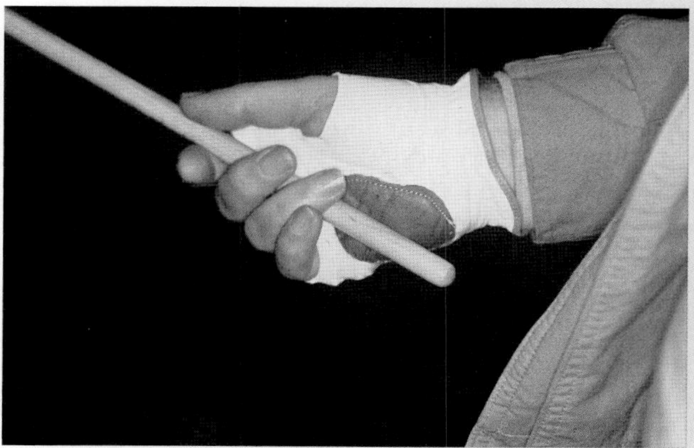

Figure 24–16 A protective glove for the right palm of a drummer.

CONCLUSION

Splinting is a vital and challenging component of treating injured musicians. To construct splints that allow the patient to make an earlier return to his or her instrument is rewarding for both the patient and the therapist (Meinke, 1998). Suitable materials and realistic goals lead the way to splints that are therapeutic and functional.

REFERENCES

Bean, C. H. G., Tencer, A. F., & Trumble T. E. (1999). The effect of thumb metacarpophalangeal ulnar collateral ligament attachment site on joint range of motion: An in vitro study. *Journal of Hand Surgery (American), 24,* 283–287.

Brandsma, J. W., Oudenaarde, E. V., & Oostendorp R. (1996). The abductores pollicis muscles: Clinical considerations based on electromyographical and anatomical studies. *Journal of Hand Therapy, 9,* 218–222.

Breger-Lee, D. E., & Buford, W. L. (1992). Properties of thermoplastic splinting materials. *Journal of Hand Therapy, 5,* 202–211.

Glickel, S. Z., Malerich, M., Pearce, S. M, & Littler, J. W. (1993). Ligament replacement for chronic instability of the ulnar collateral ligament of the metacarpophalangeal joint of the thumb. *Journal of Hand Surgery (American), 18,* 930–941.

Haelterman, J-C. (1996). Adjustable first webspace splint. *Journal of Hand Therapy, 9,* 249.

Heyman, P., Gelberman, T. H., Duncan, K., & Hip, J. A. (1993). Injuries of the ulnar collateral ligament of the thumb metacarpophalangeal joint. Biomechanical and prospective clinical studies on the usefulness of valgus stress testing. *Clinical Orthopaedics and Related Research, 252,* 165–171.

Johnson, C. D. (1992a). Splinting the injured musician. *Journal of Hand Therapy, 5,* 107–110.

Johnson, C. (1992b). Treating the hands that make music. *Journal of Hand Therapy, 5,* 58–60.

Manske, P. R. (1999). The sense of touch. *Journal of Hand Surgery (American), 24,* 213–215.

Mayer, V. A., & McCue, F.C. (1990). Rehabilitation and protection of the hand and wrist. In J. A. Nicholas, E. B. Hershman, & M. A. Posner (Eds.). *The upper extremity in sports medicine* (pp. 619–658). St. Louis: Mosby.

Meinke, W. B. (1998). Risks and realities of musical performance. *Medical Problems in the Performing Arts, 13,* 56–60.

Moberg, E. (1984). Common orthoses of low-temperature plastic material. In *Splinting in hand therapy* (pp. 36–52). Stuttgart: Thieme-Stratton.

Quarrier, N. F. (1993). Performing arts medicine: the musical athlete. *Journal of Orthopedics and Sports Therapy, 17,* 17: 90–95.

Reese, R. C., Burruss, T. P., & Patten J. (1990). Athletic taping and protective equipment. In J. A. Nicholas, E. B. Hershman, & M. A. Posner (Eds.). *The upper extremity in sports medicine* (pp. 659–670). St. Louis: Mosby.

Sadler, J. A., & Koepfer, J. M. (1992). Rehabilitation and splinting of the injured hand. In J. W. Strickland & A. C. Rettig (Eds.). *Hand injuries in athletes* (pp. 235–276). Philadelphia: Saunders.

Schenk, R. K. (1992). Biology of fracture repair. In B.D. Brown, J.B. Jupiter, A.M. Levine, & P.G. Grafton (Eds.). *Skeletal trauma* (2nd ed., pp. 33–77). Philadelphia: Saunders.

Stephens, J., Leilich, S. (1998). Overuse injuries of the upper extremity in musicians. In G. Clark, E. F. Wilgis, B. Aiello, D. Eckhaus, & L. V. Eddington (Eds.). *Hand rehabilitation* (2nd ed., pp. 401–413). New York: Churchill Livingston.

Stotko, L. (1998). Dynamically splinting the musical hand. *Medical Problems in the Performing Arts, 13,* 109–113.

Swigart, C. R., Eaton, R. G., Glickel, S. Z., & Johnson, C. (1999). Splinting in the treatment of arthritis of the first metacarpal joint. *Journal of Hand Surgery (American), 24,* 86–91.

Van Lede, P., & van Veldhoven, G. (1998). *Biological considerations. Therapeutic hand splints—Rational approach. Volume 1: Mechanical and biomechanical considerations.* Antwerp: Provan.

Wilson, F. R. (1998). *In tune and evolving prestissimo. The hand.* New York: Pantheon.

SUGGESTED READING

Amadio, P. C. (1990). Hand injuries in sports and performing artists. *Hand Clinics, 6,*(3).

Brand, P. W., & Hollister, A. (1993). *Clinical mechanics of the hand* (2nd ed.). St. Louis: Mosby Co.

Kogan, J. (1987). *Nothing but the best: The struggle for perfection at the Juilliard School.* New York: Random House.

Musicians' injuries [Special Issue]. (1992). *Journal of Hand Therapy, 5.*

Norris, R. (1993). *The musician's survival manual: A guide to preventing and treating injuries in instrumentalists.* St Louis: MMP Music.

Sataloff, R. T., Grandfonbrener, A. G., & Lederman, R. J. (1991). *Textbook of performing arts medicine* (2nd ed.). New York: Raven.

Winspur, I., & Parry, C. B. (2000). Musician's hands: A surgeon's perspective. *Medical Problems of Performing Artists, 15,* 31–33.

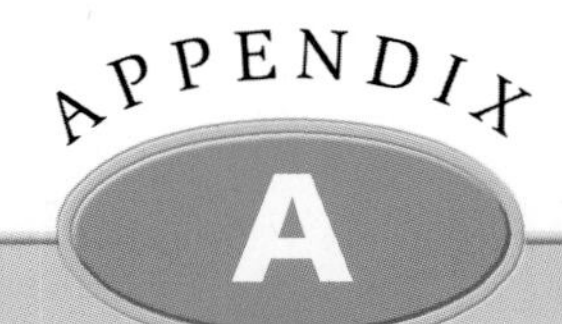

Rehabilitation Vendors

AliMed, Inc.
297 High Street
Dedham, MA 02026
800-225-2610
fax: 800-437-2966
www.alimed.com

DeRoyal/LMB, Inc.
200 DeBusk Lane
Powell, TN 37849
800-541-3992
fax: 800-327-0340
www.deroyal.com

Dynasplint
770 Ritchie highway
River Reach, W21
Severna Park, MD 21146
800-638-6771
www.dynasplint.com

Empi
599 Cardigan Road
St. Paul, MN 55126
800-367-3674
www.empi.com

Joint Active Systems
2600 South Raney Street
Effingham, IL 62401
800-879-.0117
www.jointactivesystems.com

Joint-Jack Company
108 Britt Road
East Hartford, CT 06118
860-568-7338
fax: 860-568-9588
www.jointjackcompany.com

North Coast Medical, Inc.
18305 Sutter Boulevard
Morgan Hill, CA 95037
800-821-9319
fax: 877-213-9300
www.ncmedical.com

NorthStar Therapeutics (Kinesio Tex Tape)
P.O. Box 313
Prescott, WI 54021
877-262-8484
fax: 715-262-8400
www.northstartherapeutics.com

Otto Bock HealthCare
3000 Xenium Lane North
Minneapolis, MN 55441
800-328-4058
fax: 800-962-2549
www.ottobockus.com

Sammons Preston
P.O. Box 5071
Bollingbrook, IL 60440
800-323-5547
fax: 800-547-4333
www.sammonspreston.com

Silver Ring Splint Company
P.O. Box 2856
Charlottesville, VA 22902
800-311-7028
fax: 804-971-8828
www.silverringsplint.com

Smith+Nephew, Inc.
One Quality Drive
P.O. Box 1005
Germantown, WI 53022
800-558-8633
fax: 800-545-7758
www.smith-nephew.com/us/rehab

Therakinetics
55 Carnegie Plaza
Cherry Hill, NJ 08003
800-800-4276

3-Point Products
1610 Pincay Court
Annapolis, MD 21401
888-378-7763
fax: 410-349-2648
www.3pointproducts.com

UE Tech
P.O. Box 2145
Edwards, CO 81632
800-736-1894
fax: 970-926-8870
www.uetech.com

WFR Corporation
30 Lawlins park
Wyckoff, NJ 07481
800-526-5247
fax: 800-831-.8147
www.reveals.com

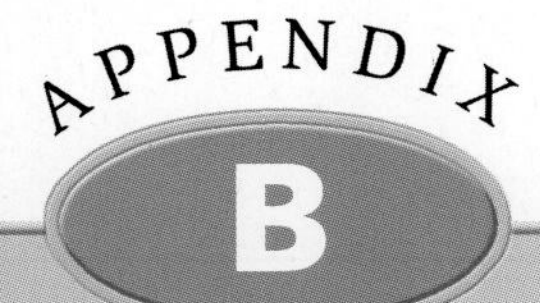

Clinical Forms

Upper Extremity Evaluation

DATE: ____________

Patient Name: ____________ DOB: ____________

Physician: ____________ DOM: R/L

Diagnosis/Surgery: R/L ____________ DOI: ____________

____________ DOS: ____________

History of Present Condition: ____________

____

____

____

Medical History/Medications: ____________

____

Social History: ____________

Vocational History: employed/work comp/light duty/currently not working/unemployed/disability/retired/student

Occupation: ____________

Job Description: ____________

____

Functional Level: (indicate min, mod, or max assist)

Self Care: ____________

____

Home Tasks: ____________

____

Leisure Activities: ____________

____

Other ____________

Pain:

____ no complaints	____ dull	Location: ____________
____ shooting	____ achy	____________
____ burning	____ tender	____________
____ sharp	Pain Scale (0-10): ____	____ Constant/Intermittent

Edema:

____ absent	____ minimal	Location: ____________
____ moderate	____ severe	____________

Measurements: ____________

____

Sensibility:

____ no complaints		
____ numbness	____ paresthesias	Location: ____________
____ hypersensitive	____ other	____________
____ see formal eval		____ Constant/Intermittent

R/L volar/dorsal

R/L volar/dorsal

Soft Tissue/Wound Status: ______________________________

____

____

Dressing: ______________________________

Range of Motion/Strength: see separate flowsheet or WNLS

Upper Extremity Problems:

________Healing Wound/Incision	________Decreased A/PROM	Other:__________
________Pain/Hypersensitivity	________Decreased Strength	__________
________Decreased Scar Mobility	________Decreased Function	__________
________Edema	________Decreased Sensation	__________

Short Term Goals:

____

____

____

____

Long Term Goals:

____

____

____

____

Rehabilitation Plan:

________Wound Care/Dressing Changes	________Scar Management	________Splints
________ROM Exercises	________Pain Control Techniques	☐ Immob
________Strengthening Exercises	________Functional Activities	☐ Mob ☐ Restrict
________Edema Management	________Modalities	________Other

Frequency/Duration: ______________________________

Today's treatment: ______________________________

____

____

The above program was discussed with and approved by the patient and/or family

______________________________ ______________________________

Patient's signature Therapist's signature

Upper Extremity Evaluation Flow Sheet

Patient: **DOB:**

Date									
ROM	**NORM**	**A/PROM**	**MMT**	**A/PROM**	**MMT**	**A/PROM**	**MMT**	**A/PROM**	**MMT**
Shoulder									
Ext/Flex									
Abd/Add									
IR/ER									
Elbow									
Ext/Flex									
Forearm									
Pro/Sup									
Wrist									
Ext/Flex									
RD/UD									
Thumb									
MP									
IP									
R/P Abd									
Opp									
Web									
Index									
MP									
PIP									
DIP									
DPC									
Middle									
MP									
PIP									
DIP									
DPC									
Ring									
MP									
PIP									
DIP									
DPC									
Small									
MP									
PIP									
DIP									
DPC									
Edema									
Strength		**Left**	**Right**	**Left**	**Right**	**Left**	**Right**	**Left**	**Right**
Grip									
Lateral Pinch									
Tip Pinch									
3-point Pinch									

Splint Evaluation

DATE: ____________

Patient Name: ______________________________ DOB: ____________

Physician: ______________________________ DOM: R/L

Diagnosis/Surgery: R/L ______________________________ DOI: ____________

______________________________ DOS: ____________

History of Present Condition: ______________________________

____

____

Medical History/Medications: ______________________________

Social/Vocation History: ______________________________

Functional Level: ______________________________

Pain: ______________________________

Edema: ______________________________

Sensibility: ______________________________

Soft Tissue/Wound Status/Dressing: ______________________________

Range of Motion/Strength: ______________________________

____

Splint Goals:

_____ Protect healing structures

_____ Increase range of motion

_____ Restrict mobility

_____ Improve joint alignment

Other: ______________________________

____

Splint Plan:

_____ Immobilization Splint

_____ Mobilization Splint

_____ Restriction Splint

_____ Nonarticular Splint

Other: ______________________________

____

Type of Splint(s) fabricated: ______________________________

____

_____ Patient/Caregiver instructed in splint wear, care, and precautions. Written splint instructions issued.

____

______________________________ Patient's Signature

______________________________ Therapist's Signature

_____ Splint only _____ Splint and HEP _____ Evaluation scheduled

Splint Follow-up Form

Patient:____________________ **DOB:**________ **DOI:**________ **DOS:**________
Diagnosis:______________________________ **DOM:** R/L
MD:____________________ **MD follow-up:**________________

Date:	Signature:	Visit #:

S:

O:

Eval/Re-eval	HP/Paraffin/CP	A/AAROM	PREs/Strengthening
Splint/Splint Adjmt	Ultrasound	PROM	Funct Activities
Wound care/Drsq	E-Stim/Ionto	Jt mob/Passive stretch	BTE/UBE__min
HEP/Review HEP	Whirlpool/Fluido	Massage/Desens	Other

A:

P:

Date:	Signature:	Visit #:

S:

O:

Eval/Re-eval	HP/Paraffin/CP	A/AAROM	PREs/Strengthening
Splint/Splint Adjmt	Ultrasound	PROM	Funct Activities
Wound care/Drsq	E-Stim/Ionto	Jt mob/Passive stretch	BTE/UBE__min
HEP/Review HEP	Whirlpool/Fluido	Massage/Desens	Other

A:

P:

Date:	Signature:	Visit #:

S:

O:

Eval/Re-eval	HP/Paraffin/CP	A/AAROM	PREs/Strengthening
Splint/Splint Adjmt	Ultrasound	PROM	Funct Activities
Wound care/Drsq	E-Stim/Ionto	Jt mob/Passive stretch	BTE/UBE__min
HEP/Review HEP	Whirlpool/Fluido	Massage/Desens	Other

A:

P:

Hand and Upper Extremity Progress Report

DATE: ____________

Patient Name: ____________ DOB: ____________

Physician: ____________ DOM: R/L

Diagnosis/Surgery: R/L ____________ DOI: ____________

____________ DOS: ____________

Initial Therapy Evaluation: ____________ # Visits: ________ FREQ: ____________

Treatment: ____________

____

Home Program: ____________

____

Progress:

____
____
____
____
____
____
____
____
____
____
____
____

Recommendations: ________Continue ________Freq/Duration ________Discharge

____________ Physician's Signature

____________ Therapist's Signature

c.c. chart

Splint Instructions

Patient Name: ______________________ Date: ______________________

The goal of your ______________________ splint is to ______________________

____

Precautions

The splint should **not** cause:

*pressure areas or redness of skin (i.e., at edges of material strapes or over bony regions)

*restriction of blood flow (noted by change in skin color i.e., deep red, purple, or white)

*skin irritation (i.e., rash or itching)

*increased pain

*increased swelling (generalized or between straps)

*increased numbness or tingling

Call your therapist for splint adjustment if experiencing any of the above symptoms.

Wearing Instructions

Your splint is to be worn:

_____ Day _____ Off for hygiene only

_____ Night _____ Off for exercise

_____ At all times Other: ______________________

____

Your therapist and physician will alter this wearing schedule when appropriate.

Splint Care

*Keep the splint away from direct sunlight and heat sources because it may melt (i.e., dashboard of your car, furnace, stove, etc.)

*Splints can be washed with luke warm water and soap or rubbing alcohol. (If the splint is lined with a foam or padding material ask the therapist for specific instructions.)

*Straps can be cleaned with soap and water using a small brush then allowed to air dry.

*Sleeves worn beneath splint should be washed daily by hand and allowed to air dry.

Therapist______________________ **Phone**______________________

c.c. chart

Hand and Upper Extremity Discharge Summary

DATE: __________

Patient Name: ______________________________ DOB: __________

Physician: ______________________________ DOM: R/L

Diagnosis/Surgery: R/L ______________________________ DOI: __________

______________________________ DOS: __________

Initial Therapy Evaluation: __________ Total # visits: ______(attended) ______(scheduled)

Goals achieved/not achieved:

	YES	NO	NA
1. Healed Wound/Incision		/	/
2. Decreased Pain/Hypersensitivity		/	/
3. Increased Scar Mobility		/	/
4. Decreased Edema		/	/
5. Increased A/PROM		/	/
6. Increased Strength		/	/
7. Increased Function		/	/
8. Increased Sensibility		/	/
9. Establish Home Program		/	/
10. Increased Patient's Awareness of Diagnosis/Treatment Plan		/	/

Discharge Status: ______________________________

____

____

____

Functional Status: ______________________________

____

Home Program: ______________________________

____

Additional Comments: ______________________________

____

____

c.c. chart

____

Therapist's Signature

Index

Page numbers in *italics* denote figures; those followed by a t denote tables.

A

D

E

F

G

N

O

P

Q

R

S

T

U

Z